Lecture Notes in Computer Science 7510

Commenced Publication in 1973
Founding and Former Series Editors:
Gerhard Goos, Juris Hartmanis, and Jan van Leeuwen

Nicholas Ayache   Hervé Delingette
Polina Golland   Kensaku Mori (Eds.)

Medical Image Computing and Computer-Assisted Intervention – MICCAI 2012

15th International Conference
Nice, France, October 1-5, 2012
Proceedings, Part I

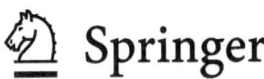 Springer

Volume Editors

Nicholas Ayache
Hervé Delingette
Inria Sophia Antipolis
Project Team Asclepios
06902 Sophia Antipolis, France
E-mail: {nicholas.ayache, herve.delingette}@inria.fr

Polina Golland
MIT, CSAIL
Cambridge, MA 02139, USA
E-mail: polina@csail.mit.edu

Kensaku Mori
Nagoya University
Information and Communications Headquarters
Nagoya, 464-8603, Japan
E-mail: kensaku@is.nagoya-u.ac.jp

ISSN 0302-9743   e-ISSN 1611-3349
ISBN 978-3-642-33414-6   e-ISBN 978-3-642-33415-3
DOI 10.1007/978-3-642-33415-3
Springer Heidelberg Dordrecht London New York

Library of Congress Control Number: 2012946929

CR Subject Classification (1998): I.4, I.5, I.3.5-8, I.2.9-10, J.3, I.6

LNCS Sublibrary: SL 6 – Image Processing, Computer Vision, Pattern Recognition, and Graphics

Typesetting: Camera-ready by author, data conversion by Scientific Publishing Services, Chennai, India

Printed on acid-free paper

Springer is part of Springer Science+Business Media (www.springer.com)

Preface

The 15th International Conference on Medical Image Computing and Computer Assisted Intervention, MICCAI 2012, was held in Nice, France, at the Acropolis Convention Center during October 1–5, 2012.

Over the past 14 years, the MICCAI conferences have become a premier international event with full articles of high standard, indexed by Pubmed, and annually attracting leading scientists, engineers and clinicians working at the intersection of sciences, technologies and medicine.

It is interesting to recall that the MICCAI conference series was formed in 1998 by the merger of CVRMed (Computer Vision, Virtual Reality and Robotics in Medicine), MRCAS (Medical Robotics and Computer Assisted Surgery) and VBC (Visualization in Biomedical Computing) conferences, and that the first CVRMed conference was held in Nice in April 1995. At that time the CVRMed conference was a single event and the proceedings, also published in Lecture Notes in Computer Science (LNCS), consisted of a single volume of 570 pages. In 2012 the MICCAI proceedings span three volumes and more than 2000 pages, and the conference was complemented by 32 MICCAI satellite events (workshops, challenges, tutorials) publishing their own proceedings, several of them in LNCS.

MICCAI contributions were selected through a rigorous reviewing process involving an international Program Committee (PC) of 100 specialists coordinated by a Program Chair and 2 Program Co-chairs from 3 continents. Decisions were based on anonymous reviews made by 913 expert reviewers. The process was double blind as authors did not know the names of the PC members/reviewers evaluating their papers, and the PC members/reviewers did not know the names of the authors of the papers they were evaluating.

We received 781 submissions and after the collection of over 3000 anonymous review forms, the final selection was prepared during a 2-day meeting in Nice (12–13 May 2012) attended by 50 PC members. They finalized the acceptation of 252 papers (i.e., acceptance rate of 32%) and also prepared a short list of candidate papers for plenary presentations. The accepted contributions came from 21 countries and 5 continents: about 50% from North America (40% USA and 8% Canada), 40% from Europe (mainly from France, Germany, the UK, Switzerland and The Netherlands), and 10% from Asia and the rest of the world.

All accepted papers were presented during 6 poster sessions of 90 minutes with the option, this year for the first time, of displaying additional dynamic material on large screens during the whole poster session. In addition, a subset of 37 carefully selected papers (mainly chosen among the short list of candidate papers recommended by PC members) were presented during 7 single-track plenary oral sessions.

Prof. Alain Carpentier, President of the French Academy of Sciences, was the Honored Guest of MICCAI 2012 for his pioneering and visionary role in several of the domains covered by MICCAI. Prof. Carpentier addressed the audience during the opening ceremony along with Prof. Michel Cosnard, the CEO of Inria, and introduced one the keynote lectures.

Prof. Jacques Marescaux, director of the Strasbourg IHU (Institut Hospitalo-Universitaire) delivered the keynote lecture "Surgery for Life Innovation: Information Age and Robotics" and Prof. Michel Haïssaguerre, director of the Bordeaux IHU, delivered the keynote lecture "Preventing Sudden Cardiac Death: Role of Structural and Functional Imaging". Both of these lectures were outstanding and inspiring.

The conference would not have been possible without the commitment and hard work of many people whom we want to thank wholeheartedly:

- The 100 Program Committee members and 913 scientific reviewers, listed in this book, who worked closely with us and prepared many written reviews and recommendations for acceptance or rejection,
- Xavier Pennec as the Chair for the organization of the 32 satellite events (workshops, challenges, tutorials) with the assistance of Tobias Heimann, Kilian Pohl and Akinobu Shimizu as Co-chairs, and all the organizers of these events,
- Agnès Cortell as the Local Organization Chair, who successfully coordinated all the details of the organization of the event with the support of a local organizing team (composed of Marc Barret, Grégoire Malandain, Xavier Pennec, Maxime Sermesant and two of us), several Inria services (involving heavily Odile Carron and Matthieu Oricelli), and the MCI company,
- Maxime Sermesant as MICCAI Website Chair,
- Grégoire Malandain for the new organization of posters including digital screens,
- Isabelle Strobant for the organization of the PC meeting in Nice, the invitations of the MICCAI guests, and her constant support during the preparation of the event,
- Gérard Giraudon, director of Inria in Sophia Antipolis, for his constant support,
- Sebastien Ourselin for his help in coordinating industrial sponsorship,
- All students and engineers (mainly from Asclepios and Athena Inria teams) who helped with the scientific and local organization,
- Emmanuelle Viau, who coordinated the team at MCI including in particular Thibault Claisse and Thibault Lestiboudois,
- Jim Duncan as the President of the MICCAI Society and its board of directors who elected MICCAI 2012 to be held in Nice,
- Janette Wallace, Johanne Guillemette and Chris Wedlake for the liaison with the MICCAI Society,
- James Stewart for his precious help with the Precision Conference System,
- All our industrial and institutional sponsors and partners for their fantastic support of the conference.

Finally, we would like to thank all the MICCAI 2012 attendees who came to Nice from 34 countries from all around the world, and we look forward to meeting them again at MICCAI 2013 in Nagoya, Japan, at MICCAI 2014 in Cambridge, Massachusetts, USA and at MICCAI 2015 in Munich, Germany.

October 2012

Nicholas Ayache
Hervé Delingette
Polina Golland
Kensaku Mori

Accepted MICCAI 2012 Papers

by Clinical Theme

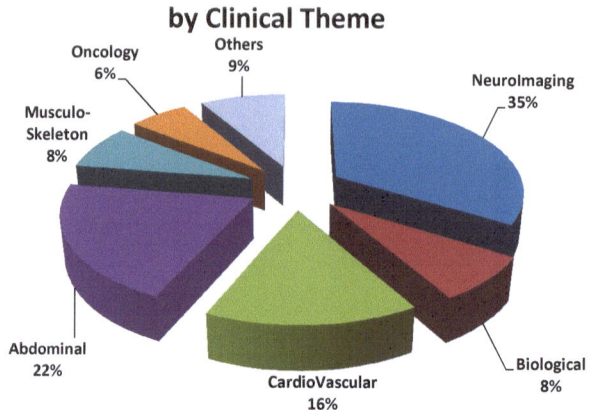

Oncology 6%
Others 9%
NeuroImaging 35%
Musculo-Skeleton 8%
Abdominal 22%
CardioVascular 16%
Biological 8%

by Technical Theme

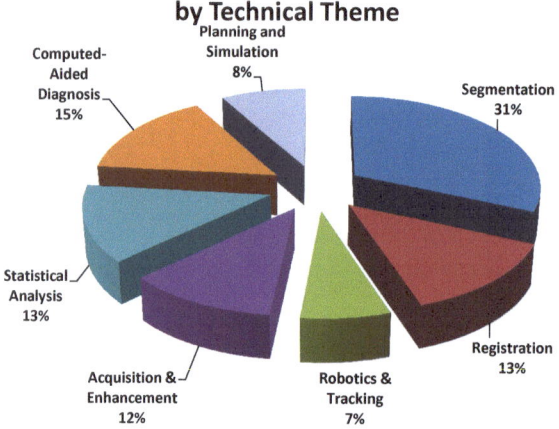

Computed-Aided Diagnosis 15%
Planning and Simulation 8%
Segmentation 31%
Statistical Analysis 13%
Acquisition & Enhancement 12%
Robotics & Tracking 7%
Registration 13%

by Country of First Author

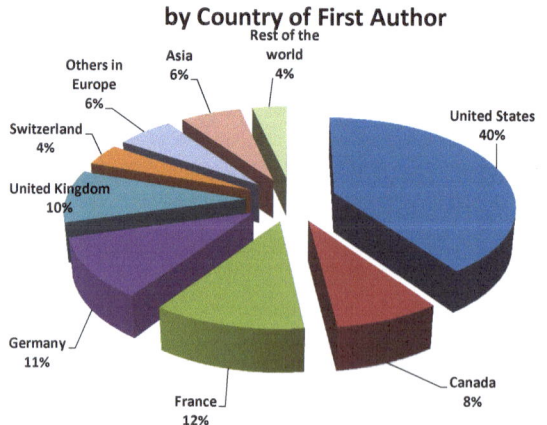

Others in Europe 6%
Asia 6%
Rest of the world 4%
Switzerland 4%
United Kingdom 10%
United States 40%
Germany 11%
France 12%
Canada 8%

Organization

General Chair

Nicholas Ayache — Inria, Sophia Antipolis, France

Program Chair and Co-chairs

Hervé Delingette — Inria, Sophia Antipolis, France
Polina Golland — MIT, Cambridge, USA
Kensaku Mori — Nagoya University, Nagoya, Japan

Workshops, Tutorials and Challenges Chair and Co-chairs

Xavier Pennec — Inria, Sophia Antipolis, France
Tobias Heimann — Cancer Research Center, Heidelberg, Germany
Kilian Pohl — University of Pennsylvania, Philadelphia, USA
Akinobu Shimizu — Tokyo University of A&T, Tokyo, Japan

MICCAI Society, Board of Directors

James Duncan (President) — Yale University, USA
Gabor Fichtinger (Treasurer) — Queen's University, Canada
Alison Noble (Exec. Director) — University of Oxford, UK
Sebastien Ourselin (Secretary) — University College London, UK
Nicholas Ayache — Inria Sophia Antipolis, France
Polina Golland — MIT, USA
David Hawkes — University College London, UK
Kensaku Mori — Nagoya University, Japan
Wiro Niessen — Erasmus MC, The Netherlands
Xavier Pennec — Inria Sophia Antipolis, France
Daniel Rueckert — Imperial College London, UK
Dinggang Shen — University North Carolina, USA
William Wells — Harvard Medical School, USA

Consultants to Board

Alan Colchester — University of Kent, UK
Terry Peters — Robarts Research Institute, Canada
Richard Robb — Mayo Clinic College of Medicine, USA

Program Committee

Purang Abolmaesumi	University of British Columbia, Canada
Daniel Alexander	University College London, UK
Amir Amini	University Louisville, USA
Elsa Angelini	Télécom ParisTech, France
Stephen Aylward	Kitware, USA
Christian Barillot	CNRS, France
Wolfgang Birkfellner	Medical University of Vienna, Austria
Oscar Camara	University Pompeu Fabra, Spain
Albert Chung	HKUST, Hong Kong
Ela Claridge	University of Birmingham, UK
Patrick Clarysse	University of Lyon, France
Louis Collins	McGill University, Canada
Olivier Colliot	ICM-CNRS, France
Dorin Comaniciu	Siemens, USA
Stéphane Cotin	Inria, France
Antonio Criminisi	Microsoft Research, UK
Christos Davatzikos	University of Pennsylvania, USA
Marleen de Bruijne	Erasmus MC, The Netherlands
Rachid Deriche	Inria, France
James Duncan	University of Yale, USA
Philip Edwards	Imperial College London, UK
Gabor Fichtinger	Queen's University, Canada
Bernd Fischer	University of Luebeck, Germany
Thomas Fletcher	University of Utah, USA
Alejandro Frangi	University Pompeu Fabra, Spain
Jim Gee	University of Pennsylvania, USA
Guido Gerig	University of Utah, USA
Leo Grady	Siemens, USA
Hayit Greenspan	Tel Aviv University, Israel
Gregory Hager	John's Hopkins University, USA
Heinz Handels	University of Luebeck, Germany
Matthias Harders	ETH Zurich, Switzerland
Nobuhiko Hata	Harvard Medical School, USA
David Hawkes	University College London, UK
Tobias Heimann	DKFZ, Germany
Ameet Jain	Philips, USA
Pierre Jannin	INSERM, France
Marie-Pierre Jolly	Siemens, USA
Leo Joskowicz	University of Jerusalem, Israel
Ioannis Kakadiaris	University of Houston, USA
Nico Karssemeijer	Radboud University, The Netherlands
Ron Kikinis	Harvard Medical School, USA

Benjamin Kimia	Brown University, USA
Rasmus Larsen	Technical University of Denmark, Denmark
Christophe Lenglet	University of Minnesota, USA
Shuo Li	General Electric, Canada
Cristian Lorenz	Philips, Germany
Anant Madabhushi	Rutgers University, USA
Frederik Maes	K.U. Leuven, Belgium
Isabelle Magnin	University of Lyon, France
Sherif Makram-Ebeid	Philips, France
Jean-François Mangin	CEA, France
Anne Martel	University of Toronto, Canada
Yoshitaka Masutani	University of Tokyo, Japan
Bjoern Menze	ETH Zurich, Switzerland
Dimitris Metaxas	Rutgers University, USA
Nassir Navab	Technical University of Munich, Germany
Poul Nielsen	University of Auckland, New Zealand
Wiro Niessen	Erasmus MC, The Netherlands
Alison Noble	Oxford University, UK
Sebastien Ourselin	University College London, UK
Nikos Paragios	Centrale & Ponts-ParisTech, France
Xavier Pennec	Inria, France
Terry Peters	Robarts Research Institute, Canada
Josien Pluim	Utrecht University MC, The Netherlands
Killian Pohl	University of Pennsylvania, USA
Richard Robb	Mayo Clinic, USA
Torsten Rohlfing	SRI, USA
Daniel Rueckert	Imperial College London, UK
Mert Sabuncu	Harvard Medical School, USA
Ichiro Sakuma	University of Tokyo, Japan
Tim Salcudean	University of British Columbia, Canada
Yoshonibu Sato	University of Osaka, Japan
Julia Schnabel	Oxford University, UK
Maxime Sermesant	Inria, France
Dinggang Shen	University of North Carolina, USA
Akinobu Shimizu	Tokyo University of A&T, Japan
Nicolas Smith	King's College London, UK
Lawrence Staib	University of Yale, USA
Colin Studholme	University of Washington, USA
Martin Styner	University of North Carolina, USA
Naoki Suzuki	Jikei University, Japan
Russell Taylor	John's Hopkins University, USA
Jean-Philippe Thiran	EPFL, Switzerland
Bertrand Thirion	Inria, France
Paul Thompson	UCLA, USA
Jocelyne Troccaz	CNRS, France

Regis Vaillant	General Electric, France
Bram van Ginneken	Radboud University, The Netherlands
Koen Van Leemput	Harvard Medical School, USA
Baba Vemuri	University of Florida, USA
Ragini Verma	University of Pennsylvania, USA
Simon Warfield	Harvard Medical School, USA
Jurgen Weese	Philips, Germany
Wolfgang Wein	Technical University of Munich, Germany
William Wells	Harvard Medical School, USA
Carl-Fredrik Westin	Harvard Medical School, USA
Guang Zhong Yang	Imperial College London, UK
Laurent Younes	John's Hopkins University, USA
Alistair Young	University of Auckland, New Zealand

Organizing Institution

This event was organized by Inria, the French Research Institute for Computer Science and Applied Mathematics.

Local Organizing Committee

Agnès Cortell	Inria, Sophia Antipolis, France
Nicholas Ayache	Inria, Sophia Antipolis, France
Marc Barret	Inria, Sophia Antipolis, France
Hervé Delingette	Inria, Sophia Antipolis, France
Grégoire Malandain	Inria, Sophia Antipolis, France
Xavier Pennec	Inria, Sophia Antipolis, France
Maxime Sermesant	Inria, Sophia Antipolis, France
Isabelle Strobant	Inria, Sophia Antipolis, France

Liaison with the MICCAI Society

| Janette Wallace | Robarts Research Institute, London, Canada |
| Johanne Guillemette | Robarts Research Institute, London, Canada |

Official Partners

Institut Océanographique de Monaco
Région Provence Alpes Côte d'Azur
Ville de Nice

Sponsors

Gold Sponsors	GE HealthCare
	Philips
	Siemens
	Canon Median
Silver Sponsors	ERC MedYMA
	Medtronic
Bronze Sponsors	Aviesan
	Dosisoft
	IHU Strasbourg
	IRCAD France
	Kitware
	Microsoft Research

Exhibitors

Camelot Biomedial systems   Claron Technology
Elsevier   NDI
Springer   Ultrasonix
VSG Visualization Sciences Group

Reviewers

Abramoff, Michael
Acar, Burak
Achterberg, Hakim
Acosta-Tamayo, Oscar
Adluru, Nagesh
Aganj, Iman
Ahmadi, Seyed-Ahmad
Aja-Fernández, Santiago
Akcakaya, Mehmet
Akhondi-Asl, Alireza
Alander, Jarmo
Alberola-López, Carlos
Alexander, Andrew
Ali, Sahirzeeshan
Aljabar, Paul
Allain, Baptiste
Allassonnière, Stephanie
Amini, Amir
An, Jungha
Anderson, Adam
Andersson, Jesper

Andres, Bjoern
Antani, Sameer
Anwander, Alfred
Arbel, Tal
Arimura, Hidetaka
Arridge, Simon R.
Ashburner, John
Astley, Sue
Atkinson, David
Audette, Michel
Augustine, Kurt
Auvray, Vincent
Avants, Brian
Avila, Rick
Awate, Suyash
Axel, Leon
Ayad, Maria
Bach Cuadra, Meritxell
Baddeley, David
Baghani, Ali
Baka, Nora

Balicki, Marcin
Ballerini, Lucia
Baloch, Sajjad
Barbu, Adrian
Barmpoutis, Angelos
Barratt, Dean
Barré, Arnaud
Basavanhally, Ajay
Batmanghelich, Nematollah
Bazin, Pierre-Louis
Beichel, Reinhard
Belongie, Serge
Ben Ayed, Ismail
Benajiba, Yassine
Benali, Habib
Bengtsson, Ewert
Bergeles, Christos
Berger, Marie-Odile
Bergtholdt, Martin
Berks, Michael
Bernal, Jorge Luis
Bernard, Olivier
Bernus, Olivier
Betrouni, Nacim
Bezy-Wendling, Johanne
Bhatia, Kanwal
Bhotika, Rahul
Biesdorf, Andreas
Bilgazyev, Emil
Bilgic, Berkin
Bishop, Martin
Bismuth, Vincent
Blaschko, Matthew
Bloch, Isabelle
Bloy, Luke
Blum, Tobias
Bogunovic, Hrvoje
Boisvert, Jonathan
Bosch, Johan
Bossa, Matias Nicolas
Bouarfa, Loubna
Bouix, Sylvain
Boukerroui, Djamal
Bourgeat, Pierrick
Bovendeerd, Peter

Brady, Michael
Breitenreicher, Dirk
Brock, Kristy
Brost, Alexander
Brun, Caroline
Burlina, Philippe
Butakoff, Constantine
Buvat, Irène
Caan, Matthan
Cahill, Nathan
Cai, Weidong
Cameron, Bruce
Camp, Jon
Cardenas, Valerie
Cardenes, Ruben
Cardoso, Manuel Jorge
Carmichael, Owen
Carson, Paul
Castaeda, Victor
Castro-Gonzalez, Carlos
Cathier, Pascal
Cattin, Philippe C.
Celebi, M. Emre
Cetingul, Hasan Ertan
Chakravarty, M. Mallar
Chan, Raymond
Chappelow, Jonathan
Chaux, Caroline
Chen, Elvis C. S.
Chen, Terrence
Chen, Ting
Chen, Xinjian
Chen, Yen-Wei
Chen, Yunmei
Cheng, Guang
Cheng, Jian
Cheriet, Farida
Chintalapani, Gouthami
Chinzei, Kiyoyuki
Chitphakdithai, Nicha
Chou, Yiyu
Chowdhury, Ananda
Christensen, Gary
Chu, Chia-Yueh Carlton
Chung, Moo K.

Chupin, Marie
Cinquin, Philippe
Ciofolo, Cybele
Ciompi, Francesco
Ciuciu, Philippe
Clark, Alys
Clarkson, Matthew
Cleary, Kevin
Clerc, Maureen
Clouchoux, Cédric
Cloutier, Guy
Combès, Benoît
Commowick, Olivier
Cootes, Tim
Corso, Jason
Coudiere, Yves
Coulon, Olivier
Coupe, Pierrick
Cowan, Brett
Crimi, Alessandro
Crum, William
Cui, Xinyi
Cuingnet, Remi
D'Alessandro, Brian
Daga, Pankaj
Dahl, Anders L.
Dai, Yakang
Daoud, Mohammad
Darkner, Sune
Darvann, Tron
Darzi, Ara
Dauguet, Julien
Dawant, Benoit
De Craene, Mathieu
Debbaut, Charlotte
Dehghan, Ehsan
Deligianni, Fani
Delong, Andrew
Demiralp, Cagatay
Demirci, Stefanie
Deng, Xiang
Dennis, Emily
Dequidt, Jeremie
Desbat, Laurent
Descoteaux, Maxime

Desvignes, Michel
Dewan, Maneesh
D'Haese, Pierre-François
DiBella, Edward
Diciotti, Stefano
Dijkstra, Jouke
Dikici, Engin
DiMaio, Simon
Ding, Kai
Dinten, Jean-Marc
Doessel, Olaf
Doignon, Christophe
Dojat, Michel
Dong, Bin
Donner, René
Douglas, Tania
Douiri, Abdel
Dowling, Jason
Doyle, Scott
Drangova, Maria
Drechsler, Klaus
Drobnjak, Ivana
Duan, Qi
Duchateau, Nicolas
Duchesnay, Edouard
Duchesne, Simon
Duriez, Christian
Durrleman, Stanley
Dzyubachyk, Oleh
Eagleson, Roy
Ebbers, Tino
Ecabert, Olivier
Ehrhardt, Jan
Elad, Michael
El-Baz, Ayman
Elen, An
Eleonora, Fornari
Elhawary, Haytham
El-Zehiry, Noha
Ennis, Daniel
Enquobahrie, Andinet
Erdt, Marius
Eskandari, Hani
Eskildsen, Simon
Eslami, Abouzar

Essert, Caroline
Fahrig, Rebecca
Fallavollita, Pascal
Fan, Yong
Farag, Aly
Fedorov, Andriy
Fei, Baowei
Felblinger, Jacques
Fenster, Aaron
Fetita, Catalin
Fiebich, Martin
Figl, Michael
Fischer, Gregory
Fishbaugh, James
Fitzpatrick, J. Michael
Fleig, Oliver
Florack, Luc
Fonov, Vladimir
Foroughi, Pezhman
Fouard, Céline
Fradkin, Maxim
Freiman, Moti
Friboulet, Denis
Fripp, Jurgen
Fritzsche, Klaus H.
Frouin, Frédérique
Frouin, Vincent
Funka-Lea, Gareth
Fuster, Andrea
Gagnon, Langis
Gangloff, Jacques
Ganz, Melanie
Gao, Mingchen
Gao, Wei
Gao, Yi
Garcia-Lorenzo, Daniel
Garvin, Mona
Gassert, Roger
Gatenby, Chris
Gee, Andrew
Georgescu, Bogdan
Georgii, Joachim
Geremia, Ezequiel
Ghanbari, Yasser
Gholipour, Ali

Ghosh, Aurobrata
Giannarou, Stamatia
Gibaud, Bernard
Gibson, Eli
Gilles, Benjamin
Gilson, Wesley
Giusti, Alessandro
Glaunès, Joan Alexis
Glocker, Ben
Gobbi, David
Goh, Alvina
Goksel, Orcun
Gonzalez Ballester, Miguel Angel
González Osorio, Fabio Augusto
Gooding, Mark
Goodlett, Casey
Gorges, Sebastien
Graham, Jim
Gramfort, Alexandre
Grass, Michael
Grau, Vicente
Grenier, Thomas
Griswold, Mark
Guerrero, Julian
Guetter, Christoph
Guevara, Pamela
Gulsun, Mehmet Akif
Gur, Yaniv
Gutman, Boris
Hacihaliloglu, Ilker
Hahn, Horst
Hajnal, Joseph
Hall, Timothy
Hamarneh, Ghassan
Hanahusa, Akihiko
Hanaoka, Shouhei
Hans, Arne
Hansen, Michael Sass
Hanson, Dennis
Hao, Xiang
Hartov, Alexander
Hastreiter, Peter
Hatt, Chuck
Haynor, David
He, Huiguang

Heberlein, Keith
Heckemann, Rolf
Heinrich, Mattias Paul
Hellier, Pierre
Heng, Pheng Ann
Hennemuth, Anja
Herlambang, Nicholas
Hernandez, Monica
Hipwell, John
Hirano, Yasushi
Hoffmann, Kenneth
Holmes, David
Hontani, Hidekata
Hoogendoorn, Corné
Hornegger, Joachim
Howe, Robert
Hsu, Li-Yueh
Hu, Yipeng
Hu, Zhihong
Huang, Heng
Huang, Junzhou
Huang, Rui
Huang, Wei
Huang, Xiaolei
Hudelot, Céline
Huisman, Henkjan
Humbert, Ludovic
Hurdal, Monica
Hyde, Damon
Iakovidis, Dimitris
Iglesias, Juan Eugenio
Imiya, Atsushi
Ingalhalikar, Madhura
Ionasec, Razvan
Irfanoglu, Mustafa Okan
Isgum, Ivana
Ishikawa, Hiroshi
Jacob, Mathews
Jacobs, Colin
Jahanshad, Neda
Janoos, Firdaus
Janowczyk, Andrew
Jbabdi, Saad
Jenkinson, Mark
Jerebko, Anna

Jian, Bing
Jiang, Tianzi
Jiang, Yifeng
Jomier, Julien
Jordan, Petr
Joshi, Anand
Joshi, Sarang
Jurrus, Elizabeth
Kabus, Sven
Kachelrie, Marc
Kadoury, Samuel
Kainmueller, Dagmar
Kallenberg, Michiel
Kamen, Ali
Kanade, Takeo
Kapoor, Ankur
Kapur, Tina
Karamalis, Athanasios
Karemore, Gopal
Krsnäs, Andreas
Karwoski, Ron
Kaster, Frederik
Katouzian, Amin
Kawata, Yoshiki
Kaynig, Verena
Kazanzides, Peter
Keeve, Erwin
Kelm, Michael
Kerrien, Erwan
Kezele, Irina
Khan, Ali R.
Kherif, Ferath
Khurd, Parmeshwar
Kim, Boklye
Kim, Kio
Kim, Minjeong
Kindlmann, Gordon
King, Andrew
Kiraly, Atilla
Kirchberg, Klaus
Kitasaka, Takayuki
Klein, Arno
Klein, Jan
Klein, Martina
Klein, Stefan

Ma, YingLiang
Machiraju, Raghu
MacLeod, Robert
Madany Mamlouk, Amir
Maddah, Mahnaz
Magee, Derek
Magnotta, Vincent
Maier-Hein, Lena
Malandain, Grégoire
Manduca, Armando
Mani, Meena
Manjón, José V.
Manniesing, Rashindra
Mansi, Tommaso
Manzke, Robert
Marchal, Maud
Marsland, Stephen
Martí, Robert
Masamune, Ken
Mattes, Julian
Maurel, Pierre
Mavroforakis, Michael
McClelland, Jamie
McCormick, Matthew
Medrano-Gracia, Pau
Meine, Hans
Meinzer, Hans-Peter
Meisner, Eric
Mekada, Yoshito
Melbourne, Andrew
Mertins, Alfred
Metz, Coert
Meyer, Chuck
Meyer, François
Michailovich, Oleg
Michel, Fabrice
Mihalef, Viorel
Miller, James
Modat, Marc
Modersitzki, Jan
Mohamed, Ashraf
Monaco, James
Montillo, Albert
Moore, John
Moradi, Mehdi

Mory, Benoit
Müller, Henning
Murgasova, Maria
Murphy, Keelin
Mylonas, George
Najman, Laurent
Nakajima, Yoshikazu
Nakamura, Ryoichi
Nassiri-Avanaki, Mohammad-Reza
Negahdar, Mohammadjavad
Negahdar, Mohammadreza
Nekolla, Stephan
Neumuth, Thomas
Ng, Bernard
Nichols, Thomas
Nicolau, Stéphane
Nie, Jingxin
Niederer, Steven
Niethammer, Marc
Noble, Jack
Noël, Peter
Nolte, Lutz
Nordsletten, David
Nuyts, Johan
O'Brien, Kieran
Oda, Masahiro
O'Donnell, Lauren
O'Donnell, Thomas
Oguz, Ipek
Okada, Kazunori
Olabarriaga, Silvia
Olesch, Janine
Oliver, Arnau
Olmos, Salvador
Oost, Elco
Orihuela-Espina, Felipe
Orkisz, Maciej
Otake, Yoshito
Ou, Yangming
Pace, Danielle
Padfield, Dirk
Padoy, Nicolas
Palaniappan, Kannappan
Pallavaram, Srivatsan
Panagiotaki, Eleftheria

Paniagua, Beatriz
Paolillo, Alfredo
Papademetris, Xenios
Papadopoulo, Theo
Park, Mi-Ae
Parthasarathy, Vijay
Passat, Nicolas
Pasternak, Ofer
Patriciu, Alexandru
Paul, Perrine
Paulsen, Keith
Paulsen, Rasmus
Pauly, Olivier
Pavlidis, Ioannis
Pearlman, Paul
Pedemonte, Stefano
Peitgen, Heinz-Otto
Pekar, Vladimir
Peng, Hanchuan
Penney, Graeme
Pernus, Franjo
Perperidis, Antonios
Perrot, Matthieu
Peters, Amanda
Petersen, Jens
Petitjean, Caroline
Peyrat, Jean-Marc
Peyré, Gabriel
Pham, Dzung
Phlypo, Ronald
Piella, Gemma
Pitiot, Alain
Pizaine, Guillaume
Pizer, Stephen
Platel, Bram
Podder, Tarun
Poignet, Philippe
Poline, Jean-Baptiste
Polzehl, Joerg
Pontre, Beau
Poot, Dirk
Popovic, Aleksandra
Poupon, Cyril
Poynton, Clare
Pozo, José Maria

Prasad, Gautam
Prastawa, Marcel
Pratt, Philip
Prima, Sylvain
Prince, Jerry
Punithakumar, Kumaradevan
Puy, Gilles
Qazi, Arish A.
Qian, Zhen
Quellec, Gwenole
Radau, Perry
Radeva, Petia
Radulescu, Emil
Rahman, Md Mahmudur
Raj, Ashish
Rajagopalan, Srinivasan
Rajagopalan, Vidya
Rajpoot, Nasir
Rangarajan, Anand
Rasoulian, Abtin
Rathi, Yogesh
Ratnanather, Tilak
Ravishankar, Saiprasad
Reichl, Tobias
Reilhac-Laborde, Anthonin
Rettmann, Maryam
Reuter, Martin
Reyes, Mauricio
Reyes-Aldasoro, Constantino
Rhode, Kawal
Ribbens, Annemie
Richa, Rogerio
Riddell, Cyrill
Ridgway, Gerard
Riklin Raviv, Tammy
Risholm, Petter
Risser, Laurent
Rit, Simon
Rittscher, Jens
Rivaz, Hassan
Riviere, Cameron
Riviere, Denis
Roche, Alexis
Rohkohl, Christopher
Rohling, Robert

Rohr, Karl
Rousseau, François
Roysam, Badrinath
Ruehaak, Jan
Russakoff, Daniel
Rusu, Mirabela
Ruthotto, Lars
Sabczynski, Jörg
Sadeghi-Naini, Ali
Sadowsky, Ofri
Saha, Punam Kumar
Salvado, Olivier
San Jose Estepar, Raul
Sanchez, Clarisa
Sanderson, Allen
Sands, Greg
Sarrut, David
Sarry, Laurent
Savadjiev, Peter
Scherer, Reinhold
Scherrer, Benoit
Schindelin, Johannes
Schmidt, Michael
Schmidt-Richberg, Alexander
Schneider, Caitlin
Schneider, Torben
Schoonenberg, Gert
Schultz, Thomas
Schweikard, Achim
Sebastian, Rafael
Seiler, Christof
Serre, Thomas
Seshamani, Sharmishtaa
Shah, Shishir
Shamir, Reuben R.
Shen, Li
Shen, Tian
Shi, Feng
Shi, Kuangyu
Shi, Pengcheng
Shi, Yonggang
Shi, Yonghong
Shi, Yubing
Sijbers, Jan
Simaan, Nabil

Simonyan, Karen
Simpson, Amber
Simpson, Ivor
Singh, Maneesh
Singh, Nikhil
Singh, Vikas
Sinkus, Ralph
Siqueira, Marcelo
Sjöstrand, Karl
Slabaugh, Greg
Slagmolen, Pieter
Smal, Ihor
Smeets, Dirk
Soeller, Christian
Sofka, Michal
Soler, Luc
Song, Sang-Eun
Song, Xubo
Sonka, Milan
Srensen, Lauge
Sotiras, Aristeidis
Sparks, Rachel
Sporring, Jon
Staal, Joes
Staring, Marius
Staroswiecki, Ernesto
Stehle, Thomas
Stewart, James
Stolka, Philipp
Stoyanov, Danail
Styles, Iain
Subramanian, Navneeth
Suinesiaputra, Avan
Sundar, Hari
Suthau, Tim
Suzuki, Kenji
Syeda-Mahmood, Tanveer
Szczerba, Dominik
Tagare, Hemant
Tahmasebi, Amir
Tai, Xue-Cheng
Tannenbaum, Allen
Tanner, Christine
Tao, Xiaodong
Tasdizen, Tolga

Tavakoli, Vahid
Taylor, Zeike
Thévenaz, Philippe
Thiriet, Marc
Tiwari, Pallavi
Tobon-Gomez, Catalina
Toews, Matthew
Tohka, Jussi
Tokuda, Junichi
Tosun, Duygu
Toth, Robert
Toussaint, Nicolas
Tristán-Vega, Antonio
Tsekos, Nikolaos V.
Turaga, Srinivas
Tustison, Nicholas
Uchiyama, Yoshikazu
Udupa, Jayaram K.
Unal, Gozde
Uzunbas, Mustafa
van Assen, Hans
van der Geest, Rob
van der Lijn, Fedde
van Rikxoort, Eva
van Stralen, Marijn
van Walsum, Theo
Vannier, Michael
Varoquaux, Gael
Vegas-Sánchez-Ferrero, Gonzalo
Venkataraman, Archana
Vercauteren, Tom
Vialard, François-Xavier
Vignon, François
Villain, Nicolas
Villard, Pierre-Frédéric
Vincent, Nicole
Visentini-Scarzanella, Marco
Visvikis, Dimitris
Viswanath, Satish
Vitanovski, Dime
Vogel, Jakob
Voigt, Ingmar
von Berg, Jens
Voros, Sandrine
Vos, Pieter

Vosburgh, Kirby
Vrooman, Henri
Vrtovec, Tomaz
Wachinger, Christian
Waechter-Stehle, Irina
Wahle, Andreas
Waldman, Lew
Wang, Chaohui
Wang, Fei
Wang, Hongzhi
Wang, Hui
Wang, Lejing
Wang, Li
Wang, Liansheng
Wang, Peng
Wang, Qian
Wang, Song
Wang, Vicky
Wang, Yalin
Wang, Yang
Wang, Ying
Wanyu, Liu
Warfield, Simon
Wassermann, Demian
Weber, Stefan
Wee, Chong-Yaw
Wei, Liu
Weiskopf, Nikolaus
Wells, William
Wels, Michael
Werner, Rene
Whitaker, Ross
Whitmarsh, Tristan
Wiles, Andrew
Wirtz, Stefan
Wittek, Adam
Wolf, Ivo
Wolz, Robin
Wörz, Stefan
Wu, Guorong
Wu, Wen
Wu, Xiaodong
Xenos, Michalis
Xie, Jun
Xiong, Guanglei

Xu, Jun
Xu, Lei
Xu, Sheng
Xu, Xiayu
Xue, Hui
Xue, Zhong
Yan, Pingkun
Yan, Zhennan
Yang, Fei
Yang, Lin
Yang, Xiaofeng
Yang, Xiaoyun
Yaniv, Ziv
Yao, Jianhua
Yap, Pew-Thian
Yaqub, Mohammad
Ye, Dong Hye
Yener, Bülent
Yeniaras, Erol
Yeo, B.T. Thomas
Yin, Zhaozheng
Ying, Leslie
Yoo, Terry
Yoshida, Hiro
Yotter, Rachel
Yushkevich, Paul
Zagorchev, Lyubomir
Zahiri Azar, Reza
Zaidi, Habib
Zeng, Wei

Zhan, Liang
Zhan, Yiqiang
Zhang, Chong
Zhang, Daoqiang
Zhang, Honghai
Zhang, Hui
Zhang, Jingdan
Zhang, Pei
Zhang, Shaoting
Zhao, Fei
Zheng, Guoyan
Zheng, Yefeng
Zheng, Yuanjie
Zhong, Hua
Zhong, Lin
Zhou, Jinghao
Zhou, Luping
Zhou, S. Kevin
Zhou, X. Sean
Zhou, Xiaobo
Zhou, Yan
Zhu, Hongtu
Zhu, Ning
Zhu, Yuemin
Zhuang, Xiahai
Zijdenbos, Alex
Zikic, Darko
Zion, Tse
Zollei, Lilla
Zwiggelaar, Reyer

Awards Presented at MICCAI 2011, Toronto

MICCAI Society Enduring Impact Award Sponsored by Philips: The Enduring Impact Award is the highest award of the MICCAI Society. It is a career award for continued excellence in the MICCAI research field. The 2011 Enduring Impact Award was presented to *Chris Taylor*, Manchester University, UK.

MICCAI Society Fellowships: MICCAI Fellowships are bestowed annually on a small number of senior members of the society in recognition of substantial scientific contributions to the MICCAI research field and service to the MICCAI community. In 2011, fellowships were awarded to:

- *Christian Barillot* (IRISA-CNRS, France)
- *Gabor Fichtinger* (Queens University, Canada)
- *Jerry Prince* (Johns Hopkins University, USA)

Medical Image Analysis Journal Award Sponsored by Elsevier: *Ola Friman*, for the article entitled: "Probabilistic 4D Blood Flow Tracking and Uncertainty Estimation", co-authored by: Ola Friman, Anja Hennemuth, Andreas Harloff, Jelena Bock, Michael Markl, and Heinz-Otto Peitgen

Best Paper in Computer-Assisted Intervention Systems and Medical Robotics, Sponsored by Intuitive Surgical Inc.: *Jay Mung*, for the article entitled "A Non-disruptive Technology for Robust 3D Tool Tracking for Ultrasound-Guided Interventions", co-authored by: Jay Mung, Francois Vignon, and Ameet Jain.

MICCAI Young Scientist Awards: The Young Scientist Awards are stimulation prizes awarded for the best first authors of MICCAI contributions in distinct subject areas. The nominees had to be full-time students at a recognized university at, or within, two years prior to submission. The 2011 MICCAI Young Scientist Awards were given to:

- *Mattias Heinrich* for his paper entitled "Non-local Shape Descriptor: A New Similarity Metric for Deformable Multi-modal Registration"
- *Tommaso Mansi* for his paper entitled "Towards Patient-Specific Finite-Element Simulation of Mitral Clip Procedure"
- *Siyang Zuo* for his paper entitled "Nonmetalic Rigid-Flexible Outer Sheath with Pneumatic Shapelocking Mechanism and Double Curvature Structure"
- *Christof Seiler* for his paper entitled "Geometry-Aware Multiscale Image Registration via OBB Tree-Based Polyaffine Log-Demons"
- *Ting Chen* for her paper entitled "Mixture of Segmenters with Discriminative Spatial Regularization and Sparse Weight Selection"

Table of Contents – Part I

Abdominal Imaging, Computer Assisted Interventions and Robotics

Reliable Assessment of Perfusivity and Diffusivity from Diffusion
Imaging of the Body 1
M. Freiman, S.D. Voss, R.V. Mulkern, J.M. Perez-Rossello,
M.J. Callahan, and Simon K. Warfield

Multi-organ Abdominal CT Segmentation Using Hierarchically
Weighted Subject-Specific Atlases 10
Robin Wolz, Chengwen Chu, Kazunari Misawa, Kensaku Mori, and
Daniel Rueckert

Radiation-Free Drill Guidance in Interlocking of Intramedullary Nails... 18
Benoit Diotte, Pascal Fallavollita, Lejing Wang, Simon Weidert,
Peter-Helmut Thaller, Ekkehard Euler, and Nassir Navab

Developing Essential Rigid-Flexible Outer Sheath to Enable Novel
Multi-piercing Surgery 26
Siyang Zuo, Takeshi Ohdaira, Kenta Kuwana, Yoshihiro Nagao,
Satoshi Ieiri, Makoto Hashizume, Takeyoshi Dohi, and
Ken Masamune

Surgical Gesture Classification from Video Data 34
Benjamín Béjar Haro, Luca Zappella, and René Vidal

Remote Ultrasound Palpation for Robotic Interventions Using Absolute
Elastography 42
Caitlin Schneider, Ali Baghani, Robert Rohling, and
Septimiu Salcudean

Computer-Aided Diagnosis and Planning I

Modeling and Real-Time Simulation of a Vascularized Liver Tissue 50
Igor Peterlík, Christian Duriez, and Stéphane Cotin

Efficient Optic Cup Detection from Intra-image Learning with Retinal
Structure Priors 58
Yanwu Xu, Jiang Liu, Stephen Lin, Dong Xu, Carol Y. Cheung,
Tin Aung, and Tien Yin Wong

Population-Based Design of Mandibular Plates Based on Bone Quality
and Morphology   66
    Habib Bousleiman, Christof Seiler, Tateyuki Iizuka,
    Lutz-Peter Nolte, and Mauricio Reyes

Thoracic Abnormality Detection with Data Adaptive Structure
Estimation   74
    Yang Song, Weidong Cai, Yun Zhou, and Dagan Feng

Domain Transfer Learning for MCI Conversion Prediction   82
    Bo Cheng, Daoqiang Zhang, and Dinggang Shen

Simulation of Pneumoperitoneum for Laparoscopic Surgery Planning . . .   91
    J. Bano, A. Hostettler, S.A. Nicolau, S. Cotin, C. Doignon,
    H.S. Wu, M.H. Huang, L. Soler, and J. Marescaux

Incremental Kernel Ridge Regression for the Prediction of Soft Tissue
Deformations   99
    Binbin Pan, James J. Xia, Peng Yuan, Jaime Gateno,
    Horace H.S. Ip, Qizhen He, Philip K.M. Lee, Ben Chow, and
    Xiaobo Zhou

Fuzzy Multi-class Statistical Modeling for Efficient Total Lesion
Metabolic Activity Estimation from Realistic PET Images   107
    Jose George, Kathleen Vunckx, Elke Van de Casteele, Sabine Tejpar,
    Christophe M. Deroose, Johan Nuyts, Dirk Loeckx, and Paul Suetens

Structure and Context in Prostatic Gland Segmentation and
Classification   115
    Kien Nguyen, Anindya Sarkar, and Anil K. Jain

Quantitative Characterization of Trabecular Bone Micro architecture
Using Tensor Scale and Muti-Detector CT Imaging   124
    Yinxiao Liu, Punam K. Saha, and Ziyue Xu

Genetic, Structural and Functional Imaging Biomarkers for Early
Detection of Conversion from MCI to AD   132
    Nikhil Singh, Angela Y. Wang, Preethi Sankaranarayanan,
    P. Thomas Fletcher, and Sarang Joshi

Robust MR Spine Detection Using Hierarchical Learning and Local
Articulated Model   141
    Yiqiang Zhan, Dewan Maneesh, Martin Harder, and
    Xiang Sean Zhou

Spatiotemporal Reconstruction of the Breathing Function   149
    D. Duong, D. Shastri, P. Tsiamyrtzis, and I. Pavlidis

A Visual Latent Semantic Approach for Automatic Analysis and
Interpretation of Anaplastic Medulloblastoma Virtual Slides 157
  Angel Cruz-Roa, Fabio González, Joseph Galaro,
  Alexander R. Judkins, David Ellison, Jennifer Baccon,
  Anant Madabhushi, and Eduardo Romero

Detection of Spontaneous Vesicle Release at Individual Synapses Using
Multiple Wavelets in a CWT-Based Algorithm 165
  Stefan Sokoll, Klaus Tönnies, and Martin Heine

Image Reconstruction and Enhancement

An Adaptive Method of Tracking Anatomical Curves in X-Ray
Sequences 173
  Yu Cao and Peng Wang

Directional Interpolation for Motion Weighted 4D Cone-Beam CT
Reconstruction 181
  Hua Zhang and Jan-Jakob Sonke

Accurate and Efficient Linear Structure Segmentation by Leveraging
Ad Hoc Features with Learned Filters 189
  Roberto Rigamonti and Vincent Lepetit

Compensating Motion Artifacts of 3D in vivo SD-OCT Scans 198
  O. Müller, S. Donner, T. Klinder, I. Bartsch, A. Krüger,
  A. Heisterkamp, and B. Rosenhahn

Classification of Ambiguous Nerve Fiber Orientations in 3D Polarized
Light Imaging 206
  Melanie Kleiner, Markus Axer, David Gräßel, Julia Reckfort,
  Uwe Pietrzyk, Katrin Amunts, and Timo Dickscheid

Non-local Means Resolution Enhancement of Lung 4D-CT Data 214
  Yu Zhang, Guorong Wu, Pew-Thian Yap, Qianjin Feng, Jun Lian,
  Wufan Chen, and Dinggang Shen

Compressed Sensing Dynamic Reconstruction in Rotational
Angiography 223
  Hélène Langet, Cyril Riddell, Yves Trousset, Arthur Tenenhaus,
  Elisabeth Lahalle, Gilles Fleury, and Nikos Paragios

Bi-exponential Magnetic Resonance Signal Model for Partial Volume
Computation 231
  Quentin Duché, Oscar Acosta, Giulio Gambarota, Isabelle Merlet,
  Olivier Salvado, and Hervé Saint-Jalmes

3D Lung Tumor Motion Model Extraction from 2D Projection Images
of Mega-voltage Cone Beam CT via Optimal Graph Search   239
  Mingqing Chen, Junjie Bai, Yefeng Zheng, and R. Alfredo C. Siochi

Atlas Construction via Dictionary Learning and Group Sparsity   247
  Feng Shi, Li Wang, Guorong Wu, Yu Zhang, Manhua Liu,
  John H. Gilmore, Weili Lin, and Dinggang Shen

Dictionary Learning and Time Sparsity in Dynamic MRI   256
  Jose Caballero, Daniel Rueckert, and Joseph V. Hajnal

Joint Reconstruction of Image and Motion in MRI:
Implicit Regularization Using an Adaptive 3D Mesh   264
  Anne Menini, Pierre-André Vuissoz, Jacques Felblinger, and
  Freddy Odille

Sparsity-Based Deconvolution of Low-Dose Perfusion CT Using
Learned Dictionaries   272
  Ruogu Fang, Tsuhan Chen, and Pina C. Sanelli

Fast Multi-contrast MRI Reconstruction   281
  Junzhou Huang, Chen Chen, and Leon Axel

Steady-State Model of the Radio-Pharmaceutical Uptake
for MR-PET   289
  Stefano Pedemonte, M. Jorge Cardoso, Simon Arridge,
  Brian F. Hutton, and Sebastien Ourselin

Analysis of Microscopic and Optical Images I

Oriented Pattern Analysis for Streak Detection in Dermoscopy
Images   298
  Maryam Sadeghi, Tim K. Lee, David McLean, Harvey Lui, and
  M. Stella Atkins

Automated Foveola Localization in Retinal 3D-OCT Images Using
Structural Support Vector Machine Prediction   307
  Yu-Ying Liu, Hiroshi Ishikawa, Mei Chen, Gadi Wollstein,
  Joel S. Schuman, and James M. Rehg

Intrinsic Melanin and Hemoglobin Colour Components for Skin Lesion
Malignancy Detection   315
  Ali Madooei, Mark S. Drew, Maryam Sadeghi, and M. Stella Atkins

Anisotropic ssTEM Image Segmentation Using Dense Correspondence
across Sections   323
  Dmitry Laptev, Alexander Vezhnevets, Sarvesh Dwivedi, and
  Joachim M. Buhmann

Apoptosis Detection for Adherent Cell Populations in Time-Lapse
Phase-Contrast Microscopy Images 331
    Seungil Huh, Dai Fei Elmer Ker, Hang Su, and Takeo Kanade

Modeling Dynamic Cellular Morphology in Images 340
    *Xing An, Zhiwen Liu, Yonggang Shi, Ning Li, Yalin Wang, and
    Shantanu H. Joshi*

Learning to Detect Cells Using Non-overlapping Extremal Regions 348
    *Carlos Arteta, Victor Lempitsky, J. Alison Noble, and
    Andrew Zisserman*

Application of the IMM-JPDA Filter to Multiple Target Tracking in
Total Internal Reflection Fluorescence Microscopy Images 357
    *Seyed Hamid Rezatofighi, Stephen Gould, Richard Hartley,
    Katarina Mele, and William E. Hughes*

Image Segmentation with Implicit Color Standardization Using
Spatially Constrained Expectation Maximization: Detection of Nuclei... 365
    *James Monaco, J. Hipp, D. Lucas, S. Smith, U. Balis, and
    Anant Madabhushi*

Detecting and Tracking Motion of *Myxococcus xanthus* Bacteria in
Swarms 373
    *Xiaomin Liu, Cameron W. Harvey, Haitao Wang,
    Mark S. Alber, and Danny Z. Chen*

Signal and Noise Modeling in Confocal Laser Scanning Fluorescence
Microscopy 381
    *Gerlind Herberich, Reinhard Windoffer, Rudolf E. Leube, and
    Til Aach*

Hierarchical Partial Matching and Segmentation of Interacting Cells 389
    Zheng Wu, Danna Gurari, Joyce Y. Wong, and Margrit Betke

Computer-Assisted Interventions and Robotics I

Hybrid Tracking and Mosaicking for Information Augmentation in
Retinal Surgery 397
    *Rogério Richa, Balázs Vágvölgyi, Marcin Balicki,
    Gregory D. Hager, and Russell H. Taylor*

Real Time Assistance for Stent Positioning and Assessment by
Self-initialized Tracking 405
    Terrence Chen, Yu Wang, Peter Durlak, and Dorin Comaniciu

Marker-Less Reconstruction of Dense 4-D Surface Motion Fields Using
Active Laser Triangulation for Respiratory Motion Management   414
  Sebastian Bauer, Benjamin Berkels, Svenja Ettl, Oliver Arold,
  Joachim Hornegger, and Martin Rumpf

Modeling of Multi-View 3D Freehand Radio Frequency Ultrasound   422
  T. Klein, M. Hansson, and Nassir Navab

Towards Intra-operative PET for Head and Neck Cancer: Lymph Node
Localization Using High-Energy Probes   430
  Dzhoshkun I. Shakir, Aslı Okur, Alexander Hartl, Philipp Matthies,
  Sibylle I. Ziegler, Markus Essler, Tobias Lasser, and Nassir Navab

Data-Driven Breast Decompression and Lesion Mapping from Digital
Breast Tomosynthesis   438
  Michael Wels, B.M. Kelm, M. Hammon, Anna Jerebko,
  M. Sühling, and Dorin Comaniciu

Real Time Image-Based Tracking of 4D Ultrasound Data   447
  Ola Kristoffer Øye, Wolfgang Wein, Dag Magne Ulvang,
  Knut Matre, and Ivan Viola

Development of an MRI-Compatible Device for Prostate Focal
Therapy   455
  Jeremy Cepek, Blaine Chronik, Uri Lindner,
  John Trachtenberg, and Aaron Fenster

Intraoperative Ultrasound Guidance for Transanal Endoscopic
Microsurgery   463
  Philip Pratt, Aimee Di Marco, Christopher Payne, Ara Darzi, and
  Guang-Zhong Yang

Robotic Path Planning for Surgeon Skill Evaluation in
Minimally-Invasive Sinus Surgery   471
  Narges Ahmidi, Gregory D. Hager, Lisa Ishii, Gary L. Gallia, and
  Masaru Ishii

Stereoscopic Scene Flow for Robotic Assisted Minimally Invasive
Surgery   479
  Danail Stoyanov

Towards Computer-Assisted Deep Brain Stimulation Targeting
with Multiple Active Contacts   487
  Silvain Bériault, Yiming Xiao, Lara Bailey, D. Louis Collins,
  Abbas F. Sadikot, and G. Bruce Pike

Image Segmentation I

Multi-object Spring Level Sets (MUSCLE) 495
  Blake C. Lucas, Michael Kazhdan, and Russell H. Taylor

Combining CRF and Multi-hypothesis Detection for Accurate Lesion
Segmentation in Breast Sonograms 504
  Zhihui Hao, Qiang Wang, Yeong Kyeong Seong, Jong-Ha Lee,
  Haibing Ren, and Ji-yeun Kim

Hierarchical Manifold Learning 512
  Kanwal K. Bhatia, Anil Rao, Anthony N. Price, Robin Wolz,
  Jo Hajnal, and Daniel Rueckert

Vertebral Body Segmentation in MRI via Convex Relaxation and
Distribution Matching 520
  Ismail Ben Ayed, Kumaradevan Punithakumar, Rashid Minhas,
  Rohit Joshi, and Gregory J. Garvin

Evaluating Segmentation Error without Ground Truth 528
  Timo Kohlberger, Vivek Singh, Chris Alvino, Claus Bahlmann, and
  Leo Grady

Rotational-Slice-Based Prostate Segmentation Using Level Set with
Shape Constraint for 3D End-Firing TRUS Guided Biopsy 537
  Wu Qiu, Jing Yuan, Eranga Ukwatta, David Tessier, and
  Aaron Fenster

Segmentation of Biological Target Volumes on Multi-tracer PET
Images Based on Information Fusion for Achieving Dose Painting in
Radiotherapy 545
  Benoît Lelandais, Isabelle Gardin, Laurent Mouchard,
  Pierre Vera, and Su Ruan

Local Implicit Modeling of Blood Vessels for Interactive Simulation 553
  A. Yureidini, E. Kerrien, J. Dequidt, Christian Duriez, and S. Cotin

Real-Time 3D Image Segmentation by User-Constrained Template
Deformation 561
  Benoît Mory, Oudom Somphone, Raphael Prevost, and
  Roberto Ardon

Prior Knowledge, Random Walks and Human Skeletal Muscle
Segmentation 569
  P.-Y. Baudin, N. Azzabou, P.G. Carlier, and Nikos Paragios

Similarity-Based Appearance-Prior for Fitting a Subdivision Mesh
in Gene Expression Images 577
  Yen H. Le, Uday Kurkure, Nikos Paragios, Tao Ju,
  James P. Carson, and Ioannis A. Kakadiaris

Learning Context Cues for Synapse Segmentation in EM Volumes   585
Carlos Becker, Karim Ali, Graham Knott, and Pascal Fua

Estimation of the Prior Distribution of Ground Truth in the STAPLE
Algorithm: An Empirical Bayesian Approach   593
Alireza Akhondi-Asl and Simon K. Warfield

Unified Geometry and Topology Correction for Cortical Surface
Reconstruction with Intrinsic Reeb Analysis   601
Yonggang Shi, Rongjie Lai, and Arthur W. Toga

Automatic Detection and Classification of Teeth in CT Data   609
*Nguyen The Duy, Hans Lamecker, Dagmar Kainmueller, and
Stefan Zachow*

Cardiovascular Imaging I

Strain-Based Regional Nonlinear Cardiac Material Properties
Estimation from Medical Images   617
*Ken C.L. Wong, Jatin Relan, Linwei Wang, Maxime Sermesant,
Hervé Delingette, Nicholas Ayache, and Pengcheng Shi*

Frangi Goes US : Multiscale Tubular Structure Detection Adapted
to 3D Ultrasound   625
Paulo Waelkens, Seyed-Ahmad Ahmadi, and Nassir Navab

Limited Angle C-Arm Tomography and Segmentation for Guidance
of Atrial Fibrillation Ablation Procedures   634
*Dirk Schäfer, Carsten Meyer, Roland Bullens,
Axel Saalbach, and Peter Eshuis*

Automatic Non-rigid Temporal Alignment of IVUS Sequences   642
*Marina Alberti, Simone Balocco, Xavier Carrillo,
Josepa Mauri, and Petia Radeva*

Stochastic 3D Motion Compensation of Coronary Arteries
from Monoplane Angiograms   651
Jonathan Hadida, Christian Desrosiers, and Luc Duong

A Fast Convex Optimization Approach to Segmenting 3D Scar Tissue
from Delayed-Enhancement Cardiac MR Images   659
*Martin Rajchl, Jing Yuan, James A. White, Cyrus M.S. Nambakhsh,
Eranga Ukwatta, Feng Li, John Stirrat, and Terry M. Peters*

Robust Motion Correction in the Frequency Domain of Cardiac
MR Stress Perfusion Sequences   667
*Vikas Gupta, Martijn van de Giessen, Hortense Kirişli,
Sharon W. Kirschbaum, Wiro J. Niessen, and
Boudewijn P.F. Lelieveldt*

Localization of Sparse Transmural Excitation Stimuli from Surface
Mapping   675
  Jingjia Xu, Azar Rahimi Dehaghani, Fei Gao, and Linwei Wang

Automated Intraventricular Septum Segmentation Using Non-local
Spatio-temporal Priors   683
  *Mithun Das Gupta, Sheshadri Thiruvenkadam,
  Navneeth Subramanian, and Satish Govind*

Active Shape Model with Inter-profile Modeling Paradigm for Cardiac
Right Ventricle Segmentation   691
  Mohammed S. ElBaz and Ahmed S. Fahmy

Brain Imaging: Structure, Function and Disease Evolution

Tractometer: Online Evaluation System for Tractography   699
  *Marc-Alexandre Côté, Arnaud Boré, Gabriel Girard,
  Jean-Christophe Houde, and Maxime Descoteaux*

A Novel Sparse Graphical Approach for Multimodal Brain Connectivity
Inference   707
  *Bernard Ng, Gaël Varoquaux, Jean-Baptiste Poline, and
  Bertrand Thirion*

From Brain Connectivity Models to Identifying Foci of a Neurological
Disorder   715
  Archana Venkataraman, Marek Kubicki, and Polina Golland

Deriving Statistical Significance Maps for SVM Based Image
Classification and Group Comparisons   723
  Bilwaj Gaonkar and Christos Davatzikos

Analysis of Longitudinal Shape Variability via Subject Specific Growth
Modeling   731
  *James Fishbaugh, Marcel Prastawa, Stanley Durrleman,
  Joseph Piven for the IBIS Network, and Guido Gerig*

Regional Flux Analysis of Longitudinal Atrophy in Alzheimer's
Disease   739
  *Marco Lorenzi, Nicholas Ayache, and Xavier Pennec
  for the Alzheimer's Disease Neuroimaging Initiative*

Erratum

Localization of Sparse Transmural Excitation Stimuli from Surface
Mapping E1
  Jingjia Xu, Azar Rahimi Dehaghani, Fei Gao, and Linwei Wang

Author Index   747

Table of Contents – Part II

Cardiovascular Imaging: Planning, Intervention and Simulation

Automatic Multi-model-Based Segmentation of the Left Atrium in
Cardiac MRI Scans 1
*Dominik Kutra, Axel Saalbach, Helko Lehmann, Alexandra Groth,
Sebastian P.M. Dries, Martin W. Krueger, Olaf Dössel, and
Jürgen Weese*

Curvilinear Structure Enhancement with the Polygonal Path Image –
Application to Guide-Wire Segmentation in X-Ray Fluoroscopy 9
*Vincent Bismuth, Régis Vaillant, Hugues Talbot, and
Laurent Najman*

Catheter Tracking via Online Learning for Dynamic Motion
Compensation in Transcatheter Aortic Valve Implantation 17
Peng Wang, Yefeng Zheng, Matthias John, and Dorin Comaniciu

Evaluation of a Real-Time Hybrid Three-Dimensional Echo and X-Ray
Imaging System for Guidance of Cardiac Catheterisation Procedures ... 25
*R.J. Housden, A. Arujuna, Y. Ma, N. Nijhof, G. Gijsbers,
R. Bullens, M. O'Neill, M. Cooklin, C.A. Rinaldi, J. Gill,
S. Kapetanakis, J. Hancock, M. Thomas, R. Razavi, and K.S. Rhode*

LBM-EP: Lattice-Boltzmann Method for Fast Cardiac
Electrophysiology Simulation from 3D Images 33
*S. Rapaka, T. Mansi, B. Georgescu, M. Pop, G.A. Wright,
A. Kamen, and Dorin Comaniciu*

Cardiac Mechanical Parameter Calibration Based on the Unscented
Transform 41
*Stéphanie Marchesseau, Hervé Delingette, Maxime Sermesant,
Kawal Rhode, Simon G. Duckett, C. Aldo Rinaldi, Reza Razavi, and
Nicholas Ayache*

Image Registration I

Temporal Shape Analysis via the Spectral Signature 49
*Elena Bernardis, Ender Konukoglu, Yangming Ou,
Dimitris N. Metaxas, Benoit Desjardins, and
Kilian M. Pohl*

Joint T1 and Brain Fiber Log-Demons Registration Using Currents
to Model Geometry   57
  Viviana Siless, Joan Glaunés, Pamela Guevara,
  Jean-François Mangin, Cyril Poupon, Denis Le Bihan,
  Bertrand Thirion, and Pierre Fillard

Automated Skeleton Based Multi-modal Deformable Registration
of Head&Neck Datasets   66
  Sebastian Steger and Stefan Wesarg

Lung Registration with Improved Fissure Alignment by Integration
of Pulmonary Lobe Segmentation   74
  Alexander Schmidt-Richberg, Jan Ehrhardt, René Werner, and
  Heinz Handels

3D Ultrasound-CT Registration in Orthopaedic Trauma Using
GMM Registration with Optimized Particle Simulation-Based Data
Reduction   82
  Ilker Hacihaliloglu, Anna Brounstein, Pierre Guy,
  Antony Hodgson, and Rafeef Abugharbieh

Hierarchical Attribute-Guided Symmetric Diffeomorphic Registration
for MR Brain Images   90
  Guorong Wu, Minjeong Kim, Qian Wang, and Dinggang Shen

Uncertainty-Based Feature Learning for Skin Lesion Matching
Using a High Order MRF Optimization Framework   98
  Hengameh Mirzaalian, Tim K. Lee, and Ghassan Hamarneh

Automatic Categorization of Anatomical Landmark-Local Appearances
Based on Diffeomorphic Demons and Spectral Clustering for
Constructing Detector Ensembles   106
  Shouhei Hanaoka, Yoshitaka Masutani, Mitsutaka Nemoto,
  Yukihiro Nomura, Takeharu Yoshikawa, Naoto Hayashi, and
  Kuni Ohtomo

A Novel Approach for Global Lung Registration Using 3D
Markov-Gibbs Appearance Model   114
  Ayman El-Baz, Fahmi Khalifa, Ahmed Elnakib, Matthew Nitzken,
  Ahmed Soliman, Patrick McClure, Mohamed Abou El-Ghar, and
  Georgy Gimel'farb

Analytic Regularization of Uniform Cubic B-spline Deformation
Fields   122
  James A. Shackleford, Qi Yang, Ana M. Lourenço,
  Nadya Shusharina, Nagarajan Kandasamy, and
  Gregory C. Sharp

Simultaneous Multiscale Polyaffine Registration by Incorporating
Deformation Statistics   130
  Christof Seiler, Xavier Pennec, and Mauricio Reyes

Fast Diffusion Tensor Registration with Exact Reorientation and
Regularization   138
  Junning Li, Yonggang Shi, Giang Tran, Ivo Dinov,
  Danny J.J. Wang, and Arthur W. Toga

Registration of Brainstem Surfaces in Adolescent Idiopathic Scoliosis
Using Discrete Ricci Flow   146
  Minqi Zhang, Fang Li, Ying He, Shi Lin, Defeng Wang, and
  Lok Ming Lui

Groupwise Rigid Registration of Wrist Bones   155
  Martijn van de Giessen, Frans M. Vos, Cornelis A. Grimbergen,
  Lucas J. van Vliet, and Geert J. Streekstra

Automated Diffeomorphic Registration of Anatomical Structures with
Rigid Parts: Application to Dynamic Cervical MRI   163
  Olivier Commowick, Nicolas Wiest-Daesslé, and Sylvain Prima

Large Deformation Diffeomorphic Registration of Diffusion-Weighted
Images   171
  Pei Zhang, Marc Niethammer, Dinggang Shen, and Pew-Thian Yap

NeuroImage Analysis I

Prediction of Brain MR Scans in Longitudinal Tumor Follow-Up
Studies   179
  Lior Weizman, Liat Ben-Sira, Leo Joskowicz, Orna Aizenstein,
  Ben Shofty, Shlomi Constantini, and Dafna Ben-Bashat

Resting-State FMRI Single Subject Cortical Parcellation
Based on Region Growing   188
  Thomas Blumensath, Timothy E.J. Behrens, and Stephen M. Smith

A Framework for Quantifying Node-Level Community Structure Group
Differences in Brain Connectivity Networks   196
  Johnson J. GadElkarim, Dan Schonfeld, Olusola Ajilore,
  Liang Zhan, Aifeng F. Zhang, Jamie D. Feusner, Paul M. Thompson,
  Tony J. Simon, Anand Kumar, and Alex D. Leow

A Feature-Based Developmental Model of the Infant Brain in Structural
MRI   204
  Matthew Toews, William M. Wells III, and Lilla Zöllei

Constrained Sparse Functional Connectivity Networks for MCI
Classification 212
    Chong-Yaw Wee, Pew-Thian Yap, Daoqiang Zhang,
    Lihong Wang, and Dinggang Shen

MR-Less Surface-Based Amyloid Estimation by Subject-Specific Atlas
Selection and Bayesian Fusion 220
    Luping Zhou, Olivier Salvado, Vincent Dore, Pierrick Bourgeat,
    Parnesh Raniga, Victor L. Villemagne, Christopher C. Rowe,
    Jurgen Fripp, and The AIBL Research Group

Hierarchical Structural Mapping for Globally Optimized Estimation
of Functional Networks 228
    Alex D. Leow, Liang Zhan, Donatello Arienzo,
    Johnson J. GadElkarim, Aifeng F. Zhang, Olusola Ajilore,
    Anand Kumar, Paul M. Thompson, and Jamie D. Feusner

Characterization of Task-Free/Task-Performance Brain States 237
    Xin Zhang, Lei Guo, Xiang Li, Dajiang Zhu, Kaiming Li,
    Zhenqiang Sun, Changfeng Jin, Xintao Hu, Junwei Han, Qun Zhao,
    Lingjiang Li, and Tianming Liu

Quantitative Evaluation of Statistical Inference in Resting State
Functional MRI... 246
    Xue Yang, Hakmook Kang, Allen Newton, and Bennett A. Landman

Identifying Sub-Populations via Unsupervised Cluster Analysis
on Multi-Edge Similarity Graphs................................. 254
    Madhura Ingalhalikar, Alex R. Smith, Luke Bloy, Ruben Gur,
    Timothy P.L. Roberts, and Ragini Verma

Geodesic Information Flows 262
    M. Jorge Cardoso, Robin Wolz, Marc Modat, Nick C. Fox,
    Daniel Rueckert, and Sebastien Ourselin

Group-Wise Consistent Parcellation of Gyri via Adaptive Multi-view
Spectral Clustering of Fiber Shapes 271
    Hanbo Chen, Xiao Cai, Dajiang Zhu, Feiping Nie,
    Tianming Liu, and Heng Huang

Diffusion Weighted Imaging

Extracting Quantitative Measures from EAP: A Small Clinical Study
Using BFOR 280
    A. Pasha Hosseinbor, Moo K. Chung, Yu-Chien Wu,
    John O. Fleming, Aaron S. Field, and Andrew L. Alexander

Sparse DSI: Learning DSI Structure for Denoising and Fast Imaging 288
    Alexandre Gramfort, Cyril Poupon, and Maxime Descoteaux

Fiber Density Estimation by Tensor Divergence 297
  Marco Reisert, Henrik Skibbe, and Valerij G. Kiselev

Estimation of Extracellular Volume from Regularized Multi-shell
Diffusion MRI 305
  Ofer Pasternak, Martha E. Shenton, and Carl-Fredrik Westin

Nonnegative Definite EAP and ODF Estimation via a Unified
Multi-shell HARDI Reconstruction 313
  Jian Cheng, Tianzi Jiang, and Rachid Deriche

Estimation of Non-negative ODFs Using the Eigenvalue Distribution
of Spherical Functions 322
  Evan Schwab, Bijan Afsari, and René Vidal

Spatial Warping of DWI Data Using Sparse Representation 331
  Pew-Thian Yap and Dinggang Shen

Tractography via the Ensemble Average Propagator in Diffusion
MRI 339
  *Sylvain Merlet, Anne-Charlotte Philippe, Rachid Deriche, and
  Maxime Descoteaux*

Image Segmentation II

A 4D Statistical Shape Model for Automated Segmentation of Lungs
with Large Tumors 347
  Matthias Wilms, Jan Ehrhardt, and Heinz Handels

Closed-Form Relaxation for MRF-MAP Tissue Classification Using
Discrete Laplace Equations 355
  Alexis Roche

Anatomical Structures Segmentation by Spherical 3D Ray Casting
and Gradient Domain Editing 363
  A. Kronman, Leo Joskowicz, and J. Sosna

Segmentation of the Pectoral Muscle in Breast MRI Using Atlas-Based
Approaches 371
  *Albert Gubern-Mérida, Michiel Kallenberg, Robert Martí, and
  Nico Karssemeijer*

Hierarchical Conditional Random Fields for Detection of
Gad-Enhancing Lesions in Multiple Sclerosis 379
  *Zahra Karimaghaloo, Douglas L. Arnold, D. Louis Collins, and
  Tal Arbel*

Simplified Labeling Process for Medical Image Segmentation 387
  Mingchen Gao, Junzhou Huang, Xiaolei Huang,
  Shaoting Zhang, and Dimitris N. Metaxas

Liver Segmentation Approach Using Graph Cuts and Iteratively
Estimated Shape and Intensity Constrains 395
  Ahmed Afifi and Toshiya Nakaguchi

Multi-Object Geodesic Active Contours (MOGAC) 404
  Blake C. Lucas, Michael Kazhdan, and Russell H. Taylor

A Pattern Recognition Approach to Zonal Segmentation of the Prostate
on MRI 413
  Geert Litjens, Oscar Debats, Wendy van de Ven,
  Nico Karssemeijer, and Henkjan Huisman

Statistical Shape Model Segmentation and Frequency Mapping
of Cochlear Implant Stimulation Targets in CT 421
  Jack H. Noble, René H. Gifford, Robert F. Labadie, and
  Benoît M. Dawant

Guiding Automatic Segmentation with Multiple Manual
Segmentations 429
  Hongzhi Wang and Paul A. Yushkevich

Atlas-Based Probabilistic Fibroglandular Tissue Segmentation
in Breast MRI 437
  Shandong Wu, Susan Weinstein, and Despina Kontos

Fast 3D Spine Reconstruction of Postoperative Patients Using a
Multilevel Statistical Model 446
  Fabian Lecron, Jonathan Boisvert, Saïd Mahmoudi,
  Hubert Labelle, and Mohammed Benjelloun

Probabilistic Segmentation of the Lumen from Intravascular Ultrasound
Radio Frequency Data 454
  E. Gerardo Mendizabal-Ruiz and Ioannis A. Kakadiaris

Precise Segmentation of Multiple Organs in CT Volumes Using
Learning-Based Approach and Information Theory 462
  Chao Lu, Yefeng Zheng, Neil Birkbeck, Jingdan Zhang,
  Timo Kohlberger, Christian Tietjen, Thomas Boettger,
  James S. Duncan, and S. Kevin Zhou

A Study on Graphical Model Structure for Representing Statistical
Shape Model of Point Distribution Model 470
  Yoshihide Sawada and Hidekata Hontani

Cardiovascular Imaging II

Quality Metric for Parasternal Long Axis B-Mode Echocardiograms 478
  Sri-Kaushik Pavani, Navneeth Subramanian, Mithun Das Gupta,
  Pavan Annangi, Satish C. Govind, and Brian Young

Hemodynamic Assessment of Pre- and Post-operative Aortic
Coarctation from MRI 486
  Kristóf Ralovich, Lucian Itu, Viorel Mihalef, Puneet Sharma,
  Razvan Ionasec, Dime Vitanovski, Waldemar Krawtschuk,
  Allen Everett, Richard Ringel, Nassir Navab, and Dorin Comaniciu

Linear Invariant Tensor Interpolation Applied to Cardiac Diffusion
Tensor MRI 494
  Jin Kyu Gahm, Nicholas Wisniewski, Gordon Kindlmann,
  Geoffrey L. Kung, William S. Klug, Alan Garfinkel, and
  Daniel B. Ennis

Morphological Analysis of the Left Ventricular Endocardial Surface
and Its Clinical Implications 502
  Anirban Mukhopadhyay, Zhen Qian, Suchendra M. Bhandarkar,
  Tianming Liu, Sarah Rinehart, and Szilard Voros

Prior-Based Automatic Segmentation of the Carotid Artery Lumen
in TOF MRA (PASCAL) 511
  Jana Hutter, Hannes G. Hofmann, Robert Grimm, Andreas Greiser,
  Marc Saake, Joachim Hornegger, Arnd Dörfler, and Peter Schmitt

A Convex Relaxation Approach to Fat/Water Separation with
Minimum Label Description 519
  Abraam S. Soliman, Jing Yuan, James A. White,
  Terry M. Peters, and Charles A. McKenzie

Regional Heart Motion Abnormality Detection via Multiview Fusion ... 527
  Kumaradevan Punithakumar, Ismail Ben Ayed, Ali Islam,
  Aashish Goela, and Shuo Li

Global Assessment of Cardiac Function Using Image Statistics
in MRI 535
  Mariam Afshin, Ismail Ben Ayed, Ali Islam, Aashish Goela,
  Terry M. Peters, and Shuo Li

Computer-Assisted Interventions and Robotics II

Ultrasound and Fluoroscopic Images Fusion by Autonomous Ultrasound
Probe Detection 544
  Peter Mountney, Razvan Ionasec, Markus Kaizer, Sina Mamaghani,
  Wen Wu, Terrence Chen, Matthias John, Jan Boese, and
  Dorin Comaniciu

Direct 3D Ultrasound to Video Registration Using Photoacoustic
Effect 552
  Alexis Cheng, Jin U. Kang, Russell H. Taylor, and Emad M. Boctor

Assessment of Navigation Cues with Proximal Force Sensing
during Endovascular Catheterization 560
  Hedyeh Rafii-Tari, Christopher J. Payne, Celia Riga, Colin Bicknell,
  Su-Lin Lee, and Guang-Zhong Yang

Data-Driven Visual Tracking in Retinal Microsurgery 568
  Raphael Sznitman, Karim Ali, Rogério Richa, Russell H. Taylor,
  Gregory D. Hager, and Pascal Fua

Real-Time Motion Compensated Patient Positioning and Non-rigid
Deformation Estimation Using 4-D Shape Priors 576
  Jakob Wasza, Sebastian Bauer, and Joachim Hornegger

Semi-automatic Catheter Reconstruction from Two Views 584
  Matthias Hoffmann, Alexander Brost, Carolin Jakob, Felix Bourier,
  Martin Koch, Klaus Kurzidim, Joachim Hornegger, and
  Norbert Strobel

Feature Classification for Tracking Articulated Surgical Tools 592
  Austin Reiter, Peter K. Allen, and Tao Zhao

Image-Based Tracking of the Teeth for Orthodontic Augmented
Reality 601
  André Aichert, Wolfgang Wein, Alexander Ladikos,
  Tobias Reichl, and Nassir Navab

Intra-op Measurement of the Mechanical Axis Deviation: An Evaluation
Study on 19 Human Cadaver Legs 609
  Lejing Wang, Pascal Fallavollita, Alexander Brand, Okan Erat,
  Simon Weidert, Peter-Helmut Thaller, Ekkehard Euler, and
  Nassir Navab

Real-Time Quantitative Elasticity Imaging of Deep Tissue Using
Free-Hand Conventional Ultrasound 617
  Ali Baghani, Hani Eskandari, Weiqi Wang, Daniel Da Costa,
  Mohamed Nabil Lathiff, Ramin Sahebjavaher,
  Septimiu Salcudean, and Robert Rohling

A Comparative Study of Correspondence-Search Algorithms in MIS
Images 625
  Gustavo A. Puerto and Gian-Luca Mariottini

3D Reconstruction in Laparoscopy with Close-Range Photometric
Stereo 634
  Toby Collins and Adrien Bartoli

Image Registration: New Methods and Results

Registration Accuracy: How Good Is Good Enough? A Statistical
Power Calculation Incorporating Image Registration Uncertainty   643
  Eli Gibson, Aaron Fenster, and Aaron D. Ward

Joint Tumor Segmentation and Dense Deformable Registration
of Brain MR Images   651
  *Sarah Parisot, Hugues Duffau, Stéphane Chemouny, and
  Nikos Paragios*

Registration Using Sparse Free-Form Deformations   659
  *Wenzhe Shi, Xiahai Zhuang, Luis Pizarro, Wenjia Bai,
  Haiyan Wang, Kai-Pin Tung, Philip Edwards, and Daniel Rueckert*

Registration of 3D Fetal Brain US and MRI   667
  *Maria Kuklisova-Murgasova, Amalia Cifor, Raffaele Napolitano,
  Aris Papageorghiou, Gerardine Quaghebeur, J. Alison Noble, and
  Julia A. Schnabel*

Author Index   675

Table of Contents – Part III

Diffusion Imaging: From Acquisition to Tractography

Accelerated Diffusion Spectrum Imaging with Compressed Sensing
Using Adaptive Dictionaries 1
    Berkin Bilgic, Kawin Setsompop, Julien Cohen-Adad, Van Wedeen,
    Lawrence L. Wald, and Elfar Adalsteinsson

Parametric Dictionary Learning for Modeling EAP and ODF in
Diffusion MRI 10
    Sylvain Merlet, Emmanuel Caruyer, and Rachid Deriche

Resolution Enhancement of Diffusion-Weighted Images by Local Fiber
Profiling 18
    Pew-Thian Yap and Dinggang Shen

Geodesic Shape-Based Averaging 26
    M. Jorge Cardoso, Gavin Winston, Marc Modat,
    Shiva Keihaninejad, John Duncan, and Sebastien Ourselin

Multi-scale Characterization of White Matter Tract Geometry 34
    Peter Savadjiev, Yogesh Rathi, Sylvain Bouix, Ragini Verma, and
    Carl-Fredrik Westin

Image Acquisition, Segmentation and Recognition

Optimization of Acquisition Geometry for Intra-operative Tomographic
Imaging 42
    Jakob Vogel, Tobias Reichl, José Gardiazabal, Nassir Navab, and
    Tobias Lasser

Incorporating Parameter Uncertainty in Bayesian Segmentation
Models: Application to Hippocampal Subfield Volumetry 50
    Juan Eugenio Iglesias, Mert Rory Sabuncu, Koen Van Leemput, and
    The Alzheimer's Disease Neuroimaging Initiative

A Dynamical Appearance Model Based on Multiscale Sparse
Representation: Segmentation of the Left Ventricle from 4D
Echocardiography 58
    Xiaojie Huang, Donald P. Dione, Colin B. Compas,
    Xenophon Papademetris, Ben A. Lin, Albert J. Sinusas, and
    James S. Duncan

Automatic Detection and Segmentation of Kidneys in 3D CT Images
Using Random Forests   66
  Rémi Cuingnet, Raphael Prevost, David Lesage, Laurent D. Cohen,
  Benoît Mory, and Roberto Ardon

Neighbourhood Approximation Forests   75
  Ender Konukoglu, Ben Glocker, Darko Zikic, and Antonio Criminisi

Recognition in Ultrasound Videos: Where Am I?   83
  Roland Kwitt, Nuno Vasconcelos, Sharif Razzaque, and
  Stephen Aylward

Image Registration II

Self-similarity Weighted Mutual Information: A New Nonrigid Image
Registration Metric   91
  Hassan Rivaz and D. Louis Collins

Inter-Point Procrustes: Identifying Regional and Large Differences in
3D Anatomical Shapes   99
  Karim Lekadir, Alejandro F. Frangi, and Guang-Zhong Yang

Selection of Optimal Hyper-Parameters for Estimation of Uncertainty
in MRI-TRUS Registration of the Prostate   107
  Petter Risholm, Firdaus Janoos, Jennifer Pursley, Andriy Fedorov,
  Clare Tempany, Robert A. Cormack, and William M. Wells III

Globally Optimal Deformable Registration on a Minimum Spanning
Tree Using Dense Displacement Sampling   115
  Mattias P. Heinrich, Mark Jenkinson, Sir Michael Brady, and
  Julia A. Schnabel

Unbiased Groupwise Registration of White Matter Tractography   123
  Lauren J. O'Donnell, William M. Wells III,
  Alexandra J. Golby, and Carl-Fredrik Westin

Regional Manifold Learning for Deformable Registration of Brain MR
Images   131
  Dong Hye Ye, Jihun Hamm, Dongjin Kwon,
  Christos Davatzikos, and Kilian M. Pohl

Estimation and Reduction of Target Registration Error   139
  Ryan D. Datteri and Benoît M. Dawant

A Hierarchical Scheme for Geodesic Anatomical Labeling of Airway
Trees   147
  Aasa Feragen, Jens Petersen, Megan Owen, Pechin Lo,
  Laura H. Thomsen, Mathilde M.W. Wille, Asger Dirksen, and
  Marleen de Bruijne

Initialising Groupwise Non-rigid Registration Using Multiple
Parts+Geometry Models   156
    Pei Zhang, Pew-Thian Yap, Dinggang Shen, and Timothy F. Cootes

An Efficient and Robust Algorithm for Parallel Groupwise Registration
of Bone Surfaces   164
    *Martijn van de Giessen, Frans M. Vos, Cornelis A. Grimbergen,
    Lucas J. van Vliet, and Geert J. Streekstra*

NeuroImage Analysis II

Realistic Head Model Design and 3D Brain Imaging of NIRS Signals
Using Audio Stimuli on Preterm Neonates for Intra-Ventricular
Hemorrhage Diagnosis   172
    *Marc Fournier, Mahdi Mahmoudzadeh, Kamran Kazemi,
    Guy Kongolo, Ghislaine Dehaene-Lambertz, Reinhard Grebe, and
    Fabrice Wallois*

Hemodynamic-Informed Parcellation of fMRI Data in a Joint Detection
Estimation Framework   180
    L. Chaari, F. Forbes, T. Vincent, and P. Ciuciu

Group Analysis of Resting-State fMRI by Hierarchical Markov Random
Fields   189
    Wei Liu, Suyash P. Awate, and P. Thomas Fletcher

Metamorphic Geodesic Regression   197
    *Yi Hong, Sarang Joshi, Mar Sanchez, Martin Styner, and
    Marc Niethammer*

Eigenanatomy Improves Detection Power for Longitudinal Cortical
Change   206
    *Brian Avants, Paramveer Dhillon, Benjamin M. Kandel,
    Philip A. Cook, Corey T. McMillan, Murray Grossman, and
    James C. Gee*

Optimization of fMRI-Derived ROIs Based on Coherent Functional
Interaction Patterns   214
    Fan Deng, Dajiang Zhu, and Tianming Liu

Topology Preserving Atlas Construction from Shape Data without
Correspondence Using Sparse Parameters   223
    *Stanley Durrleman, Marcel Prastawa, Julie R. Korenberg,
    Sarang Joshi, Alain Trouvé, and Guido Gerig*

Dominant Component Analysis of Electrophysiological Connectivity
Networks   231
    *Yasser Ghanbari, Luke Bloy, Kayhan Batmanghelich,
    Timothy P.L. Roberts, and Ragini Verma*

Tree-Guided Sparse Coding for Brain Disease Classification   239
    Manhua Liu, Daoqiang Zhang, Pew-Thian Yap, and Dinggang Shen

Improving Accuracy and Power with Transfer Learning Using a
Meta-analytic Database   248
    Yannick Schwartz, Gaël Varoquaux, Christophe Pallier,
    Philippe Pinel, Jean-Baptiste Poline, and Bertrand Thirion

Radial Structure in the Preterm Cortex; Persistence of the Preterm
Phenotype at Term Equivalent Age?   256
    Andrew Melbourne, Giles S. Kendall, M. Jorge Cardoso,
    Roxanna Gunney, Nicola J. Robertson, Neil Marlow, and
    Sebastien Ourselin

Temporally-Constrained Group Sparse Learning for Longitudinal Data
Analysis   264
    Daoqiang Zhang, Jun Liu, and Dinggang Shen

Feature Analysis for Parkinson's Disease Detection Based on
Transcranial Sonography Image   272
    Lei Chen, Johann Hagenah, and Alfred Mertins

Longitudinal Image Registration with Non-uniform Appearance
Change   280
    Istvan Csapo, Brad Davis, Yundi Shi, Mar Sanchez,
    Martin Styner, and Marc Niethammer

Cortical Folding Analysis on Patients with Alzheimer's Disease and
Mild Cognitive Impairment   289
    David M. Cash, Andrew Melbourne, Marc Modat, M. Jorge Cardoso,
    Matthew J. Clarkson, Nick C. Fox, and Sebastien Ourselin

Inferring Group-Wise Consistent Multimodal Brain Networks via
Multi-view Spectral Clustering   297
    Hanbo Chen, Kaiming Li, Dajiang Zhu, Tuo Zhang, Changfeng Jin,
    Lei Guo, Lingjiang Li, and Tianming Liu

Test-Retest Reliability of Graph Theory Measures of Structural Brain
Connectivity   305
    Emily L. Dennis, Neda Jahanshad, Arthur W. Toga,
    Katie L. McMahon, Greig I. de Zubicaray, Nicholas G. Martin,
    Margaret J. Wright, and Paul M. Thompson

Registration and Analysis of White Matter Group Differences with a
Multi-fiber Model   313
    Maxime Taquet, Benoît Scherrer, Olivier Commowick,
    Jurriaan Peters, Mustafa Sahin, Benoît Macq, and
    Simon K. Warfield

Analysis of Microscopic and Optical Images II

Scalable Tracing of Electron Micrographs by Fusing Top Down and
Bottom Up Cues Using Hypergraph Diffusion...................... 321
    *Vignesh Jagadeesh, Min-Chi Shih, B.S. Manjunath, and
Kenneth Rose*

A Diffusion Model for Detecting and Classifying Vesicle Fusion and
Undocking Events... 329
    Lorenz Berger, Majid Mirmehdi, Sam Reed, and Jeremy Tavaré

Efficient Scanning for EM Based Target Localization 337
    *Raphael Sznitman, Aurelien Lucchi, Natasa Pjescic-Emedji,
Graham Knott, and Pascal Fua*

Automated Tuberculosis Diagnosis Using Fluorescence Images from a
Mobile Microscope 345
    *Jeannette Chang, Pablo Arbeláez, Neil Switz, Clay Reber,
Asa Tapley, J. Lucian Davis, Adithya Cattamanchi,
Daniel Fletcher, and Jitendra Malik*

Image Segmentation III

Accurate Fully Automatic Femur Segmentation in Pelvic Radiographs
Using Regression Voting 353
    *C. Lindner, S. Thiagarajah, J.M. Wilkinson, arcOGEN Consortium,
G.A. Wallis, and Timothy F. Cootes*

Automatic Location of Vertebrae on DXA Images Using Random
Forest Regression 361
    M.G. Roberts, Timothy F. Cootes, and J.E. Adams

Decision Forests for Tissue-Specific Segmentation of High-Grade
Gliomas in Multi-channel MR 369
    *Darko Zikic, Ben Glocker, Ender Konukoglu, Antonio Criminisi,
C. Demiralp, J. Shotton, O.M. Thomas, T. Das, R. Jena, and
S.J. Price*

Efficient Global Optimization Based 3D Carotid AB-LIB MRI
Segmentation by Simultaneously Evolving Coupled Surfaces 377
    Eranga Ukwatta, Jing Yuan, Martin Rajchl, and Aaron Fenster

Sparse Patch Based Prostate Segmentation in CT Images 385
    Shu Liao, Yaozong Gao, and Dinggang Shen

Anatomical Landmark Detection Using Nearest Neighbor Matching
and Submodular Optimization 393
    David Liu and S. Kevin Zhou

Integration of Local and Global Features for Anatomical Object
Detection in Ultrasound 402
  Bahbibi Rahmatullah, Aris T. Papageorghiou, and J. Alison Noble

Spectral Label Fusion 410
  Christian Wachinger and Polina Golland

Multi-Organ Segmentation with Missing Organs in Abdominal
CT Images 418
  Miyuki Suzuki, Marius George Linguraru, and Kazunori Okada

Non-local STAPLE: An Intensity-Driven Multi-atlas Rater Model 426
  Andrew J. Asman and Bennett A. Landman

Shape Prior Modeling Using Sparse Representation and Online
Dictionary Learning 435
  Shaoting Zhang, Yiqiang Zhan, Yan Zhou, Mustafa Uzunbas, and
  Dimitris N. Metaxas

Detection of Substantia Nigra Echogenicities in 3D Transcranial
Ultrasound for Early Diagnosis of Parkinson Disease................. 443
  Olivier Pauly, Seyed-Ahmad Ahmadi, Annika Plate,
  Kai Boetzel, and Nassir Navab

Prostate Segmentation by Sparse Representation Based Classification ... 451
  Yaozong Gao, Shu Liao, and Dinggang Shen

Co-segmentation of Functional and Anatomical Images 459
  Ulas Bagci, Jayaram K. Udupa, Jianhua Yao, and Daniel J. Mollura

Diffusion Weighted Imaging II

Using Multiparametric Data with Missing Features for Learning
Patterns of Pathology 468
  Madhura Ingalhalikar, William A. Parker, Luke Bloy,
  Timothy P.L. Roberts, and Ragini Verma

Non-local Robust Detection of DTI White Matter Differences with
Small Databases 476
  Olivier Commowick and Aymeric Stamm

Group-Wise Consistent Fiber Clustering Based on Multimodal
Connectional and Functional Profiles 485
  Bao Ge, Lei Guo, Tuo Zhang, Dajiang Zhu, Kaiming Li,
  Xintao Hu, Junwei Han, and Tianming Liu

Learning a Reliable Estimate of the Number of Fiber Directions in
Diffusion MRI 493
  Thomas Schultz

Computer-Aided Diagnosis and Planning II

Finding Similar 2D X-Ray Coronary Angiograms 501
Tanveer Syeda-Mahmood, Fei Wang, R. Kumar, D. Beymer,
Y. Zhang, Robert Lundstrom, and Edward McNulty

Detection of Vertebral Body Fractures Based on Cortical Shell
Unwrapping 509
Jianhua Yao, Joseph E. Burns, Hector Munoz, and
Ronald M. Summers

Multiscale Lung Texture Signature Learning Using the Riesz
Transform 517
Adrien Depeursinge, Antonio Foncubierta–Rodriguez,
Dimitri Van de Ville, and Henning Müller

Blood Flow Simulation for the Liver after a Virtual Right Lobe
Hepatectomy 525
Harvey Ho, Keagan Sorrell, Adam Bartlett, and Peter Hunter

A Combinatorial Method for 3D Landmark-Based Morphometry:
Application to the Study of Coronal Craniosynostosis................ 533
Emeric Gioan, Kevin Sol, and Gérard Subsol

A Comprehensive Framework for the Detection of Individual Brain
Perfusion Abnormalities Using Arterial Spin Labeling 542
Camille Maumet, Pierre Maurel, Jean-Christophe Ferré, and
Christian Barillot

Automated Colorectal Cancer Diagnosis for Whole-Slice
Histopathology 550
Habil Kalkan, Marius Nap, Robert P.W. Duin, and Marco Loog

Patient-Adaptive Lesion Metabolism Analysis by Dynamic
PET Images... 558
Fei Gao, Huafeng Liu, and Pengcheng Shi

A Personalized Biomechanical Model for Respiratory Motion
Prediction 566
B. Fuerst, T. Mansi, Jianwen Zhang, P. Khurd, J. Declerck,
T. Boettger, Nassir Navab, J. Bayouth, Dorin Comaniciu, and
A. Kamen

Endoscope Distortion Correction Does Not (Easily) Improve
Mucosa-Based Classification of Celiac Disease 574
Jutta Hämmerle-Uhl, Yvonne Höller, Andreas Uhl, and
Andreas Vécsei

Gaussian Process Inference for Estimating Pharmacokinetic Parameters
of Dynamic Contrast-Enhanced MR Images   582
  Shijun Wang, Peter Liu, Baris Turkbey, Peter Choyke,
  Peter Pinto, and Ronald M. Summers

Automatic Localization and Identification of Vertebrae in Arbitrary
Field-of-View CT Scans...   590
  Ben Glocker, J. Feulner, Antonio Criminisi, D.R. Haynor, and
  E. Konukoglu

Pathology Hinting as the Combination of Automatic Segmentation
with a Statistical Shape Model   599
  Pascal A. Dufour, Hannan Abdillahi, Lala Ceklic,
  Ute Wolf-Schnurrbusch, and Jens Kowal

An Invariant Shape Representation Using the Anisotropic Helmholtz
Equation..   607
  A.A. Joshi, S. Ashrafulla, D.W. Shattuck, H. Damasio, and
  R.M. Leahy

Microscopic Image Analysis

Phase Contrast Image Restoration via Dictionary Representation of
Diffraction Patterns   615
  Hang Su, Zhaozheng Yin, Takeo Kanade, and Seungil Huh

Context-Constrained Multiple Instance Learning for Histopathology
Image Segmentation..   623
  Yan Xu, Jianwen Zhang, Eric I-Chao Chang, Maode Lai, and
  Zhuowen Tu

Structural-Flow Trajectories for Unravelling 3D Tubular Bundles   631
  Katerina Fragkiadaki, Weiyu Zhang, Jianbo Shi, and Elena Bernardis

Online Blind Calibration of Non-uniform Photodetectors: Application
to Endomicroscopy   639
  Nicolas Savoire, Barbara André, and Tom Vercauteren

Author Index   647

Reliable Assessment of Perfusivity and Diffusivity from Diffusion Imaging of the Body[*]

M. Freiman[1], S.D. Voss[2], R.V. Mulkern,
J.M. Perez-Rossello[2], M.J. Callahan[2], and Simon K. Warfield[1]

[1] Computational Radiology Laboratory, Boston Children's Hospital,
Harvard Medical School, MA, USA
[2] Department of Radiology, Boston Children's Hospital, Harvard Medical School,
MA, USA

Abstract. Diffusion-weighted MRI of the body has the potential to provide important new insights into physiological and microstructural properties. The Intra-Voxel Incoherent Motion (IVIM) model relates the observed DW-MRI signal decay to parameters that reflect perfusivity (D^*) and its volume fraction (f), and diffusivity (D). However, the commonly used voxel-wise fitting of the IVIM model leads to parameter estimates with poor precision, which has hampered their practical usage. In this work, we increase the estimates' precision by introducing a model of spatial homogeneity, through which we obtain estimates of model parameters for all of the voxels at once, instead of solving for each voxel independently. Furthermore, we introduce an efficient iterative solver which utilizes a model-based bootstrap estimate of the distribution of residuals and a binary graph cut to generate optimal model parameter updates. Simulation experiments show that our approach reduces the relative root mean square error of the estimated parameters by 80% for the D^* parameter and by 50% for the f and D parameters. We demonstrated the clinical impact of our model in distinguishing between enhancing and nonenhancing ileum segments in 24 Crohn's disease patients. Our model detected the enhanced segments with 91%/92% sensitivity/specificity which is better than the 81%/85% obtained by the voxel-independent approach.

1   Introduction

Diffusion-weighted MRI (DW-MRI) of the body is a non-invasive imaging technique sensitive to the incoherent motion of water molecules inside the body. This motion is be a combination of the thermally-driven random motion of water molecules and blood flow in the randomly oriented tissue micro capillaries. These phenomena are characterized through the so-called, intra-voxel incoherent

[*] This investigation was supported in part by NIH grants R01 EB008015, R01 LM010033, R01 EB013248, and P30 HD018655 and by a research grant from the Boston Children's Hospital Translational Research Program.

N. Ayache et al. (Eds.): MICCAI 2012, Part I, LNCS 7510, pp. 1–9, 2012.

motion (IVIM) model with the diffusion (D), and the pseudo-diffusion (D^*) as the decay rate parameters, and the fractional contribution (f) of each motion to the DW-MRI signal decay [1,7].

IVIM model parameters have recently shown promise as quantitative imaging biomarkers for various clinical applications in the body, including differential analysis of tumors [4] and the assessment of liver cirrhosis [9]. However, IVIM parameter estimates are often unreliable, and thus are not widely utilized in the clinic [7]. Reliable estimates of IVIM model parameters are difficult to achieve because of 1) the non-linearity of the IVIM model, 2) the limited number of DW-MRI images as compared to the number of the IVIM model parameters; and 3) the low signal-to- noise ratio (SNR) observed in body DW-MRI.

While commonly used methods for IVIM parameter estimation fit the model to the signal at each voxel independently, they typically ignore the spatial context of the signal and thus produce highly unreliable estimates, especially for the pseudo-diffusion (D^*) and the fractional contribution (f) parameters [7]. In current practice, the DW-MRI signal is averaged over a region of interest (ROI) to increase the SNR, effectively yielding more reliable IVIM parameter estimates [12]. Unfortunately, by averaging the signal over a ROI, the estimated parameters do not reflect critical heterogeneous environments such as the necrotic and viable parts of tumors. An alternative approach is to average several DW-MRI acquisitions to increase the SNR [7]. While this retains the spatial sensitivity of the estimated parameters, it also increases the overall image acquisition time, which is not feasible in clinical practice. However, the overall image acquisition time increases, preventing this approach to be feasible in clinical practice.

Other groups have suggested incorporating spatial knowledge as a prior term to increase the reliability of parameters estimates in quantitative dynamic contrast enhanced MRI [6,10]. However, these models are difficult to optimize as compared to the simple voxel-wise approaches, and have not been successfully applied to incoherent motion quantification from body DW-MRI.

In this work, we increase the precision of the incoherent motion parameters estimates by introducing a model of spatial homogeneity, through which we obtain estimates of model parameters for all of the voxels at once, instead of solving for each voxel independently. Furthermore, we introduce an efficient iterative solver in order to obtain precise parameter estimates with this new model. Our solver utilizes a model-based bootstrap estimate of the distribution of residuals and a binary graph cut to generate optimal model parameter updates.

In our simulation experiments, we have shown a reduction in the relative root mean square (RRMS) error of parameter estimates in clinical SNR conditions by 80% for the D^* parameter and by 50% for the D and f parameters. In addition, we have assessed clinical impact, namely, the ability of incoherent motion parameters to distinguish enhancing from non-enhancing ileal segments in a study cohort of 24 Crohn's disease (CD) patients. Our results demonstrated that the incoherent motion parameters estimated with our method yielded a sensitivity of 91% and specificity of 92%, while the traditional voxel-independent approach only produced a sensitivity of 81% and specificity of 85%.

2   Method

2.1   DW-MRI Signal Decay Model

The IVIM model of DW-MRI signal decay assumes a function of the form [1]:

$$m_i = s_0 \left(f \exp(-b_i(D^* + D)) + (1 - f) \exp(-b_i(D)) \right) \tag{1}$$

where m_i is the expected signal at b-factor=b_i, s_0 is the baseline signal (without any diffusion effect); f is the pseudo-diffusion fraction; D^* is the so-called, pseudo-diffusion coefficient characterizing the perfusion component; and D is the apparent diffusion coefficient associated with extravascular water.

Given the DW-MRI data acquired with multiple b-factors, the observed signal (S_v) at each voxel v is a vector of the observed signal at the different b-factors: $S_v = \{s_i\}, i = 1 \ldots N$. We model the IVIM model parameters at each voxel v as a continuous-valued four-dimensional random variable (i.e. $\Theta_v = \{s_0, f, D^*, D\}$). Taking a Bayesian perspective, our goal is to find the IVIM parametric maps $\hat{\Theta}$ that maximizes the posterior probability associated with the maps given the observed DW-MRI images (S) and the spatial prior knowledge ($p(\Theta)$):

$$\hat{\Theta} = \underset{\Theta}{\operatorname{argmax}}\, p(\Theta|S) \propto p(S|\Theta)p(\Theta) \tag{2}$$

By using a spatial prior in the form of a continuous-valued Markov random field, the posterior probability $p(S|\Theta)p(\Theta)$ decomposes into the product of maximal node and clique potentials:

$$p(S|\Theta)p(\Theta) \propto \prod_v p(S_v|\Theta_v) \prod_{v_p, v_q \in \Omega} p(\Theta_{v_p}, \Theta_{v_q}) \tag{3}$$

where Θ_v is the IVIM model parameters at voxel v, $p(S_v|\Theta_v)$ is the data term representing the probability of voxel v to have the DW-MRI signal S_v given the model parameters Θ_v, Ω is the collection of the neighboring voxels according to the employed neighborhood system, and $p(\Theta_{v_p}, \Theta_{v_q})$ is the spatial smoothness prior in the model.

The maximum *a posteriori* (MAP) estimate $\hat{\Theta}$ is then found by minimizing:

$$E(\Theta) = \sum_v \phi(S_v; \Theta_v) + \sum_{v_p, v_q \in \Omega} \psi(\Theta_{v_p}, \Theta_{v_q}) \tag{4}$$

where $\phi(S_v; \Theta_v)$ and $\psi(\Theta_{v_p}, \Theta_{v_q})$ are the compatibility functions:

$$\phi(S_v; \Theta_v) = -\log p(S_v|\Theta_v), \quad \psi(\Theta_{v_p}, \Theta_{v_q}) = -\log p(\Theta_{v_p}, \Theta_{v_q}) \tag{5}$$

Assuming a noncentralized χ-distribution noise model for parallel MRI acquisition [3] as used in DW-MRI, the data term takes the following form:

$$\phi(S_v; \Theta_v) = -\sum_{i=1}^{N} \frac{m_i}{\sigma^2} + \log \left(\frac{m_i}{s_i} \right)^{n-1} - \left(\frac{m_i^2 + s_i^2}{2\sigma^2} \right) + \log I_{n-1} \left(\frac{s_i m_i}{\sigma^2} \right) \tag{6}$$

where s_i is the observed signal at b-factor b_i, m_i is the expected signal at b_i given the model parameters Θ_v calculated with Eq. 1, σ being the noise standard deviation of the Gaussian noises present on each of the acquisition channels, n being the number of channels used in the acquisition and I_{n-1} being the $(n-1)$th order modified Bessel function of the first kind.

The robust L1-norm is used as the spatial smoothness term:

$$\psi(\Theta_{v_p}, \Theta_{v_q}) = \alpha W |\Theta_{v_p} - \Theta_{v_q}| \tag{7}$$

where $\alpha \geq 0$ is the spatial coupling factor, and W is a diagonal weighting matrix which accounts for the different scales of the parameters in Θ_v.

2.2   Optimization Scheme

Direct minimization of the energy in Eq. 4 is a challenging optimization problem due to the very high dimensionality of the parameters vector Θ. For example a clinical 3D DW-MRI data of $192 \times 156 \times 40$ voxels would result in a parameter vector Θ of $\sim 5 \cdot 10^6$ dimensions.

To overcome this challenging optimization problem, we developed a new solver to robustly minimize the energy in Eq. 4.

Our "fusion bootstrap moves (FBM)" algorithm, inspired by the fusion-moves algorithm [8], iteratively applies the following two steps until the improvement in the optimized energy is smaller than some epsilon. First, we draw a new possible proposal of the incoherent motion model parameters values from the parameters distribution using model-based statistical bootstrapping [2]. Next, given the current assignment and the drawn sample, we use the binary graph-cut technique to fuse the two possible assignments of the IVIM values at each voxel in an optimal manner [8] to an assignment that reduces the model energy.

Since the fusion of the two possible proposals at each iteration is optimal, the reduction in the overall model energy (Eq. 4) is guaranteed. By applying the proposal drawing and optimal fusion steps iteratively, the algorithm will robustly converge, at least to a local minimum. We will describe these steps in detail next.

Proposal Drawing: We utilize the model-based bootstrap technique [2] to draw a new proposal from the empirical distribution of the incoherent motion parameters values as follows: For each voxel v, the raw residuals between the observed signal (S_v) and the expected signal ($M_v = \{m_i\}, i = 1, \ldots N$) at each b-factor b_i, given the current model estimate (Θ_v^0), are defined as: $\epsilon_i = m_i - s_i$. The model-based bootstrap resampling is defined as:

$$S_v^*(\Theta_v^0) = M_v + t_i \hat{\epsilon} \tag{8}$$

where $S_v^*(\Theta_v^0)$ is the resampled measures at the b-factors $b_i, i = 1 \ldots N$, $\hat{\epsilon}$ are the rescaled version of ϵ that accounts for heterogeneous error leverages [5], and t_i is a two-point Rademacher distributed random variable with $p(t = 1) = 0.5$ and $p(t = -1) = 0.5$ defined for each b-factor independently. The IVIM model parameters Θ_v^1 are then estimated for each voxel independently [7].

Binary Optimization: We use the binary graph-cut technique [8] to find the optimal combination of the current assignment Θ^0 and the new proposal Θ^1 for the IVIM model parameters values at each voxel as follows:

Let $G = (V, E)$ be an undirected graph, where each voxel v is represented as a graph node, the two proposals Θ^0 and Θ^1 are represented by the terminal nodes v_s and v_t, and graph edges consist of three groups: $E = \{(v_p, v_q), (v_p, v_s), (v_p, v_t)\}$.

Edge weights $w(v_p, v_s)$ and $w(v_p, v_t)$ represent the likelihood of the model parameters Θ^0 and Θ^1 given the observed signal S_{v_p}, respectively:

$$w(v_p, v_s) = \phi(S_v; \Theta_v^0), \qquad w(v_p, v_t) = \phi(S_v; \Theta_v^1) \tag{9}$$

Edge weights $w(v_p, v_q)$ penalize for adjacent voxels that have different model parameters: $w(v_p, v_q) = \psi(\Theta_{v_p}, \Theta_{v_q})$. The optimal fusion between Θ^0 and Θ^1 is then found by solving the corresponding graph min-cut problem. Finally, the result $\hat{\Theta}$ is assigned as Θ^0 for the next iteration.

3   Experimental Results

3.1   Simulation Experiment

We conducted a Monte-Carlo simulation study to analyze the estimation errors. We constructed a simulated heterogeneous tumor example [6] as follows. We defined three-dimensional reference parametric maps with $100 \times 100 \times 5$ voxels with the following parameters: Border: $\Theta = \{200, 0.35, 0.03, 0.003\}$, middle part: $\Theta = \{200, 0.25, 0.02, 0.002\}$, innermost part: $\Theta = \{200, 0.15, 0.01, 0.001\}$. We computed simulated DW-MRI images from the parametric maps using Eq. 1 with 7 b-values in the range $[0, 800]$ s/mm^2. We then corrupted the simulated data by noncentralized χ-distributed noise with single coil noise σ values of 2-16.

We estimated the model parameters $\hat{\Theta}$ from the noisy DW-MRI data for each voxel, using the voxel-independent approach (IVIM) [7] and using our model (IM). The optimization algorithm parameters were determined experimentally and were set as follows: α was set to 0.01, the rescaling matrix W diagonal was set to: $\{1.0, 0.001, 0.0001, 0.01\}$. The noise parameter σ was estimated using a pre-defined background region. Stopping criteria was defined as an energy improvement of less than 0.1% from the initial energy or 500 iterations. We calculated the RRMS error between the reference and estimated parameters [6].

Fig. 1 depicts the middle slice of the reference parametric maps and the model parameters estimates using the two methods along with the RRMS error of each estimator as a function of the SNR$_{b0}$ defined as the baseline signal s_0 divided by the noise level σ. Visually, the parametric maps computed using the IVIM model (2nd column) exhibit very noisy estimates, in which the heterogeneous environment is hardly detectable, mainly for the D^* and f parameters (1st and 2nd rows). However, the maps computed using our IM method are much smoother, and the heterogeneous environment is more detectable. Quantitatively, our IM model decreases the overall RRMS of the D^* parameter by 80% and of the f and D parameters by 50% as compared to the IVIM model for SNR$_{B0} = 25$ which represents the actual noise level observed in clinical imaging studies.

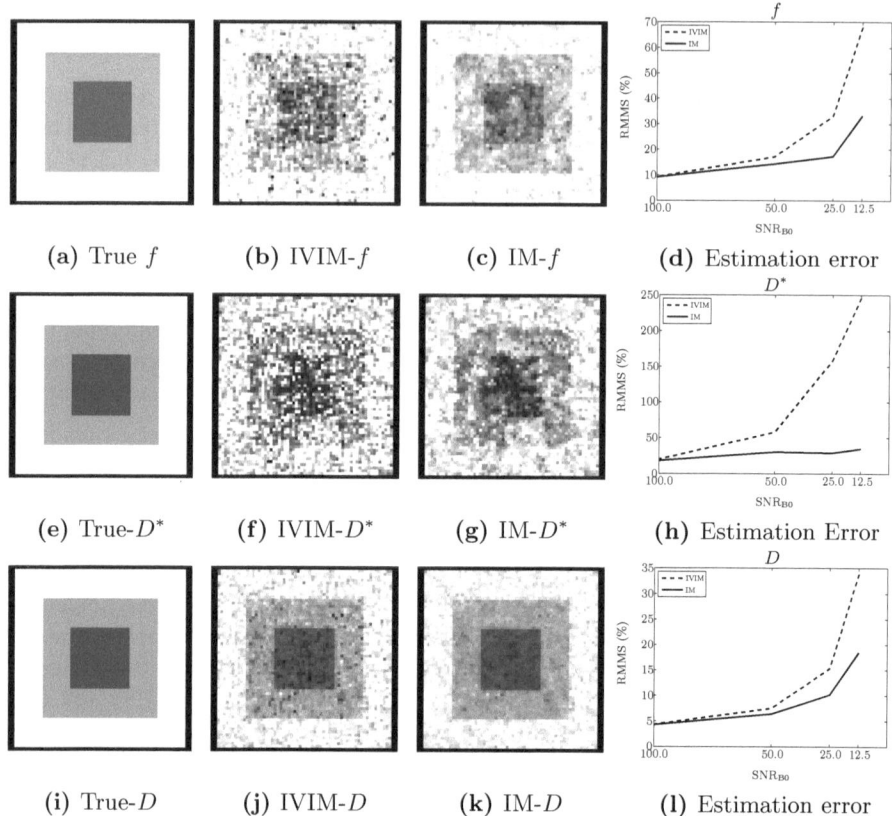

Fig. 1. Simulated heterogeneous tumor example. The first column presents the "ground-truth" values used to simulate the DW-MRI data. The second and third columns present the estimated parameters using the IVIM, and our IM approaches, respectively. The fourth column presents the RRMS errors for each parameter for the different noise levels.

3.2   Clinical Impact

To demonstrate the actual clinical impact of using our IM model instead of the voxel-independent IVIM model, we assessed the discriminatory performance of the incoherent motion model parameters, in discerning enhancing from nonenhancing ileal segments of CD patients. CD is a chronic inflammatory disorder of the bowel, in which involvement of the ileum is common. Characterization of perfusivity and diffusivity in the ileum has a promising role in patient-specific management of the disease.

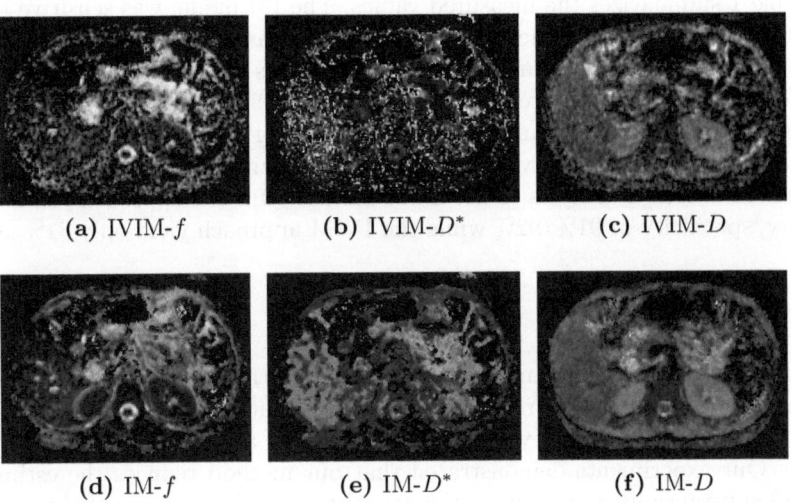

(a) IVIM-f **(b)** IVIM-D^* **(c)** IVIM-D

(d) IM-f **(e)** IM-D^* **(f)** IM-D

Fig. 2. Representative upper abdomen slice of the parametric maps reconstructed by the IVIM method (1st row), and by our method (2nd row). Our method yields smoother, more realistic maps, with sensitivity to details.

Table 1. Quantitative analysis of incoherent motion parameters for the nonenhancing and enhancing ileal segments. All values are in mean(std). Significant differences (two-tailed Student's t-test, $n_1=11$, $n_2=13$, $p<0.05$) are in bold.

	IVIM			IM		
	Nonenhancing	Enhancing	p-value	Nonenhancing	Enhancing	p-value
f	0.55 (0.24)	0.28 (0.16)	**0.004**	0.66(0.43)	0.32(0.15)	**0.02**
D^*	24.2(16.3)	36.1(20.6)	0.13	28.7(22.9)	42.5(32.7)	0.24
D	1.6 (0.6)	1.3 (0.4)	0.17	1.7(0.4)	1.2(0.3)	**0.002**

We acquired DW-MRI from 24 consecutive patients with confirmed CD using a 1.5-T unit (Magnetom Avanto, Siemens Medical Solutions, Erlangen, Germany). We performed free-breathing single-shot echo-planar imaging using the following parameters: repetition/echo time (TR/TE) = 6800/59 ms; matrix size = 192×156; field of view = 300×260 mm; slice thickness/gap = 5 mm/0.5 mm; 40 axial slices; 8 b-values = 5,50,100,200,270,400,600,800 s/mm^2. We defined reference standard classification of the ileal segments as the consensus of two independent radiologists' qualitative review of the clinical MR enterography data as enhancing (n=11) or nonenhancing (n=13). We fitted the signal-decay model to the DW-MRI using both the IVIM and IM approaches and we averaged the parameters values over the manually annotated ileum region.

Fig. 2 depicts a representative parametric maps of the upper abdomen. The IM model yields smoother, more realistic maps, especially for the f parameter.

Table 1 summarizes the measured values. The IM model was sensitive to the actual differences in both the tissue cellularity (D) and blood-flow (f) [11], while the IVIM model was not sensitive to the differences in tissue cellularity.

We constructed generalized linear models (GLM) from the parameters values to distinguish between enhancing and nonenhancing ileal segments. We assessed the sensitivity and specificity of the models by utilizing the optimal cutoff values calculated by ROC analysis of the GLM models. Our IM approach yield a sensitivity/specificity of 91%/92% while the IVIM approach yield only 81%/85%.

4 Conclusions

We have presented a new model and method for the reliable quantification of perfusivity and diffusivity from body DW-MRI that features the incorporation of spatial prior knowledge, with a new robust and accurate optimization technique. Our experiments demonstrated that our method reduces the estimates' RRMS substantially and improve the actual diagnostic accuracy of the incoherent motion parameters as compared to the voxel-independent approach.

References

1. Le Bihan, D., Breton, E., Lallemand, D., Aubin, M.L., Vignaud, J., Laval-Jeantet, M.: Separation of diffusion and perfusion in intravoxel incoherent motion MR imaging. Radiology 168(2), 497–505 (1988)
2. Davidson, R., Flachaire, E.: The wild bootstrap, tamed at last. J. of Econometrics 146(1), 162–169 (2008)
3. Dietrich, O., Raya, J.G., Reeder, S.B., Ingrisch, M., Reiser, M.F., Schoenberg, S.O.: Influence of multichannel combination, parallel imaging and other reconstruction techniques on mri noise characteristics. Magn. Reson. Imaging 26(6), 754–762 (2008)
4. Döpfert, J., Lemke, A., Weidner, A., Schad, L.R.: Investigation of prostate cancer using diffusion-weighted intravoxel incoherent motion imaging. Magn. Reson. Imaging 29(8), 1053–1058 (2011)
5. Freiman, M., Voss, S., Mulkern, R., Perez-Rossello, J., Warfield, S.: Quantitative Body DW-MRI Biomarkers Uncertainty Estimation Using Unscented Wild-Bootstrap. In: Fichtinger, G., Martel, A., Peters, T. (eds.) MICCAI 2011, Part II. LNCS, vol. 6892, pp. 74–81. Springer, Heidelberg (2011)
6. Kelm, B.M., Menze, B.H., Nix, O., Zechmann, C.M., Hamprecht, F.A.: Estimating kinetic parameter maps from dynamic contrast-enhanced mri using spatial prior knowledge. IEEE Trans. Med. Imaging 28(10), 1534–1547 (2009)
7. Koh, D.M., Collins, D.J., Orton, M.R.: Intravoxel incoherent motion in body diffusion-weighted mri: Reality and challenges. AJR Am. J. Roentgenol. 196(6), 1351–1361 (2011)
8. Lempitsky, V., Rother, C., Roth, S., Blake, A.: Fusion moves for markov random field optimization. IEEE Trans. Pattern Anal. Mach. Intell. 32(8), 1392–1405 (2010)
9. Luciani, A., Vignaud, A., Cavet, M., Van Nhieu, J.T., Mallat, A., Ruel, L., Laurent, A., Deux, J.F., Brugieres, P., Rahmouni, A.: Liver cirrhosis: intravoxel incoherent motion mr imaging–pilot study. Radiology 249(3), 891–899 (2008)

10. Schmid, V.J., Whitcher, B., Padhani, A.R., Taylor, N.J., Yang, G.Z.: Bayesian methods for pharmacokinetic models in dynamic contrast-enhanced magnetic resonance imaging. IEEE Trans. Med. Imaging 25(12), 1627–1636 (2006)
11. Targan, S., Shanahan, F., Karp, L.: Inflammatory bowel disease: from bench to bedside. Springer (2005)
12. Zhang, J.L., Sigmund, E.E., Rusinek, H., Chandarana, H., Storey, P., Chen, Q., Lee, V.S.: Optimization of b-value sampling for diffusion-weighted imaging of the kidney. Magn. Reson. Med. 67(1), 89–97 (2012)

Multi-organ Abdominal CT Segmentation Using Hierarchically Weighted Subject-Specific Atlases

Robin Wolz[1], Chengwen Chu[2], Kazunari Misawa[3],
Kensaku Mori[2,4,*], and Daniel Rueckert[1,*]

[1] Imperial College London, London, UK
[2] Department of Media Science, Nagoya University, Nagoya, Japan
[3] Aichi Cancer Center, Nagoya, Japan
[4] Information and Communications Headquarters, Nagoya University, Japan

Abstract. A robust automated segmentation of abdominal organs can be crucial for computer aided diagnosis and laparoscopic surgery assistance. Many existing methods are specialised to the segmentation of individual organs or struggle to deal with the variability of the shape and position of abdominal organs. We present a general, fully-automated method for multi-organ segmentation of abdominal CT scans. The method is based on a hierarchical atlas registration and weighting scheme that generates target specific priors from an atlas database by combining aspects from multi-atlas registration and patch-based segmentation, two widely used methods in brain segmentation. This approach allows to deal with high inter-subject variation while being flexible enough to be applied to different organs. Our results on a dataset of 100 CT scans compare favourable to the state-of-the-art with Dice overlap values of 94%, 91%, 66% and 94% for liver, spleen, pancreas and kidney respectively.

1 Introduction

The accurate segmentation of organs like the liver, pancreas and kidneys on abdominal computed tomography (CT) scans form an important input to computer aided didagnosis (CAD) systems and to laparoscopic surgery assistance. The detailed segmentation and rendering of such structures can crucially assist clinicians in surgery planning and navigation. Further applications include cancer detection and staging, especially of pancreatic cancer [1]. Most previous work is based on either statistical shape models or probabilistic atlases learned on a training set and applied in combination with post-processing steps based on image intensities and morphology that are often specialized to a particular organ [2–5]. However, the high inter-subject variability in shape and location of abdominal organs, especially the pancreas, poses a challenge to generalized, population-based models and requires more subject-specific prior knowledge. In [1], a subject-specific segmentation model based on statistical shape models is presented. While this method achieves good segmentation results, it is specific

---

* Supported by RS-JSPS Research Cooperative Program, MEXT/JSPS KAKENHI.

N. Ayache et al. (Eds.): MICCAI 2012, Part I, LNCS 7510, pp. 10–17, 2012.

and limited to pancreas segmentation. Linguraru et al.[5] propose a 4D graph model that incorporates patient-specific data for multi-organ segmentation.

Subject-specific, automated segmentation methods based on multi-atlas registration have been pioneered and are now widely used for brain segmentation of magnetic resonance (MR) imaging [6],[7]. Other application areas include cardiac segmentation on CT [8]. With multi-atlas registration, high accuracies are achieved for the segmentation of cortical and subcortical brain structures [6],[7]. A comparatively low variation between subjects in overall brain shape generally allows a good global alignment, providing atlas-patient correspondences that allow the generation of target specific segmentation priors [7]. The high shape and position variability in abdominal organs as well as the differences in global abdominal shape and potentially differences in field of view, forms a significant challenge to the pairwise image registration of abdominal scans. This hampers correspondence estimation on a localized voxel level but also the organ level which is a key requirement for atlas-based propagation strategies.

Patch-based segmentation [9] has recently been proposed as an alternative to multi-atlas registration in brain imaging. In this approach, a coarse alignment is sought between the target and atlas images, and patch-comparison between target and atlases is carried out in a local window to obtain the target labelling.

Previous work for abdominal segmentation based on spatial atlases employed general, population-based probabilistic models, e.g., [2]. Here, we propose an approach that is more sensitive to inter-subject variation. We generate a subject-specific probabilistic atlas for an unlabelled subject by selecting and aligning suitable atlases from a database, combining multi-atlas registration and patch-based refinement. We have evaluated the proposed method on a set of 100 abdominal CT scans for the segmentation of the liver, spleen, kidneys and pancreas and achieve a segmentation accuracy that compares favourably to existing methods.

2 Method

In the proposed approach, the final segmentation is obtained by establishing correspondences between every target voxel and multiple, manually labelled atlas images. Atlases are weighted on three scales: on a global level, the organ level and the voxel level. In the first step, the set of most suitable atlases from a database is selected for a new subject by measuring global image appearance. After aligning all pre-selected atlases with the target image, a local atlas weighting is carried out on an organ by organ basis. Finally, a patch-based segmentation refinement is applied to identify atlas labels at the voxel level.

Given a target image $\mathcal{I}$, the segmentation problem is formulated by assigning each voxel $x_i \in \mathcal{I}$, a label $l \in \{l_0, l_1, ..., l_L\}$ with L anatomical labels and a background label l_0. The labelling procedure is defined as a weighted fusion of expert votes defined on a database of N atlases $\mathbf{A} = \{\mathcal{A}_1, ..., \mathcal{A}_N\}$:

$$l(x_i) = \frac{\sum_{n=1}^{N} w_n^g \sum_{x_j \in \mathcal{A}_n} w_j^o w_j^v l(x_j)}{\sum_{n=1}^{N} w_n^g \sum_{x_j \in \mathcal{A}_n} w_j^o w_j^v} \tag{1}$$

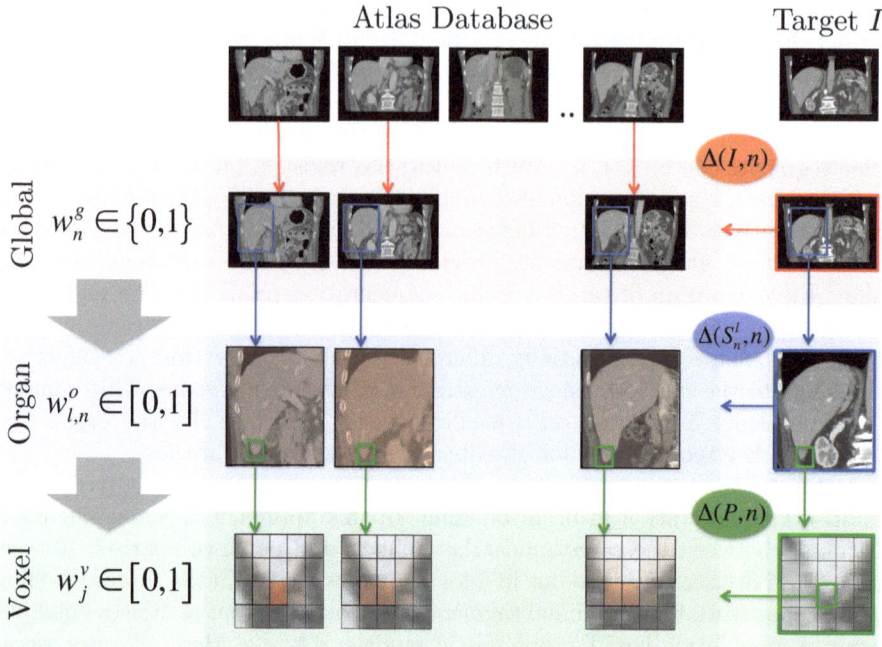

Fig. 1. In the proposed method, atlases are weighted on the global, organ, and voxel level. This scheme specifies the expert knowledge used during the segmentation in a coarse to fine approach, allowing an improved correspondence estimation. On the global level, a binary weighting is applied while a continuous weighting is used in organ- and voxel levels (indicated in red tone).

with weights w_n^g defined on the global atlas level and local weights w_j^o and w_j^v that are assigned on an organ- and voxel-level respectively.

Based on this hierarchical weighting scheme, the target segmentation is inferred from all available atlases. The proposed method is illustrated in Fig. 1: at the **global** stage, a set of atlases is selected based on overall appearance. After pairwise alignment, an individual atlas weighting is defined for every **organ**. Finally, the labelling at the most localized level is inferred after non-linearly aligning atlases on an organ level and by evaluating image-atlas similarities on a voxel-by **voxel** basis.

Weights on all levels are based on the sum of squared intensity differences $\Delta(R, n)$ between image $\mathcal{I}$ and atlas $\mathcal{A}_n$, defined over a region of interest R measuring image appearance on the relevant level of locality:

$$\Delta(R, n) = \sum_{j \in R} \|\mathcal{I}(x_j) - \mathcal{A}_n(x_j)\|^2 \qquad (2)$$

In Sections 2.1, 2.2 and 2.3, the atlas weighting schemes applied at the global- organ- and voxel levels are described respectively.

2.1   Global Atlas Weighting

For a given target image $\mathcal{I}$, binary weights w^g are assigned on a global atlas level. This weight defines a pre-selection of atlases based on global appearance in order to deal with significant differences in body size and field of view. No pairwise registration is performed before computing global atlas weights. By doing so, local minima that may arise from a mis-registration of very different images does not influence the measurement. The ROI R in Eq. 2 spans the whole CT scan and weights are defined as follows:

$$w_n^g = \begin{cases} 1 \text{ if } \Delta(\mathcal{I}, n) < \Delta_\delta \\ 0 \text{ , otherwise.} \end{cases} \tag{3}$$

where Δ_δ is a threshold on the global image distance.

2.2   Organ Level Atlas Weighting

Atlases $\mathcal{A}_n$ that show a high similarity with the target image $\mathcal{I}$ at a global scale are thus weighted with $w_n^g = 1$. These atlases are then aligned with the target image to perform atlas selection on the localized organ, and voxel levels. After pairwise alignment, the atlas label maps S_n^l for label l from atlas n are transformed to the target space. The organ-wide atlas weight $w_{l,n}^o$ is the product of a term $w_{l,n}^{\mathcal{I}}$ that is defined by atlas-target similarities as well as a term $w_{l,n}^S$ that is defined by the agreement between individual atlas label maps:

$$w_{l,n}^o = w_{l,n}^{\mathcal{I}} w_{l,n}^S \tag{4}$$

The similarity-based term $w_{l,n}^{\mathcal{I}}$ is defined after affine alignment of $\mathcal{A}_n$ to $\mathcal{I}$ and measures similarities over the transformed organ label:

$$w_{l,n}^{\mathcal{I}} = \exp\left(-\frac{\Delta(S_n^l, n)}{h}\right) \tag{5}$$

where h is a user-set variable that defines the number of atlases supporting the segmentation of organs with label l. $w_{l,n}^S$ measures the agreement between transformed label maps after applying a non-rigid atlas-target alignment:

$$w_{l,n}^S = \frac{1}{N-1} \sum_{k \in N, k \neq n} JI(S_k^l, S_n^l) w_k^g \tag{6}$$

where JI is the Jaccard index.

This term is based on a similar principle to the one proposed in the STAPLE algorithm [10] where raters that show good agreement with others are weighted higher. The main difference being that in STAPLE the confidence vote is evaluated on the voxel-level while in our approach confidence is evaluated over the whole label of a given structure, allowing independent intensity-based corrections at the voxel level.

2.3   Local Voxel Weighting

Label weights on a voxel level are assigned based on the similarity of a patch surrounding a given voxel $x_i \in \mathcal{I}$ and patches in a local neighbourhood of all aligned atlas images $\mathcal{A}_n$. This nonlocal means fusion strategy was recently adapted from image-denoising to the labelling of brain MR scans [9]. A 3-D patch of size s_p x s_p x s_p is defined around every voxel $x_i \in \mathcal{I}$. The image similarity between this patch and patches of the same size defined around the voxels in a local neighbourhood of size s_n, is evaluated in all available atlases. This results in weights defined by patches P around x_i and the voxels $x_{n,j}$ in all atlases $\mathcal{A}_n$ and in the defined search window. Following [9], the weights are defined as

$$w_j^v(x_i, x_j) = \exp\left(-\frac{\Delta(P, n)}{h^v}\right) \tag{7}$$

where x_j is a voxel in atlas $\mathcal{A}_n$ as defined in Eq. 1 and h^v defines the weighting in relation to patch distance.

3   Experiments and Results

Our method was evaluated on 100 3D abdominal CT scans acquired from 21 female and 79 male subjects. Subjects were aged between 26 and 83 with a mean age of 63. Scans have a resolution of 512 x 512 voxels in plane and contain between 263 and 538 slices depending on the field of view and the slice thickness. Voxel sizes range between 0.55 and 0.82 mm and the slice spacing varied between 0.4 and 0.8 mm. For each scan a manual segmentation generated by a single trained rater is available for the liver, spleen, pancreas and the kidneys.

3.1   Experiments

A leave-one-out strategy was applied, where one scan in turn was segmented by using the remaining 99 subjects as atlas database. The threshold Δ_δ was defined in a way that 30 atlases where weighted with $w_n^g = 1$ by the global similarity measure in Eq. 3. Correspondence is sought between atlases and target image before extracting organ- and voxel level similarities in Eqs. 4 and 7. A rigid and affine registration step was followed by a multi-level non-rigid registration step using free-form deformations with B-spline control-point spacings of 20 mm, 10 mm and 5 mm [11]. The registration is driven by the normalized mutual information between target and source in the relevant region of interest.

In the patch-based segmentation procedure used to obtain voxel-level weights defined in Eq. 7 a patch-size of $s_p = 5$ and a neighbourhood size of $s_n = 9$ where used and h^v was set to the minimum patch distance as proposed in [9].

The results obtained with the proposed approach are compared to results based on a direct application of atlas-registration with atlas selection as proposed in [6],[7]. For direct fusion, a set of 30 atlases is selected for each organ from the atlas database based on image similarites and non-rigidly aligned with the target. The final label at the voxel label is obtained by performing a majority voting strategy as widely used in brain segmentation [6],[7].

Table 1. Average Jaccard index (JI), Dice overlap (similarity index, SI) and Recall/
Precision for 100 subjects. Compared are reference segmentations with the proposed
method and a standard mulit-atlas segmentation technique.

Structure	Proposed method			Direct fusion		
	Dice	Jaccard	Rec./Prec.	Dice	Jaccard	Rec./Prec.
Liver	94.4	89.5	95.3/93.9	93.0	87.1	93.5/92.9
Spleen	90.9	84.6	92.4/90.7	78.4	68.0	77.0/82.9
Pancreas	65.5	49.6	62.9/70.7	43.6	29.3	33.6/71.9
Kidneys	94.3	88.1	93.4/93.9	88.3	79.6	84.9/92.3

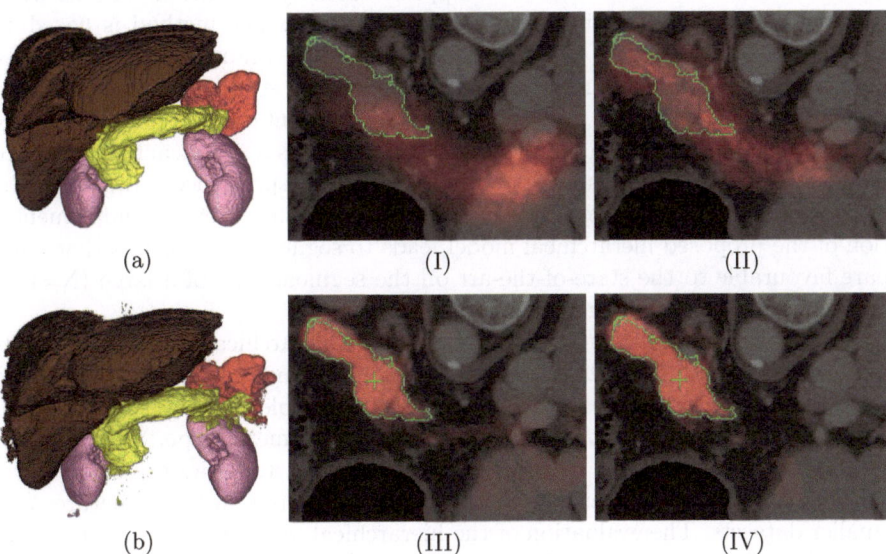

(a)   (I)   (II)

(b)   (III)   (IV)

Fig. 2. Panels (a) and (b) show renderings for the liver (brown), kidneys (pink), pancreas (yellow) and spleen (red) based on the manual reference and the proposed method
respectively. Panels I-IV illustrate the automated, hierarchical pancreas segmentation
on an axial slice with manual labels outlined in green and atlas probabilities in red
tone. Panel (I) shows the overall distribution of all atlases in the database. In panel
(II), shows the subject-specific probabilistic atlas at the global scale. Panel (III) shows
the refined atlas after pairwise registration and organ-wide intensity-based weighting.
Panel (IV) also incorporates the proposed confidence-based weighting.

3.2   Results

Automated and manual segmentations were compared by widely used measures
that all are defined by the true positive (TP) and false negative (FN) rates and
that range from 0 to 100. The Jaccard index (JI), the Dice overlap (Similarity
index, SI) as well as recall (REC) and precision (PRE) values between structural
labels obtained with the proposed method and direct fusion as well as manual
reference labels are presented in Tab. 1.

Fig. 2 shows example for the automated segmentation procedure. Panels (a) and (b) compare volume renderings obtained from automated and manual segmentations. Panels (I) - (IV) present exemplarily the different steps of the proposed hierarchical atlas weighting scheme for pancreas segmentation.

4   Discussion and Conclusion

In this paper we propose a novel, atlas-based segmentation technique for multi-organ abdominal segmentation. The strength of the presented method is its general nature which allows it to be applied robustly to multiple organs without specialisation and individual parameter settings. The method is based on multi-atlas registration, a technique widely used in brain imaging. Here, we present a hierarchical coarse-to-fine atlas weighting strategy that is designed to deal with the challenges found in abdominal segmentation. Especially, a large inter-subject variation in abdominal appearance poses a significant challenge to image registration algorithms and therefore to correspondence estimation, the essence of atlas-based segmentation techniques. We show how the implementation of the proposed hierarchical model leads to segmentation results that compare favourable to the state-of-the-art on the segmentation of a large (N=100) and relatively diverse image database.

The results in Tab. 1 show how the proposed hierarchical model clearly outperforms multi-atlas selection and registration schemes as originally proposed for brain segmentation [7]. Especially for highly variable structures like the pancreas, a substantial improvement is achieved. The method performs at least as good as state-of-the-art multi-organ segmentation strategies presented in recent years [3],[5]. Both methods, however, are evaluated on less structures and smaller datasets. The evaluation of the hierarchical model in [3], is restricted to the liver and the work in [5] does not provide results for the pancreas which is the most challenging structure due to a high variability in shape and also position. Shimizu et. al [1] recently describe a method based on shape models that addresses this challenge, achieving a satisfactory accuracy for pancreas segmentation on a database of 20 subjects. While our method gives stable results for pancreas segmentation, such more specialized models can improve the segmentation accuracy. Adding some shape knowledge may further improve the presented results for more challenging organs and is a direction of future work.

The run-time of our method is defined by that of the non-rigid registration step. In the current research implementation, one registration runs for approximately one hour for a whole abdominal scan, resulting in an overall runtime for all organs of around three hours on a machine with eight Intel Xeon cores clocked at 3GHz and 32GB RAM. A recent implementation [12] of the used registration algorithm [11], however, allows speed ups of around 10 fold, making the method relevant for an application in a clinical environment.

Future work needs to be done to evaluate the full potential of the proposed method. As can be seen from the volume rendering in Fig. 2, the lack of topological constraints in our voxel-level weighting may produce sometimes fuzzy and anatomically unplausible or even subdivided segmentations. A way to address this problem is to incorporate smoothness constraints into the final label assignment instead of independently thresholding the weight at the 50% level as described in the current model in Eq. 1. One way to include such constraints is via graph cuts, an optimization technique widely used for labelling problems in medical imaging [13]. Furthermore, to assess inter-observer variability, all reference segmentations will be performed by a second independent, trained rater.

References

1. Shimizu, A., Kimoto, T., Kobatake, H., Nawano, S., Shinozaki, K.: Automated pancreas segmentation from three-dimensional contrast-enhanced computed tomography. Int. J. CARS 5, 85–98 (2010)
2. Park, H., Bland, P., Meyer, C.: Construction of an abdominal probabilistic atlas and its application in segmentation. IEEE TMI 22(4), 483–492 (2003)
3. Okada, T., Yokota, K., Hori, M., Nakamoto, M., Nakamura, H., Sato, Y.: Construction of Hierarchical Multi-Organ Statistical Atlases and Their Application to Multi-Organ Segmentation from CT Images. In: Metaxas, D., Axel, L., Fichtinger, G., Székely, G. (eds.) MICCAI 2008, Part I. LNCS, vol. 5241, pp. 502–509. Springer, Heidelberg (2008)
4. Rusko, L., Bekes, G., Fidrich, M.: Automatic segmentation of the liver from multi- and single-phase contrast-enhanced CT images. MedIA 13(6), 871–882 (2009)
5. Linguraru, M., Pura, J., Chowdhury, A., Summers, R.: Multi-organ Segmentation from Multi-phase Abdominal CT via 4D Graphs Using Enhancement, Shape and Location Optimization. In: Jiang, T., Navab, N., Pluim, J.P.W., Viergever, M.A. (eds.) MICCAI 2010, Part III. LNCS, vol. 6363, pp. 89–96. Springer, Heidelberg (2010)
6. Heckemann, R.A., Hajnal, J.V., Aljabar, P., Rueckert, D., Hammers, A.: Automatic anatomical brain MRI segmentation combining label propagation and decision fusion. NeuroImage 33(1), 115–126 (2006)
7. Artaechevarria, X., Munoz-Barrutia, A., Ortiz-de Solorzano, C.: Combination Strategies in Multi-Atlas Image Segmentation: Application to Brain MR Data. IEEE TMI 28(8), 1266–1277 (2009)
8. Isgum, I., Staring, M., Rutten, A., Prokop, M., Viergever, M., van Ginneken, B.: Multi-Atlas-Based Segmentation With Local Decision Fusion - Application to Cardiac and Aortic Segmentation in CT Scans. IEEE TMI 28(7), 1000–1010 (2009)
9. Coupe, P., Manjón, J.V., Fonov, V., Pruessner, J., Robles, M., Collins, D.L.: Patch-based segmentation using expert priors: Application to hippocampus and ventricle segmentation. NeuroImage 54(2), 940–954 (2011)
10. Warfield, S.K., Zou, K.H., Wells III, W.M.: Simultaneous truth and performance level estimation (STAPLE): an algorithm for the validation of image segmentation. IEEE TMI 23(7), 903–921 (2004)
11. Rueckert, D., Sonoda, L.I., Hayes, C., Hill, D.L.G., Leach, M.O., Hawkes, D.J.: Nonrigid registration using free-form deformations: Application to breast MR images. IEEE TMI 18(8), 712–721 (1999)
12. Modat, M., Ridgway, G.R., Taylor, Z.A., Lehmann, M., Barnes, J., Hawkes, D.J., Fox, N.C., Ourselin, S.: Fast free-form deformation using graphics processing units. Computer Methods and Programs in Biomedicine 98(3), 278–284 (2010)
13. Boykov, Y., Veksler, O., Zabih, R.: Fast approximate energy minimization via graph cuts. IEEE PAMI 23(11), 1222–1239 (2001)

Radiation-Free Drill Guidance
in Interlocking of Intramedullary Nails

Benoit Diotte[1], Pascal Fallavollita[1], Lejing Wang[1], Simon Weidert[2],
Peter-Helmut Thaller[2], Ekkehard Euler[2], and Nassir Navab[1]

[1] Chair for Computer Aided Medical Procedures (CAMP), TU Munich, Germany
[2] Trauma Surgery Department, Klinikum Innenstadt, LMU Munich, Germany

Abstract. Intramedullary nailing is a technically demanding procedure
which involves an excessive amount of X-ray acquisitions; one study lists
as many as 48 to successfully complete the procedure. In this work, a
novel low cost radiation-free drilling guide is designed to assist surgeons
in completing the distal locking procedure without any X-ray acquisitions. Using an augmented reality fluoroscope that coregisters optical and
X-ray images, we exploit solely the optical images to detect the drilling
guide in order to estimate the tip position in real-time in X-ray. We
tested over 200 random drill guide poses showing a mean tip-estimation
error of 1.72 ± 0.7 mm which is significantly robust and accurate for the
interlocking. In a preclinical study on dry bone phantom, three expert
surgeons successfully completed the interlocking 56 out of 60 trials with
no X-ray acquisition for guidance and an average time of 2 min.

1 Introduction

Modern trauma and orthopedic surgeries such as fracture reduction and osteosynthesis use C-arm X-ray or standard X-ray radiography for interventional
guidance, especially in minimally invasive surgery. As X-ray is displayed in 2D,
the surgeon relies on their skill set to mentally transfer the bone configuration
shown in the image onto the patient location. This requires added mental effort
and may lead to distraction, possibly resulting in procedural errors compromising quality of surgery. Tibial fractures are among the most common lower limb
injuries to be treated by an orthopedic & trauma surgeon. In the early 1990s,
tibial fractures accounted for 77.000 hospitalizations per year. Today, the incidence has increased to approximately 500.000 cases in the United States per
year. On average, almost 26 tibia fractures occur per 100.000 population per
year[1]. Intramedullary nailing is a common surgical procedure mostly used in
fracture reduction of the tibial and femoral shaft. After successful insertion of
the nail into the medullary canal, the nail has to be fixed in its position in
order to prevent rotation and dislocation by inserting screws perpendicular to
the nail through the provided proximal and distal holes inside the nails shaft.

---

[1] Epidemiology at `http://emedicine.medscape.com/article/`
`1248857-overview#a0199`

N. Ayache et al. (Eds.): MICCAI 2012, Part I, LNCS 7510, pp. 18–25, 2012.
© Springer-Verlag Berlin Heidelberg 2012

The insertion of the screws near the entrance point of the nail is achieved using an aiming bow attached to the nail. In the distal part of the nail, locking is commonly performed freehand with a radiolucent drill attachment or similar aiming devices. Various techniques and devices developed for facilitating locking procedures are reviewed in [7]. The conclusions from this work are that interlocking of intramedullary nails is a technically demanding procedure. Several ingenious computer aided methods and devices were developed recently, e.g. robot based guide positioning [8] and 3D optical tracking [1] however these have not yet gained worldwide acceptance in clinical practice due to the higher learning curve and additional cumbersome hardware involved in the operating room. The amount of radiation exposure is excessive due to the intricacy of drilling a screw inside a 5mm nailing hole solely by X-ray image acquisition and guidance.

Intraoperative Radiation Exposure: Much experimental work has been performed to evaluate the amount of radiation exposure to surgeons during interlocking procedures. Müller *et al.* [2] showed that the average X-ray time per procedure, mainly spent with distal locking, was 4.63 min and the primary surgeon received a 2.02 mSv mean radiation exposure to his hand. On the other hand, Suhm *et al.* showed that when using a computer aided surgery navigation system, the radiation time exposure decreased from 108 sec to 7 sec, but took significantly longer operation time from 13.7 min to 17.9 min when compared to a standard mobile C-arm fluoroscope [5]. In a more recent study by Rohilla *et al.*, authors document that the average number of images taken for the complete procedure to be 48.27 [4]. In an effort to reduce radiation exposure, Navab *et al.* have attempted an augmented reality (AR) fluoroscopy system for orthopedic surgery that allows to facilitate the surgical procedure and to reduce the radiation exposure. They augment a regular mobile C-arm by a video camera and a X-ray/video image overlay [3]. Through a mirror construction and one time calibration of the device, the acquired X-ray images are coregistered with the video images without any further calibration or registration during the intervention. The surgeon can thus visualize on the same video both soft tissue and bone position. Such system allows them to better plan the scar positioning and the screw insertion point. Moreover, the surgeon can better target using the real-time video view where the X-ray image is taken, and therefore avoid unnecessary radiation. This technology has been described to reduce radiation; a decrease from 17.05 ± 4.61 X-ray shots to 9.85 ± 3.10 using the system in [3]. However, two immediate limitations of the overlay are observed. First, none of these works use the optical video image effectively as the optics provides a simple raw image to the surgeon; in other words, they often revert back to the X-ray image for decision making and navigation completion. Secondly, the instrument tip (i.e. scalpel tip, drill tip, etc.) is not visible to the surgeon when it is positioned inside the patient anatomy of interest.

Contribution: In this paper, a radiation-free guide is designed and used to enable surgeons to complete the interlocking of intramedullary nailing procedure

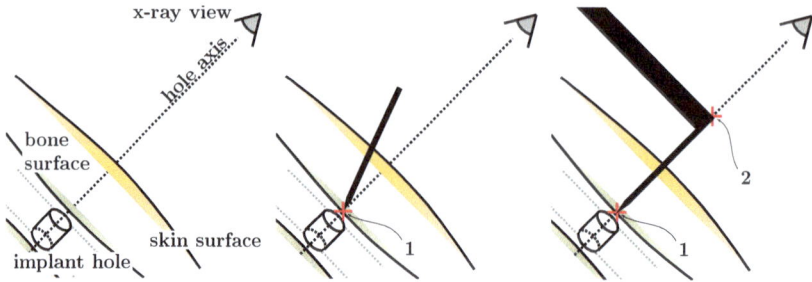

Fig. 1. (Left) The down-beam positioning technique for distal locking aligns the hole axis of the nail with the camera center to guide the drilling process. (Center) The center punch marks point 1. (Right) The drill top is aligned on the axis at point 2. Points 1 and 2 are required to be kept on the axes by the surgeon in order to guarantee the success of drilling.

without any X-ray acquisitions. Motivated from the technologies in [3], for the very first time we propose to use the optical video images for full procedure guidance and navigation, thereby becoming the first such interlocking system using single view optical video input data. The radiation-free guide is detected by the optical camera and its tip is measured in real-time and displayed to the surgeon in both the X-ray and video images. In contrast to commercially available optical tracking tools we need no additional light sources or navigation base, and the cameras data is not solely dedicated to navigation. The camera is viewing inside the C-arm working volume, usually free of occlusions. Our hypothesis is the complex interlocking of intramedullary nails procedure will be simplified. Via a computer-simulation and dry bone phantom study, we evaluate the precision and success rate of the interlocking of intramedullary nails.

2   Methodology

2.1   The Surgical Workflow in Interlocking of Intramedullary Nails

The typical distal locking workflow (WF) is divided into seven surgical steps [6]:

WF 1) **X-ray Positioning:** Moving the C-arm on top of the patient and ends after the X-ray image shows the distal part of the nail inside the bone.
WF 2) **Adjustment of Hole:** Position the C-arm until the hole is perfectly round in order to allow for orthogonal drilling (i.e. down-beam positioning, fig. 1)
WF 3) **Skin Incision:** Finding the incision position and cutting the skin. The correct incision position is confirmed by images showing the scalpel tip located inside the locking hole on the X-ray image or using augmented fluoroscopy as in [3].
WF 4) **Center Punch:** Alignment of a Schanz screw with the target hole. Then, with the help of a hammer, a small dimple is formed on the bone surface in which

the tip of the drill will be positioned. This step is required to prevent slipping of the drill. To ensure alignment X-ray images are acquired.

WF 5) Alignment of the Tip of the Drill: Alignment of the drill bit with the target hole. It ends when X-ray images show that the projection of the tip is located inside the circle of the target hole.

WF 6) Drilling: Drilling the bone until the drill bit passes through the locking hole of the nail and the bone cortex on the other side. It ends after confirmation by X-rays.

WF 7) Locking Screw Insertion: Inserting a locking screw into the hole. X-ray is required to confirm the success of the insertion, which indicates the end of the procedure.

The challenge for the surgeon lies in aligning the drill along the down the beam axis to ensure a successful drilling process (fig. 1). This is achieved using an average of 9.15 ± 6.65 X-ray images [6] in WF 4-WF 6. Our objective is to eliminate X-ray guidance completely during these steps by designing a radiation-free drilling guide.

2.2 Radiation-Free Drill Guide Model

We modified a 200 mm long, 5 mm diameter Schanz screw by fixing seven fluorescent coated spherical markers (fig. 2). The top ball has the largest size at 2.0 cm. An upper branch containing 3 spherical markers is attached to the pin at position B. These three spherical markers have a size of 1.2 cm in diameter. A lower branch containing 3 spherical markers is attached to the pin at position C. These three spherical markers have a size of 1.0 cm in diameter. The reason for choosing different sized markers was for the correct ordering between the top ball, and upper, lower branch markers. The distances on the upper branch are: **ab:** 3.0 cm, **ac:** 5.7 cm, **aB:** 8.9 cm. The lower branch has the same dimensions. Lastly, the metrics for the main axis of the Schanz screw are: **AB:** 4.7 cm, **AC:** 10.7 cm, **AD:** 18.8 cm.

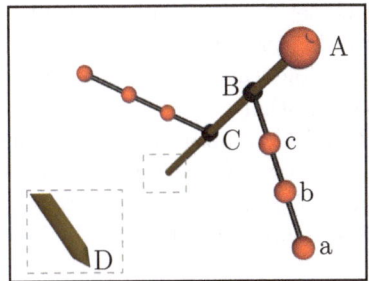
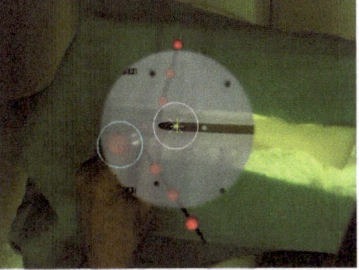

Fig. 2. (Left) The design of the radiation-free drill guide. (Right) The overlay of X-ray and video image. The target hole is bounded by a white circle marked with an (x) for its center. The estimated tip position for the radiation-free drill guide is visualized by a yellow (+) icon.

Tip Estimation Using the Cross-Ratio. Having collinear markers detected in an image we are able to compute the tip-position of the radiation-free drill guide. Given the 3D geometry of our instrument, (i.e. the position of the distal end of the guide with respect to the other markers) we compute the tip based on the cross-ratio:

$$d_{AD} = \frac{(S \cdot d_{AB}) - d_{AC}}{S - 1} \quad \text{where} \quad S = \frac{crossratio \cdot d_{AC}}{d_{AB}} \tag{1}$$

$$crossratio = \frac{AB \cdot CD}{AC \cdot BD} \tag{2}$$

Here d_{ij} are the image distances between the markers i and j respectively. The same idea is applied to estimate the image position of B and C on the main axis of the pin from the upper and lower branches; using the three collinear balls on each branch.

Real-Time Detection of the Seven Spherical Markers in Video Image. We observed that using red fluorescent pigmentation peaked the saturation channel of HSV in such a way that thresholding the S image with a very high cutoff value results in the spherical markers being seen by the video camera as bright ellipses (i.e. close to a circular shape), which can be easily segmented. From the binary image all contours are extracted using the OpenCV library. In a post-processing step we filter those contours having a low compactness value and those having a smaller area than a threshold (i.e. in our setup the default values are 0.5 for the compactness and 100 px for the area). For all contours being retained by the filtering routine, the sub-pixel centroids are computed based on grayscale image moments. From the possible blob candidates we select the largest blob as being the most likely candidate for the top ball of the radiation free drill guide. From the remaining blobs, we choose two disjoint sets yielding an optimal least squares line fitting and least size variance. We now have the seven best estimates for the spherical marker center locations. From equation (1), we solve for B and C points located on the main axis of the Schanz screw by applying the same side axis cross ratio to the 2 branches. For each set we get 2 possible solutions (i.e. because cross ratio is based on a ball ordering process, and we don't have any point correspondences). To rectify this, we find the combination of estimated points that have the smallest distance to each other (i.e. assign them as possible B and C points). Lastly, we order the B and C combination on the main axis according to their distances from the top ball on a fitted line. Having ABC we can estimate the tip-position of the radiation-free drill guide (fig. 2). A note: we observe that turning the white balancing off in video stabilizes the blob detection based on our fluorescent colored markers.

2.3   Quantification Experiments for Tip Estimation Accuracy

We first performed an experiment to quantify the accuracy of the estimated tip position. We print a binary circle with 5 mm diameter on a sheet of paper that is placed about 20 cm away and parallel to the image intensifier. The image center of the circle is extracted with sub-pixel accuracy from the video image; defining ground-truth of the tip image position. We physically fix the tip of pin at the center of the circle for all pose variations. We rotated the radiation-free drill guide about the tip position to generate 200 video images of random different poses. We computed the difference between the estimated tip position and ground-truth to quantify the accuracy of the tip detection. The metric error in mm can be calculated from image error in px, since the ratio between px and mm is known. The rotational values spanned a cone angle range between $\pm 30°$.

2.4 Dry Bone Phantom Experiment

In this pre-clinical phantom study, we used dry bones having similar shape and size, and common surgical instruments, including an AO radiolucent drill attachment, and a 10 mm solid Titanium Femoral Nail (Synthes, Oberdorf, Switzerland). The dry bones were placed inside a plastic box in a horizontal position and then fixed on the C-arm intensifier. In order to simulate the rigidity of a normal leg, the dry bones were fixed inside the box. Each dry bone was drilled open from the proximal joint and the nail was inserted in the medullary cavity of the bone prior to the beginning of the experiment (fig. 3).

Visualization in X-ray and Video Image. For our method, we employ the system calibration method described in [3] in order to align the projection geometry of an X-ray and video image. The estimated tip of the radiation-free drill guide is directly registered to the X-ray images. The target hole of the nail seen in X-ray is bounded by a white circle and marked with an x for its center. The radiation-free drill guide tip is marked with a yellow + and the top ball of the guide is bounded with a blue circle (fig. 2). The visualization colors and details were suggested by the surgeons participating in our study. The AR fluoroscopy system used was built by attaching a video camera (Flea2, from Point Grey Research Inc., Vancouver, BC, Canada) and mirror construction, covered by an X-ray source housing, to a mobile C-arm (Powermobile, isocentric

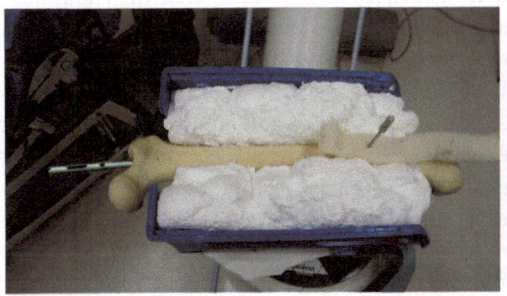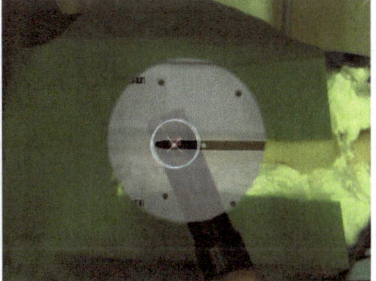

Fig. 3. (Left) The dry bone phantom setup with a nail inside the bone. (Right) The top ball of the drill guide is bounded by a blue circle.

C-arm, from Siemens Healthcare, Erlangen, Germany). The mean error of the calibration computed on about 200 control points was 1.59 ± 0.87 px with a maximum error of 5.02; approximately 0.5 mm on the plane of the calibration pattern.

Surgical Protocol for Radiation-Free Interlocking. Two expert surgeons and one resident surgeon from the orthopedic and trauma surgery department participated in a total of 60 interlocking of intramedullary nails. 30 trials were performed with video and X-ray overlay visualization, and the remaining trials were performed by looking at augmented X-ray images. To begin with, an X-ray image of the nail within the dry bone was acquired along the down the beam position. The target entry point of the hole was automatically thresholded via a circular Hough transform. Then by visualizing the X-ray and video overlay, the surgeons maneuver the radiation-free drill guide until the tip was superimposed on the center of the target hole. The guide is then positioned along the down beam position prior to center punching. Using a hammer, the bone is notched by hammering down on top of our guide. Lastly, the drill tip is positioned on the notch by the surgeon and the drill top is detected in real-time in video and maneuvred until it is superimposed with the target center in X-ray (fig. 3). The surgeon lastly drills through the nail hole.

3   Results and Discussion

For the quantification study with 200 trials and ± 30° cone angle rotation of the radiation free guide we obtain the following errors for tip estimation when compared to ground-truth: 3.93 ± 1.6 px which is equivalent to 1.72 ± 0.7 mm; 57% of the samples were below the mean error, 98% below 4 mm. These errors indicate the accuracy and robustness of our detection and tip estimation algorithm and are within the clinical tolerances for interlocking procedures since the hole diameter of the nail is 5 mm. For the preclinical dry bone phantom study, a success rate of 93% (56 out of 60 trials) was achieved by the surgeons. The average time for completion was 2 min. No X-ray images were acquired or requested outside of one X-ray needed to confirm whether the drill missed or hit the hole of the nail. Therefore, by detecting the radiation-free drill guide only in video, the surgeons effectively guided the interlocking workflow steps WF 4-WF 6 defined in 2.1. This is considered the first attempts of using video guidance for augmented reality fluoroscopy systems as in [3]. Of the 4 failed trials, one was due to the nail moving out of position when the surgeon hammered the radiation-free drill guide to notch the bone. This was a design issue for our phantom setup. The three surgeons confirmed that in clinical practice the interlocking nail is fixed by external jigs and that the nail would not move out of position. The remaining 3 failed trials were attributed to the resident surgeon. Interestingly, when compared to the two expert surgeons, the resident surgeon did not perform a *deep enough* notch on the bone surface during the center punching step, thereby not being able to position properly the drill tip prior to drilling. He remedied his approach accordingly and succeeded in the remaining trials. The final results in both studies indicate that our radiation-free drill guide has the potential to eliminate a large number of X-ray acquisitions to complete the interlocking of intramedullary nails procedure. The immediate feedback received by the three surgeons was listing a potential orthopedic and trauma procedures that can immediately benefit from such a guide: interlocking nailing of humeral shaft fractures or plate osteosynthesis fixation.

4 Conclusions

In this paper, a radiation-free guide is designed and used to assist surgeons in completing the interlocking of intramedullary nailing procedure without additional X-ray acquisitions. This is the very first video guided study for completing the interlocking procedure. Our radiation-free guide has its tip estimated in real-time and displayed to the surgeon at all instances regardless if they are visualizing only augmented X-ray images. Our hypothesis is that the complex interlocking of intramedullary nails procedure will be simplified by our elegant radiation-free solution. Our results demonstrate potential for this.

References

1. Leloup, T., El Kazzi, W., Schuind, F., Warzee, N.: A novel technique for distal locking of intramedullary nail based on two non-constrained fluoroscopic images and navigation. IEEE Transactions on Medical Imaging 27(9), 1202–1212 (2008)
2. Müller, L.P., Suffner, J., Wenda, K., Mohr, W., Rommens, P.M.: Radiation exposure to the hands and the thyroid of the surgeon during intramedullary nailing. Injury 29(6), 461–468 (1998)
3. Navab, N., Heining, S.M., Traub, J.: Camera augmented mobile c-arm (camc): Calibration, accuracy study and clinical applications. IEEE Transactions on Medical Imaging 29(7), 1412–1423 (2009)
4. Rohilla, R., Singh, R., Magu, N., Devgan, A., Siwach, R., Sangwan, S.: Simultaneous use of cannulated reamer and schanz screw for closed intramedullary femoral nailing. ISRN Surg. (2011) (published online)
5. Suhm, N., Messmer, P., Zuna, I., Jacob, L.A., Regazzoni, P.: Fluoroscopic guidance versus surgical navigation for distal locking of intramedullary implants. a prospective, controlled clinical study. Injury 35(6), 567–574 (2004)
6. Wang, L., Landes, J., Weidert, S., Blum, T., von der Heide, A., Euler, E., Navab, N.: First Animal Cadaver Study for Interlocking of Intramedullary Nails under Camera Augmented Mobile C-arm. In: Navab, N., Jannin, P. (eds.) IPCAI 2010. LNCS, vol. 6135, pp. 56–66. Springer, Heidelberg (2010)
7. Whatling, G., Nokes, L.: Literature review of current techniques for the insertion of distal screws into intramedullary locking nails. Injury 37(2), 109–119 (2006)
8. Yaniv, Z., Joskowicz, L., Member, S.: Precise robot-assisted guide positioning for distal locking of intramedullary nails. IEEE Transactions on Medical Imaging 24(5), 624–635 (2005)

Developing Essential Rigid-Flexible Outer Sheath to Enable Novel Multi-piercing Surgery

Siyang Zuo[1], Takeshi Ohdaira[2], Kenta Kuwana[1], Yoshihiro Nagao[2], Satoshi Ieiri[2], Makoto Hashizume[2], Takeyoshi Dohi[1], and Ken Masamune[1]

[1] Graduate School of Information Science and Technology, University of Tokyo, Japan
[2] Departments of Advanced Medicine and Innovative Technology,
Kyushu University Hospital, Japan
sa.siyou@atre.t.u-tokyo.ac.jp

Abstract. We have developed a new generation device called rigid-flexible outer sheath with multi-piercing surgery (MPS) to solve the issues of tissue closure, triangulation, and platform stability in natural orifice transluminal endoscopic surgery (NOTES), and the problems of restricted visual field, organ damage, and removing a resected organ from body in needlescopic surgery (NS). The shape of the flexible outer sheath can be selectively locked by a novel pneumatic shapelocking mechanism. Major features include four directional flexion at the distal end, four working channels, and suction and water jet functions. The insertion part of the prototype is 330 mm long with a 25 mm maximum outer diameter. The outer sheath system has successfully preformed *in vivo* experiment using a swine on partial gastrectomy. The advanced outer sheath system has shown great promise for solving NOTES and NS issues.

Keywords: Outer sheath, Pneumatic shapelocking mechanism, NS, NOTES, MRI-compatible.

1   Introduction

Natural orifice transluminal endoscopic surgery (NOTES) is minimally invasive surgical procedure using a flexible endoscope to access to the abdominal cavity via transoral, transcolonic or transvaginal routes [1-3]. The major advantages of this method are the absence of associated abdominal wall complications, and providing cosmetic benefits. However, some problems remain unsolved in NOTES. Firstly, although many devices are under development to enable closure procedure [4-5], the closure of the internal entry point for NOTES presents a significant challenge. Secondly, usually the dual-channel endoscope is used in NOTES allowing procedures to be performed in a manner as laparoscopic surgery. The channels are close and parallel to the camera, leading to loss of triangulation and a more technically challenging procedure. Some devices have been developed to solve triangulation problem [6-7]. However, triangulation is still minimal by these devices. Finally, because the endoscope is flexible, attempting to manipulate tissues and organs may lead the endoscope to create an

N. Ayache et al. (Eds.): MICCAI 2012, Part I, LNCS 7510, pp. 26–33, 2012.

unstable operative platform. The TransPort (USGI Medical, San Capistrano, CA, USA) was designed for NOTES using ShapeLock technology [8]. However, because the TransPort uses wire tension to lock the shape of the shaft, they often suffer from problems of wire breakage and thus cannot be used safely. Additionally the mechanisms and structures of TransPort are complicated, costly, and difficult to achieve MRI compatibility. Needlescopic surgery (NS) is a laparoscopic surgical technique using instruments and ports smaller than 3 mm in diameter. NS can reduce the surgical incisions in the abdominal wall to a size which is difficult to detect macroscopically. However, NS has not been widely adopted for minimally invasive surgery as involving some limitations. Firstly, observations are restricted by the poor scope visualization and instantaneous loss of visual field due to blood and fat mist. Secondly, instruments used in NS are easy bending of the shaft caused by its small diameter and leading to risk of organ damage because the instruments themselves act as needle. Finally, it is difficult to remove a resected organ from the needlescopic ports which smaller than 3 mm in diameter.

We invented a novel procedural concept called multi-piercing surgery (MPS) [9]. MPS is defined as NOTES-assisted NS. Our new proposal in this paper is an ideal rigid-flexible outer sheath to solve the issues of access, and platform stability in NOTES. The outer sheath could provide a clear visual field, assist to resect the lesion, and remove a resected organ from the body. On the other hand, the tasks of NS in MPS are to perform the surgery itself, and open and close the incision safely in the gastrointestinal tract for NOTES. The outer sheath combined with NS could also solve the problems of triangulation in NOTES, and organ damage problems in NS. The outer sheath can exchange between flexible and rigid modes, and make instrumental path to the abdominal cavity. In MPS, an entrance wound is first created in the intestinal tract for the outer sheath by NS. Then, in flexible mode, the outer sheath is inserted through the entrance wound in the intestinal tract, and locates an internal organ. When the outer sheath approaches the target in the abdominal cavity, the surgeon locks the shape of the outer sheath and then inserts flexible instruments easily through the path created by the sheath. Then, NS can be performed easily with the outer sheath assisted. Once in place, variety of flexible instruments can be inserted again and again without damaging the tissues around the outer sheath.

In this paper, a new prototype of the outer sheath with lockable operating part is presented. In addition, the paper reports the analysis of working space of the bending distal end and shape holding torque of the rigid-flexible shaft. Especially, the outer sheath system was first tested in *in vivo* partial gastrectomy experiments, and successfully preformed *in vivo* experiment using a swine.

2   Method

The outer sheath consists of a bending distal end for local treatment and route selection, and a rigid-flexible shaft for selective shapelocking of the shaft, and an operating part for simple operation by surgeon.

2.1   Bending Distal End Structure

The bending distal end consists of six aligned frames that mutually rotate 90° around their axes. The frames are driven by four wires that are 90° apart. For each frame, the rotating angle in the vertical and horizontal direction is ± 40° and ±45°, respectively, because of which the bending distal end can achieve a curvature of ±120° and ±90° in the vertical and horizontal directions, respectively (Fig. 1(A)). The workspace as an end effector of the outer sheath is given in Fig. 1(B). Furthermore, the bending distal end is manufactured in an integrated manner, and therefore, assembly of the frames is not necessary. The resin material (FullCure720, Objet Geometries Ltd., Israel) which used in the prototype was authorized as biocompatible material by FDA (the U.S. Food and Drug Administration). Because the breakdown limit of the bending distal end is about 58 N, it should be strong enough to be used in clinical practice.

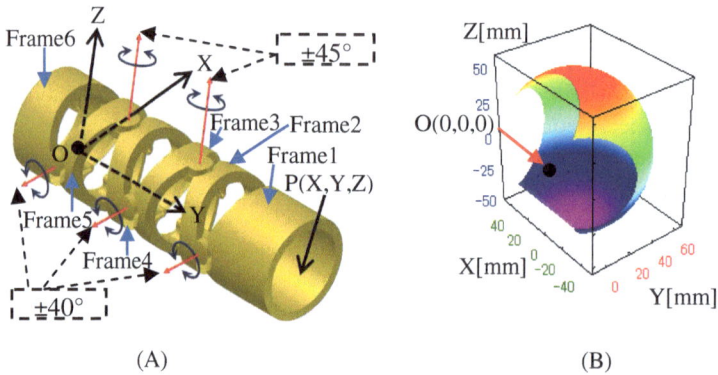

(A)   (B)

Fig. 1. Structure of bending distal end. (A) Mechanism of bending distal end. (B) Workspace of the bending distal end P(X,Y,Z).

2.2   Rigid-Flexible Shaft Mechanism

The pneumatic shapelocking mechanism exchanging between a flexible and a rigid mode have been represented in [10]. The design consists of flexible toothed links, a bellows tube and sealed cover (Fig. 2(A)). The bellows tube and toothed link mechanism can be easily locked as well as relaxed by control of the vacuum, providing a smooth transition between flexible and rigid modes. An approximate model is built for design the toothed links (Fig. 2(A)). The relationship among the tooth top angle α, area S per tooth, atmospheric pressure P, coefficient of friction μ, number of teeth n per toothed link, distance d, and shape holding torque M are described by equation (1) and (2) with relations in Fig. 2(A). When n is 60, d is 9.5 mm, relationship among α, S, and M is shown in Fig. 2(B). Fig. 2(B) shows that, in rigid mode, the shape holding torque is decide by tooth top angle and area per tooth. The shape of the toothed links is designed base on this calculated value.

$$F = PS \sin(\frac{\alpha}{2})(\cos(\frac{\alpha}{2}) - \mu \sin(\frac{\alpha}{2})) \quad (1), \qquad\qquad M = 3 \times F \times d \times n \quad (2)$$

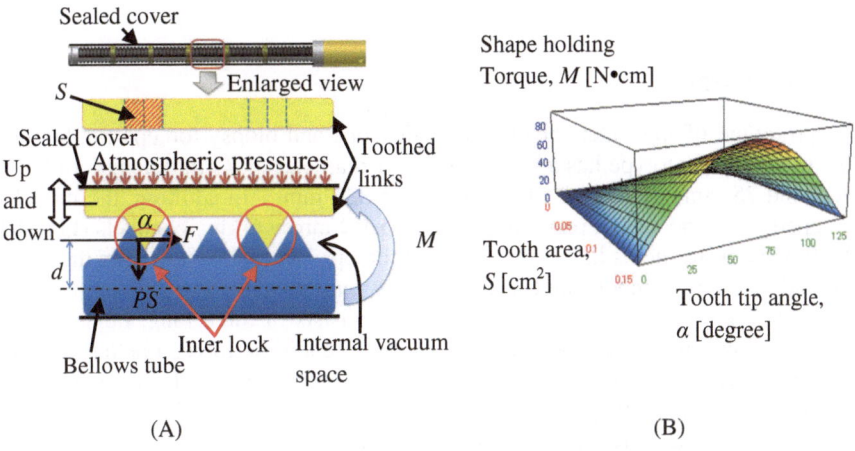

Fig. 2. Design of the toothed links. (A) Image of toothed link and bellows tube. (B) Relationship of shape holding torque, tooth area and tooth tip angle.

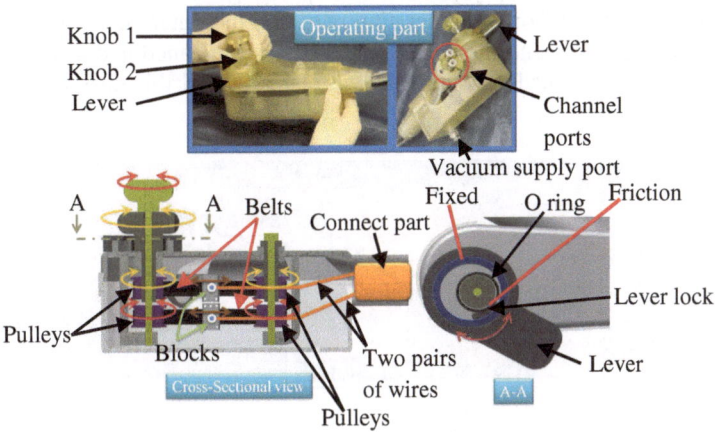

Fig. 3. Operating part of the outer sheath

2.3 Operating Part Structure

The operating part is shown in Fig. 3. To achieve smooth rotational movement and reduce backlash, belt and pulley structure is designed to control the bending angle of the distal end. Two pairs of wires (Fig. 3) for control of the bending angle are fixed on the Blocks (Fig. 3). Two sets of belt and pulley structure (two pulleys in common to one belt) allow for transmitting rotary movement of the pulleys to translatory movement of the Blocks (Fig. 3). Therefore surgeons can easily control the bending angle of distal end by rotating two knobs. Bending angles of ±120° in the vertical direction and ±90° in the horizontal direction can be achieved by Knob 1 (Fig. 3) and Knob 2 (Fig. 3), respectively. Furthermore, Surgeons can turn the lever to lock the rotation of the knob by the friction between rubber O ring (Fig. 3) and Lever lock (Fig. 3), and then the bending angle of distal end can be locked.

2.4   Prototype

The prototype of the outer sheath with endoscope and biopsy forceps can be seen in Fig. 4(A). The prototype has a maximum outer diameter of 25 mm, length of bending distal end 75 mm, and length of inserting part 330 mm.   In addition, the model was equipped with one 7 mm, one 3 mm, and two 1.9 mm working channels (Fig. 4(B)). The flexible instruments like endoscope and forceps can be inserted from the 7 mm, 3 mm and 1.9 mm channels, and one of the 1.9 mm channels is used for suction and water jet (Fig. 4(C)). The rigid-flexible shaft consists of three long, flexible toothed links, a bellows tube, and a polyethylene cover. In addition, to get a better lock on the elementary part of rigid-flexible shaft, two short flexible toothed links are added on the base side of shaft (Fig. 4(D)). The outer sheath is connected to a vacuum pump (DTC-41, ULVAC KIKO Inc., Japan) and a vacuum controller to alternate between flexible and rigid modes by pushing a button. The sheath is also connected to a roller pump (RP-2100, Tokyo Rikakikai Co., Ltd., Japan) to jet water. Suction can be applied through vacuum supply ports in the operating room. The disposable inserting part can be separated from the operating part, and the outer sheath is separated from the vacuum controller and the vacuum source, to be cleaned and sterilized. All parts of the prototype are made of nonmagnetic material, and this ensures excellent MRI compatibility.

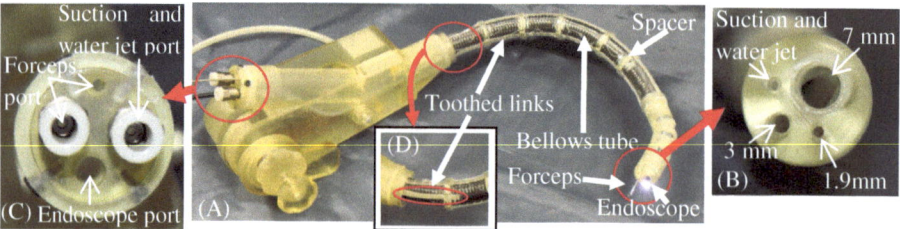

Fig. 4. Prototype of the outer sheath. (A) Image of prototype. (B) Enlarged view of bending distal end. (C) Enlarged view of channel ports. (D) Toothed links for locking base side of shaft.

3   Results

Using the outer sheath, MPS *in vivo* experiment using a swine (female, 43.5 kg) has been performed for partial gastrectomy (Fig. 5(A)). The needle devices were inserted through two 3 mm access ports in the upper abdominal region. We inserted the outer sheath through lower abdominal region as much as possible to near rectal route.

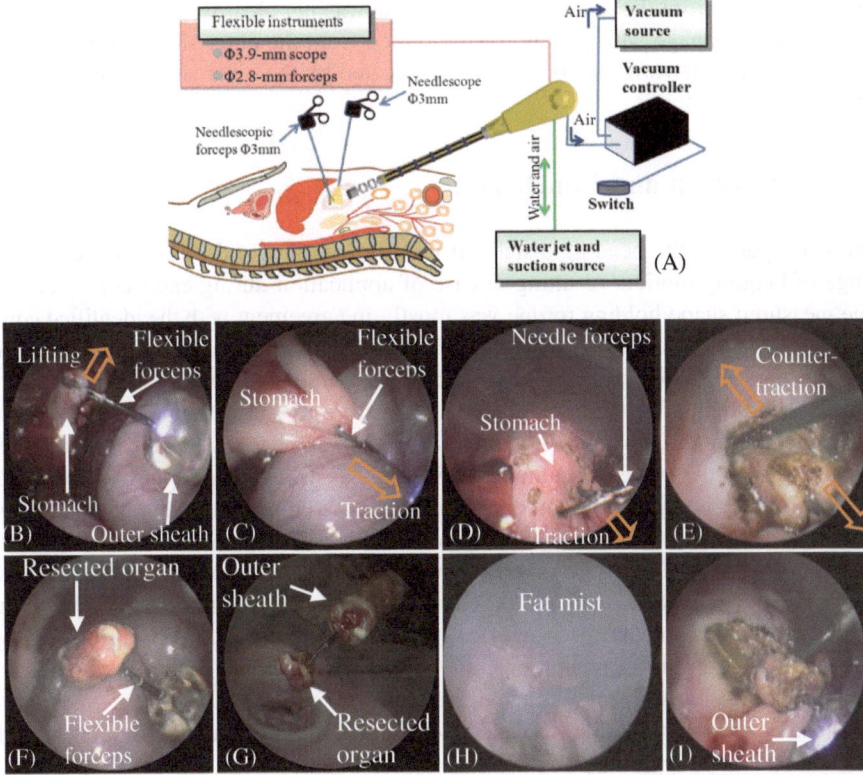

Fig. 5. 3 mm laparoscopic broad views of the abdominal cavity of a swine. (A) Outer view of *in vivo* experiment (B) Stomach clamping. (C) Stomach traction. (D) Gastric resection with traction. (E) Gastric resection with counter-traction. (F) Resected tissue clamping. (G) Removal of the resected stomach from body. (H) Image without suction from the outer sheath. (I) Image with suction from the outer sheath.

The incision part during insertion of the outer sheath was protected with a LAP DISK (Hakko Medical Inc., Japan). The instruments inserted into the outer sheath were a 3.9 mm industrial endoscope and a 2.8 mm flexible forceps. Fig. 5 (B) ~ (I) were views from a 3 mm needle scope (Karl Storz, Munich, Germany). Firstly, the outer sheath threaded its way through the large intestines and small intestines to locate stomach. We clamped the stomach surface (Fig. 5(B)), and exerted traction on stomach (Fig. 5(C)) to expose the hypothetical affected area for treatment using the 2.8 mm forceps inserted from the outer sheath. Secondly, we resected the hypothetical affected area by radiofrequency 3 mm needle forceps with traction on stomach using the 2.8 mm flexible forceps (Fig. 5(D)). Thirdly, we clamped the hypothetical affected area directly by 2.8 mm flexible forceps, and continued resection with counter-traction achieved by the outer sheath (Fig. 5(E)). The hypothetical affected area was successfully resected with the outer sheath assisted (Fig. 5(F)). Finally, we removed the resected organ from the outer sheath incision (Fig. 5(G)). Moreover, we tested the suction performance of the outer sheath. Fig. 5(H) was image of resection moment without suction from the outer sheath. The view was not clear by the fat mist. On the other hand, the image which suction was applied from the outer sheath was shown in Fig. 5(I). The clear view means that suction created by the outer sheath took effective action against fat mist.

4   Discussion and Conclusion

The workspace of the bending distal end was shown that the distal end cover a large range of bending motion, resulting in ease of application during endoscopic surgery. The measured shape holding torque was mostly in agreement with the identified equation in the straight condition. Because the number of engaged teeth diminished in curved condition, the shape holding torque was impaired as compared with the straight condition. The major distinguishing feature of the pneumatic shapelocking mechanism, besides its simple structure, is ability to achieve high shape locking power by inputting low power vacuum which is less than 1 kPa. The rupture of the sealed cover should be possible problem during inserting the outer sheath into body. However, the tissues near the outer sheath are protected from damage even in the event of air leakage (1 kPa), and the outer sheath can be removed easily from the body as it is flexible. Actually the air leakage problem has not occurred in *in vivo* experiment. Therefore, the design concept is an effective principle to produce high rigidity safely. The locking capability of bending distal end and rigid-flexible shaft allows the outer sheath to be positioned at the target field. Thus, the surgeon's hands are free. These features, combined with the flexible endoscope's four-directional flexion, enable more complex manipulation.

In *in vivo* experiment, the partial gastrectomy was successfully performed. The outer sheath has been easily located the target, and manipulated tissues stably, in comparison with conventional endoscope using in [9]. These results showed that the outer sheath has strong potential for solving access problems and stability issues in NOTES. Its robust size with 2.8 mm flexile forceps makes it easy to manipulate tissues or even to retract and lift the stomach, which are necessary maneuvers during partial gastrectomy. Because the large angle is achieved between the needlescopic devices and flexible instruments inserted from channels of the outer sheath, triangulation with separate optics and instrumentation is easy to realize. Therefore, the risk of impaired visual field, damaging tissue due to the unforeseen movements of forceps caused by clashing of devices can be minimized. In particular, two flexible instruments inserted from the outer sheath, combined with two needlescopic devices gave the surgeon the ability to manipulate tissue with traction and counter-traction almost in all planes. Furthermore, the suction from the outer sheath was very useful to draw in fat mist, which provided a clear visual field. The low resolution of the 3.9 mm industrial endoscope was not adequate for observing local fields. A high-resolution medical endoscope is scheduled for introduction. Because the flexible endoscope are inserted though the channel of the outer sheath, this makes the outer sheath itself less complex and therefore more cost effective. Furthermore, the performance of the prototype was tested in an MR environment by phantom experiment. The S/N decreasing ratio is 4.6% from introduction of the outer sheath into the phantom [10]. We will continue development of the outer sheath device focusing on a smaller diameter and better shapelocking capabilities including partially-lockable mechanism by changing the material and structure. Furthermore, the outer sheath with ultrasonic motor control system will be evaluated in an MR environment. MRI navigation and shape tracking technologies for the outer sheath will also be developed.

References

1. Rattner, D., Kalloo, A.: ASGE/SAGES Working Group on Natural Orifice Translumenal Endoscopic Surgery. J. Surg. Endosc. 20, 329–333 (2006)
2. Marescaux, J., Dallemagne, B., Perretta, S., Wattiez, A., Mutter, D., Coumaros, D.: Surgery without scars: report of transluminal cholecystectomy in a human being. J. Arch. Surg. 142, 823–826 (2007)
3. Pearl, J.P., Ponsky, J.L.: Natural orifice translumenal endoscopic surgery: a critical review. J. Gastrointest. Surg. 12, 1293–1300 (2008)
4. Vitale, G.C., Davis, B.R., Tran, T.C.: The advancing art and science of endoscopy. J. Am. J. Surg. 190, 228–233 (2005)
5. Hu, B., Chung, S.C., Sun, L.C., Lau, Y.J., Kawashima, K., Yamamoto, T., Cotton, P.B., Gostout, C.J., Hawes, R.H., Kaloo, A.N., Kantsevoy, S.V., Pasricha, P.J.: Endoscopic suturing without extracorporeal knots: a laboratory study. J. Gastrointest. Endosc. 62, 230–233 (2005)
6. Suzuki, N., Sumiyama, K., Hattori, A., Ikeda, K., Murakami, E.A.Y., Suzuki, S., Hayashibe, M., Otake, Y., Tajiri, H.: Development of an endoscopic robotic system with two hands for various gastric tube surgeries. Medicine Meets Virtual Reality 11, 349–353 (2003)
7. Phee, S.J., Low, S.C., Huynh, V.A., Kencana, A.P., Sun, Z.L., Yang, K.: Master and slave transluminal endoscopic robot (MASTER) for natural orifice transluminal endoscopic surgery (NOTES). In: Proc. 31st IEEE Engineering in Medicine and Biology Society, vol. 1, pp. 1192–1195 (2009)
8. Swanstrom, L., Kozarek, R., Pasricha, P.F., Gross, S., Birkett, D., Park, P.O., Saadat, V., Ewers, R., Swain, P.: Development of a new access device for transgastric surgery. J. Gastrointest. Surg. 9, 1129–1137 (2005)
9. Ohdaira, T., Tsutsumi, N., Xu, H., Mori, M., Uemura, M., Ieiri, S., Hashizume, M.: Ultra-minimally invasive local immune cell therapy and regenerative therapy by multi-piercing surgery for abdominal solid tumor: therapeutic simulation by natural orifice translumenal endoscopic surgery-assisted needlescopic surgery using 3-mm diameter robots. J. Hepato-biliary Pancreat Sci. 18(4), 499–505 (2011)
10. Zuo, S., Masamune, K., Kuwana, K., Dohi, T.: Nonmetallic Guide Sheath with Negative Pressure Shapelocking Mechanism for Minimally Invasive Image-Guided Surgery. In: Dohi, T., Liao, H. (eds.) ACCAS 2011. PICT, vol. 3, pp. 1–9. Springer, Heidelberg (2012)

Surgical Gesture Classification from Video Data

Benjamín Béjar Haro*, Luca Zappella*, and René Vidal

Center for Imaging Science, Johns Hopkins University

Abstract. Much of the existing work on automatic classification of gestures and skill in robotic surgery is based on kinematic and dynamic cues, such as time to completion, speed, forces, torque, or robot trajectories. In this paper we show that in a typical surgical training setup, video data can be equally discriminative. To that end, we propose and evaluate three approaches to surgical gesture classification from video. In the first one, we model each video clip from each surgical gesture as the output of a linear dynamical system (LDS) and use metrics in the space of LDSs to classify new video clips. In the second one, we use spatio-temporal features extracted from each video clip to learn a dictionary of spatio-temporal words and use a bag-of-features (BoF) approach to classify new video clips. In the third approach, we use multiple kernel learning to combine the LDS and BoF approaches. Our experiments show that methods based on video data perform equally well as the state-of-the-art approaches based on kinematic data.

Keywords: surgical gesture classification, time series classification, dynamical system classification, bag of features, multiple kernel learning.

1 Introduction

Recent technological advances have contributed to, and changed, the way in which surgery can be performed. One of them is Robotic Minimally Invasive Surgery (RMIS), which has several advantages over traditional surgery, such as better precision, smaller incisions and reduced recovery time. However, the steep learning curve together with the lack of fair and effective criteria for judging the skills acquired by a trainee, may reduce the benefits of this technology.

This has motivated a number of approaches for automatic RMIS skill assessment and gesture classification. One of the most natural approaches is to decompose a surgical task into a series of pre-defined 'atomic' gestures or *surgemes* [1–3], such as 'insert a needle', 'grab a needle', 'position a needle', etc. (Fig. 1 shows sample frames from three different surgemes). The problem then becomes how these surgemes can be segmented in time, recognized, and finally assessed.

Most of the prior work on surgical gesture recognition (see, e.g., [4–6]) uses hidden Markov models (HMMs) to analyze kinematic data stored by the robot, such as the position of the robot tools, angles between robot joints, velocity measurements and force/torque signatures. All these approaches model each surgeme

---

* Equal contribution.

N. Ayache et al. (Eds.): MICCAI 2012, Part I, LNCS 7510, pp. 34–41, 2012.
© Springer-Verlag Berlin Heidelberg 2012

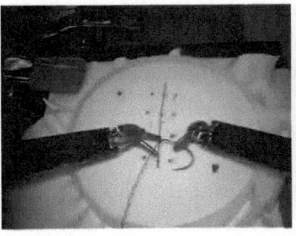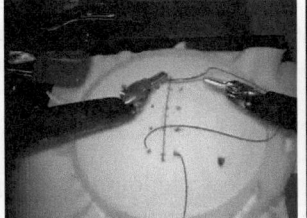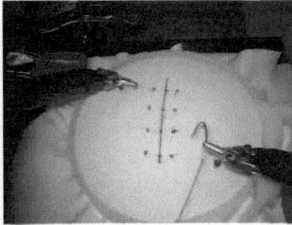

(a) S2: positioning needle   (b) S4: transferring needle from (c) S5: moving to center with
                              left to right   needle in grip

Fig. 1. Examples of three different surgemes in a suturing task

as one or more states of an HMM. The main difference is in how these approaches model the observations within each surgeme. For example, [5] vector-quantizes the observations into discrete symbols, [7] uses a Gaussian model combined with linear discriminant analysis (LDA), [6] assumes that the observations are generated from a lower-dimensional latent space using Factor Analyzed HMMs (FA-HMMs) and Switched Linear Dynamical Systems (SLDSs), [8] uses a Gaussian mixture model (GMM), and [9] models the observations as a linear combination of atomic motions with sparse coefficients. All of these methods have significantly improved surgical gesture classification over a standard HMM.

In addition to kinematic measurements, RMIS systems are also typically equipped with cameras that record the entire procedure. The work in [10, 11] propose to recognize the different phases of a surgery (e.g. CO_2 inflation, abdominal suturing, etc.) using laparoscopic videos. Other works on video data analysis [12, 13] focus on recognizing the phases of a surgery by also observing surgeons and nurses in the operating room. To the best of our knowledge, the only existing work on automatic skill and surgical gesture (rather than coarse phases as in [10–13]) classification from video is [14], which uses basic visual cues based on optical flow and concludes that kinematic-based approaches are generally more accurate.

In this paper, we propose and evaluate three approaches to surgical gesture classification from video. The first approach uses linear dynamical systems (LDSs) to model each video clip from each surgeme. Distances between the parameters of the LDSs are then used to classify new video clips. The second approach is a bag-of-features (BoF) approach in which a dictionary of spatio-temporal words is learned from spatio-temporal features extracted from all video clips. Each video clip is then represented with a histogram of such words and distances between histograms are used to classify new video clips. The third approach combines the LDS and BoF approaches using multiple kernel learning (MKL). Our experiments on kinematic data from a typical surgical training setup show that methods based on LDSs already outperform state-of-the-art approaches based on HMMs [9]. For video data, the BoF approach performs better than the LDS approach, while the MKL approach performs equally well in terms of accuracy, but is typically more robust. Overall, our main conclusion is that methods based on video data perform equally well as methods based on kinematic data for a typical surgical training setup. This result should encourage further investigation of video based techniques for surgical gesture classification as videos potentially carry more unexploited information than kinematic data.

2   Video-Based Methods for Classifying Surgical Gestures

In this section we describe three techniques for surgical gesture classification based on video data. We assume that each video is segmented into *video surgemes*, i.e., video clips corresponding to a single execution of one out of a pre-defined set of surgemes. All three methods use labeled video surgemes to learn a model for each of them. We then show how these models can be compared and used for classifying gestures in new video surgemes.

2.1   Classification Using Linear Dynamical Systems

In this approach, we model the raw pixel intensities of each frame in a video surgeme as the output of a Linear Dynamical System (LDS). More specifically, the raw pixel intensities at time instant k, $\mathbf{z}_k \in \mathbb{R}^p$, with $p \gg n$, are given by

$$\mathbf{x}_{k+1} = \mathbf{A}\mathbf{x}_k + \mathbf{B}\mathbf{u}_k, \tag{1}$$

$$\mathbf{z}_k = \mathbf{C}\mathbf{x}_k + \mathbf{n}_k, \tag{2}$$

where $\mathbf{x}_k \in \mathbb{R}^n$ is an unobserved (latent) continuous state, $\mathbf{u}_k$ is the state driving process (assumed to be Gaussian) with zero mean and identity covariance, i.e., $\mathbf{u}_k \sim \mathcal{N}(\mathbf{0}, \mathbf{I})$, and $\mathbf{n}_k$ represents the measurement noise, also Gaussian with $\mathbf{n}_k \sim \mathcal{N}(\mathbf{0}, \mathbf{R})$ and independent from $\mathbf{u}_k$. The matrices $\mathbf{A}$, $\mathbf{B}$ and $\mathbf{C}$ describe, respectively, the dynamics of the state variable, the correlation among the driving process samples and the mapping of the latent state to the observed signal.

Given a video surgeme, we identify the system's parameters $\mathbf{A}, \mathbf{B}, \mathbf{C}$ and $\mathbf{R}$ using a sub-optimal, but computationally efficient, method based on Principal Component Analysis proposed in [15]. Once, we have identified an LDS for each video surgeme, we need a distance to asses how close two given surgeme models are. A survey of different metrics that could be used can be found in [16]. We tried different distances on the space of LDSs based on subspace angles [17] (Finsler, Frobenius and Martin) and Binet-Cauchy kernels (Trace, Determinant and Max Singular Value) [17, 18]. Since the Martin and Frobenius distances performed best, we will present the results obtained with these two distances. More specifically, let $\theta_1, \dots, \theta_{2n}$ be the subspace angles between the observability subspaces of two nth order LDS models $\mathcal{M}_1$ and $\mathcal{M}_2$. The (squared) Martin and Frobenius distances between the models $\mathcal{M}_1$ and $\mathcal{M}_2$ are, respectively, given by:

$$d_M^2(\mathcal{M}_1, \mathcal{M}_2) = -\log \prod_{i=1}^{2n} \cos^2(\theta_i) \quad \text{and} \quad d_F^2(\mathcal{M}_1, \mathcal{M}_2) = 2\sum_{i=1}^{2n} \sin^2(\theta_i). \tag{3}$$

These distances can be used to classify new surgemes using a nearest neighbor approach. In our experiments we have used them to train a Support Vector Machine (SVM) classifier with a Radial Basis Function (RBF) kernel. That is $k(\mathcal{M}_i, \mathcal{M}_j) = e^{-\gamma d_X^2(\mathcal{M}_i, \mathcal{M}_j)}$, where $d_X = d_M$ or d_F and $\gamma > 0$ is a parameter.

2.2   Classification Using Bag of Spatio-Temporal Features

The second approach is based on the Bag of Features (BoF) approach, a widely used technique for object recognition [19]. In the standard BoF approach, some salient features (e.g., SIFT features [20]) are first extracted from images of different objects. These features are then clustered to learn a dictionary of visual words given by the cluster centers. Each image is then represented in terms of the dictionary using a histogram, and classifiers are trained to recognize new images based on their histograms. The BoF approach can also be extended to action recognition tasks. The most direct way to do so is to build a histogram for each video, where the features are extracted from groups of frames rather than from a single image (see, e.g., [21–23]).

In the case of surgical gesture recognition, we extract Space-Time Interest Points (STIP) [21] from each video surgeme. STIP are salient points where the video has significant variations both in space and in time (as opposed to uniform regions). Hence, STIP can be seen as an extension of space corners to the space-time domain. Moreover, STIP are always detected in correspondence of motion, thus most of the information contained in the static background is automatically discarded. A 3D cuboid is then centered around each of the detected STIP and the local information contained in the cuboid is used to build a 72-bin histogram of oriented gradients (HOG) and a 90-bin histogram of optical flow (HOF), as described in [24]. Therefore, each STIP is described with a vector of size 162 that contains gradient and motion information. The HOG-HOF features extracted from a training set of videos are then clustered by K-means to form a dictionary of N words and histograms of words are built for each video surgeme. Given these histograms, we compute the χ^2-kernel and train an SVM classifier for each surgeme.

2.3   Classification Using Multiple Kernel Learning

Both the LDS and BoF techniques previously described use visual data. However, while the LDS approach tries to capture the dynamics of the scene, the BoF approach is based on sparse (due to feature detection) local structures of the frame (captured by HOG) and very small and sparse motion (captured by HOF). Hence, it seems natural to think about a strategy that integrates these complementary techniques.

One way of combining the LDS and BoF approaches is to exploit the fact that both techniques use a kernel to train an SVM classifier. Therefore, we can combine the kernels using a Multiple Kernel Learning (MKL) framework [25]. In this framework, the SVM optimization problem is solved with respect to a new kernel obtained as a weighted linear combination of a set of given kernels. Thus, the principle behind MKL is to simultaneously solve for the classifier parameters and the kernel weights. Specifically, given a training set of features $\{\mathbf{x}_i\}$ and their labels $\{y_i\}$, the objective is to learn a classification function of the form $f(\mathbf{x}) = \mathbf{w}^t\phi(\mathbf{x}) + b$, where the kernel is given by $\phi^t(\mathbf{x}_i)\phi(\mathbf{x}_j) = \sum_k d_k\phi_k(\mathbf{x}_i)^t\phi_k(\mathbf{x}_j)$, with d_k being the weight of each kernel k. The problem, therefore, is:

$$\min_{\mathbf{w},b,\mathbf{d}} \frac{1}{2}\mathbf{w}^\top\mathbf{w} + C\sum_i l(y_i, f(\mathbf{x}_i)) + r(\mathbf{d}), \quad \text{subject to } d_k \geq 0, \tag{4}$$

where $r(\cdot)$ is a regularizer (ℓ_1 or ℓ_2 norm), $l(y_i, f(\mathbf{x}_i)) = \max(0, 1 - y_i f(\mathbf{x}_i))$ is the loss function and $C > 0$ is a parameter that sets the trade-off between maximizing the margin and minimizing the loss [25].

3   Experiments

Surgical Data. For our tests we used the California dataset [3]. The dataset consists of three different tasks: suturing (SU, 39 trials), needle passing (NP, 26 trials) and knot tying (KT, 36 trials). Each task is performed by 8 surgeons with different skill levels. Typically each surgeon performed around 3 to 5 trials for each task. Each trial lasts, on average, 2 minutes and both kinematic and video data are recorded at a rate of 30 frames per second. Kinematic data consists of 78 motion variables (positions, rotation angles, and velocities of the master/patient side manipulators), whereas video data consists of JPEG images of size 320×240.

The data was manually segmented based on the surgeme's definition of [3]. Specifically, the vocabulary of possible atomic actions consisted of 14 surgemes: 1) reaching for needle with right hand, 2) positioning needle, 3) pushing needle through tissue, 4) transferring needle from left to right, 5) moving to center with needle in grip, 6) pulling suture with left hand, 7) pulling suture with right hand, 8) orienting needle, 9) using right hand to help tighten suture, 10) loosening more suture, 11) dropping suture at end and moving to end points, 12) reaching for needle with left hand, 13) making 'C' loop around right hand, 14) right hand reaches for suture and 15) both hands pull.

Results. In order to compare the accuracy of the surgeme recognition task using kinematic versus visual data, we created two different test setups. The first setup is the *leave-one-super-trial-out* (LOSO), where we leave one trial for each one of the users out for testing. The second setup is the *leave-one-user-out* (LOUO), where we leave all the trials from one user out for testing. For each task we performed a training and a test phase using only the surgemes that appeared in that task.

Note that the LDS approach is not restricted to video data, in fact we also present here the results of LDS with kinematic data. For kinematic data, an additional approach based on sparse dictionary learning (KSVD) [9] is evaluated. With the exception of [9], all other techniques use the SVM classifier (one-versus-one multi-class classification) [26]. The SVM penalty parameter C is estimated using 3-fold cross validation. We empirically set $\gamma = 10^{-3}$ for the RBF kernel, $n = 15$ for the order of the LDS, and $N = 300$ for the size of the BoF dictionary. For MKL, we use ℓ_2 norm regularization on the kernel weights. In order to avoid over-fitting in favor of the most frequent surgemes, we randomly sample no more than 40 surgemes per class and average the results over 20 repetitions.

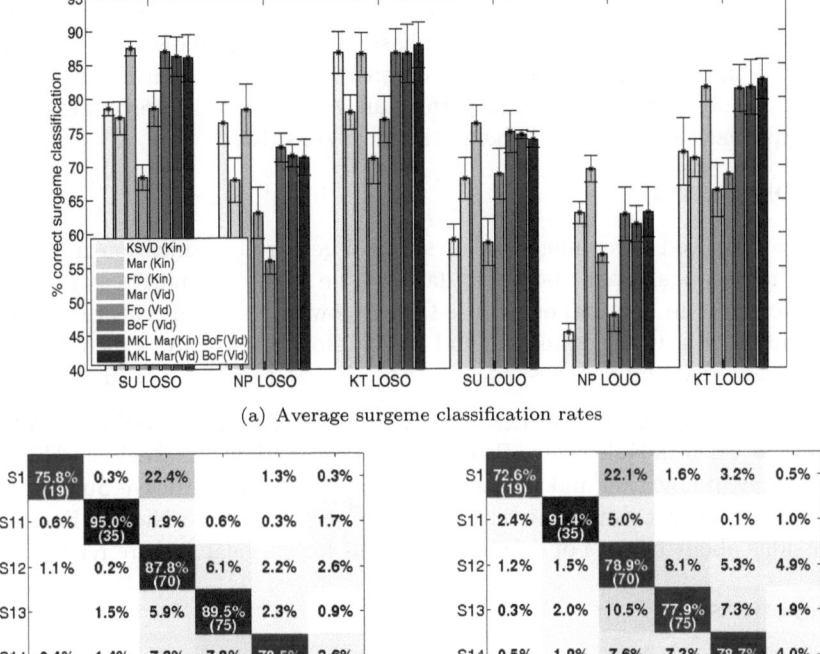

(a) Average surgeme classification rates

(b) Confusion matrix KT task MKL Mar (Vid) BoF (Vid) - LOSO

(c) Confusion matrix KT task MKL Mar (Vid) BoF (Vid) - LOUO

Fig. 2. Results of Kinematic- (Kin) and Video- (Vid) based techniques

The performance is measured as the percentage of correctly identified surgemes averaged over all tests and repetitions for each setup (see Fig. 2). The intervals at the top of the bars of Fig. 2(a) correspond to the average standard deviation for that experiment. Fig. 2(b) and 2(c) show the confusion matrices for Knot Tying (with video data) for the LOSO and LOUO setups, respectively. The numbers in parentheses along the main diagonal represent the number of times that the corresponding surgeme appeared in the dataset.

Among the kinematic-based algorithms the LDS technique with the Frobenius distance outperforms the LDS with Martin distance and the KSVD approach of [9] in almost all of the cases. The combination of gradient and optical flow features extracted by BoF leads to higher accuracy than LDS on video in all of the cases. When merging LDS and BoF using the MKL framework, the average accuracy seems to be slightly improved although not in all of the tested cases. However, as shown in Fig. 2(b) and 2(c), the errors become almost equally spread among classes.

Particularly interesting is the LOUO test, which provides an insight into the ability of the algorithms to generalize and recognize actions performed by users that were unseen during the training phase. The results show that kinematic- and video-based algorithms are able to generalize equally well in this setting. Overall, we observe a decrease in performance of around 10 percentage points for all approaches, with KSVD being the most sensitive.

4   Conclusion

We have proposed three methods for surgical gesture classification from video data. The results showed that video data can be as discriminative as kinematic data. However, in this paper we used fairly low-level visual features, such as image intensities, image gradients and optical flow. Future work includes using more advanced visual features, such as detection and tracking of surgical tools.

Acknowledgments. This work was funded by NSF grants 0931805 and 0941362, and by the Talentia Fellowships Programme of the Andalusian Regional Ministry of Economy, Innovation and Science. The authors thank Intuitive Surgical and Carol Reiley for providing the dataset, and Greg Hager and Nicolas Padoy for discussions about the use of dynamical models for surgical gesture recognition.

References

1. Rosen, J., Solazzo, M., Hannaford, B., Sinanan, M.: Task decomposition of laparoscopic surgery for objective evaluation of surgical residents' learning curve using hidden Markov model. Computer Aided Surgery 7(1), 49–61 (2002)
2. McKenzie, C., Ibbotson, J., Cao, C., Lomax, A.: Hierarchical decomposition of laparoscopic surgery: A human factors approach to investigating the operating room environment. Journal of Minimally Invasive Therapy and Allied Technologies 10(3), 121–127 (2001)
3. Reiley, C.E., Lin, H.C., Varadarajan, B., Vagolgyi, B., Khudanpur, S., Yuh, D.D., Hager, G.D.: Automatic recognition of surgical motions using statistical modeling for capturing variability. In: Medicine Meets Virtual Reality, pp. 396–401 (2008)
4. Dosis, A., Bello, F., Gillies, D., Undre, S., Aggarwal, R., Darzi, A.: Laparoscopic task recognition using hidden Markov models. Studies in Health Technology and Informatics 111, 115–122 (2005)
5. Reiley, C.E., Hager, G.D.: Task versus Subtask Surgical Skill Evaluation of Robotic Minimally Invasive Surgery. In: Yang, G.-Z., Hawkes, D., Rueckert, D., Noble, A., Taylor, C. (eds.) MICCAI 2009, Part I. LNCS, vol. 5761, pp. 435–442. Springer, Heidelberg (2009)
6. Varadarajan, B.: Learning and inference algorithms for dynamical system models of dextrous motion. PhD thesis, Johns Hopkins University (2011)
7. Varadarajan, B., Reiley, C., Lin, H., Khudanpur, S., Hager, G.: Data-Derived Models for Segmentation with Application to Surgical Assessment and Training. In: Yang, G.-Z., Hawkes, D., Rueckert, D., Noble, A., Taylor, C. (eds.) MICCAI 2009, Part I. LNCS, vol. 5761, pp. 426–434. Springer, Heidelberg (2009)
8. Leong, J.J.H., Nicolaou, M., Atallah, L., Mylonas, G.P., Darzi, A.W., Yang, G.-Z.: HMM Assessment of Quality of Movement Trajectory in Laparoscopic Surgery. In: Larsen, R., Nielsen, M., Sporring, J. (eds.) MICCAI 2006. LNCS, vol. 4190, pp. 752–759. Springer, Heidelberg (2006)

9. Tao, L., Elhamifar, E., Khudanpur, S., Hager, G.D., Vidal, R.: Sparse Hidden Markov Models for Surgical Gesture Classification and Skill Evaluation. In: Abolmaesumi, P., Joskowicz, L., Navab, N., Jannin, P. (eds.) IPCAI 2012. LNCS, vol. 7330, pp. 167–177. Springer, Heidelberg (2012)
10. Blum, T., Feußner, H., Navab, N.: Modeling and Segmentation of Surgical Workflow from Laparoscopic Video. In: Jiang, T., Navab, N., Pluim, J.P.W., Viergever, M.A. (eds.) MICCAI 2010, Part III. LNCS, vol. 6363, pp. 400–407. Springer, Heidelberg (2010)
11. Padoy, N., Blum, T., Ahmadi, S., Feussner, H., Berger, M., Navab, N.: Statistical modeling and recognition of surgical workflow. Medical Image Analysis 16(3), 632–641 (2012)
12. Lalys, F., Riffaud, L., Bouget, D., Jannin, P.: An Application-Dependent Framework for the Recognition of High-Level Surgical Tasks in the OR. In: Fichtinger, G., Martel, A., Peters, T. (eds.) MICCAI 2011, Part I. LNCS, vol. 6891, pp. 331–338. Springer, Heidelberg (2011)
13. Miyawaki, F., Masamune, K., Suzuki, S., Yoshimitsu, K., Vain, J.: Scrub nurse robot system - intraoperative motion analysis of a scrub nurse and timed-automata-based model for surgery. Transactions on Industrial Electronics 52(5), 1227–1235 (2005)
14. Lin, H.: Structure in surgical motion. PhD thesis, Johns Hopkins University (2010)
15. Doretto, G., Chiuso, A., Wu, Y., Soatto, S.: Dynamic textures. Int. Journal of Computer Vision 51(2), 91–109 (2003)
16. Chaudhry, R., Vidal, R.: Recognition of visual dynamical processes: Theory, kernels and experimental evaluation. Technical Report 09-01, Department of Computer Science, Johns Hopkins University (2009)
17. Cock, K.D., Moor, B.D.: Subspace angles and distances between ARMA models. System and Control Letters 46(4), 265–270 (2002)
18. Martin, A.: A metric for ARMA processes. IEEE Trans. on Signal Processing 48(4), 1164–1170 (2000)
19. Dance, C., Willamowski, J., Fan, L., Bray, C., Csurka, G.: Visual categorization with bags of keypoints. In: European Conference on Computer Vision (2004)
20. Lowe, D.G.: Object recognition from local scale-invariant features. In: IEEE Conf. on Computer Vision and Pattern Recognition, pp. 1150–1157 (1999)
21. Laptev, I.: On space-time interest points. Int. Journal of Computer Vision 64(2-3), 107–123 (2005)
22. Willems, G., Tuytelaars, T., Van Gool, L.: An Efficient Dense and Scale-Invariant Spatio-Temporal Interest Point Detector. In: Forsyth, D., Torr, P., Zisserman, A. (eds.) ECCV 2008, Part II. LNCS, vol. 5303, pp. 650–663. Springer, Heidelberg (2008)
23. Chaudhry, R., Ravichandran, A., Hager, G., Vidal, R.: Histograms of oriented optical flow and Binet-Cauchy kernels on nonlinear dynamical systems for the recognition of human actions. In: IEEE Conference on Computer Vision and Pattern Recognition (2009)
24. Wang, H., Ullah, M.M., Klaser, A., Laptev, I., Schmid, C.: Evaluation of local spatio-temporal features for action recognition. In: British Machine Vision Conference, pp. 1–11 (2009)
25. Varma, M., Babu, R.: More generality in efficient multiple kernel learning. In: International Conference on Machine Learning, pp. 1065–1072 (2009)
26. Chang, C.C., Lin, C.J.: LIBSVM: a library for support vector machines (2001), Software http://www.csie.ntu.edu.tw/~cjlin/libsvm

Remote Ultrasound Palpation for Robotic Interventions Using Absolute Elastography

Caitlin Schneider[1], Ali Baghani[1], Robert Rohling[1,2], and Septimiu Salcudean[1]

[1] Department of Electrical and Computer Engineering,
University of British Columbia, Vancouver, BC, Canada
[2] Department of Mechanical Engineering,
University of British Columbia, Vancouver, BC, Canada

Abstract. Although robotic surgery has addressed many of the challenges presented by minimally invasive surgery, haptic feedback and the lack of knowledge of tissue stiffness is an unsolved problem. This paper presents a system for finding the absolute elastic properties of tissue using a freehand ultrasound scanning technique, which utilizes the da Vinci Surgical robot and a custom 2D ultrasound transducer for intra-operative use. An external exciter creates shear waves in the tissue, and a local frequency estimation method computes the shear modulus. Results are reported for both phantom and *in vivo* models. This system can be extended to any 6 degree-of-freedom tracking method and any 2D transducer to provide real-time absolute elastic properties of tissue.

Keywords: Ultrasound, Absolute Elastography, Robotic Surgery.

1 Introduction

During laparoscopic procedures, surgeons face challenges such as limited vision of the surgical site and lack of dexterity and haptic feedback. In this type of surgery, the organs are only touched with the distal ends of long surgical instruments that must pass through the patient's abdominal wall. While the da Vinci Surgical System (Intuitive Surgical, Sunnyvale, CA) has overcome with some of the issues that make laparoscopic surgery difficult, including stereoscopic vision and improved tool dexterity [7], the issue of haptic feedback remains unsolved.

Ultrasound elastography has the potential to offer an alternative to providing haptic feedback by instead providing a full image of tissue stiffness and viscosity - the very properties that surgeons try to measure during manual palpation. Ultrasound imaging is relatively inexpensive, non-ionizing and real-time, making it an advantageous imaging modality for intra-operative navigation. Conventional ultrasound has been integrated previously into the da Vinci Surgical System using multiple types of ultrasound transducers [14,15].

Previous ultrasound elastography has been primarily based on *strain* imaging. Ultrasound strain imaging, which provides images of relative tissue deformation in response to various compression levels applied by the ultrasound transducer

N. Ayache et al. (Eds.): MICCAI 2012, Part I, LNCS 7510, pp. 42–49, 2012.

[12], has also been integrated with the da Vinci Surgical System [4]. That system uses the 'Read-Write' Application Programming Interface (API) to overlay a palpation motion onto the movements of the surgeon. This removes some of the user-related difficulties of creating quality strain images by moving the transducer with a known amplitude and frequency. Strain imaging can be used to determine the tumour extent and for image registration [16], but is more affected by boundary conditions.

Acoustic radiation force imaging (ARFI) has shown promising results, and been tested *in vivo* [10,5]. This method of imaging uses the acoustic force produced by the ultrasound transducer to create a shear wave in the tissue, whose speed is then captured through fast imaging techniques and correlation based methods. Unfortunately, this method requires high powered ultrasound machines.

This paper proposes a novel freehand *absolute* elastography method for the da Vinci robot. The method uses an external exciter to induce vibrations into the patient's body, while a 2D intra-operative transducer, manoeuvred by the surgeon, is used to acquire 1D axial vibration amplitude and phase over a volume. These vibration phasors are acquired at known 3D locations by using the da Vinci 'Read' API to determine the position and orientation of the transducer. In the paper, 'axial' will refer to the direction in the image away from the transducer face.

To the best of our knowledge, this is the first time that an absolute elastography approach with external excitation has been developed using the position and orientation of a 2D transducer for freehand sampling of a tissue volume. Contributions of this paper include the novel use of 2D tracked ultrasound to create 3D absolute elastograms, the use of external excitation which does not require specialized ultrasound hardware and the integration of elastography with robotic surgery.

2   Methods

2.1   Elastography

Absolute ultrasound elastography is based on the measurement of shear wave propagation in tissue in response to a mechanical excitation. The excitation can be generated by an acoustic impulse radiation force [10] or by an external vibrator [11]. We use an external vibrator in our work because there are no issues related to penetration depth and tissue heating and because we can use a standard, limited power ultrasound machine. For a harmonic excitation, shear wave propagation in a homogeneous elastic solid, for small strain and linear approximations, is described in the frequency domain by the following wave equation:

$$\rho(j\omega)^2 \hat{\boldsymbol{u}}(x, j\omega) = \mu \nabla^2 \hat{\boldsymbol{u}}(x, j\omega) \ . \tag{1}$$

We make the assumptions that the density of tissue ρ is homogeneous and equal to that of water, although tissue density does change with tissue type and effects the wave speed slightly, this assumption is common in the elastography community. We also make the assumption that the displacement phasors $\hat{\boldsymbol{u}}(x, j\omega)$

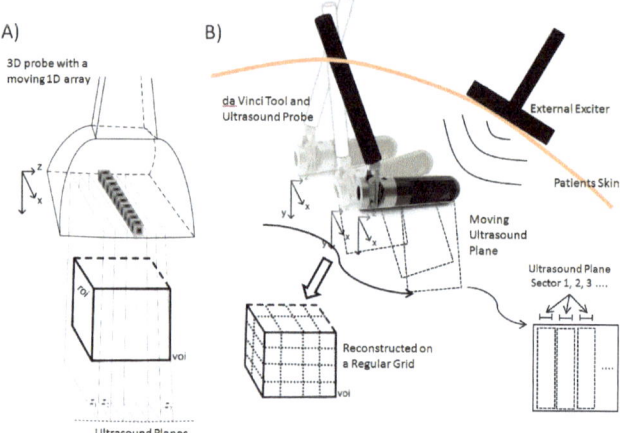

Fig. 1. A) Elastography set-up for the 3D probe method. B) Set-up for the extension to freehand scanning using a 2D transducer and the da Vinci robot. In both cases, sector subdivision high-frame rate imaging is applied.

generated in tissue by the vibrator have only a shear wave component. Then, if one component of the displacement phasors $\hat{u}(x, j\omega)$ is known over a region of interest, the shear wave equation (1) can be used to find the shear modulus μ. The phasors are then interpolated over a regular 3D grid covering the acquisition volume, and the distribution of shear moduli over the tissue is estimated by using a local spatial frequency estimator [9]. The estimation method is based on directional filtering of the displacement image using a set of filter banks, for which the ratio of the outputs determines the local frequency of the image.

The shear modulus provided with this system is an *absolute* measure of elasticity that, unlike strain imaging, is less dependent on boundary conditions. Strain is inversely proportional to elasticity under certain conditions, such as uniform stress. Changing boundaries, violates this assumption, which results in image artifacts which do not represent the elasticity of tissue, but are a result of non-uniform stress field within the tissue. The presented method however measures the local wavelength of the waves traveling in the tissue, which is dependent on the local intrinsic elasticity of the tissue, and not the boundary conditions.

With a steady state excitation, the axial displacement phasors can be estimated over a volume at a high effective frame rate using a sector-based approach [Figure 1] [1]. With this method each sector is imaged several times. Because this sector is small, imaging can be completed at a frame rate 16 times higher than if the image lines were acquired in sequence, in this case, about 1.25 kHz. The image acquisition is synchronized with the external excitation such that the sectors can be reconstructed to create a single frame using time delay compensation [1].

Our system uses an external mechanical exciter (LDS Model V203, B&K, Denmark) driven by waveforms created by a signal generator (Agilent 33220A) controlled by a standard PC. The excitation is applied using a 3.5 cm diameter circular plate. No particular positioning of the exciter with respect to the transducer is used.

2.2   Freehand Technique

A mechanical 3D probe has been used previously to capture a 3D volume of tissue displacements [Figure 1A] [2]. Such a probe mechanically sweeps a 1D crystal array to create regularly spaced ultrasound planes, but can be large and bulky. In this paper, we use a tracked 2D transducer to create the same type of 3D volume [Figure 1B].

The custom-designed transducer creates a static and repeatable transform between the da Vinci tool (Prograsp) and the ultrasound image. The transducer has 128 elements, is 28 mm long and is operated at 7 to 10 MHz. Image sector size was 8 lines. The tool-to-image transform was found using the single-wall phantom method implemented in Stradwin [13].

To synchronize the external exciter with the ultrasound image acquisition, the surgeon using the transducer triggers the image capture by using the clutch pedal in the robot console, an event captured by the da Vinci API. This approach has the benefit of keeping the ultrasound transducer still while imaging takes place but has the drawback that it interferes with the natural, smooth motion of ultrasound scanning. See Section 4 for methods of improving upon the natural movement limitation.

Image acquisition begins with the collection of radio frequency (RF) data along the axial direction of the ultrasound image. The RF data is used to compute the displacement phasors $\hat{u}(x, j\omega)$ at all depths in the image with respect to the transducer face. When a full volume of displacements phasors is captured, typically 15-30 frames, the real and imaginary parts of the axial displacement phasors (scalar values) are reconstructed into a volume on a regular grid. The volume reconstruction is performed using the PLUS software architecture [8] and uses linear interpolation between points for the real part and the imaginary part of the estimated displacement phasors. The field of view with an intra-operative transducer is small, about 30 mm by 40 mm, which means the computational time required for reconstruction is minimal. The absolute elastic properties of the samples are found from the grid displacements using local frequency estimation [Section 2.1]. This final volume of elasticity can be displayed to the operating surgeon or used to create a local model for haptic feedback.

3   Experimental Set-Up and Results

3.1   Elastography Phantom

A CIRS Elastic Quality Assurance (QA) Phantom, model 049 (Computerized Imaging Reference Systems, Norfolk, VA), was used to evaluate the accuracy of the elastic properties found using this method. The soft (6 kPa) and stiff (54 kPa) shallow lesions were imaged against a neutral background (29 kPa). Image

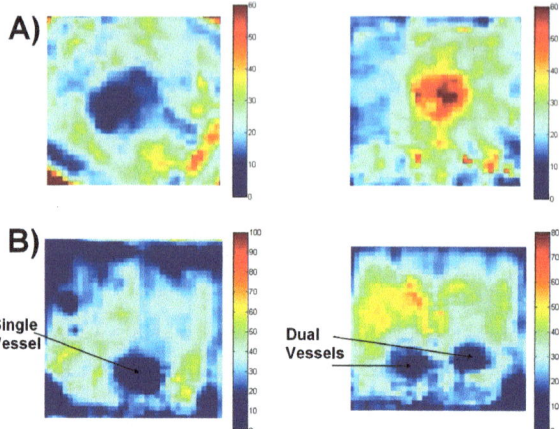

Fig. 2. A) Left: Image of 6 kPa CIRS phantom lesion. Right: Image of the 54 kPa CIRS phantom lesion. The colour bar shows the elasticity in kilopascals (kPa). B) Cross-sectional elastograms of the flow phantom. Left: Single vessel. Right: dual vessels after bifurcation. The colour bar shows the elasticity in kilopascals.

acquisition was performed simultaneously at four different frequencies: 180, 210, 230 and 270 Hz.

The soft and stiff lesions were imaged at a depth of 4 cm and a frequency of 7 MHz and the resulting elastograms are shown in Figure 2A. The diameter and average elasticity were measured in two images (corresponding to the middle of the lesion) for 5 trials for each lesion. The diameters of each lesion were also measured using the caliper function of the ultrasound software [Table 1]. The results for the stiff lesion were within 6% error of the manufacturer's specifications and within 4% of the values found using magnetic resonance elastography (MRE) on the same phantom model [3]. The softer lesion was stiffer than the manufacturer specified value but within 2% of the values reported with MRE. The results achieved through freehand ultrasound elastography are repeatable, with narrow standard deviations in both the diameter measurements and the elastic properties.

3.2 Vessel/Flow Phantom

A vessel phantom (Blue Phantom, Redmond, WA) with a single incoming vessel that branches in two halfway through the phantom was used to demonstrate the ability to highlight vessels. Because fluid does not support the transmission of shear waves, the shear wave amplitude drops significantly within the vessels. Areas within the image that show no presence of shear waves at the frequencies of excitation correspond to vessels or cysts or other fluid-filled cavities. See Section 4 for further discussion of flow imaging.

The results of these scans are shown in Figure 2B. The vessels before and after the bifurcation point can be clearly seen in the elastograms.

Table 1. Results from the CIRS QA Elastography Phantom

	Diameter of Soft Lesion	Diameter of Stiff Lesion
B-Mode	8.9 ± 0.6 mm	10.8 ± 0.2 mm
Elastogram	10.4 ± 1.6 mm	10.7 ± 1.6 mm
	Elasticity of Soft Lesion	Elasticity of Stiff Lesion
Manufacturer Specifications	6 kPa	54 kPa
MR Elastography [3]	11.1 ± 2.1 kPa	49.4 ± 16.9 kPa
Freehand Elastography	10.9 ± 0.6 kPa	51.1 ± 5.2 kPa

3.3 *In vivo* Feasibility

In order to determine if this type of absolute elastography imaging is feasible *in vivo*, experiments were performed on a healthy volunteer. In this case only, we used a 3D motorized ultrasound transducer to image a healthy kidney. The purpose of this experiment was to prove that an external exciter will sufficiently transmit waves into the body to create quality elastograms. The results of the *in vivo* kidney scans are shown in Figure 3. The kidney is circled in both images. The outline of the kidney can be approximately delineated in the elastogram, as well as the contrasting internal collecting system.

In addition to the use with kidneys, studies have shown that B-mode and strain imaging are useful for prostatectomy [6], and the system described in this paper could easily be applied to this procedure. The surgeon would also have the option to combine information from a trans-rectal ultrasound transducer and the da Vinci controlled transducer.

4 Discussion and Future Work

This paper presents the method and associated results for 3D absolute elastography with a freehand scanning technique. Specifically, a small 2D intra-operative probe allows robotic laparoscopic surgeons access to the elastic values of tissue. The results with freehand imaging are comparable to both those achieved with a mechanical 3D probe [2] and within 5% of the results achieved with magnetic resonance imaging techniques [3]. We have demonstrated this system's accuracy in a phantom model and feasibility in an *in vivo* setting.

The method is currently implemented using the da Vinci robotic system but can easily be extended to any 2D probe and any tracking system, such as electromagnetic or optical tracking systems. This would allow absolute elasticity values to be found in nearly every clinical setting. We have used the da Vinci robot as an initial platform for integration for several reasons; the robotic environment has the most room for improvement with regards to haptic feedback, and at the same time provides a stable and accurate platform for transducer tracking. The quality of the elastogram is dependent on the tracking error, which in turn depends on the tracker involved. Generally speaking though, if the planes are dense, a better elastogram is obtained, because of the higher signal to noise ratio due to averaging.

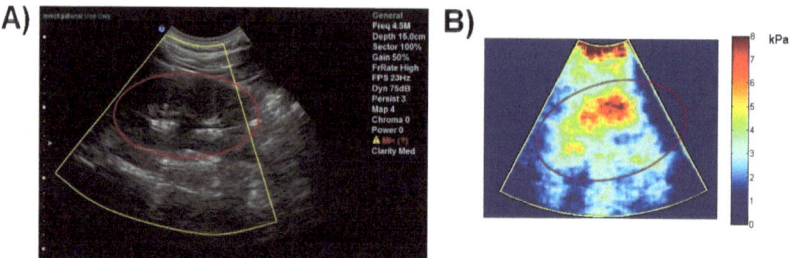

Fig. 3. Images of a healthy kidney circled in red. Left: B-Mode image. Right: Elastogram.

One current limitation of the system is synchronization of the imaging and the external exciter. This is currently addressed by using the clutch pedal in the surgeon's console to trigger imaging at a specified phase of the exciter. With accurate time stamps on the image acquisition and knowledge of the exciter phase, each sector or image could be placed in a temporal and spatial location within the end volume. This information would allow the surgeon to move the transducer in the same smooth manner that is used while scanning with only B-mode.

As mentioned above, elastic imaging could be used to visualize vessels as well as elastic properties. Shear waves do not propagate in fluid causing a marked decrease in the wave amplitude at the frequencies of the external exciter. Interestingly, the methods that are used to track the tissue motion are the same techniques that are used to create traditional Doppler images that measure the flow velocity in vessels [11]. Given that the decrease in amplitude can be visualized clearly, it is possible to localize these areas and then use Doppler techniques to measure the flow velocity. With this cascade of image processing, it would be possible to automatically locate the vessels within an image and optimally position the gate for Doppler imaging. Surgeons would also be able to image both elastic properties and flow at the same time. Additionally, because the elastography algorithms are similar in multiple modalities, it is possible to register absolute ultrasound elastograms directly to other elastic imaging modalities, in particular pre-operative MRE images. Because MRE and US elastograthy measure the same quantity, the registration may become more straight forward, considerably simplifying a generally difficult problem.

In this paper, we present an absolute elastography method for a tracked 2D ultrasound transducer. Absolute elastography methods provide new quantitative information over the previous strain imaging methods. Our methods are user and exciter independent and less affected by boundary conditions. These qualities make it easy to use and possibly more repeatable than strain imaging. We implemented this system on the da Vinci in order to address its lack of haptic feedback but this method can be extended to any 2D transducer and tracking system.

References

1. Baghani, A., Brant, A., Salcudean, S., Rohling, R.: A high-frame-rate ultrasound system for the study of tissue motions. IEEE Ultrasonics, Ferroelectrics and Frequency Control 57(7), 1535–1547 (2010)
2. Baghani, A., Eskandari, H., Wang, W., Da Costa, D., Nabil, N., Sahebjavaher, R., Salcudean, S., Rohling, R.: Real-time quantitative elasticity imaging of deep tissue using free-hand conventional ultrasound. In: MICCAI: ACCEPTED (2012)
3. Baghani, A., Salcudean, S., Honarvar, M., Sahebjavaher, R., Rohling, R., Sinkus, R.: Travelling wave expansion: A model fitting approach to the inverse problem of elasticity reconstruction. IEEE Medical Imaging (99), 1 (2011)
4. Billings, S., Deshmukh, N., Kang, H., Taylor, R., Boctor, E.: System for robot-assisted real-time laparoscopic ultrasound elastography. In: SPIE Medical Imaging (2012)
5. Evans, A., Whelehan, P., Thomson, K., McLean, D., Brauer, K., Purdie, C., Jordan, L., Baker, L., Thompson, A.: Quantitative shear wave ultrasound elastography: initial experience in solid breast masses. Breast Cancer Res. 12(6) (2010)
6. Han, M., Kim, C., Mozer, P., Schafer, F., Badaan, S., Vigaru, B., Tseng, K., Petrisor, D., Trock, B., Stoianovici, D.: Tandem-robot assisted laparoscopic radical prostatectomy to improve the neurovascular bundle visualization: A feasibility study. Urology (2010)
7. Hubens, G., Coveliers, H., Balliu, L., Ruppert, M., Vaneerdeweg, W.: A performance study comparing manual and robotically assisted laparoscopic surgery using the da Vinci system. Surgical Endoscopy 17(10), 1595–1599 (2003)
8. Lasso, A., Heffter, T., Pinter, C., Ungi, T., Chen, T.K., Boucharin, A., Fichtinger, G.: Plus: An open-source toolkit for developing ultrasound-guided intervention systems. In: 4th Image Guided Therapy Workshop, vol. 4, p. 103 (2011)
9. Manduca, A., Muthupillai, R., Rossman, P., Greenleaf, J., Ehman, R.: Local wavelength estimation for magnetic resonance elastography. In: Int. Conf. on Image Processing, vol. 3, pp. 527–530. IEEE (1996)
10. Nightingale, K., Soo, M., Nightingale, R., Trahey, G.: Acoustic radiation force impulse imaging: in vivo demonstration of clinical feasibility. Ultrasound in Medicine & Biology 28(2), 227–235 (2002)
11. Ophir, J., Alam, S., Garra, B., Kallel, F., Konofagou, E., Krouskop, T., Varghese, T.: Elastography: ultrasonic estimation and imaging of the elastic properties of tissues. Journal of Engineering in Medicine 213(3), 203 (1999)
12. Ophir, J., Cespedes, I., Ponnekanti, H., Yazdi, Y., Li, X.: Elastography: a quantitative method for imaging the elasticity of biological tissues. Ultrasonic Imaging 13(2), 111–134 (1991)
13. Prager, R., Rohling, R., Gee, A., Berman, L.: Rapid calibration for 3-D freehand ultrasound. Ultrasound in Medicine & Biology 24(6), 855–869 (1998)
14. Schneider, C.M., Dachs II, G.W., Hasser, C.J., Choti, M.A., DiMaio, S.P., Taylor, R.H.: Robot-Assisted Laparoscopic Ultrasound. In: Navab, N., Jannin, P. (eds.) IPCAI 2010. LNCS, vol. 6135, pp. 67–80. Springer, Heidelberg (2010)
15. Schneider, C., Guerrero, J., Nguan, C., Rohling, R., Salcudean, S.: Intra-operative "Pick-Up" Ultrasound for Robot Assisted Surgery with Vessel Extraction and Registration: A Feasibility Study. In: Taylor, R.H., Yang, G.-Z. (eds.) IPCAI 2011. LNCS, vol. 6689, pp. 122–132. Springer, Heidelberg (2011)
16. Stolka, P., Keil, M., Sakas, G., McVeigh, E., Allaf, M., Taylor, R., Boctor, E.: A 3D-elastography-guided system for laparoscopic partial nephrectomies. In: SPIE Medical Imaging (2010)

Modeling and Real-Time Simulation of a Vascularized Liver Tissue

Igor Peterlík, Christian Duriez, and Stéphane Cotin

Inria

Abstract. In Europe only, about 100,000 deaths per year are related to cirrhosis or liver cancer. While surgery remains the option that offers the foremost success rate against such pathologies, several limitations still hinder its widespread development. Among the limiting factors is the lack of accurate planning systems, which has been a motivation for several recent works, aiming at better resection planning and training systems, relying on pre-operative imaging, anatomical and biomechanical modelling. While the vascular network in the liver plays a key role in defining the operative strategy, its influence at a biomechanical level has not been taken into account.

In the paper we propose a real-time model of vascularized organs such as the liver. The model takes into account separate constitutive laws for the parenchyma and vessels, and defines a coupling mechanism between these two entities. In the evaluation section, we present results of *in vitro* porcine liver experiments that indicate a significant influence of vascular structures on the mechanical behaviour of tissue. We confirm the values obtained in the experiments by computer simulation using standard FEM. Finally, we show that the conventional modelling approach can be efficiently approximated with the proposed composite model capable of real-time calculations.

1 Introduction

The liver is one of the major organs in the human body and is in charge of more than a hundred vital functions. Because of its many functions, its pathologies are varied, numerous and often lethal. The most advanced state of evolution of these pathologies is cirrhosis or cancer, with nearly 100,000 related deaths in 2008. Surgical procedures remain the option that offers the best success rates against such pathologies, with a 5-year survival rate above 50% for surgery. Yet, surgery is not always performed due to several limitations, in particular the pre-operative estimation of the liver volume remaining after resection. This volume depends highly on the choice of the operative strategy as well as anatomical constraints defined by the vascular network.

Such limitations could be overcome by improving the quality of the planning, which relies on a combination of components, mostly image processing and biomechanical modelling. Several works have addressed this problem. A tool for liver resection planning and training is described in [1] where a model of the liver including the vascular system is reconstructed from CT data and visualized in a

N. Ayache et al. (Eds.): MICCAI 2012, Part I, LNCS 7510, pp. 50–57, 2012.
© Springer-Verlag Berlin Heidelberg 2012

virtual environment. In [2], a resection map is developed to enhance the resection accuracy by visualizing the structures near to the resection plane. mainly the tumour boundaries and main veins. In [3], techniques for geometrical and structural analysis of vessels are presented. Besides the vessel segmentation and skeletonization based on graph algorithms, the liver parenchyma is segmented into non-overlapping regions according to the supply areas which are visualized during the resection planning. A real-time vascular visualization method is developed in [4]. The vessels are modelled as tubular structures and the complete vascular model is projected onto the patient's liver during surgery.

While an important body of work exists regarding the biomechanical properties of the liver parenchyma, only few studies focus on the role of vascularization inside the tissue. In [5], visco-elastic model of the liver is proposed as well as material parameters experimentally measured *ex vivo* on perfused liver. In [6], a patient specific model of hepatic vasculature is proposed. The material properties of vessels are modelled by non-linear constitutive law. Nevertheless, the model does not allow for real-time performance as the vessel walls are modelled with large number of finite elements.

In this paper a real-time composite model of vascularized organs such as the liver is proposed. The model takes into account separate constitutive laws for the parenchyma and vessels, and defines a coupling mechanism between the two components. As an illustration of mechanical influence of vascularization inside a tissue sample, results conducted on vascularized and non-vascularized tissue samples *in vitro* are reported. The measured values are further confirmed by a simulation using dense meshes needed for correct discretization of the thin vessel wall. Finally, it is shown that the proposed composite model provides a very good approximation of the conventional model with dense mesh, at the same time being sufficiently fast to run in real-time even for complex geometry.

2   Methods

2.1   Parenchyma Model

While most studies concerning the material properties of liver parenchyma agree on a viscoelastic behaviour (see [5] or [7] for instance), we employ a simpler non-linear elastic model. This is essentially motivated by the fact that we are not focusing on the transient part of the deformation but rather the static equilibrium under some specific loading conditions.

The parenchyma is modeled using a finite element co-rotational method. This allows for large displacements or rotations in the model, while relying on a linear expression of the stress-strain relationship. Different methods exist for computing the local rotation of each element; in this paper we use a geometric approach proposed in [8]. In a co-rotational model the stiffness matrix $\mathbf{K}$ depends on the deformation $\mathbf{u}$ and the equation relating the external forces to the displacements can be written as $\mathbf{f} = \mathbf{K}(\mathbf{u})\mathbf{u}$. The system of equations is solved by direct LU solver.

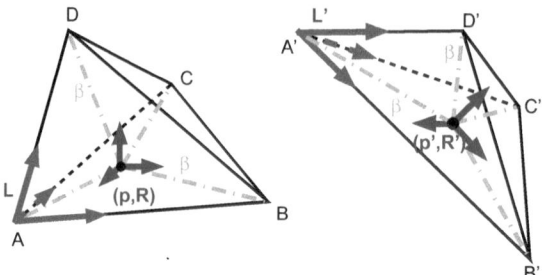

Fig. 1. Mapping between 6DoF beam node and tetrahedron in initial and rotated positions. The positions of beam and tetrahedron nodes do not coincide.

2.2   Vessel Model

As a first step towards a mechanical model of vessels, a continuous representation of vascular structures is constructed. Using segmented data of a vessel tree, points along centerlines of each vessel branch are selected. This task can be performed either manually or automatically, e.g. with VMTK[1]. Each branch can be represented as a series of cubic Bezier curves fitted to the centerline points: the series begins in a starting point of the branch and ends either in another branching point or in the endpoint of the branch.

A set of interpolated points is constructed using the Bezier curves; positions of the interpolated points can be chosen arbitrarily along each branch dividing it into intervals with a constant or varying length. For each interpolated point we calculate its orientation given by the tangent and normal of the Bezier curve in that point.

The interpolated points are used as nodes of serially linked beam elements, in a similar way as proposed by Duriez *et al.* [9] for simulating catheters and guidewires. This model shares some similarities with the co-rotational model described above, and in particular allows for geometrically non-linear deformations. We introduce some modifications to the model to take into account the particular nature of vessels, in particular through specific cross section profiles and moments of inertia (see [10] for details). The static formulation for the deformation of a beam is described by a system similar to the one used for the paranchyme, with the difference that each node is described with six degrees of freedom, three of which correspond to the spatial position, and three to the angular position of the node in a global reference frame (see Fig.1).

2.3   Mechanical Coupling between Vessel and Parenchyma

We propose a mapping between the mesh nodes of the vessels and parenchyma to create the vascularized model. Since no relative motion between the vessels and parenchyma is observed in reality, the mapping between the two can be modeled as a constraint. In each step of the simulation, the actual displacements

---

[1] www.vmtk.org

of the parenchyma mesh nodes are mapped to the vessel nodes and reciprocally, the force contribution due to the deformation of the vessel is propagated to the parenchyma. The mapping of forces is based on a principle of virtual work. Using the corotational model, the parenchyma is discretized by a mesh composed of linear P_1 tetrahedral elements given by four nodes with three degrees of freedom. The vessel is modeled with beam elements where each beam is given by two end points each having 6 degrees of freedom (positions and rotations). We focus on mapping between an arbitrary beam node b and tetrahedron T.

Let us denote $\mathbf{p}$ the initial position and $\mathbf{R}$ initial rotation of the beam node b. Before the simulation starts, we select the tetrahedron $T = \{\mathbf{t}_A, \mathbf{t}_B, \mathbf{t}_C, \mathbf{t}_D\}$ which is closest to the beam node b. Then, the barycentric coordinates $\boldsymbol{\beta}_T = \{\beta_A, \beta_B, \beta_C\}$ of the position $\mathbf{p}$ are computed w.r.t. the tetrahedron T and stored. Similarly, the initial rotation $\mathbf{R}$ is transformed to a matrix $\mathbf{O}_T$ which defines the orientation of the point b w.r.t. the local basis $\mathbf{L}$ defined by the edges of the tetrahedron, i.e. $\mathbf{O}_T = \mathbf{L}^{-1}\mathbf{R}$ (see Fig. 1). According to the initial assumption (no relative motion between parenchyma and vessel), both the barycentric coordinates $\boldsymbol{\beta}_T$ and orientation $\mathbf{O}_T$ are constant during the simulation. Let's suppose that in the actual step, the tetrahedron is rotated and deformed as shown in Fig. 1. Denoting the nodal positions of the deformed tetrahedron $T' = \{\mathbf{t}'_A, \mathbf{t}'_B, \mathbf{t}'_C, \mathbf{t}'_D\}$, new actual position $\mathbf{p}'$ of the beam node is computed using the barycentric coordinates $\boldsymbol{\beta}_T$ as

$$\mathbf{p}' = \mathbf{t}'_A \beta_A + \mathbf{t}'_B \beta_B + \mathbf{t}'_C \beta_C + \mathbf{t}'_D (1 - \beta_A - \beta_B - \beta_C). \tag{1}$$

The updated orientation $\mathbf{R}'$ of the beam node is computed using the basis $\mathbf{L}'$ given by the actual displacement of the tetrahedron nodes and pre-computed orientation $\mathbf{O}_T$. First, $\tilde{\mathbf{R}}' = \mathbf{L}'\mathbf{O}_T$ is computed. However, since besides the rotation a deformation of the tetrahedron must be taken into account, the matrix $\tilde{\mathbf{R}}$ is not necessarily orthogonal. Therefore, the updated orientation $\mathbf{R}'$ is calculated as orthogonal component of polar decomposition of $\tilde{\mathbf{R}}'$. As the positional mapping is applied in each step of the simulation, the positions of the beams are kinematically linked to the positions of tetrahedra.

After the updated position is mapped from the tetrahedron to the beam point, the forces acting in the beam point must be mapped onto the vertices of the associated tetrahedron. For the beam point, we have linear forces $\mathbf{f} = \{f_x, f_y, f_z\}$ as well as torques $\boldsymbol{\tau} = \{\tau_x, \tau_y, \tau_z\}$, whereas for the tetrahedron, there are only linear nodal forces $\mathbf{F} = \{\mathbf{F}_A, \mathbf{F}_B, \mathbf{F}_C, \mathbf{F}_D\}$. The force contribution to each node given by linear forces $\mathbf{f}$ is computed using the barycentric coordinates, required by the positional mapping. The torques are transformed to linear forces acting in the tetrahedron nodes using the equation $\boldsymbol{\tau} = \mathbf{r} \times \mathbf{F}$ where $\mathbf{r}$ is vector connecting the beam and tetrahedron nodes. Putting it together, the force in tetrahedron node $I \in \{A, B, C, D\}$ is computed as $\mathbf{F}_I = \beta_I \mathbf{f} - (\mathbf{t}'_I - \mathbf{p}') \times \boldsymbol{\tau}$.

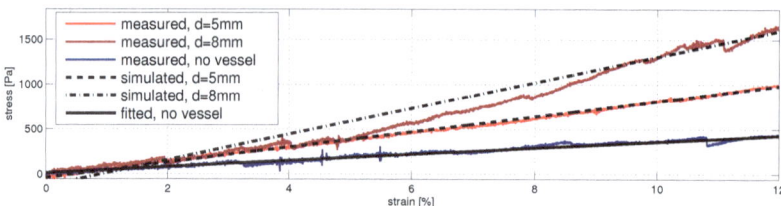

Fig. 2. Experimental and fitted stress-strain curves for three selected samples

3   Results

3.1   *In Vitro* Measurements of Vascularized Sample Response

While many studies on liver tissue have been conducted in the past, almost none focused on the evaluation of mechanical properties of hepatic veins. Recently, tensile tests on porcine hepatic veins were performed and reported in [11]. The stiffness of vessel wall was experimentally measured and compared to parameters known for other vascular structures in the human body. Nevertheless, to our best knowledge, there has been no experiments evaluating the influence of vessel walls on mechanical behaviour and elastic response of the soft tissue.

To address this gap, we conducted a series of tensile tests on fresh porcine liver using a Bose ElectroForce 3330 Test Instrument. The liver was cut into cube-shaped samples of size approximately $9\,cm^3$. Two main types of samples were extracted: homogeneous and heterogeneous samples with single straight vessel of diameter $d > 4\,mm$. Using cyanoacrylate, the samples were glued on top and bottom face to small wooden plates attached to the test device. The orientation of the vessel was aligned with the direction of the tension.

The top face of the sample was displaced up to 3.5 mm (about 12% strain) and the speed of motion was restricted to 1 mm per minute to emulate quasi-static conditions (the experimental setup is shown in Fig. 3a). During loading, either tissue damage or glue failure occurred in many samples, decreasing the number of reliable measurements. Three representatives were chosen so that during the experiment, none of the issues mentioned above were observed: one homogeneous sample and two vascularized samples having vessels segments with diameters 5 mm and 8 mm. As mechanical properties of vessel wall was measured, the vessel segments were filled with air. As the gravitational load applied due to the mass of each sample is not negligible w.r.t. the forces being measured, zero-strain state was approximately determined for each tissue and recorded force — displacement data were converted into stress — strain curves. For each sample, the stiffness coefficient was obtained using linear fitting: for the homogeneous tissue, the resulting value is an estimation of Young's modulus of the paranchyme (3.5 kPa), whereas for the vascularized samples, the values represent a measure of an *apparent stiffness* (8.54kPa, 14.41kPa). The measured data (depicted in Fig. 2) indicates that the presence of the vein inside the sample affects significantly the force response of the tissue and the increase in apparent stiffness is proportional to the size of the vessel.

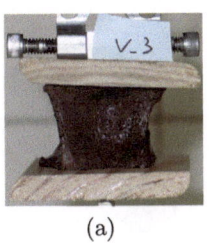 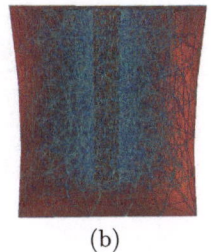 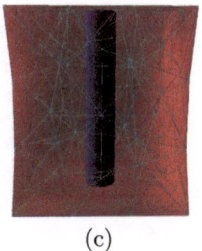

(a) (b) (c)

Fig. 3. Vascularized sample tensile test: (a) Experimental setup, (b) standard FEM with graded mesh, (c) composite model with beams

3.2 Numerical Simulation of Vascularized Tissue

In the next step, we reproduced the experiments described above by a numerical simulation in SOFA[2] where both the parenchyma and the vessel wall were discretized with tetrahedral mesh and deformed using standard FEM. Three parameters were needed to set up the model: stiffness of the paranchyme (known from the experiment with homogeneous sample), stiffness and thickness of the vessel wall. As only the apparent stiffness of vascularized samples was known, it was not possible to determine the two unknown parameters uniquely. In [12] the average thickness of human veins is reported to be $150 - 250\,\mu m$ depending on the diameter of the vein. We use the value $250\,\mu m$ as we are interested mainly in large veins with diameter of 5 mm and more.

We generated tetrahedral mesh of the vascularized samples; to discretize the thin vessel wall correctly, graded meshes having 37,000 and 52,000 elements (samples with smaller and larger vessel, respectively) were generated (see the mesh depicted in Fig. 3b). The last parameter, vessel wall stiffness, was determined by the simulation: we performed a series of computations for different values of the wall stiffness. Finally, we chose the one that resulted in response force closest to the values measured *in vitro*. The obtained values of the wall stiffness were determined as 1.1 MPa and 1.4 MPa for the sample with smaller and large vessel, respectively. The Young's modulus of hepatic vein wall reported in [11] is 0.62±0.41 MPa, so our values are slightly higher, but still in the range reported by other studies.

3.3 Composite Model Evaluation

The conventional FEM used above requires a huge number of elements even to model a small sample with simple vascularization. We show that a good approximation of the conventional FEM requiring detailed meshes can be achieved by the composite model that we have implemented in SOFA according to section 2, keeping the number of elements much lower and allowing for real-time calculations. First, in order to perform a numerical validation of the composite model,

---

[2] www.sofa-framework.org

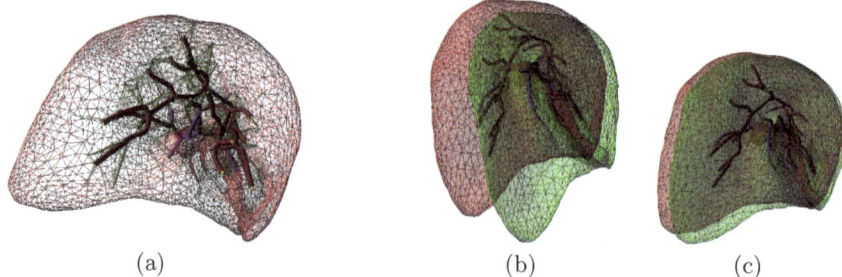

Fig. 4. Vascularized model of the liver: (a) initial position with mapped vascular trees; (b) comparison of deformation under gravitational loading in vascularized liver with E_1=3.5 kPa (red) and non-vascularized liver (green); (c) comparison of vascularized liver with $E_2 = 15$ kPa (red) and non-vascularized liver (green)

we performed the same type of simulation as above, however, we used a homogeneous corotational FEM to model the parenchyma and mapped beam FEM to model the mechanical contribution of the vein. In all computations, the vessel was modelled with two beams coupled to the parenchyma. First, the parenchyma was discretized by a mesh having 1160 elements: the relative errors between the force responses computed by standard and composite FEM was 6.5% and 2.45% for smaller and larger vein, respectively. Second, mesh having 170 elements was used for parenchyma, resulting in relative error in force responses of 9% and 4.6% for smaller and larger veins. The accuracy of the composite model is emphasized by the fact that the error was significantly lower for samples with large vascularization that has more important influence on the overall elastic response.

In order to demonstrate the efficiency of the algorithm, we performed a simulation of the entire liver: the parenchyma was discretized into 2620 tetrahedra and two vascular trees were modelled inside the liver: hepatic veins composed of 257 beams and hepatic portal veins modelled with 57 beams (Fig.4a). The tetrahedral mesh was fixed on the surface close to the entrance of the hepatic vein. Gravitational loading was applied on the liver, resulting in large displacements.

Two comparisons of vascularized liver (in red) and non-vascularized liver (in green) are presented in Fig.4 for two different values of Young's modulus of the parenchyma: E_1=3.5 kPa (Fig.4b) and E_2=15 kPa (Fig.4c). The influence of vascularization is more significant in liver with lower stiffness (difference of more than 5 cm in deformation between vascularized and non-vascularized model), nevertheless in case of E_2 the difference in deformation remains over 1 cm for some parts of the liver. In all experiments, refresh rate of 60 FPS was achieved on PC with CPU Intel CPU i7-2630QM running at 2.00 GHz.

4   Conclusion

In the paper we focused on mechanical modeling of vascularized tissues. We introduced a novel approach based on modelling the parenchyma and vessels as two separated entities, mechanically coupled with a mapping of position and forces. The experiments presented in the evaluation section confirmed that vascular structures play important role in tissue behaviour. We also evaluated the composite model, comparing the relative error w.r.t. standard detailed FEM. Finally, we demonstrated that proposed model can be used in real-time even for complicated structures, such as liver organ with two vascular trees.

In future work, we plan to employ the composite model in inverse problems that appear in elastography. Also, we want to propose similar approach for mapping between parenchyma and thin two-dimensional structures to model Glisson capsule on the surface of the liver.

References

1. Sojar, V., Stanisavljevic, D., Hribernik, M., Glusic, M., Kreuh, D., Velkavrh, U., Fius, T.: Liver surgery training and planning in 3d virtual space. International Congress Series, vol. 1268, pp. 390–394 (2004)
2. Lamata, P., Jalote-Parmar, A., Lamata, F., Declerck, J.: The resection map, a proposal for intraoperative hepatectomy guidance. International Journal of Computer Assisted Radiology and Surgery 3(3-4), 299–306 (2008)
3. Selle, D., Preim, B., Schenk, A., Peitgen, H.: Analysis of vasculature for liver surgical planning. IEEE Trans. on Medical Imaging 21(11), 1344–1357 (2002)
4. Ritter, F., Hansen, C., Dicken, V., Konrad, O., Preim, B., Peitgen, H.O.: Realtime illustration of vascular structures. IEEE Trans. on Visual. and Computer Graphics 12, 877–884 (2006)
5. Kerdok, A.E., Ottensmeyer, M.P., Howe, R.D.: Effects of perfusion on the viscoelastic characteristics of liver. Journal of Biomechanics 39, 2221–2231 (2006)
6. Nguyen, B.P., Yang, T., Leon, F., Chang, S., Ong, S.H., Chui, C.K.: Patient Specific Biomechanical Modeling of Hepatic Vasculature for Augmented Reality Surgery. In: 4th International Workshop on Medical Imaging and Augmented Reality (2008)
7. Gao, Z., Kim, T., James, D.L., Desai, J.P.: Semi-automated soft-tissue acquisition and modeling forsurgical simulation. In: CASE 2009: Proceedings of the Fifth Annual IEEE International Conference on Automation Science and Engineering, Piscataway, NJ, USA, pp. 268–273. IEEE Press (2009)
8. Nesme, M., Payan, Y., Faure, F.: Efficient, physically plausible finite elements. In: Dingliana, J., Ganovelli, F. (eds.) Eurographics 2005, Short papers, Trinity College, Dublin, Irlande (August 2005)
9. Duriez, C., Cotin, S., Lenoir, J., Neumann, P.F.: New approaches to catheter navigation for interventional radiology simulation. Computer Aided Surgery 11, 300–308 (2006)
10. Przemieniecki, J.S.: Theory of Matrix Structural Analysis (1985); reprint of McGraw Hill (1968)
11. Umale, S., Chatelin, S., Bourdet, N., Deck, C., Diana, M., Dhumane, P., Soler, L., Marescaux, J., Willinger, R.: Experimental in vitro mechanical characterization of porcine glisson's capsule and hepatic veins. J. of Biomech. 44, 1678–1683 (2011)
12. Forauer, A., Theoharis, C.: Histologic changes in the human vein wall adjacent to indwelling central venous catheters. J. of Vasc. and Interv. Rad. 14, 1163–1168 (2003)

Efficient Optic Cup Detection from Intra-image Learning with Retinal Structure Priors*

Yanwu Xu[1], Jiang Liu[1], Stephen Lin[2], Dong Xu[3],
Carol Y. Cheung[4], Tin Aung[4,5], and Tien Yin Wong[4,5]

[1] Institute for Infocomm Research, Agency for Science, Technology and Research, Singapore
[2] Microsoft Research Asia, P.R. China
[3] School of Computer Engineering, Nanyang Technological University, Singapore
[4] Singapore Eye Research Institute, Singapore
[5] Department of Ophthalmology, National University of Singapore, Singapore

Abstract. We present a superpixel based learning framework based on retinal structure priors for glaucoma diagnosis. In digital fundus photographs, our method automatically localizes the optic cup, which is the primary image component clinically used for identifying glaucoma. This method provides three major contributions. First, it proposes processing of the fundus images at the superpixel level, which leads to features more descriptive and effective than those employed by pixel-based techniques, while yielding significant computational savings over methods based on sliding windows. Second, the classifier learning process does not rely on pre-labeled training samples, but rather the training samples are extracted from the test image itself using structural priors on relative cup and disc positions. Third, we present a classification refinement scheme that utilizes both structural priors and local context. Tested on the $ORIGA^{-light}$ clinical dataset comprised of 650 images, the proposed method achieves a 26.7% non-overlap ratio with manually-labeled ground-truth and a 0.081 absolute cup-to-disc ratio (CDR) error, a simple yet widely used diagnostic measure. This level of accuracy is comparable to or higher than the state-of-the-art technique [1], with a speedup factor of tens or hundreds.

1 Introduction

Glaucoma is the second leading cause of blindness, with a mean prevalence of 2.4% for all age groups and 4.7% for ages 75 years and above [2]. It is critical to detect this degeneration of the optic nerve as early as possible in order to stall its progression; however, studies suggest that more than 90% of the afflicted are unaware of their condition [3,4]. To facilitate widespread testing, much recent work has focused on computer-assisted glaucoma diagnosis techniques based on inexpensive and widely used digital color fundus images.

Two major image structures used in glaucoma diagnosis are the optic disc, where optical nerve fibers join at the retina, and the optic cup, which is a depression within the optic disc where the fibers exit the retina. The cup and disc boundaries are common features used for identifying glaucoma, via measures such as the cup-to-disc ratio

---

* This work is funded by Singapore A*STAR SERC Grant (092-148-00731).

N. Ayache et al. (Eds.): MICCAI 2012, Part I, LNCS 7510, pp. 58–65, 2012.

(CDR), defined as the ratio of the vertical cup diameter to the vertical disc diameter [5]. Typically, the CDR value is determined from a manually outlined optic disc and cup. But since manual annotation is labor intensive, researchers have sought automatic methods for disc and cup segmentation.

Research in this area has primarily focused on segmentation of the optic disc, using various techniques such as intensity gradient analysis, Hough transforms, template matching, pixel feature classification [6], vessel geometry analysis, deformable models and level sets [7][8]. In this paper, we address the challenging problem of cup detection [1][9][10], using a large clinical dataset called $ORIGA^{-light}$ [11] in which the ground-truth of discs and cups is marked by a team of graders from a hospital.

Previous cup detection techniques are based either on classifying pixels as part of the cup or rim (the disc area outside the cup) [6][10] or on an analysis of sliding windows [1]. In contrast to these methods, our technique identifies a cup via classification at an intermediate superpixel scale. This allows for richer classification features than pixel-based methods, and faster processing than sliding window techniques without loss of accuracy. Our method also takes advantage of prior information on retinal structure to infer cup/rim training data directly from the test image, without needing a pre-labeled training set. This property is significant in that manual labeling of training sets is avoided, and the training data is specifically suited for the given test image. We furthermore utilize the structural priors, as well as local context, to refine the cup/rim labels. This optic cup detection approach provides accuracy comparable to or better than the current state-of-the-art optic cup detection method [1] with a substantial increase in computation speed. This detection framework indicates much promise for developing practical automated/assisted glaucoma diagnosis systems with low-cost and widespread digital fundus cameras.

2   Intra-image Learning with Retinal Structure Priors

In this work, we start with a disc image which may be obtained using methods such as [7]. Described in the remainder of this section, our method segments the input disc image into superpixels, removes superpixels that correspond to blood vessels, classifies each remaining superpixel to the cup or rim, refines the superpixel classification labels, and then determines a cup location by ellipse fitting.

2.1   Superpixel Segmentation

Superpixels are becoming increasingly popular in computer vision applications because of improved performance over pixel-based methods. In this work, we utilize the state-of-the-art SLIC (Simple Linear Iterative Clustering) algorithm [12] to segment the fundus disc image into compact and nearly uniform superpixels. Unlike dividing an image into a grid of regular patches, superpixels have the important property of preserving local boundaries, as exemplified by the typical segmentation result shown in Fig. 1. This segmentation is processed rapidly, in only 21ms for a GPU implementation or 354ms for a CPU implementation on a 640×480 image [13].

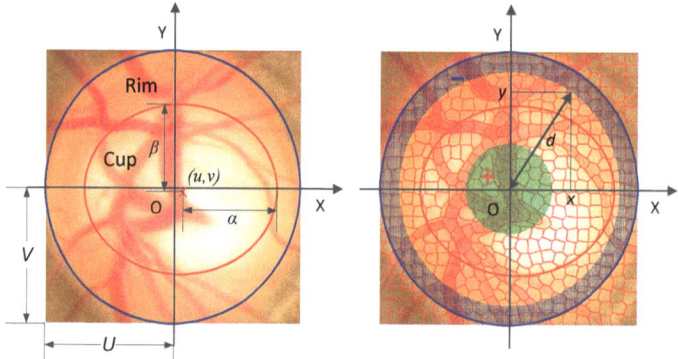

Fig. 1. Illustration of a fundus disc image segmented into 512 superpixels. Left: outline of rim and cup in the original disc image. Right: segmentation into superpixels.

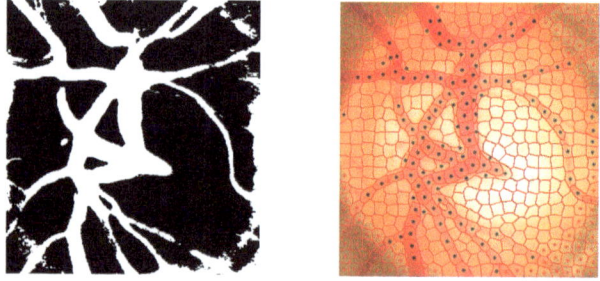

Fig. 2. Blood vessel extraction and removal. Left: blood vessel mask. Right: superpixels on blood vessels (marked with black dots) or out of disc (with red dots).

2.2 Blood Vessel Removal

Since blood vessels appear approximately the same in both the rim and cup regions, many algorithms have been proposed for blood vessel extraction in retina images to avoid their effects on rim/cup classification accuracy. In our case, extraction results need not be very precise, since images are processed at the level of superpixels. So we use the bottom-hat filtering algorithm [14], which trades off some precision for speed, to rapidly generate a rough blood vessel mask, and then identify superpixels that overlap the mask by at least 75% (Fig. 2). These superpixels, as well as those that lie outside the disc, are eliminated from further processing.

2.3 Feature Representation for Superpixels

Various features have been used for modeling superpixels, including shape, location, texture, color, and thumbnail appearance [15]. In our application, only location and color information are relevant for cup/rim classification. For the i-th superpixel, we extract a feature vector $\mathbf{f}_i$ that consists of position information (denoted by (x_i, y_i, d_i) as shown in Fig. 1), mean RGB colors (r_i, g_i, b_i) and a 256-bin histogram (h_i^r, h_i^g, h_i^b) for each color channel. To avoid magnitude differences among the features, they are each normalized to the range of $[0, 1]$, with L_1-normalization of each histogram.

We note that for classification with pre-labeled training samples from different images, additional normalization would be needed to reduce the influence of illumination change among the images. In this case, r, g and b are divided by average RGB values of the disc image (denoted as $(\bar{r}, \bar{g}, \bar{b})$), and the histograms h^r, h^g and h^b are aligned to $\bar{r}$, $\bar{g}$ and $\bar{b}$, respectively.

2.4   Superpixel Classification

To learn a classifier without pre-labeled samples, we capitalize on prior knowledge of retinal structure. As illustrated in Fig. 1, a superpixel is essentially certain to lie in the rim region if it is very close to the disc outer boundary. On the other hand, we can be assured that a superpixel exists within the cup region if it is very close to the disc center. Based on discussions with professional graders, we have conservatively modeled this structural prior such that superpixels within 1/5 of the disc radius from the disc center (green area in Fig. 1) are considered to be definitely in the cup, while superpixels beyond 9/10 of the disc radius from the center (blue area) are definitely in the rim region.

With this structural prior we obtain cup/rim training samples from *within the test image* for classifier learning. This technique not only avoids manual labeling of training sets, but also generates training data *specific to the given retina*, without requiring any ad hoc image manipulations to conform the test data to the training data (*e.g.* illumination normalization). From these cup/rim samples, we train a classifier to label each superpixel as belonging to the cup or rim. An equal number of positive and negative samples are used for balanced training. For efficiency, the simple linear support vector machine (SVM) classifier is employed, with a weight vector ω trained to estimate the class label l_i (+1 for cup and -1 for rim) of a given superpixel with feature vector $\mathbf{f}_i$, according to $l_i = \omega^T \mathbf{f}_i$. For SVM training, we use the LIBLINEAR toolbox [16].

2.5   Classification Label Refinement

To reduce classification errors, we employ a refinement scheme that accounts for the retinal structure prior as well as local context. To reflect label confidence with respect to the structural prior, we increase/decrease classification values according to how near/far a superpixel is located from the disc center:

$$l_i' = l_i(d - [l_i > 0])^2, \tag{1}$$

where d is the radial distance from the center, and $[l_i > 0] = 1$ when $l_i > 0$, otherwise $[l_i > 0] = 0$.

Contextual information is then introduced by filtering of superpixel labels with respect to feature similarity among superpixels within a certain range (*e.g.*, 1/10 of the disc radius). This yields the final label l'' of a superpixel:

$$l_i'' = l_i' + \frac{1}{N} \sum_{j=1}^{N} l_{i,j}' \cdot s_{i,j}, \tag{2}$$

where $l'_{i,j}$ denotes the label of the j-th neighbor of the i-th superpixel and $s_{i,j}$ denotes the similarity between i-th superpixel and its j-th neighbor, defined as

$$s_{i,j} = e^{-\frac{(f_i - f_{i,j})^2}{2\sigma_f^2}} \tag{3}$$

in which σ_f controls the sensitivity to feature noise.

After obtaining the final labels of all superpixels, the minimum ellipse that encompasses all the superpixels with positive labels is computed to produce the detection result, represented by ellipse center/elongation parameters $(\hat{u}, \hat{v}, \hat{\alpha}, \hat{\beta})$.

3   Experiments

We evaluate our technique through an experimental comparison of four labeling methods based on our framework. The first is our proposed method of intra-image learning with refinement (referred to as *intra-image+refinement*). The second method learns instead from pre-labeled training samples, followed by our refinement scheme (referred to as *pre-learned+refinement*). In the third method (referred to as *refinement only*), we use the retinal structure priors to label definite cup (+1) and rim (-1) superpixels, with the others initialized to 0, and then apply our refinement scheme. The fourth method (called *intra-image only*) excludes the refinement stage from our proposed intra-image learning method. Additionally, we compare our superpixel based approach to state-of-the-art pixel [7][10] and sliding window [1] based methods. We also report how the algorithm parameters affect performance.

3.1   Cup Detection Evaluation Criteria

In this work, we use the same three evaluation criteria as in [1] to measure cup detection accuracy, namely non-overlap ratio (m_1), relative absolute area difference (m_2) and absolute CDR error (δ), defined as

$$m_1 = 1 - \frac{area(E_{dt} \bigcap E_{gt})}{area(E_{dt} \bigcup E_{gt})}, \ m_2 = \frac{|area(E_{dt}) - area(E_{gt})|}{area(E_{gt})}, \ \delta = \frac{|D_{dt} - D_{gt}|}{2} \tag{4}$$

where E_{dt} denotes a detected cup region, E_{gt} denotes the ground-truth ellipse, D_{dt} is the vertical diameter of the detected cup, D_{gt} is the vertical diameter of the ground-truth cup. The vertical diameter of the disc is set to 2, so $0 < D_{dt}, D_{gt} \leq 2$.

3.2   Experimental Setup

The settings in [1] are also adopted in this work to facilitate comparisons. For testing we use the $ORIGA^{-light}$ dataset, comprised of 168 glaucoma and 482 normal images. Besides the image sets S_A and S_B used in [1], which consist of 150 images and 175 images respectively, another set S_C comprised of 325 additional images is also tested. Among the four labeling methods based on our framework, only the pre-learned+refinement method requires a separate training set. For this, we also follow [1] by using S_A for classifier training, using the illumination-normalized feature described in Sec. 2.3.

Table 1. Performance comparisons on different image sets

Method	$S_A \& S_B$			S_C			$S_A \& S_B \& S_C$		
Evaluation criteria	m_1	m_2	δ	m_1	m_2	δ	m_1	m_2	δ
intra-image+refinement	**0.265**	**0.313**	**0.079**	**0.269**	**0.267**	**0.082**	**0.267**	**0.290**	**0.081**
pre-learned+refinement	0.277	0.314	0.087	0.301	0.285	0.091	0.289	0.300	0.089
refinement only	0.331	0.341	0.105	0.325	0.318	0.112	0.328	0.329	0.109
intra-image only	0.269	0.324	0.084	0.277	0.283	0.087	0.273	0.303	0.086
pixel based [10]	0.476	0.702	0.140	0.471	0.663	0.157	0.474	0.683	0.149
window based [1]	0.268	0.315	0.091	0.299	0.297	0.101	0.284	0.306	0.096
Error reduction relative to [10]	44.4%	55.5%	43.6%	42.9%	59.7%	47.6%	**43.6%**	**57.5%**	**45.8%**
Error reduction relative to [1]	1.3%	0.8%	13.3%	10.0%	10.0%	18.6%	**5.9%**	**5.3%**	**16.1%**

3.3 Comparison of Labeling Methods in our Framework

A comparison of the four methods demonstrates the effectiveness of our superpixel based framework. The same parameters (superpixel number $SP = 2048$, propagation range $R_p = 0.1$, regularization parameter $C = 100$ for linear SVM training, $\delta_f = 0.8$ for similarity measurement) are used for all the methods, and the results are listed in Table 1. The following observations can be made about the proposed method:

1. The comparison to *pre-learned+refinement* shows that intra-image learning with retinal structure priors has the following advantages: 1) higher accuracy, 2) no need of extra training samples, 3) no need of specific feature normalization and alignment to deal with the inconsistency between training and testing images;
2. The results of *refinement only* indicate that labeling with a trained classifier is essential for minimizing errors;
3. The comparison to *intra-image only* shows that the refinement scheme provides some reduction in error.

3.4 Comparison to Pixel Based Segmentation and Window Based Learnig

We also compared our superpixel based approach to state-of-the-art pixel and window based methods. The pixel based level-set segmentation method of [10] first identifies pixels that belong to the cup region, and then fits an ellipse to the convex hull. The results show that all four methods based on superpixel labeling lead to significant improvements in cup localization accuracy, which indicates the advantage of superpixel based features over pixel based methods, as also observed in previous work [12].

The state-of-the-art sliding window based method [1] identifies a cup as a whole, by ranking all the cup candidate regions obtained with sliding windows and then producing a single detection result. Our proposed method is shown in Table 1 to yield improvements over [1]. We note that [1] in some sense implicitly uses a structural prior as well, since it searches for cup ellipses only within a certain range of the disc. By contrast, our technique uses the structural priors for intra-image learning of a classifier specific to the retina, which we believe contributes to the higher performance.

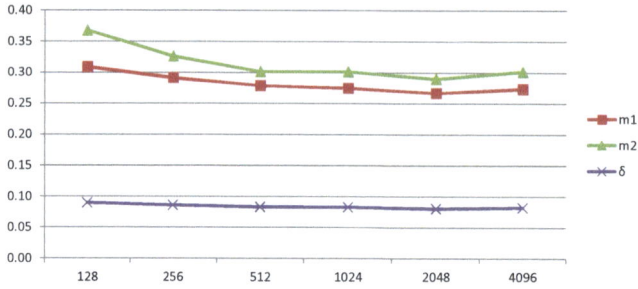

Fig. 3. Cup detection errors with different numbers of superpixels

3.5 Influence of Parameter Settings on Accuracy and Speed

We examined the performance and stability of the proposed method with different parameter settings. For superpixel based approaches, the number of superpixels (SP) is a key parameter that affects performance in terms of both accuracy and speed. As shown in Fig. 3, one can observe that the errors become almost stable when $SP \geq 512$, with the lowest errors at $SP = 2048$ (about 80 pixels per superpixel). When superpixels are too large, the resulting under-segmentation can lead to ambiguously-labeled boundary superpixels that require further segmentation. When superpixels are too small, the resulting features computed from the over-segmented regions may become somewhat less distinctive, making it more difficult to infer the correct labels.

Computation speed was also evaluated, using a four-core $3.4GHz$ PC with $12GB$ RAM. Superpixel segmentation is very fast, requiring less than 200ms for a 400×400 image. Training and testing of linear SVM classifiers is also quick. The most time consuming part is feature extraction for each superpixel, and the overall processing time increases almost linearly with the number of superpixels. For 256, 512 and 2048 superpixels, the computation takes only 1.7, 3.2 and 20.2 seconds per image, respectively. The speed is comparatively slower than that of pixel based segmentation [10], which costs about 1.5 seconds per image; however, our method is much more accurate. Compared to the window based method [1] which takes about 6 minutes per image, ours is much more efficient (tens to hundreds of times faster) with comparable or higher accuracy. We moreover note that our method was implemented with only a single thread, while [1] employs parallel computation.

We also investigated the influence of the propagation range (R_p). Little change in accuracy was found when R_p varies from 0.1 to 0.2; however, the errors become larger when R_p is set much larger (e.g., 0.5). This can be expected, as long range context is less applicable for a superpixel and may introduce error.

4 Conclusion

For cup detection in glaucoma diagnosis, we proposed an intra-image learning framework based on superpixels and retinal structure priors. Tested on a large clinical dataset with three evaluation criteria, it achieves a 26.7% non-overlap ratio (m_1) with manually-labeled ground-truth, a 29.0% relative absolute area difference (m_2) and a 0.081 absolute CDR error (δ). In future work, we plan to improve contextual label refinement by utilizing a Markov random field (MRF), and elevate system performance using an online learning algorithm which combines intra-image and pre-learned training.

References

1. Xu, Y., Xu, D., Lin, S., Liu, J., Cheng, J., Cheung, C.Y., Aung, T., Wong, T.Y.: Sliding Window and Regression Based Cup Detection in Digital Fundus Images for Glaucoma Diagnosis. In: Fichtinger, G., Martel, A., Peters, T. (eds.) MICCAI 2011, Part III. LNCS, vol. 6893, pp. 1–8. Springer, Heidelberg (2011)
2. Klein, B., Klein, R., Sponsel, W., Franke, T., Cantor, L., Martone, J., Menage, M.: Prevalence of glaucoma: the beaver dam eye study. Ophthalmology 99(10), 1499–1504 (1992)
3. Foster, P., Oen, F., Machin, D., Ng, T., Devereux, J., Johnson, G., Khaw, P., Seah, S.: The prevalence of glaucoma in Chinese residents of Singapore: a cross-sectional population survey of the Tanjong Pagar district. Arch Ophthalmology 118(8), 1105–1111 (2000)
4. Shen, S., Wong, T.Y., Foster, P., Loo, J., Rosman, M., Loon, S., Wong, W., Saw, S.M., Aung, T.: The prevalence and types of glaucoma in Malay people: the Singapore Malay eye study. Invest Ophthalmol. Vis. Sci. 49(9), 3846–3851 (2008)
5. Jonas, J., Budde, W., Panda-Jonas, S.: Ophthalmoscopic evaluation of the optic nerve head. Survey of Ophthalmology 43, 293–320 (1999)
6. Abramoff, M., Alward, W., Greenlee, E., Shuba, L., Kim, C., Fingert, J., Kwon, Y.: Automated segmentation of the optic disc from stereo color photographs using physiologically plausible features. Invest Ophthalmol. Vis. Sci. 48(4), 1665–1673 (2007)
7. Liu, J., Wong, D.W.K., Lim, J.H., Li, H., Tan, N.M., Zhang, Z., Wong, T.Y., Lavanya, R.: ARGALI: an automatic cup-to-disc ratio measurement system for glaucoma analysis using level-set image processing. In: Int. Conf. Biomed. Eng. (2008)
8. Li, C., Xu, C., Gui, C., Fox, M.: Level set evolution without re-initialization: A new variational formulation. In: CVPR, pp. 430–436 (2005)
9. Merickel, M., Wu, X., Sonka, M., Abramoff, M.: Optimal segmentation of the optic nerve head from stereo retinal images. In: Med. Imag.: Phys., Func., and Struct. from Med. Im. (2006)
10. Wong, D.W.K., Lim, J.H., Tan, N.M., Zhang, Z., Lu, S., Li, H., Teo, M., Chan, K., Wong, T.Y.: Intelligent fusion of cup-to-disc ratio determination methods for glaucoma detection in ARGALI. In: Int. Conf. Engin. in Med. and Biol. Soc., pp. 5777–8570 (2009)
11. Zhang, Z., Yin, F., Liu, J., Wong, D.W.K., Tan, N.M., Lee, B.H., Cheng, J., Wong, T.Y.: Origa-light: An online retinal fundus image database for glaucoma analysis and research. In: IEEE Int. Conf. Engin. in Med. and Biol. Soc., pp. 3065–3068 (2010)
12. Achanta, R., Shaji, A., Smith, K., Lucchi, A., Fua, P., Susstrunk, S.: SLIC Superpixels. EPFL Technical report (2010)
13. Ren, C.Y., Reid, I.: gSLIC: a real-time implementation of SLIC superpixel segmentation. Technical report. University of Oxford, Department of Engineering Science (2011)
14. Onkaew, D., Turior, R., Uyyanonvara, B., Akinori, N., Sinthanayothin, C.: Automatic Vessel Extraction with combined Bottom-hat and Matched-filter. In: Int. Conf. Information and Communication Technology for Embedded Systems (ICICTES), pp. 101–105 (2011)
15. Tighe, J., Lazebnik, S.: SuperParsing: Scalable Nonparametric Image Parsing with Superpixels. In: Daniilidis, K., Maragos, P., Paragios, N. (eds.) ECCV 2010, Part V. LNCS, vol. 6315, pp. 352–365. Springer, Heidelberg (2010)
16. Fan, R.E., Chang, K.W., Hsieh, C.J., Wang, X.R., Lin, C.J.: LIBLINEAR: A Library for Large Linear Classification. Journal of Machine Learning Research 9, 1871–1874 (2008)

Population-Based Design of Mandibular Plates Based on Bone Quality and Morphology

Habib Bousleiman[1,*], Christof Seiler[1,2], Tateyuki Iizuka[3],
Lutz-Peter Nolte[1], and Mauricio Reyes[1]

[1] Institute for Surgical Technology and Biomechanics,
University of Bern, Stauffacherstrasse 78, 3014 Bern, Switzerland
{habib.bousleiman,mauricio.reyes}@istb.unibe.ch
[2] INRIA, Sophia-Antipolis, France
[3] Department of Cranio- Maxillofacial Surgery, University of Bern,
Inselspital, 3010 Bern, Switzerland

Abstract. In this paper we present a new population-based implant design methodology, which advances the state-of-the-art approaches by combining shape and bone quality information into the design strategy. The method enhances the mechanical stability of the fixation and reduces the intra-operative in-plane bending which might impede the functionality of the locking mechanism. The method is presented for the case of mandibular locking fixation plates, where the mandibular angle and the bone quality at screw locations are taken into account. Using computational anatomy techniques, the method automatically derives, from a set of computed tomography images, the mandibular angle and the bone thickness and intensity values at the path of every screw. An optimisation strategy is then used to optimise the two parameters of plate angle and screw position. Results for the new design are presented along with a comparison with a commercially available mandibular locking fixation plate. A statistically highly significant improvement was observed. Our experiments allowed us to conclude that an angle of 126° and a screw separation of $8mm$ is a more suitable design than the standard 120° and $9mm$.

Keywords: Orthopaedic implant design, population-based analysis, computational anatomy, mandibular locking fixation plate.

1 Introduction

The human mandible is a complex structure and a site of high incidence of traumatic or pathologic defects. Reconstruction of defects of the mandible using internal fixators is a common procedure in the general and specialised orthopaedic wards. Similar to other sites, mandibular fixation plates are selected from a limited range of manufactured models [1]. Therefore the need to intra-operatively adapt the implant to the patient-specific anatomy is almost always present.

---

* Corresponding author.

N. Ayache et al. (Eds.): MICCAI 2012, Part I, LNCS 7510, pp. 66–73, 2012.
© Springer-Verlag Berlin Heidelberg 2012

Recent research presented population-based methods to improve the design of the shape of pre-contoured fixation plates [2,3]. In [2], an alteration of a commercially available proximal tibial implant was proposed based on optimisation of surface distances using level-set segmentation in a statistical shape space. In [3], an articulated model of the implant was used to minimise more clinically relevant metrics, namely the amount of bending and torqueing required to adapt the implant to the anatomy of the patient being operated (as opposed to minimising surface distances). However, neither one of the approaches include bone quality information into the design. Moreover, they both focus on the out-of-plane deformations and do not address the in-plane bending of the plates.

For the specific case of locking mandibular plates, in-plane bending is the most important type of deformation since it affects the shape of the screw holes and locking mechanism. Out-of-plane deformations are less important in this case because mandibular plates are thinner, hence much easier to adapt to the patient anatomy. Therefore, for mandibular plates the angle between the mandibular body and ramus, referred to hereafter as mandibular or plate angle, is of major importance.

In addition to the surface morphology, the mechanical properties of bone are a major criterion in the design of implants [4], especially in structures such as the mandible where the amount of bone is not in large supply. A well designed implant must present reduced risk of screw pullout and higher mechanical stability. Bone thickness and bone mineral density can be inferred from computed tomography (CT) images where bone porosity, bone density, and image intensity values are well correlated [5,6]. Moreover, it has been shown that the quality of cortical bone has a considerable positive influence on the stability of the implant [7]. For the particular case of the mandibular reconstruction plate, the AO Foundation (Davos, Switzerland) recommends to flush the implant to the inferior edge of the body and posterior edge of the ramus. These regions are almost entirely composed of cortical bone.

In this paper we present a population-based design methodology of orthopaedic fixators, which advances the state-of-the-art approaches by combining shape and bone quality information into the design strategy. The proposed methodology is presented for the specific case of mandibular locking plates. Of special interest is the in-plane pre-contouring and the bone thickness and intensity values at screw insertion sites. The implant parameters that we optimise are the plate angle and the distance between adjacent screw holes. In addition we present a comparison between the proposed design and a commercially available model.

2 Methods

2.1 Experimental Data

A population of 43 CT images of the adult mandible (gender: $m = 25, f = 18$ — age: $mean = 56, st.dev = 11.37, median = 66$) was used in this study. Each image is composed of $99 \times 147 \times 145$ voxels and a voxel spacing of $1.25mm$.

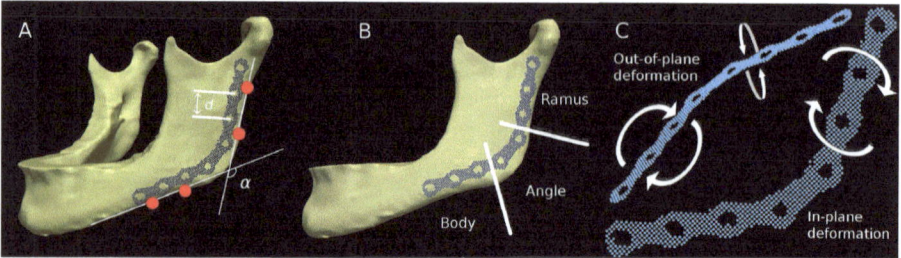

Fig. 1. 3D view of the reference mandible with the standard fixation plate placed in its correct location. (*A*) Visible landmarks (*red circles*) used to measure the mandibular angle. (*B*) Anatomical grouping of the mandible and plate into three regions, namely, ramus, angle, and body of the mandible. (*C*) Illustration of the in-plane and out-of-plane deformations relative to the plate.

All images were initially rigidly aligned and resampled to the resolution specified above. Non-rigid registration was then applied in order to establish a voxelwise correspondence between every image and a predefined reference. We used the algorithm described in [8] that was initially designed for mandibles and final aim towards implant design. It is a non-linear log-domain demons-based image registration method that uses a hierarchy of locally affine transformations as a regularisation model. The algorithm results in a deformation vector field (DVF) for every image relating voxels in the image to those in the reference via an anatomically meaningful correspondence.

2.2   Measurement of the Mandibular Angle

A well-designed angle reduces the need of intra-operative in-plane bending and hence the risk of deforming the locking screw holes. For this reason, we measured the mandibular angle within the population of images in our database. A set of four landmark points was manually placed on the reference mandible. Two landmarks were aligned with the left posterior edge of the ramus and the other two with the left inferior edge of the body of the mandible. The computed DVF was used to propagate the coordinates of the landmarks to all other images in the population. For every instance, the angle between the line connecting the two ramal landmarks and that connecting the landmarks on the mandibular body was automatically measured. Fig. 1A illustrates this process graphically.

2.3   Measurement of Bone Thickness and Intensity Values

Similarly, a set of eight landmarks (analogous to the eight screw holes in the standard plate and consistent with AO guidelines, i.e., at least three screws on either side of the fracture) was placed at the screw entry points on the reference image. A corresponding set was also placed on the interior side of the mandible to delineate the paths of the screws.

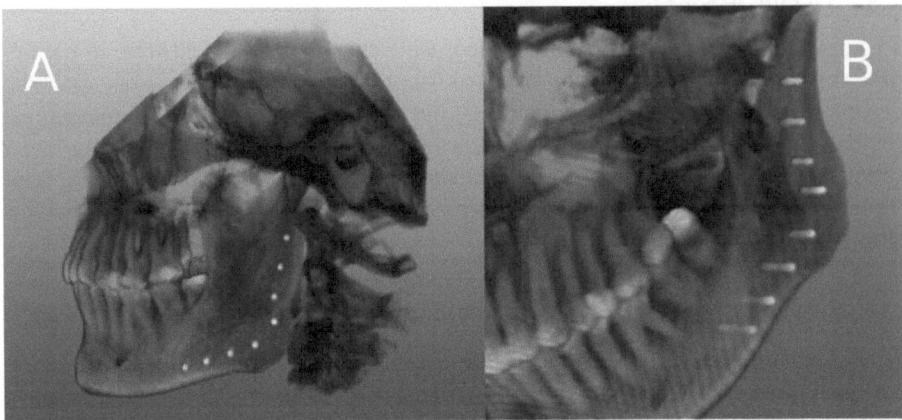

Fig. 2. Volume rendering of the reference image showing the (A) landmarks corresponding to the screw sites of a $120°$ plate and (B) the paths of the screws along which the intensity values are sampled

For any particular combination of implant parameters, the landmark configuration is modified accordingly and propagated to all instances of the population using the computed DVF. Geometrical constraints were used in order to ensure that the screw holes remain equidistant, that they are not misaligned, and that the plate angle is not affected by the varying mandibular angle due to the DVF propagation. Additionally, a safety margin of $3mm$ (consistent with the implant dimensions) was set around the screws in order to prevent any parts of the implant from being placed outside the bone.

The Euclidean distance between each pair of corresponding landmarks was computed. This represents the bone thickness at that particular screw insertion site. A $2mm$ tube (diameter of a typical mandibular screws) was used to sample voxels between the same landmarks. The average intensity value was used to represent the cortical bone quality at that location. Fig. 2 shows a 3D view of the landmark configuration and the sampled volumes.

2.4 Anatomical Grouping

Based on recommendations of the AO Foundation and standards of anatomy, the plate and mandible were divided into three anatomically distinct regions, namely, the ramus, the angle, and the body of the mandible. The regions contain three, two, and three screw holes, respectively. Each region was treated separately and considered as a single unit during the optimisation process and the analysis of the results. The two screws of the angle region were used to anchor the plate in place and remain fixed during the optimisation. Therefore, changes in intensity values or bone thickness are not expected for that region. The configuration of the regions is illustrated in Fig. 1B.

2.5   Design Process

The mandibular plate was parametrised using two geometric features, in particular the plate angle α and the distance separating two adjacent screws d. The design criteria were the bone thickness and the intensity values per anatomical region $R = \{Ramus, Angle, Body\}$.

For every image in the database, the algorithm scans through the two-dimensional search space and for every pair of parameters computes the intermediate energy function

$$E(\alpha, d)_{im} = w_\Theta \sum_{r \in R} \Theta_r^{\alpha,d} + w_I \sum_{r \in R} I_r^{\alpha,d}. \tag{1}$$

$E(\alpha, d)$ is composed of two components, namely, the thickness and the intensity components. Both terms are weighted according to their relative significance. In Eq. (1), w_Θ and w_I are the respective weighting factors. Both terms are normalised by their respective ranges to a unitless scale with values within $[0, 1]$ in order allow linear combination.

The thickness component is the average of the bone thickness measured at all screw sites within one region and can be written as

$$\Theta_{r \in R} = \frac{1}{N_r} \sum_{i=1}^{N_r} \tilde{T}_{r,i}, \tag{2}$$

where N_r is the number of screws in one particular region and $\tilde{T}$ the normalised local bone thickness.

Similarly, the intensity component is the mean of the intensity values sampled along all screws within one region, or equivalently

$$I_{r \in R} = \frac{1}{N_r} \sum_{i=1}^{N_r} \left[\frac{1}{n} \sum_{j=1}^{n} \tilde{H}_j \right]_{r,i}, \tag{3}$$

where n is the number of sampled voxels for every screw, and $\tilde{H}$ the normalised individual voxel intensity.

Calculating Eq. (1) for all images results in a vector of length equal to the total number of images p for every combination of α and d. The final energy function to be maximised is but the magnitude of the obtained vectors. A traceable extensive search was used, thus eliminating the need for an optimisation strategy such as gradient-based approaches. A formal representation of the total energy function is given as

$$E(\alpha, d)_{total} = \sqrt{\sum_{im=1}^{p} [E(\alpha, d)_{im}]^2}$$

$$= \sqrt{\sum_{im=1}^{p} [w_\Theta \sum_{r \in R} \Theta_r^{\alpha,d} + w_I \sum_{r \in R} I_r^{\alpha,d}]^2}. \tag{4}$$

3   Results

The first step was to measure the mandibular angle in the population using the approach described above. The mean mandibular angle was found to be 127.30° with a standard deviation of 6.66° and a median of 126.56°. These findings were used to initialise and set the domain of the optimisation along the angle parameter. This was chosen to be two standard deviations around the mean mandibular angle of the population with unit steps. The distance between the screws was limited by the screw hole geometry ($6mm$) and an arbitrarily larger value ($16mm$) with unit steps. Different weighting combinations for the energy function were tested. Stable and optimal results were obtained for $\omega_\Theta \geq 0.5$ (i.e., $\omega_I \leq 0.5$). These combinations are consistent with our design strategy to assign higher importance to the available thickness of the bone. We applied the optimisation algorithm on the whole population. Eq. (4) reached its maximum value at $\alpha = 126°$ and $d = 8mm$. The energy function is plotted in Fig. 3 against the 2D space of design parameters.

In order to evaluate the new design, we generated an implant configuration with the obtained parameters and compared it with that generated using the parameters of the standard design (low-profile MODUS® TriLock® 2.0/2.3/2.5, Medartis AG, Basel, Switzerland. $\alpha = 120°$ and $d = 9mm$). We applied the same method in both cases and measured the resulting distribution of bone thickness along the screw insertion paths. We carried out two-tailed t-tests to calculate the statistical significance of the differences in the obtained results using a significance level of 0.05. The results are shown in Fig. 4 with the statistical significance

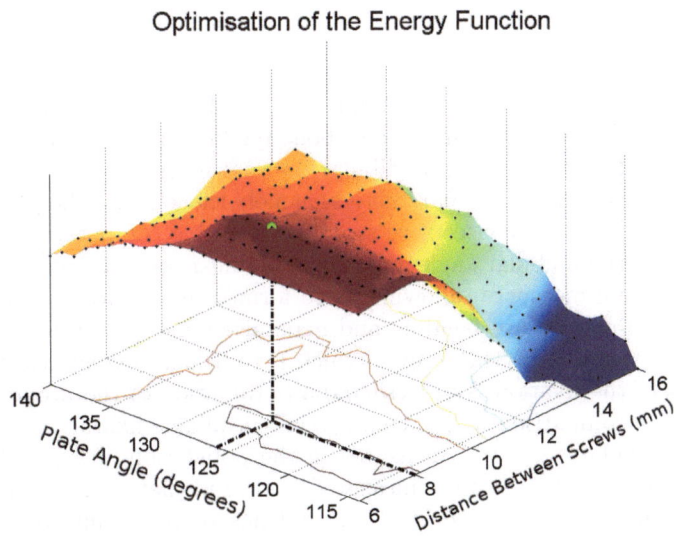

Fig. 3. Surface plot of the energy function against the 2-dimensional optimisation space spanned by the design parameters α and d. The green circle is the maximum value.

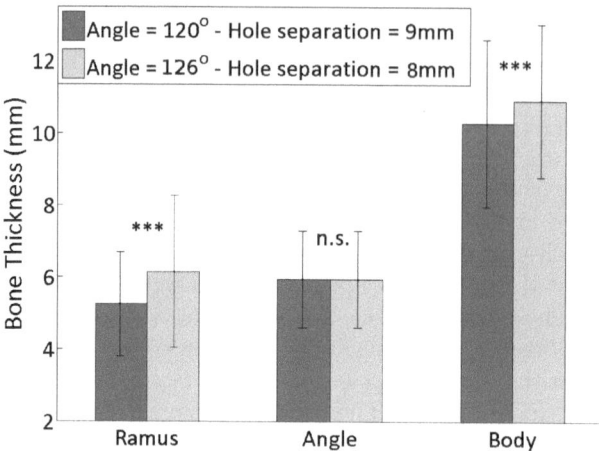

Fig. 4. Comparison of the distribution of bone thickness at the screw insertion paths for the commercially available plate and the proposed new design. The graph shows the results for the three anatomical regions. The statistical significance of the difference between the means of the populations is indicated on the graph (n.s.: not significant, ***: $p < 0.001$).

marked with asterisks. A net increase in the sampled intensity values of 7.87% and 23.19% was also observed for the ramus and body regions, respectively.

4   Discussion

In this paper we presented a new population-based orthopaedic implant design methodology that combines shape and bone quality information. The method was presented for the case of mandibular internal reconstruction plates. Of interest to the design were two parameters, namely the angle of the plate and the distance separating two consecutive screw holes. Using computational anatomy techniques, the mandibular angle and the bone thickness and intensity values at screw paths were measured, allowing us to formulate an optimisation strategy to minimise in-plane plate bending and maximise bone quality in the volumes that will be occupied by the screws, which is to a large extent responsible for the success of the fixation. We presented an evaluation of the proposed design by means of a comparison with a commercially available fixator.

The mandibular angle was measured in the population of available CT images. The difference between the measured angle and that of the standard plate indicates that the latter is not optimal and has room for improvement. The proposed and the standard designs were compared and the bone thickness and intensity values at screw locations were recorded. A statistically highly significant increase was measured for the new design in both the ramus and the body regions of the mandible. As expected, and since the screws of the mandibular angle were fixed, no change was observed.

The method presented herein can be extended to be applied on other implant types and for various anatomical sites. The length of the implant is not as important as its shape since in practice a plate longer than needed is intra-operatively cut to size. Therefore the length of the fixator was excluded from our analysis. The overall length of the plate will increase with increasing distance between the screw holes. Therefore, the respective effects will be correlated and redundant. We are aware that the length of the fixation might have a direct effect on the mechanical properties of the reconstruction and the force distribution over the locking mechanism. However we have plans to examine this topic in a study involving mechanical and finite element analysis that are outside the scope of this paper.

Acknowledgments. This work was carried out within the frame of the National Centre of Competence in Research, Computer-Aided and Image-Guided Medical Interventions (NCCR Co-Me), supported by the funds of the Swiss National Science Foundation (SNSF).

References

1. Nagamune, K., Kokubo, Y., Baba, H.: Computer-assisted designing system for fixation plate. In: IEEE International Conference on Fuzzy Systems - FUZZ IEEE, Jeju Island, Korea, pp. 975–980 (2009)
2. Kozic, N., Weber, S., Büchler, P., Lutz, C., Reimers, N., González, M., Reyes, M.: Optimisation of orthopaedic implant design using statistical shape space analysis based on level sets. Medical Image Analysis 14, 265–275 (2010)
3. Bou-Sleiman, H., Ritacco, L.E., Nolte, L.-P., Reyes, M.: Minimization of Intra-Operative Shaping of Orthopaedic Fixation Plates: A Population-Based Design. In: Fichtinger, G., Martel, A., Peters, T. (eds.) MICCAI 2011, Part II. LNCS, vol. 6892, pp. 409–416. Springer, Heidelberg (2011)
4. Schiuma, D., Brianza, S., Tami, A.E.: Development of a novel method for surgical implant design optimization through noninvasive assessment of local bone properties. Medical Engineering & Physics 33, 256–262 (2011)
5. Merheb, J., Van Assche, N., Coucke, W., Jacobs, R., Naert, I., Quirynen, M.: Relationship between cortical bone thickness or computerized tomography-derived bone density values and implant stability. Clinical Oral Implants Research 21, 612–617 (2010)
6. Zhang, J., Yan, C.-H., Chui, C.-K., Ong, S.H.: Accurate measurement of bone mineral density using clinical CT imaging with single energy beam spectral intensity correction. IEEE Transactions on Medical Imaging 29, 1382–1389 (2010)
7. Hong, J., Lim, Y.-J., Park, S.-O.: Quantitative biomechanical analysis of the influence of the cortical bone and implant length on primary stability. Clinical Oral Implants Research, 1–5 (2011)
8. Seiler, C., Pennec, X., Reyes, M.: Geometry-Aware Multiscale Image Registration via OBBTree-Based Polyaffine Log-Demons. In: Fichtinger, G., Martel, A., Peters, T. (eds.) MICCAI 2011, Part II. LNCS, vol. 6892, pp. 631–638. Springer, Heidelberg (2011)

Thoracic Abnormality Detection
with Data Adaptive Structure Estimation

Yang Song[1], Weidong Cai[1], Yun Zhou[2], and Dagan Feng[1]

[1] Biomedical and Multimedia Information Technology (BMIT) Research Group,
School of Information Technologies, University of Sydney, Australia
[2] The Russell H. Morgan Department of Radiology and Radiological Science,
Johns Hopkins University School of Medicine

Abstract. Automatic detection of lung tumors and abnormal lymph nodes are useful in assisting lung cancer staging. This paper presents a novel detection method, by first identifying all abnormalities, then differentiating between lung tumors and abnormal lymph nodes based on their degree of overlap with the lung field and mediastinum. Regression-based appearance model and graph-based structure labeling are designed to estimate the actual lung field and mediastinum from the pathology-affected thoracic images adaptively. The proposed method is simple, effective and generalizable, and can be potentially applicable to other medical imaging domains as well. Promising results are demonstrated based on our evaluations on clinical PET-CT data sets from lung cancer patients.

1 Introduction

Lung cancer is currently the leading cause of cancer deaths; and staging plays a critical role in defining the prognosis and the best treatment approaches. Imaging-based staging with positron emission tomography – computed tomography (PET-CT) is now widely accepted as the best non-invasive technique.

Since the existence of primary lung tumors and disease spread in regional lymph nodes are the most important factors for classifying the stage of lung cancer, our aim of this study is to develop a computerized method to detect the lung tumors and abnormal lymph nodes from PET-CT thoracic images automatically. PET highlights abnormal areas with high uptake values (Fig. 1b), but it is difficult to identify the type of the abnormality from PET without well-depicted anatomical structures. While such information can be viewed from the integrated CT (Fig. 1a), it is still quite challenging to differentiate lung tumors and abnormal lymph nodes, especially for complex cases with lung tumors invading into the mediastinum or lymph nodes abutting the lung field.

The prior works mainly focus on detecting either lung tumors [1,2] or lymph nodes [3,4] only. They avoid handling the influence from the other type of abnormality by assuming its non-existence [2,4] or with user-defined region of interest [1,3]. For simultaneous detection of both lung tumors and abnormal lymph nodes, a multi-level inference method has recently been proposed [5]. While the proposed local-, spatial- and object-level features are demonstrated effective for

N. Ayache et al. (Eds.): MICCAI 2012, Part I, LNCS 7510, pp. 74–81, 2012.
© Springer-Verlag Berlin Heidelberg 2012

the detection, the feature design appears to be based on empirical study, and hence might be limited to the available scenarios in the data sets and difficult to generalize to a larger variation of cases.

In this work, we propose a new and intuitive idea to the detection problem – after attempting to detect all abnormalities, if we can identify the actual lung field (tumors inclusive), then we can differentiate lung tumors and abnormal lymph nodes based on the degree of overlap between the detected abnormality and the lung field. The main problem is thus how to estimate the pathology-affected lung field. Limited studies exist in this area, and are mostly based on statistical shape models [6,7], with time-consuming registration [6] or complex landmark detections [7]. Since our problem does not require a very precise lung segmentation, but only a fair estimation of the overlap, we design a simpler yet effective atlas-based approach. Our design can be considered similar to [8], which unlike local-level computation [9], obtains brain segmentation mask by minimizing the weighted difference for the whole image with a regression-based approach. However, its direct derivation of segmentation from multiple weak segmenters might impose a stringent requirement on the weight learning, which would be difficult to optimize in our problem domain due to the large variety of thoracic patterns caused by abnormalities. This thus motivates us to opt for an indirect approach, with intermediate multi-atlas modeling of the feature space and a further classification for final labeling.

Our main contributions of this work are five-fold: (i) we approach the detection problem with a more intuitive and generalizable method, based on estimation of the actual lung field and mediastinum; (ii) the estimation is adaptive to each image, by weighted approximation of appearance model and then structure labeling; (iii) we design a regression approach for the appearance model, with enhanced local weights, supervised labeling information, and sparse regularization; (iv) we construct a customized conditional random field (CRF) [10] for globally-optimal structure labeling, encoding global and pairwise contrast information; and (v) simple features are used for structure estimation and abnormality classification, to keep the method adaptable for other imaging domains.

2   Proposed Method

2.1   Initial Abnormality Detection

The PET-CT thoracic images are first preprocessed to remove the background and soft tissues outside of the lung and mediastinum with morphological operations. All images are then aligned based on the carina of tracheae, and rescaled to the same size [4]. Next, the abnormalities are detected by classification of lung field (L), mediastinum (M) or abnormalities (O) (Fig. 1c), based on PET uptake values and CT densities. This classification method is the same as the *local-level modeling* described in [5], and lung tumors and lymph nodes are not differentiated. The high-uptake myocardium is masked out based on its size, spatial location within the thorax and the shape of the left lung field.

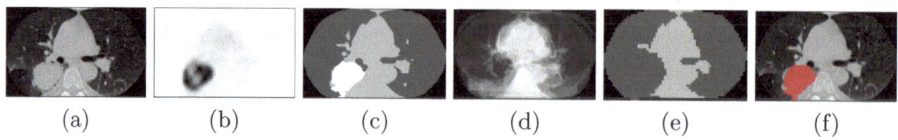

(a)   (b)   (c)   (d)   (e)   (f)

Fig. 1. Method illustration. (a) An axial CT slice (after preprocessing). (b) The co-registered PET slice, where the dark region indicates a lung tumor. (c) Output of the initial abnormality detection, showing the lung field, mediastinum and abnormality with increasing grayscale values. (d) The appearance model generated with regression, approximating the CT intensities if without the lung tumor. (e) Output of the graph-based structure labeling for lung field and medaistinum. (f) The detection output after tumor/lymph node classification, with tumor highlighted in red on CT image.

2.2   Adaptive Structure Estimation

To differentiate between lung tumors and abnormal lymph nodes, a general rule is that lung tumors should be inside the lung field, while lymph nodes are outside. However, as shown in Fig. 1c, due to the lung tumor, only a portion of the right lung field is correctly identified. Such problems are especially common for cases with tumors adjacent to or invading into the mediastinum. Therefore, we need to estimate the actual lung field before the tumor growth (Fig. 1e). Given a 3D PET-CT thoracic volume I, our objective is thus to label each voxel i (excluding the background) to the lung field or mediastinum type. To do this, the thoracic appearance is first modeled from a set of reference images, then the voxels are classified as L/M.

Regression-Based Appearance Model. Although patient-specific conditions introduce variational factors, there is still great similarity between images for the normal structures. It is thus a fair assumption that one image can be approximated by a weighted combination of multiple images. Therefore, at a first stage, we model the CT appearance of the original thoracic structure (Fig. 1d) based on other reference images. PET data is not used here due to its limited capability in depicting the anatomical structures.

We first introduce a basic formulation for the appearance model. Let $y \in \mathbb{R}^{n \times 1}$ be the n-dimensional feature vector (i.e. voxel-wise CT intensities) of I, and $D \in \mathbb{R}^{n \times K}$ be the matrix of K feature vectors from K reference images I_k ($n \gg K$). The difference between y and the weighted combination of D should then be minimized: $\min_x \| y - Dx \|_2^2$, where $x \in \mathbb{R}^{K \times 1}$ is the weight vector; and Dx is the original appearance of I approximated.

With the derived x, each reference image I_k is assigned one weight x_k, and hence all voxels in I_k contribute equally to the approximated appearance. However, due to the non-rigid structure of the thorax and presence of the abnormalities, it is normal that only a portion of I_k is similar to I and the rest should take lower weights. Therefore, we incorporate a voxel-wise similarity-based weight vector for each I_k. For voxel i_k of image I_k, the weight $w_{i,k}$ is computed as:

$$w_{i,k} = \frac{1}{\alpha_i} \exp(-\frac{1}{\beta_i} \parallel i - i_k \parallel_2), \ \beta_i = \sum_{k=1}^{K} \parallel i - i_k \parallel_2 \qquad (1)$$

where α_i is to normalize $\sum_k w_{i,k} = 1$. With the weight matrix $W = \{w_{i,k}\} \in \mathbb{R}^{n \times K}$, the regression formulation thus becomes: $\min_x \parallel y - (W \circ D)x \parallel_2^2$.

Furthermore, while the above formulation is sufficient for obtaining a closely matching appearance model, the L/M labeling information is not utilized. Since the final objective is to achieve accurate structure labeling, it is natural to integrate the supervised information to enhance the discriminative power:

$$\min_x \parallel y - (W \circ D)x \parallel_2^2 + \parallel h - (W \circ A)x \parallel_2^2$$
$$= \min_x \parallel \begin{pmatrix} y \\ h \end{pmatrix} - \begin{pmatrix} W \circ D \\ W \circ A \end{pmatrix} x \parallel_2^2 \qquad = \min_x \parallel f - \Omega x \parallel_2^2 \qquad (2)$$

where $h \in \{1, 2, 1.5\}^{n \times 1}$ is the label vector of I from the initial detection outputs (1=L, 2=M, and 1.5=O), and $A \in \{1, 2\}^{n \times K}$ for the reference images from the ground truth. The value 1.5 is chosen to have equal distance between O/L and between O/M, to assign no preference for matching such areas with L or M . Both h and A are normalized to the same range as y and D, and the approximated appearance model is then $(W \circ D)x$ and the labeling $(W \circ A)x$.

Finally, to avoid overfitting, we choose not to have all reference images contributing to the appearance approximation, with a sparse regularization:

$$\min_x \parallel f - \Omega x \parallel_2^2, \ s.t. \parallel x \parallel_0 \leq C \qquad (3)$$

where C is the constant number of reference images we limit to (set to 5 in this study). The OMP algorithm [11] is then used to solve x.

Implementation details. Due to small correlations between voxels of large distances, and to improve computational efficiency, we divide I into multiple sections, each with three slices, and y is then derived for each section. To construct D, the annotated tumor voxels are replaced with the average intensity of the lung field labeled at the initial detection step.

Graph-Based Structure Labeling. Next, based on the appearance model (Fig. 1d), we would like to classify the lung fields and mediastinum (Fig. 1e). A straightforward idea is to use the approximated labeling $(W \circ A)x$ as the classification output. However, such labelings are sometimes erroneous especially for the boundary areas, as shown in Fig. 2c. Therefore, we design a further graph-based classification step for the structure labeling (Fig. 2d).

We first define a notation for the appearance model: $G = \{g_i\} = (W \circ D)x$, where g_i is the approximated intensity for voxel i. The problem is thus to derive a label set $V = \{v_i \in \{L, M\}\}$, to classify each voxel to category L or M.

Based on the example, we can tell that the mislabeled part in Fig. 2c does appear lighter in G (Fig. 2b), but still darker than the real mediastinum. It thus motivates us to encode contrast information for the labeling. To do this, from G, we first calculate the mean values (m) and the graylevel histograms (d, range 1 to 256)

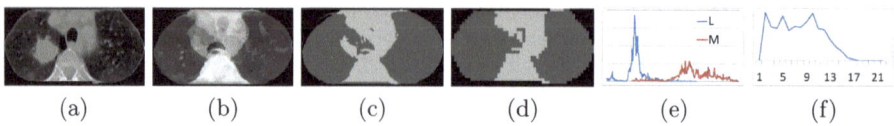

| (a) | (b) | (c) | (d) | (e) | (f) |

Fig. 2. Illustration of structure labeling. (a) An axial CT slice. (b) The appearance model. (c) The approximated labeling; compared with (d), a part of the right lung field is misclassified as mediastinum. (d) The structure labeling output. (e) The graylevel histograms of (b) for lung field and mediastinum. (f) The distribution of spatial distances between voxel pairs with nonzeros $s_{i,j}$ in (b).

of the lung field and mediastinum (labeled during the initial abnormality detection). As shown in Fig. 2e, a quite clear separation can be observed between the intensity distributions of L and M; and the probability density of g_i relative to d_L and d_M can be a good indicator of its structure category. A 5-dimensional feature vector q_i is thus computed for each voxel i: (i) g_i; (ii) g_i/m_L; (iii) g_i/m_M; (iv) $Pr[g_i \leq d_L \leq 256]$; and (v) $Pr[1 \leq d_M \leq g_i]$.

In addition to q_i, which incorporates the global-level information m and d, contrast information can also be described in a pairwise fashion. Specifically, for two voxels i and j, if g_i and g_j are similar and they are spatially close, they would likely take the same label. Hence we define the difference $s_{i,j}$ between i and j based on their intensity $| g_i - g_j |$ and spatial $\| i - j \|_2$ distances:

$$s_{i,j} = \log(\| i - j \|_2 + 1) \times \log(| g_i - g_j | + 1) \qquad (4)$$

A lower $s_{i,j}$ would imply a higher probability of $v_i = v_j$.

We then design a CRF construct to integrate both q_i and $s_{i,j}$ to label G, with the following energy function:

$$E(V|G) = \sum_i \phi(v_i) + \sum_{i,j} \psi(v_i, v_j) \qquad (5)$$

Here $\phi(v_i)$ represents the cost of i taking the label v_i, computed as $1 - p(v_i|q_i)$; and $p(.)$ is the probability estimate from a binary linear-kernel support vector machine (SVM) classifier based on q_i. The pairwise term $\psi(v_i, v_j)$ penalizes the labeling difference between i and j, with a cost value of $\exp(-0.5\gamma^{-1}s_{i,j})\mathbf{1}(v_i \neq v_j)$, where γ is the normalization factor as the average of all $s_{i,j}$ in G.

The pairwise term connects longer distance (beyond neighboring) voxels to encourage consistent labelings for similar voxels. And to ensure a sparse graph, we introduce a constant threshold tr, so that $s_{i,j} = 0$, if $| g_i - g_j |> tr$ with $tr = 3$; and Fig. 2f indicates that most pairwise terms are formed from non-neighboring voxels. The labeling set V is then derived by minimizing $E(V|G)$ using graph cut [12].

Implementation Details. Since the L/M labeling during the initial abnormality detection is quite accurate for the normal areas of the thorax, we only need to reclassify the detected abnormalities and their surrounding areas. Therefore, the graph-based labeling is conducted for the bounding box volume enclosing the detected abnormality and with an extended contour (of constant width of 20 voxels) of the bounding box to cover the surrounding areas (denoted as B). For memory efficiency, the image I is rescaled to 1/4 (not too small to affect detection of small lymph nodes) of the size (in xy dimension) and divided into multiple sections (three slices per section), for minimizing $E(V|G)$.

2.3 Feature Extraction and Classification

Based on the estimated thoracic structure V (Fig. 1e), we then classify the detected abnormalities (O) into tumors (T) or abnormal lymph nodes (N) (Fig. 1f). A simple 4-dimensional feature vector is designed: (i) size of O; (ii) size of overlap between O and lung field labeled in V; (iii) size of overlap between O and mediastinum labeled in V; and (iv) size of overlap between O and the convex hull of lung field detected during initial abnormality detection. Features (ii)–(iv) are also normalized by the size of O. A binary linear-kernel SVM is then trained to classify O to T or N. To enhance the error tolerance, the classification is performed on a section basis as well, and the final T/N label is produced based on a weighted averaging of the probability estimates from each section. The weights are computed as $\exp(-d/\eta)$, where d is the distance between the section and center of O, and η is the maximum distance possible for O.

3   Experimental Results

Data Sets. The experiment is performed on 50 sets of 3D PET-CT thoracic images from patients with non-small cell lung cancer (NSCLC), provided by the Royal Prince Alfred Hospital, Sydney. A total of 54 lung tumors and 35 abnormal lymph nodes are annotated as the ground truth. For each data set, the contour of lung field is also roughly delineated. Five images representing the typical cases are selected manually as the training set for both structure labeling and classification between tumors and lymph nodes. The data sets are then randomly divided into five sets; and within each set, each image is used as the testing image, with the other nine as the reference images.

Initial Detection. The initial abnormality detection results in a total of 4 false negatives (2 tumors and 2 lymph nodes), and 5 false positives. This is equivalent to a recall of 95.5% and precision of 94.4% for all abnormalities. These measurements are very similar to the detection rates reported in [5].

Table 1. The labeling accuracy comparing various components of our method. R-* are variations of the regression-based appearance model, and L-* are variations of the graph-based structure labeling. Refer to the text for details.

	R-basic	R-weight	R-label	R-sparse	L-approx	L-global	L-neigh	L-long
Acc (%)	83.9	87.9	89.2	89.7	86.8	88.2	87.4	89.7

Structure Estimation. The usefulness of each component in the structure estimation can be seen from Table 1. The accuracy is computed as *# voxels with correct labeling/ size of the bounding box volume B*. First, with the proposed graph-based structure labeling, we evaluate the appearance model with: basic regression, including voxel-wise weights, labeling information, and sparse regularization, to confirm the benefits over the basic regression model. Next, with the fixed regression-based appearance model, we then evaluate the structure labeling by: using the regression-approximated labeling, classification on global contrast features, and CRF with standard neighboring pairwise terms or long-distance pairwise terms. The results suggest the advantages of the global and pairwise contrast information; and that the standard pairwise terms actually cause lower performance than the non-structured classification. Note that R-sparse and L-long both represent our proposed method.

Table 2. The detection recall and precision

	Tumor (Proposed)	Node (Proposed)	Tumor [5]	Node [5]
Recall (%)	90.7	88.6	84.4	77.8
Precision (%)	89.1	88.6	83.8	76.9

Final Detection. Among the detected abnormalities, three tumors and two lymph nodes are misclassified as the other type. The mislabelings are mainly due to the close resemblance between tumors and lymph nodes at the hilum; and one lymph node is mistaken as tumor due to it connecting into an adjacent tumor volume. Together with the five false positive detections, four of which classified as tumors and one as lymph node, the overall detection recall and precision are shown in Table 2. The results show significant improvement over [5], especially for the abnormal lymph nodes; and it suggests the effectiveness of our approach for differentiating the two abnormalities, by mainly analyzing the degree of overlap between the detected abnormality and the estimated lung structures. Fig. 3 shows three examples with tumors near to the mediastinum and lymph nodes attaching to the lung field, to demonstrate the capability of our proposed method in handling such cases.

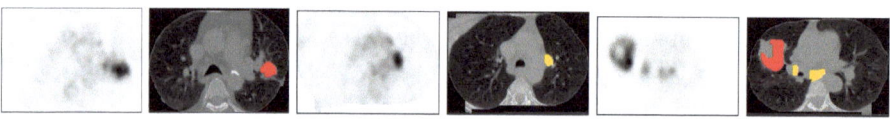

Fig. 3. Three example detection results, with each showing a PET axial slice and the detected tumor or abnormal lymph node highlighted on the CT slice (red for tumors and orange for lymph nodes)

4   Conclusions

We proposed a new detection method for lung tumors and abnormal lymph nodes from PET-CT thoracic images. The actual lung field and mediastinum are estimated with a regression-based appearance model and graph-based structure labeling, and the detected abnormalities are then classified based on their degree of overlap with the estimated structures. We have also shown improved detection performance compared to the existing method. The proposed method would assist the physicians in the image interpretation process and potentially also provide a second opinion for staging.

References

1. Saradhi, G., Gopalakrishnan, G., Roy, A., Mullick, R., Manjeshwar, R., Thielemans, K., Patil, U.: A Framework for Automated Tumor Detection in Thoracic FDG PET Images Using Texture-based Features. In: ISBI, pp. 97–100 (2009)
2. Gubbi, J., Kanakatte, A., Kron, T., Binns, D., Srinivasan, B., Mani, N., Palaniswami, M.: Automatic tumour volume delineation in respiratory-gated PET images. J. Med. Imag. Radia. Oncol. 55, 65–76 (2011)
3. Feulner, J., Zhou, S.K., Huber, M., Hornegger, J., Comaniciu, D.: Lymph Nodes Detection in 3-D Chest CT Using a Spatial Prior Probability. In: CVPR, pp. 2926–2932 (2010)
4. Feuerstein, M., Glocker, B., Kitasaka, T., Nakamura, Y., Iwano, S., Mori, K.: Mediastinal Atlas Creation from 3-D Chest Computed Tomography Images: Application to Automated Detection and Station Mapping of Lymph Nodes. Med. Image Anal. 16(1), 63–74 (2011)
5. Song, Y., Cai, W., Eberl, S., Fulham, M.J., Feng, D.: Discriminative Pathological Context Detection in Thoracic Images Based on Multi-level Inference. In: Fichtinger, G., Martel, A., Peters, T. (eds.) MICCAI 2011, Part III. LNCS, vol. 6893, pp. 191–198. Springer, Heidelberg (2011)
6. Sluimer, I., Prokop, M., van Ginneken, B.: Toward Automated Segmentation of the Pathological Lung in CT. IEEE Trans. Med. Imag. 24(8), 1025–1038 (2005)
7. Sofka, M., Wetzl, J., Birkbeck, N., Zhang, J., Kohlberger, T., Kaftan, J., Declerck, J., Zhou, S.K.: Multi-stage Learning for Robust Lung Segmentation in Challenging CT Volumes. In: Fichtinger, G., Martel, A., Peters, T. (eds.) MICCAI 2011, Part III. LNCS, vol. 6893, pp. 667–674. Springer, Heidelberg (2011)
8. Chen, T., Vemuri, B.C., Rangarajan, A., Eisenschenk, S.J.: Mixture of Segmenters with Discriminative Spatial Regularization and Sparse Weight Selection. In: Fichtinger, G., Martel, A., Peters, T. (eds.) MICCAI 2011, Part III. LNCS, vol. 6893, pp. 595–602. Springer, Heidelberg (2011)
9. Rousseau, F., Habas, P.A., Studholme, C.: Human Brain Labeling Using Image Similarities. In: CVPR, pp. 1081–1088 (2011)
10. Wu, D., Lu, L., Bi, J., Shinagawa, Y., Boyer, K., Krishnan, A., Salganicoff, M.: Stratified Learning of Local Anatomical Context for Lung Nodules in CT Images. In: CVPR, pp. 2791–2798 (2010)
11. Tropp, J.: Greed Is Good: Algorithmic Results for Sparse Approximation. IEEE Trans. Inform. Theory 50, 2231–2242 (2004)
12. Kolmogorov, V., Zabih, R.: What Energy Functions Can Be Minimized via Graph Cuts? IEEE Trans. Pattern Anal. Machine Intell. 26(2), 147–159 (2004)

Domain Transfer Learning for MCI Conversion Prediction

Bo Cheng[1,2], Daoqiang Zhang[1,2], and Dinggang Shen[2]

[1] Dept. of Computer Science and Engineering,
Nanjing University of Aeronautics and Astronautics, Nanjing 210016, China
[2] Dept. of Radiology and BRIC, University of North Carolina at Chapel Hill, NC 27599
{cb729,dqzhang}@nuaa.edu.cn, dgshen@med.unc.edu

Abstract. In recent studies of Alzheimer's disease (AD), it has increasing attentions in identifying mild cognitive impairment (MCI) converters (MCI-C) from MCI non-converters (MCI-NC). Note that MCI is a prodromal stage of AD, with possibility to convert to AD. Most traditional methods for MCI conversion prediction learn information only from MCI subjects (including MCI-C and MCI-NC), not from other related subjects, e.g., AD and normal controls (NC), which can actually aid the classification between MCI-C and MCI-NC. In this paper, we propose a novel domain-transfer learning method for MCI conversion prediction. Different from most existing methods, we classify MCI-C and MCI-NC with aid from the domain knowledge learned with AD and NC subjects as auxiliary domain to further improve the classification performance. Our method contains two key components: (1) the cross-domain kernel learning for transferring auxiliary domain knowledge, and (2) the adapted support vector machine (SVM) decision function construction for cross-domain and auxiliary domain knowledge fusion. Experimental results on the Alzheimer's Disease Neuroimaging Initiative (ADNI) database show that the proposed method can significantly improve the classification performance between MCI-C and MCI-NC, with aid of domain knowledge learned from AD and NC subjects.

1   Introduction

Alzheimer's disease (AD) is the most common form of dementia in elderly people worldwide. Early diagnosis of AD is very important for possible delay of the disease. Mild cognitive impairment (MCI) is a prodromal stage of AD, which can be further categorized into MCI converters (MCI-C) and MCI non-converters (MCI-NC). The former will convert into AD in follow-up time, while the latter will not convert. Thus, accurate diagnosis of MCI converters is of great importance. Nowadays, many machine learning methods have been proposed for the classification of AD or MCI [1-3]. More recently, an increasing number of studies in AD research begin to address MCI conversion prediction, i.e., the classification between MCI-C and MCI-NC based on the baseline imaging data [2-7].

One challenge in MCI conversion prediction is that the number of MCI (including both MCI-C and MCI-NC) subjects available for training is generally very small and

N. Ayache et al. (Eds.): MICCAI 2012, Part I, LNCS 7510, pp. 82–90, 2012.

thus the generalization ability of the classifier is limited. The same problem also exists in the classification between AD and NC, where the number of AD and NC subjects are also limited. Recently, to enhance the classification between AD and NC, several studies have used semi-supervised learning (SSL) methods [8] in AD diagnosis, where MCI subjects are treated as unlabeled data to aid AD classification [9-11]. Semi-supervised learning methods can efficiently utilize unlabeled samples to improve classification and regression performance, but it requires unlabeled samples and labeled samples coming from the same data distribution [8], which is usually not satisfied in practice. For example, Fig. 1 plots the distributions of AD, MCI-C, MCI-NC and NC from ADNI. As can be seen from Fig. 1, the distribution of MCI is different from that of AD and NC.

On the other hand, in the machine learning areas, a new learning methodology called transfer learning has been developed for dealing with problems involving cross-domain learning. Unlike SSL, transfer learning does not assume the auxiliary data (unlabeled data in SSL) have the same distribution as target data (labeled data in SSL), and can effectively adopt those auxiliary data from the related domain for improving classification performance, as validated in several successful applications in computer vision [12-13]. However, to the best of our knowledge, transfer learning has not been used for addressing brain disease classification problems in medical imaging, although intuitively the inclusion of additional AD and NC subjects as auxiliary data may be beneficial for the classification between MCI-C and MCI-NC. For example, as we can see from Fig. 1, although the distributions of MCI-C and MCI-NC are different from those of AD and NC, they are very related and the domain knowledge for diagnosing AD and NC may help diagnose MCI conversion.

In this paper, we propose a new transfer learning method called Domain Transfer Support Vector Machines (DTSVMs) to classify MCI-C and MCI-NC, with the aid from auxiliary AD and NC subjects. Specifically, we first construct a cross-domain kernel to transfer auxiliary domain knowledge, and then we utilize the adapted SVM to fuse cross-domain and auxiliary domain knowledge for better helping MCI-C and MCI-NC classification. We validate our method on single-modality and multi-modality biomarkers, including magnetic resonance imaging (MRI), fluorodeoxy-glucose positron emission tomography (FDG-PET), and quantification of specific proteins measured through cerebrospinal fluid (CSF), from the Alzheimer's Disease Neuroimaging Initiative (ADNI) database.

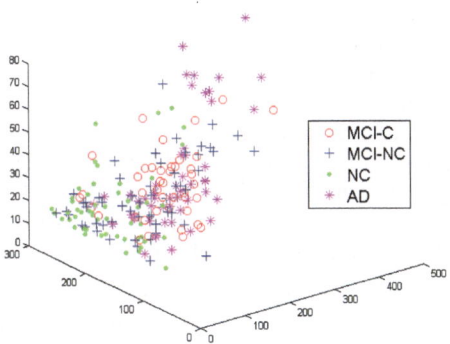

Fig. 1. Distributions of AD, NC, MCI-C, and MCI-NC subjects with CSF features

2   Domain Transfer Support Vector Machines (DTSVMs)

Transfer learning aims to apply knowledge learned from one or more related auxiliary domain to improve the performance on the target domain. In this section, we propose a new method called DTSVM for MCI-C and MCI-NC classification. There are two main steps in DTSVM, i.e., cross-domain kernel learning for transferring auxiliary domain knowledge, and the adapted SVM decision function construction for cross-domain and auxiliary domain knowledge fusion. Fig. 2 shows the flow chart of our proposed DTSVM classification method.

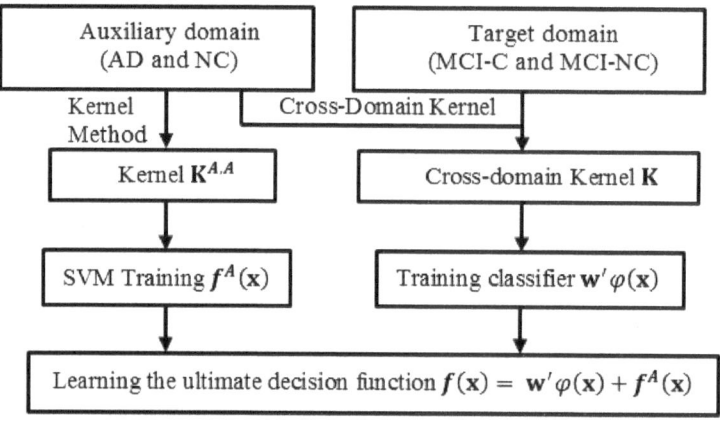

Fig. 2. Flow chart of the proposed DTSVM classification method

2.1   Cross-Domain Kernel for Transferring Knowledge of the Auxiliary Domain

Because of distribution difference between the auxiliary and the target domains, training with samples from the auxiliary domain may degrade the classification performance in another target domain. So, we cannot directly add auxiliary data to target domains for training. In cross-domain learning, it is crucial to reduce the difference between data distributions of the auxiliary and target domains. To avoid such differences, we use *cross-domain kernel learning* for transferring auxiliary domain knowledge [13]. Briefly, the auxiliary and target domains are first mapped to the Reproducing Kernel Hilbert Space (RKHS), and then the cross-domain kernel approach is used to build a new kernel function that can reduce the difference between data distributions of the auxiliary and target domains.

In the following, we formally address the problem of the cross-domain kernel approach by building a new kernel function. Firstly, we define the kernel matrices from the auxiliary domain A and from the target domain T as: $\mathbf{K}^{A,A} = k(\mathbf{x}_i^A, \mathbf{x}_j^A) \in R^{n_A \times n_A}$ and $\mathbf{K}^{T,T} = k(\mathbf{x}_i^T, \mathbf{x}_j^T) \in R^{n_T \times n_T}$, respectively, where $\mathbf{x}_i^A$ and $\mathbf{x}_j^A$ are samples in the auxiliary domain A, and n_A is the number of samples in domain A. Then, we define the cross-domain kernel matrices from the auxiliary domain to the target domain and from the target domain to the auxiliary domain as:

$\mathbf{K}^{A,T} = k(\mathbf{x}_i^A, \mathbf{x}_j^T) \in R^{n_A \times n_T}$ and $\mathbf{K}^{T,A} = k(\mathbf{x}_i^T, \mathbf{x}_j^A) \in R^{n_T \times n_A}$, respectively, where $\mathbf{x}_i^T$ and $\mathbf{x}_j^T$ are samples in the target domain T, and n_T is the number of samples in domain T. Finally, the kernel matrix $\mathbf{K} = k(\mathbf{x}_i, \mathbf{x}_j)$ is obtained as:

$$\mathbf{K} = \begin{bmatrix} \mathbf{K}^{A,A} & \mathbf{K}^{A,T} \\ \mathbf{K}^{T,A} & \mathbf{K}^{T,T} \end{bmatrix} \in R^{n \times n} \qquad (1)$$

Where $n = n_T + n_A$.

2.2 Adapted SVM for Knowledge Fusion

Assume we have n_A samples and corresponding class labels in the auxiliary domain as $\{\mathbf{x}_i^A, y_i^A\}_{i=1}^{n_A}$, where $\mathbf{x}_i{}^A \in R^d$ is a sample and $y_i^A \in \{+1, -1\}$ is the class label (i.e., AD as 1 and NC as -1). Also, assume we have n_T samples and corresponding class labels as $\{\mathbf{x}_j^T, y_j^T\}_{j=1}^{n_T}$, where $\mathbf{x}_j^T \in R^d$ is a sample and $y_j^T \in \{+1, -1\}$ is the class label (i.e., MCI-C as 1 and MCI-NC as -1). For the convenience of description in the following, we can also define $y = \{y_l\}_{l=1}^n = y^A \cup y^T = \{y_i^A\}_{i=1}^{n_A} \cup \{y_j^T\}_{j=1}^{n_T}$. According to Section 2.1, we can learn the cross-domain kernel $\mathbf{K}$ from both auxiliary and target domains. In addition, since AD and NC subjects are sitting in the auxiliary domain while MCI-C and MCI-NC subjects are sitting in the target domain, we can assign the cross-domain label so that the MCI-NC label will be the same as the NC label and the MCI-C label will be the same as the AD label, considering that the learning tasks for the MCI-C vs. MCI-NC classification and the AD vs. NC classification are very related [9]. Here, we adopt the adapted SVM method in [12] to learn the cross-domain classifier $f(\mathbf{x})$, which is the ultimate decision function of our adapted SVM method. This ultimate decision function $f(\mathbf{x})$ is first learned from the cross-domain classifier $\mathbf{w}'\varphi(\mathbf{x})$ as:

$$f(\mathbf{x}) = \mathbf{w}'\varphi(\mathbf{x}) + b \qquad (2)$$

Where $\varphi(\mathbf{x})$ is a kernel-induced nonlinear implicit mapping, $\mathbf{w}$ is the parameter vector of the classifier, b is the bias term, and $\mathbf{x}$ is the cross-domain data obtained by $\mathbf{x} = \mathbf{x}^A \cup \mathbf{x}^T$. Also, $\mathbf{w}'$ denotes the transpose of $\mathbf{w}$.

Because the ultimate decision function $f(\mathbf{x})$ can also be learned from the auxiliary domain classifier $f^A(\mathbf{x}^A)$, Eq. 2 can thus be written as:

$$f(\mathbf{x}) = \mathbf{w}'\varphi(\mathbf{x}) + f^A(\mathbf{x}^A) \qquad (3)$$

To learn the weight vector $\mathbf{w}$ in Eq. 3, we use the following objective function, similar to the SVM:

$$\min_{\mathbf{w}} \frac{1}{2}\|\mathbf{w}\|^2 + C \sum_{i=1}^n \zeta_l$$
$$s.t. \ \zeta_l \geq 0, \ \text{with} \ y_l \mathbf{w}' \varphi(\mathbf{x}_l) + y_l f^A(\mathbf{x}_l^A) \geq 1 - \zeta_l \qquad (4)$$

Where l is the l-th sample in the cross-domain $y = y^A \cup y^T$ with range of $1 \leq l \leq n$, ζ_l is the corresponding slack variable, and $n_T + n_A$ represents the total number of samples in y as indicated above.

According to [12], we can solve this objective function (in Eq. 4) to obtain the solution for the weight vector $\mathbf{w}$. Then, we can obtain the final solution for $f(\mathbf{x})$.

3   Experiments

In this section, we evaluate the effectiveness of our proposed DTSVM method on multimodal data, including MRI, PET and CSF, from the Alzheimer's disease Neuroimaging Initiative (ADNI) database.

3.1   Experimental Settings

In our experiments, the baseline ADNI subjects with all corresponding MRI, PET, and CSF data are included, which leads to a total of 202 subjects (including 51 AD patients, 99 MCI patients, and 52 normal controls (NC)). For 99 MCI patients, it includes 43 MCI converters and 56 MCI non-converters. We use 51 AD and 52 NC subjects as auxiliary domains, and 99 MCI subjects as target domains.

The same image pre-processing as used in [1] is adopted here. First, for all structural MR images, we correct their intensity inhomogeneity by the N3 algorithm, perform skull-stripping, and remove the cerebellum. Then, we use the FSL package to segment each structural MR image into three different tissue types: gray matter (GM), white matter (WM), and cerebrospinal fluid (CSF). We further use an atlas warping algorithm [14] to partition each structural MR brain image into 93 ROIs. For each of the 93 ROIs, we compute GM volume in that ROI as a feature; For PET image, we use a rigid transformation to align it to its corresponding structural MR image of the same subject, and then compute the average PET value of each ROI as a feature. Accordingly, for each subject, we can acquire 93 features from the structural MR image, another 93 features from the PET image, and 3 features ($A\beta_{42}$, t-tau, and p-tau) from the CSF biomarkers.

To evaluate the performance of different classification methods, we use a 10-fold cross-validation strategy to compute the classification AUC (areas under the ROC curve), accuracy, sensitivity and specificity. Specifically, the whole set of subject samples are equally partitioned into 10 subsets, and then one subset is successively selected as the testing samples and all remaining subsets are used for training classifiers. This process is repeated 10 times. The SVM classifier training of standard SVM and DTSVM are implemented using LIBSVM toolbox [15], with a linear kernel and a default value for the parameter C (i.e., C=1). For comparison, LapSVM is also adopted in this paper. LapSVM is a typical semi-supervised learning method based on manifold hypothesis [8]. For LapSVM settings, we use linear kernel, and the graph Laplacian L with $n_T + n_A$ nodes are connected using k (i.e., k=5) nearest neighbors, and their edge weights are calculated using the Euclidean distance among samples. We use both multi-modality and single-modality biomarkers to validate our method. For combining multimodality data in DTSVM, standard SVM, and LapSVM methods, we specifically use a linear multi-kernel combination technique, with the weights learned from the training samples through a grid search, using the range from 0 to 1 at a step size of 0.1. Also, for features of each modality, the same feature normalization scheme as used in [1] is adopted here.

3.2   Results

We compare DTSVM with LapSVM and standard SVM (i.e., SVM) for both multi-modality and single-modality cases. Table 1 shows the classification performance measures of DTSVM, LapSVM, and SVM on different modalities. Note that Table 1 shows the averaged results of 10 independent experiments. As we can see from Table 1, DTSVM can consistently achieve better results than LapSVM and SVM methods on each performance measure, which validates the efficacy of our DTSVM method on using AD and NC subjects as auxiliary domains for helping classification. Specifically, for multi-modality case, DTSVM can achieve a classification accuracy of 69.4%, which is significantly better than LapSVM and SVM that achieve only 60.8% and 63.8%, respectively. In addition, for multi-modality case, if using the leave-one-out evaluation strategy, DTSVM can achieve a classification accuracy of 70.7%.

On the other hand, AUC and ROC are further used to validate the classification performance of DTSVM, LapSVM, and SVM. Table 1 also gives the AUC values of the three methods, and Fig. 3 plots their ROC curves with respect to different modalities. Both Table 1 and Fig. 3 indicate that DTSVM is superior to LapSVM and SVM for MCI-C and MCI-NC classification. Specifically, in the multi-modality case, the AUC value is 0.736 for DTSVM, while the AUC values for LapSVM and SVM are only 0.626 and 0.683, respectively.

Table 1. Comparison of performance measures of DTSVM, LapSVM, and SVM for MCI-C vs. MCI-NC classification using different modalities. (ACC= Accuracy, SEN=Sensitivity, SPE= Specificity).

Modality	Methods	ACC %	SEN %	SPE %	AUC
MRI+CSF+PET	**DTSVM**	**69.4**	**64.3**	**73.5**	**0.736**
	LapSVM	60.8	55.3	65.0	0.626
	SVM	63.8	58.8	67.7	0.683
MRI	**DTSVM**	**63.3**	**59.8**	**66.0**	**0.700**
	LapSVM	56.8	50.6	61.5	0.563
	SVM	53.9	47.6	57.7	0.554
CSF	**DTSVM**	**66.2**	**60.3**	**70.8**	**0.701**
	LapSVM	60.8	55.3	65.0	0.626
	SVM	60.8	55.2	65.0	0.647
PET	**DTSVM**	**67.0**	**59.6**	**72.7**	**0.732**
	LapSVM	55.0	48.7	59.8	0.558
	SVM	58.0	52.1	62.5	0.612

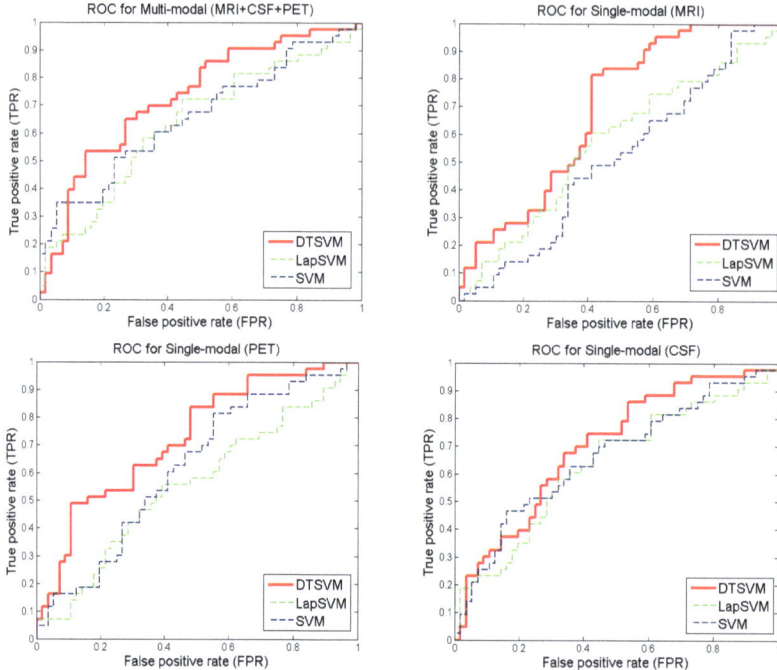

Fig. 3. ROC curves of DTSVM, LapSVM, and SVM, using multi-modality and single-modality data, respectively

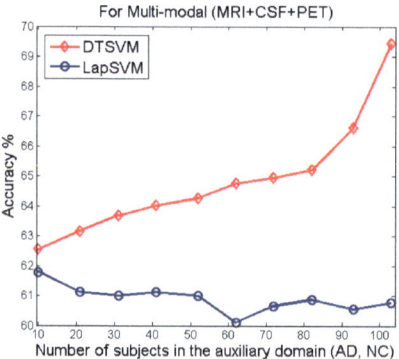

Fig. 4. Comparison of classification accuracy of DTSVM and LapSVM with respect to the use of different number of subjects in the auxiliary domain

Finally, in Fig. 4, we compare DTSVM with LapSVM for classification accuracy, with respect to the use of different number of subjects in the auxiliary domain. As we can see from Fig. 4, in most cases, the performance of DTSVM is significantly better than LapSVM as the number of subjects in the auxiliary domain increases. This validates the usefulness of adopting domain transfer learning method (i.e. DTSVM) to learn AD and NC domain knowledge, compared to the semi-supervised learning method (i.e., LapSVM). This result further demonstrates that the distribution of MCI is different from that of AD and NC.

4   Conclusion

This paper addresses the problem of exploiting the use of auxiliary domain data (AD and NC subjects) for helping MCI-C vs. MCI-NC classification. By integrating the cross-domain kernel learning and the adapted SVM methods, we propose a Domain Transfer SVM classification method, namely DTSVM. Our method does not require the auxiliary domain data and the target domain data to be from the same distribution. Experimental results on ADNI dataset validate the efficacy of our proposed method.

Acknowledgements. This work was partially supported by NIH grants (EB006733, EB008374, EB009634, AG041721 and MH088520), NSFC grant (60875030), and CQKJ (KJ121111).

References

1. Zhang, D., Wang, Y., Zhou, L., Yuan, H., Shen, D.: Multimodal classification of Alzheimer's disease and mild cognitive impairment. NeuroImage 55(3), 856–867 (2011)
2. Davatzikos, C., Bhatt, P., Shaw, L.M., Batmanghelich, K.N., Trojanowski, J.Q.: Prediction of MCI to AD conversion, via MRI, CSF biomarkers, and pattern classification. Neurobiology of Aging 32, 2322.e19-2322.e27 (2011)
3. Cho, Y., Seong, J.K., Jeong, Y., Shin, S.Y.: Individual subject classification for Alzheimer's disease based on incremental learning using a spatial frequency representation of cortical thickness data. NeuroImage 59, 2217–2230 (2012)
4. Aksu, Y., Miller, D.J., Kesidis, G., Bigler, D.C., Yang, Q.X.: An MRI-derived definition of MCI-to-AD conversion for long-term, automatic prognosis of MCI patients. PLoS One 6, e25074 (2011)
5. Misra, C., Fan, Y., Davatzikos, C.: Baseline and longitudinal patterns of brain atrophy in MCI patients, and their use in prediction of short-term conversion to AD: results from ADNI. NeuroImage 44, 1415–1422 (2009)
6. Leung, K.K., Shen, K.K., Barnes, J., Ridgway, G.R., Clarkson, M.J., Fripp, J., Salvado, O., Meriaudeau, F., Fox, N.C., Bourgeat, P., Ourselin, S.: Increasing power to predict mild cognitive impairment conversion to Alzheimer's disease using hippocampal atrophy rate and statistical shape models. Med. Image Comput. Comput. Assist. Interv. 13, 125–132 (2010)
7. Risacher, S.L., Saykin, A.J., West, J.D., Shen, L., Firpi, H.A., McDonald, B.C.: Baseline MRI predictors of conversion from MCI to probable AD in the ADNI cohort. Curr. Alzheimer. Res. 6, 347–361 (2009)
8. Belkin, M., Niyogi, P., Sindhwani, V.: Manifold Regularization: A Geometric Framework for Learning from Labeled and Unlabeled Examples. Journal of Machine Learning Research 7, 2399–2434 (2006)
9. Filipovych, R., Davatzikos, C.: Semi-supervised pattern classification of medical images: Application to mild cognitive impairment (MCI). NeuroImage 55(3), 1109–1119 (2011)

10. Filipovych, R., Resnick, S.M., Davatzikos, C.: Semi-supervised cluster analysis of imaging data. NeuroImage 54(3), 2185–2197 (2011)
11. Zhang, D., Shen, D.: Semi-supervised multimodal classification of Alzheimer's disease. In: IEEE International Symposium on Biomedical Imaging, pp. 1628–1631 (2011)
12. Yang, J., Yan, R., Hauptmann, A.G.: Cross-Domain Video Concept Detection Using Adaptive SVMs. ACM Multimedia (2007)
13. Duan, L., Xu, D., Tsang, I., Luo, J.: Visual Event Recognition in Videos by Learning from Web Data. In: IEEE Int'l Conf. Computer Vision and Pattern Recognition, pp. 1959–1966 (2010)
14. Shen, D., Davatzikos, C.: HAMMER: Hierarchical attribute matching mechanism for elastic registration. IEEE Transactions on Medical Imaging 21, 1421–1439 (2002)
15. Chang, C.C., Lin, C.J.: LIBSVM: a library for support vector machines (2001)

Simulation of Pneumoperitoneum
for Laparoscopic Surgery Planning

J. Bano[1,2], A. Hostettler[1], S.A. Nicolau[1], S. Cotin[3], C. Doignon[2], H.S. Wu[4],
M.H. Huang[4], L. Soler[1], and J. Marescaux[1]

[1] IRCAD, Virtual-Surg, Place de l'Hopital 1, 67091 Strasbourg Cedex, France
[2] LSIIT (UMR 7005 CNRS), University of Strasbourg, Parc d'Innovation,
Boulevard S. Brant, BP 10412 67412 Illkirch Cedex, France
[3] SHACRA Group, Inria, France
[4] IRCAD Taiwan, Medical Imaging Team, 1-6 Lugong Road, Lukang 505, Taiwan
jordan.bano@etu.unistra.fr

Abstract. Laparoscopic surgery planning is usually realized on a preoperative image that does not correspond to the operating room conditions. Indeed, the patient undergoes gas insufflation (pneumoperitoneum) to allow instrument manipulation inside the abdomen. This insufflation moves the skin and the viscera so that their positions do no longer correspond to the preoperative image, reducing the benefit of surgical planning, more particularly for the trocar positioning step. A simulation of the pneumoperitoneum influence would thus improve the realism and the quality of the surgical planning. We present in this paper a method to simulate the movement of skin and viscera due to the pneumoperitoneum. Our method requires a segmented preoperative 3D medical image associated to realistic biomechanical parameters only. The simulation is performed using the SOFA simulation engine. The results were evaluated using computed tomography [CT] images of two pigs, before and after pneumoperitoneum. Results show that our method provides a very realistic estimation of skin, viscera and artery positions with an average error within 1 cm.

Keywords: simulation, surgical planning, pneumoperitoneum.

1   Introduction

1.1   Clinical Context

Laparoscopic surgery has become a common procedure in the sugical community. It involves inserting an endoscopic camera and several instruments through small incisions made on the abdomen. In order to create a working space, gas is injected into abdominal cavity (pneumoperitoneum). Surgical planning is usually performed on a preoperative image, or in the best case, using a three-dimensional model. Part of the planning requires determining the trocar positioning so that the surgeon has a good triangulation between his instruments as well as good camera viewpoint. However, the preoperative model does not take deformation

N. Ayache et al. (Eds.): MICCAI 2012, Part I, LNCS 7510, pp. 91–98, 2012.
© Springer-Verlag Berlin Heidelberg 2012

due to gas injection into consideration. Since the pneumoperitoneum shifts the skin up and moves the abdominal viscera by several centimeters [9], the planned trocar positioning becomes inconsistent with the true position in the operating room, which drastically reduces the usefulness of the preoperative planning.

In this paper, we propose a individualized simulation of pneumoperitoneum and viscera motion using a preoperative medical image (CT) that can be used for laparoscopic surgery planning. The realism of the simulation method is evaluated with ground truth data and we show our method can even predict real pneumoperitoneum with an accuracy close to 0.5 cm which is accurate enough for trocar positioning planning. We highlight that in case the CT is injected with contrast medium, the abdominal wall arteries (cf. Fig. 1 for abdominal wall artery definition) are visible in the CT image and their position after pneumoperitoneum can also be simulated. This information can be crucial to avoid injury of abdominal wall arteries during trocar insertion, which is a common complication in laparoscopic surgery [2,10,7,4].

1.2   Previous Work

To our knowledge, only Kitasaka et al. [3,5] have explored pneumoperitoneum simulation for surgical planning. They simulated the deformation due to gas injection by applying forces that seem to be antero-posterior, on the inner surface of a portion of the abdominal wall. Recently, they evaluated the accuracy of their results on eight patients by comparing thirteen skin landmark positions after pneumoperitoneum and with simulation results [6]. Their simulation method uses two parameters which are empirically chosen to fit the *in vivo* data. With an optimally chosen set of parameters, the minimal mean error obtained was 13.8mm. Although their simulation provides interesting results, its usefulness is still limited since they do not take the viscera motion into account. Moreover the parameters of their model have no biomechanical meaning and cannot be adapted for a particular patient shape.

Soler et al. [11] have presented a patient-specific simulator for laparoscopic surgery. However in this paper, skin and viscera motions due to gas injection are also not taken into account. Viscera shape corresponds to viscera segmentation in the preoperative image (without pneumoperitoneum), and trocar positions are chosen without being related to skin position after pneumoperitoneum. Therefore, integrating realistic skin simulation after pneumoperitoneum would improve the realism of such simulator.

This paper proposes a method to simulate a pneumoperitoneum from a preoperative image, using realistic biomechanical parameters. In Section 2, we present the anatomical structures that we need to model from the preoperative image and how we choose the biomechanical parameters. In Section 3, we explain how the influence of gas pressure on the abdominal cavity is modeled and how we account for multiple contacts between moving structures in the abdomen. Finally, we evaluate in Section 4 our simulation realism using porcine data and we show our simulation accuracy is within 4mm on average for the abdominal wall and viscera and 5mm for abdominal wall arteries.

2   Model Generation

The input model of our simulation is created from an abdo-thoracic CT in three steps: segmentation, mesh generation and mechanical parameterization.

Segmentation Step. The preoperative image is segmented by dividing it into three regions: the abdo-thoracic wall, the abdominal viscera and the thoracic viscera (Fig. 1). In case they are visible, the arteries in the abdominal wall are also segmented. Note that they are not mandatory for the model. These segmentations are done semi-manually using custom-developed software and take one hour on average. Improvements are planned in future works to reduce the required time.

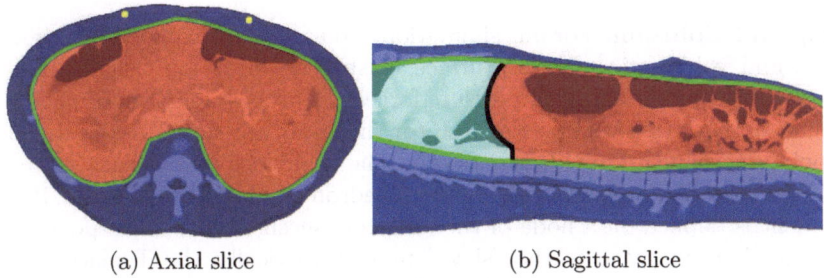

(a) Axial slice   (b) Sagittal slice

Fig. 1. On these two slices extracted from a preoperative pig CT acquisition, one can see the anatomical structures of our simulation model: the abdo-thoracic wall (blue), its internal surface (green line), the abdominal viscera (red), the thoracic viscera (cyan) and the diaphragm (black line). On the left figure, the abdominal wall arteries, located in the abdo-thoracic wall, are colored in yellow.

Mesh Generation. Volume and surface meshes are generated using the CGAL library[1] for the abdo-thoracic wall, the abdominal viscera and the thoracic viscera. Volumetric meshes are required for the finite element approach used in the computation of soft tissue deformation, while surface meshes are used for collision detection. The mesh generation needs a few seconds only from the segmented images.

Mechanical Parameters. Our simulation is based on a finite-element approach using a geometrically non-linear elastic law and a co-rotational formulation. The simulation is parametrized by associating Young's modulus [YM] and Poisson ratio to each volume mesh: the abdominal wall volume mesh is associated with a YM equal to 24 kPa (cf. Song et al. paper [12]) and a Poisson ratio of 0.49 (we assume that the abdominal wall is almost incompressible). Although abdominal viscera contain various organs with different stiffnesses, we chose, for simplicity reasons, to consider it as a homogeneous set associated to standard

---

[1] Computational Geometry Algorithms Library, http://www.cgal.org

YM of liver (15 kPa found in [8]). The thoracic viscera, containing the lungs and the heart (which reduces the mobility of the diaphragm), was assumed as a homogeneously elastic set (YM of 7 kPa). Moreover, a diaphragm was added to the model with a tenfold YM as for the abdominal wall.

3   Simulation

Our approach consists in simulating the realistic phenomena occuring during pneumoperitoneum. Our simulation is performed with SOFA [1] which provides a set of methods for modeling and simulating soft tissues and their interactions. We describe here only the main elements of the simulation, in particular gravity (and its compensation) and the effect of gas pressure in the abdominal cavity.

Mapping and Collision. For our simulation, we use an intricate combination of surface and volumetric meshes. Surface meshes are used for visualization, collision detection or for applying pressure forces. To propagate the information from a surface mesh to a volumetric mesh (or the other way around) we rely on the mapping mechanism provided by SOFA. The basic idea is that each vertex of a surface mesh is associated with a tetrahedron of the volume mesh. If a displacement is applied on a node of the "master" mesh, then a corresponding displacement is propagated to the "slave" mesh (practically, the displacement of a node is distributed to the vertices of the element it maps, according to its barycentric coordinates within that element). Similarly, if a force is applied on a node of a mapped mesh, then the force is propagated to the "master" mesh and distributed over the nearby nodes. The relationship between the initial and mapped forces is given by the transpose of the Jacobian of the mapping: $f_{initial} = J^T f_{mapped}$

Inverse Gravitational Deformation. To accurately simulate the deformation of the abdominal wall, or to correctly handle contacts between various anatomical structures, we need to include gravitational forces in our simulation. However, the different meshes used in the simulation are extracted from a CT image that has been acquired while gravity was applied to the tissues. Therefore, we cannot naively apply gravitational forces again onto the anatomical models. Although this problem is common in patient-specific simulations, it is not often mentioned and compensated except for some works, as that of Whiteley [13].

The main idea is to create a model representing the patient if he was not subject to gravity. Then, gravity is applied onto this model in order to obtain a new model, including the constraints due to gravity, and having a shape as similar as possible to the preoperative model.

The model without gravity is obtained by applying a negative gravity on the preoperative model. Therefore, a negative gravity is applied while the model is fixed on the table via the contact surface between the table and the pig.

Gas Pressure. A small part of the posterior skin is fixed all along the cranio-caudal direction to simulate the contact with the operating table (Fig. 2). Then, the simulation of the abdominal wall lift is done by applying forces on the abdominal wall internal surface. The force value corresponds to the gas injection pressure of 12mmHg commonly used in laparoscopic surgery and which direction is normal to the surface. The abdominal wall volume mesh is then expanded due to its mapping, resulting in deformations of its associated surface mesh. Moreover, the abdominal wall internal surface collides with the thoracic viscera surface mesh, which is pushed in the cranial direction. The simulation takes about 30 seconds (Intel Core i7 920 2.67GHz).

Abdominal Wall Artery Simulation. The artery surface mesh is mapped with the abdo-thoracic volume mesh. Therefore, it will be consistently deformed, following the deformation of the abdo-thoracic mesh due to the simulated pressure in the abdominal cavity.

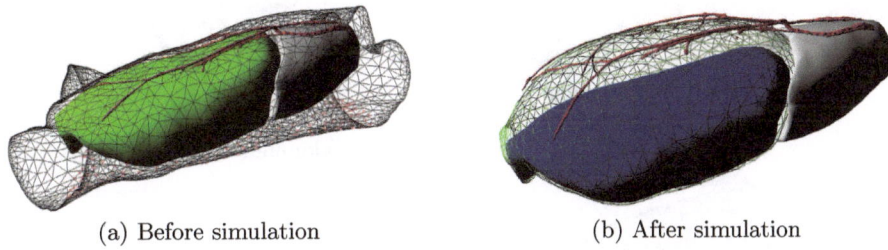

(a) Before simulation   (b) After simulation

Fig. 2. One can see our pneumoperitoneum simulation with skin (black wireframe, on the left only), abdominal cavity (green), thoracic viscera (white), abdominal viscera (blue) and abdominal wall arteries (red). On the left figure, constrained vertices are colored in pink.

4   Evaluations on Porcine Data

The assessement of our method was performed using two sets of CT images, acquired before and after creating a pneumoperitoneum for each pig. To evaluate the quality of our simulation, we compare the simulated abdominal wall, viscera and artery positions to the actual ones extracted from the CT data after pneumoperitoneum.

4.1   Evaluation of the Abdo-Thoracic Wall and Abdominal Viscera Position Simulation

For each simulated structure, the corresponding ground truth is a very dense point cloud extracted from the binary segmented mask of the CT image after

Table 1. The euclidian distance existing between each vertex of the simulated surface meshes and the actual ones is computed and sorted in four groups. Each group contains a quartile of the vertex total number.

Skin (mm)	Internal surface (mm)	Abdominal viscera (mm)	Color range
0 - 1.3	0 - 1.0	0 - 0.6	Blue to Turquoize
1.3 - 2.7	1.0 - 2.4	0.6 - 1.5	Turquoize to Green
2.7 - 5.1	2.4 - 4.9	1.5 - 3.8	Green to Yellow
5.1 - 10.6	4.9 - 16.5	3.8 - 20.1	Yellow to Red
3.2 (± 2.2)	3.4 (± 3.0)	2.9 (± 3.5)	Mean (± Std.Dev.)

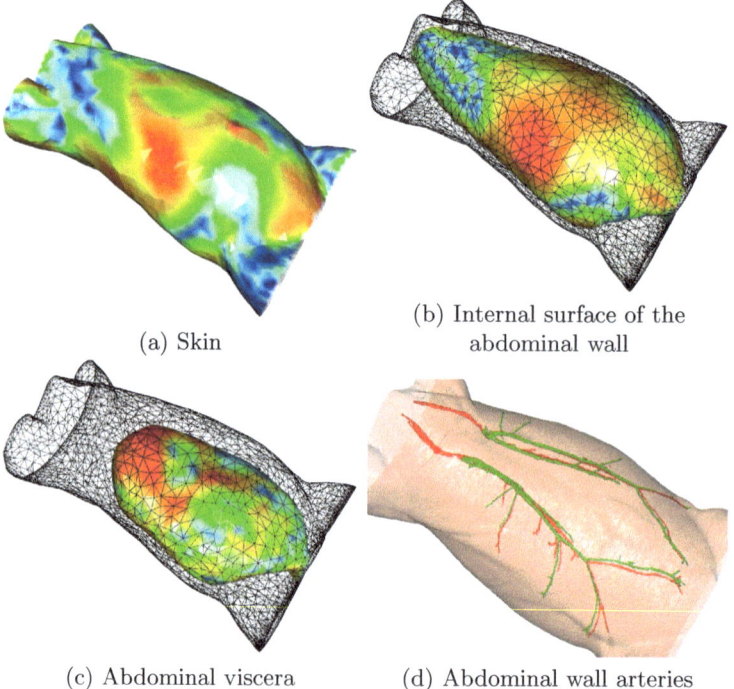

(a) Skin

(b) Internal surface of the abdominal wall

(c) Abdominal viscera

(d) Abdominal wall arteries

Fig. 3. These meshes represent the distance between our abdo-thoracic wall internal surface estimation and the ground truth using the scale from Tab. 1. On the lower right, one can see our artery position prediction (red) and the arteries segmented after pneumoperitoneum (green) with pig skin in transparency.

pneumoperitoneum. We compute the distance between each vertex of the simulated structure surface to the closest point of the ground truth point cloud. The same method is used for the internal surface of the abdominal wall, its external surface (namely the skin) and the abdominal viscera.

The average error of our simulation on the first pig is detailed in Tab.1. Regarding the second pig, we have approximately the same results for the abdominal wall

(3.8 mm ±3.3 mm for the internal surface and 3.4 mm ±3.5 mm for the skin), but for the abdominal viscera, we obtain a worse result (5.7 mm ±4.9 mm). A lack of realism due to the gas inside viscera distorts the results. Surface error of the viscera mainly occurs close to liver since the viscera are constrained by the pelvis. Moreover, reaching a perfect accuracy does not seem crucial for trocar insertion and the knowledge of abdominal viscera surface is enough. To visually assess the error, we display in Fig. 3 the simulated surfaces with a color code described in Tab.1.

4.2 Evaluation of our Artery Position Simulation

Contrary to previous evaluations, we decide to evaluate artery simulation by computing the distance between artery bifurcations. Indeed, providing average distance between artery surfaces will not highlight translation error along the main direction of arteries. Six bifurcation points have been selected manually in simulated and ground truth arteries, and an average error of 5.1 mm on pig 1 and 5.6 mm on pig 2 have been reported.

5 Conclusion

In this paper, we have presented a method to predict abdominal wall and viscera positions after pneumoperitoneum using only a preoperative medical image and realistic biomechanical parameters. Three structures are generated from the preoperative CT data and are associated to different biomechanical parameters. Then, the pneumoperitoneum is simulated by applying realistic pressure on the abdominal wall (after properly taking gravity into account in our modeling approach). An evaluation has been performed using medical CT acquisitions of two pigs before and after pneumoperitoneum, allowing us to quantitatively measure the realism of our method. Results show that our method provides very realistic simulation of skin, abdominal wall and artery, with a reported accuracy below 0.5 cm. Although the viscera simulation is less accurate (around 0.6 cm on average), it can still be useful to help surgical planning of laparoscopic procedures. We point out that our model does not depend on empirical values, and thus should provide reproducible accuracy and realism. In a future work, we plan to improve viscera simulation by integrating different Young's moduli to the viscera structure. We also plan to register our simulated model in the operating room using an augmented reality technique to help surgeons during trocar positioning.

References

1. Allard, J., Cotin, S., Faure, F., Bensoussan, P.J., Poyer, F., Duriez, C., Delingette, H., Grisoni, L., et al.: Sofa-an open source framework for medical simulation. Medicine Meets Virtual Reality 15, 13–18 (2007)
2. Geraci, G., Sciumè, C., Pisello, F., Li Volsi, F., Facella, T., Modica, G.: Trocar-related abdominal wall bleeding in 200 patients after laparoscopic cholecistectomy: Personal experience. World Journal of Gastroenterology 12(44), 7165 (2006)

3. Kitasaka, T., Mori, K., Hayashi, Y., Suenaga, Y., Hashizume, M., Toriwaki, J.-I.: Virtual Pneumoperitoneum for Generating Virtual Laparoscopic Views Based on Volumetric Deformation. In: Barillot, C., Haynor, D.R., Hellier, P. (eds.) MICCAI 2004. LNCS, vol. 3217, pp. 559–567. Springer, Heidelberg (2004)
4. Lam, A., Kaufman, Y., Khong, S.Y., Liew, A., Ford, S., Condous, G.: Dealing with complications in laparoscopy. Best Practice & Research Clinical Obstetrics & Gynaecology 23(5), 631–646 (2009)
5. Mori, K., Kito, M., Kitasaka, T., Misawa, K., Fujiwara, M.: Patient-specific laparoscopic surgery planning system based on virtual pneumoperitoneum technique. International Journal of Computer Assisted Radiology and Surgery 4, S140–S142 (2009)
6. Oda, M., Di Qu, J., Nimura, Y., Kitasaka, T., Misawa, K., Mori, K.: Evaluation of deformation accuracy of a virtual pneumoperitoneum method based on clinical trials for patient-specific laparoscopic surgery simulator. In: Proceedings of SPIE, vol. 8316, p. 83160G (2012)
7. Saber, A.A., Meslemani, A.M., Davis, R., Pimentel, R.: Safety zones for anterior abdominal wall entry during laparoscopy: a ct scan mapping of epigastric vessels. Annals of Surgery 239(2), 182 (2004)
8. Samur, E., Sedef, M., Basdogan, C., Avtan, L., Duzgun, O.: A robotic indenter for minimally invasive characterization of soft tissues. International Congress Series, vol. 1281, pp. 713–718. Elsevier (2005)
9. Sanchez-Margallo, F.M., Moyano-Cuevas, J.L., Latorre, R., Maestre, J., Correa, L., Pagador, J.B., Sanchez-Peralta, L.F., Sanchez-Margallo, J.A., Usan-Gargallo, J.: Anatomical changes due to pneumoperitoneum analyzed by mri: an experimental study in pigs. Surg. Radiol. Anat. 33(5), 389–396 (2011)
10. Shamiyeh, A., Wayand, W.: Laparoscopic cholecystectomy: early and late complications and their treatment. Langenbeck's Archives of Surgery 389(3), 164–171 (2004)
11. Soler, L., Marescaux, J.: Patient-specific surgical simulation. World Journal of Surgery 32(2), 208–212 (2008)
12. Song, C., Alijani, A., Frank, T., Hanna, G.B., Cuschieri, A.: Mechanical properties of the human abdominal wall measured in vivo during insufflation for laparoscopic surgery. Surgical Endoscopy 20(6), 987–990 (2006)
13. Whiteley, J.P.: The solution of inverse non-linear elasticity problems that arise when locating breast tumours. Journal of Theoretical Medicine 6(3), 143–149 (2005)

Incremental Kernel Ridge Regression
for the Prediction of Soft Tissue Deformations

Binbin Pan[1,2], James J. Xia[1], Peng Yuan[1], Jaime Gateno[1], Horace H.S. Ip[3],
Qizhen He[3], Philip K.M. Lee[4], Ben Chow[4], and Xiaobo Zhou[1]

[1] The Methodist Hospital Research Institute, Houston, Texas, USA
{JXia,PYuan,JGateno,XZhou}@tmhs.org
[2] School of Mathematics and Computational Science, Sun Yat-Sen University, China
alt26cn@gmail.com
[3] Department of Computer Science, City University of Hong Kong, Hong Kong, China
{Horace.ip,qizhen.he}@cityu.edu.hk
[4] Hong Kong Dental Implant & Maxillofacial Centre, Hong Kong, China
{kmleeoms,kcbchow}@netvigator.com

Abstract. This paper proposes a nonlinear regression model to predict soft tissue deformation after maxillofacial surgery. The feature which served as input in the model is extracted with Finite Element Model (FEM). The output in the model is the facial deformation calculated from the preoperative and postoperative 3D data. After finding the relevance between feature and facial deformation by using the regression model, we establish a general relationship which can be applied to all the patients. As a new patient comes, we predict his/her facial deformation by combining the general relationship and the new patient's biomechanical properties. Thus, our model is biomechanical relevant and statistical relevant. Validation on eleven patients demonstrates the effectiveness and efficiency of our method.

Keywords: kernel ridge regression, finite element model, maxillofacial surgery, soft tissue deformation.

1   Introduction

Craniomaxillofacial (CMF) deformities affect human's head and facial appearance. CMF surgery is designed to reconstruct such condition. This type of the surgery usually requires extensive presurgical planning. Currently we are able to accurately simulate osteotomies. However, soft-tissue-change simulation still remains a challenge. The most widely used method to simulate soft tissue change is biomechanical relevant Finite Element Model (FEM) [1] and its improvements [2-5]. However, a major disadvantage of FEM methods is that they are individually-based. Population-based statistical information was not considered. On the other hand, a statistical based method [6] is efficient but does not consider the biomechanical properties and thus it is less-than-accurate. To this end, we hypothesized that the soft tissue change could be accurately simulated if we could combine the FEM and statistical model into

N. Ayache et al. (Eds.): MICCAI 2012, Part I, LNCS 7510, pp. 99–106, 2012.
© Springer-Verlag Berlin Heidelberg 2012

one model. This integrated model should not only maintain the integrity of biomechanical information, but also be computational efficient. In this study, we developed an Incremental Kernel Ridge Regression (IKRR) model to effectively utilize the biomechanical information and statistical information. Kernel Ridge Regression (KRR) model was first established from the training data which consisted of a set of preoperative and postoperative 3D images. When a new patient arrived, the KRR model was adjusted incrementally to incorporate the new patient's biomechanical information. Compared to [6], our method combined different information, the statistical information and biomechanical information, into one model. Eleven patients were used for validation. The average prediction error of IKRR was found to be lower than other evaluated algorithms. Comparison of running time revealed that IKRR was more efficient than KRR.

2   Methodology

2.1   Data Acquisition and Pre-Processing

Eleven sets of patient's preoperative and postoperative CT scans and facial surface scans, obtained from a 3D surface camera, were acquired. The only reason of using facial surface scans was to prevent any unintended soft tissue strain during the CT scanning. The 3D camera was operated by a doctor who ensured the patient's facial expression was neutral. During the computation, the CT soft tissues were replaced with the 3D surface scans. Both preoperative and postoperative surface scans were rigidly registered to the preoperative CT images with the Mimics software (Materialise, Belgium). The bones of preoperative and postoperative CT images were segmented in Mimics which would be further used to determine surgical plan.

2.2   Feature Extraction

Biomechanical properties, including stress, strain and displacement, were computed from FEM. We used stress as a feature. In order to execute FEM, the following two components were utilized: the mesh and the surgical plan.

Mesh Generation. A Visible Human Female Dataset was used to generate an anatomic detailed mesh as a template. From the CT data, the following muscles contributed in facial soft tissue deformation were segmented from the dataset: Buccinator, Depressor anguli oris, Depressor labii, Levator anguli oris, Levator labii, Levator labii alaeque nasi, Mentalis, Orbicularis oris, Zygomaticus major, Zygomaticus minor and Masseter [7]. The remaining soft tissue tissues between the skin and mucosa were considered as a homogenous material. In order to generate a mesh structure applicable to all the patients, the segmented structures were then export as Stereolithography (STL) files and subsequently imported into TrueGrid (XYZ Scientific Applications, Inc., Livermore, CA). Finally, a hexahedral block mesh of this dataset was generated. It served as a template to map the detailed anatomic structures to real patients.

For real patient data, the segmented CT bones and registered 3D surface scan were imported into TrueGrid as facial geometries. The facial landmarks of each patient were manually marked. A surface projection technique of TrueGrid can change the template shape into patient shape by matching the corresponding landmarks.

Determination of Surgical Plan. The postoperative skull was firstly manually registered to the preoperative one based on an unaltered part at cranium. Afterwards, the preoperative skull was osteotomized into pieces according to the postoperative CT. Then, the bony segments were separately aligned to the postoperative counterparts. The Iterative Closest Point (ICP) algorithm [8] was used to compute the displacement between the preoperative and postoperative skull parts. After finding the displacement of all skull parts, we get surgical plan.

Calculation of Stress with FEM. For each node, it had the following quantity:

$$\begin{cases} \text{displacement}: & \boldsymbol{u} = \left(u, v, w\right)^{\mathrm{T}} \\ \text{stress}: & \boldsymbol{\sigma} = (\sigma_{xx}, \sigma_{yy}, \sigma_{zz}, \tau_{xy}, \tau_{xz}, \tau_{yz})^{\mathrm{T}} \\ \text{strain}: & \boldsymbol{\varepsilon} = (\varepsilon_{xx}, \varepsilon_{yy}, \varepsilon_{zz}, \gamma_{xy}, \gamma_{xz}, \gamma_{yz})^{\mathrm{T}} \end{cases} \quad (1)$$

Linear FEM (LFEM), based on linear elasticity to characterize the deformation behavior of soft tissues, was used to calculate the stress of the node [9]. Since we were interested in facial appearance, only the nodes lying on the outer skin were selected. There were totally 2652 nodes, and each node had a stress vector of length six. We stacked the stress of the selected 2652 nodes together to form a vector $\boldsymbol{\sigma}_i \in \mathfrak{R}^{15912}$ for the ith patient, $i = 1, \dots, n$. We called $\boldsymbol{\sigma}_i$ the feature of the ith patient.

2.3   Training Kernel Ridge Regression Model

The feature was served as input in regression model. The true displacement of the selected 2652 nodes was calculated from the preoperative and postoperative meshes. These nodal displacements were stacked together to form a vector $\mathbf{u}_i$ of length 7956. Given input-output pairs $(\boldsymbol{\sigma}_i, \mathbf{u}_i) \in \mathfrak{R}^{15912} \times \mathfrak{R}^{7956}$, $i = 1, \dots, n$, we could learn a prediction function f such that $f(\boldsymbol{\sigma}_i) \approx \mathbf{u}_i$ for each i.

KRR model was adopted [10]. This was a nonlinear regression model. The input was first embedded into a higher dimensional space H via a nonlinear mapping ϕ. Space H induced a kernel function which characterized the inner product in H and was given by the relation $k(\mathbf{x}, \mathbf{y}) = \phi^{\mathrm{T}}(\mathbf{x}) \cdot \phi(\mathbf{y})$, where $\mathbf{x}$ and $\mathbf{y}$ were in the input space. The kernel function adopted here was the widely used Gaussian kernel

$$k(\mathbf{x}, \mathbf{y}) = \exp\left(-\frac{\|\mathbf{x} - \mathbf{y}\|^2}{2\omega^2}\right) \tag{2}$$

with the width $\omega > 0$. KRR performed linear regression in H which was equivalent to performing nonlinear regression in input space. KRR assumed that the prediction function was of the form $f(\boldsymbol{\sigma}) = \mathbf{W}^{\mathrm{T}}\phi(\boldsymbol{\sigma})$, where $\mathbf{W}$ was the coefficients to be determined. By minimizing an objective function

$$L(\mathbf{W}) = \frac{1}{2}\sum_{i=1}^{n}\left\|\mathbf{u}_i - \mathbf{W}^{\mathrm{T}}\phi(\boldsymbol{\sigma}_i)\right\|^2 + \frac{\lambda}{2}\mathrm{tr}(\mathbf{W}^{\mathrm{T}}\mathbf{W}), \tag{3}$$

where $\lambda > 0$, we could find solution

$$\mathbf{W}^* = \boldsymbol{\Phi}(\boldsymbol{\Phi}^{\mathrm{T}}\boldsymbol{\Phi} + \lambda\mathbf{I}_n)^{-1}\mathbf{U} \tag{4}$$

with $\boldsymbol{\Phi} = \left(\phi(\boldsymbol{\sigma}_1), \ldots, \phi(\boldsymbol{\sigma}_n)\right)$ and $\mathbf{U} = (\mathbf{u}_1, \ldots, \mathbf{u}_n)^{\mathrm{T}}$.

For any $\boldsymbol{\sigma}$, the prediction of KRR model could be expressed as

$$\tilde{\mathbf{u}} = \left(\mathbf{W}^*\right)^{\mathrm{T}}\phi(\boldsymbol{\sigma}) = \mathbf{U}^{\mathrm{T}}(\mathbf{K} + \lambda\mathbf{I}_n)^{-1}\mathbf{k}(\boldsymbol{\sigma}), \tag{5}$$

where $\mathbf{k}(\boldsymbol{\sigma}) = \left(k(\boldsymbol{\sigma}_1, \boldsymbol{\sigma}), \ldots, k(\boldsymbol{\sigma}_n, \boldsymbol{\sigma})\right)^{\mathrm{T}}$, $\mathbf{K} = (k(\boldsymbol{\sigma}_i, \boldsymbol{\sigma}_j))_{i,j}$, $i, j = 1, \ldots, n$. In (5), the kernel function was sufficient for calculating the prediction. Therefore, it was not necessary to know the nonlinear mapping ϕ. This could reduce the computational complexity since we could avoid the operations in high dimensional space.

2.4   Prediction of Soft-Tissue Deformations with Incremental KRR Model

We incrementally modified KRR model by adding pair $(\tilde{\boldsymbol{\sigma}}, \tilde{\mathbf{u}}_{\mathrm{FEM}})$ to the training set, where $\tilde{\boldsymbol{\sigma}}$ was the stress for the new patient and $\tilde{\mathbf{u}}_{\mathrm{FEM}}$ was the displacement computed from linear FEM. Compared with KRR, our method predicted the output with biomechanical information $\tilde{\mathbf{u}}_{\mathrm{FEM}}$. We called it Incremental KRR (IKRR).

From (5), we could compute the prediction of IKRR as

$$\begin{aligned}\tilde{\mathbf{u}} &= \begin{pmatrix}\mathbf{U} \\ \tilde{\mathbf{u}}_{\mathrm{FEM}}^{\mathrm{T}}\end{pmatrix}^{\mathrm{T}}\begin{pmatrix}\mathbf{K} + \lambda\mathbf{I}_n & \mathbf{k}(\tilde{\boldsymbol{\sigma}}) \\ \mathbf{k}^{\mathrm{T}}(\tilde{\boldsymbol{\sigma}}) & k(\tilde{\boldsymbol{\sigma}}, \tilde{\boldsymbol{\sigma}}) + \lambda\end{pmatrix}^{-1}\begin{pmatrix}\mathbf{k}(\tilde{\boldsymbol{\sigma}}) \\ k(\tilde{\boldsymbol{\sigma}}, \tilde{\boldsymbol{\sigma}})\end{pmatrix} \\ &= t\tilde{\mathbf{u}}_{\mathrm{FEM}} + (1-t)\tilde{\mathbf{u}}_{\mathrm{KRR}},\end{aligned} \tag{6}$$

where the prediction of KRR $\tilde{\mathbf{u}}_{\mathrm{KRR}} = \mathbf{U}^{\mathrm{T}}(\mathbf{K} + \lambda \mathbf{I}_n)^{-1}\mathbf{k}(\tilde{\sigma})$, $t = (e - \lambda)/e$, $e = k(\tilde{\sigma}, \tilde{\sigma}) + \lambda - \mathbf{k}^{\mathrm{T}}(\tilde{\sigma})(\mathbf{K} + \lambda \mathbf{I}_n)^{-1}\mathbf{k}(\tilde{\sigma})$. By using the positive semi-definiteness of $\mathbf{K}$, we could proof that $t \in [0,1)$.

Equation (6) showed that the prediction of IKRR was a convex combination of the prediction of KRR and prediction of FEM. There were three major advantages in IKRR. First, IKRR was more general. It contained KRR as a special case by setting $t = 0$. Second, IKRR was more flexible. It combined two parts together, one from the KRR, the other from the FEM. The contribution of each part could be tuned by changing t . Finally, IKRR was more efficient. It did not need repetitive training when adding new training data. The computational complexity of KRR for training $n+1$ data was $O(n^3)$ (See (5)). However, the complexity of IKKR reduced to $O(n^2)$ by updating the results of KRR (See (6)).

2.5   Implementation Issues

One key point in statistical model was the corresponding relationship amongst all the data. Since all the meshes were generated from the same template, a natural corresponding relationship was established. The input of statistical model was normalized to have a zero mean and one standard deviation for each feature. The computations of FEM and statistical analysis were implemented in Matlab on a 64 bit Windows PC with 1.6GHz CPU and 24GB RAM. The regularization parameter λ and the width of Gaussian kernel ω were selected via grid search. The best values of the parameters were those that gave the best performance.

3   Results

3.1   Predictions with Different Number of Training Data

We tested different number of training data, from 6 to 10, to generate IKRR models. The prediction accuracy of these five IKRR was recorded. The difference between the prediction and ground truth was calculated as

$$E = \frac{1}{2652}\sum_{i=1}^{2652}\left\|\mathbf{d}_i - \tilde{\mathbf{d}}_i\right\|, \qquad (7)$$

where $\mathbf{d}_i$ was the true displacement of the ith node, $\tilde{\mathbf{d}}_i$ was the predicted displacement of the ith node. Table 1 showed the results.

Table 1. Prediction difference v.s. number of training data

Number of training	6	7	8	9	10
E (mm)	0.7845	0.7817	0.7814	0.7811	0.7756

The above table clearly showed that the prediction was improved when more training data were available. The statistical information gained from the added training data was beneficial to the prediction of soft-tissue deformations.

3.2   Empirical Comparisons

We carried out leave-one-out cross-validation using eleven patients' datasets. The algorithms to be evaluated included LFEM [9], KRR and IKRR. Table 2 tabulated the prediction difference as defined in (7).

Table 2. Bmax (mm) is the maximal skull displacement during surgery. E_{LFEM}, E_{KRR} and E_{IKRR} are the prediction differences of corresponding methods. Surgical plans are described in the second column: M represents mandible, X represents maxilla, A represents advance, B represents back, R represents right, L represents left.

Patient	Surgery	B_{max}	E_{LFEM}	E_{KRR}	E_{IKRR}
1	MB	11.6847	1.3241	2.9955	1.1963
2	MB+XB	6.1581	0.8054	1.3840	0.7756
3	MB	7.3624	1.2456	4.5722	1.0467
4	MB +XA	7.2343	0.7389	2.4249	0.7082
5	MR	8.3622	0.8567	1.6896	0.7870
6	MA	10.5866	0.9391	2.6338	0.8739
7	MB+XB	13.4578	1.1490	2.6418	0.9551
8	MB+XA	7.3898	0.8845	3.4110	0.8090
9	ML	10.5032	0.9978	2.3010	0.9783
10	MR	6.1608	0.9531	2.1136	0.9209
11	MB+XA	13.6617	0.9821	2.1602	0.9626
mean		9.3238	0.9888	2.5752	0.9103

KRR underperformed LFEM because of its lack of the new patient's biomechanical information. As a biomechanical based model, LFEM provided accurate predictions [9]. However, IKRR method outperformed all other algorithms by combining the statistical information learned from the training data and the test patient's biomechanical information. The results indicated that the test patient's biomechanical information was critical to the prediction performance.

The visualization was achieved by using inverse distance weighted interpolation [11] (Figure 1). This patient underwent a surgery to setback the mandible (bilateral sagittal split osteotomies) and advance the maxilla (Le Fort I osteotomy). As shown in Fig. 1, IKRR produced more accurate visualization than LFEM. The lower lip was prominent in LFEM prediction. While the lower lip was aligned with upper lip in IKRR prediction, which accorded with the postoperative image.

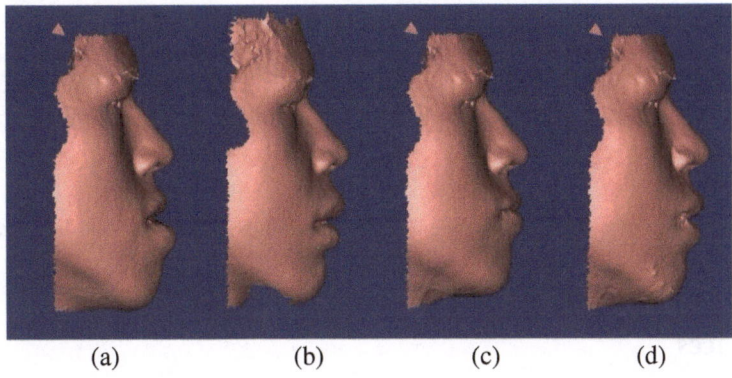

| (a) | (b) | (c) | (d) |

Fig. 1. (a) preoperative image (b) postoperative image (c) prediction of LFEM (d) prediction of IKRR

3.3   Computation Time

We compared the computational time of IKRR and KRR side by side. Once an initial KRR model was generated, re-training process could be achieved by two methods. The first was to recompute KRR entirely when a new patient was added as shown in (5). The running time of repetitive KRR was the elapsed time for the computation of (5) by replacing n with $n+1$. The second method was IKRR approach in which it only incrementally updated the existing KRR model as shown in (6). The running time of IKRR was the elapsed time for the computation of (6). The larger the n is, the more meaningful the comparison is. The experimental results in Table 3 clearly showed that IKRR was much more efficient than KRR for large number of training data.

Table 3. Computation time (s) for repetitive KRR and IKRR. "Speedup" means the factor that IKRR gained in CPU time over KRR

Number of training	1000	2000	3000	4000	5000
KRR	0.8542	3.3293	7.6927	14.1571	22.6551
IKRR	0.0089	0.0203	0.0357	0.0477	0.0629
Speedup	96.0	164.0	215.5	296.8	360.2

4   Conclusions and Discussions

We applied IKRR for the soft-tissue-change simulation after maxillofacial surgery. Unlike previous purly biomechanical based FEM [9] and statistical based model [6], our model integrated the statistical information and biomechanical information together. The results empirically showed our method outperformed the others.

Possible future work is discussed. In the future, a varity of preoperative and postoperative data with different types of deformities should be included in the training model. The limitation for the application is the deficiency of postoperative images. In contrast, the preoperative images is easier to obtain. To this end, we will investigate a semi-supervised learning approach to use two types of data: paired pre- and postoperative data, and purely preoperatively data. We will determine whether the performance would be improved by adding the second type of data into the training model.

Acknowledgements. This work is partially funded by TMHRI scholar award and NIH/NIDCR grant R01DE022676-01 (Xia & Zhou).

References

1. Zachow, S., Gladiline, E., Hege, H.C., Deuflhard, P.: Finite-element simulation of soft tissue deformation. In: Lemke, H.U. (ed.) Computer Assisted Radiology and Surgery (CARS), pp. 23–28. Elsevier (2000)
2. Chabanas, M., Payan, Y., Marécaux, C., Swider, P., Boutault, F.: Comparison of linear and non-linear soft tissue models with post-operative CT scan in maxillofacial surgery. Medical Simulation, 19–27 (2004)
3. Chabanas, M., Luboz, V., Payan, Y.: Patient specific finite element model of the face soft tissues for computer-assisted maxillofacial surgery. Medical Image Analysis 7, 131–151 (2003)
4. Barbarino, G.G., Jabareen, M., Trzewik, J., Nkengne, A., Stamatas, G., Mazza, E.: Development and validation of a three-dimensional finite element model of the face. Journal of Biomechanical Engineering 131, 1–11 (2009)
5. Marchetti, C., Bianchi, A., Bassi, M., Gori, R., Lamberti, C., Sarti, A.: Mathematical modeling and numerical simulation in maxillo-facial virtual surgery (VISU). Journal of Craniofacial Surgery 17, 661–667 (2006)
6. Meller, S., Nkenke, E., Kalender, W.: Statistical Face Models for the Prediction of Soft-Tissue Deformations After Orthognathic Osteotomies. In: Duncan, J.S., Gerig, G. (eds.) MICCAI 2005, Part II. LNCS, vol. 3750, pp. 443–450. Springer, Heidelberg (2005)
7. Schünke, M., Schulte, E., Schumacher, U., Voll, M., Wesker, K.: Prometheus Lernatlas der Anatomie. Georg Thieme Verlag (2009)
8. De Groeve, P., Schutyser, F., Van Cleynenbreugel, J., Suetens, P.: Registration of 3D Photographs with Spiral CT Images for Soft Tissue Simulation in Maxillofacial Surgery. In: Niessen, W.J., Viergever, M.A. (eds.) MICCAI 2001. LNCS, vol. 2208, pp. 991–996. Springer, Heidelberg (2001)
9. Mollemans, W., Schutyser, F., Nadjmi, N., Maes, F., Suetens, P.: Predicting soft tissue deformations for a maxillofacial surgery planning system: from computational strategies to a complete clinical validation. Medical Image Analysis 11, 282–301 (2007)
10. Bishop, C.M.: Pattern recognition and machine learning. Springer, New York (2006)
11. Watson, D.F., Philip, G.M.: A refinement of inverse distance weighted interpolation. Geo-processing 2, 315–327 (1985)

Fuzzy Multi-class Statistical Modeling for Efficient Total Lesion Metabolic Activity Estimation from Realistic PET Images

Jose George[1,2,3], Kathleen Vunckx[1,4], Elke Van de Casteele[1,2,3],
Sabine Tejpar[5], Christophe M. Deroose[4], Johan Nuyts[1,4],
Dirk Loeckx[1,3,6], and Paul Suetens[1,2,3]

[1] Medical Imaging Research Center, UZ Leuven, Belgium
[2] IBBT-KU Leuven Future Health Department, Belgium
[3] Medical Image Computing (ESAT/PSI/MIC)
[4] Nuclear Medicine
[5] Gastroenterology
[3,4,5] KU, Leuven, Belgium
[6] icoMetrix NV, Leuven, Belgium

Abstract. ^{18}F-fluorodeoxyglucose (FDG) positron emission tomography (PET) has become the de facto standard for current clinical therapy follow up evaluations. In pursuit of robust biomarkers for predicting early therapy response, an efficient marker quantification procedure is certainly a necessity. Among various PET derived markers, the clinical investigations indicated that the total lesion metabolic activity (TLA) of a tumor lesion has a good prognostic value in several longitudinal studies. We utilize a fuzzy multi-class modeling using a stochastic expectation maximization (SEM) algorithm to fit a finite mixture model (FMM) to the PET image. We then propose a direct estimation formula for TLA and SUV_{mean} from this multi-class statistical model. In order to evaluate our proposition, a realistic liver lesion is simulated and reconstructed. All results were evaluated with reference to the ground truth knowledge. Our experimental study conveys that the proposed method is robust enough to handle background heterogeneities in realistic scenarios.

Keywords: ^{18}F-FDG PET, SEM, FMM, TLA, fuzzy partial volume modeling, convex combination of random variables.

1 Introduction

^{18}F-FDG PET has become the de facto standard in current clinical therapy follow up evaluations. PET can record the metabolic response of several trillions of cells in the human body by the use of radiotracers such as ^{18}F-FDG. The tumor lesion, being more metabolically active, shows a higher tracer uptake in the PET scan, thereby enabling quantification of metabolic activity information in contrast to anatomic imaging modalities like magnetic resonance imaging (MRI), computed tomography (CT), etc. Due to its ability to visualize the functional

N. Ayache et al. (Eds.): MICCAI 2012, Part I, LNCS 7510, pp. 107–114, 2012.

information in the metabolic change, PET has been widely used in therapy response evaluations. PET images are typically normalized for injected dose and patient weight to a scale known as the standardized uptake value (SUV) in g/mL. Several PET derived markers [3, 7, 12] have been used in the literature for the longitudinal evaluation of tumor proliferation. SUV_{max} (maximum lesion activity uptake), SUV_{mean} (average lesion activity uptake), SUV_{peak} (activity uptake in $1cc$ spherical region of interest (ROI) around the SUV_{max}) [12], TLV (total lesion volume) and TLA (total lesion activity uptake) or TLG (total lesion glycolysis), in the context of ^{18}F-FDG PET, are some of them. However, TLA was found to be clinically relevant in [3, 7]. TLA calculation typically involves tumor delineation, to find TLV, followed by the quantification $\text{TLA} = \text{SUV}_{\text{mean}} \times \text{TLV}$.

The aforementioned functional markers computed from the PET image are corrupted by partial volume effects and acquisition blur. Nonetheless, we recently proposed a direct statistical estimation method, statistical lesion activity computation (SLAC), in [6] for computing TLA, in the presence of blur. SLAC only incorporated a fuzzy two class model to fit a Gaussian mixture of tumor, background and its combinations. However, in realistic scenarios, due to the presence of background heterogeneities, such a model may not be sufficient. In this paper, this direct estimation approach is extended to a fuzzy multi-class model to handle more realistic scenarios. A 3-class fuzzy model to handle heterogeneous tumors was introduced in [8]. Nevertheless, this model ignored the possibility of fuzzy mixing all 3 classes in the model. The main contributions of this paper include a fuzzy multi-class statistical modeling of the PET data with fuzzy mixing of all 'hard' classes involved in the model (in order to handle lesion as well as background heterogeneities) along with a direct estimation formula for TLA and SUV_{mean} from the statistical model parameters.

2   Materials and Methods

2.1   Fuzzy Multi-class Modeling

Let the observed PET image and the hidden statistical structure be realizations $\mathbf{y} = \{y_s\}_{s \in \mathcal{S}}$ and $\mathbf{x} = \{x_s\}_{s \in \mathcal{S}}$ of the random fields $\mathcal{Y} = \{\mathcal{Y}_s\}_{s \in \mathcal{S}}$ and $\mathcal{X} = \{\mathcal{X}_s\}_{s \in \mathcal{S}}$ respectively, where $\mathcal{S} = \{1, \ldots, N\}$ is the set of voxels. The unsupervised learning problem consists of estimating the unknown model parameters and the hidden $\mathcal{X}$ from the observed noisy version of $\mathcal{X}$ in $\mathcal{Y}$. In the fuzzy multi-class modeling, each voxel s is associated with a $\mathcal{K}$-dimensional vector $\boldsymbol{\epsilon}_s = [\epsilon_{ks}]_{1 \leq k \leq \mathcal{K}}$ denoting % allocation of each of the $\mathcal{K}$ 'hard' classes. E.g., in the case of a liver lesion falling close to the liver boundary, $\mathcal{K}$ could be 3 due to the contributions from the lesion itself, liver background and normal background. While the statistical part models the uncertainty in the classification, the fuzzy part models the imprecision in voxel membership. Now $\mathcal{X}_s$ in the model takes its value from $\boldsymbol{\epsilon} = [\epsilon_k]_{1 \leq k \leq \mathcal{K}}$ with ϵ_k in the closed interval $[0, 1]$ such that $\sum_k \epsilon_k = 1$. This is achieved by simultaneously using Dirac and Lebesgue measures in the fuzzy model. Then the measure will be $\boldsymbol{\nu} = \sum_i \boldsymbol{\zeta}_i + \sum_j \boldsymbol{\mu}_j$, where $\boldsymbol{\zeta}_i$'s are the Dirac measures on

$\mathcal{K}$ 'hard' classes and μ_j is the Lebesgue measure with elements on the fuzzy interval $[0, 1]$ formed by fuzzy mixing $\mathcal{K}$ 'hard' classes.

To find the conditional density of $\mathcal{Y}_s$ given the hidden classification $\mathcal{X}_s$, consider $\mathcal{K}$ independent and identically distributed (iid) random variables, $\{\mathcal{Y}_k\}_{1 \leq k \leq \mathcal{K}}$ associated to $\mathcal{K}$ 'hard' classes with densities $f_{\mathcal{Y}_s}(\xi \mid \mathcal{X}_s = \delta_k)$ defining the distributions of $\mathcal{Y}_s$ conditional to $\mathcal{X}_s = \delta_k$ respectively, where the $\mathcal{K}$-dimensional class labels $\delta_k = [\epsilon_j]_{1 \leq j \leq \mathcal{K}}$ such that $\epsilon_j = 1$ for $j = k$. Then the partial volume activities can be modeled by convex combinations of these independent random variables as $\mathcal{Y}_s = \sum_k \epsilon_k \mathcal{Y}_k$, for $\mathcal{X}_s = \epsilon$, and $\epsilon = [\epsilon_k]_{1 \leq k \leq \mathcal{K}}$ is the $\mathcal{K}$-dimensional fuzzy mixture class with $\epsilon_k \in]0, 1[$, $\sum_k \epsilon_k = 1$. Here the $\mathcal{Y}_k$'s and $\mathcal{Y}_s$ model the noise associated with the kth 'hard' class (for e.g., tumor, lesion background, normal background, etc) and the 'fuzzy' partial volume activities (mixture of 'hard' classes) respectively. If $f_{\mathcal{Y}_s}(\xi \mid \mathcal{X}_s = \delta_k)$'s are Gaussian distributed with densities $\mathcal{N}(\mu_k, \sigma_k^2)$, then $\mathcal{Y}_s$ is again Gaussian distributed with density $\mathcal{N}(\mu_\epsilon, \sigma_\epsilon^2)$ conditional to $\mathcal{X}_s = \epsilon$, $f_{\mathcal{Y}_s}(\xi \mid \mathcal{X}_s = \epsilon)$, such that $\mu_\epsilon = \sum_k \epsilon_k \mu_k$ and $\sigma_\epsilon^2 = \sum_k \epsilon_k^2 \sigma_k^2$.

Given $\mathcal{K}$ 'hard' classes, there are $2^{\mathcal{K}} - 1$ ways of fuzzy mixing the activities, of which $\mathcal{K}$ are purely belonging to 'hard' classes and the remaining $2^{\mathcal{K}} - \mathcal{K} - 1$ are 'fuzzy'. For $\mathcal{K} = 3$, there are 7 possibilities of mixing viz. '001', '010', '011', '100', '101', '110' and '111' of which the 1st, 2nd and 4th represent 'hard' classes ($\mathcal{H}_i$) and the remaining 4 denote 'fuzzy' classes ($\mathcal{F}_j$). Also, for each of the fuzzy mixing possibilities, we can assign infinite combinations for ϵ_k. However, in our investigations, we use a tolerance of 10% for ϵ_k along with an equal weightage class ($\frac{100}{3}$%), making it a total of $66 + 1$ class labels including 'hard' as well as 'fuzzy' classes for $\mathcal{K} = 3$. Here onwards, 'class' in general denotes those $2^{\mathcal{K}} - 1 = 7$ combinations, where as 'class label' denotes those 67 mixing possibilities in the model.

In our modeling, we assume $\mathcal{X}_s$ to be non stationary and use an adaptive support window to estimate the *a priori* information locally. Let $\mathcal{Z} = \{\mathcal{Z}_s\}_{s \in \mathcal{S}}$ be the learned hidden classification map at a particular iteration, then the local prior is

$$\gamma_{\mathcal{C}}^{(s)} \leftarrow \frac{\sum_{r \in \mathcal{W}_s} \delta(\mathcal{Z}_r, \mathcal{C})}{Card(\mathcal{W}_s)}, \text{ for } \mathcal{C} \in \{\mathcal{H}_i, \mathcal{F}_j\} \tag{1}$$

where $\mathcal{W}_s$ is a $w \times w \times w$ local support window around voxel s, δ is the Kronecker delta function and $Card(\mathcal{W}_s)$ is the cardinality of $\mathcal{W}_s$. That means for $\mathcal{K} = 3$, there will be a $\gamma_{\mathcal{C}}$ for each of the 7 classes $\{\mathcal{H}_i, \mathcal{F}_j\}$. Now, the *a posteriori* distribution of $\mathcal{X}_s$ with respect to ν given the noisy observation $\mathcal{Y}_s = y_s$ is given by

$$p_{\mathcal{X}_s}^{(s)}(\epsilon \mid y_s) = \frac{\gamma_\epsilon^{(s)} f(y_s \mid \epsilon)}{\sum_i \gamma_i^{(s)} f(y_s \mid \mathcal{H}_i) + \sum_j \gamma_j^{(s)} f(y_s \mid \mathcal{F}_j)} \tag{2}$$

where $f(y_s \mid \mathcal{F}_j)$ in the denominator are obtained by numerical integration.

The SEM algorithm [2] is used for iteratively estimating the parameters of the model. It is a stochastic version of the EM algorithm [4] making use of stochastic expectation and maximization steps to efficiently model the PET image. In each iteration, $p_{\mathcal{X}_s}^{(s)}(\epsilon \mid y_s)$ are estimated as in (2). This forms the expectation part of the SEM module. At iteration q, $p_{\mathcal{X}_s}^{(s)}(\epsilon \mid y_s)$ are sampled to estimate the intermediate labels $\mathcal{Z}_s^q$. The maximization part involves the direct estimation of distribution parameters from $\mathcal{Z}_s^q$ and the local adaptive prior computation using (1). The parameters $\{\mu_k, \sigma_k^2\}$ of the density functions $f_{\mathcal{Y}_s}(\xi \mid \mathcal{X}_s = \delta_k)$ are updated from the 'hard' classes in $\mathcal{Z}_s^q$. Then fuzzy parameters $\{\mu_\epsilon, \sigma_\epsilon^2\}$ are computed.

In order to obtain the hidden variable $\mathcal{Z} = \{\mathcal{Z}_s\}_{s\in\mathcal{S}}$, we sample the posterior distribution $p_{\mathcal{X}_s}^{(s)}(\epsilon \mid y_s)$ taking values from $\mathcal{C} = \{\mathcal{H}_i, \mathcal{F}_j\}$ and making use of the maximum posterior likelihood (MPL) method [1]. MPL integrates a dual sampling stage as follows. If $p_{\mathcal{X}_s}^{(s)}(\mathcal{H}_i \mid y_s)$ and $p_{\mathcal{X}_s}^{(s)}(\mathcal{F}_j \mid y_s)$ are the *a posteriori* densities associated with the $\mathcal{K}$ 'hard' classes and $2^{\mathcal{K}} - \mathcal{K} - 1$ 'fuzzy' classes respectively, then the classification rule assigns to each voxel s the label η in $\{\mathcal{H}_i, \mathcal{F}_j\}$ which has the maximum *a posteriori* density. i.e. $\mathcal{Z}_s = \arg\max_{\eta \in \{\mathcal{H}_i, \mathcal{F}\}} p_{\mathcal{X}_s}^{(s)}(\eta \mid y_s)$. If $\mathcal{Z}_s \in \mathcal{H}_i$, i.e. when the classifier opts for hard class labels, the decision rule halts. Otherwise, i.e. when $\mathcal{Z}_s \in \mathcal{F}_j$, the classification proceeds to the second stage decision rule given by $\mathcal{Z}_s = \arg\max_{\eta \in \{\epsilon_k\}} p_{\mathcal{X}_s}^{(s)}(\eta \mid y_s)$ to sample one of the fuzzy labels ϵ_k in $\mathcal{F}_j$.

To deal with initialization, we use random starts. In each of these random starts, a fuzzy C-means clustering routine looks for the initial feasible solution consisting of $2^{\mathcal{K}} - 1$ clusters representing 'hard' as well as 'fuzzy' classes. The model parameters are estimated to compute the message length [5]. The one giving the minimum message length is selected to initialize the SEM algorithm. The initial parameters of $\mathcal{N}(\mu_k, \sigma_k^2)$ and $\mathcal{N}(\mu_\epsilon, \sigma_\epsilon^2)$ are thus obtained. The local adaptive priors are initialized to $(2^{\mathcal{K}} - 1)^{-1}$ for each voxel. The SEM is run for utmost 100 iterations or until the total absolute relative change in the model parameters as well as the prior between consecutive iterations falls below $1e^{-3}$.

2.2   Direct TLA and SUV_{mean} Estimation

Once the fuzzy multi-class modeling is complete, the functional markers TLA and SUV_{mean} can be directly computed. A statistical direct computation formula to compute TLA for a fuzzy 2-class model is discussed in [6]. Here, we extend this idea to a fuzzy multi-class model. Total lesion activity (TLA) is the integral of metabolic activity over the whole lesion. It represents the weight of the metabolic lesion in gram (g). For a given ROI, starting from the total PET activity (TPA), constituting contributions from the lesion (TLA) and the background activities, we deduce the relationship between TLA and the SEM model parameters. From the observed PET image voxels $\{y_s\}_{s\in\mathcal{S}}$, $\text{TPA} := \sum_{s\in\mathcal{S}} y_s = \sum_{j\in\mathcal{J}} j\, h(j)$, where $\mathcal{S} = \{1, \ldots, N\}$, $h(j)$ is the observed histogram and $\mathcal{J}$ is the set of observed PET activity levels, $y_s \in \mathcal{J}$. In other words, the total activity in $\mathcal{S}$ is the same as the sum of all activity levels j scaled by respective frequencies of occurrence $h(j)$. Based on the fact that normalization of the observed histogram $h(j)$ gives the associated probability mass function $p(j) = P[\mathcal{Y}_s = j]$, without the loss of generality, $\text{TPA} := \sum_{s\in\mathcal{S}} y_s = N \sum_{j\in\mathcal{J}} j\, p(j)$, where N is the number of voxels. Extending it to the continuous domain and integrating the activity over the whole $\mathcal{S}$, the total PET activity, TPA can be related to the density $f_{\mathcal{Y}_s}(\xi)$ defining the distribution of $\mathcal{Y}_s = \xi$ as well as the 1st moment of $\mathcal{Y}_s$, $E(\mathcal{Y}_s)$ from the Riemann-Stieltjes integral by TPA $:= N \int \xi f_{\mathcal{Y}_s}(\xi)d\xi = N \times E(\mathcal{Y}_s)$. However, the density $f_{\mathcal{Y}_s}(\xi)$ is a finite mixture $\sum_i \alpha_i f_{\mathcal{Y}_s}(\xi \mid \epsilon_i)$, where α_i stands for the mixing probabilities $P[\mathcal{X}_s = \epsilon_i]$ for each of the class labels (67 labels for $\mathcal{K} = 3$) after modeling. If $E(\mathcal{Y}_s \mid \epsilon_i)$ represents the conditional expectation of $\mathcal{Y}_s$ given $\mathcal{X}_s = \epsilon_i$, then the TPA $:= N \sum_i \alpha_i \int \xi f_{\mathcal{Y}_s}(\xi \mid \epsilon_i)d\xi = N \sum_i \alpha_i E(\mathcal{Y}_s \mid \epsilon_i)$.

In the fuzzy modeling, $\mathcal{Y}_s$ is a convex combination of *iid* random variables $\mathcal{Y}_k$'s such that $\mathcal{Y}_s = \sum_k \epsilon_k \mathcal{Y}_k$. Then, the conditional expectation of $\mathcal{Y}_s$ given $\mathcal{X}_s = \epsilon_i$ is $E(\mathcal{Y}_s \mid \epsilon_i) = \sum_k \epsilon_{ki} E(\mathcal{Y}_k)$, where ϵ_{ki} is the fraction of the kth 'hard' class in the ith class label. applying the linearity property of the expectation operator and the statistical independence between the random variables $\mathcal{Y}_k$'s. Then the total PET activity is modified as TPA $:= N \sum_i \alpha_i \sum_{k \in \mathcal{K}} \epsilon_{ki} E(\mathcal{Y}_k)$. Now, we have an expression for TPA depending only on the 'hard' class model parameters $(E(\mathcal{Y}_k))$. If among the $\mathcal{K}$ 'hard' classes used for modeling the PET image, only $\mathcal{M}$ classes belong to the tumor, then the total lesion activity (TLA) is given by TLA $:= N \sum_i \alpha_i \sum_{k \in \mathcal{M}} \epsilon_{ki} E(\mathcal{Y}_k)$. Let's go back to the previous case of a liver lesion with 3 dominant classes viz. lesion $(\mathcal{Y}_1)$, liver background $(\mathcal{Y}_2)$ and normal background $(\mathcal{Y}_3)$, the TLA $= N \sum_i \alpha_i \epsilon_{1i} E(\mathcal{Y}_1)$, where ϵ_{1i} is the fraction of lesion class in the ith class label used in the modeling. After modeling, the delineation is made from the fuzzy class labels by selecting voxels with 50% or more allocation of the lesion class as belonging to the lesion. The lesion volume, TLV is the voxel count in that delineation. Once TLA and TLV are accurately estimated, the mean activity can be computed by $\text{SUV}_{\text{mean}} = \frac{\text{TLA}}{\text{TLV}}$.

2.3 Simulated Lesions

To evaluate the performance, an NCAT phantom [11] with a hot liver lesion was simulated. Realistic FDG uptake values were assigned to the various organs and tissues of the NCAT phantom. A non spherical tumor $(27.67mL)$ was inserted in the liver (see Fig. 1). In the tumor, the activity was set to $18.2kBq/cc$. The activity in the liver, spleen, lungs and body was $6.3kBq/cc$, $5.5kBq/cc$, $0.9kBq/cc$ and $2.5kBq/cc$ respectively. The voxel size used to generate the phantom was $1mm \times 1mm \times 1mm$. 30 $3min$ scans of the NCAT phantom were simulated using a Monte Carlo simulator (PET-SORTEO [10]) which models among others the spatially variant point spread function (PSF) of the ECAT Exact HR+ scanner. Attenuation and scatter were also modeled. During reconstruction of both datasets, the system PSF resolution was recovered by modeling as an isotropic Gaussian with $5mm$ FWHM. The projection data were reconstructed using the maximum likelihood expectation maximization (MLEM) algorithm [9] with ordered subsets. As in clinical routine, 4 iterations over 16 subsets were performed. The reconstruction voxel size was set to $2mm \times 2mm \times 2mm$. The images were post-smoothed with $5mm$ Gaussian FWHM.

3 Experiments and Results

Fig. 1(a) illustrates transverse slices of the liver lesion along with the binary delineation mask (whose integral gives TLV) obtained by 50% threshold as discussed in Section 2.2, as well as the lesion falling inside the delineation (commonly integrated for TLA). The liver lesion under study has voxels belonging to the lesion, liver background as well as normal background. So, we model fuzzy multi-class SEM with $\mathcal{K} = 3$ consisting of 67 class labels (see Section 2.1) and $w = 3$. Fig. 1(b) depicts respective transverse slices of images reconstructed from 30 different noise realizations. Fig. 1(c) shows the % allocation of each of the 3 'hard' classes in each voxel location. Fig. 1(d) plots the histogram modeled with 3 'hard' classes and its 'fuzzy' mixtures. Table 1 lists the SUV_{mean} as well

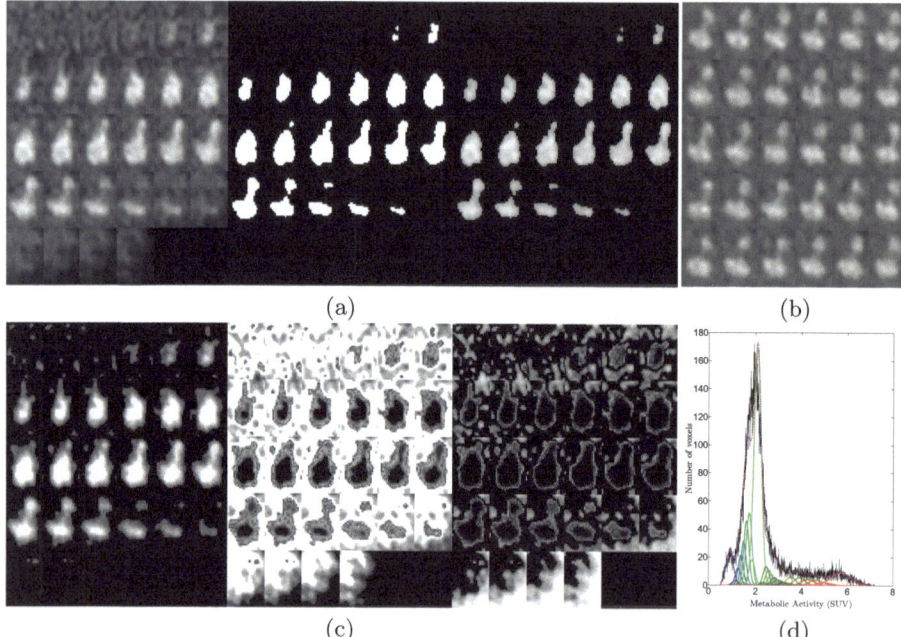

(a)   (b)

(c)   (d)

Fig. 1. (a)-Transverse slices of the simulated liver lesion (left), the delineated mask estimated from the model (middle) and the delineated lesion (right) from which TLA is commonly estimated. (b)-Respective slices of the MLEM reconstructed PET images from 30 noise realizations. (c)-Slices showing the percentage allocation of each of the 3 classes viz. the tumor class (left), the liver background class (middle) and the normal background class (right), used in the model. (d)-Actual histogram (in black) modeled as a finite mixture of 3 hard classes (the tumor class in red, the liver background in green and the normal background in blue shade) and a mixture of fuzzy classes (in a combination of red, green and blue shades) representing partial volume voxels; TLA being contributed from the tumor class and the fuzzy classes.

as the TLA obtained using our direct estimation method (dir) and computation from delineation ($deli$). In the first case, TLA^{dir} is directly computed as discussed in Section 2.2. Once the delineation is achieved, TLV is computed from it. Then $SUV_{mean}^{dir} = \frac{TLA^{dir}}{TLV}$. In the latter case, SUV_{mean}^{deli} is estimated as the mean activity in the delineation. Afterwards, TLA^{deli} is estimated as $\text{TLA}^{deli} = \text{SUV}_{\text{mean}}{}^{deli} \times \text{TLV}$. The TLV estimated at (5, 50, 95) percentile were (24.62, 25.74, 26.68) in mL with % error (-11.04, -6.97, -3.58) resp. Actual TLA and SUV_{mean} from the ground truth knowledge is $166.03g$ and $6g/mL$ resp. The median estimates ($\text{TLA}^{dir} = 162.62g$, $\text{SUV}_{\text{mean}}{}^{dir} = 6.33g/mL$) denote that our method provided the best estimate for both of these markers, whereas the delineation-based method yields an underestimation of the tumor uptake.

Table 1. 5, 50 (median) and 95 percentiles of the mean lesion activity (SUV_{mean}) and the total lesion activity (TLA) estimated using delineation-based (*deli*) and direct (*dir*) approaches from 30 noise realizations, with 3-FLAB [8] and proposed approach

Percentile		3-FLAB estimator [8]				Proposed multi-class estimator			
		deli		*dir*		*deli*		*dir*	
		Value	(% error)	Value	(% error)	Value	(% error)	Value	(% error)
SUV_{mean}	5	4.98	(-17.0%)	6.28	(4.7%)	4.86	(-19.0%)	6.16	(2.6%)
	50	**5.08**	**(-15.4%)**	**6.43**	**(7.1%)**	**4.96**	**(-17.2%)**	**6.33**	**(5.5%)**
(g/mL)	95	5.39	(-10.2%)	8.03	(33.8%)	5.06	(-15.7%)	6.48	(8.1%)
TLA	5	92.47	(-44.3%)	137.71	(-17.1%)	123.53	(-25.6%)	157.39	(-5.2%)
	50	**120.19**	**(-27.6%)**	**152.19**	**(-8.3%)**	**127.77**	**(-23.0%)**	**162.62**	**(-2.1%)**
(g)	95	125.38	(-24.5%)	157.83	(-4.9%)	131.40	(-20.9%)	168.08	(1.2%)

4   Discussion and Conclusion

The experimental studies done with 30 noise realizations of a realistic liver lesion showed again that the current trend of estimating TLA and SUV_{mean} from the delineation lead to underestimation in those PET derived markers. Moreover this underestimation is more pronounced for smaller lesions due to the influence of blur [6] and hence the quantification of these markers for longitudinal lesion evolution studies could be heavily compromised. At this point, our direct computation approach is beneficial. To our best knowledge, there are only few methods developed taking into consideration the need to estimate actual metabolic activity. Moreover, due to the limitation imposed by the PET acquisition system, any approach to delineate the actual tumor lesion will potentially end up underestimating the actual activity. This is in fact substantiated in the relative % errors. The proposed fuzzy multi-class SEM model is computationally fast and relatively robust to initialization compared to the conventional EM algorithm. Basic EM requires better initialization and more iterations to reach convergence. However, SEM achieves that with less iterations. Moreover due to direct parameter estimation, SEM is less computationally intensive. The advantages with fuzzy modeling is that it takes into account the spatially varying resolution automatically within the model. On the contrary, typical partial volume correction schemes assume that the PSF is Gaussian, which is not always the case. We put a tolerance of 10% allocation so that this spatial variability is aptly modeled irrespective of the noise realizations. To a good extent, this is handled as indicated by the 90% confidence interval (see Table 1). By providing multiple classes in the model, heterogeneous lesion as well as heterogeneous background can be efficiently modeled. The future work includes modeling with other probability distributions, analyzing clinical PET images, application to heterogeneous tumors and robustness study for varying reconstruction parameters.

Acknowledgments. The authors gratefully acknowledge the financial support by KU Leuven's Concerted Research Action GOA/11/006, IWT - TBM project 070717 and Research Foundation - Flanders (FWO).

References

1. Caillol, H., Pieczynski, W., Hillion, A.: Estimation of fuzzy Gaussian mixture and unsupervised statistical image segmentation. IEEE Trans. Image Process. 6(3), 425–440 (1997)
2. Celeux, G., Diebolt, J.: L'algorithme SEM: Un algorithme d'apprentissage probabiliste pour la reconnaissance de mélanges de densités. Revue de Statistique Appliquée 34(2), 35–52 (1986)
3. Costelloe, C.M., Macapinlac, H.A., Madewell, J.E., Fitzgerald, N.E., Mawlawi, O.R., Rohren, E.M., Raymond, A.K., Lewis, V.O., Anderson, P.M., Bassett Jr., R.L., Harrell, R.K., Marom, E.M.: ^{18}F-FDG PET/CT as an indicator of progression-free and overall survival in osteosarcoma. J. Nucl. Med. 50(3), 340–347 (2009)
4. Dempster, A.P., Laird, N.M., Jain, D.B.: Maximum likelihood from incomplete data via the EM algorithm. J. Roy. Stat. Soc. B Stat. Meth. 39(1), 1–38 (1977)
5. Figueiredo, M.A.T., Jain, A.K.: Unsupervised learning of finite mixture models. IEEE Trans. Pattern Anal. Mach. Intell. 24(3), 381–396 (2002)
6. George, J., Vunckx, K., Tejpar, S., Deroose, C.M., Nuyts, J., Loeckx, D., Suetens, P.: Fuzzy Statistical Unsupervised Learning Based Total Lesion Metabolic Activity Estimation in Positron Emission Tomography Images. In: Suzuki, K., Wang, F., Shen, D., Yan, P. (eds.) MLMI 2011. LNCS, vol. 7009, pp. 233–240. Springer, Heidelberg (2011)
7. Hatt, M., Le Rest, C.C., Aboagye, E.O., Kenny, L.M., Rosso, L., Turkheimer, F.E., Albarghach, N.M., Metges, J.P., Pradier, O., Visvikis, D.: Reproducibility of ^{18}F-FDG and 3'-Deoxy-3'-^{18}F-Fluorothymidine PET tumor volume measurements. J. Nucl. Med. 51(9), 1368–1376 (2010)
8. Hatt, M., Le Rest, C.C., Descourt, P., Dekker, A., Ruyssscher, D.D., Oellers, M., Lambin, P., Pradier, O., Visvikis, D.: Accurate automatic delineation of heterogeneous functional volumes in positron emission tomography for oncology applications. Int. J. Radiation Oncology 77(1), 301–308 (2010)
9. Hudson, H.M., Larkin, R.S.: Accelerated image reconstruction using ordered subsets of projection data. IEEE Trans. Med. Imag. 13(4), 601–609 (1994)
10. Reilhac, A., Lartizien, C., Costes, N., Sans, S., Comtat, C., Gunn, R.N., Evans, A.C.: PET-SORTEO: A Monte Carlo-based simulator with high count rate capabilities. IEEE Trans. Nucl. Sci. 51(1), 46–52 (2004)
11. Segars, W.P.: Development of a new dynamic NURBS-based cardiac-torso (NCAT) phantom. PhD Dissertation, The University of North Carolina (2001)
12. Wahl, R.L., Jacene, H., Kasamon, Y., Lodge, M.A.: From RECIST to PERCIST: evolving considerations for PET response criteria in solid tumors. J. Nucl. Med. 50(suppl. 1), 122S–150S (2009)

Structure and Context in Prostatic Gland Segmentation and Classification

Kien Nguyen[1], Anindya Sarkar[2], and Anil K. Jain[1]

[1] Michigan State Unversity, East Lansing, MI 48824, USA
[2] Ventana Medical Systems, Inc., Sunnyvale, CA 94085, USA
{nguye231,jain}@cse.msu.edu, anindya.sarkar@ventana.roche.com

Abstract. A novel gland segmentation and classification scheme applied to an H&E histology image of the prostate tissue is proposed. For gland segmentation, we associate appropriate nuclei objects with each lumen object to create a gland segment. We further extract 22 features to describe the structural information and contextual information for each segment. These features are used to classify a gland segment into one of the three classes: artifact, normal gland and cancer gland. On a dataset of 48 images at 5× magnification (which includes 525 artifacts, 931 normal glands and 1,375 cancer glands), we achieved the following classification accuracies: 93% for artifacts v. true glands; 79% for normal v. cancer glands, and 77% for discriminating all three classes. The proposed method outperforms state of the art methods in terms of segmentation and classification accuracies and computational efficiency.

1 Introduction

In detecting prostate cancer on a digitized tissue slide, the pathologist relies on: (i) structural information; glands in a cancer region (cancer glands) appear to have structural properties (e.g. nuclei abundance, lumen size) different from glands in a normal region (normal glands) and (ii) contextual information; cancer glands typically cluster into groups and are of similar shape and size[1], while shape and size of normal glands vary widely. These two sources of information can be observed in Fig. 1b. Hence, a reasonable approach to assist a pathologist in finding cancer regions includes segmenting out glandular regions, examining their structural and contextual information and finally classifying them.

The cancer detection problem in prostate tissue images has been studied in the literature. Monaco et al. [2] (Table 1) segmented glands and classified individual glands into normal or cancer by (i) using gland size feature to assign initial gland labels and (ii) applying a probabilistic pairwise Markov model (PPMM) to update gland labels. On the other hand, Nguyen et al. [3] and Doyle et al. [4] detected cancer regions by classifying individual image patches and image pixels, respectively, by using a combination of cytological and textural features [3],

---

[1] It was also mentioned in [1] that cancer glands tend to appear close to other cancer glands, which is a biological motivation for this contextual information.

N. Ayache et al. (Eds.): MICCAI 2012, Part I, LNCS 7510, pp. 115–123, 2012.

or textural features alone [4]. Unlike [2,3,4], other studies focused on the tissue image classification problem, i.e. they classified every prostatic tissue image (which is a region in the whole slide tissue) into normal or cancer or into different cancer grades. This problem was addressed by either segmentation-based approaches [5,6] (Table 1) or texture-based approaches [7,8,9].

Table 1. Studies on gland segmentation and gland feature extraction reported in the literature. Note that each study used a different database.

Study	Segmentation algorithm	Gland feature	Use of context	Final goal	Dataset
Monaco et al. [2]	Region growing	Gland size	PPMM method	Detect cancer regions	40 images at 1.23×
Peng et al. [5]	Region growing	Gland size	No	Classify tissue images	62 images at 100×
Naik et al. [6]	Level set	Shape features of lumen and gland	No	Classify tissue images	44 images at 40×
Proposed method	Nuclei lumen association	Structural features	Contextual features	Classify glands	48 images at 5×

Similar to [6], we also address artifacts[2] (Fig. 1c) in this paper by including them into the gland classification step, leading to a three-class classification problem: artifact, normal gland and cancer gland. The contributions of the paper include: (i) The proposed segmentation algorithm is computationally efficient and is able to successfully segment out appropriate gland regions, (ii) we explore features related to nuclei which are distinctive for classification, (iii) we introduce robust features to capture contextual information of a gland.

2   Gland Segmentation

Gland Structure: A gland consists of nuclei, cytoplasm and lumen (Fig. 1c, [6], [9]). Hence, a gland segmentation algorithm should capture these components in the results. We achieve this goal by employing the following two steps.

Tissue Component Identification: For each image, we perform k-means clustering algorithm ($k = 4$) in the RGB color space of 10,000 randomly selected pixels (Fig. 1d) to find 4 cluster centers. By finding the nearest cluster center, each pixel in the image is assigned a label corresponding to one of the 4 tissue components (stroma, nuclei, cytoplasm and lumen). We apply a connected component algorithm [10] on nuclei pixels and lumen pixels to generate nuclei objects and lumen objects, respectively, which are used for segmentation. Since the colors of nuclei and lumen are quite salient, the k-means algorithm on RGB space is sufficient to identify them despite the intensity variation among images.

---

[2] The term "artifact" denotes broken tissue areas, and has been used in [9].

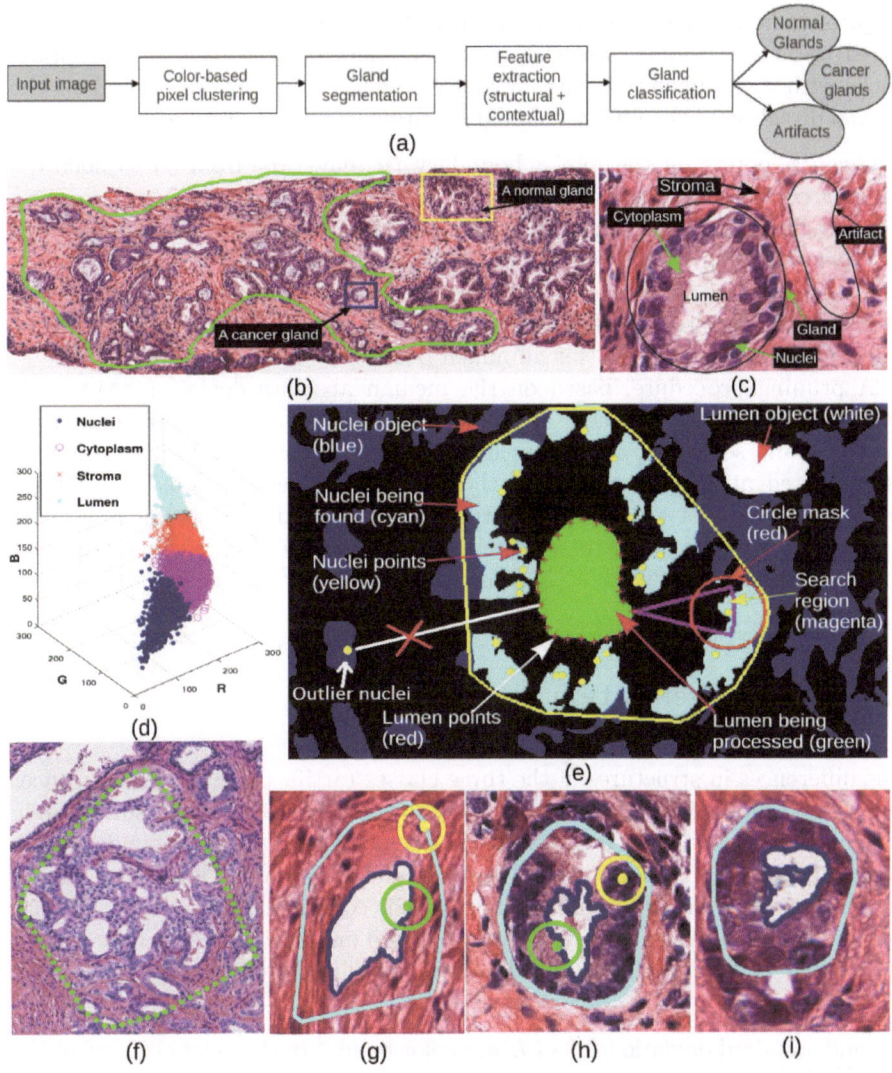

Fig. 1. The proposed method for gland segmentation and classification. (a) Flowchart. (b) Input image showing the cancer glands in a cancer region annotated by a pathologist (**green contour**); normal glands are present in the region outside the green contour. (c) A gland with basic components (nuclei, cytoplasm and lumen) and an artifact. (d) Clustering result of the image pixels in the *RGB* color space. (e) The gland segmentation process, where the segmentation result is depicted by a convex hull enclosing the detected nuclei. (f) Glands are assigned into a group (dotted contour) to compute contextual features. Segmentation results for three classes of interest: (g) Artifact, (h) normal gland and (i) cancer gland. Green and yellow circles in (g), (h) denote the neighborhood of a lumen point and a nuclei point, respectively.

Segmentation Algorithm. The proposed algorithm (Fig. 1e), which is referred to as nuclei-lumen association (NLA) algorithm, associates appropriate nuclei with each lumen to create a gland segment. Nuclei are searched along the normal direction of the lumen boundary contour. The algorithm has three steps:

1. Given n points on the lumen boundary (n may vary from 30 to 3000 depending on the lumen size), by considering the trade-off between a sparse (for computational efficiency) and dense set (adequate search coverage), we sample $n/3$ points uniformly, and refer to them as lumen points.
2. A search region, of a conical shape, centered at each lumen point, is expanded to find nuclei. A circle mask is used to limit nuclei regions to be merged to the gland. This step is repeated for all lumen points.
3. A pruning procedure, based on the median absolute deviation (MAD), is applied to remove outlier nuclei and generate smoother segmentation boundary[3]. Besides gland segments, the algorithm also produces a set of points located at the detected nuclei, referred to as the nuclei point set. The nuclei point set and lumen point set are used for feature extraction. Although some non-gland segments created by artifacts are present (Fig. 1g), we do not detect them at this step. Instead, we will identify them in the classification procedure.

3   Gland Classification

The differences in structures of the three classes (artifact, normal gland, cancer gland) are as follows. An artifact (Fig. 1g) does not have cytoplasm surrounding the lumen and has very few associated nuclei. Nuclei on the boundary of a normal gland (Fig. 1h) are more abundant and have darker blue color than a cancer gland (Fig. 1i). Lumina of cancer glands commonly appear more circular and smaller than normal glands (Fig. 1b). Based on these differences, we extract the following four sets of *structural features*, including 19 features, for each gland:

1. **Set 1 (8 nuclei features)**: For each nuclei point (NP), we compute the mean (μ) and standard deviation (σ) of L, a, b color bands[4] in the neighborhood of NP (Ω_{NP}). In addition, we compute μ and σ of percentage of Ω_{NP} that contains nuclei pixels, i.e. nuclei abundance on the gland boundary and its variation. Ω_{NP} is a circular region centered at NP (yellow circle in Fig. 1g, 1h), and has a radius R_{NP}. Since cancer glands usually have one nuclei layer (NL) on the boundary, while normal glands have more than one NL (mostly 2 NL), we choose $R_{NP} = 10$ pixels, which corresponds to the 2-NL thickness (the diameter of a nucleus is

---

[3] MAD = $\text{median}_i(|d_i - \text{median}_j(d_j)|)$, where d is the distance between a lumen point and a nuclei point. A nuclei point k with $d_k > 3\sigma + mean(d)$ ($\sigma = 1.48MAD$) is considered an outlier and being discarded. All pixel distances (used in the paper) can be converted to physical distances when the magnification is known.

[4] The *Lab* color space, which separates luminance and chrominance, is suitable to describe the color intensity of the tissue components.

approximately 5 pixels in $5\times$ images). Hence, Ω_{NP} is sufficient to capture most nuclei of the gland, while excluding nuclei of neighbor glands.

2. **Set 2 (6 cytoplasm features)**: For each lumen point (LP), we compute μ and σ of L, a, b color bands in the neighborhood of LP (Ω_{LP}). Ω_{LP} is a circular region (green circle in Fig. 1g, 1h), which is centered at LP and excludes lumen area. The radius of Ω_{LP} is the distance between LP and the corresponding NP. Hence, in a true gland segment, Ω_{LP} mostly contains cytoplasm.

3. **Set 3 (3 lumen shape features)**: Area, solidity (ratio of the lumen area to its convex hull area) and circularity ($(4\pi\text{area})/\text{perimeter}^2$) of the lumen.

4. **Set 4 (2 global features)**: μ and σ of the distance between a LP and a NP.

To explore contextual information, we first assign gland segments into groups (Fig. 1f) by using the connected component (CC) algorithm in graph theory. Let $\{Lu^i\}_{i=1}^n$ denote the n lumen objects used to represent n gland segments, and let $(Lu_{x_o}^i, Lu_{y_o}^i)$ denote the centroid of Lu^i. A graph is built where each node is a gland. If $\|(Lu_{x_o}^i - Lu_{x_o}^j, Lu_{y_o}^i - Lu_{y_o}^j)\| < t_d,$[5] there is an edge connecting Lu^i and Lu^j. Each CC is considered a group of gland. So groups are disjoint and the grouping is unique. Once groups are formed, we compute the following 3 *contextual features* for each gland segment Lu^i (which belongs to group O):

1. **Neighborhood crowdedness**: $|O|$ or the no. of elements in O.

2. **Shape similarity**: $\frac{1}{|O|}\sum_{j=1}^{|O|} \|LV_i - LV_j\|$, where LV denotes the 3-dimensional lumen shape feature vector described above.

3. **Size similarity**: $\frac{1}{|O|}\sum_{j=1}^{|O|} \frac{min(|Lu^i|,|Lu^j|)}{max(|Lu^i|,|Lu^j|)}$, where $|Lu|$ denotes the lumen size.

Finally, each gland segment can be represented by a full feature vector of dimensionality 22 (19 + 3). We use a SVM classifier (linear kernel, C = 1) with this feature vector to classify the gland segment[6].

4   Experiments

a. Data Set: The dataset includes 48 images at $5\times$ magnification (average image size is $900 \times 1,500$ pixels), which come from 20 patients. Glands in images of the same patient still have very large variability in structures. Given the pathologist's annotation on each image, we manually label 525 artifacts, 931 normal glands and 1,375 cancer glands to form the (ground truth) gland dataset. We also implemented the methods in [2] and [6] to compare them with the proposed method. Since all three methods perform segmentation by starting at the same

---

[5] We choose $t_d = 65$, which minimizes the cross validation error in classifying the 3 different gland types. However, when minimizing the training error on an independent training set, we also obtain $t_d = 65$.

[6] The code for gland segmentation and feature extraction, along with the details of the experiments can be found at www.cse.msu.edu/~nguye231/GlandSegClass.html

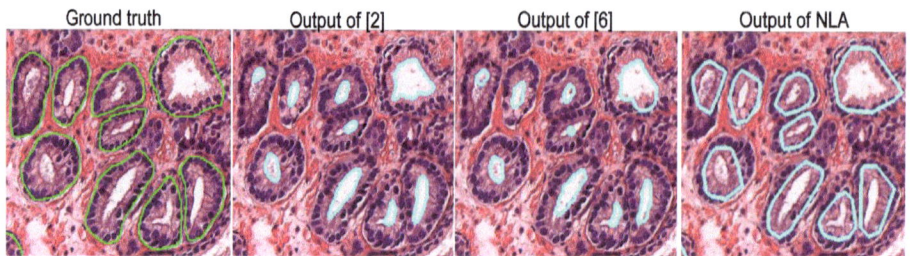

Fig. 2. Comparison of the NLA algorithm with [2] and [6] for gland segmentation. Glands are segmented more completely by the NLA algorithm

Table 2. Gland classification accuracies (s.d.) for the method in [6], method in [2], SVM-SF, PPMM-SF, PPMM-SCF, and SVM-SCF by cross validation

Classification problem	Method in [6]	Method in [2]	SVM-SF	PPMM-SF	PPMM-SCF	SVM-SCF
Artifact v. true gland	0.78 (0.09)	-	0.93 (0.03)	0.93 (0.06)	0.93 (0.04)	**0.93** (0.04)
Normal v. cancer	0.67 (0.13)	0.68 (0.13)	0.75 (0.07)	0.73 (0.11)	0.75 (0.11)	**0.79** (0.08)
All three classes	0.54 (0.12)	-	0.74 (0.06)	0.75 (0.10)	0.73 (0.08)	**0.77** (0.07)

lumen objects (identified in section 2), and use the same ground truth (which is not affected by lumen objects), the comparison is unbiased.

b. Gland Segmentation Evaluation: We manually select 309 glands whose boundaries are well-defined, and create segmentation ground truth for each gland (G_i^0) by outlining its area. We use the Jaccard Index (JI) to evaluate the output of a segmentation algorithm. Given a gland segment G_i^m produced by the algorithm m for the ith gland (with ground truth G_i^0), JI is computed as $J(G_i^0, G_i^m) = |G_i^0 \cap G_i^m|/|G_i^0 \cup G_i^m|$. Higher JI values (range is [0,1]) indicate better segmentation results. *The average JI value per gland segment obtained by the algorithms in [2], [6] and the proposed NLA algorithm are 0.31, 0.43 and 0.66, respectively.* Since the NLA algorithm aims at detecting nuclei surrounding the lumen (while the algorithms in [2] and [6] mostly detect lumen and cytoplasm), it segments more complete gland regions than [2] and [6] (Fig. 2). The computational complexity of the three segmentation algorithms is measured by their running time on a 369×1213 image, containing 64 glands. *The total computation time of [2], [6] and the NLA algorithm for the image are 242.0s, 256.5s and 2.7s, respectively (all algorithms, implemented in Matlab, were run on a 2.93GHz machine with 16GB memory).* While the NLA algorithm processes pixels by only considering their labels (see Fig. 1d and section 2), the algorithms in [2] and [6] perform complicated operations on the grayscale intensities of the pixels. More precisely, the level set algorithm [6] needs to iteratively evolve a zero level curve by minimizing both the internal energy and the external energy of the curve,

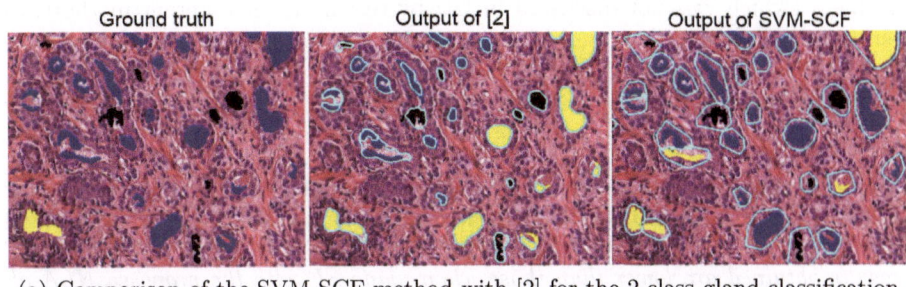

(a) Comparison of the SVM-SCF method with [2] for the 2-class gland classification

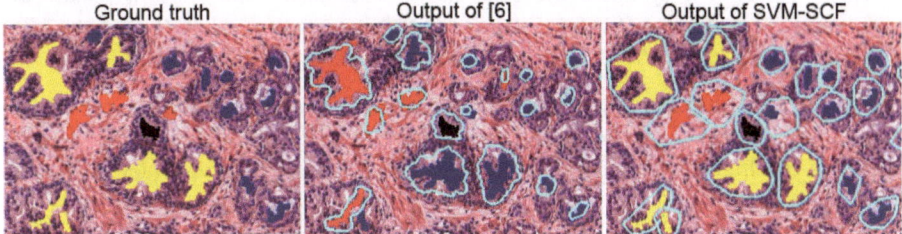

(b) Comparison of the SVM-SCF method with [6] for the 3-class gland classification

Fig. 3. Gland classification comparison. Cyan contours denote segmentation results, and color of the lumen corresponds to gland label (black, red, yellow and blue denote non-labeled glands, artifacts, normal glands and cancer glands, respectively)

and the region growing algorithm [2] needs to, at every step, add one pixel to the growing region and recompute the boundary strength of the region. Hence, the NLA algorithm is better than [2] and [6] in both accuracy and complexity.

c. Gland Classification Evaluation: We perform a 10-fold cross validation on the gland dataset, and report the average classification accuracy. First, we solve the two 2-class classification problems, i.e. (i) artifacts v. true glands and (ii) normal glands v. cancer glands. Next, we perform the 3-class classification by combining the previous two 2-class classification problems in a hierarchical fashion. In Table 2, besides the methods in [6], [2] and the proposed method (denoted by SVM-SCF, i.e. applying SVM classifier on the structural-contextual features (SCF)), we also report the results of the SVM-SF method (applying SVM classifier on the structural features (SF)), the results of the PPMM-SF method (applying the PPMM (Table 1) on the SF), and the results of the PPMM-SCF method (applying the PPMM on the SCF). Since artifacts were not addressed in [2], we only report normal v. cancer result for this method.

From Table 2, we can see that: (i) The SVM-SCF method obtains the highest accuracy, (ii) the superior performance of PPMM-SF over [2] shows that the SF are robust, and (iii) it is better to use SCF with SVM classifier than with PPMM. A drawback of the PPMM is that it requires a density estimation $p(y|x)$ (y is the feature vector, and x is the class label), which is difficult when y is high dimensional like the SF or SCF. Here, we address this "curse of dimensionality" problem (which was not discussed in [2]) by testing three different methods to estimate $p(y|x)$, i.e. (i) parzen window density estimator (PWDS), Naive Bayes model with assumption that each feature follows a (ii) Gaussian distribution, and (iii) Gamma distribution. The best results among them are obtained by PWDS, which are reported in Table 2 (columns 5 and 6).

The Role of Segmentation: To evaluate how segmentation results affect classification results, we extract the proposed SF of the gland segments resulted from the level set algorithm in [6], and perform classification using these features. *The results obtained are lower than those when using SF with the proposed NLA algorithm (column 4 of Table 2). This shows that good segmentation results are necessary for good classification results, as we discuss in section 4b that the NLA algorithm performs better than the level set algorithm in [6].*

Feature Weight: By applying linear SVM to compute weights for all 22 features, we observe that the nuclei abundance (on the gland boundary) feature receives the highest weight. This shows the important role of nuclei in classification.

Classifier Selection: We also conduct experiments using other classifiers such as: Neural Network, KNN, and Adaboost. However, the accuracies obtained by those classifiers were lower than SVM. Moreover, performing classification by a linear SVM is fast while the time-consuming training part is an offline process.

5   Conclusions and Future Work

We have presented a novel method to segment and classify glands in a prostate histology image. The proposed method outperforms state of the art methods for both gland segmentation and classification. The detected cancer glands can facilitate the Gleason scoring task performed by either a pathologist or an automated system. Since the proposed segmentation algorithm relies on lumen, it is not applicable to regions with occluded lumina. However, occluded lumina are seldom observed in prostate tissue images. In our future work, we will address this limitation. Moreover, we will improve the accuracy of the normal v. cancer glands classification by further research on contextual information, and textural information of the glands.

References

1. Kumar, V., Abbas, A., Fausto, N.: Robbins and Cotran Pathologic Basis of Disease. Saunders (2004)
2. Monaco, J., Tomaszewski, J., Feldman, M., Hagemann, I., Moradi, et al.: High-throughput detection of prostate cancer in histological sections using probabilistic pairwise markov models. Medical Image Analysis 14, 617–629 (2010)
3. Nguyen, K., Jain, A., Sabata, B.: Prostate cancer detection: Fusion of cytological and textural features. Journal of Pathology Informatics 2, 2–3 (2011)

4. Doyle, S., Feldman, M., Tomaszewski, J., Madabhushi, A.: A boosted Bayesian multi-resolution classifier for prostate cancer detection from digitized needle biopsies. IEEE Trans. Biomed. Eng. 59, 1205–1218 (2012)
5. Peng, Y., Jiang, Y., Eisengart, L., et al.: Segmentation of prostatic glands in histology images. In: IEEE Int. Symp. on Biomedical Imaging, pp. 2091–2094 (2011)
6. Naik, S., Doyle, S., Madabhushi, A., Tomaszewski, J., et al.: Automated gland segmentation and Gleason grading of prostate histology by integrating low-, high-level and domain specific information. In: MIAAB Workshop, Piscataway, NJ (2007)
7. Yoon, H.J., Li, C.C., Christudass, C., Veltri, R., et al.: Cardinal multiridgelet-based prostate cancer histological image classification for Gleason grading. In: IEEE Int. Conf. Bioinformatics and Biomedicine, pp. 315–320 (2011)
8. Khouzani, K.J., Zadeh, H.S.: Multiwavelet grading of pathological images of prostate. IEEE Trans. Biomed. Eng. 50, 697–704 (2003)
9. Tabesh, A., Teverovskiy, M., et al.: Multifeature prostate cancer diagnosis and gleason grading of histological images. IEEE Trans. Med. Img. 26, 1366–1378 (2007)
10. Haralick, R., Shapiro, L.: Computer and robot vision, vol. 2, pp. 28–48. Addison-Wesley (1992)

Quantitative Characterization
of Trabecular Bone Micro-architecture
Using Tensor Scale and Multi-Detector CT Imaging

Yinxiao Liu, Punam K. Saha, and Ziyue Xu

Iowa Institute of Biomedical Imaging, Departments of ECE and Radiology
University of Iowa, Iowa City, IA, US 52242
{yinxiao-liu,punam-saha,ziyue-xu}@uiowa.edu

Abstract. Osteoporosis, characterized by low bone mineral density (BMD) and micro-architectural deterioration of trabecular bone (TB), increases risk of fractures associated with substantial morbidity, mortality, and financial costs. A quantitative measure of TB micro-architecture with high reproducibility, large between-subjects variability and strong association with bone strength that may be computed via *in vivo* imaging would be an important indicator of bone quality for clinical trials evaluating fracture risks under different clinical conditions. Previously, the notion of tensor scale (t-scale) was introduced using an ellipsoidal model that yields a unified representation of structure size, orientation and anisotropy. Here, we develop a new 3-D t-scale algorithm for fuzzy objects and investigate its application to compute quantitative measures characterizing TB micro-architecture acquired by *in vivo* multi-row detector CT (MD-CT) imaging. Specifically, new measures characterizing individual trabeculae on the continuum of a perfect plate and a perfect rod and their orientation are directly computed in a volumetric BMD representation of a TB network. Reproducibility of these measures is evaluated using repeat MD-CT scans and also by comparing their correlation between MD-CT and μ-CT imaging. Experimental results have demonstrated that the t-scale-based TB micro-architectural measures are highly reproducible with strong association of their values at MD-CT and μ-CT resolutions. Results of an experimental mechanical study have proved these measures' ability to predict TB's bone strength.

Keywords: Trabecular bone, structural micro-architecture, quantitative geometry, tensor scale, skeletonization, CT imaging, biomechanics.

1   Introduction

Osteoporosis increases risk of fractures associated with substantial morbidity, mortality, and financial costs. Approximately, 30% of postmenopausal white women in the United States suffer from osteoporosis [1] and the prevalence in Europe and Asia is similar. Approximately one in two women and one in four men over age 50 will have an osteoporosis-related fracture in their remaining lifetime. Clinically, osteoporosis is defined by low bone mineral density (BMD). However, increasing evidence suggests that micro-architectural quality of trabecular bone (TB) is an important determinant of

N. Ayache et al. (Eds.): MICCAI 2012, Part I, LNCS 7510, pp. 124–131, 2012.
© Springer-Verlag Berlin Heidelberg 2012

bone strength and fracture risk [2-5]. BMD only explains about 65% to 75% of the variance in bone strength [6,7], while the remaining variance is due to the cumulative and synergistic effect of various factors including bone macro- and micro-architecture, tissue composition, and micro-damage [8,9]. Therefore, a quantitative measure of TB micro-architecture with high reproducibility, large between-subjects variability and strong association with bone strength that may be computed via *in vivo* imaging would be an important indicator of bone quality for clinical trials evaluating fracture risks under different clinical conditions.

Saha *et al.* developed digital topological analysis (DTA) [10,11]which classifies surfaces (plates), curves (rods), junctions, and edges in a skeletal representation of a TB network using local topological parameters [10,12,13]. Although DTA is widely applied [5,6,14,15], a major limitation of the method is that resulting classifications are inherently discrete failing to distinguish between narrow and wide plates. Later, Saha *et al.* developed volumetric topological analysis algorithm (VTA) [16] characterizing the topology of individual trabeculae on the continuum between a perfect plate and a perfect rod. Although VTA provides an effective measure of TB micro-architecture, its premise is built on digital topology and path propagation approaches and misses some important information related to structure orientation and anisotropy.

Here, a simultaneous solution to estimate TB plateness/rodness and orientation is presented using a geometric approach of representing local structures with tensor scale (t-scale) [17]; initial results of application of t-scale in TB micro-architectural analyses were reported in [18]. T-scale provides a parametric representation of local structures using an ellipsoidal model. A new 3-D t-scale algorithm is developed for fuzzy objects and its application is studied to characterize TB micro-architecture acquired by *in vivo* multi-row detector CT (MD-CT) imaging. Other applications of t-scale may include assessment of vessel and airway wall geometry and detection and segmention of lung fissures in pulmonary CT imaging, and also, assessment of gyri and polyps geomtery in neuro-imaging and in virtyal colonoscopy, respectively. In the following section, we briefly present the algorithms for computation of t-scale and TB measures which will be followed by description of experimental plans and methods. Finally, we discuss the results and draw our conclusion.

2   Methods and Algorithms

2.1   3-D T-Scale Computation

T-scale-based quantitative micro-architectural assessment algorithm may be applied on fuzzy representation of an object where the membership value at each image voxel is interpreted as local object content or density. Here, we intend to apply the algorithm on TB bone images where the value at each voxel p represents the bone mineral content (BMC) at p and is denoted by $BMC(p)$. In the rest of this section, fuzzy membership and BMC will be used synonymously. T-scale computation is performed by locally tracing an object along m pairs of mutually opposite sample lines selected at an approximately uniform distribution over the entire 3-D angular space ensuring that the final t-scale is not skewed in any direction. Here, we have used 22.5^o of angular interval between every two neighboring sample lines. Interval length between two successive sample points on each sample line is chosen equal to image voxel resolution. The extent of a fuzzy object along an individual sample line is determined by tracing the first sample points where the interpolated membership value is zero and an edge point is located at that sample point location. These edge points are intended to roughly describe the boundary of the t-scale ellipse centered at the candidate voxel, denoted as p. Following the axial symmetry of an ellipse, for each pair of opposite sample lines, the edge points are repositioned so that each pair of two edge points on the opposite direction are equidistant from the center point p. Finally, an ellipsoid is fit to those repositioned edge points; in the rest of this section, "edge point" will refer to "repositioned edge point". The literature on ellipsoid fitting is quite mature where, essentially, an error between the observed data (here, the edge points) and the computed ellipsoid is minimized. Here, the geometric distance error is used and the algorithm is summarized as follows.

Step 1. Translate all edge points to move the candidate point p at the origin.
Step 2. Apply principle component analysis (PCA) to edge points computing eigenvectors ($\mathbf{i}_1$, $\mathbf{i}_2$, $\mathbf{i}_3$) and eigenvalues (λ_1, λ_2, λ_3) of the point-distribution.
Step 3. Rotate the edge points to align $\mathbf{i}_1$, $\mathbf{i}_2$ and $\mathbf{i}_3$ with the three coordinate axes.
Step 4. Determine the smallest box enclosing all edge points and use it to determine the initial guess for the best-fit ellipsoid.
Step 5. Compute the final ellipsoid by applying iterative minimization of the sum of geometric distance errors using the Newton's optimization algorithm.

See Fig. 1 for illustration of steps in t-scale computation; here, 2-D illustrations are used to improve the quality of presentation.

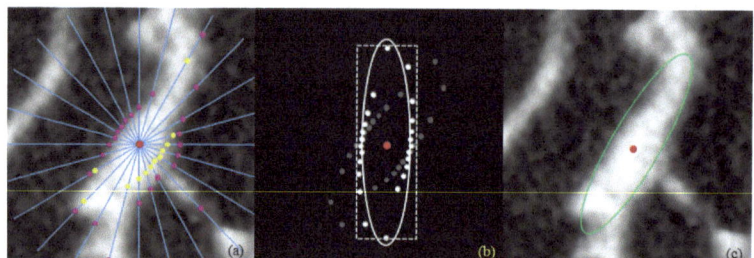

Fig. 1. Steps in t-scale computation. (a) Edge points (pink) on radial sample lines (blue) and repositioned edge points (yellow). (b) Bounding box (dotted) and the best-fit ellipse (grey) after rotating repositioned edge points (grey) using PCA. (c) Final t-scale ellipsoid (green).

2.2   Trabecular Bone Quality Analysis

As described in the previous section, t-scale produces three eigenvectors ($\mathbf{i}_1$, $\mathbf{i}_2$, $\mathbf{i}_3$) and corresponding eigenvalues (λ_1, λ_2, λ_3) parametrically representing local structures. The idea here is to use these parameters to characterize micro-architecture of individual trabeculae. Let $\mathbf{i}_j(p)$ and $\lambda_j(p)$, where $j = 1,2,3$, denote the three eigenvectors and eigenvalues, respectively, at a given TB voxel p. The local structure width at p, denoted by $TS_W(p)$, may be defined in the millimeter unit using the length of the second largest eigenvalue $\lambda_2(p)$ as shown in Fig. 2b; local structure measure using the VTA algorithm is presented in in Fig. 2c which has been thorough evaluated in [16]. The agreement of the TB width measures using the two different approaches as shown in Fig. 2b,c is encouraging. The motivation of investigating the t-scale method is two-folded – (1) t-scale computes the local structure width measure using a geometric approach as compared to the VTA method based on digital topology and path propagation and (2) simultaneous measures of local structure orientation and thickness. Here, we study the orientation measure of TB. The orientation of the structure, denoted by $TS_O(p)$, is defined by the cosine of the angle between the eigenvector $i_1(p)$ corresponding to the largest eigenvalue and the bone's longitudinal axis; color-coded illustration of the orientation measure is shown in Fig. 2e. As observed in the figure, the t-scale-based orientation measure successfully distinguishes between the longitudinal (green) and transverse (red) trabeculae. Also, the normalized plateness measure over the [0,1] interval, denoted by $TS_P(p)$, is classically defined using the anisotropy between the length of the second largest eigenvalue $\lambda_2(p)$ and the smallest eigenvalue $\lambda_3(p)$ as follows:

$$TS_P(p) = \sqrt{1 - (\lambda_3(p)/\lambda_2(p))^2}. \qquad (1)$$

It may be noted that the above plateness measure does not require threshold values as needed in VTA [16]. The normalized rodness measure $TS_R(p)$ is defined as:

$$TS_R(p) = 1 - TS_P(p). \qquad (2)$$

The above measures at an individual voxel location may be directly computed from its local t-scale. However, it can be shown that these measures suffer from edge artifacts when the target voxel is far from the skeleton due to the failure of covering the entire geometry of the local structure within its t-scale. Therefore, we define our algorithm as follows using an initialization and feature propagation approach.

1) Compute the surface skeleton S for the TB structure O where O is set of all voxels with nonzero BMC value.
2) For each voxel $p \in S$, initiate the TB measures values: $TS_W(p)$, $TS_O(p)$, $TS_P(p)$ and $TS_R(p)$ as defined above.
3) At each non-skeletal voxel $q \in O - S$, inherit the TB measures: $TS_W(q)$, $TS_O(q)$, $TS_P(q)$ and $TS_R(q)$ from the nearest skeletal voxel p using a feature propogation algorithm.

In the above steps, the surface skeletonization is computed using the algorithm by Saha et al. [19] and the noise removal procedure presented in [16]. The feauture propagation is accomplished using the classical algorithm introduced in [16]. Finally, the following TB measures are computed over a VOI V as a parameter representing the micro-architectural properties of the TB over V:

1. Bone mineral density: $BMD = \sum_{p \in V} BMC(p)/\|V\|$,
2. Surface width: $SW_{TS} = \sum_{p \in V} TS_W(p)BMC(p)/\sum_{p \in V} BMC(p)$,
3. Surface curve ratio: $SCR_{TS} = \sum_{p \in V} TS_P(p)BMC(p)/\sum_{p \in V} TS_R(p)BMC(p)$,
4. Longitude bone mineral density: $BMD_{Long} = \sum_{p \in V} TS_O(p)BMC(p)/\|V\|$,
5. Transverse bone mineral density: $BMD_{Tran} = \dfrac{\sum_{p \in V}(1 - TS_O(p))BMC(p)}{\|V\|}$.

3   Experimental Plans and Methods

The experiment was performed on 15 fresh-frozen human cadaveric ankle specimens harvested from 11 body donors. Six steps were performed on each ankle specimen in the following order – (1) MD-CT imaging, (2) Soft-tissue removal and tibia dislocation, (3) μ-CT imaging, (4) specimen preparation, (5) mechanical testing, and (6) image processing and computation of TB measurements. All ankle specimens were kept frozen until the performance of MD-CT imaging.

High resolution MD-CT scans of the distal tibia were acquired at the I-CLIC center, University of Iowa on a 128 slice SOMATOM Definition Flash scanner at 120 kV, 200 effective mAs, and reconstructed at 0.2 mm slice thickness using a special U70u kernel achieving high structural resolution. An INTable™ Calibration Phantom Couch Pad was scanned to calibrate CT Hounsfield units into BMC (mg/cm^3). Three repeat MD-CT scans of each distal tibia specimen were acquired after repositioning the specimen on the CT table before each scan. Each specimen was also scanned on an Imtek Micro-cat II scanner at 28.8μm isotropic resolution after removing soft tissue and dislocating tibia from the ankle joint.

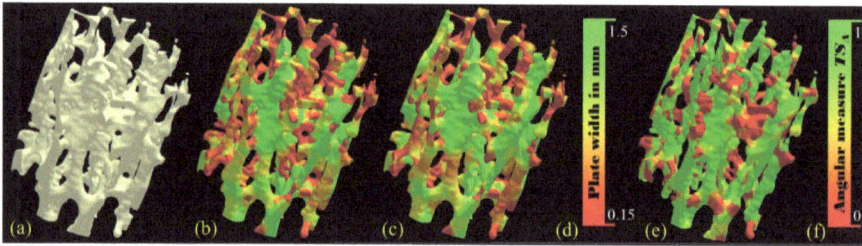

Fig. 2. Characterization of TB micro-architecture using the t-scale. (a) A TB region selected from μ-CT image of a human ankle specimen. (b,c) TB characterization on the continuum between a perfect plate (green) and a perfect rod (red) using the t-scale- VTA-based algorithms. (d) Color-coding for (b,c). (e) TB orientation analysis using t-scale. (f) Color-coding for (e).

To determine actual TB strength, a cylindrical TB core of nominally 8 mm in diameter and 20.9±3.3 mm in length were cored from distal tibia *in situ* along the proximal-distal direction. The TB cores were mechanically tested in compression using an electromechanical materials testing machine. To minimize specimen end effects, strain was measured with a 6 mm gage length extensometer attached directly to the midsection of the bone. A compressive preload of 10 N was applied and strains then set to zero. At a strain rate of 0.005 sec^{-1}, each specimen was preconditioned to a low strain with at least ten cycles and then loaded to failure. Yield stress was determined as the intersection of the stress-strain curve and a 0.2% strain offset of the modulus.

Finally, each TB MD-CT data was processed through the following cascade of image processing steps – (1) computation of bone mineral content or BMC image using a step-up ramp function, (2) re-sampling of BMC images at 0.15 mm isotropic voxel using the linear interpolation method, (3) do surface skeletonization and (4) application of t-scale to each skeleton and propagate back to TB volume. MD-CT Hounsfield number at each voxel was converted to a BMC (mg/cc) value using average MD-CT values in three calibration rods in the INTable™ Calibration Phantom at concentrations of 0, 75 and 150 mg/cc of calcium hydroxyapatite homogeneously (CaHA) blended into the CT-Water™ compound. For a μ-CT scan, bone volume fraction (BVF) image was used instead of BMC due to lack of a calibration phantom for μ-CT. Therefore, BV/TV was computed over a VOI instead of BMD.

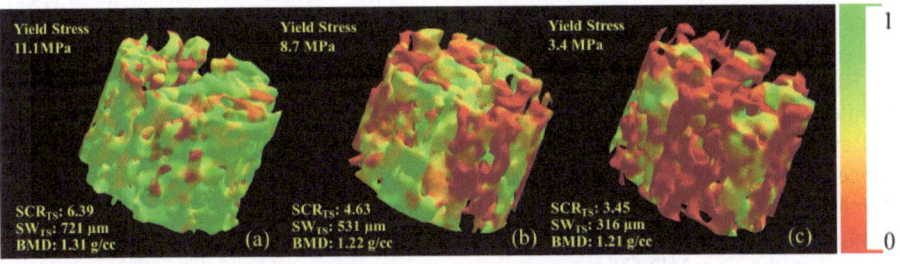

Fig. 3. Illustration of the t-scale plate measure for three different TB specimens – (a) strong (Yield stress: 11.1MPa), (b) moderate (7.1MPa) and (c) weak (3.4 MPa).

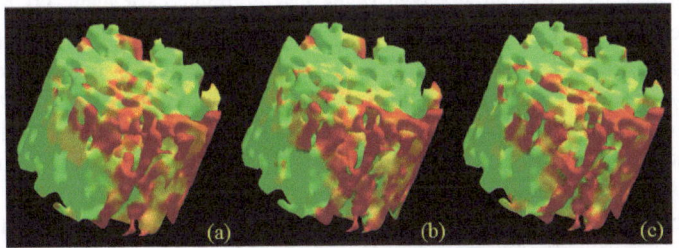

Fig. 4. Illustration of reproducibility for t-scale-based plateness classification of a TB specimen in three repeat MD-CT scans (a-c) shown using the same color coding scheme of   Fig. 3.

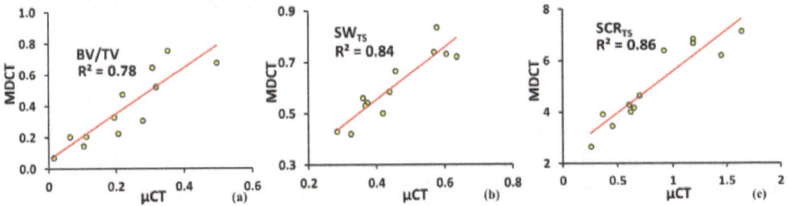

Fig. 5. Correlation of different TB measures, namely BV/TV (a), SW_{TS} (b) and SCR_{TS} (c), computed via MD-CT and μ-CT imaging.

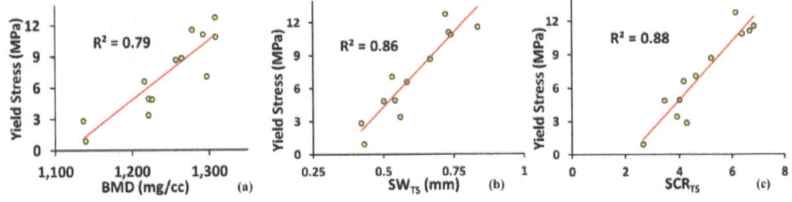

Fig. 6. Ability of different TB measures to predict bone strength shown in terms of R^2 values of linear correlation between Yield stress and each of BMD (a), SW_{TS} (b) and SCR_{TS} (c).

4   Results and Conclusion

Results of t-scale based classification of TB micro-architecture are illustrated in Fig. 2 and the plateness/rodness classification results are visually compared with VTA results. Results of t-scale-based plateness classification of TB network for three specimens with different experimental mechanical strengths are shown in Fig. 3. As shown in the figure, a 8% difference in BMD from a strong bone (a) to a weak bone (c) leads to 70% loss in bone strength and manifests into 60% difference in TB micro-architectural measure SCR_{TS} establishing its high sensitivity in bone degeneration.

Repeat scan MD-CT reproducibility of the method under *in vivo* condition was determined for BMD and all five t-scale measures. Color-coded illustration of t-scale plateness measure over a matching region in three repeat scans MD-CT data is shown in Fig. 4. For this study, ten spherical VOIs each of 3.75 mm radius were randomly selected in the first MD-CT scan of each specimen above the position 8mm proximal to the distal endplate leading to a total of 150 VOIs. Post-registration algorithm was used to locate the matching VOIs in the second and the third scans. Finally, the intra-class correlation (ICC) of three repeat scans was computed for each TB measure and the observed results are – (1) **BMD**: 0.997, (2) BMD_{Long}: 0.983, (3) BMD_{Tran}: 0.987, (4) SW_{VTA}: 0.966 and (5) SCR_{VTA}: 0.953. Although the two t-scale-based measures SW_{TS} SCR_{TS} have demonstrated slightly lower ICC values than the BMD measures, which are expected to be highly reproducible in CT imaging modality, the observed ICC values are satisfactory considering the fact that the measures were computed over small VOIs and less averaging of errors.

Linear correlations of three different TB measures derived from MD-CT and μ-CT imaging are graphically illustrated in Fig. 5. For these experiments, 15 VOIs were used from 15 specimens and same VOIs are used for correlation study with TB pressure experiments. The t-scale-based measure SCR_{TS} shows higher linear correlation between *in vivo* (MD-CT) and *ex vivo* (μ-CT) resolutions as compared to the BMD measure; note that BV/TV measure was used for μ-CT.

For correlation analysis with TB's experimental Yield stress, the image-based measures were computed over a cylindrical VOI with its axis aligned with that of distal tibia and its length and position were selected as per the data recorded during specimen preparation. The results of correlation analysis between Yield stress and different TB measures are shown in Fig. 6. Both t-scale measures have demonstrated better strength to predict TB's Yield stress as compared to BMD.

In this paper, we have developed a new 3-D t-scale algorithm for fuzzy object and have investigated its role in computing quantitative TB micro-architecture measures through MD-CT imaging under an *in vivo* condition. Results of an extensive study on fifteen cadaveric ankle specimens evaluating the new t-scale-based method are presented. Observed results have demonstration satisfactory repeat scan reproducibility of method. High correlation of t-scale measures derived via *in vivo* and *ex vivo* imaging modalities is observed. Also, t-scale-based TB micro-architectural measures have demonstrated higher ability to predict trabecular bone's experimental mechanical properties under an *in vivo* condition.

References

[1] Melton, 3rd.: Epidemiology of spinal osteoporosis. Spine 22, 2S–11S (1997)
[2] Benito, et al.: Deterioration of trabecular architecture in hypogonadal men. J. Clin. Endocr. Metab. 88, 1497–1502 (2003)
[3] Chesnut, 3rd., et al.: Effects of salmon calcitonin on trabecular microarchitecture as determined by magnetic resonance imaging:results from the QUEST study. J. Bone Miner. Res. 20, 1548–1561 (2005)
[4] Kleerekoper, et al.: The role of three-dimensional trabecular microstructure in the pathogenesis of vertebral compression fractures. Cal. Tis. Int. 37, 594–597 (1985)
[5] Wehrli, et al.: In vivo magnetic resonance detects rapid remodeling changes in the topology of the trabecular bone network after menopause and the protective effect of estradiol. J. Bone Miner. Res. 23, 730–740 (2008)
[6] Wehrli, et al.: Role of magnetic resonance for assessing structure and function of trabecular bone. Topics in Mag. Res. Imag. 13, 335–356 (2002)
[7] Ammann, et al.: Bone strength and its determinants. Osteoporos Int. 14, S13–S18 (2003)
[8] Chapurlat, et al.: Bone microdamage: a clinical perspective. Ost. Int. 20, 1299–1308 (2009)
[9] Seeman, et al.: Bone quality–the material and structural basis of bone strength and fragility. N. Engl. J. Med. 354, 2250–2261 (2006)
[10] Saha, Chaudhuri: 3D digital topology under binary transformation with applications. Comp. Vis. Image Und. 63, 418–429 (1996)
[11] Saha, et al.: Three-dimensional digital topological characterization of cancellous bone architecture. Int. J. Imag. Sys. Tech. 11, 81–90 (2000)
[12] Saha, Chaudhuri: Detection of 3D simple points for topology preserving transformation with application to thinning. IEEE TPAMI 16, 1028–1032 (1994)
[13] Saha, et al.: Topology preservation in 3D digital space. Pat. Rec. 27, 295–300 (1994)
[14] Liu, et al.: Individual trabecula segmentation (ITS)-based morphological analysis of microscale images of human tibial trabecular bone at limited spatial resolution. J. Bone Miner Res. 26, 2184–2193 (2011)
[15] Chang, et al.: Adaptations in trabecular bone microarchitecture in Olympic athletes determined by 7T MRI. J. Mag. Res. Imag. 27, 1089–1095 (2008)
[16] Saha, et al.: Volumetric topological analysis: a novel approach for trabecular bone classification on the continuum between plates and rods. IEEE TMI 29, 1821–1838 (2010)
[17] Saha: Tensor scale: a local morphometric parameter with applications to computer vision and image processing. Com. Vis. Imag. Und. 99, 384–413 (2005)
[18] Saha, et al.: In vivo assessment of trabecular bone architecture via three-dimensional tensor scale. In: SPIE, pp. 750–760 (2004)
[19] Saha, et al.: A new shape preserving parallel thinning algorithm for 3D digital images. Pat. Rec. 30, 1939–1955 (1997)

Genetic, Structural and Functional Imaging Biomarkers for Early Detection of Conversion from MCI to AD

Nikhil Singh, Angela Y. Wang, Preethi Sankaranarayanan,
P. Thomas Fletcher, and Sarang Joshi
for the Alzheimer's Disease Neuroimaging Initiative*

University of Utah, Salt Lake City, UT
nikhil@cs.utah.edu

Abstract. With the advent of advanced imaging techniques, genotyping, and methods to assess clinical and biological progression, there is a growing need for a unified framework that could exploit information available from multiple sources to aid diagnosis and the identification of early signs of Alzheimer's disease (AD). We propose a modeling strategy using supervised feature extraction to optimally combine high-dimensional imaging modalities with several other low-dimensional disease risk factors. The motivation is to discover new imaging biomarkers and use them in conjunction with other known biomarkers for prognosis of individuals at high risk of developing AD. Our framework also has the ability to assess the relative importance of imaging modalities for predicting AD conversion. We evaluate the proposed methodology on the Alzheimer's Disease Neuroimaging Initiative (ADNI) database to predict conversion of individuals with Mild Cognitive Impairment (MCI) to AD, only using information available at baseline.

1 Introduction

Mild cognitive impairment (MCI) is an intermediate stage between healthy aging and dementia. Patients diagnosed with MCI are at high risk of developing Alzheimer's disease (AD), but not everyone with MCI will convert. Accurate prognosis for MCI patients is an important prerequisite for providing the optimal treatment and management of the disease. The complex anatomical shape changes that occur during disease progression can be extracted from magnetic resonance images (MRI) of the brain. Decreased synaptic response and brain

---

* Data used in preparation of this article were obtained from the Alzheimer's Disease Neuroimaging Initiative (ADNI) database (adni.loni.ucla.edu). As such, the investigators within the ADNI contributed to the design and implementation of ADNI and/or provided data but did not participate in analysis or writing of this report. A complete listing of ADNI investigators can be found at: http://adni.loni.ucla.edu/wp-content/uploads/how_to_apply/ADNI_Acknowledgement_List.pdf

N. Ayache et al. (Eds.): MICCAI 2012, Part I, LNCS 7510, pp. 132–140, 2012.
© Springer-Verlag Berlin Heidelberg 2012

function can be measured using functional imaging modalities, such as $[^{18}F]$-fluorodeoxyglucose Positron Emission Tomography (FDG-PET). Additional potential risk biomarkers include blood and cerebrospinal fluid (CSF) markers, including genetic susceptibility assessed by apolipoprotein E (APOE) genotype and plaque deposition assessed by concentration of $A\beta$-42 and ptau$_{181}$. The challenge for predicting conversion is to combine these heterogeneous data sources, some of which are high-dimensional (MRI and PET) and some low-dimensional (clinical, CSF, APOE carrier), by selecting features that optimally weight the relative contribution from each modality.

Recent studies have examined the role of different classes of biomarkers, cognitive measures, and genetic risk factors either in combination with a single imaging modality or independently for predicting conversion from MCI to AD [1,2]. Weiner et. al [3] offer a comprehensive review of this ongoing research. Despite evidence for the predictive capability of individual biomarkers, cognitive measures, or neuroimaging data, relatively little attention has been given to combining information available from multiple imaging modalities with the biomarkers [4]. In one such study, Kohannim et. al [4] combine FDG-PET-derived numerical summaries, MRI-derived volume measures, CSF biomarkers, APOE genotype, and subject demographics for the task of discriminating MCI from AD. However, their work did not address prediction of conversion to AD.

In this article, we present a unified framework to combine the high-dimensional information available from multiple imaging modalities, anatomical shape atrophy (derived from MRI) and neuronal hypometabolism (derived from FDG-PET), with other low-dimensional biomarkers, such as APOE carrier status, $A\beta$-42 and ptau$_{181}$ concentration. We use Partial Least Squares as a supervised dimensionality-reduction technique to fuse the weighted combination of the two imaging modalities together with the clinical information. This data-driven formulation finds the optimal combination of these high-dimensional modalities that best characterize the disease progression. The focus of this work is to assess the combined predictive capability of this model for early detection of conversion of MCI to AD by using only the information available at baseline.

2   Methodology

We use the general framework of computational anatomy [5] to characterize the anatomical shape variation. Since the anatomical shape and neuronal metabolic activity are two separate measures obtained from independent imaging modalities, we combine the two to form a product space of the joint imaging modalities. To make pattern analysis robust, we propose a supervised dimensionality reduction to represent this high-dimensional data in terms of a few features, specifically selected to best explain factors relevant to dementia. Further, the extracted imaging features are used in conjunction with APOE genotype and/or CSF biomarkers for assessing the risk of conversion of an MCI individual to AD. Fig. 1 summarizes our feature selection and classification framework.

Anatomical Shape Variations—Deformation Momenta: We follow the now well-established framework of large deformation diffeomorphic

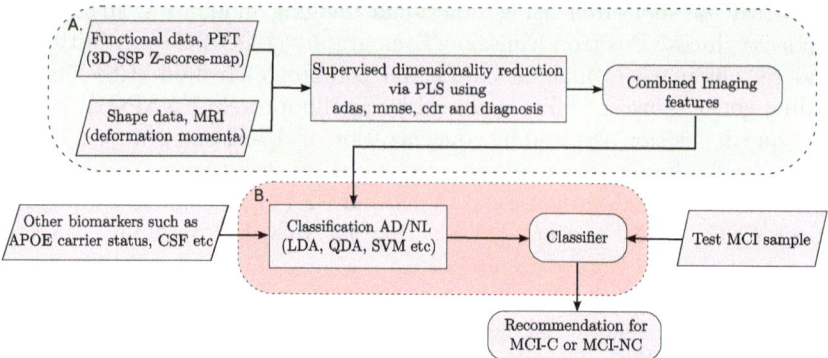

Fig. 1. MCI-C/MCI-NC prediction framework. Block A: Feature extraction process from high-dimensional imaging data. Block B: Classification.

transformations (LDDMM [5]) for capturing structural variation. A convenient and natural machinery for generating diffeomorphic transformations is by the integration of ordinary differential equations (ODE) on underlying coordinate space, Ω defined via the smooth time-indexed velocity vector fields $v(t, y) : (t \in [0, 1], y \in \Omega) \to \mathbb{R}^3$. The function $\phi^v(t, x)$ given by the solution of the ODE $\frac{dy}{dt} = v(t, y)$ with the initial condition $y(0) = x$ defines a diffeomorphism of Ω.

Following [6], we use a group-wise approach and build the mean population-based atlas, $\bar{I}$. We quantify the structural variability of the individual by registering the atlas to each image via estimating geodesic diffeomorphic transformations. Given a collection of anatomical images $\{I^i, i = 1, \cdots, N\}$, the minimum mean squared energy atlas construction problem is that of jointly estimating an image $\bar{I}$ and N individual deformations:

$$\bar{I} = \arg\min_{I, \phi_i} \frac{1}{N} \sum_{i=1}^{N} \int_{\Omega} ||I \circ \phi_i^{-1} - I^i||^2 dx + d(id, \phi_i)^2, \qquad (1)$$

where d is the Riemannian metric defined on the space of diffeomorphisms and id is the identity diffeomorphism. For each of the N LDDMM image matching problems the geodesic evolution are given in terms of deformation momenta, $\alpha^i(t)$, by:

$$v^i(t) + K \star \nabla I_t \alpha^i(t) = 0, \ \ \partial_t \alpha^i(t) + \nabla \cdot (\alpha^i(t) v^i(t)) = 0 \text{ and } \partial_t I_t + \nabla I_t \cdot v^i(t) = 0$$

where K is the kernel associated with the metric d. The second equation is the conservation of momenta while the third is the infinitesimal action of the velocity field, v on the image. This results in the estimate of N geodesics emanating from the atlas towards each image. The geodesic equations are completely determined via the scalar initial momenta, $\alpha^i(0)$ in the atlas space corresponding to each individual image deformation direction. The LDDMM image matching problem is solved using the iterative backward-integration based gradient descent algorithm. The gradient of the energy functional in (1) is expressed in terms of time-dependent Lagrangian multiplier or adjoint variables over the path of geodesics resulting in a set of adjoint equations (details in [7]).

FDG-PET Metabolism Activity—SSP: As the disease advances the progressive neurodegeneration is accompanied by reduced neuronal metabolism and increased synaptic dysfunction. This results in decreased uptake of $[^{18}F]$-fluorodeoxyglucose (FDG) measured by Positron Emission Tomography (PET) functional imaging. ADNI FDG-PET images are co-registered to the talaraich atlas space using Neurostat [8]. Peak pixel values are selected and 3D-stereotactic surface projection (3D-SSP) maps of glucose metabolism are computed relative to pons. Corresponding statistical maps of Z-scores, $p_i(i = 1, \cdots, N)$, are generated in comparison to cognitively normal control subjects ($\mu_{age} = 69.6 \pm 7.7$).

Combining Structure & Function: The shape space represented by the space of deformation momenta, $\mathcal{S}$, and the space of neuronal metabolic activity represented by 3D-SSP, $\mathcal{P}$, are both high-dimensional spaces. Since the anatomical shape and metabolic activity are two separate measures obtained from independent imaging modalities, we combine the two spaces to form a product space that defines the combined space of imaging modalities, $\mathcal{M}$ such that: $M = \mathcal{S} \times \mathcal{P}$. Inner product between a pair $m_i = (\alpha_i, p_i) \in \mathcal{M}$ and $m_j = (\alpha_j, p_j) \in \mathcal{M}$ is defined via a their convex combination as: $\langle m_i, m_j \rangle_{\mathcal{M}} = \eta \langle \alpha_i, \alpha_j \rangle_{\mathcal{S}} + (1 - \eta) \langle p_i, p_j \rangle_{\mathcal{P}}$. The factor, η is interpretable as a relative weight when both the modalaties are normalized to have unit variance.

Supervised Dimensionality Reduction via Partial Least Squares: The structural and functional information extracted from two imaging modalities results in a feature space with much higher dimension than the population size. Although classifiers utilizing kernel approaches such as Support Vector Machines (SVM) could work in the high-dimensional imaging feature space, for Linear Discriminant Analysis (LDA), dimensionality reduction has to be performed. We adopt a well known methodology for regression called Partial Least Squares (PLS) [9][10]. The Partial Least Squares can be interpreted as a supervised dimensionality reduction technique based on latent decomposition model. We adapt the PLS methodology for the purpose of extracting relevant features from the combination of shape and 3D-SSP data supervised by the clinical scores such as MMSE, ADAS, CDR and clinical cognitive status that are treated as global measures of dementia. We find directions $\hat{m}$ in the combined product space of imaging modalities, $\mathcal{M}$, and directions $\hat{y}$ in the clinical response space, $\mathcal{Y}$, that explain their association in the sense of their common variance. The projections of shape and pet data along the directions, $\hat{m}_i$ are treated as the features for the classifier. The PLS problem is given by:

$$\max \ \text{cov}(\langle \hat{m}, m^i \rangle, \langle \hat{y}, y^i \rangle) \text{ subject to } \|\hat{m}\| = 1 \ , \ \|\hat{y}\| = 1 \qquad (2)$$

The subsequent directions are found by removing the component extracted (deflating the data) both in space, $\mathcal{M}$ and the clinical response space, $\mathcal{Y}$ as:

$$m^i \leftarrow m^i - \langle \hat{m}, m^i \rangle_{\mathcal{M}} \hat{m} \text{ and } y^i \leftarrow y^i - \langle \hat{y}, y^i \rangle_{\mathcal{Y}} \hat{y}$$

The solution to this covariance maximization problem is the Singular Value Decomposition (SVD) of the cross covariance matrix. The corresponding direction vectors $\hat{m}$'s and $\hat{y}$'s are the respective left and right singular vectors. The maximum number of possible latent vectors are limited by the inherent dimensionality of the two spaces, i.e., by $\min(\dim(\mathcal{M}), \dim(\mathcal{Y}))$.

Note that the efficient implementations of solution to the PLS via SVD uses the Gram matrix of inner products of the data. If we denote the Gram matrix of momenta by G_S and that of 3D-SSP by G_P, the fused Gram matrix for the product space weighted by η can be written as: $G_M = \eta G_S + (1 - \eta)G_P$. The projection scores, thus obtained by PLS, have combined information of anatomical shape and glucose metabolic activity that is used as features together with low-dimensional modalities such as genetic biomarkers of APOE carrier status and/or CSF biomarker available from spinal tap tests.

APOE Carrier Status—Genetic Biomarker: A confirmed risk factor for Alzheimer's disease is the status of apolipoprotein E (APOE) gene in an individual. APOE exhibit polymorphisms with three major isomorphisms or alleles: APOE $\varepsilon 2$, APOE $\varepsilon 3$ and APOE $\varepsilon 4$. Majority of the population with late-onset of AD is found to be dominant in APOE $\varepsilon 4$ allele. APOE carrier status is computed based on the allele copy inherited from parents in an individual. We consider the binary status for APOE genetic risk based on whether the individual has at least one copy of allele $\varepsilon 4$ and treat those subjects as APOE-carrier.

Prediction of Conversion to AD: Distinguishing the probable convertors from the population of MCI is a binary classification problem. While there are several ways to look at this problem, we present here a formulation of the classifier supervised by the AD group and healthy control group (NL). In other words, the classifier is trained on the AD and NL but is used as a "recommender" for the test MCI subject. Based on the classification score obtained on the MCI subject, the prediction of the classifier is interpreted. We denote the test MCI subject as "AD-like" when the classifier recommends AD and treated as predicted MCI-C otherwise termed as "Stable-MCI" or predicted MCI-NC. The classifier accuracy is assessed by comparing the predicted MCI-C or MCI-NC status with the conversion status from the follow-up study for that test MCI subject. The proposed methodology is evaluated using the LDA, its quadratic variant–Quadratic Discriminant Analysis (QDA), and SVM as binary classifiers.

3   Results and Discussion

Data Preprocessing: All the baseline and screening T1 weighted, bias-field-corrected and N3 scaled structural Magnetic Resonance Images were downloaded from the Alzheimer's Disease Neuroimaging Initiative (ADNI) database. Preprocessing the MRI involved skull stripping and registration to talairach coordinates as a part of the ADNI preprocessing pipeline. Tissue-wise intensity normalization for white matter, gray matter, and cerebrospinal fluid was performed using the

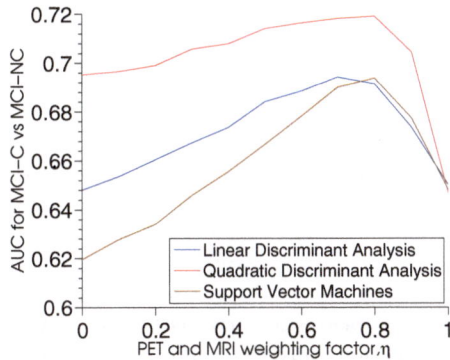

Fig. 2. Shape and PET weighting factor, η for different classifiers based on AUC

Table 1. ADNI data details

Diagnosis	54 Stable NL controls, 127 MCI, 61 AD
Education	$\mu = 15.27$ and $\sigma = 3.23$
Age	$\mu = 75.56$ and $\sigma = 6.65$
Gender	98 Females and 144 Males
Handedness	229 Right and 13 Left
APOE positive	13 NL's, 70 MCI's, 41 AD's
Follow-up	From baseline upto 48 months
MCI-C/NC status	54 out of 127 MCI converted to AD

Table 2. MCI-C vs. MCI-NC classification results for η_{OPT}

	AUC	Acc (%)	Sen(%)	Spec(%)	η
QDA	0.72	66.14	64.81	67.12	0.7
LDA	0.69	63.78	74.07	56.16	0.8
SVM	0.69	64.57	72.20	58.90	0.8

expectation maximization based segmentation followed by the piecewise polynomial histogram matching algorithm. The FDG-PET data was processed to get 3D-SSP as detailed in Section 2. The corresponding clinical test score, the CSF-biomarker data and the APOE genotype information were also retrieved. The baseline subjects that had all the clinical, APOE genotyping, FDG-PET imaging and MRI imaging data from the ADNI database comprised of a total of 242 individuals. Table 1 reports the details about the subject demographics, diagnosis, apoe carrier status and future conversion status.

To extract the anatomical shape features, the unbiased atlas, $\bar{I}$ is constructed from the preprocessed baseline MR brain images on the Graphical Processing Unit (GPU) [6]. The geodesics emanating from this estimated atlas towards each subject are estimated by warping $\bar{I}$ to each of the baseline subjects to give initial deformation momenta, $\alpha^i(0)(i = 1, \cdots, N)$ [7]. The corresponding 3D-stereotactic surface projection (3D-SSP) maps, $p_i(i = 0, \cdots, N)$, of glucose metabolism from FDG-PET are computed using Neurostat [8] to give Z-score maps. The supervised PLS dimensionality reduction is applied on combined imaging data of AD and NL subjects. Since the response is 4-D, the resulting feature space is 4-D and is represented by $\hat{m}_i$ $(i = 1, \cdots, 4)$. The imaging features are then combined together with low-dimensional biomarkers such as APOE carrier status to train the binary classifier for AD/NL classification.

The independent test MCI subject is projected into the shape and PET feature space defined by the training AD and NL group in terms of $\hat{m}_i$'s. The imaging

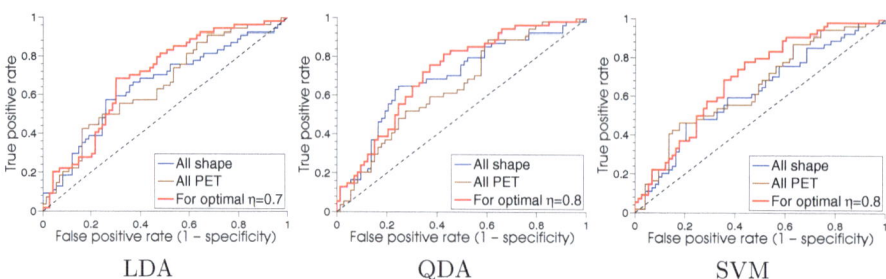

Fig. 3. Receiver operating characterstic curves (ROC) for MCI-C/MCI-NC classification with only shape information, only PET information and optimal combination of shape and PET as per η_{OPT}

features for the test MCI subject are combined with its APOE carrier status. The trained AD/NL-classifier's prediction on MCI baseline features is then used as a recommendation for future conversion to AD. Note that, for the test MCI subject, no clinical scores such as ADAS, MMSE, CDR or diagnostic information in any form is used during feature extraction from imaging data or classifier prediction. The accuracy of prediction is evaluated by comparing against the actual conversion status using the follow-up diagnosis data.

Fig. 2 shows area under the receiver operating characterstic curve (AUC) as a function of the weighting factor, η, for the three separate classifiers discriminating MCI-C vs MCI-NC. The accuracy of prediction of MCI to AD conversion and the associated η is given in Table 2. The reported numbers correspond to optimal η, based on AUC. QDA performed the best with accuracy of 66% and AUC of 0.72 at $\eta = 0.8$. Also, the optimal combination of PET and shape performed much better as compared to only using PET or anatomical shape information irrespective of the choice of classifier used (Fig. 3). Besides APOE carrier status, the above analysis was also done after adding log transformed CSF-biomarkers: $A\beta$-42 and ptau$_{181}$ concentration, which reduced the study sample-size to only: 29 NL, 36 AD and 59 MCI. With CSF-biomarkers, a slight increase in accuracy was observed for QDA: accuracy=68% and AUC= 0.72 ($\eta = 0.8$).

The log Jacobians of the deformation, overlayed on atlas image $\bar{I}$, resulting from evolving $\bar{I}$ along the geodesic represented by the classifier weights are shown in Fig. 4. The selected slices from this 3D overlay shown here capture relevant regions of the neuro-anatomical structures, such as hippocampus, pertinent to cognitive impairment in Alzheimer's and related dementia. Similarly, the PET classifier weights are translated back in the Z-score space of 3D-SSP (Fig. 5).

The major contribution of this article is the ability to extract, in order of relevance, the disease-characterizing patterns from multiple imaging modalities. The presented framework has broad applicability to data analysis studies involving heterogeneous data sources, both in terms of modalities and dimensions. We observed that the shape component dominated the model with up to 80% contribution compared to only 20% contribution from the PET component, irrespective of the classifier used. The spatial patterns of anatomical shape changes

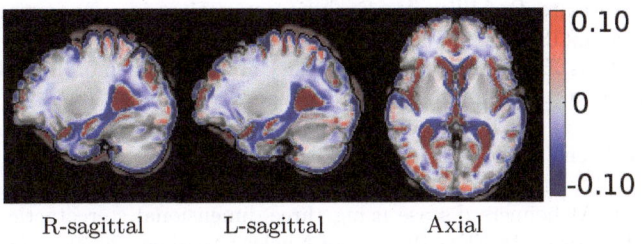

R-sagittal   L-sagittal   Axial

Fig. 4. Shape: Discriminating regions obtained from classifier weights for prediction of MCI conversion to AD. Log of Jacobians overlayed on atlas. Red denotes regions of local expansion and blue denotes regions of local contraction.

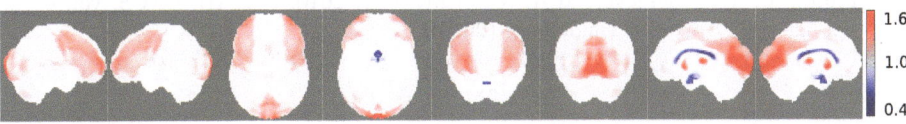

R-Lateral L-Lateral Superior   Inferior   Anterior Posterior R-Medial L-Medial

Fig. 5. FDG-PET: Discriminating regions obtained from classifier weights for prediction of MCI conversion to AD in 3D-SSP Z-score space.

were primarily the expansion of lateral ventricles and CSF, together with the shrinkage of the cortical surface.Another critical observation was the clearly evident shrinkage of the hippocampus and cortical and sub-cortical gray matter along the discriminating directions. Such patterns of atrophy are well known to characterize the disease progression in AD and related dementia.

Acknowledgements: Data collection and sharing for this project was funded by the Alzheimer's Disease Neuroimaging Initiative (ADNI) (NIH Grant U01 AG024904). The research in this paper was supported by NIH grant 5R01EB007688, the University of California, San Francisco (NIH grant P41 RR023953), NSF grant CNS-0751152), and NSF CAREER Grant 1054057.

References

1. Davatzikos, C., Bhatt, P., Shaw, L.M., Batmanghelich, K.N., Trojanowski, J.Q.: Prediction of MCI to AD conversion, via MRI, CSF biomarkers, and pattern classification. Neurobiology of Aging 32(12), 2322.e19–2322.e27 (2011)
2. Lemoine, B., Rayburn, S., Benton, R.: Data Fusion and Feature Selection for Alzheimer's Diagnosis. In: Yao, Y., Sun, R., Poggio, T., Liu, J., Zhong, N., Huang, J. (eds.) BI 2010. LNCS, vol. 6334, pp. 320–327. Springer, Heidelberg (2010)
3. Weiner, M.W., et al.: The Alzheimers Disease Neuroimaging Initiative: A review of papers published since its inception. Alzheimer's and Dementia, S1–S68 (2012)
4. Kohannim, O., et al.: Boosting power for clinical trials using classifiers based on multiple biomarkers. Neurobiology of Aging 31(8), 1429–1442 (2010)

5. Younes, L., Arrate, F., Miller, M.: Evolutions equations in computational anatomy. NeuroImage 45(1S1), 40–50 (2009)
6. Joshi, S., Davis, B., Jomier, M., Gerig, G.: Unbiased diffeomorphic atlas construction for computational anatomy. NeuroImage 23, 151–160 (2004)
7. Vialard, F.X., et al.: Diffeomorphic 3D image registration via geodesic shooting using an efficient adjoint calculation. IJCV, 1–13 (2011)
8. Minoshima, S., Frey, K.A., Koeppe, R.A., Foster, N.L., Kuhl, D.E.: A diagnostic approach in Alzheimers disease using three-dimensional stereotactic surface projections of Fluorine-18-FDG PET. J. of Nuclear Medicine 36(7), 1238–1248 (1995)
9. Bookstein, F.L.: Partial Least Squares: A dose-response model for measurement in the behavioral and brain sciences. Psycoloquy 5(23) (1994) (revised)
10. Singh, N., Fletcher, P.T., Preston, J.S., Ha, L., King, R., Marron, J.S., Wiener, M., Joshi, S.: Multivariate Statistical Analysis of Deformation Momenta Relating Anatomical Shape to Neuropsychological Measures. In: Jiang, T., Navab, N., Pluim, J.P.W., Viergever, M.A. (eds.) MICCAI 2010, Part III. LNCS, vol. 6363, pp. 529–537. Springer, Heidelberg (2010)

Robust MR Spine Detection Using Hierarchical Learning and Local Articulated Model

Yiqiang Zhan[1], Dewan Maneesh[1], Martin Harder[2], and Xiang Sean Zhou[1]

[1] Siemens Medical Solutions USA, Inc., Malvern, USA
[2] Siemens Healthcare Imaging MR, Erlangen, German

Abstract. A clinically acceptable auto-spine detection system, i.e., localization and labeling of vertebrae and inter-vertebral discs, is required to have high robustness, in particular to severe diseases (e.g. scoliosis) and imaging artifacts (e.g. metal artifacts in MR). Our method aims to achieve this goal with two novel components. *First*, instead of treating vertebrae/discs as either repetitive components or completely independent entities, we emulate a radiologist and use a *hierarchial* strategy to learn detectors dedicated to anchor (distinctive) vertebrae, bundle (non-distinctive) vertebrae and inter-vertebral discs, respectively. At run-time, anchor vertebrae are detected concurrently to provide redundant and distributed appearance cues robust to local imaging artifacts. Bundle vertebrae detectors provide candidates of vertebrae with subtle appearance differences, whose labels are mutually determined by anchor vertebrae to gain additional robustness. Disc locations are derived from a cloud of responses from disc detectors, which is robust to sporadic voxel-level errors. *Second*, owing to the non-rigidness of spine anatomies, we employ a *local articulated* model to effectively model the spatial relations across vertebrae and discs. The local articulated model fuses appearance cues from different detectors in a way that is robust to abnormal spine geometry resulting from severe diseases. Our method is validated by 300 MR spine scout scans and exhibits robust performance, especially to cases with severe diseases and imaging artifacts.

1 Introduction

As one of the major organs in the human body, spine relates to various neurological, orthopaedic and oncological studies. Magnetic resonance imaging (MR) is often preferred for spine imaging due to the high contrast between soft tissues. However, MR imaging quality is highly dependent on the position and orientation of the slice group. For example, a high-res transversal slice group should be positioned in parallel to inter-vertebral disc and centered at the junction of spinal cord. In current MR workflow, high-res slice group positioning is performed manually in a 2D/3D scout scan. Compared to 2D scout, 3D scout provides comprehensive anatomical context, which facilitates slice group positioning even in strong scoliotic cases (c.f., Fig. 3a). However, the manual positioning in 3D scout also takes more time due to cross slice navigation. Therefore,

N. Ayache et al. (Eds.): MICCAI 2012, Part I, LNCS 7510, pp. 141–148, 2012.

automatic spine detection in 3D scout becomes very desirable to improve MR spine workflow.

Automatic spine detection work in MR can be traced back to the 1980's [1], where a heuristic algorithm is designed to detect lumbar discs in 2D MR slices. Alomari et.al. [2] proposed a 2D lumbar vertebrae labeling system incorporating appearance and geometrical priors. However, more complicated spine geometry in 3D (especially for disease cases), and smaller/challenging appearance of cervical vertebrae, would make this approach limiting for 3D MR whole spine labeling. One of the first 3D whole spine detection methods was proposed by Schmidt et. al. [3]. Local appearance cues learned by random trees are combined with non-local geometrical priors modeled by a parts-based graphical model. Another interesting method presented in [4] focuses on learning disc location in a nine dimensional transformation space. Iterative marginal space learning is proposed to generate candidates comprising position, orientation, and scale, which are further pruned by an anatomical network. In general, state-of-the-art methods did achieve certain robustness by combining low-level appearance and high-level geometry information. However, in the presence of severe imaging artifacts or spine diseases (see Fig.3a), which are more common in 3D MR scout scans, none of existing methods provides evidence of handling these cases robustly. (Note that spine detection algorithms for other imaging modalities [5] may not be borrowed to MR owing to the intrinsically different appearances.)

In fact, two unique characteristics of spine anatomies are mostly ignored in previous works. First, although spine is composed of repetitive components (vertebrae and discs), these components have different distinctiveness and reliability in terms of detection. Second, spine is a non-rigid structure, where local articulations exist in-between vertebrae and discs. This articulation can be quite large in the presence of certain spine diseases. An effective geometry modeling should not consider vertebrae detections from scoliotic cases as errors just because of the abnormal geometry. Building upon these ideas, in this paper, we propose a spine detection method by exploiting these two characteristics. Instead of learning a general detector for vertebrae/discs or treating them as completely independent entities, we use a hierarchical strategy to learn "distinctiveness adaptive" detectors dedicated to anchor vertebrae, bundle vertebrae and inter-vertebral discs, respectively. These detectors are fused with a local articulated model to propagate information from different detectors handling abnormal spine geometry. With the hallmarks of *hierarchical learning* and *local articulated model*, our method becomes highly robust to severe imaging artifacts and spine diseases.

2   Method

2.1   Problem Statement

Notations: Human spine usually consists of 24 articulated vertebrae, which can be grouped as cervical (C_1-C_7), thoracic (T_1-T_{12}) and lumbar (L_1-L_5) sections. These 24 vertebrae plus the fused sacral vertebrae (S_1) are the targets of spine labeling in most clinical practices.

We define vertebrae and inter-vertebral discs as $V = \{v_i | i = 1 \cdots N\}$ and $D = \{d_i | i = 1 \cdots N - 1\}$, where v_i is the i-th vertebra and d_i is the inter-vertebral disc between the i-th and $i+1$-th vertebra. Here, $v_i \in \mathbb{R}^3$ is the vertebra center and $d_i \in \mathbb{R}^9$ includes the center, orientation and size of the disc. It is worth noting that i is not a simple index but bears anatomical definition. In this paper, without loss of generality, v_i is indexed in the order of vertebrae from head to feet, e.g., v_1, v_{24}, v_{25} represent C_1, L_5 and S_1, respectively.

Formulation: Given an image I, spine detection problem can be formulated as the maximization of a posterior probability with respect to V and D as:

$$(V^*, D^*) = arg \max_{V,D} P(V, D | I) \tag{1}$$

Certain vertebrae that appear either at the extremity of the entire vertebrae column, e.g., C_2, S_1, or at the transition regions of different vertebral sections, e.g., L_1 , have much better distinguishable characteristics (red ones in Fig. 1(a)). The identification of these vertebrae helps in the labeling of others, and are defined as *"anchor vertebrae"*. The remaining vertebrae (blue ones in Fig. 1(a)) are grouped into a set of continuous "bundles" and hence defined as *"bundle vertebrae"*. Vertebrae characteristics are different across bundles but similar within a bundle, e.g., C_3-C_7 look similar but are very distinguishable from T_8-T_{12}.

Denoting V_A and V_B as anchor and bundle vertebrae, the posterior in Eq. 1 can be rewritten and further expanded as:

$$P(V, D | I) = P(V_A, V_B, D | I) = P(V_A | I) \cdot P(V_B | V_A, I) \cdot P(D | V_A, V_B, I) \tag{2}$$

In this study, we use Gibbs distributions to model the probabilities. The logarithm of Eq. 2 can be then derived as Eq. 3.

$$\begin{aligned} \log[P(V, D | I)] &= A_1(V_A | I) &\Leftarrow P(V_A | I) \quad (3) \\ &+ A_2(V_B | I) + S_1(V_B | V_A) &\Leftarrow P(V_B | V_A, I) \\ &+ A_3(D | I) + S_2(D | V_A, V_B) &\Leftarrow P(D | V_A, V_B, I) \end{aligned}$$

Here, A_1, A_2 and A_3 relate to the appearance characteristics of anchor, bundle vertebrae and inter-vertebral discs. S_1 and S_2 describe the spatial relations of anchor-bundle vertebrae and vertebrae-disc, respectively. It is worth noting that the posterior of anchor vertebrae solely depends on the appearance term, while those of bundle vertebrae and inter-vertebral discs depend on both appearance and spatial relations. This is in accordance to the intuition: while anchor vertebrae can be identified based on its distinctive appearance, bundle vertebrae and inter-vertebral discs have to be identified using both appearance characteristics and the spatial relations to anchor ones.

Fig. 1(b) gives a schematic explanation of Eq. 3. Our framework consists of three layers of appearance models targeting to anchor, bundle vertebrae and discs.

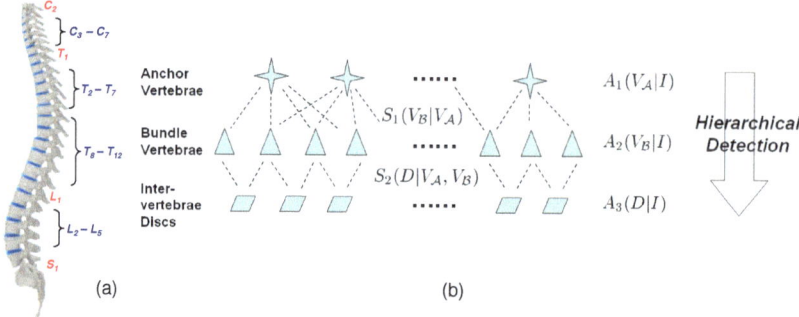

Fig. 1. (a) Schematic explanation of anchor(red) and bundle(blue) vertebrae. (b) Proposed spine detection framework.

The spatial relations across different anatomies "bridge" different layers (lines in Fig. 1). Note that this framework is completely different from the two-level model of [2], which separates pixel- and object-level information. Instead, different layers of our framework target to anatomies with different appearance distinctiveness.

2.2   Hierarchical Learning Framework

Building upon the the success of learning-based anatomy detection work [6], we employ the *Adaboost* cascade classification framework along with over-complete Haar wavelets features to model appearance characteristics of vertebrae and discs. However, in order to model the different characteristics of vertebrae and discs, we employ different training strategies for each scenario as discussed below.

Anchor Vertebrae: Distinctive characteristics of anchor vertebrae (red ones in Fig.1(a)) warrant that their detectors be trained in a very discriminative way with high response only around the center of that specific vertebra.

Bundle Vertebrae: Bundle vertebrae look similar to their neighbors but different from remote ones. Therefore, both the extremes of training a general detector for *all* bundle vertebrae (including distal ones), or specific detectors for neighboring vertebrae, would adversely affect the detector robustness and reliability. For example, consider a scenario where two specific detectors are trained to differentiate similar appearance T_9 and T_{10} vertebrae. If local imaging artifacts are present around T_9, T_9 detector might have highest response at T_{10}, since T_{10} is more salient than T_9 in this situation. This problem is also observed in [4], where "(standard) MSL approach may end up with detections for the most salient disks only". To avoid these issues, we employ a strategy in the middle to group similar neighboring vertebrae as several "bundles" (blue ones in Fig.1(a)). Each bundle has one detector that learns the commonality of corresponding vertebrae and distinguishes them from other bundles.

Inter-Vertebral Discs: Compared to vertebrae detection, disc detection has a high dimensional configuration space with 9 parameters. Different from [4],

Table 1. Training scheme of detectors for anchor vertebrae, bundle vertebrae and inter-vertebral discs

Detector	Positive Samples	Negative Samples	Image Alignment
Anchor vertebrae	Voxels close to the center of the *specific* vertebrae	Remaining voxels in the *entire* volume image	No alignment
Bundle vertebrae	Voxels close to the centers of *any* vertebrae within the bundle	Remaining voxels in the *local* volume image covering neighboring bundles	Aligned by anchor vertebrae
Inter-vertebral Discs	Voxels located on the disc	Remaining voxels in the *local* volume image covering the two neighboring vertebrae	Aligned by two neighboring vertebrae

which learns/detects a disc as a whole, we treat each voxel on the disc as an individual sample. Disc locations are derived by fitting disc response maps with principal component analysis. In this way, disc detection becomes robust to sporadic classification errors at voxel-level. Since voxels on the same disc are almost indistinguishable, similar to bundle vertebrae, all of them are "bundled" in the training stage.

To summarize, the differences in training strategies primarily exist in the selection of positive/negative samples and image alignment before feature extraction, which are outlined in Table 1. Moving down the table from anchor vertebrae to inter-vertebral discs, as the targeted anatomies become less and less distinctive, more positive samples are extracted in a more local fashion, and the image alignment becomes more and more sophisticated.

Using the above strategy, we train detectors for anchor vertebrae, bundle vertebrae and inter-vertebral discs as $A_i(\mathfrak{F}(p))$, $B_j(\mathfrak{F}(p))$, and $D_k(\mathfrak{F}(p))$. Here, $\mathfrak{F}(p)$ denotes the over-complete Haar features extracted around voxel p, and A_i, B_j and D_k are the trained Adaboost classifiers, which select and combine a small proportion of $\mathfrak{F}(p)$ to achieve best anatomy detection. The appearance terms in Eq. 3 are eventually concretized as $A_1(V_A|I) = \sum_{v_i \in V_A} A_i(\mathfrak{F}(v_i))$, $A_2(V_B|I) = \sum_{v_j \in V_B} B_j(\mathfrak{F}(v_j))$ and $A_3(D|I) = \sum_{d_k \in D} \sum_{p \in d_k} D_k(\mathfrak{F}(p))$.

2.3   Local Articulated Spine Model

Recall the definition of Eq. 3, $S_1(V_B|V_A)$ and $S_2(D|V_A, V_B)$ model the spatial relations between anchor-bundle vertebrae and vertebrae-discs, respectively. Spine is a flexible structure where each vertebra has freedom of local articulation (see Fig. 2). The local rigid transformation can be quite large in the presence of certain spine diseases, e.g., scoliosis. Shape/gemetry modeling methods [7] that treats the object as a whole can not effectively model these local variations of the spine geometry. In our study, we employ a local articulated spine model [8][9] to describe the spatial relations across vertebrae. Assume v_i is an anchor vertebra and $\{v_{i+1}, \cdots, v_{i+M}\}$ are the subsequent bundle vertebrae. As shown in Fig. 2, the spatial relations between anchor and bundle vertebrae are modeled as

$[T_i, T_i \circ T_{i+1}, \ldots, T_i, \circ T_{i+1} \circ \ldots \circ T_{i+M-1}]$, where T_i defines a local similarity transformation between v_i and v_{i+1}. $S_1(V_\mathcal{B}|V_\mathcal{A})$ is defined as:

$$S_1(V_\mathcal{B}|V_\mathcal{A}) = \sum_i e^{-(\psi(T_i)-\mu_{T_i})^T \Xi_{T_i}(\psi(T_i)-\mu_{T_i})} + 2/(1 + e^{\gamma\|\psi(T_i)-\psi(T_{i+1})\|^2}) \quad (4)$$

Here, $\psi(.)$ is an operator that converts T_i to a vector space, i.e., the rotation part of T_i is converted to its quaternion. μ_{T_i} and Ξ_{T_i} are the Frechet mean and generalized covariance of local transformation T_i, calculated as [8]. The first term contains the prior information of local transformations across *population*. The second term evaluates the difference between local T_i across the same *spine*. These two terms complement each other, such that a scoliotic spine still gets a high value of S_1 , due to the continuity of its local transformations.

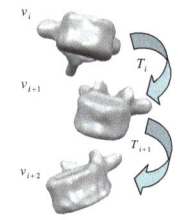

Spatial configurations between vertebrae and discs, $S_2(D|V_\mathcal{A}, V_\mathcal{B})$, is modeled with two assumptions: 1) A vertebral disc is roughly perpendicular to the line connecting its neighboring vertebrae centers; and 2) Center of an intervertebral disc is close to the mid point of the two neighboring vertebrae centers. $S_2(D|V_\mathcal{A}, V_\mathcal{B})$ is then defined in the similar fashion as Eq. 4.

Fig. 2. Local articulation model

2.4   Hierarchical Spine Detection

As a high-dimensional and non-linear function, Eq. 3 is optimized using a multi-stage algorithm. Different stages target to anchor vertebrae, bundle vertebrae and inter-vertebral discs, respectively. In each stage, we alternatively optimize the appearance terms and spatial terms.

Fig. 1 (a) gives a more schematic explanation of the optimization procedure. This hierarchial detection scheme emulates a radiologists and guarantees the robustness in three aspects: 1) Anchor vertebrae are detected *concurrently* to provide redundant and distributed appearance cues. Even when some anchor vertebrae are missed due to severe local imaging artifacts, others still provide reliable clues for spine detection. 2) Detectors of bundle vertebrae and discs provide support cues. More specifically, instead of trying to directly derive vertebrae labels, bundle vertebrae detectors provide a set of candidates whose labels are *mutually* assigned according to relative positions to anchor vertebrae. Note that labels assigned by different anchor vertebrae might be different, and are fused through the maximization of S_1. Disc detectors return a cloud of responses for disc localization, which is robust to individual false classifications as well. 3) Local articulated model propagates these appearance cues in a way robust to abnormal spine geometry resulting from severe diseases.

Table 2. Evaluations of spine detections. LS: LSpine, CS: CSpine, WS: WholeSpine

	W/O Hierarchy			W/O Articulation			Proposed Method		
	Perfect	Accept	Reject	Perfect	Accept	Reject	Perfect	Accept	Reject
LS	85	10	5	93	5	2	98	2	0
CS	65	11	4	76	3	1	79	0	1
WS	97	16	7	106	8	6	116	2	2
All	247	37	16	275	16	9	**293**	4	3
	82.4 %	12.3%	5.3%	91.7%	5.3%	3.0%	**97.7%**	1.3%	1.0%

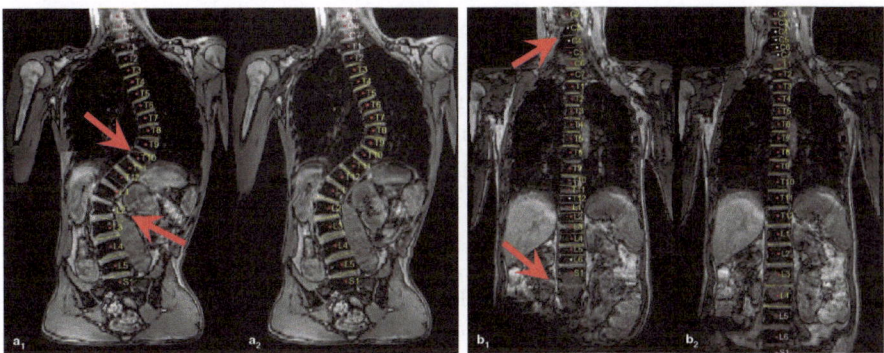

Fig. 3. Comparisons of spine detection using different methods. Curved coronal MPRs are shown for better illustration. (a): A scoliotic case using Method2 (a1) and the proposed method (a2). (b): An artifact case using Method1 (b1) and the proposed method (b2).

3   Results

Our experimental data includes 405 LSpine, CSpine and WholeSpine scout scans with isotropic resolution 1.7mm. (105 for training and 300 for testing). These datasets come from different clinical sites and were generated by different types of Siemens MR Scanners (Avanto 1.5T, Verio 3T, Skyra 3T, etc.). Quantitative evaluation is carried on 355 discs and 340 vertebrae from 15 WholeSpine scans. The average translation errors of discs and vertebrae are $1.91\,mm$ and $3.07\,mm$. The average rotation error of discs is $2.33°$.

A larger scale evaluation is performed on 300 scans (80 CSpine, 100 LSpine and 120 WholeSpine), including 43 (14.3%) with severe pathology and 36 (12.0%) with strong imaging artifacts. Three experienced radiologists rated spine detection results as "perfect" (no manual editing required), "acceptable" (minor manual editing required) and "rejected" (major manual editing required). For comparison, we also evaluate results from two adapted versions of the proposed method, **Method1**: without hierarchical learning and **Method2**: without local articulated model. As shown in Table 2, the proposed method generates "perfect" results in more than **97%** cases, which is significantly better than the others (Two examples are shown in Fig. 3.). In general , Method2 is better than Method1, since the lack of articulated model mainly affects cases with abnormal spine geometry, e.g., scoliosis, which has a small proportion in our datasets. Another interesting observation is that Method1 has larger impacts on CSpine than LSpine, but Method2 is in the other way around. This phenomenon in fact results from the different sizes of cervical and lumbar vertebrae. Due to the smaller size of cervical vertebrae, it is prone to error detections using non-hierarchical detectors. On the other hand, the larger size of lumbar vertebrae makes the detection more sensitive to abnormal spine geometry, which can only be tackled with the local articulated model.

4   Conclusion

In this paper, we proposed a robust method to detect spine in 3D MR scout scans. Using hierarchical learning framework and local articulated model, our method exhibits accurate and robust performance on 300 testing datasets.

References

1. Chwialkowski, M., Shile, P., Peshock, R., Pfeifer, D., Parkey, R.: Automated detection and evaluation of lumbar discs in mr images. In: IEEE EMBS, pp. 571–572 (1989)
2. Alomari, R., Corso, J., Chaudhary, V.: Labeling of lumbar discs using both pixel- and object-level features with a two-level probabilistic model. IEEE Trans. Med. Imaging 30, 1–10 (2011)
3. Schmidt, S., Kappes, J.H., Bergtholdt, M., Pekar, V., Dries, S.P.M., Bystrov, D., Schnörr, C.: Spine Detection and Labeling Using a Parts-Based Graphical Model. In: Karssemeijer, N., Lelieveldt, B. (eds.) IPMI 2007. LNCS, vol. 4584, pp. 122–133. Springer, Heidelberg (2007)
4. Kelm, M., Zhou, S., Sühling, M., Zheng, Y., Wels, M., Comaniciu, D.: Detection of 3d spinal geometry using iterated marginal space learning. In: MCV, pp. 96–105 (2010)
5. Klinder, T., Ostermann, J., Ehm, M., Franz, A., Kneser, R., Lorenz, C.: Automated model-based vertebra detection, identification, and segmentation in ct images. Medical Image Analysis 13, 471–482 (2009)
6. Zhan, Y., Dewan, M., Harder, M., Krishnan, A., Zhou, X.S.: Robust automatic knee mr slice positioning through redundant and hierarchical anatomy detection. IEEE Trans. Med. Imaging 30, 2087–2100 (2011)
7. Zhang, S., Zhan, Y., Dewan, M., Huang, J., Metaxas, D.N., Zhou, X.S.: Towards robust and effective shape modeling: Sparse shape composition. Medical Image Analysis 16, 265–277 (2012)
8. Boisvert, J., Cheriet, F., Pennec, X., Labelle, H., Ayache, N.: Geometric variability of the scoliotic spine using statistics on articulated shape models. IEEE Trans. Med. Imaging 27, 557–568 (2008)
9. Kadoury, S., Labelle, H., Paragios, N.: Automatic inference of articulated spine models in ct images using high-order markov random fields. Medical Image Analysis 15, 426–437 (2011)

Spatiotemporal Reconstruction
of the Breathing Function

D. Duong[1], D. Shastri[2], P. Tsiamyrtzis[3], and I. Pavlidis[1]

[1] Department of Computer Science, University of Houston, Houston, TX 77024, USA
[2] Department of Computer and Mathematical Sciences, University of
Houston-Downtown, Houston, TX 77002, USA
[3] Department of Statistics, Athens University of Economics and Business,
Athens 10434, Greece
dcduong@cs.uh.edu, shastrid@uhd.edu, pt@aueb.gr, ipavlidis@uh.edu

Abstract. Breathing waveform extracted via nasal thermistor is the
most common method to study respiratory function in sleep studies. In
essence, this is a temporal waveform of mean temperatures in the nostril
region that at every time step collapses two-dimensional data into a
single point. Hence, spatial heat distribution in the nostrils is lost along
with valuable functional and anatomical cues. This article presents the
construction and experimental validation of a spatiotemporal profile for
the breathing function via thermal imaging of the nostrils. The method
models nasal airflow advection by using a front-propagating level set
algorithm with optimal parameter selection. It is the first time that the
full two-dimensional advantage of thermal imaging is brought to the fore
in breathing computation. This new multi-dimensional measure is likely
to bring diagnostic value in sleep studies and beyond.

Keywords: Breathing, data visualization, sleep studies, thermal imaging.

1 Introduction

Sleep studies require overnight monitoring of the patient's breathing function
which is typically accomplished via contact-sensors. A widely used sensor is the
nasal thermistor which extracts the temporal breathing waveform by sensing
the average temperatures in the nostril region at every point in time. The sensor
is placed inside the nostril, a non-comfortable arrangement for patients who
have problems with breathing and sleep in the first place. As an alternative
to this clinical practice, a thermal imaging method has been proposed recently
[1][2]. The method could be characterized as a 'virtual thermistor', because it
produces a temporal breathing waveform by averaging emission values in the
nostrils at every time step. The comparative advantage lies only in its non-
contact nature. Although thermal imaging carries inherently spatial information,
this is never recovered and used. Evolution of spatial heat distribution in the
nostrils can reveal subtle breathing abnormalities that may hint at anatomical

N. Ayache et al. (Eds.): MICCAI 2012, Part I, LNCS 7510, pp. 149–156, 2012.

and functional problems. These problems by and large go undetected due to the averaging nature of the existing measurement methods [3]. Relevant examples include small nasal polyps that locally affect airflow or hypopnea, where airflow is curtailed but not totally suppressed [4].

In this article, we describe a method for spatiotemporal reconstruction of the breathing function via thermal imaging.[1] A level set algorithm captures the spatial evolution of nostril emission, as affected by inspiratory and expiratory airflow. A registration algorithm that accounts for nostril motion ensures the meaningful application of the level set computation. The soundness of the method is verified experimentally. Interestingly, the method captures subtle pathophysiological incidents in the data set that escape detection by the 'virtual thermistor', thus, bringing to the fore its potential clinical value.

2   Methodology

2.1   Temporal Registration

Breathing is a physiological process that continuously modulates the spatial heat distribution inside the nostrils (see Fig. 1). We capture this spatial evolution by employing the Chan-Vese active contour without edge model [5] (see Section 2.2). Prior this step though, we nullify the subject's head motion that gradually translates and rotates the nostril region over time, introducing artifacts in the spatiotemporal visualization. We correct the motion error by registering the perinasal region in every frame to a global reference frame. We use the FFT-based phase correlation algorithm proposed by Reddy *et.al* [6] for that purpose. The main advantage of this algorithm is that it computes any amount of translation and rotation in fixed time for images of the same size. The algorithm has been designed for visual images where low-level features, such as object boundaries, are clearly distinguishable. Boundaries in thermal images, however, are fuzzy because of thermal diffusion. For this reason we support Reddy's algorithm with a Laplacian boundary enhancement function.

Translation. Let f represent the thermal image of the perinasal region (see the insets of Fig 1). Let also the perinasal image f_1 be translated by the vector (x_0, y_0), producing the image f_2 (i.e., $f_2(x, y) = f_1(x - x_0, y - y_0)$). As per the Fourier shift theorem, their corresponding Fourier transforms F_1 and F_2 are related via the following equation:

$$F_2(\xi, \eta) = e^{-j2\pi(\xi x_0 + \eta y_0)} F_1(\xi, \eta). \tag{1}$$

The cross-power spectrum of the images is defined as:

$$\frac{F_1(\xi, \eta) F_2^*(\xi, \eta)}{|F_1(\xi, \eta) F_2^*(\xi, \eta)|} = e^{-j2\pi(\xi x_0 + \eta y_0)}, \tag{2}$$

---

[1] Spatiotemporal visualization clips of breathing function from the experimental set can be accessed at:http://www.cpl.uh.edu/miccai-2012/

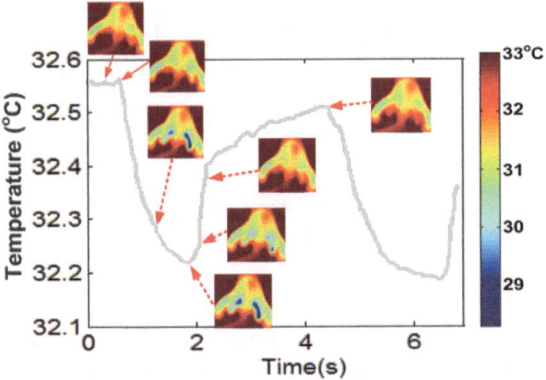

Fig. 1. Spatiotemporal heat distribution at the nostril region

where F^* is the complex conjugate of F. Taking the inverse Fourier transform of this representation will yield an impulse function at the displacement (x_0, y_0) and zero everywhere else.

Rotation. Let the image f_1 be translated by the vector (x_0, y_0) and rotated by angle θ_0, producing the image f_2 (i.e., $f_2(x, y) = f_1(x \cos \theta_0 + y \sin \theta_0 - x_0, -x \sin \theta_0 + y \cos \theta_0 - y_0)$). According to the Fourier translation and rotation property, their Fourier transforms F_1 and F_2 are related by:

$$F_2(\xi, \eta) = e^{-j2\pi(\xi x_0 + \eta y_0)} F_1(\xi \cos \theta_0 + \eta \sin \theta_0,$$
$$-\xi \sin \theta_0 + \eta \cos \theta_0). \tag{3}$$

The rotation without translation can be represented as a translation displacement in polar coordinates. Using phase correlation, one can find the angle θ_0 easily. Let us denote f_2' to be the motion corrected image.

2.2 Nostril Segmentation

In this step we localize the left and right nostrils inside the perinasal region of interest. The nostril region features a non-uniform heat distribution of the breathing function which evolves over time. This dynamic nature of the spatiotemporal heat distribution poses a modeling challenge to the segmentation task. In particular, the nostrils' temperature elevates during the breathing expiration phase because the expired air absorbs heat in the lungs and respiratory passageways. In contrast, their temperature lowers during the breathing inspiration phase. We have adopted the active contour model framework because it is suitable for tracking this kind of spatiotemporal dynamic behavior [7]. In particular, we use the Chan-Vese active contour without edge modeling algorithm that is appropriate for fuzzy thermal boundaries [5].

Let $f_1', f_2', ..., f_n'$ be continuous thermal images of the perinasal region that are corrected for motion error as discussed in Section 2.1. Given a feature vector $\mathbf{I}$, the Chan-Vese active contour model is defined by:

$$\frac{\partial \phi}{\partial t} = \delta_\epsilon \left(\phi \right) \left[\mu \nabla \cdot \left(\frac{\nabla \phi}{\|\nabla \phi\|} \right) \right.$$

$$- \frac{1}{N} \sum_{i=1}^{N} \lambda_i^+ \left(I_i \left(x, y \right) - c_i^+ \right)^2$$

$$+ \frac{1}{N} \sum_{i=1}^{N} \lambda_i^- \left(I_i \left(x, y \right) - c_i^- \right)^2$$

$$\left. - \upsilon \right], \tag{4}$$

where c^+ and c^- are mean values of regions inside and outside the evolving curve and N is the length of the feature vector. λ_i^+ and λ_i^- are the scaling parameters. μ controls the smoothness of the contour. υ refines the level of the contour.

We construct a feature vector of size $N = 2$ that includes the pixel temperature in the current frame and temporal variation of pixel temperature in previous frames. Specifically, for a pixel at location (x, y) in frame n, the feature vector $\mathbf{I_n} \left(x, y \right) = \left(f_n' \left(x, y \right), \alpha \sigma_n^2 \left(x, y \right) \right)$, where α is the weight that we set dynamically using an exponential decaying function [8]. The decay constant of the function is set to 0.0743, which takes into account the temperature variation of half the normal breathing cycle (at the data acquisition rate of 25 frames per second). This arrangement guarantees that the contour evolution in the current frame takes into account the most recent temporal changes due to breathing.

2.3   Spatiotemporal Construction

Outcomes from the segmentation step are collected into a 3D array. Each X-Y plane of the array stores the segmented nostril region. The planes are stacked along the Z-axis of the array. To comply with sleep study metrics, every 30 seconds of data (i.e., 1 epoch), is stacked into one array. Finally, the 3D sets are supplied as a time-series model to the Avizo 6.2 software visualization tool.

3   Validation Analysis

3.1   Registration Validation

Thermal imaging records both physical motion (e.g., head motion) and physiological process (e.g., breathing). To find out how well our registration algorithm corrects the motion error in presence of breathing, we performed a simulation study. To build the simulation we used as a reference frame the thermal image of a subject's face. Within the reference frame we modulated the nostrils' temperature by applying a spatiotemporal evolution of a normal breathing cycle. We generated 20 simulated images equidistantly spaced across the breathing cycle. Each image was then translated and rotated by randomly generated values $((x_0, y_0), \theta_0)$. The values were treated as ground truth. The transformed images were supplied to our registration algorithm for motion correction. The resultant images were compared with the corresponding reference frames for qualitative analysis (see Fig. 2). The translation and rotation parameters estimated through the algorithm were compared against their respective ground truth values. The ANOVA test performed on the data shows that there no statistically significant difference between the estimated translations and their ground truth values ($P > 0.01$) as well as the estimated rotations and their ground truth values ($P > 0.01$). This validates the registration algorithm.

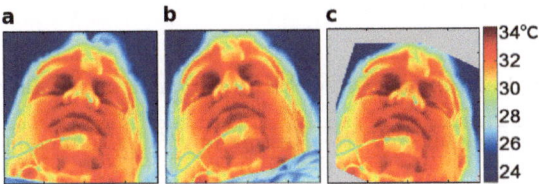

Fig. 2. (a)Reference image. (b) Simulated image. (c) Registered image. The orientation and position of the registered image is in agreement with that of the reference image.

3.2   Segmentation Validation

In a heterogeneous region, such as the perinasal region in the thermal imagery, a zero-level contour of convergence ϕ often leads to suboptimal delineation of the region of interest. Therefore, it is required to train the regulating parameter v to achieve optimal delineation.

Training the Parameter v: We used manual segmentations of the nostril region and a probabilistic scoring mechanism for training the parameter. In particular, three experts were asked to manually delineate in the thermal images the breathing evolution inside the left and right nostrils. A total of six sets of the thermal images were prepared from the six subjects. Each set comprised of 100 consecutive thermal images that represented 2-3 normal breathing cycles. Each expert repeated the delineation task twice per set. Thus, we acquired a total of six ground truth sets of manual segmentation per subject.

The performance of the segmentation algorithm was assessed against these ground truth sets by computing the Probabilistic Rand Index (PRI) [10]. PRI finds a common agreement between the multiple ground truth values and the segmentation output. Higher PRI indicates better performance of the segmentation algorithm. For every thermal image we varied v from 0 to 4 in steps of 0.05 and computed the PRI for each v value. The v value corresponding to the highest PRI was recorded as the optimal value for that particular image. The process was repeated for all 100 images in each set. Their optimal v values were averaged and designated as the tuned parameter v_t for that set. Corresponding PRI values were also averaged and recorded for comparison with the testing dataset. (see column-1 in Table 1).

Testing the Trained Parameter: The trained parameter was tested on different sets of manual segmentations generated by three experts different from the one used in the parameter training. This time however, the six sets were pre-pared from randomly selected 100 images from the thermal videos. We supplied every set of images along with its tuned v value to the segmentation algorithm and computed the PRI.

Table 1 summarizes the mean and standard deviation of the PRI values for every subject. The ANOVA test performed on the data concludes that there are no statistically significant difference between the PRIs of training and testing images ($P > 0.01$). This confirms that the regulating parameter v was trained optimally for every subject.

Table 1. Mean and Std. of PRI for training and testing sets

	$\mu(PRI)$ (Training)	$\mu(PRI)$ (Testing)	$\sigma(PRI)$ (Training)	$\sigma(PRI)$ (Testing)
Subject 1	0.88	0.78	0.07	0.13
Subject 2	0.88	0.82	0.04	0.05
Subject 3	0.95	0.96	0.05	0.05
Subject 4	0.92	0.96	0.03	0.05
Subject 5	0.90	0.85	0.02	0.09
Subject 6	0.87	0.76	0.05	0.13

4   Experiments

4.1   Experimental Setup

The experiment was conducted in a controlled room environment at a Sleep Research Center. Six subjects (1 female and 5 males) participated in the experiment. The mean age of the subject pool was 25 ± 1.86 years. The experiment lasted 45 minutes. During the experiment the subjects were fitted with the standard polysomnography sensors to ground truth the imaging measurements. The subjects were asked to lay prostrate in a comfortable bed for the experiment period. They were positioned $2.5\ m$ away from a thermal imaging system focused on their faces (see Fig. 2). The thermal imaging system consisted of a Thermo Vision SC6000 Mid-Wave Infrared (MWIR) camera from FLIR [9], a MWIR 100 mm lens, and a HP Pavilion m9040n desktop.

4.2   Experimental Results

Fig. 3 illustrates the spatiotemporal reconstruction of the breathing function. The 3D clouds in the figure represent the inhalation phases. The clouds' inhomo-geneous colors depict the nonuniformity of the breathing function. In particular, the core of each cloud has marginally higher temperature than the peripheral region. The temperature gradient exists because the nasal cavities get narrower as they run from the mandibular to the periorbital region. This progressive steno-sis amplifies heat convection which elevates the core's temperature. The gap in between two clouds represents the exhalation phase that our algorithm is unable

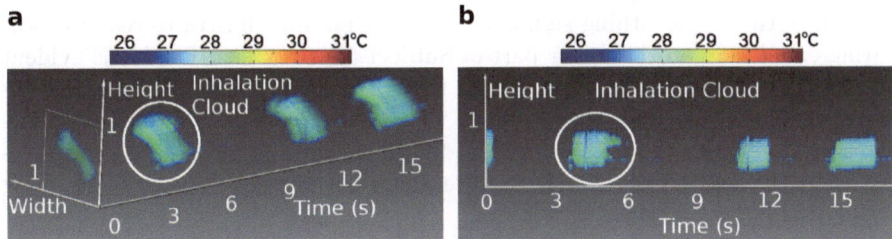

Fig. 3. The plot illustrates an angular view (a) and a projection view (b) of Subject 1's breathing function

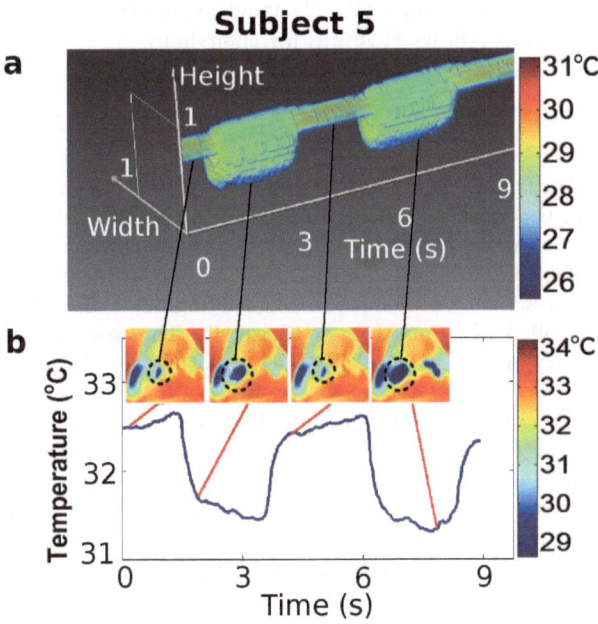

Fig. 4. (a) Angular view of the multi-dimensional visualization. (b) 1D breathing waveform. Conditions of reduced air-flow during exhalation on the upper part of the right nostril are evident by the bridging 'pipe' between the successive exhalation clouds. This spatiotemporal pattern is lost in the 1D breathing signal.

to capture at this point. This happens because the hot air from the exhalation phase has similar thermal profile as the nostril cartilage. In the future we plan on applying probabilistic methods, such as Bayesian classification, to separate the more dynamic breathing function from the relatively stationary thermal profile of the nostril cartilage.

An advantage of the spatiotemporal reconstruction of the breathing function over the mean temperature waveform [1][2] is the localization of subtle pathological patterns. These patterns are usually obliterated by the averaging process at work in the 1D-breathing signal formation. Fig. 4(a) illustrates reduced flow during exhalation on the upper part of Subject 5's right nostril. This is evident by a bridging 'pipe' in the visualization that connects the two inhalation clouds and reveals that in the upper part of the nasal cavity, inhalation conditions persist even during exhalation. This finding is all but obscured if one considers Fig. 4(b) that shows the classic 1D breathing waveform, where the breathing waveform appears normal.

Acknowledgments. This material is based upon work supported by a National Science Foundation (NSF) grant (# IIS-1049004) titled 'EAGER: Improving Human Engagement and Enjoyment in Routine Activities.' We are grateful to Dr. Max Hirshkowitz, and Dr. Amir Sharafkhaneh from the Baylor Sleep Research Center of the Veterans Affairs Hospital for their help.

References

1. Murthy, J., Van Jaarsveld, J., Fei, J., Pavlidis, I., Harrykissoon, R., Lucke, J., Faiz, S., Castriotta, R.: Thermal Infrared Imaging: A Novel Method to Monitor Airflow During Polysomnography. Sleep 32(11), 1521–1527 (2009)
2. Fei, J., Pavlidis, I.: Thermistor at a Distance: Unobtrusive Measurement of Breathing. IEEE Transactions on Biomedical Engineering 57(4), 988–998 (2010)
3. Rappai, M., Collop, N., Kemp, S., de Shazo, R.: The Nose and Sleep-disordered Breathing: What We Know and What We Do Not Know. Chest 124(6), 2309–2323 (2003)
4. Farre, R., Montserrat, J.M., Rotger, M., Ballester, E., Navajas, D.: Accuracy of Thermistors and Thermocouples as Flow-measuring Devices for Detecting Hypopnoeas. European Respiratory Journal 11(1), 179–182 (1998)
5. Chan, T.F., Vese, L.A.: Active Contours Without Edges. IEEE Transactions on Image Processing 10(2), 266–277 (2001)
6. Reddy, B., Chatterji, B.: An FFT-based Technique for Translation, Rotation, and Scale-invariant Image Registration. IEEE Transactions on Image Processing 5(8), 1266–1271 (1996)
7. Kass, M., Witkin, W., Terzopoulos, D.: Active Contour Models. International Journal of Computer Vision 1(4), 321–331 (1988)
8. Nowlan, S.: Soft Competitive Adaptation: Neural Network Learning Algorithms Based on Fitting Statistical Mixtures. PhD thesis, School of Computer Science, Carnegie Mellon University, Pittsburgh (1991)
9. FLIR Systems, http://www.flir.com
10. Unnikrishnan, R., Pantofaru, C., Hebert, M.: Toward Objective Evaluation of Image Segmentation Algorithms. IEEE Transactions on Pattern Analysis and Machine Intelligence 29(1), 929–944 (2007)

A Visual Latent Semantic Approach for Automatic Analysis and Interpretation of Anaplastic Medulloblastoma Virtual Slides

Angel Cruz-Roa[1], Fabio González[1], Joseph Galaro[2], Alexander R. Judkins[3], David Ellison[4], Jennifer Baccon[5], Anant Madabhushi[2], and Eduardo Romero[1]

[1] BioIngenium Research Group, Universidad Nacional de Colombia, Bogotá, Colombia
[2] Rutgers, Department of Biomedical Engineering, Piscataway, NJ, USA
[3] Children Hospital of L.A., Department of Pathology Lab Medicine, Los Angeles, CA, USA
[4] St. Jude Children's Research Hospital from Memphis, TN, USA
[5] Penn State College of Medicine, Department of Pathology, Hershey, PA, USA

Abstract. A method for automatic analysis and interpretation of histopathology images is presented. The method uses a representation of the image data set based on bag of features histograms built from visual dictionary of Haar-based patches and a novel visual latent semantic strategy for characterizing the visual content of a set of images. One important contribution of the method is the provision of an interpretability layer, which is able to explain a particular classification by visually mapping the most important visual patterns associated with such classification. The method was evaluated on a challenging problem involving automated discrimination of medulloblastoma tumors based on image derived attributes from whole slide images as anaplastic or non-anaplastic. The data set comprised 10 labeled histopathological patient studies, 5 for anaplastic and 5 for non-anaplastic, where 750 square images cropped randomly from cancerous region from whole slide per study. The experimental results show that the new method is competitive in terms of classification accuracy achieving 0.87 in average.

1 Introduction

This paper presents a new method, ViSAI, for automatic analysis and interpretation of histopathological images. The method comprises three main stages: learning of an image representation based on bag of features (BOF), characterization of the rich visual variety of a histopathological image collection using visual latent topic analysis, and connection of visual patterns with the semantics of the problem using a probabilistic classification model. The learnt probabilistic model is applied to new images, and the class posterior probability is used to determine the corresponding class. The method is applied to the classification of a type of brain cancer called medulloblastoma, which is one of the most common types of malignant brain tumors [10]. In adults, the disease is rare whereas in children the incidence amounts to a 25% of all pediatric brain tumors. Tumor classification of medulloblastoma is currently performed by microscopical examination and no quantitative image analysis and classification tools are so far available for this task. Different histologic types of medulloblastoma have different prognosis.

N. Ayache et al. (Eds.): MICCAI 2012, Part I, LNCS 7510, pp. 157–164, 2012.

The differential diagnosis is a hard task and tends to be qualitative. Determine the subtypes of medulloblastoma are difficult to establish and subject to inter-observer variability because of the similarity between the two basic histologic subclasses: anaplastic and non-anaplastic and their similarity with a long list of differential diagnoses. The anaplastic medulloblastoma have worse prognosis and this is mostly characterized by the presence of large, irregular cells that lack organization and in some cases attempt to wrap around each other. The therapeutical management changes radically depending on the subtype of medulloblastoma so that histopathological diagnosis is useful in determining the potential outcome of the disease. Hence computerized and quantitative image analysis tools are useful in this kind of problem for better estimation of medulloblastoma subtype allowing potentially make better prognostic decisions.

Recent investigations [9] have pointed out the importance of provide computerized and automatic image analysis tools as support to diagnosis and prognosis for different types of cancer. Recent work in histologic image analysis has explored the use of automated methods for breast cancer and prostate cancer diagnosis and grading [4,8] using other images modalities. Galaro et al. [6] classified anaplastic and non-anaplastic medulloblastoma subtypes, using a BOF of Haar wavelet coefficients as local pixel-based descriptors. The authors of [6] reported on average a classification accuracy of 0.80. The above works have essentially developed tools to improve the quality of diagnosis in terms of objective support and some level of quantification. Bag of features approach is an image content representation commonly used in computer vision area which comprises three main stages: local feature extraction, dictionary construction, and image representation. This approach have been successful adapted and applied in histology images previously in image analysis and classification tasks [2,3]. On the other hand, latent topic analysis is an approach widely used in text document collection analysis to find the semantic topics related with these documents. The representative techniques are latent semantic analysis (LSA), pLSA [7] and latent Dirichlet analysis (LDA) [1]. Both pLSA and LDA suppose a generative model for documents. The main assumptions here are: first, the image content of image could be represented by an appropriate set of visual words from dictionary learnt from whole image collection represented by a good visual word representation, and second, the large visual variability in the image collection is generated from a relatively small set of visual latent factors. Under our analysis, visual latent factors correspond to high-level patterns that mix sets of visual words that co-occur with high frequency in the collection. Semantics is then linked to visual latent factors coding the relationship between the visual appearance and particular classes.

The new method in this paper addresses the problem of automated classification of histological slides. The method provides higher accuracy coupled with an interpretation of classification results for the expert in terms of semantic domain, rather than being a black-box approach. In particular, the main contributions of the present work are:

- A strategy to characterize the rich visual content of histology images combining an image representation, based on BOF, and a texture local descriptor for image patches based on a Haar wavelet transform.
- A visual latent-topic analysis model for finding higher-level visual patterns that combine multiple visual words.

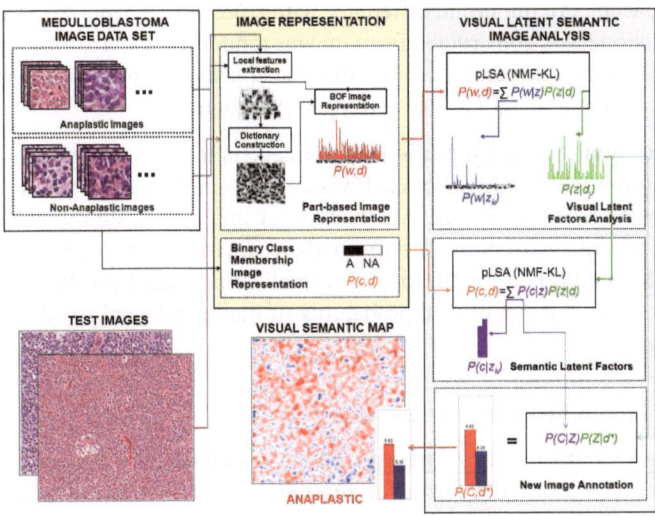

Fig. 1. Overall scheme for the visual latent semantic analysis for automatic classification and interpretation method

- A method that is able, not only to globally classify a virtual slide, but also provides interpretability determining the most important visual patterns associated with such classification, and identifying their location in the original image.

2   Visual Latent Semantic Analysis of Medulloblastoma Images

ViSAI method performs an implicit semantic identification of the visual patterns that characterize each class (anaplastic and non-anaplastic). The strategy is built upon an image representation, based on BOF, and a visual latent semantics analysis, based on probabilistic latent semantic analysis (pLSA). The overall scheme is depicted in Figure1.

2.1   Image Representation

Step 1: Local Features Extraction. square patches of 50 pixels, that is the minimum spatial resolution that covers a cellular unit (nucleus and cytoplasm), are extracted using a dense grid strategy with an overlap of 80%. Each patch is represented by two different local descriptors, raw-blocks (block) and Haar wavelet coefficients (haar). The raw-block descriptor corresponds to luminance values of pixels in the patch, whereas the Haar descriptor corresponds to the filter responses of two scales of a Haar-wavelet-based wavelet transform. Luminance differences are reduced by applying, before feature extraction, a mean-zero-variance-one normalization.

Step 2: Dictionary Construction. the dictionary is built by applying a conventional k-means clustering strategy to a sample of image patches from the training set. The number of clusters, k, corresponds to the dictionary size, and each centroid corresponds to a visual concept. An important difference with a previous texton-based approach [6] is that our dictionary is constructed from images randomly selected from both classes, regardless of whether it belongs to the class anaplastic or not, by which the visual concepts are mixed up within a very heterogeneous dictionary.

Step 3: Novel Image Representation. each image is then represented by a k-bin histogram, capturing the frequency of each visual word in the image given the local descriptor and the visual dictionary. A collection of images can be represented then by a matrix, X, where each column corresponds to an image and each row to a visual word. If each column is normalized (L1 normalization), each position in the matrix, $X_{i,j}$, corresponds to the conditional probability of finding a visual word w_i in an image d_j, i.e., $p(w_i|d_j)$.

2.2   Visual Latent Semantic Image Analysis

Step 1: Visual Latent Factors Analysis. The new method uses an approach similar to pLSA that assumes that the presence of different terms (visual words) in a set of documents (images) can be explained by the presence of a reduced set of hidden variables called latent factors. Specifically, the conditional probability $P(w_i|d_j)$ can be represented as:

$$P(w_i|d_j) \approx \sum_k P(w_i|z_k)P(z_k|d_j) \tag{1}$$

where $P(w_i|z_k)$ is the conditional probability of visual word w_i given latent factor z_k and $P(z_k|d_j)$ is the conditional probability of a latent factor z_k given the image d_j. The latent factors can be found by solving an optimization problem that looks for $P(W|Z)$ and $P(Z|D)$ that minimizes the Kullback-Leibler divergence between the left and right sides of Equation 1 [5]. In our case, we solve the optimization problem by modeling it as a matrix factorization problem: $P(W|D) = P(W|Z)P(Z|D)$, where $P(W|D) = X$ is the histogram representation of the image collection discussed in Subsection 2.1, $P(W|Z)$ contains the latent factors represented in terms of visual words, and $P(Z|D)$ contains the representation of the images in the collection, in terms of latent factors.

Step 2: Semantic Latent Factors. Given a set of annotated training images, each image, d_i, is associated with one of two classes: anaplastic ($C_1 = A$) or non-anaplastic ($C_2 = NA$). If, for instance, the image is anaplastic then $P(C_1|d_i) = 1$ and $P(C_2|d_i) = 0$. Following the same reasoning as in previous subsection this probability can be expressed in terms of the latent factors as follows:

$$P(C_i|d_j) \cong \sum_k P(C_i|z_k)p(z_k|d_j) \tag{2}$$

The probability $P(C_i|z_k)$ effectively connects each latent factor with the semantics of the problem represented in terms of the biological concept associated with each class. These probabilities can be found applying a matrix factorization algorithm [5] that fixes $P(Z|D)$ from the previous step and looks for $P(C|Z)$ such that: $P(C|D) = P(C|Z)P(Z|D)$.

Step 3: New Image Classification. A new image, d^*, is first represented using the strategy discussed in Subsection 2.1. This produces a normalized histogram $P(W|d^*)$.

The image is then represented in terms of latent factors (z_k) finding $P(Z|d^*)$ such that: $P(W|d^*) \cong P(W|Z)P(Z|d^*)$, where $P(W|Z)$ was previously found in step 1 solving Equation 1. Then, the posterior class probability of the image $P(C|d^*)$ is calculated using: $P(C|d^*) \cong P(C|Z)P(Z|d^*)$, where $P(C|Z)$ was previously calculated in step 2 solving Equation 2 and obtained $P(Z|d^*)$. Finally, the class assigned to the new image is the one with the maximum class posterior probability.

3   Experimental Results and Discussion

3.1   Experimental Design

The dataset comprises 10 labeled histopathological cases from St. Jude Children's Research Hospital, which 5 are anaplastic and 5 are non-anaplastic. Each slide is a whole virtual slide of 80000×80000 pixels with one or more cancerous regions with a large tumoral variability, manually annotated by a neuro-pathologist. For every slide, 750 individual images of 200×200 pixels non-overlapping where extracted uniformly at random from these cancerous regions, resulting in a database of 7500 different images: half of them anaplastic. The local feature extraction is carried out as was described in Subsection 2.1 for two local descriptors *block* and *haar*. The dictionary size was tested with different sizes, 10, 20, 40, 80, 160 and 320 visual words. Finally the number of latent factors was fixed to the dictionary size since this amounts to a maximum number of elemental building blocks (visual words) to be represented by visual semantic concepts (latent factors). The probabilistic analysis described in Subsection 2.2 provides a probability value associated with the semantic importance of each of the initial visual features so that these can be grouped together (into latent factors) by similar levels of relevance per class (Equations 1 and 2).

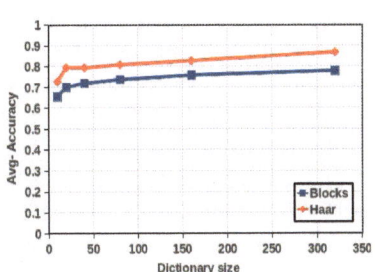

Fig. 2. Dictionary size vs average accuracy for both local features (block and haar)

In this sense, three different experiments were proposed to evaluate each parameter of the proposed method. First, determine the visual words appearance from dictionaries and impact of dictionary size for each local descriptor (block or haar) evaluation average accuracy in test data set over multiple trials of cross-validation. Second, evaluate the classification performance of the proposed image representation (Subsection 2.1) for each local descriptor using the proposed method (Subsection 2.2) compared with a k-NN classifier. Third, a visual mapping of high-level concepts to identify spatial regions associated by each one (anaplastic and non-anaplastic).

3.2   Visual Dictionary Construction

Figure 2 shows the impact of the dictionary size on the validation average accuracy. Overall, haar-based dictionary outperforms the raw-block representation by about 7%.

For both representations the best performances were obtained with the largest dictionary size obtaining 0.77 (blocks) and 0.86 (haar) in average accuracy. Visual words can be related to a particular class calculating the posterior class probability. Table 1 shows the 20 visual words with highest posterior class probability for both classes, for the two types of representation. In all the cases the visual dictionary is composed basically of smooth samples of nuclei and cells in different orientations and arrangements, a result that matches perfectly with a very basic principle in pathology analysis which introduces the cell as the basic unit of information. Also some differences between the visual words associated to each class can be observed, for both (block and haar), non-anaplastic patterns are more homogeneous. This is consequent with the biological definition of anaplasia, where cells are undifferentiated and nuclei shapes and sizes have high variability.

Table 1. A sample of the visual dictionaries obtained using different local features. Second column shows the 20 visual words with highest probability by class (A:anaplastic, NA:non-anaplastic) for each kind of local feature in a dictionary size of 160.

3.3 Classification Performance

For each of multiple trials of cross-validation, we used 4 anaplastic and 4 non-anaplastic slides for training the visual semantic model and 1 anaplastic and 1 non-anaplastic slides for testing. For comparison, the k-NN classifier was employed. An optimal value for k, 10, was found by cross validation such as was suggested in [6]. Different dictionary sizes and patch representations were evaluated to determine the best configuration for this classification task in terms of classifier accuracy, specificity, and sensitivity. The results are presented in Table 2, which shows the performance obtained with each image representation strategy and classification algorithm. Clearly the haar-based representation outperforms the block-based representation, independent of classifier choice. The new classification method is competitive with respect to the k-NN, a classical classifier used in [6], the improvement was 3.6% in accuracy (haar), 12.7% in sensitivity (block) and 10.1% in specificity (haar).

Table 2. Classification performance in terms of accuracy, specificity and sensitivity for dictionary size of 320

	ViSAI			k-NN		
	Accuracy	Sensitivity	Specificity	Accuracy	Sensitivity	Specificity
block	0.78	**0.89**	0.67	0.80	0.79	0.81
haar	**0.87**	0.86	**0.87**	0.84	0.88	0.79

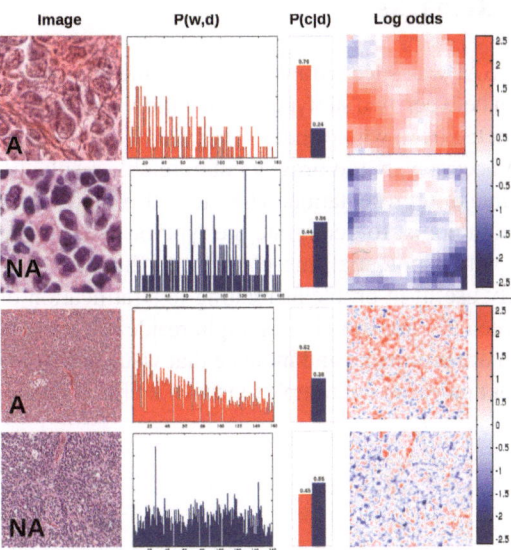

Fig. 3. Visual semantic maps for test images from a cross validation trial. Images in the first column were correctly classified (A-anaplastic and NA-non-anaplastic). See Subsection 3.4 for description.

3.4 Visual Pattern Mapping and Interpretation

The methodology presented in this paper allows for new unknown images to determine the spatial probability maps for each class using conditional probabilities. Figure 3 illustrates the semantic visual maps generated for two unknown test images in a particular trial of cross validation. Rows one and two show images of the same size used in training (200×200), whereas rows three and four show a larger field of view (2000×2000). The center column shows the corresponding BOF histogram representation for each image (i.e. occurrence frequency of each visual word of the dictionary in the image) . Bin (visual words) has been sorted according to the posterior class probabilities: visual words with a higher class probability of being anaplastic are at the left, and visual words with a higher class probability for non-anaplastic are at the right. The third column shows the posterior class probability. The fourth column shows a map that indicates how likely a particular region of the image is to be related to one of the semantic classes. This is depicted by the log-odds of the posterior class probabilities to emphasize the differences. A positive value (*red*) indicates a higher probability for class anaplastic, a negative value (*blue*) indicates a higher probability for class non-anaplastic. An advantage of the BOF image representation is that new method is able to scale towards larger image size as shown in the rows three and four of Figure 3, where the correct prediction of classes and spatial location of semantic regions is more challenging.

4   Concluding Remarks

The new method ViSAI was successfully applied to the challenging problem of automatic discrimination between two subtypes of medulloblastoma using computer derived image features extracted from whole slides. The goal of our method was not just to improve classification accuracy, but to provide interpretable results using latent semantic analysis and BOF image representation. The method provides an interpretation layer that helps out the pathologist to determine the type of patterns present in the sample under examination with a potential improvement of diagnostic significance. This attribute is particularly useful in problems relating to stratification of the disease where the distinction between disease sub-classes might reside in very subtle visual cues. The experimental results are promising and indicate that visual latent semantic analysis has potential as a tool for analyzing the complex visual patterns exhibited by histopathology images.

References

1. Blei, D.M., Ng, A.Y., Jordan, M.I.: Latent dirichlet allocation. Mach. Learn. 3, 993–1022 (2003)
2. Cruz-Roa, A., Caicedo, J., González, F.: Visual pattern mining in histology image collections using bag of features. Artif. Intell. Med. 52(2), 91–106 (2011)
3. Cruz-Roa, A., Díaz, G., Romero, E., González, F.: Automatic Annotation of Histopathological Images Using a Latent Topic Model Based on Non-negative Matrix Factorization. J. Path Inform. 2(1), 4 (2011)
4. Dalle, J.R., Leow, W.K., Racoceanu, D., Tutac, A.E., Putti, T.C.: Automatic breast cancer grading of histopathological images. In: EMBS 2008, pp. 3052–3055 (2008)
5. Ding, C., Li, T., Peng, W.: On the equivalence between non-negative matrix factorization and probabilistic latent semantic indexing. Comput. Stat. Data An. 52(8), 3913–3927 (2008)
6. Galaro, J., Judkins, A., Ellison, D., Baccon, J., Madabhushi, A.: An integrated texton and bag of words classifier for identifying anaplastic medulloblastomas. In: EMBC 2011, pp. 3443–3446 (2011)
7. Hofmann, T.: Unsupervised learning by probabilistic latent semantic analysis. Mach. Learn. 42, 177–196 (2001)
8. Kwak, J.T., Hewitt, S.M., Sinha, S., Bhargava, R.: Multimodal microscopy for automated histologic analysis of prostate cancer. BMC Cancer 11(1), 62 (2011)
9. Madabhushi, A., Agner, S., Basavanhally, A., Doyle, S., Lee, G.: Computer-aided prognosis: Predicting patient and disease outcome via quantitative fusion of multi-scale, multi-modal data. Comput. Med. Imag. Grap. 35, 506–514 (2011)
10. Roberts, R.O., Lynch, C.F., Jones, M.P., Hart, M.N.: Medulloblastoma: A population-based study of 532 cases. J. Neuropath. Exp. Neur. 50(2), 134–144 (1991)

Detection of Spontaneous Vesicle Release at Individual Synapses Using Multiple Wavelets in a CWT-Based Algorithm

Stefan Sokoll[1,2], Klaus Tönnies[2], and Martin Heine[1]

[1] Group Molecular Physiology, Leibniz Inst. for Neurobiology, Magdeburg, Germany
[2] Dept. of Simulation and Graphics, Otto-von-Guericke Univ., Magdeburg, Germany

Abstract. In this paper we present an algorithm for the detection of spontaneous activity at individual synapses in microscopy images. By employing the optical marker pHluorin, we are able to visualize synaptic vesicle release with a spatial resolution in the nm range in a non-invasive manner. We compute individual synaptic signals from automatically segmented regions of interest and detect peaks that represent synaptic activity using a continuous wavelet transform based algorithm. As opposed to standard peak detection algorithms, we employ multiple wavelets to match all relevant features of the peak. We evaluate our multiple wavelet algorithm (MWA) on real data and assess the performance on synthetic data over a wide range of signal-to-noise ratios.

Keywords: multiple wavelets, continuous wavelet transform, peak detection, pHluorin, individual synaptic activity, microscopy.

1 Introduction

Neuronal signal transmission relies on the release of neurotransmitters from vesicles at chemical synapses. Efficacy of synaptic transmission is highly variable, and thereby participating in controlling the information flow in the brain. Therefore, the estimation of biophysical parameters modulating transmission efficacy is of great interest for neurobiologists.

Due to the nanometer-sized structures of chemical synapses, optical methods based on fluorescence microscopy are preferable for the analysis of neurotransmitter release. The most direct method uses pH-sensitive variants of green fluorescent protein (pHluorins) coupled to the inside of synaptic vesicles [1]. As depicted in Fig. 1, pHluorins change their fluorescence during vesicle recycling due to the pH gradient between the in- and outside of vesicles. These changes can be detected and have been used to analyze the kinetics of endocytosis [2], the quantification of different vesicle release pools [3] and involved molecules [4]. However, the computational procedures to detect activity still require manual interaction. Neurobiologists evoke single action potentials, that may lead to vesicle fusion, by image-locked electrical stimulation. Small regions with in-focus synapses are selected and difference images at the time of stimulation are calculated.

N. Ayache et al. (Eds.): MICCAI 2012, Part I, LNCS 7510, pp. 165–172, 2012.
© Springer-Verlag Berlin Heidelberg 2012

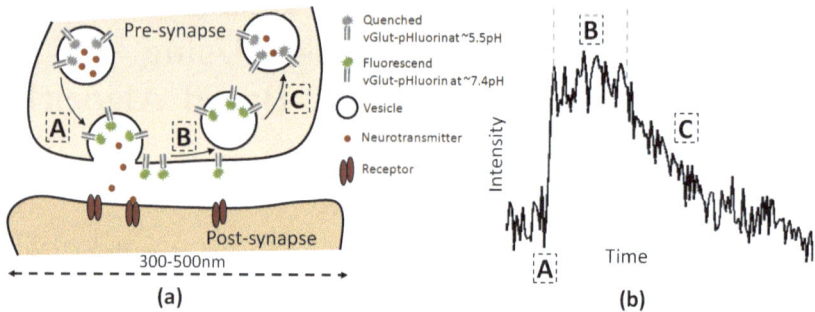

Fig. 1. Neuronal signal transmission at chemical synapses (a). At the low pH inside vesicles, pHluorins are quenched and thus hardly fluorescent. Upon vesicle fusion with the pre-synaptic membrane (exocytosis), pHluorins undergo a conformational change and their fluorescence increases (A). At the beginning of endocytosis, vesicles get recycled (B) and reacidify (C), thus, pHluorins get quenched again. The resulting intensity signal (b) is characterized by an immediate increase of intensity (A), followed by a dwell until endocytosis (B) and an intensity decay due to vesicle reacidification (C).

To our knowledge, there is no automated approach for the detection of individual synaptic communication. We present an algorithm based on the continuous wavelet transform (CWT) that also detects spontaneous events of active synapses[1]. This is particularly important for the analysis of changes in transmission efficacy and must be robust to varying signal strengths due to off-focus synapses and variations in the number of released vesicles per action potential.

2   Related Work

Peak detection in one-dimensional signals is challenging due to measurement noise and the lack of unique discriminating features. The most basic method is amplitude thresholding. Template matching is more robust with respect to noise since it also analyzes the shape of the peak. For a known shape, matched filtering [5] provides optimal detection under Gaussian noise. If only estimates are available, thresholding can be performed on similarity measures of the signal [6]. However, performance decreases if the peaks significantly vary in shape or size.

On the other hand, algorithms that use no prior shape information and perform blind equalization instead [7,8], require sufficiently large amounts of data and are highly sensitive to artifacts. Assuming that basic peak properties are preserved over all peaks, the wavelet transform is another alternative. Here, the signal is correlated with a mother wavelet at different scales, which enhances peak properties in the wavelet coefficients. Thresholding can then be applied on sets of wavelet coefficients [9–11].

---

[1] The software, including a GUI, is available at `http://sourceforge.net/projects/isad/`

A major drawback of CWT-based analysis is the usage of a single, probably suboptimal, wavelet for all peaks. We, therefore, propose the combination of multiple wavelets in a CWT-based algorithm referred to as MWA to match shape properties that cannot be addressed by a single wavelet.

3 Method

Our MWA peak detection method operates on intensity responses of individual synapses in microscopy images. Active synapses appear as elliptic spots in the mean intensity image of all acquired pHluorin time lapse images and are detected using the top hat filter. These candidates are fitted with an elliptical Gaussian function using a restricted region around synapses. The support regions are computed using an inverse watershed algorithm. This allows for the separation of nearby synapses and application of constraints on the size of synapses. Furthermore, we co-transfect any culture with synapsinRFP, which serves as a marker for the pre-synapse and include only those synapses that are double positive for pHluorin and synapsin. The individual intensity response for each point in time is then computed from the mean intensities within a fixed region centered over each synapse (see Fig. 2a). The region must be as small as possible to optimize the signal-to-noise ratio (SNR) but large enough to contain both sites of vesicle recycling. Experiments show that both requirements are robustly fulfilled taking a diameter of three times the size of the point spread function of the microscope. The wavelet transform decomposes a signal $s(t)$ into shifted and scaled versions $\psi_{a,b}(t)$ of a mother wavelet $\psi(t)$ to project it into the wavelet space:

$$C(a,b) = \int_{\mathbb{R}} s(t)\psi_{a,b}(t)dt, \ \psi_{a,b}(t) = \frac{1}{\sqrt{a}}\psi\left(\frac{t-b}{a}\right) \ a,b \in \mathbb{R}, \ a > 0. \quad (1)$$

The wavelet coefficients $C(a,b)$ determine the similarity between the signal and the mother wavelet at different scales a and translations b.

The immediate increase of intensity, the variation in the dwell time, and the intensity decay are the characterizing peak shape features even though the kinetics are superimposed by photobleaching. For successful CWT-based peak detection, the mother wavelet must match the basic peak shape. Unfortunately, the major wavelet families provide no wavelet that supports all features. We, therefore, propose to cover the peak features by different wavelets and fuse their information after processing in the wavelet space. By visual inspection, we find that a combination of the Haar and the Bior3.1 wavelet describes the major peak shape characteristics (see Fig. 2b). Here, the Haar wavelet detects the intensity increase in a small support region and Bior3.1 adjusts to the dwell time, limited by the local discontinuities at the intensity increase and the onset of the decay. The actual peak detection method basically comprises six steps that are illustrated in Fig. 3 using a section from signal A in Fig. 2a. In step I, the signal is projected twice into the wavelet space using the two wavelets independently and resulting in C_{haar} and C_{bior}. The projections are directly applied on the signal without prior baseline removal as the influence of photobleaching is minor and monotonically decreasing in the peak support region [11].

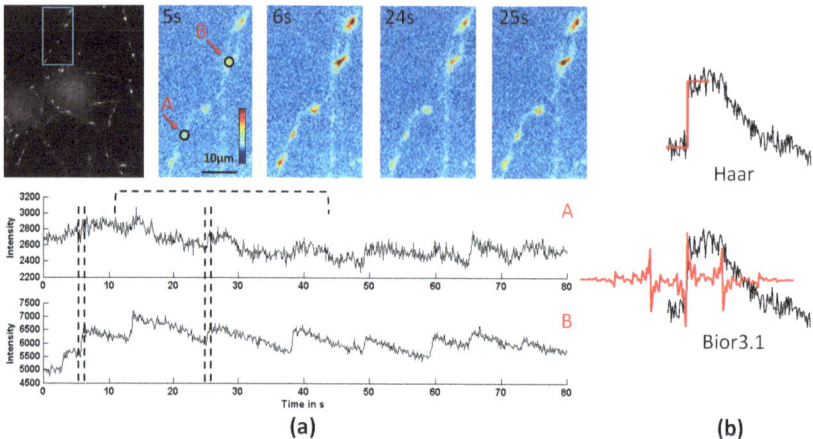

Fig. 2. The change in intensity during synaptic activity is highlighted using a false colored region of the microscopy image (a). Below, the two intensity signals illustrate that synapses in the same image can have different SNR and baseline intensity. (b) depicts the use of the two wavelets, presenting the decomposing wavelet functions ψ in red and an almost ideal intensity response in black. The wavelets are mirrored at the x axis for illustration.

In step II, the most significant coefficients are selected using the thresholding strategy, proposed for wavelet denoising by Donoho and Johnstone [12]:

$$C_t(a,b) = \begin{cases} C(a,b) & \text{if } C(a,b) \geq t_a \\ 0 & \text{otherwise} \end{cases}.$$ (2)

The threshold t_a for each scale a is derived from the noise coefficients at that scale. As they are unknown, a reasonably unbiased estimate can be obtained from the median absolute deviation $\tilde{\sigma}_a$, giving $t_a = \tilde{\sigma}_a/0.6745$ [13]. If the variation in peak size is known from biophysical properties, then the relevant coefficients can also be restricted from the support range of the mother wavelet [9, 10]. In our application, the current dwell time of a peak is unknown but follows an exponential distribution with a mean lifetime of ∼14s [2]. For any point in time we, therefore, continuously select all remaining coefficients up to the scale $a_{dwell}(b)$ that has the highest coefficient $\hat{c}(b)$, or is a defined maximal scale $\hat{a}$. This selects the most useful scales for a peak, as significant signal structures propagate across scales [14] and at the location of a peak wavelet coefficients continuously increase over scales until the match is optimal. Thus, our scale selection aims at estimating from $\hat{c}(b)$ the scale $a_{dwell}(b)$ that correlates to the dwell time of a peak. The maximal scale $\hat{a}$ is independently defined for the two wavelets. Since the Haar wavelet matches a narrow local discontinuity it is set to $\hat{a}_{haar} = 20$, corresponding to 2s time interval. The Bior wavelet covers the whole peak and we therefore define $\hat{a}_{bior} = (2\tau f_s)/r_{bior} = 94$. Here, τ is the mean dwell time, r_{bior} the support range of the Bior wavelet and f_s the sampling rate.

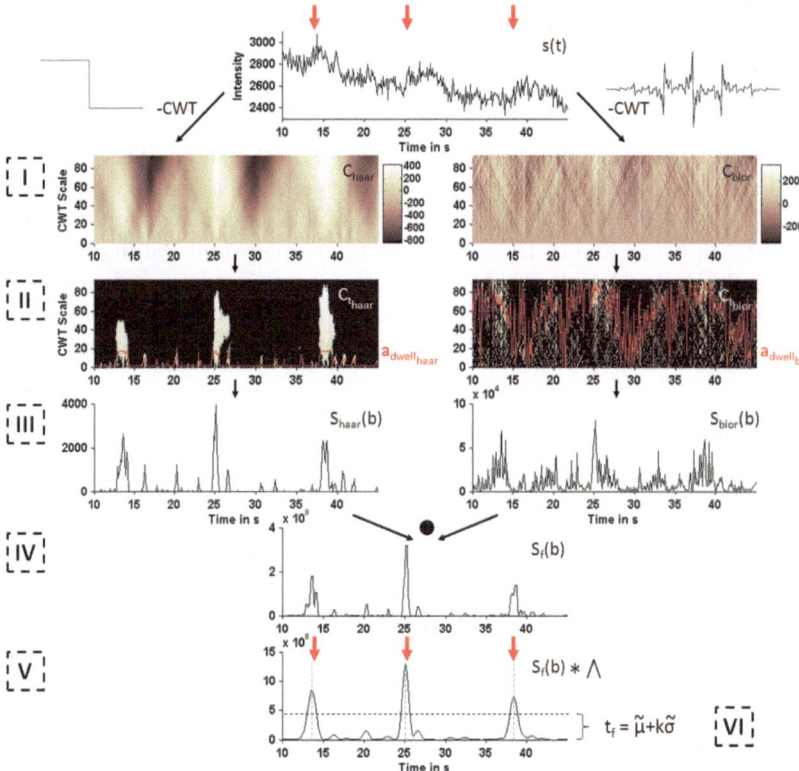

Fig. 3. Steps of MWA: I multiple signal projection into the wavelet space, II selection of relevant coefficients, III combination of coefficients, IV fusion of multi wavelet information, V Bartlett window smoothing and VI peak thresholding

In step III the selected coefficients are combined to the signal $S(b)$:

$$S(b) = \sum_{a=1}^{a_{dwell}(b)} C_t(a,b). \qquad (3)$$

This is similar to computing the ridge lines in the wavelet coefficients [11] as it also favors continuous scale combinations and tolerates gaps between scales. However, it is computationally much more efficient and requires no additional parameters to be set.

The information from the two wavelets are fused in step IV. In contrast to the multispectra algorithm [15], where Hsueh et al. propose the merging of redundant signals directly in the wavelet coefficients we fuse the complementary signals $S_{haar}(b)$ and $S_{bior}(b)$ by pointwise multiplication ($\bullet$) into $S_f(b)$. This can be interpreted as a logical AND operation between two individual peak indications. Further, a third order local maximum filter is applied to each signal before fusion to account for the fact that the Haar and Bior wavelet have a location shift at the same peak. Hence, the data fusion becomes:

$$S_f(b) = \max_{b-1\leq b^*\leq b+1} S_{haar}(b^*) \bullet \max_{b-1\leq b^*\leq b+1} S_{bior}(b^*). \qquad (4)$$

Finally, local maxima are found and compared to a threshold. Therefore in step V, $S_f(b)$ is first smoothed by convolution with the Bartlett window [9] to remove spurious peaks in the vicinity of real peaks as well as plateaus of similar values in $S_f(b)$ that can occur due to the maximum filter operation. We finally compute the threshold in step VI using robust statistics: $t_f = \tilde{\mu}_{S_f} + k\tilde{\sigma}_{S_f}$, where $\tilde{\mu}$ is the median and $\tilde{\sigma}$ the median absolute deviation. Hence, under constant imaging conditions, t_f is applicable for all synapses without individual adjustment of k.

4   Evaluation

To evaluate the detection performance of our method, we analyzed real data[2] that comprises 123 synapse signals from four images acquired at 10Hz for 2-3min. To distinguish between evoked and spontaneous activity, six action potentials have been evoked by single pulse electrical stimulation during each acquisition. Three biological experts individually detected peaks in the data. The inter-rater reliability was surprisingly low. The neurobiologists' ground truths exhibited only a mutual similarity of 34±10% (approximated with the Jaccard index) and thus, did not allow a quantitative performance assessment.

As an indirect correctness measure, we instead show in larger data sets that detected peaks exhibit a quantized distribution of peak intensities [2,4]. As we include off-focus synapses and combine acquisitions from cell preparations with different expression levels, peaks from different synapses have different absolute intensity quanta. Hence, we estimate the individual absolute quantal intensity from the peaks of each synapse by hierarchical clustering. This allows for computing relative peak intensities, which can be combined with other synapses. The distributions for spontaneous activity are shown in Fig. 4a-c. There is only one significant peak in Fig. 4a indicating that all peaks at a synapse originate from the same amount of released vesicles. In comparison, there are several evenly spaced peaks under high Ca^{2+} concentration suggesting that at single synapses peaks with different intensities did occur. We conclude that correct peaks have been detected, because, as expected, applying high Ca^{2+} concentration (5mM $CaCl_2$, 0.6mM $MgCl_2$) increases the probability for higher numbers of released vesicles per action potential. Analysis of evoked peaks yields equal results.

For a more rigorous test, we applied MWA on synthetic data and compared its performance with amplitude thresholding (AT). The data were created from 60 clearly identifiable evoked and spontaneous peaks that were repeatedly placed on signals of length 3min. To test the performance over different SNRs, we added

---

[2] Rat Hippocampal neurons were transfected to couple pHluorin to the vesicle protein vGlut. We performed recordings after 14-18 DIV while perfusing with normal extracellular solution and standard calcium concentration (2mM $CaCl_2$, 2mM $MgCl_2$).

scaled noise from real signals that showed no activity. The noise between peaks was also adjusted to match the SNR of the peaks. Similar to the receiver operating characteristic curve, we assess the performance by plotting true positive rate (TPR) and false discovery rate (FDR) for different thresholds k (see Fig. 4d-e). Clearly, the detection capability of MWA is superior at any SNR for evoked and spontaneous peaks. The relative improvement even increases towards low SNR.

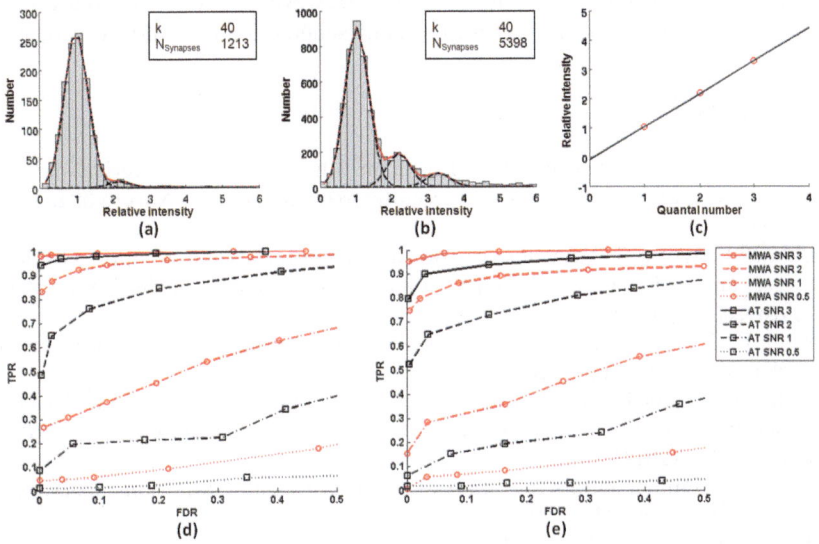

Fig. 4. Relative intensity distributions for standard (a) and high (b) Ca^{2+} concentration. The red curve is the overall fit to a set of Gaussians of the same width. The black curve shows the individual Gaussians. The line fit to the fitted peak positions visualizes the integer multiples of the quantal distribution (c). (d) and (e) show the performance assessment over varying SNR for evoked and spontaneous activity, respectively. Each curve is computed from 500 peaks.

5   Conclusion

We proposed a multi wavelet algorithm for the improved detection of in particular spontaneous activity that has not been investigated yet. The application of two different wavelets is novel and allows to match the most important peak features. On synthetic data, our method shows superior performance to amplitude thresholding at any SNR and, thus, addresses the requirement for high temporal resolution up to 100Hz [3]. On real data, we showed that detected peaks reveal the quantal nature of vesicle release, indicating the correctness of our method. A ground truth evaluation failed due to the poor inter-rater reliability. This underlines the need for automatic approaches. Notably, our method is not limited to two wavelets, but can be used with any number of wavelets, yielding a great potential for the detection of even more varying peak shapes.

For unsupervised detection, there are still two problems to solve. First, the SNR depends on the size of the synaptic region which itself depends on the setup, particularly the objective and emission wavelength. Instead of computing the intensity signal using a fixed region, 2D Gaussian functions could be fitted to the intensity profile of synapses to track the optimal intensity, which also counteracts motion artefacts. Second, we will investigate the choice of the threshold parameter k more rigorously. In fact, the chosen values k are reasonably robust for imaging synapses in a wider field of view. However, the expression level of cell preparations often varies and an adjustment scheme for k would be preferable.

References

1. Miesenböck, G., De Angelis, D.A., Rothman, J.E.: Visualizing secretion and synaptic transmission with pH-sensitive green fluorescent proteins. Nature 394, 192–195 (1998)
2. Balaji, J., Ryan, T.A.: Single-vesicle imaging reveals that synaptic vesicle exocytosis and endocytosis are coupled by a single stochastic mode. PNAS 104(51), 20576–20581 (2007)
3. Ariel, P., Ryan, T.A.: Optical mapping of release properties in synapses. Frontiers in Neural Circuits 4(18) (2010)
4. Sinha, R., Ahmed, S., Jahn, R., Klingauf, J.: Two synaptobrevin molecules are sufficient for vesicle fusion in central nervous system synapses. PNAS 108(34), 14318–14323 (2011)
5. Kay, S.M.: Fundamentals of statistical signal processing: detection theory, pp. 94–140. Prentice Hall PTR (1998)
6. Jain, A.K., Duin, R.P.W., Mao, J.: Statistical Pattern Recognition: A Review. IEEE Trans. Pattern Anal. Mach. Intell. 22(1), 4–37 (2000)
7. Shahid, S., Walker, J., Smith, L.S.: A New Spike Detection Algorithm for Extracellular Neural Recordings. IEEE Trans. Biomed. Eng. 57(4), 853–866 (2010)
8. Natora, M., Obermayer, K.: An Unsupervised and Drift-Adaptive Spike Detection Algorithm Based on Hybrid Blind Beamforming. EURASIP J. Adv. Signal Process. (2011)
9. Kim, K.H., Kim, S.J.: A Wavelet-Based Method for Action Potential Detection From Extracellular Neural Signal Recording With Low Signal-to-Noise Ratio. IEEE Trans. Biomed. Eng. 50(8), 999–1011 (2003)
10. Benitez, R., Nenadic, Z.: Robust Unsupervised Detection of Action Potentials With Probabilistic Models. IEEE Trans. Biomed. Eng. 55(4), 1344–1354 (2008)
11. Du, P., Kibbe, W.A., Lin, S.M.: Improved Peak Detection in Mass Spectrum by Incorporating Continuous Wavelet Transform-based Pattern Matching. Bioinformatics 22, 2059–2065 (2006)
12. Donoho, D.L., Johnstone, I.M.: Ideal Spatial Adaptation by Wavelet Shrinkage. Biometrika 81, 425–455 (1994)
13. Nenadic, Z., Burdick, J.W.: Spike Detection Using the Continuous Wavelet Transform. IEEE Trans. Biomed. Eng. 52(1), 74–87 (2005)
14. Mallat, S., Zhong, S.: Characterization of Signals from Multiscale Edges. IEEE Trans. Pattern Anal. Mach. Intell. 14(7), 710–732 (1992)
15. Hsueh, H., Kuo, H., Tsai, C.: Multispectra CWT-based algorithm (MCWT) in mass spectra for peak extraction. J. Biopharm. Stat. 18, 869–882 (2008)

An Adaptive Method of Tracking Anatomical Curves in X-Ray Sequences

Yu Cao[1] and Peng Wang[2]

[1] Department of Computer Science and Engineering, University of South Carolina, Columbia, SC 29208, USA
[2] Corporate Research and Technology, Siemens Corporation, 755 College Road East, Princeton, NJ 08540, USA

Abstract. Tracking anatomical structures in X-Ray sequences has broad applications, such as motion compensation for dynamic 3D/2D model overlay during image guided interventions. Many anatomical structures are curve-like such as ribs and liver dome. To handle various types of anatomical curves, a generic and robust tracking framework is needed to track shapes of different anatomies in noisy X-ray images. In this paper, we present a novel tracking framework, which is based on adaptive measurements of structures' shape, motion, and image intensity patterns. The framework does not need offline training to achieve robust tracking results. The framework also incorporates an online learning method to robustly adapt to anatomical structures of different shape and appearances. Experimental results on real-world clinical sequences confirm that the presented anatomical curve tracking method improves the tracking performance compared to a baseline performance.

1 Introduction

Anatomical curve tracking in X-ray sequences have important applications in image guided surgery, such as motion compensations for 3D/2D dynamic model overlap, and needle insertion guidance. In such applications, it is desirable to compensate organ motions, in order that models can be properly visualized on X-ray images to guide the interventional procedures. Since many anatomical structures are curve-like, e.g., ribs and liver dome, as shown in Fig. 1, this paper presents a generic framework that tracks a wide variety of anatomical curve structures in a fluoroscopic sequence, to provide motion compensation information for image guided interventions.

The generic anatomical curve tracking in X-ray sequences is challenging. Shown in Fig. 1, the image quality is usually poor due to preferred low radiation dose. Anatomical structures have different shapes which undergo continuous changes due to breathing and cardiac motions during interventions. The motion could cause image blurs, and occlusions between different structures. Traditional tracking methods that are based on the constant image intensity assumptions, such as optical flow based method [1], will suffer from severe drifting when being used in such challenging situations. A variety of curve tracking methods have

N. Ayache et al. (Eds.): MICCAI 2012, Part I, LNCS 7510, pp. 173–180, 2012.

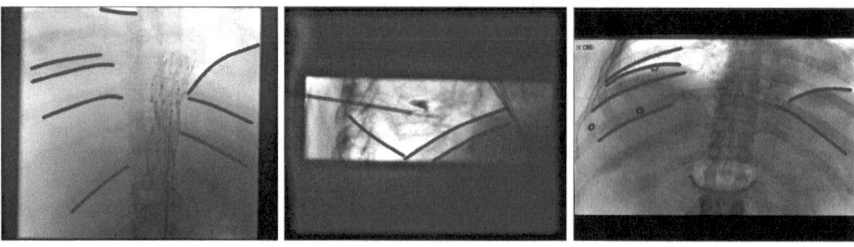

Fig. 1. Exemplar anatomical curves in X-ray image sequences, denoted by blue curves. The curves include ribs, liver dome, and diaphragm.

been developed for tracking anatomical structure in [2,5,10] or devices in [9,7,4]. In [2], an endocardium tracking method based on fusing optical flows with learning based shape subspace is used. In [5], a shape-based segmentation and tracking of deformable anatomical structures method is presented. In [9], a probabilistic tracking method is presented in order to track the guidewire in fluoroscopy images. This method requires offline learning to build classifiers specifically for guidewires. In [7], a deformable guidewire tracking method is proposed based on offline training. [4] proposed a graph-based guidewire tracking method which relies on B-spline curve model and strong geometric interests points. However, all the above methods focus on tracking specific anatomical structures or devices, rather than a generic form of anatomical structures.

In this paper, we present a probabilistic framework for anatomical curves tracking in X-ray image sequences. Through novel measurement models and probabilistic measurements fusion, the framework can capture the shape and image intensity variations of generic anatomical curves, and adapt to different tracking situations. Compared with existing methods [2,5,9,7,4], the presented framework makes the following contributions: 1) It is a generic approach and can be applied to track a variety of anatomical curve structures; 2) It introduces novel measurements in a Bayesian framework, including a novel formalization of combining optical flow, binary image patterns, and an online learning method as measurements for curve tracking; and 3) by the fusion of multiple measurements, the method is adaptive to motions, shapes and intensity pattern changes during tracking. The details of the tracking framework are explained in Section 2, and the experimental results in Section 3 demonstrates the effectiveness of presented tracking method.

2   Anatomical Curve Tracking Framework

2.1   Framework Overview

In this paper, the anatomical curve tracking is formalized with a Bayesian inference framework. A spline Γ is used to represent an anatomical curve structure to be tracked. To simplify the representation, a spline curve is sampled and noted as $\Gamma(\mathbf{x})$, where $\mathbf{x} = \{x_1, \ldots, x_N\}$ are the set of N uniformly sampled landmarks.

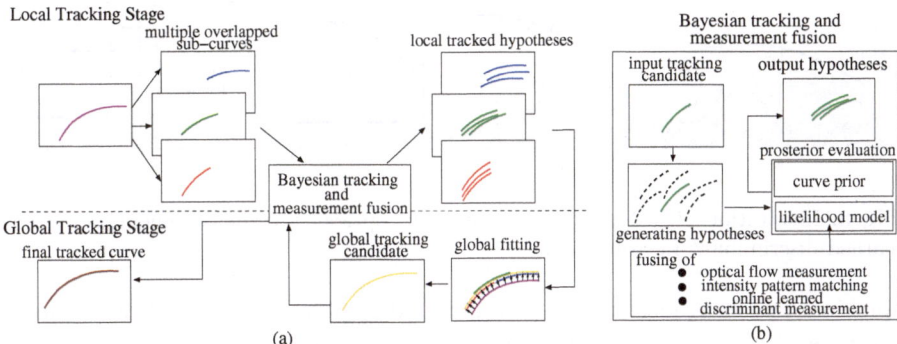

Fig. 2. (a) The hierarchical tracking framework; (b) The Bayesian framework for curve tracking

At the t-th frame, a curve candidate is noted as $\Gamma_t(\mathbf{x}_t^k)$ and the landmarks are $\mathbf{x}_t^k$. Base on the Bayesian rule and a commonly assumed Markov property for tracking, the posterior probability of a curve to be tracked has the form of

$$P(\Gamma_t(\mathbf{x}_t^k)|\mathbf{Z}_t) \propto P(\Gamma_t(\mathbf{x}_t^k))P(\mathbf{Z}_t|\Gamma_t(\mathbf{x}_t^k)) \tag{1}$$

where $\mathbf{Z}_t$ is the image observation on the t-th frame. The tracking result $\hat{\Gamma}_t(\mathbf{x}_t)$ is the curve that maximizes the posterior probability, i.e.,

$$\hat{\Gamma}_t(\mathbf{x}_t) = \arg \max_{\Gamma_t(\mathbf{x}_t^k)} P(\Gamma_t(\mathbf{x}_t^k)|\mathbf{Z}_t) \tag{2}$$

In Eqn. (1), $P(\Gamma_t(\mathbf{x}_t^k))$ is a prior probability of a curve candidate $\Gamma_t(\mathbf{x}_t^k)$. The prior probability imposes a constraint on 2D motions between a curve candidate $\Gamma_t(\mathbf{x}_t^k)$ and the previous tracked curve $\hat{\Gamma}_{t-1}(\mathbf{x}_{t-1})$. The likelihood model $P(\mathbf{Z}_t|\Gamma_t(\mathbf{x}_t^k))$ measures the likelihood of the tracking candidate $\Gamma_t(\mathbf{x}_t^k)$ based on the observation at the t-frame. To adaptively track anatomical curves in X-ray images, carefully designed prior models and likelihood measurement models are applied in our framework, with more details provided in Section 2.2 and Section 2.3, respectively.

Our tracking framework follows a hierarchical scheme, i.e, from a local scale to a global scale, as illustrated in Fig. 2.(a). At the local scale, a curve is divided into several sub-curves (each two neighbouring sub-curves have 50% overlaps with each other), and then each sub-curve is independently tracked. The local tracking provides multiple candidates for each local curve, and their combinations (using global fitting, Fig. 2.(a)) provide hypotheses for the subsequent global tracking, which is to maximize the posterior probability of the whole curve. Both local and global tracking follow the same Bayesian tracking framework, as shown in Fig. 2.(b). The hierarchical tracking scheme allows the adaptive and effective tracking of an anatomical curve: first, the local tracking allows flexible affine deformation for each sub-curve whose motion may be different from the other part of the curve; second, the global tracking combines all the possible

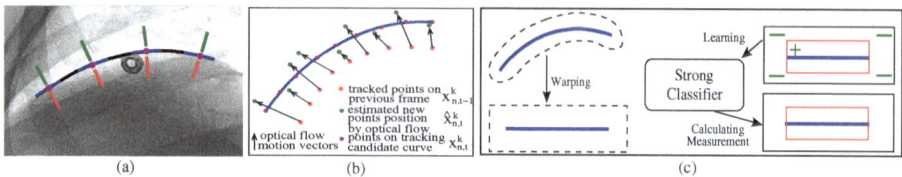

Fig. 3. Illustration of: (a) intensity pattern; (b) optical flow measurement; (c) online learned discriminant measurement

combinations from local tracking results and impose constraints from a global shape, so it can prevent possible drifting of local sub-curves.

2.2   Curve Prior

Most motions of anatomical structures such as ribs and livers, are mainly caused by breathing motions, and less impacted by cardiac motions. So we can conveniently assume that the motion can be approximated by an affine transformation. At the t-th frame, a curve candidate $\Gamma_t(\mathbf{x}_t^k)$ is transformed from the tracked curve at a previous frame $\hat{\Gamma}_{t-1}(\mathbf{x}_{t-1})$, via an affine transformation:

$$\Gamma_t(\mathbf{x}_t^k) = A_k \hat{\Gamma}_{t-1}(\mathbf{x_{t-1}}) \tag{3}$$

A_k is an affine transformation matrix. Through our experiments, we find such motions can well describe the anatomical curve movements in X-ray images.

By further decomposing A_k with the QR decomposition $A_k = Q_k R_k$ [8], we can retrieve the affine motion parameters set $\mathbf{M}_k$. Based on $\mathbf{M}_k$ of each curve candidate, we define the curve prior as:

$$P(\Gamma_t(\mathbf{x_t^k})) \propto G(\mathbf{M}_k|\mathbf{0}, \Sigma) \tag{4}$$

where $G(\mathbf{M}_k|\mathbf{0}, \Sigma)$ is a Gaussian distribution with zero mean. Σ is the diagonal covariance matrix. Without sacrificing the generalization of the algorithm, Σ is empirically set and the same parameters are applied to all the data.

2.3   Likelihood Measurements

It is challenging to robustly and adaptively model the shape and appearance of a generic curve, as it can be of a variety of continuously changing shapes and image intensities. In this work, we achieve the robust tracking in two ways: 1) designing novel measurements that can effectively model curves' shape and appearance during tracking; 2) fusing multiple measurements. The measurement models used in this framework include optical flow measurement noted as $P^O(\mathbf{Z}_t|\Gamma_t(\mathbf{x}))$, intensity pattern matching noted as $P^I(\mathbf{Z}_t|\Gamma_t(\mathbf{x}))$, and online learned discriminant measurement noted as $P^B(\mathbf{Z}_t|\Gamma_t(\mathbf{x}))$. Each of the measurement models is explained at subsequent sections. By fusing multiple measurements, the likelihood measurement model can be written as

$$P(\mathbf{Z}_t|\Gamma_t(\mathbf{x}_t)) = P_O P^O(\mathbf{Z}_t|\Gamma_t(\mathbf{x}_t)) + P_I P^I(\mathbf{Z_t}|\Gamma_t(\mathbf{x}_t)) + P_B P^B(\mathbf{Z}_t|\Gamma_t(\mathbf{x}_t)) \tag{5}$$

where P_O, P_I, P_B are the prior probability of each measurement model, and $P_O + P_I + P_B = 1$. In the experiments, P_O, P_I and P_B can be equally weighted.

Optical Flow Measurement. Optical flow assumes constant image intensity of corresponding pixels, and provides motion estimation of individual pixels. However, optical flow suffers "aperture" and "drifting" problems on a homogeneous region, thus we use the optical flow results as one of measurements, instead of fully depending on optical flow results. Assuming that the new position of a point $x_{n,t-1}^k$ in the curve $\hat{\Gamma}_{t-1}(\mathbf{x}_{t-1}^k)$ estimated by the optical flow method is $\hat{x}_{n,t}^k$, illustrated in Fig. 3.(b), we can define the likelihood of $x_{n,t}^k$, the new position of $x_{n,t-1}^k$, as:

$$P(\mathbf{Z}_t|x_{n,t}^k) = G[\hat{x}_{n,t}^k; \sigma_o](x_{n,t}^k) \tag{6}$$

where $G[\hat{x}_{n,t}^k; \sigma_o]$ is a Gaussian distribution with $\hat{x}_{n,t}^k$ as the mean, and σ_o as the standard deviation. The measurement of the a curve is therefore the integration of the measurements of all the N points along the curve $\mathbf{Z}_t$, given that the landmarks are uniformly sampled along the curve:

$$P^O(\mathbf{Z}_t|\Gamma_t(\mathbf{x}_t^k)) = \frac{1}{N} \sum_{n=1}^{N} P(\mathbf{Z}_t|x_{n,t}^k) \tag{7}$$

Intensity Pattern Matching. In the anatomical curve tracking, it is observed that the intensity patterns of a curve needs to remain similar between two successive images. However, directly using image intensity for template matching leads to poor results due to low image quality of X-ray. In this method, three intensity patterns, similar to the LBP (Local Binary pattern) [6], are defined to describe the curve intensity. For simplicity, we name them SLBP, Spline and Bar pattern. As shown in Fig. 3.(a), given a tracking candidate $\Gamma_t(\mathbf{x}_t^k)$ shown as the black curve and its landmarks shown as magenta points, then for each landmark $x_{n,t}^k$ on the curve, we define three profiles: (1) along positive curve norm with average intensity $I_n^{\mathcal{P}}$ (green bar); (2) along $\Gamma_t(\mathbf{x}_t^k)$ and centered at $x_{n,t}^k$ with average intensity $I_n^{\mathcal{S}}$ (blue curve); and (3) along negative curve norm with average intensity $I_n^{\mathcal{N}}$ (red bar). Then a binary 3-tuple (a_n^1, a_n^2, a_n^3) can be defined as

$$a_n^1 = \begin{cases} 1, & I_n^{\mathcal{P}} > I_n^{\mathcal{N}} \\ 0, & \text{else} \end{cases} \qquad a_n^2 = \begin{cases} 1, & I_n^{\mathcal{N}} > I_n^{\mathcal{S}} \\ 0, & \text{else} \end{cases} \qquad a_n^3 = \begin{cases} 1, & I_n^{\mathcal{P}} > I_n^{\mathcal{S}} \\ 0, & \text{else} \end{cases} \tag{8}$$

Then we can define SLPB, Spline and Bar intensity patterns (I_L, I_S and I_B) as follows respectively:

$$\mathbf{I}_L(\Gamma_t(\mathbf{x}_t^k)) = (a_1^1, a_1^2, a_1^3, \cdots, a_N^1, a_N^2, a_N^3), \quad \mathbf{I}_S(\Gamma_t(\mathbf{x}_t^k)) = (I_1^{\mathcal{S}}, \cdots, I_N^{\mathcal{S}}),$$
$$\mathbf{I}_B(\Gamma_t(\mathbf{x}_t^k)) = (I_1^{\mathcal{P}}, I_1^{\mathcal{S}}, I_1^{\mathcal{N}}, \cdots, I_N^{\mathcal{P}}, I_N^{\mathcal{S}}, I_N^{\mathcal{N}}). \tag{9}$$

The measurement of intensity pattern $P^I(\mathbf{Z}_t|\Gamma_t(\mathbf{x}_t^k))$ is then defined based on the correlation between each curve and the template (tracked curves at a previous frame) as:

$$P^I(\mathbf{Z}_t|\Gamma_t(\mathbf{x}_t^k)) = 0.5 * (\frac{|\mathbf{I}(\Gamma_t(\mathbf{x}_t^k)) \cdot \mathbf{I}_{template}|}{|\mathbf{I}(\Gamma_t(\mathbf{x}_t^k))| \cdot |\mathbf{I}_{template}|} + 1) \qquad (10)$$

Online Learned Discriminant Measurement. To further improve the tracking robustness, we introduce a discriminative measurement model. Different from previous two measurement models, the discriminant measurement further distinguish the curve from backgrounds. Since we aim at tracking generic anatomical curves, we use the online boosting method [3] (rather than offline methods) to build the online discriminant model. Given a tracked curve $\hat{\Gamma}_{t-1}(\mathbf{x})$ in $(t-1)$-th frame, its neighboring region in a X-ray image can be warped into a straightened image, as illustrated in Fig. 3.(c). The straightened image together with positive (sampled within upper red box in Fig. 3.(c)) and negative samples (randomly sampled surround the red box) are used to train an online-boost tracker during the tracking [3]. Through online updating, the discriminant measurement model enables itself to adapt to the appearance changes during tracking. During tracking, for each curve candidate, we input its straightened image patch (lower red box in Fig. 3.(c)) to online-boost tracker. The probabilistic score from the online-boost tracker is used as the online discriminant measurement:

$$P^B(\mathbf{Z}_t|\Gamma_t(\mathbf{x}_t)) = \sum_{i=1}^{N'} \alpha_i \cdot h_i^{sel} \qquad (11)$$

where h_i^{sel} are the selectors of the online boost tracker, α_i are the linear combination weights, and N' is the number of selectors in the tracker [3].

3   Experiments

Our framework is validated on a set of X-ray image sequences acquired in clinical scenarios. The dataset includes 22 sequences, more than 2,000 frames in total. The anatomical structures in the dataset include lung, ribs, diaphragm, and liver. The frame sizes range from 512×512 to 1024×1024 where the physical distance between neighbouring pixels is 0.1mm. The dataset is further divided into two sub-datasets: Dataset-1 and Dataset-2. Dataset-1 contains 22 sequences which are acquired under normal radiation dose and have reasonably distinguishable curves. Dataset-2 is only consist of challenging sequences (11 sequences) in Dataset-1, where the images are acquired under lower radiation dose which makes curves even hard for human to observe.

For each sequence, we annotate multiple (2 to 8) curves along anatomical structures throughout the image sequence as the ground-truth. The annotation on the first frame is used to initialize tracking (physicians we collaborated with agree to manually specify the curves of interests to track), and the annotations

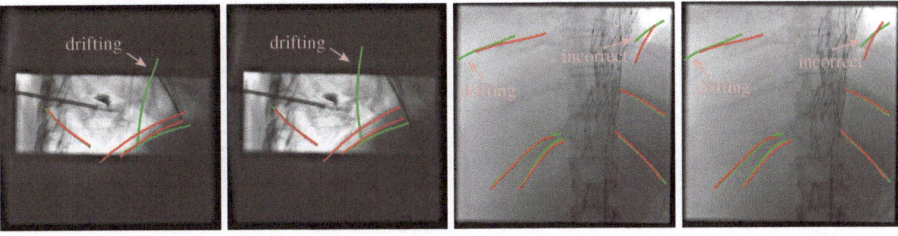

Fig. 4. Qualitative tracking results comparison between only using optical flow measurement (green curves) and using SLBP+optical flow measurements+discriminative online-learned measurement (red curves)

Table 1. Comparison of tracking error rates of different methods and combinations: (I)SLBP+Spline, (II)SLBP+Bar, (III)Spline+Bar, and (IV)SLBP+Spline+Bar

Evaluation on Dataset-1									
Threshold τ	Physical Distance	Optical flow	SLBP	Spline	Bar	(I)	(II)	(III)	(IV)
10	1mm	10.0%	7.7%	9.5%	8.1%	7.7%	8.6%	8.5%	8.9%
Evaluation on Dataset-2									
Threshold τ	Physical Distance	Optical flow	SLBP	Spline	Bar	(I)	(II)	(III)	(IV)
10	1mm	12.3%	8.6%	10.9%	9.2%	8.7%	9.5%	9.6%	10.4%

on the rest frames are used for quantitative evaluations. We define the following quantitative evaluation metrics. For a landmark on a curve, we calculate the shortest distance d from this landmark to the corresponding ground-truth curve. For a pre-defined threshold τ, if $d <= \tau$, we consider the landmark as being correctly tracked. We use the averaged tracking error rate (rate of incorrectly tracked landmarks number over total landmarks number) as tracking performance.

We tested the proposed framework and compared the tracking performance between different measurement combinations. Figure 4 shows some visual tracking results. We notice that the results from only using optical flow measurement suffer from drifting problem, especially when the image quality is low. The average tracking error rate curves of using different measurement combinations are shown in Fig. 5. From the figure, using SLBP+optical flow+online-learned discriminative measurements achieves the best performance on both Dataset-1 and Dataset-2 from thresholds 5 to 15, except only a few thresholds.

Further from Table 1, at $\tau = 10$ where the physical distance is 1mm, using SLBP+optical flow+online-learned discriminative measurements achieves the best performances on Dataset-1 and Dataset-2 with error rates 7.7% and 8.6%, respectively. This is much better than only using optical measurements whose tracking error rates are 10% and 12.3%, respectively. This demonstrates that the presented tracking framework improves the baseline performance (when only using optical flow) by a significant amount.

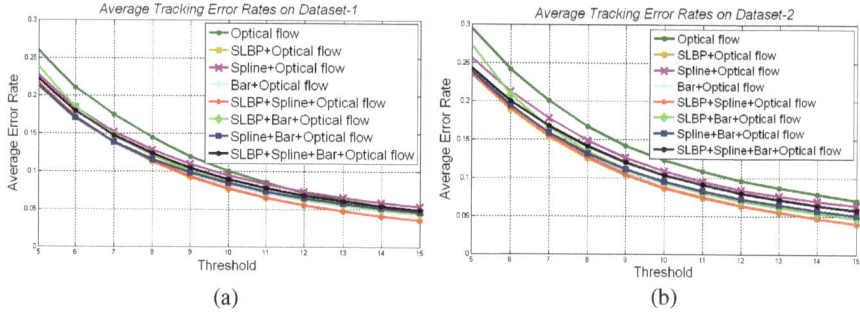

Fig. 5. The quantitative comparisons between the results of using different measurement combinations on: (a)Dataset-1 and (b)Dataset-2

4   Conclusion

In this paper, we present a probabilistic framework for adaptively tracking generic anatomical curve structures in X-ray images. We demonstrate the effectiveness of integrating appearance pattern, shape and motion information in tracking curve structures. We plan to extend the method to other image modalities such as ultrasound, and to further explore its usages in clinical applications.

References

1. Comaniciu, D.: Nonparametric information fusion for motion estimation. In: CVPR (2003)
2. Georgescu, B., Zhou, X.S., Comaniciu, D., Rao, B.: Real-Time Multi-model Tracking of Myocardium in Echocardiography Using Robust Information Fusion. In: Barillot, C., Haynor, D.R., Hellier, P. (eds.) MICCAI 2004, Part II. LNCS, vol. 3217, pp. 777–785. Springer, Heidelberg (2004)
3. Grabner, H., Grabner, M., Bischof, H.: Real-time tracking via on-line boosting. BMVC 1, 47–56 (2006)
4. Honnorat, N., Vaillant, R., Paragios, N.: Graph-Based Geometric-Iconic Guide-Wire Tracking. In: Fichtinger, G., Martel, A., Peters, T. (eds.) MICCAI 2011, Part I. LNCS, vol. 6891, pp. 9–16. Springer, Heidelberg (2011)
5. Mignotte, M., Meunier, J., Tardif, J.C.: Endocardial Boundary Estimation and Tracking in Echocardiographic. Pattern Analysis & Applications 4, 256–271 (2001)
6. Ojala, T., Pietikainen, M., Harwood, D.: Performance evaluation of texture measures with classification based on kullback discrimination of distributions. In: ICPR, pp. 582–585 (1994)
7. Pauly, O., Heibel, H., Navab, N.: A Machine Learning Approach for Deformable Guide-Wire Tracking in Fluoroscopic Sequences. In: Jiang, T., Navab, N., Pluim, J.P.W., Viergever, M.A. (eds.) MICCAI 2010, Part III. LNCS, vol. 6363, pp. 343–350. Springer, Heidelberg (2010)
8. Shoemake, K., Duff, T.: Matrix animation and polar decomposition. In: Proceedings of the Conference on Graphics Interface 1992, pp. 258–264. Morgan Kaufmann Publishers Inc. (1992)
9. Wang, P., Chen, T., Zhu, Y., Zhang, W., Zhou, S.K., Comaniciu, D.: Robust guidewire tracking in fluoroscopy. In: CVPR, pp. 691–698 (2011)
10. Wang, P., Zhou, S., Szucs, M.: Endocardium tracking by fusing optical flows in straightened images with learning based detections. In: ISBI (2011)

Directional Interpolation for Motion Weighted 4D Cone-Beam CT Reconstruction

Hua Zhang and Jan-Jakob Sonke*

Department of Radiation Oncology, The Netherlands Cancer Institute - Antoni van
Leeuwenhoek Hospital, Plesmanlaan 121, 1066 CX Amsterdam, The Netherlands
{h.zhang,j.sonke}@nki.nl

Abstract. Image quality of four dimensional cone-beam computed tomography (4D CBCT) is limited by streaking artifacts due to insufficient projections after respiratory sorting. In this paper, a framework is proposed to combine improved motion and stationary regions of CBCT together to enhance the final reconstructed image. Firstly, streaking artifacts are decreased in the 4D CBCT by directional interpolation for additional cone-beam projections. Secondly, motion is estimated through deformable image registration of the 4D CBCT and motion proportional weights are assigned to each voxel. Finally, the weighted combination of the 3D and an interpolated 4D image is calculated. The proposed method is validated by both phantom and clinical data. Experiments demonstrate this method decreases streaking artifacts as well as image blur, and then improves image quality.

Keywords: 4D CBCT, directional interpolation, phase-correlated reconstruction.

1 Introduction

Cone-beam (CB) computed tomography (CT) is used to obtain patient images immediately before radiotherapy delivery. For patients with lesions in the thoracic and upper abdominal region, respiratory induced organ motion degrades reconstructed image quality. Phase-correlated four dimensional (4D) CBCT [1,2,3,4] was introduced to decrease respiratory induced blur and obtain time-resolved image information. These methods sorted acquired projections into nearly motion-free subsets according to a respiratory signal, and reconstructed each subset with FDK algorithm [5]. Since view-aliasing artifacts emerged due to insufficient number of projections after sorting, slowing gantry rotation [4] and multiple rotations [3] schemes were introduced to acquire more projections and improve image quality. McKinnon *et al.* [6] incorporated forward projection step to increase sampling projection number, while Bergner *et. al.* [7] introduced AAPC to distinguish the motion between respiratory and gantry-rotation on projection data, and applied a projectionwise phase-dependent weighting function. Then a phase-correlated

---

* This research was sponsored by CTMM, project Breast CARE (grant 03O-104).

N. Ayache et al. (Eds.): MICCAI 2012, Part I, LNCS 7510, pp. 181–188, 2012.

4D CBCT was reconstructed by combining high temporal resolution regions with strong motion and motionless regions with improved image quality. On the other hand, Betram *et al.*[8] employed directional interpolation to calculate intermediate views in 3D CBCT for skull imaging. Directional interpolation uses a structure tensor to estimate the local orientation of extracted sinograms, and interpolates pixels by applying the orientation. This method increases the number of projections and improves the reconstructed image quality. A complete comparison of different 4D methods is discussed in the paper [9].

In this paper, we introduce and evaluate a strategy called motion weighted 4D CBCT reconstruction. We firstly sort all projections into subsets according to respiratory signal after image acquisition. Directional interpolation is applied to each subset to increase projection number. All acquired original projections are reconstructed to a 3D CBCT, and both interpolated and acquired projections are reconstructed to an interpolated 4D CBCT. Finally, according to the motion estimation results on this 4D data, we combine the 3D and 4D image by a weighting function. The proposed method is evaluated on both phantom and patient data.

2   Methods

The flow chart of our method is depicted in Fig.1. Directional interpolation is to reduce view aliasing artifacts and thus increase the image quality of 4D data. Motion estimation distinguishes moving and stationary anatomy in 4D CBCT. Finally, a new CBCT is generated based on the 3D CBCT reconstructed from all the original acquired projections for the stationary part, and based on the 4D interpolated reconstruction for the moving part.

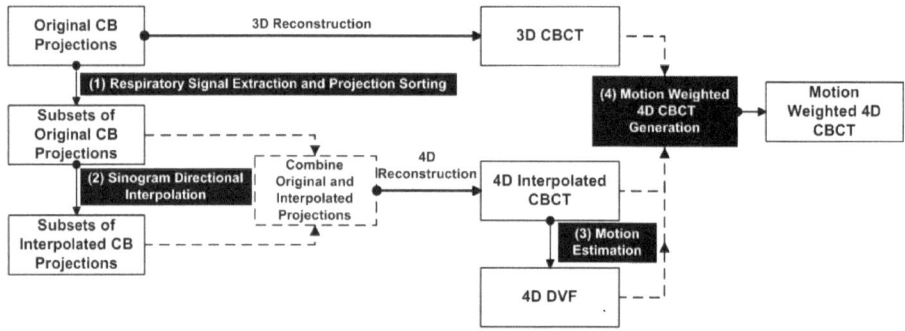

Fig. 1. Flow chart of our method. Rectangles are data and dashed rectangle means combining data from different source. The dark rectangles are main processing steps. FDK [5] is for 3D or 4D reconstruction (after sorting).

2.1   Respiratory Signal Extraction and Projection Sorting

Phase-correlated 4D CBCT reconstruction requires a respiratory signal to sort projections into subsets according to the respiratory phase. This signal is extracted from the series of acquired original CB projections through image processing following the diaphragm motion [4]. According to the phase of respiratory signal, we sort the projections into ten phase bins. In each bin, we collect a subset of projections which from the same respiratory phase. This process is illustrated in Fig.2.(a) where the bigger dots in phase graph represent the projections from the same phase bin.

2.2   Sinogram Directional Interpolation

Directional interpolation [8] is used to increase projection number. After projection sorting, all projections from the same phase bin are stacked together as a

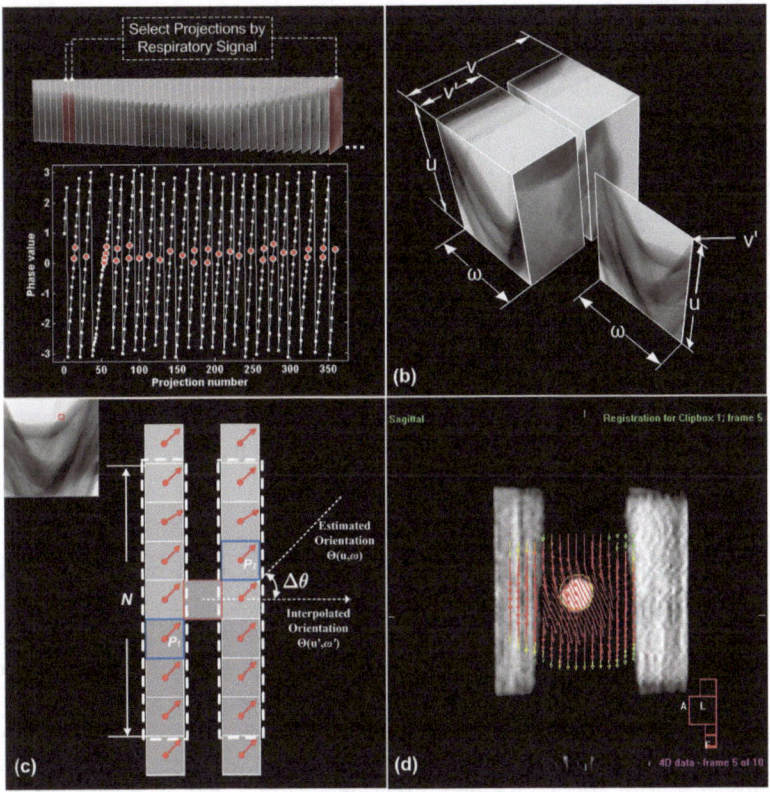

Fig. 2. (a) Selected cone-beam projections according to the respiratory signal. (b) The projections are stacked together and the sinogram is extracted. (c) The interpolated weight calculation. The dotted arrow represents the interpolated orientation $\theta_{(u',\omega')\rightarrow(u,\omega)}$, and the line arrows indicate the estimated orientations $\theta(u,\omega)$. (d) 4D deformation vector fields.

cube $C(u, v, \omega)$ (Fig.2.(b)), where u and v represent the detector panel coordinate axes, and the axis ω is perpendicular to plane (u, v) representing the gantry angle. Then a slice is extracted to form a sinogram. Since the respiratory motion is minimized by projection sorting, the projection pixel motion distance $|\boldsymbol{u}|$ is larger than $|\boldsymbol{v}|$ ($|\boldsymbol{u}|$ is from gantry rotation and $|\boldsymbol{v}|$ is from respiratory motion). Therefore, the 2D sinogram (u, ω) is adequate to implement interpolation. The local orientation of the sinogram is defined as the directional axis which has the minimum pixel value variation in a local region. This direction is sought by calculating the eigenvectors of a structure tensor. Mixed-orientation-parameters [10] are used to detect multiple orientations, and a final single orientation is generated by setting threshold. A more detailed description on its implementation is introduced in paper [10].

Different weights $\{\eta(u, \omega), (u, \omega) \in \Omega\}$ are given to neighboring original pixels $(u, \omega) \in \Omega$ according to the orientation results. Ω is a region of all the neighboring pixels contributing to the interpolated pixel. Then the interpolated pixel value is calculated as

$$i(u', \omega') = \frac{\sum_{(u,\omega)\in\Omega} \eta(u, \omega) \cdot i(u, \omega)}{\sum_{(u,\omega)\in\Omega} \eta(u, \omega)}. \tag{1}$$

The weight η is from $\eta(u, \omega) = \varepsilon \cdot [\cos(\Delta\theta)]^4 \cdot \lambda$. Fig.2.(c) illustrates our interpolation weighting strategy. In this figure, (u', ω') is the interpolated location, (u, ω) is the neighboring pixel position, and $\Delta\theta = \theta(u, \omega) - \theta_{(u',\omega')\rightarrow(u,\omega)}$. The difference between estimated and interpolated orientation is quantified by $\Delta\theta$. When $\Delta\theta$ is closer to 0, the interpolated pixel is closer to the local orientation, and higher weight is given to this neighbor pixel. We use $\cos(\Delta\theta)$ to smooth the weighting distribution in a none-linear shape. An indicator ε is introduced as

$$\varepsilon(x) = \begin{cases} 1 & \text{if } \cos(\triangle\theta) \geq 0 \\ 0 & \text{otherwise} \end{cases} \tag{2}$$

to eliminate these neighbor pixels where $\cos(\Delta\theta)$ is negative. This means the local orientation and interpolation direction are quite different. $\lambda = (1 - e_1/e_2)$ is a ratio to specify local single orientation accuracy, and it means that the orientation estimation is more accurate when λ is closer to 1. e_1 and e_2 are two eigenvalues from local orientation estimation [10] and $e_1 < e_2$.

The interpolation function (1) also strongly depends on the interpolation neighborhood Ω. The size of Ω is defined by $d = (s_1 \cdot \Psi)/(m \cdot 2\pi)$, where s_1 is the object motion distance along direction u (Fig.2.(b)), Ψ is total acquisition rotation angle, and m is total acquired projection number for interpolation. During a full rotation acquisition, it is assumed that $\Psi = 2\pi$, s_1 equals to detector size. Then the average motion distance between adjacent projections is s_1/m. In Fig.2.(c), the neighborhood size $N = d/0.16$ pixels, and 0.16 cm is detector pixel size.

2.3   Motion Estimation

The motion estimation algorithm analyzes the deformation between each phase of a 4D CBCT. The peak-inhale phase 3D CBCT is chosen as the reference, and other phases are registered to the reference. For the phantom data, local rigid registration by a shaped region of interest around a moving insert is used. For clinical data, an optical flow motion estimation method [11] was applied to calculate deformation vector fields (DVFs) between the reference image and other phase image. Then a 4D DVF is generated to express the respiratory motion of each voxel in a respiratory cycle.

2.4   Motion Weighted 4D CBCT Reconstruction

Our motion weighted reconstruction utilizes the 4D DVF to distinguish the moving and static part in the 4D CBCT, and combines these parts together according to the motion weight. From the 4D DVF, we calculate the displacement $\beta_i = \sqrt{v_{i1}^2 + v_{i2}^2 + v_{i3}^2}$ for each voxel. v_{i1}, v_{i2}, v_{i3} are the motion in left-right (LR), cranial-caudal (CC) and anterior-posterior (AP) directions. In the 4D DVF, we find the largest displacement $\mathbf{B}_j = \max(\beta_i)$ in current phase j, and the motion weighted 4D CBCT is defined as $t(i,j) = (1 - \omega_i) \cdot t_s(i) + \omega_i \cdot t'(i,j)$, where t_s is the 3D CBCT, t' is the interpolated CBCT, j is current phase number, and $\omega_i = \beta_i/\mathbf{B}$.

3   Experiments and Results

3.1   Data and Image Analysis

In our experiments, the Dynamic Thorax Phantom (CIRC, Norfolk, USA) was scanned over an arc of $200°$ with the acquisition times of 2, 4 and 8 minutes. The phantom had a 3 cm diameter solid water sphere moving with 2 cm peak-to-peak amplitude in the CC direction and 4s period within lung density equivalent material. For the clinical study, a patient with respiratory tumor peak-to-peak amplitude of 1.1 cm in CC direction was scanned in 1 and 4 minutes. CB projections were acquired by a Synergy CBCT scanner (Elekta Oncology Systems, Crawley, UK). The flat imager has the specifications: 5.5 fps, 40.96^2 cm^2, 1024^2 pixels; source-to-isocenter distance: 100 cm, and source-to-panel distance 153.6 cm. For computation efficiency, CB images were downsized to 256^2 pixels 0.16^2 cm^2. CBCT volumes were reconstructed by FDK [5] with a resolution 0.2^3 cm^3 in a grid 128^3. All voxel values were approximately normalized to Hounsfield Unit (HU).

For image analysis, a shaped region of interest (ROI) was manually defined from a 3D planning CT in phantom data, and the CBCT scan was subsequently registered to the planning CT. To assess streaking artifacts, root-mean-square-error (RMSE) between CBCT and planning CT was calculated as $E = \sqrt{\frac{1}{n}\sum(t_k - t'_k)^2}$, where $k \in \Omega_1$, t_k was a voxel from reconstructed CBCT, t'_k

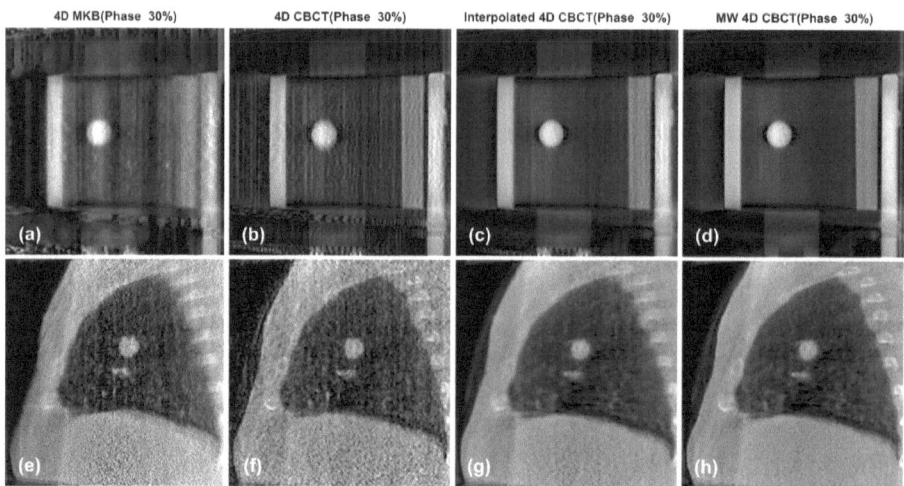

Fig. 3. Sagittal central slices of reconstructed images. (a)-(d) Phantom 4 min acquisition time. (e)-(h) Patient with 1.1 cm tumor motion, 4 min acquisition time. (a)-(h) Phase of 30% inhale-exhale cycle for the different time resolved reconstruction methods.

was a voxel from CT after it was resampled to the the grid of CBCT, and n was the total voxel number inside Ω_1. Ω_1 was a manually segmented mask with setting threshold [1000, 1100] (HU) and erosion post-processing, and it comprised homogenous voxel values. The voxels from 3D CBCT (or each phase of 4D CBCT) were extracted in Ω_1, and RMSE was calculated. Furthermore, image blur was defined in an extracted region $\Omega_2 > 1300$ (HU) of CT. Then Ω_2 was mapped to the CBCT through image registration, and the average voxel value $\bar{t} = \frac{1}{k} \sum t_k, k \in \Omega_2$ was calculated. Region Ω_2 contained high-contrast objects, and the decrement of $\bar{t}$ suggested the increment of image blur. For clinical study, the patient's gross tumor volume (GTV) was rigidly registered from CT to CBCT (or each 4D CBCT phase). After registration, the correlation ratio [12] in GTV was used to quantify the image similarity of planning CT and reconstructed CBCT. FDK and MKB [6] were implemented to compare to our methods. 3D CBCT was reconstructed from full acquired projections by FDK. 4D CBCT and 4D interpolated CBCT were sorted into 10 respiratory bins. MKB was implemented by only one forward projection step and two backward projection steps.

3.2   Results

Fig.3 displays the sagittal slice of reconstructed CBCT by 4 minutes image acquisition time. 4D MKB (Fig.3 is blurred by forward interpolation.(a)(e)). Fig.3.(b)(f) belong to phase-correlated 4D CBCT and streaking artifacts are obvious, because only about 10% of the projections are used to reconstruct each phase. Interpolated 4D CBCT decreases streaking artifacts but induces image

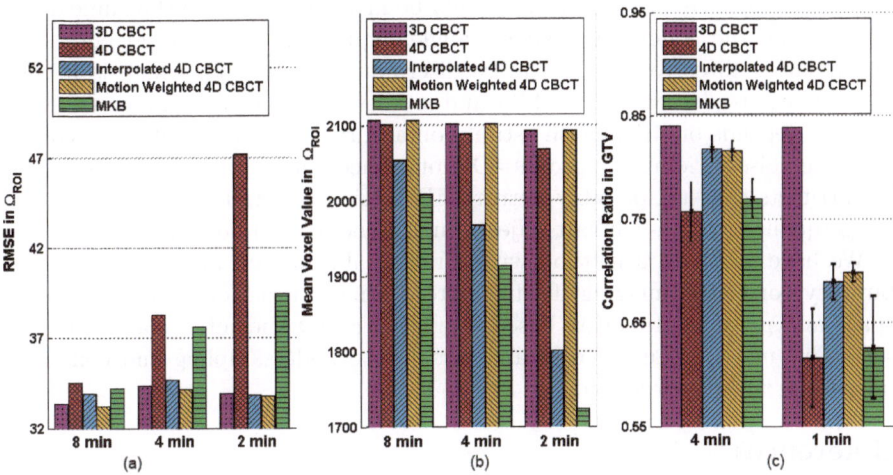

Fig. 4. (a) Streaking artifacts of phantom. (b) Image blur of phantom. (c) Correlation ratio of patient in GTV. Error bars are standard deviation calculated from 10 correlation ratios between 4D images and CT.

blur. And finally motion weighted 4D CBCT preserves the sharpness of motionless bony structure and decreases the streaking artifacts.

The quantitative results are depicted in Fig.4, and the results of 4D images are the mean value of all 10-phase images. In Fig.4.(a), streaking artifacts are compared between different acquisition protocols and methods. Interpolated and motion weighted 4D CBCT decrease the artifacts caused by undersampling of 4D CBCT. For highly undersampled 2 min scan, the streaking artifacts reduction is most pronounced. Image blur induced by interpolation is reduced by motion weighting strategy (Fig.4.(b)). Finally, Fig.4.(c) illustrates the correlation ratio of patient data. Since tumor motion is small, the correlation ratio between 3D CBCT and CT is close between different scanning times. The correlation ratio between interpolated and motion weighted CBCT is similar, but the decrease of standard deviations (error bars in Fig.4.(c)) suggests the improved image quality.

4   Discussion and Conclusion

In this paper, we have presented a motion weighted 4D CBCT reconstruction approach to cope with streaking artifacts and image blur. Streaking artifacts from undersampling were decreased by directional interpolation in sinogram space. MKB can be considered as an interpolation from all acquired projections, and our methods only utilize adjacent projections. Interpolation by more projections causes more image blur, and MKB has more blur than our method. Image blurring is a common phenomenon after interpolation, and depends on either the interpolation filter size or weights. Consequently, MKB and our method blur both interpolated projection and reconstructed images. The balance between image blur and streaking artifacts should be made according to the clinical purpose. Under the condition of sparse angle acquisition, our method boosts the interpolation filter to generate more discriminative weights, which is a effective strategy to decrease image blur and preserve the sharpness. Meanwhile, our method depends on 4D motion estimation accuracy. Our interpolation strategy decrease noise ratio and improves 4D motion accuracy. However, severe streaking artifacts can still possibly perturb 4D motion estimation and decrease the image quality of high-contrast objects such as bones and fiducial markers.

We have proposed a method with directional sinogram interpolation of respiratory correlated imaging, feeding into motion estimation in reconstruction space and motion estimation based weighting of 3D and interpolated 4D data sets. This method can decrease artifacts due to undersampling and constrains image blur after interpolation.

References

1. Dietrich, L., Jetter, S., Tücking, T., Nill, S., Oelfke, U.: Linac-integrated 4D cone beam CT: first experimental results. Physics in Medicine and Biology 51, 2939–2952 (2006)
2. Kriminski, S., Mitschke, M., Sorensen, S., Wink, N.M., Chow, P.E., Tenn, S., Solberg, T.D.: Respiratory correlated cone-beam computed tomography on an isocentric C-arm. Physics in Medicine and Biology 50, 5263–5280 (2005)
3. Li, T., Xing, L., Munro, P., McGuinness, C., Chao, M., Yang, Y., Loo, B., Koong, A.: Four-dimensional cone-beam computed tomography using an on-board imager. Medical Physics 33, 3825–3833 (2006)
4. Sonke, J.J., Zijp, L., Remeijer, P., van Herk, M.: Respiratory correlated cone beam CT. Medical Physics 32, 1176–1186 (2005)
5. Feldkamp, L.A., Davis, L.C., Kress, J.W.: Practical cone-beam algorithm. J. Opt. Soc. Am. A 1, 612–619 (1984)
6. Mckinnon, G.C., Bates, R.H.T.: Towards imaging the beating heart usefully with a conventional CT. IEEE Transactions on Biomedical Engineering BME-28(2), 123–127 (1981)
7. Bergner, F., Berkus, T., Oelhafen, M., Kunz, P., Pan, T., Kachelrieß, M.: Autoadaptive phase-correlated (AAPC) reconstruction for 4D CBCT. Medical Physics 36, 5695–5706 (2009)
8. Betram, M., Wiegert, J., Schäfer, D., Aach, T., Rose, G.: Directional view interpolation for compensation of sparse angular sampling in cone-beam CT. IEEE Transactions on Medical Imaging 28, 1011–1021 (2009)
9. Bergner, F., Berkus, T., Oelhafen, M., Kunz, P., Pan, T., Grimmer, R., Ritschl, L., Kachelrieß, M.: An investigation of 4D cone-beam CT algorithms for slowly rotating scanners. Medical Physics 37, 5044–5053 (2010)
10. Aach, T., Mota, C., Stuke, I., Mühlich, M., Barth, E.: Analysis of superimposed oriented patterns. IEEE Transactions on Image Processing 15, 3690–3700 (2006)
11. Wolthaus, J., Sonke, J.J., van Herk, M., Damen, E.: Reconstruction of a time-averaged midposition CT scan for radiotherapy planning of lung cancer patients using deformable registration. Medical Physics 35, 3998–4011 (2008)
12. Roche, A., Malandain, G., Pennec, X., Ayache, N.: The Correlation Ratio as a New Similarity Measure for Multimodal Image Registration. In: Wells, W.M., Colchester, A.C.F., Delp, S.L. (eds.) MICCAI 1998. LNCS, vol. 1496, pp. 1115–1124. Springer, Heidelberg (1998)

Accurate and Efficient Linear Structure Segmentation by Leveraging Ad Hoc Features with Learned Filters

Roberto Rigamonti and Vincent Lepetit*

CVLab, École Polytechnique Fédérale de Lausanne, Lausanne, Switzerland
{roberto.rigamonti,vincent.lepetit}@epfl.ch
http://cvlab.epfl.ch

Abstract. Extracting linear structures, such as blood vessels or dendrites, from images is crucial in many medical imagery applications, and many handcrafted features have been proposed to solve this problem. However, such features rely on assumptions that are never entirely true. Learned features, on the other hand, can capture image characteristics difficult to define analytically, but tend to be much slower to compute than handcrafted features. We propose to complement handcrafted methods with features found using very recent Machine Learning techniques, and we show that even few filters are sufficient to efficiently leverage handcrafted features. We demonstrate our approach on the STARE, DRIVE, and BF2D datasets, and on 2D projections of neural images from the DIADEM challenge. Our proposal outperforms handcrafted methods, and pairs up with learning-only approaches at a fraction of their computational cost.

1 Introduction

The extraction of linear or tubular structures has received a lot of attention from the medical imaging community, as it is the first step to recover the structure of blood vessels and neurons from images. Such extraction can be reliable if a human operator uses a semi-automated system [13]. However, imaging nowadays efficiently generates images with increasingly higher resolution, and the amount of data to analyse is overwhelming. Manually processing images thus becomes infeasible, even with very efficient semi-automated systems, and as such there is a need for automatic, reliable and fast, ways of extracting linear structures.

In order to fully automatize this extraction, many handcrafted approaches have been proposed. A common technique is to rely on the eigenvalues of the image Hessian matrix [11], which can be computed from the responses of a few separable filters [19,21], as in the multiscale vessel enhancement filtering (EF) method [7]. Other approaches rely on differential kernels [1], look for parallel

* This work has been supported in part by the Swiss National Science Foundation. The authors would like to thank C. Becker and F. Benmansour for their help in the experiments.

N. Ayache et al. (Eds.): MICCAI 2012, Part I, LNCS 7510, pp. 189–197, 2012.

edges [6], or fit superellipsoids to the image stack. A recent successful approach is the Optimally Oriented Flux (OOF) [12], computed by convolving the second derivatives of the image with the N-dimensional unit ball.

While these handcrafted methods are typically fast, the quality of their results is limited. This is because actual linear structures do not necessarily conform to the assumptions they make. For example, OOF sometimes provides weak responses, especially at bifurcations and crossovers, and yet these locations are crucial for the automated tracing of the tree structure underlying the input image. Moreover, its effectiveness on noisy data is rather poor.

Several authors used Machine Learning techniques to avoid making strong assumptions. [18,8] apply a Support Vector Machine to the responses of *ad hoc* filters. [18] considers the Hessian's eigenvalues, while the Rotational Features of [8] use steerable filters. More recently, [17] used a dictionary learning method to learn a set of linear filters on images of linear structures, by contrast with hard-coding them. In particular, it shows that convolving images with this filter bank gives responses that, when fed to an SVM, outperform state-of-the-art methods including EF, OOF, and the Rotational Features. Unfortunately, it requires a large number of filters—more than one hundred—which makes it impractical for large images.

In this paper we show that handcrafted methods and learned filters complement each other very well, as depicted in Fig. 1-right. We can therefore take advantage of both types of approaches to extract quickly and reliably linear structures. More precisely, we apply a classifier—we use Random Forests (RFs) [3] and ℓ_1-regularized logistic regression (ℓ_1-reg) [10] for efficiency—to the responses of several filters. For the handcrafted methods, we consider the EF and OOF methods. The other filters are learned with sparsity constraints, and by contrast with [17], we use a very small number of them, typically less than 10. Thanks to this small number, we save a great amount of time not only when extracting the features from the image, but also during training and testing, as the vectors to be classified are much more compact.

In short, our approach is significantly more accurate than handcrafted methods, and much faster than learning-based-only methods, bringing the accuracy advantage of learning to practical applications. In the remainder of the paper, we first describe our method, and then give a summary of our experiments comparing it against state-of-the-art approaches on challenging data.

2   Method

In this section we describe how we compute linear filters from training images, how we apply these filters to extract features from images, and how we use these features to extract linear structures.

2.1   Learning Linear Filters

We learn our linear filters by modeling the distribution of images representative of the problem at hand. This is done by assuming that there exists a sparse

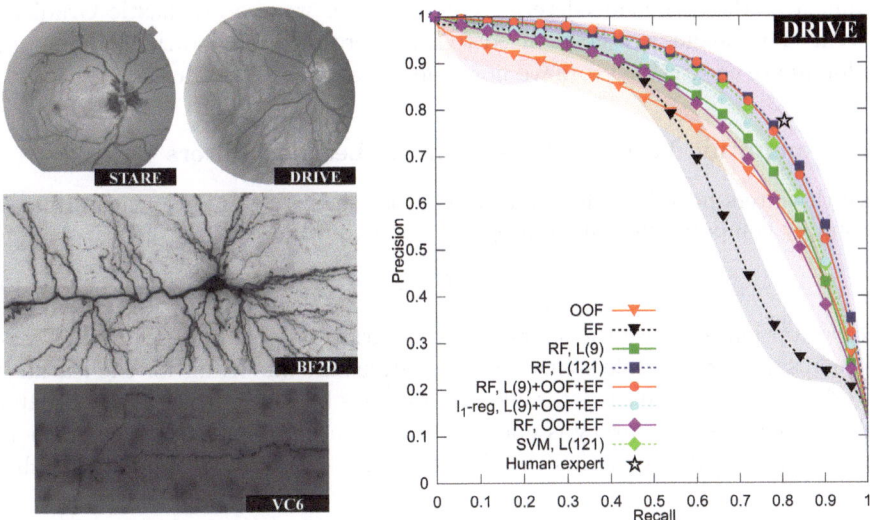

Fig. 1. Left: Sample images from the datasets we used to evaluate our approach. **Right:** Evaluation of different approaches on the DRIVE dataset. The state-of-the-art OOF and EF methods are significantly outperformed by learned features. However, this is only true when the number of learned features is very large, which makes this prohibitive in real medical imaging applications. We show that the handcrafted methods can be complemented by a very small number of learned features to obtain the same quality as learning only approaches, but at a fraction of their computational cost.

representation of the images, from which these images can be retrieved by applying a linear transformation. Such model was originally proposed in [14], and has been shown to be useful for image denoising and object recognition.

More exactly, we optimize the following objective function:

$$\underset{\{\mathbf{f}^j\},\{\mathbf{m}_i^j\}}{\mathrm{argmin}} \sum_i \left(\left\| \mathbf{x}_i - \sum_{j=1}^N \mathbf{f}^j * \mathbf{m}_i^j \right\|_2^2 + \lambda \sum_{j=1}^N \left\| \mathbf{m}_i^j \right\|_1 + \xi \sum_{j=1}^N \sum_{k \neq j} \left(\langle \mathbf{f}^j, \mathbf{f}^k \rangle \right)^2 \right). \quad (1)$$

The $\mathbf{x}_i$s are training images and the $\mathbf{f}^j$s are the learned filters. For each training image $\mathbf{x}_i$ the set $\{\mathbf{m}_i^j\}_{j=1...N}$ is the corresponding representation. Each element $\mathbf{m}_i^j$ has the same size as $\mathbf{x}_i$. The $*$ symbol represents the convolution product. The second term in Eq. (1) forces the $\{\mathbf{m}_i^j\}$ representations to be sparse, while the third term was used in [17] to counteract the natural tendency of the filters to sometimes converge to similar solutions.

The minimization process alternates between the optimization with respect to the representations and the optimization with respect to the filters. For the former we adopt a proximal method [2], which in the case of ℓ_1-norm regularization simply consists in performing a step in the direction opposite to the gradient of the ℓ_2-regularized term, followed by a component-wise soft-thresholding of the argument of the ℓ_1-penalized term. For the latter we use Stochastic Gradient Descent. The images are normalized to have zero mean and variance one, and the filters are constrained to have norm one to avoid trivial solutions [14].

2.2   Computing Feature Maps with the Learned Filters

Once the filters have been learned, we can use them to compute feature maps. We simply compute our feature maps by plain convolution:

$$\mathbf{L}_j = \mathbf{f}^j * \mathbf{x} . \tag{2}$$

Another option is to use the sparse representation $\{\mathbf{m}^j\}$ of the image $\mathbf{x}$ as feature maps. However, while sparse representations are important for the learning procedure, their effectiveness for classification has been recently questioned [16], and [17] shows that accuracy is not improved by using them as feature maps at run-time. Unreported experiments yield the same conclusion for our approach.

2.3   Description Vector and Classification

For a given input image, we compute several feature maps, namely one for EF, one for OOF, and one for each learned filter. For each image location (u, v), we obtain the vector:

$$\Big[\text{EF}[u, v], \text{OOF}[u, v], \mathbf{L}_1[u, v] \ldots \mathbf{L}_N[u, v] \Big]^T \tag{3}$$

we call descriptor below. We then apply a Random Forest or a ℓ_1-regularized logistic regressor on such descriptors to classify each image location as lying on a linear structure or on the background. Compared to a traditional logistic regressor, the optimized functional for the ℓ_1-regularized logistic regressor includes a ℓ_1 penalty on the weights, forcing them to be sparse [10].

3   Results and Discussion

In this section we first introduce the datasets we have adopted for the evaluation of our method, we then describe our evaluation setup, and we finally present our results and how they compare to existing approaches [1]. Note that the Rotational Features [8] were shown to be outperformed by [17] and, as such, we do not compare against this method.

3.1   Datasets

We use four datasets in our evaluations (see Figure 1-left):

The STARE dataset [9] is composed of 20 RGB retinal fundus slides, along with two different ground truth sets traced by two different human experts.

---

[1] The code, the datasets, and the extensive experimental results are available on the website http://cvlab.epfl.ch/~rigamont

Half of the images come from healthy patients and are therefore rather clean, while the other half present pathologies which partly occlude the underlying vasculatures and alter their appearances. Moreover, some images are affected by severe illumination changes which challenge automated algorithms.

The DRIVE dataset [20] is a set of 40 retinal scans captured for the diagnosis of systematic diseases. It is simpler than the STARE dataset in that the pathologies affecting the patients compromise less the image quality. The dataset is splitted in 20 training images and 20 test images, and ground truth data is available for both sets.

The BF2D dataset is made by minimum intensity projections of bright-field micrographs that capture neurons. The images have a very high resolution but exhibit a low signal-to-noise ratio, because of irregularities in the staining process, and the dendrites often appear as point-like structures which can be easily mistaken for the structured and unstructured noise affecting the images. As a consequence, the quality of the annotations is poor. Also, only two images have been annotated by a human expert. For this reason we have selected the image with the best ground truth as test image, and used the other image for training.

We created the VC6 dataset from a subset of the images composing the publicly available Visual Cortical Layer 6 Neuron dataset [4], which consists of 25 separated dendritic and axonal subtrees from one primary visual cortical neuron, sectioned into five physical slices. We have taken three image stacks from this dataset and computed their minimum intensity projections. These projections exhibit numerous artifacts and have a poor contrast. Their segmentation therefore represents a challenging undertaking for automated systems. We selected the first two images for the training of the algorithms, and retained the third one for testing. Ground truth data has been reconstructed from the traces made by the experts.

3.2   Experimental Setup

We first pre-processed the images in the datasets, converting them to grayscale and rescaling pixel values to zero-mean, unit-variance. For the retinal scans we only considered the green channel, since it has been shown to present the highest contrast between vessels and background [15]. We then computed the multiscale OOF and EF responses.

We also learned several filter banks of different cardinalities, at a single scale. The size of each filter has been fixed to 21×21 pixels to be consistent with the filter banks used in [17] [2]. We have experimented with smaller filter sizes, and the results show little influence. The gradient step, the regularization parameter, and all the other parameters involved in the filter learning were manually tuned.

---

[2] Learning a bank of 121 filters posed some problems in the VC6 dataset case, as low contrast and high noise prevented the learning process to get more than few dozens of meaningful filters, leading to poor performances (only slightly superior to those of 16 filters). To make a fair comparison, and for the 121 filters/VC6 case only, we have weighted the training images inversely proportionally to the OOF response, easing the learning process by focusing only on the parts where OOF responds weakly.

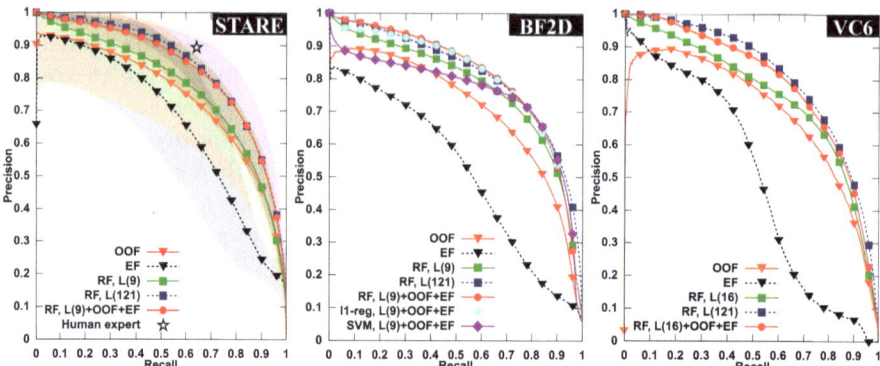

Fig. 2. Comparing EF,OOF, the method of [17] with few learned filters only, our approach, and the original method of [17] with 121 learned filters on the STARE, BF2D, and VC6 datasets (the results on DRIVE are given in Fig. 1-right). The cardinality of the learned filter banks (denoted as **L**) is given between parentheses. Note that the learning-based approaches outperform handcrafted methods even on the STARE dataset, where the used filters are not specifically tuned to the characteristics of the images, but are instead tuned to those of the DRIVE images. The results are averaged on 10 random trials and over the images of the different datasets. The shades represent 1 standard deviation around the mean value.

To test the generalization power of the learned filter banks, the results reported here for the STARE dataset were obtained with the filters learned on the DRIVE dataset, even though the former exhibits pathologies and illumination issues which are not present in the latter.

For classification, except when specifically noted, we have used 600 random trees learned on 10,000 positive and 10,000 negative samples. Comparisons between binary masks have been used as a metric in the evaluations.

3.3   Results and Discussion

The Precision/Recall curves [5] averaged over 10 random trials for different approaches are given in Figs 1-right and 2, while Fig. 3 depicts qualitative results for a randomly sampled region of a retinal scan. These figures show that our method and the method of [17] outperform the other methods, but ours is significantly faster: Table 1 details the average timings on the DRIVE dataset for the method we propose, and compares them with those of [17]. Because we use fewer filters and because the OOF and EF can be implemented in a very efficient, multi-threaded way, extracting the features is much faster in our approach. The gap widens considerably as higher-resolution images are considered.

Moreover, our descriptors are much more compact than [17]'s, as their sizes are divided by more than a factor of 10. This substantially speeds up the training and testing stages. While [17] considered only SVMs for classification, we found Random Forests and ℓ_1-regularized logistic regression well suited for the task at

Table 1. Average timings recorded for [17] and our approach on the 565×584 images of the DRIVE dataset. The time is expressed in seconds, except for the filter learning stage, and includes the time spent in reading/writing from disk ([17]: training 0.08s, testing 20s; our approach: training 0.01s, testing 2.8s). Although strongly parallelizable, implementations were restricted to use a single core to provide a fair evaluation. The OOF, which accounts for almost 50% of the time spent by our approach in the feature extraction phase, does not use an optimized implementation. The recorded SVM training timings do not include the time spent for the grid search on the parameters.

Method	Filter Learning	Feature Extraction	Training			Testing		
			RF	ℓ_1-reg	SVM	RF	ℓ_1-reg	SVM
[17]	several days	10.52	354.02	0.26	950.70	152.40	20.33	2568.53
our approach	several mins	2.12	55.91	0.05	210.56	86.70	2.84	455.97

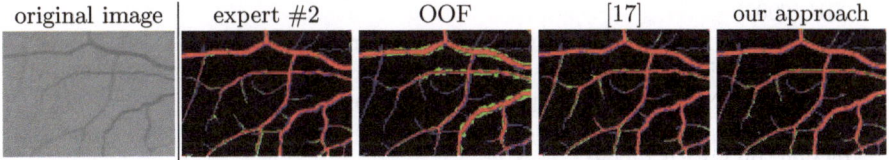

original image   expert #2   OOF   [17]   our approach

Fig. 3. Qualitative segmentation results on a randomly selected part of an image randomly chosen from the DRIVE dataset. True positives are outlined in red, false positives in green, and false negatives in blue. The segmentation accuracies for [17] and our approach are comparable, while our approach is much more efficient.

hand, obtaining comparable if not superior results in a fraction of the time (see Fig. 1-right), and without any need for a precise parameter tuning.

While the performance of logistic regression is inferior to that of Random Forests, it is still interesting to keep it into account: Its execution time is several orders of magnitude smaller, which can be appealing in practical applications.

Reducing the number of learned filters yields important speedups not only at run-time, but also during the learning of the filter banks themselves. A few minutes are typically required to learn a bank of 9 filters, which have to be compared with days for the larger filter banks in [17]. This, together with the reduced computational times, allows the practitioner to set up the segmentation pipeline from scratch and get state-of-the-art results within few dozens of minutes.

4   Conclusion

Through extensive experiments we showed that handcrafted and learned features can complement each other very well for the extraction of linear structures. This results in an efficient implementation, useful for practical applications. Our approach is general and could be used in domains where handcrafted methods exist, as is the case for the initial steps of many medical image processing algorithms, benefitting from improvements in the latter.

References

1. Al-Kofahi, K., Lasek, S., Szarowski, D., Pace, C., Nagy, G., Turner, J., Roysam, B.: Rapid Automated Three-Dimensional Tracing of Neurons from Confocal Image Stacks. ITB (2002)
2. Bach, F., Jenatton, R., Mairal, J., Obozinski, G.: Convex Optimization with Sparsity-Inducing Norms. MIT Press (2011)
3. Breiman, L.: Random Forests. Machine Learning (2001)
4. Brown, K., Barrionuevo, G., Canty, A., Paola, V.D., Hirsch, J., Jefferis, G., Lu, J., Snippe, M., Sugihara, I., Ascoli, G.: The DIADEM data sets: representative light microscopy images of neuronal morphology to advance automation of digital reconstructions. Neuroinformatics (2011)
5. Davis, J., Goadrich, M.: The Relationship Between Precision-Recall and ROC Curves. In: ICML (2006)
6. Dima, A., Scholz, M., Obermayer, K.: Automatic Segmentation and Skeletonization of Neurons from Confocal Microscopy Images Based on the 3D Wavelet Transform. TIP (2002)
7. Frangi, A.F., Niessen, W.J., Vincken, K.L., Viergever, M.A.: Multiscale Vessel Enhancement Filtering. In: Wells, W.M., Colchester, A.C.F., Delp, S.L. (eds.) MICCAI 1998. LNCS, vol. 1496, pp. 130–137. Springer, Heidelberg (1998)
8. González, G., Fleuret, F., Fua, P.: Learning Rotational Features for Filament Detection. In: CVPR (2009)
9. Hoover, A., Kouznetsova, V., Goldbaum, M.: Location Blood Vessels in Retinal Images by Piecewise Threshold Probing of a Matched Filter Response. TMI (2000)
10. Koh, K., Kim, S.J., Boyd, S.: An Interior-Point Method for Large-Scale ℓ_1-Regularized Logistic Regression. JMLR (2007)
11. Krissian, K., Malandain, G., Ayache, N., Vaillant, R., Trousset, Y.: Model Based Detection of Tubular Structures in 3D Images. CVIU (2000)
12. Law, M.W.K., Chung, A.C.S.: Three Dimensional Curvilinear Structure Detection Using Optimally Oriented Flux. In: Forsyth, D., Torr, P., Zisserman, A. (eds.) ECCV 2008, Part IV. LNCS, vol. 5305, pp. 368–382. Springer, Heidelberg (2008)
13. Meijering, E., Jacob, M., Sarria, J.C., Steiner, P., Hirling, H., Unser, M.: Design and Validation of a Tool for Neurite Tracing and Analysis in Fluorescence Microscopy Images. Cytometry A (2004)
14. Olshausen, B., Field, D.: Sparse Coding with an Overcomplete Basis Set: A Strategy Employed by V1? Vision Res. (1997)
15. Patasius, M., Marozas, V., Jegelevicius, D., Lukoševičius, A.: Ranking of Color Space Components for Detection of Blood Vessels in Eye Fundus Images. In: EMBEC (2009)
16. Rigamonti, R., Brown, M., Lepetit, V.: Are Sparse Representations Really Relevant for Image Classification? In: CVPR (2011)
17. Rigamonti, R., Türetken, E., González, G., Fua, P., Lepetit, V.: Filter Learning for Linear Structure Segmentation. Tech. rep., EPFL (2011)
18. Santamaría-Pang, A., Colbert, C.M., Saggau, P., Kakadiaris, I.A.: Automatic Centerline Extraction of Irregular Tubular Structures Using Probability Volumes from Multiphoton Imaging. In: Ayache, N., Ourselin, S., Maeder, A. (eds.) MICCAI 2007, Part II. LNCS, vol. 4792, pp. 486–494. Springer, Heidelberg (2007)

19. Sato, Y., Nakajima, S., Shiraga, N., Atsumi, H., Yoshida, S., Koller, T., Gerig, G., Kikinis, R.: 3D Multi-Scale Line Filter for Segmentation and Visualization of Curvilinear Structures in Medical Images. Med. Image Anal. (1998)
20. Staal, J., Abràmoff, M., Niemeijer, M., Viergever, M., van Ginneken, B.: Ridge-Based Vessel Segmentation in Color Images of the Retina. TMI (2004)
21. Streekstra, G., van Pelt, J.: Analysis of Tubular Structures in Three-Dimensional Confocal Images. Network-Comp. Neural (2002)

Compensating Motion Artifacts
of 3D *in vivo* SD-OCT Scans

O. Müller[1], S. Donner[2,3], T. Klinder[4], I. Bartsch[3], A. Krüger[2,3],
A. Heisterkamp[2,3], and B. Rosenhahn[1,⋆]

[1] Institut für Informationsverarbeitung, Leibniz Universität Hannover, Germany
{omueller,rosenhahn}@tnt.uni-hannover.de
[2] Laser Zentrum Hannover e.V., Germany
[3] CrossBIT, Hannover Medical School, Germany
[4] Philips Research Hamburg, Germany

Abstract. We propose a probabilistic approach for compensating motion artifacts in 3D in vivo SD-OCT (spectral-domain optical coherence tomography) tomographs. Subject movement causing axial image shifting is a major problem for in vivo imaging. Our technique is applied to analyze the tissue at percutaneous implants recorded with SD-OCT in 3D. The key challenge is to distinguish between motion and the natural 3D spatial structure of the scanned subject. To achieve this, the motion estimation problem is formulated as a conditional random field (CRF). For efficient inference, the CRF is approximated by a Gaussian Markov random field. The method is verified on synthetic datasets and applied on noisy in vivo recordings showing significant reduction of motion artifacts while preserving the tissue geometry.

1 Introduction

Optical coherence tomography (OCT) is a rapidly evolving non-invasive imaging modality used for high-resolution imaging of biological tissue structures. OCT measures the backscattering profile (over time) of a light beam penetrating the sample in axial direction. Spectral-domain OCT (SD-OCT) acquires the backscattering profile in spectral domain rather than time domain, enabling shorter acquisition time. For 3D volume acquisition, single axial scan (A-scan) acquisition is combined with a lateral scanning mechanism. 2D scans (B-scans) are composed by a series of A-scans along the x-axis (fast scanning axis). 3D volume scans in turn consist of a series of B-scans along the y-axis (slow scanning axis). In our setting we are confronted with severe axial motion shift due to heart beat or breathing during in vivo SD-OCT (spectral-domain OCT) volume acquisition of mouse skin tissue around a percutaneous implant (see Fig. 1). Along the fast scanning axis, motion artifacts are illustrated by averaging three consecutive B-scans, resulting in noticeable image blur. In slow scanning direction, motion artifacts manifest itself in dithering in axial direction.

⋆ This work is supported by funding from the DFG (German Research Foundation) for the Cluster of Excellence REBIRTH.

N. Ayache et al. (Eds.): MICCAI 2012, Part I, LNCS 7510, pp. 198–205, 2012.
© Springer-Verlag Berlin Heidelberg 2012

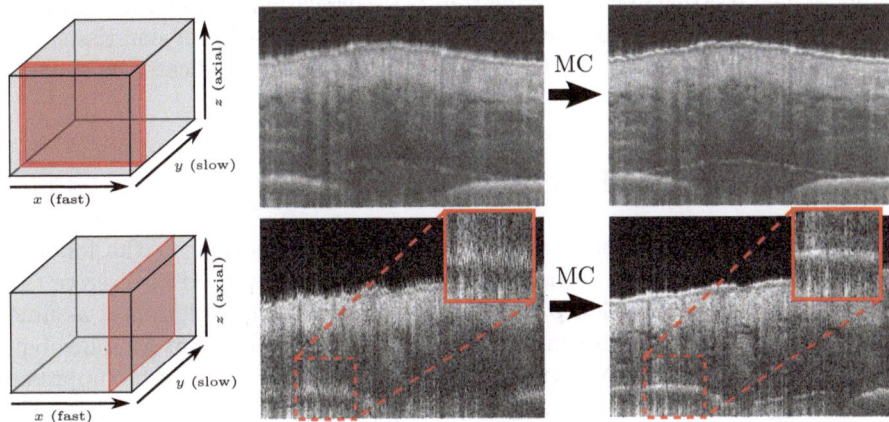

Fig. 1. In vivo SD-OCT scan (cropped) and its motion compensated (MC) result. Top: Slice along the fast scanning axis. Three slices are averaged for visualization of the motion distortion. Bottom: One reslice along the slow scanning axis.

Yun et al. [1] have investigated motion artifacts of SD-OCT occurring during a single A-scan capturing such as signal fading, spatial distortion and blurring. These artifacts can be reduced by increasing the A-scan acquisition rate. However, image shifts in axial direction of several pixels occurring during acquisition of several thousands of A-scans (e.g. for volume acquisition) are still an issue. Later works [2,3] focus on compensating such image shifts in full volume scans using reference measures. While Ricco et al. [2] compensate transverse motion in retinal volume scans using scanning laser ophthalmoscopy (SLO) images as a reference measure, Lee et al. [3] correct motion shift in dynamic SD-OCT imaging, periodically capturing the same region over several seconds, using one of such captures as reference. Recent work in [4] correct motion artifacts by estimating a displacement vector for each A-scan using orthogonal OCT scan patterns. The method works without having a reference measure. Inference of the displacement field is done by minimizing an objective function using a gradient-descent method combined with a multi-resolution approach. Our work extends this approach by transferring the objective function to CRF notation and adding additional priors, allowing better tissue structure preservation and fast global optimization.

Contributions: We propose a probabilistic method for estimation and compensation of axial motion shift in *in vivo* SD-OCT without requiring a reference measure. The key challenge is to distinguish between motion shift and the natural spatial structure of the subject tissue. We tackle this problem by combining two different lateral scanning schemes for volume acquisition: The motion shift of multiple taken A-scans at the same lateral position (but at various time points) differ whereas the tissue structure remains unchanged. The motion compensation problem is formulated as an energy minimization problem using a conditional random field (CRF) notation, allowing both estimation of the motion field and the tissue structure. For inference, the CRF is simplified to a Gaussian Markov random field (GMRF) by approximating crosscorrelation terms with a Gaussian pdf. Finally, our method is applied on in vivo SD-OCT scans of skin tissue with a percutaneous implant (see Fig. 1, dashed red rectangles indicate the subcutaneous implant base).

2   Motion Field Model

For estimation and compensation of in vivo subject movement, the following assumptions are made: A sequence of A-scans $\{d_t\}$ is captured at discrete time points t and lateral position $\boldsymbol{p}_t = (x_t, y_t)$. For image acquisition, it is assumed that the scanned subject is somehow fixed (e.g. no freehand capturing involving transverse motion drift). Nevertheless, subject movements can not be suppressed completely, e.g., slight up-down movements caused by breathing or heart beating can still occur, but are limited in amplitude. Thus, for each A-scan d_t, we have a corresponding axial *motion shift* f_t. Since axial shift is not solely determined by f_t due to spatial tissue structure changes, the true axial shift is defined by $f_t + s_{\boldsymbol{p}_t}$, where $s_{\boldsymbol{p}_t}$ is the tissue surface height at lateral position $\boldsymbol{p}_t$. In the following, we derive a CRF model $E(f, s \mid d) = E(d \mid f, s) + E(f, s)$ given an observation model $E(d \mid f, s)$ and regularizer $E(f, s)$ with $f = \{f_t\}$ as described below. $E(f, s \mid d)$ is defined over a graph $\mathcal{G} = (\mathcal{V}, \mathcal{E})$ given the vertex set $\mathcal{V}$ containing model instances and the edge set $\mathcal{E}$ representing dependencies between instances.

Observation Model: The observation model is based on the assumption of structural similarity of (i) spatial neighbored A-scans d_i and d_j with $(i, j) \in \mathcal{E}^R$, where the structure of $\mathcal{E}^R$ depends on the scanning scemes used (see Fig. 3(c) in Sect. 3) and (ii) A-scans taken at the same spatial position but at different time points d_i and d_j with $(i, j) \in \mathcal{E}^c = \{(i, j) \mid \boldsymbol{p}_i = \boldsymbol{p}_j\}$. As a similarity measure of adjacent A-scans, we use the crosscorrelation $R[\tilde{d}_i, \tilde{d}_j](z) = \int \tilde{d}_i(\tau) \cdot \tilde{d}_j(z + \tau) \, d\tau$ of two adjacent volume gradient columns $\tilde{d}_i, \tilde{d}_j$, with $z = f_i - f_j$ denoting the relative motion shift (see Fig. 2(a)). Actually, the axial shift does not only depend on the motion shift itself, but also on the spatial change of the tissue surface structure. Therefore, we introduce new model variables $\{s_{\boldsymbol{p}_i}\}_{\boldsymbol{p}_i \in \mathcal{V}^s}$ denoting the subject surface change. Then, the relative axial shift is now determined by $f_i + s_{\boldsymbol{p}_i}$, rather than only by f_i, i.e. z becomes $(f_i + s_{\boldsymbol{p}_i}) - (f_j + s_{\boldsymbol{p}_j})$. If s is not known a priori, the problem is ill-posed because of ambiguities in the sum of relative motion and surface change. We solve this ambiguity by correlating A-scans taken at the same sample position at different time points. For such A-scans, it is $z = f_i + s_{\boldsymbol{p}_i} - f_j - s_{\boldsymbol{p}_j} = f_i - f_j$, because $s_{\boldsymbol{p}_i} = s_{\boldsymbol{p}_j} \; \forall (i, j) \in \mathcal{E}^c$. Thus, we have

$$E(d \mid f, s) = \gamma \sum_{(i,j) \in \mathcal{E}^R} R_{ij}(f_i + s_{\boldsymbol{p}_i} - f_j - s_{\boldsymbol{p}_j}) + \sum_{(i,j) \in \mathcal{E}^c} R_{ij}(f_i - f_j) \quad (1)$$

where $R_{ij}(\,\cdot\,) := -\log R[\tilde{d}_i, \tilde{d}_j](\,\cdot\,)$ and γ is a weighting factor.

Motion Field Prior: For regularizing the motion estimation problem, additional assumptions are encoded in the prior energy term. Due to mass inertia of the subject, the motion field has to be smooth in time direction. In our model,

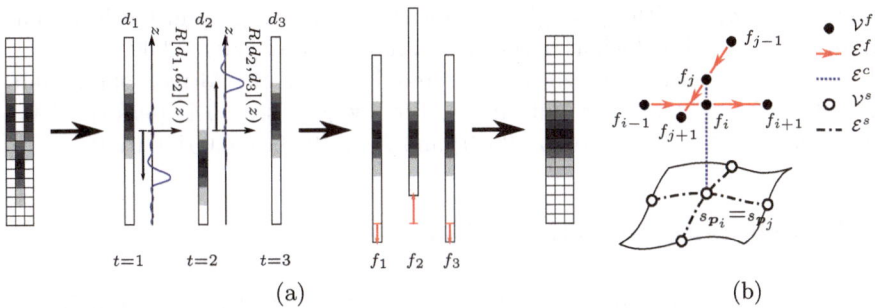

Fig. 2. Proposed model: (a) Motion correction workflow: Motion field $\{f_i\}_i$ (red arrows) is estimated by maximizing the crosscorrelation $R[d_i, d_j](z = f_i - f_j)$ (blue curves) of adjacent image rows d_i, d_j, (b) Graphical model structure (red arrows indicate temporal scanning direction).

we use first order smoothness. Additionally, we assume a Gaussian motion shift prior with zero mean, i.e. $f_t \sim \mathcal{N}(0, \sigma_f^2)$. The tissue surface s is regularized analogously. Thus, the prior is:

$$E(f, s) = \theta_1 \sum_{i \in \mathcal{V}^f} \frac{f_i^2}{2} + \theta_2 \sum_{(i,j) \in \mathcal{E}^f} (f_i - f_j)^2 + \theta_3 \sum_{i \in \mathcal{V}^s} \frac{s_{\boldsymbol{p}_i}^2}{2} + \theta_4 \sum_{(i,j) \in \mathcal{E}^s} (s_{\boldsymbol{p}_i} - s_{\boldsymbol{p}_j})^2 \tag{2}$$

with $\mathcal{E}^f = \{(t, t+1) \mid t \in [0, 1, \ldots, T]\}$ and $\theta_1 = 1/\sigma_f^2$, $\theta_2 = \lambda_f$, $\theta_3 = 1/\sigma_s^2$, $\theta_4 = \lambda_s$, $\theta_5 = \gamma$ are the model parameters. The composed graph structure $\mathcal{G} = (\mathcal{V}^f \cup \mathcal{V}^s, \mathcal{E}^f \cup \mathcal{E}^R \cup \mathcal{E}^s \cup \mathcal{E}^c)$ is depicted in Fig. 2(b).

2.1 Inference

To efficiently find a configuration $\{f^*, s^*\}$ minimizing $E(f, s \mid \theta)$, we have decided to simplify $E(f, s \mid \theta)$. The only terms in $E(f, s \mid \theta)$ which makes efficient inference difficult are the crosscorrelations $R[d_i, d_j](\,\cdot\,)$. Assuming that the A-scan intensities follow an edge-step model and is augmented with additive white Gaussian noise, the crosscorrelation of the first derivative of the A-scan intensities has a Gaussian shape with additive white Gaussian noise. For model parameter estimation, nonlinear least-squares Gaussian fitting is applied. Thus we obtain $R[d_i, d_j](z) \approx \hat{R}[d_i, d_j](z) = \mathcal{N}(\mu_{ij}, \sigma_{ij}^2, z)$, where μ_{ij} and σ_{ij}^2 are the mean and variance of the estimated Gaussian distribution $\mathcal{N}(\mu, \sigma^2, \,\cdot\,)$.

Using this approximation, the CRF energy function $E(f, s \mid d)$ simplifies to a Gaussian Markov random field (GMRF), i.e. $E(f, s \mid d)$ is a quadratic function in $\{f, s\}$ and can be rewritten as $E(x \mid \theta) = \frac{1}{2} x^\mathsf{T} A_\theta x + x^\mathsf{T} b_\theta + c_\theta$, where $x = \{f, s\}$ and A_θ is sparse due to the Markov property. Its minimizer is $x^* = -A_\theta^{-1} b_\theta$. This can be efficiently solved by (sparse) Cholesky decomposition of A_θ [5].

Estimation of the optimal parameter vector θ^* is done by minimizing the mean-square-error (MSE) of f with $\theta^* = \arg\min_\theta \|f_\theta^* - f_{\text{correct}}\|_2^2$, where $x_\theta^* =$

$\arg\min_x E(x \mid d, \theta)$ with $x_\theta^* = \{f_\theta^*, s_\theta^*\}$ and f_{correct} is the ground truth motion field. In practice, it is sufficient to set σ_s, λ_s and γ fixed (e.g. $\sigma_s = 500$, $\lambda_s = 0.01$ and $\gamma = 1$) and only optimize over σ_f and λ_f, since the former parameters don't affect the estimation results much. Finally, grid search is performed for estimation of $\sigma_f \in \{10, 100, 1000, 10000\}$ and $\lambda_f \in \{0.0001, 0.001, 0.01, 0.1\}$.

3   Experiments and Discussion

In this section, we compare three different settings of our proposed method. The first setting uses $\gamma = 1$, $\sigma_s = 500$ and $\lambda_s = 0.01$. In the second setting, the tissue surface is ommited, enforcing $s \equiv 0$, i.e. $\sigma_s \to 0$ and $\lambda_s \to \infty$. The third setting additionally omits the spatial crosscorrelation ($\mathcal{E}^R$) term, i.e. $\gamma = 0$, leading to a configuration most similar to the approach of Kraus et al. [4].

We present two different experiments involving synthetic data and real OCT acquisitions. The first experiments are done on synthetic datasets, where ground truth surface and motion fields are available. In a second part, real OCT scans of both post mortem (with artificial motion field) and in vivo (without prior known motion field) are evaluated. For synthetic data, as well as real OCT measures, the subjects are scanned consecutively with two scanning schemes for ensuring that enough surface points are scanned twice. The first scheme is a spoke pattern scanning scheme with N_{spoke} B-scans, each B-scan consists of N_A A-scans as shown in Fig. 3(a). The second scanning scheme is a dense 3D (cuboidal) scanning scheme with N_{3D} B-scans. Figure 3(b) shows a schematic of the lateral scanning positions over time of a complete subject scan. Figure 3(c) shows the spatial structure of neighboring, crosscorrelated A-scans (encoded in $\mathcal{E}^R$).

Synthetic data is generated with $N_{\text{spoke}} = 16$, $N_{\text{3D}} = 100$, $N_A = 100$ and axial resolution of $Z = 600$ px. The tissue is modeled as a uniformly scattered medium with the tissue-air interface modeled by a step edge function convolved with a Gaussian kernel with $\sigma_{\text{step}} = 5$. The image intensities (with range $[0, 1]$)

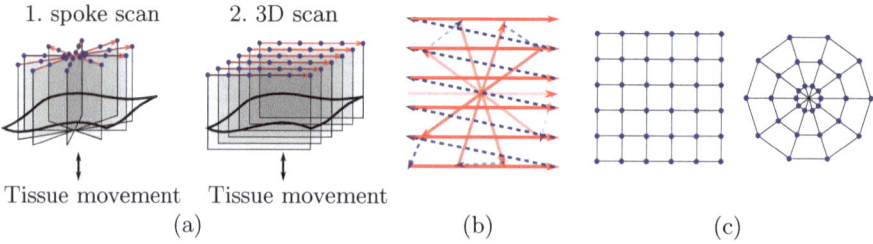

Fig. 3. Scanning schemes: (a) spoke and dense 3D pattern, (b) lateral positions of B-scans (red lines) over time. Dashed blue lines: connection of consecutive B-scans. Color shading and arrows depict temporal direction, (c) spatial structure of $\mathcal{E}^R$ for spoke and 3D pattern. Blue points: A-scans d_i, black lines: neighborhood relations $(i, j) \in \mathcal{E}^R$.

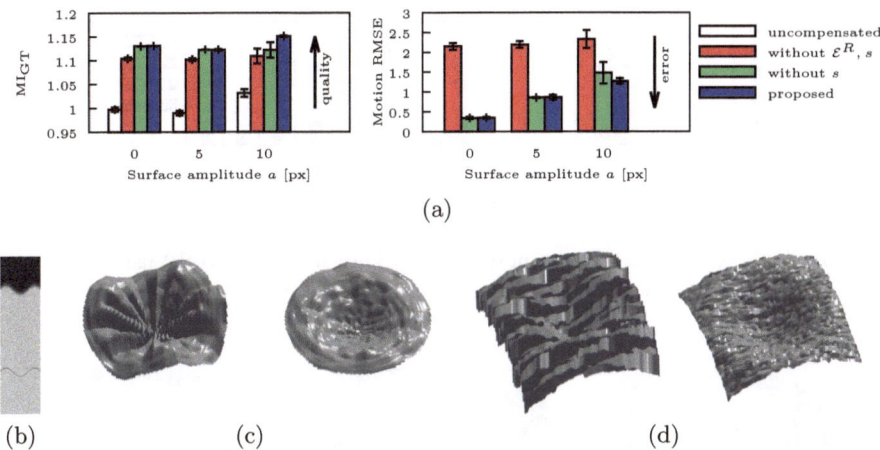

Fig. 4. Synthetic data results: (a) Evaluation of the mutual information towards the ground truth ($\mathrm{MI_{GT}}$, left) and the RMSE of the motion fields towards ground truth for different surface amplitudes (right) and (b)–(d) example surface segmentation of a synthetic dataset with non-planar surface. (b) Example B-scan slice, (c) Spoke scans and (d) dense 3D volume scans. Left: with motion artifacts, right: motion compensated.

are corrupted with additive Gaussian noise with $\sigma^2_{\mathrm{noise}} = 0.07$. Artificial motion artifacts were generated by adding two sine waves of random amplitude and phase to simulate periodic movement. Low-frequency random shift of up to $\pm 20\,\mathrm{px}$ is added for simulation of non-periodic movement. We evaluated our motion compensation algorithm on data with sinusoidal tissue surface of amplitude a as shown in Fig. 4(b). Performance evaluation is done using mutual information (MI) inspired by [4], i.e. measuring the similarity between spoke scan volume and 3D scan volume (resliced to capture the same regions as the spoke scan), denoted with $\mathrm{MI_{sp\text{-}3D}}$. Since ground truth volumes for synthetic data is available, we can also compute the MI of the ground truth volume scans to its motion compensated volume, denoted with $\mathrm{MI_{GT}}$. Figure 4(a) shows $\mathrm{MI_{GT}}$ and motion RMSE results of 30 randomly generated datasets with varying tissue surface amplitudes (10 datasets for $a = 0$, 5, and 10 respectively) with errorbars indicating the standard deviation. The results show best performance on the first configuration, showing most increase of MI and least motion RMSE. The configuration ommiting $\mathcal{E}^R$ and s performs worst on every dataset. $\mathrm{MI_{sp\text{-}3D}}$ gives nearly similar results for every configuration, since this measure only captures intra-volume similarity enforced by the $\mathcal{E}^c$ term and cannot capture the tissue structure preservation, as noticed in [4]. Figure 4(c)–(d) shows a comparison of extracted tissue surface renderings of uncompensated to compensated volumes.

Real OCT Scans: Our real world application uses in vivo and post mortem SD-OCT scans of the percutaneous implant of an anesthetized (and fixed) mouse from [6]. The setting has following parameters: $N_{\mathrm{spoke}} = 72$, $N_{\mathrm{3D}} = 800$, $N_A =$

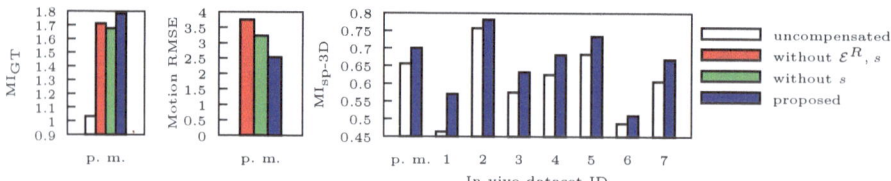

Fig. 5. Evaluation on post mortem data (with known ground truth) using MI_{GT} and motion RMSE and in vivo data (without known ground truth) using $MI_{sp\text{-}3D}$

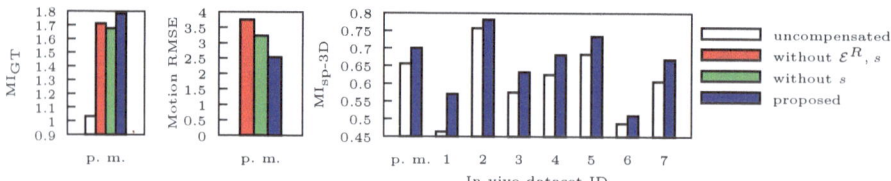

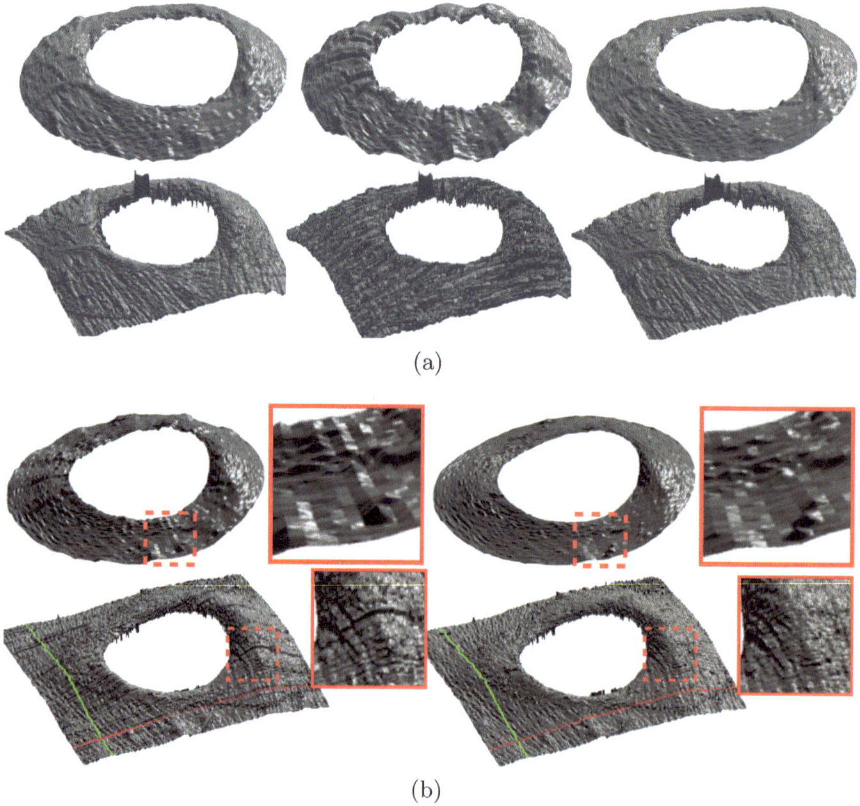

(a)

(b)

Fig. 6. Motion compensation results: (a) post mortem dataset with ground truth (left), artificial motion (middle), and motion compensated (right) and (b) in vivo data with motion artifacts (left) and motion compensated (right). Red and green lines indicating the position of slices and reslices respectively shown in Fig. 1. Top row: spoke pattern scan, bottom row: dense 3D scan respectively.

800 and an axial resolution of $Z = 600$ px. Acquisition time was approx. 0.1 s per B-scan. For enhancement of computation time and memory usage, a downsampling along the fast scanning axis by a factor of 8 is applied and the motion field is upsampled afterwards for providing motion compensation in full resolution. In Fig. 5, the evaluation results of one post mortem dataset (p. m.) corrupted with artificial motion (thus known ground truth) and several in vivo datasets (without known ground truth) are shown. For both post mortem and in vivo scans a increase of MI_{GT} and $MI_{sp\text{-}3D}$, respectively, is observed, showing a significant reduction of motion artifacts. This finding can also be observed in the surface segmentation visualization of the post mortem dataset (see Fig. 6(a)) and a typical in vivo data example as shown in Fig. 6(b) and Fig. 1.

4   Conclusion

In this work, we propose a novel probabilistic approach for motion compensation of in vivo SD-OCT volume scans. The motion estimation problem is reformulated as a CRF energy function and approximated by a GMRF for efficient inference. Our method reliably separates axial motion from tissue structure change by combining two scanning schemes. We use multiple A-scans taken at the same lateral position but different time points as anchor points to estimate the tissue morphology. The method is verified on synthetic data as well as in vivo SD-OCT volume scans. Motion artifacts are significantly reduced while the geometry of the tissue is preserved.

References

1. Yun, S.H., Tearney, G.J., de Boer, J.F., Bouma, B.E.: Motion artifacts in optical coherence tomography with frequency-domain ranging. Optics Express 12, 2977 (2004)
2. Ricco, S., Chen, M., Ishikawa, H., Wollstein, G., Schuman, J.: Correcting Motion Artifacts in Retinal Spectral Domain Optical Coherence Tomography via Image Registration. In: Yang, G.-Z., Hawkes, D., Rueckert, D., Noble, A., Taylor, C. (eds.) MICCAI 2009, Part I. LNCS, vol. 5761, pp. 100–107. Springer, Heidelberg (2009)
3. Lee, J., Srinivasan, V., Radhakrishnan, H., Boas, D.A.: Motion correction for phase-resolved dynamic optical coherence tomography imaging of rodent cerebral cortex. Optics Express 19(22), 21258–21270 (2011)
4. Kraus, M.F., Potsaid, B., Mayer, M.A., Bock, R., Baumann, B., Liu, J.J., Hornegger, J., Fujimoto, J.G.: Motion correction in optical coherence tomography volumes on a per A-scan basis using orthogonal scan patterns. Biomedical Optics Express 3(6), 1182–1199 (2012)
5. Rue, H., Held, L.: Gaussian Markov Random Fields: Theory and Applications. Chapman & Hall/CRC, Boca Raton (2005)
6. Müller, O., Donner, S., Klinder, T., Dragon, R., Bartsch, I., Witte, F., Krüger, A., Heisterkamp, A., Rosenhahn, B.: Model Based 3D Segmentation and OCT Image Undistortion of Percutaneous Implants. In: Fichtinger, G., Martel, A., Peters, T. (eds.) MICCAI 2011, Part III. LNCS, vol. 6893, pp. 454–462. Springer, Heidelberg (2011)

Classification of Ambiguous Nerve Fiber Orientations in 3D Polarized Light Imaging

Melanie Kleiner[1], Markus Axer[1,2], David Gräßel[1], Julia Reckfort[1], Uwe Pietrzyk[1,2], Katrin Amunts[1,3], and Timo Dickscheid[1]

[1] Institute of Neuroscience and Medicine (INM-1, INM-4),
Research Center Jülich,Germany
[2] Department of Physics, University of Wuppertal, Germany
[3] Department of Psychiatry, Psychotherapy and Psychosomatics,
RWTH Aachen University, Germany

Abstract. 3D Polarized Light Imaging (3D-PLI) has been shown to measure the orientation of nerve fibers in post mortem human brains at ultra high resolution. The 3D orientation in each voxel is obtained as a pair of angles, the direction angle and the inclination angle with unknown sign. The sign ambiguity is a major problem for the correct interpretation of fiber orientation. Measurements from a tiltable specimen stage, that are highly sensitive to noise, extract information, which allows drawing conclusions about the true inclination sign. In order to reduce noise, we propose a global classification of the inclination sign, which combines measurements with spatial coherence constraints. The problem is formulated as a second order Markov random field and solved efficiently with graph cuts. We evaluate our approach on synthetic and human brain data. The results of global optimization are compared to independent pixel classification with subsequent edge-preserving smoothing.

1 Introduction

Fiber tracts are composed of axons, which connect nerve cells between each other, and thus transmit information between brain areas. The exact courses of fiber tracts are still far from being fully understood. Several methods for mapping fiber tracts have been developed to approach a complete model of all fiber tracts, the *connectome*. 3D-PLI is a method that measures the birefringence of lipids surrounding single axons (myelin sheath) by transmitting polarized light through histological sections [1], [2]. 3D fiber orientations can be reconstructed at micro scale resolution (Fig. 1(a)). For comparison, the measurement of water diffusion by Diffusion Weighted Magnetic Resonance Imaging (DW-MRI) can resolve fiber orientations in vivo [3], but on scales of millimeters.

In 3D-PLI measurements, the sign of the fiber inclination angle is unknown. This ambiguity has been addressed previously by Larsen et al. [4], who used a simulated annealing technique to optimize a smoothness criterion, but did not collect additional measurements about the inclination sign at each individual pixel. Pajdzik et al. [5] developed a microscope tilting-stage to identify the sign

N. Ayache et al. (Eds.): MICCAI 2012, Part I, LNCS 7510, pp. 206–213, 2012.

of the optical indicatrix of birefringent, uniaxial crystals, which corresponds to the inclination sign in the context of 3D-PLI.

The inclination sign ambiguity can be regarded as a binary labeling problem, similar to segmentation or denoising in digital imaging, that can be solved efficiently by Markov random field (MRF) theory [6], [7].

2   3D Polarized Light Imaging

Polarimeter Setup. Linearly polarized light is transmitted through a brain section, a retarder, an analyzer and then imaged by a digital camera (Fig. 1(b)). The polarizing filters are rotated simultaneously to generate a series of intensity images. The measured signal can be modeled as a sine curve with phase φ and amplitude r [8]. Referring to the histological sectioning plane, the parameter φ (*direction*) corresponds to the in-plane angle of measured fibers in relation to the polarizing filters. The parameter r (*retardation*) is correlated nonlinearly with the out-of-plane angle α (*inclination*). The pair of angles (φ, α) represents a 3D

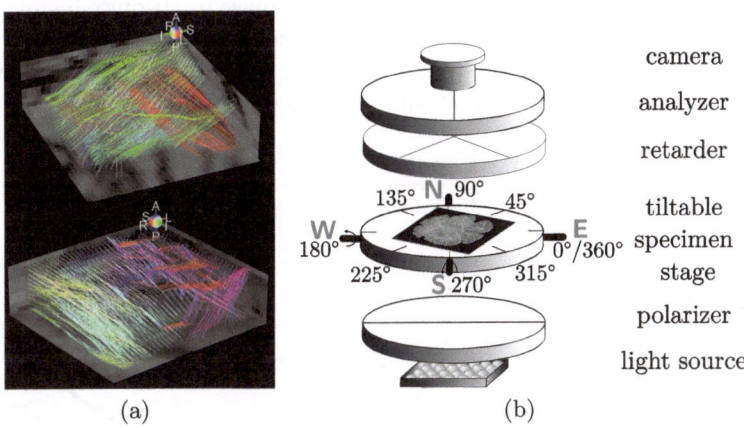

(a)   (b)

Fig. 1. (a) Reconstructed fiber tracts from 3D-PLI as presented in [2, Fig. 6] (b) The 3D-PLI setup shows a specimen stage, which is tiltable in four directions (N, W, E, S). The measured in-plane fiber direction φ is related to the polarizing filters and annotated in degrees. The inclination sign can be derived most reliably, when the tilting direction and the in-plane fiber direction are similar.

fiber orientation with unknown direction. To avoid alternating notations for the same orientation, we restrict φ to $[0°, 180°]$ and α to $[-90°, 90°]$. According to [8, Eq. 6], α can be approximated as

$$|\alpha| = \arccos\left(\sqrt{\frac{2 \cdot \arcsin(r)}{\pi \cdot d_{\mathrm{rel}}}}\right) \tag{1}$$

with a reference value d_{rel} depending on section thickness, wavelength and bire-fringence. Assuming a constant value of d_{rel} ignores the inhomogeneity of the examined tissue, and limits the accuracy of (1). The restriction to slice thick-nesses with $d_{\text{rel}} \leq 1$ is necessary for a bijective relation between $|\alpha|$ and r. Equation (1) shows that only the absolute value of α can be determined from r, which leads to the *inclination sign ambiguity* in 3D-PLI.

Tilting Setup. In addition to the measurement of the flat specimen stage, fur-ther measurements can be acquired in four tilting directions $\psi \in \{\text{north}(N){=}90°,$ west(W)=180°, east(E)=0°, south(S)=270°$\}$ by tilting the stage along one of two perpendicular axes. All tilted images are registered to the flat image by a pro-jective linear transformation. The specimen stage is tilted by the angle $\tau \leq 4°$ to avoid strong distortions. The relation between tilting directions and fiber in-plane directions is illustrated in Fig. 1(b). We denote the tilted measurements by α^ψ and r^ψ in contrast to α and r on a flat specimen stage. For each tilting direc-tion ψ, the *opposite* direction is $\psi \pm 180°$. If the fiber in-plane direction and the tilting direction are similar, fibers with positive inclination can be distinguished from those with negative inclination by their decrease in absolute inclination af-ter tilting (Fig. 2(a)). Otherwise, the change is less significant or even inversed. Generally, these changes are marginal and hence very sensitive to noise. We can formalize this relationship for fiber directions $\varphi \in (\psi - 90°, \psi + 90°)$ as

$$\alpha \geq 0 \Leftrightarrow |\alpha^\psi| \leq |\alpha^{\psi \pm 180°}| \,. \tag{2}$$

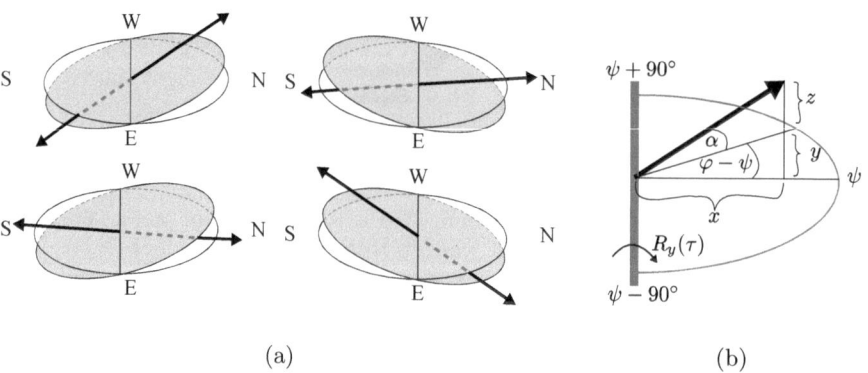

(a)   (b)

Fig. 2. (a) The absolute inclination, i. e. steepness, of fibers with a positive inclination sign (top row) decreases when tilting from S to N. If the inclination sign is negative (bottom row), the steepness increases. (b) The fiber orientation can be represented as a vector $v = (x, y, z)^{\mathrm{T}}$. A tilt by the angle τ can be modeled as a rotation $R_y(\tau)$ applied to v.

3   Solving the Inclination Sign Ambiguity

The classification of the inclination sign can be considered as a labeling problem. Given the image domain Ω and a binary set of labels $\mathcal{S} = \{-1, +1\}$ reflecting the unknown inclination sign, we want to find a *labeling function* $s : \Omega \to \mathcal{S}$ that assigns one of two possible values to every $i \in \Omega$. A second order MRF can take spatial coherence into account and leads to an energy function of the form

$$E(s) = \sum_i \theta_i(s_i) + \lambda \cdot \sum_{(i,j) \in \mathcal{N}} \theta_{i,j}(s_i, s_j) . \tag{3}$$

for any non-negative potentials θ_i (*data potential*), $\theta_{i,j}$ (*smoothness potential*) and a neighborhood relation $\mathcal{N}$.

Data Potential. A large difference between oppositely tilted, unsigned inclination angles $|\alpha^\psi| - |\alpha^{\psi \pm 180°}|$ indicates high reliability of a positive inferred inclination sign. We therefore require the data potential to be proportional to the sum of these differences for all tilting directions, i. e.

$$\theta_i \propto \sum_\psi |\alpha_i^\psi| - |\alpha_i^{\psi \pm 180°}| . \tag{4}$$

However, due to the reference value d_{rel} in (1), the inclination values possess limited accuracy. Therefore, we develop an alternative formulation that does not require d_{rel}. We achieve this by deriving the sign and the absolute value of the given difference separately.

First, we take advantage of the dependency

$$|\alpha_i^\psi - \alpha_i^{\psi \pm 180°}| \approx 2 \cdot \cos(\varphi_i - \psi) \cdot \sin(\tau) , \tag{5}$$

which is restricted to small angles τ, such that $\tau \approx \sin(\tau)$. Equation (5) is obtained by rotating the flat fiber orientation vector as shown in Fig. 2(b). Second, we need the sign of $|\alpha_i^\psi| - |\alpha_i^{\psi \pm 180°}|$ to distinguish positive and negative inclination signs. Again, we avoid the approximation of inclination angles by (1). Instead, we consider the difference of retardation values $r_i^\psi - r_i^{\psi \pm 180°}$. The nonlinear relation between inclination α_i and retardation r_i, is strictly decreasing (for $d_{\text{rel}} \leq 1$, see (1)), so we expect

$$\text{sgn}(\alpha_i^\psi - \alpha_i^{\psi \pm 180°}) = \text{sgn}(r_i^{\psi \pm 180°} - r_i^\psi) . \tag{6}$$

Equations (6) and (5) finally lead to the data potential

$$\theta_i \propto \sum_\psi \cos(\varphi_i - \psi) \cdot \sin(\tau) \cdot \text{sgn}(r_i^{\psi \pm 180°} - r_i^\psi) \tag{7}$$

that does not require d_{rel}. By inserting $\psi \in \{\text{E=0°, N=90°, W=180°, S=270°}\}$, and applying a normalization term, (7) becomes

$$\theta_i(s_i) = \frac{1}{2} + s_i \cdot \frac{\sin(\varphi_i) \cdot \text{sgn}(r_i^N - r_i^S) + \cos(\varphi_i) \cdot \text{sgn}(r_i^E - r_i^W)}{2\sqrt{2}} . \tag{8}$$

Smoothness Potential. We assume that neighboring pixels tend to belong to the same anatomical structure with a similar fiber orientation. Hence, if neighboring pixels have similar in-plane fiber directions, their inclination signs are very likely to be the same as well. This leads to a *contrast-sensitive Potts model* [9, Eq. 3], where the contrast is defined as the absolute difference of neighboring in-plane angles.

$$\theta_{i,j}(s_i, s_j) = \left(1 - \frac{|\varphi_i - \varphi_j|}{180°}\right) \cdot \begin{cases} 1 & \text{, if } s_i \neq s_j \\ 0 & \text{, else} \end{cases} \tag{9}$$

This function is regular and graph-representable according to [7, Theorem 4.1]. Therefore, the minimization of (3) can be computed efficiently via graph cuts.

4   Evaluation

The inclination sign and the resulting vector fields are evaluated on synthetic images and selected regions of various human brain sections. The presented approach by MRF optimization (GLOBALOPT) is compared to the direct determination of the inclination sign by tilted measurements (DATAONLY), which corresponds to GLOBALOPT without a smoothness potential ($\lambda = 0$). The third approach to be compared is DATAONLY with subsequent median filtering with variable radius (DATAMEDIAN).

Synthetic Data. A synthetic data set consisting of a direction image $\tilde{\varphi}$ and an inclination image $\tilde{\alpha}$ was created. The structure consists of rounded and crossing fiber tracts (Fig. 4(a)). The corresponding direction measurements φ were simulated by adding noise with $\sigma_\varphi = 0.5$. The retardation measurements r were simulated in several steps. First, the tilted inclination angles $\tilde{\alpha}^\psi$ were calculated by rotation as shown in Fig. 2(b). Second, retardation values were calculated from $\tilde{\alpha}$ according to (1) with $d_{\text{rel}} = 0.4$. Finally, noise was added with $\sigma_r = 0.006$. The simulated inclination measurements α were obtained from the absolute inclination $|\alpha|$ calculated from r and an inclination sign $s \in \{s^\lambda,\ s^R \text{ or } s'\}$. s^λ was determined by GLOBALOPT and weighting factor λ, s' was determined by DATAONLY, and s^R was determined by DATAMEDIAN with radius $R \in \{1, 2, 3\}$. The noise levels σ_r and σ_φ were determined in 30 repeated measurements.

For evaluation, the true orientation vector $\tilde{v}$ was composed from the synthetic orientation angles $\tilde{\varphi}$ and $\tilde{\alpha}$. Accordingly, the orientation vector $v \in \{v^\lambda, v^R, v'\}$ was composed from the simulated measurements φ and α. The difference between the true and the simulated vector field was measured by the root mean squared deviation (RMSD) of both vectors at each pixel location. Background pixels displayed in black in Fig. 4(a) are not considered. Fig. 3(a) shows that GLOBALOPT achieves an RMSD of 2.5° (optimum at $\lambda = 0.32$) compared to DATAONLY with an RMSD of 3.36° and DATAMEDIAN with RMSD values above 6°. The sensitivity of GLOBALOPT to determine the correct inclination sign at pixels that are not classified correctly by DATAONLY was examined in Fig. 3(b).

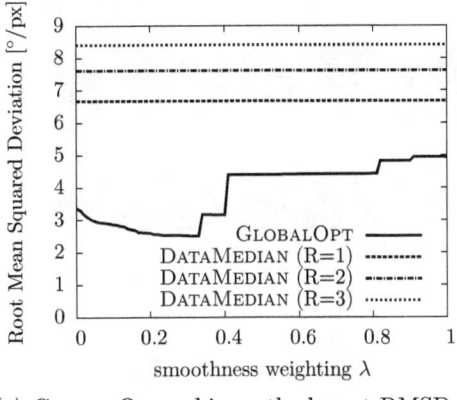

(a) GLOBALOPT achieves the lowest RMSD values with an optimum at $\lambda = 0.32$.

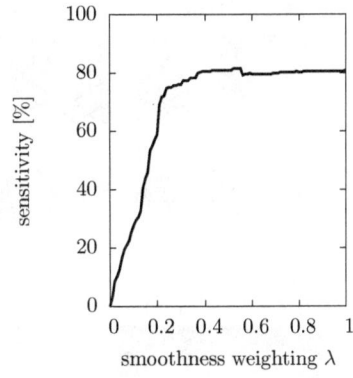

(b) GLOBALOPT can detect wrong classification to 80 %.

Fig. 3. evaluation of the determined inclination signs on synthetic data

Human Brain Data. Regions in histological sections of three post mortem brains without pathological findings were selected to demonstrate the different behavior of all approaches (Fig. 4(b)–(d)). The manual evaluation of inclination signs requires an appropriate visualization of the vector field. The resulting 3D orientations were visualized in HSV color space, but brightness was reduced where local differences were high in terms of the mean absolute deviation (MAD) in the local 8-neighborbood of each pixel i. The color coding (Fig. 4(e)) emphasizes abrupt changes in a vector field by dark pixels or edges. Accordingly, unexpected changes in the vector fields, which could be caused by wrong inclination signs, are made visible. For GLOBALOPT, the results appeared best with $\lambda = 0.2$. This is not equal to the optimum for synthetic data ($\lambda = 0.32$), which reflects the lack of realistic noise modeling in the simulation.

Both GLOBALOPT and DATAMEDIAN are able to remove isolated deviating inclination signs in DATAONLY, which is shown in the white matter beneath the cerebellar cortex, containing mainly parallel fibers (Fig. 4(b)). DATAMEDIAN introduces severe artifacts into the vector field, which is demonstrated in the optic radiation (Fig. 4(c)). The inhomogeneous vector field in the corpus callosum (Fig. 4(d)), where fibers of both hemispheres cross to the contralateral side, also clearly benefits from regularization. GLOBALOPT with $\lambda = 0.2$ and DATAMEDIAN with $R = 1$ eliminate noise on an equal level, while GLOBALOPT with $\lambda = 0.32$ slightly oversmoothes the vector field. The influence of λ is strong and therefore must be determined carefully.

5   Discussion

The classification of ambiguous inclination signs is an essential step, when determining the fiber orientation in 3D-PLI. Until now, the inclination sign ambiguity

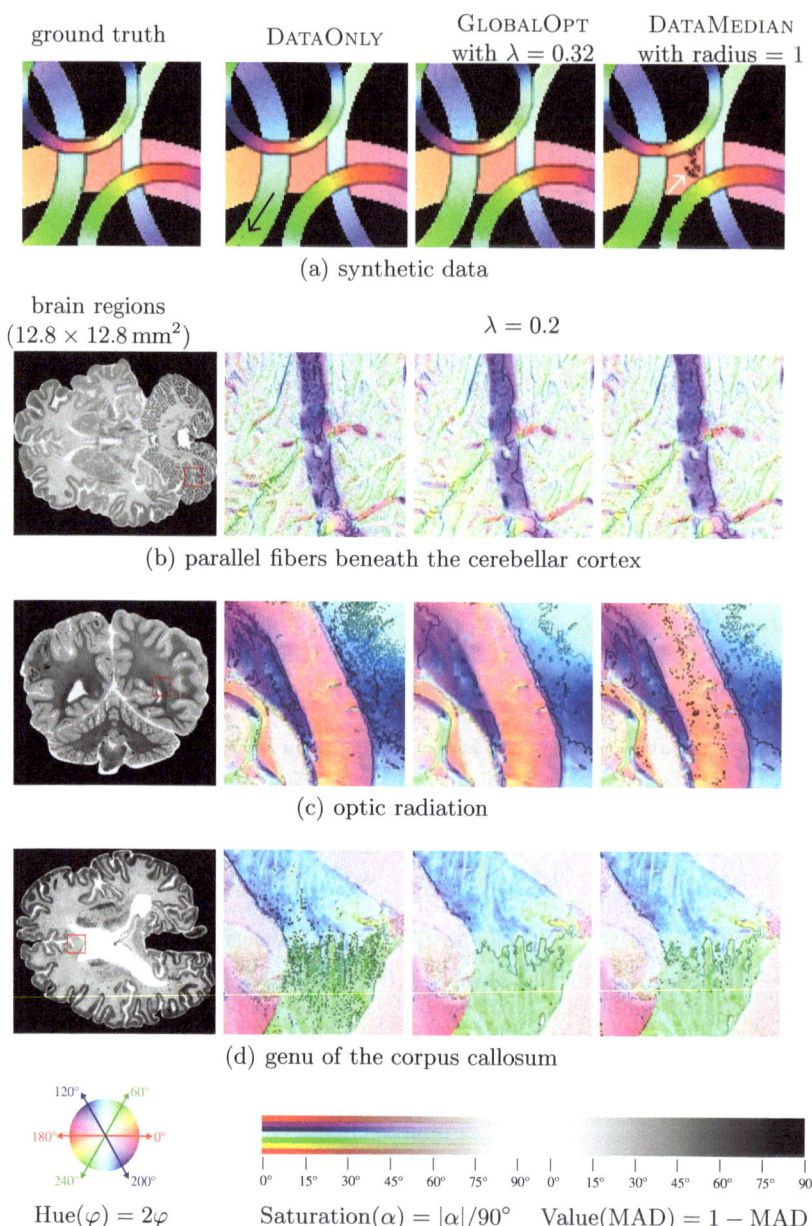

ground truth   DataOnly   GlobalOpt with $\lambda = 0.32$ DataMedian with radius = 1

(a) synthetic data

brain regions $(12.8 \times 12.8\,\text{mm}^2)$ $\lambda = 0.2$

(b) parallel fibers beneath the cerebellar cortex

(c) optic radiation

(d) genu of the corpus callosum

$\text{Hue}(\varphi) = 2\varphi$ $\text{Saturation}(\alpha) = |\alpha|/90°$ $\text{Value(MAD)} = 1 - \text{MAD}$

(e) HSV color coding. The mean absolute deviation (MAD) of each vector to its neighbors was emphasized as decreased brightness to visualize the homogeneity of the resulting vector fields.

Fig. 4. On brain data, the apparently best results were achieved with GlobalOpt for $\lambda = 0.2$. The quantitative evaluation on synthetic images determined the optimum for GlobalOpt at $\lambda = 0.32$. The parallel fibers beneath the cerebellar cortex and the corpus callosum demonstrate the benefit of regularization opposed to DataOnly. The optic radiation shows that DataMedian introduces undesired artifacts.

has been tackled by using either tilted measurements [5] or context information [4] separately. We have presented a global solution for this problem based on a second order Markov random field, which considers both sources of information simultaneously. In contrast to DW-MRI, which aims at identifying fiber pathways with a millimeter resolution, 3D-PLI aims at ultra-high resolution up to a few microns. Working with such high spatial accuracy demands for eliminating as much noise as possible. In our experiments, the new method better conserves the true inclination sign than sole tilted measurements with subsequent edge-preserving smoothing by a median filter, which has shown to introduce artifacts. These problems especially appear where the fiber direction angle changes from $0°$ to $180°$ and vice versa. In contrast to the proposed contrast-sensitive smoothness term, the median sorting criterion cannot adequately handle these changes. The global optimization leaves a single parameter controlling the influence of context information. In the synthetic data set, $\lambda = 0.32$ is optimal, while $\lambda = 0.2$ seems optimal for real data. Future work will include further validation with reference tissue samples to enable more precise analysis of errors. With a well-balanced smoothness term, the presented method shows significant improvements, but only on a small fraction of pixels. However, considering the envisaged accuracy, we believe that such a small fraction is still crucial for meaningful fiber tracking.

References

1. Larsen, L., Griffin, L.D., Graessel, D., Witte, O.W., Axer, H.: Polarized light imaging of white matter architecture. Microsc. Res. Techniq. 70(10), 851–863 (2007)
2. Axer, M., Gräßel, D., Kleiner, M., Dammers, J., Dickscheid, T., Reckfort, J., Hütz, T., Eiben, B., Pietrzyk, U., Zilles, K., Amunts, K.: High-resolution fiber tract reconstruction in the human brain by means of three-dimensional polarized light imaging (3d-pli). Front. Neuroinform. 5 (2011)
3. Hagmann, P., Jonasson, L., Maeder, P., Thiran, J.P., Wedeen, V.J., Meuli, R.: Understanding diffusion mr imaging techniques: From scalar diffusion-weighted imaging to diffusion tensor imaging and beyond. Radiographics 26(suppl. 1), S205–S223 (2006)
4. Larsen, L., Griffin, L.: Can a Continuity Heuristic Be Used to Resolve the Inclination Ambiguity of Polarized Light Imaging? In: Sonka, M., Kakadiaris, I.A., Kybic, J. (eds.) CVAMIA/MMBIA 2004. LNCS, vol. 3117, pp. 365–375. Springer, Heidelberg (2004)
5. Pajdzik, L.A., Glazer, A.M.: Three-dimensional birefringence imaging with a microscope tilting-stage. i. uniaxial crystals. J. Appl. Crystallogr. 39(3), 326–337 (2006)
6. Chen, S.Y., Tong, H., Cattani, C.: Markov models for image labeling. Math. Probl. Eng., Article ID 814356, 18 pages (2012)
7. Kolmogorov, V., Zabih, R.: What energy functions can be minimized via graph cuts? IEEE TPAMI 26(2), 147–159 (2004)
8. Axer, M., Amunts, K., Gräßel, D., Palm, C., Dammers, J., Axer, H., Pietrzyk, U., Zilles, K.: A novel approach to the human connectome: Ultra-high resolution mapping of fiber tracts in the brain. NeuroImage 54(2), 1091–1101 (2011)
9. Boykov, Y.Y., Jolly, M.P.: Interactive graph cuts for optimal boundary & region segmentation of objects in n-d images. In: IEEE ICCV 2004 (2001)

Non-local Means Resolution Enhancement
of Lung 4D-CT Data

Yu Zhang[1, 2], Guorong Wu[2], Pew-Thian Yap[2], Qianjin Feng[1], Jun Lian[3],
Wufan Chen[1], and Dinggang Shen[2,*]

[1] School of Biomedical Engineering, Southern Medical University, Guang Zhou, China
[2] Department of Radiology and BRIC, University of North Carolina, Chapel Hill, U.S.A.
[3] Department of Radiation Oncology, University of North Carolina, Chapel Hill, U.S.A.

Abstract. Image resolution in 4D-CT is a crucial bottleneck that needs to be overcome for improved dose planning in radiotherapy for lung cancer. In this paper, we propose a novel patch-based algorithm to enhance the image quality of 4D-CT data. Our premise is that anatomical information missing in one phase can be recovered from complementary information embedded in other phases. We employ a patch-based mechanism to propagate information across phases for reconstruction of intermediate slices in the axial direction, where resolution is normally the lowest. Specifically, structurally-matching and spatially-nearby patches are combined for reconstruction of each patch. For greater sensitivity to anatomical nuances, we further employ a quad-tree technique to adaptively partition each slice of the image in each phase for more fine-grained refinement. Our evaluation based on a public 4D-CT lung data indicates that our algorithm gives very promising results with significantly enhanced image structures.

1   Introduction

4D-CT is becoming increasingly popular in lung cancer treatment for providing respiratory-related information that is essential for guiding radiation therapy effectively. However, due to the risk of radiation [1], only a limited number of CT segments are usually acquired, which often results in very low resolution along the inferior-superior direction. This low-resolution (LR) data are usually plagued with visible imaging artifacts such as vessel discontinuity and partial volume effect. More importantly, insufficient resolution further distorts the shape of a tumor. This distortion might finally interfere with optimal dose planning.

Super-resolution (SR) reconstruction is an effective approach for improving image resolution. Classical SR methods can be divided into two major categories: interpolation-based and model-based. The main advantage of interpolation-based methods is their simplicity. However, blurred edges and undesirable artifacts are inevitable. Currently, more attention has been directed to model-based SR approach. The general assumption of model-based SR approaches is that the LR image is a degraded version

---

* Corresponding author. The work was done while Dr. Yu Zhang was with UNC Chapel Hill.

N. Ayache et al. (Eds.): MICCAI 2012, Part I, LNCS 7510, pp. 214–222, 2012.
© Springer-Verlag Berlin Heidelberg 2012

of the SR image. The degradation can be represented using matrix representation such as $Z = DBM$, where D is the down-sampling matrix, B is the blur matrix, and M is the transformation matrix, which can be used to characterize the effect of motion. More recent SR works aim at constraining the model with regularization terms, e.g. total variation, non-local means, etc. Matrix Z has direct influence on the SR reconstruction, and yet its estimation is non-trivial and often error-prone.

A more recent alternative is the learning based methods. The key idea of these methods is to utilize the relationship between the high-resolution (HR) and the LR images, learned via training images, to help recover details in the target LR images. Freeman et al. [2], Chang et al. [3], and Yang et al. [4] showed that state-of-the-art performance can be achieved by using various learning-based methods. The major limitation of these methods is that a significant amount of HR images are required for learning. In many instances, such as in the case of lung 4D-CT SR reconstruction, the required HR dataset might not even be available.

In this paper, we propose a different method for enhancing the resolution of 4D-CT lung data, based on our observation that, in 4D-CT, complementary anatomical information is distributed throughout images acquired at different phases. Generally, the 4D-CT captures 10-20 phases, corresponding to different stages of motion of the lung. Therefore, information can be propagated from various phases to recover the structural details that are missing in one particular phase.

The core of our proposed method is fuzzy patch matching, which is inspired by recent advances in non-local image processing, e.g., for denoising [5], labeling [6], segmentation [7]. First, a new patch distance measure is proposed for determining matching patches. Then, a non-local strategy is employed to combine the matching patches. Finally, for achieving greater sensitivity to anatomical nuances, we further perform a quadtree-based algorithm to adaptively partition CT slices into patches of different sizes. Compared with conventional linear and cubic-spline interpolation methods, we will show that our method yields superior performance both qualitatively and quantitatively.

2   Methods

2.1   Overview

Given an acquired 4D-CT image $I = \{I_i(s)|i = 1,..,N, s = 1,...,S\}$, where N is the number of phases and S is the total number of slices in each phase image I_i, the goal is to reconstruct an intermediate high-resolution slice between two consecutive slices $I_i(s)$ and $I_i(s + 1)$ in image I_i. Our proposed solution is illustrated in Fig. 1. The larger red dashed square denotes the intermediate slice to be reconstructed between slice s and $s + 1$ in phase 1. The smaller red box (denoted by y in Fig. 1) denotes a patch in the intermediate slice that needs to be estimated. For each patch y, we intend to employ a set of structurally-similar patches, i.e., $y_1', y_2', ..., y_j'$ (shown in blue boxes in Fig. 1), that are obtained from other phases (i.e., Phase 2, Phase 3,..., Phase N), to reconstruct it. Two questions immediately arise: 1) How do we determine the suitable patches to form the patch set? 2) How do we combine matching patches effectively? Proposed solutions to these two problems will be discussed next.

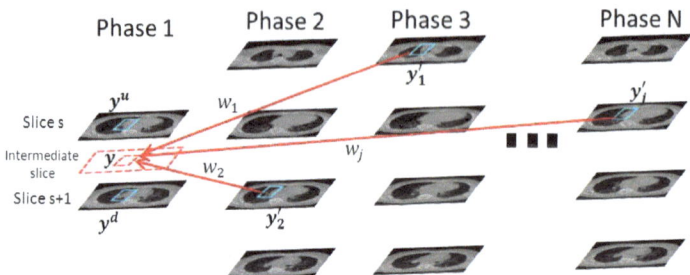

Fig. 1. Method overview

2.2   Patch Distance Measurement

To determine patches that can be used to reconstruct y, we search for patches with similar structures in a limited spatial region in all other phases. Patch similarity with respect to a candidate patch y' is simply evaluated based on the Euclidean distance:

$$D(y, y') = ||y - y'||_2^2. \tag{1}$$

Based on the distance measurement, similar patches can be found. However, in our case, y is not known beforehand. A possible approach is to first obtain an interpolated version of y such as based on y^u and y^d, which are the patches immediately superior and inferior to (See Fig. 1), using either linear interpolation or cubic-interpolation. However, as aforementioned, interpolation will result in undesirable artifacts in y, which will subsequently influence patch matching significantly, as will be illustrated in Section 3.

In this work, y^u and y^d are used as constraints for the reconstruction of y First, we expect that the reconstructed patch y should resemble y^u and y^d. In this way, a joint distance between y' and y^u and between y' and y^d is defined:

$$D(y^u, y^d, y') = ||y^u - y'||_2^2 + ||y^d - y'||_2^2 \tag{2}$$

In addition, we require that the reconstructed patch is not biased towards any of the consecutive patches, i.e., $||\bar{y}^u - \bar{y}'||_2^2$ and $||\bar{y}^d - \bar{y}'||_2^2$ should be balanced:

$$\frac{1}{\varepsilon} \le \frac{||y^u - y'||_2^2}{||y^d - y'||_2^2} \le \varepsilon \tag{3}$$

where ε is a tolerance factor. For better characterization of structural patterns, we use both intensity and derived features to represent each patch. Thus, Equations (2) and (3) can be combined as:

$$D(\bar{y}^u, \bar{y}^d, \bar{y}') = ||\bar{y}^u - \bar{y}'||_2^2 + ||\bar{y}^d - \bar{y}'||_2^2 \quad s.t. \quad \frac{1}{\varepsilon} \le \frac{||\bar{y}^u - \bar{y}'||_2^2}{||\bar{y}^d - \bar{y}'||_2^2} \le \varepsilon \tag{4}$$

where $\bar{y}^u$, $\bar{y}^d$ and $\bar{y}'$ are the new patches, as defined by $\bar{y}^u = \begin{bmatrix} y^u \\ \lambda F y^u \end{bmatrix}$, $\bar{y}^d = \begin{bmatrix} y^d \\ \lambda F y^d \end{bmatrix}$, $\bar{y}' = \begin{bmatrix} y' \\ \lambda F y' \end{bmatrix}$. Here, F is the feature operator. We use gradients as features in our approach. λ is a tuning parameter controlling the balance between the contributions of image intensity and image feature.

2.3   Non-local Approach

Upon obtaining the matching patches for y, the next task is to determine a suitable reconstruction strategy to combine them together. In a recent work, Buades *et al.* [5] shows that non-local means filtering gives state-of-the-art performance in structure-preserving image denoising. The strategy has also been applied to brain image labeling [6], image registration [8], and MR image super-resolution [9]. We employ non-local averaging for combining all matching patches that have been determined based on the distance measure as described in Section 2.2. The non-local averaging is performed as below:

$$y = \frac{\sum_{y' \in \Omega} w(\bar{y}^u, \bar{y}^d, \bar{y}') \, y'}{\sum_{y' \in \Omega} w(\bar{y}^u, \bar{y}^d, \bar{y}')} \tag{5}$$

where Ω is the patch set composed with all matching patches. w is the weight that is associated with the distance $D(\bar{y}^u, \bar{y}^d, \bar{y}')$, and is computed as follows:

$$w(\bar{y}^u, \bar{y}^d, \bar{y}') = \exp\left(-\frac{D(\bar{y}^u, \bar{y}^d, \bar{y}')}{2\sigma^2}\right) \tag{6}$$

Where σ controls the decay of the exponential function.

2.4   Quadtree-Based Patch Partition

A commonly used approach to partition a slice is to divide it into identically sized patches. However, this approach fails to take into account the fact that anatomical structures manifest in different scales. Consequently, we employ a quadtree-based strategy [10] to partition the slice into structurally adaptive patches. Since the intermediate slice is not available beforehand, we partition the slices immediately superior and inferior to the intermediate slice. A standard top-down approach to construct the quadtree is performed for each slice. Starting with the entire slice, we test each superior-inferior patch-pair (e.g., y^u *and* y^d — simultaneously to see if they meet a predefined homogeneity criterion. If the superior-inferior patch-pair meet the criterion, the division is halted. Otherwise, the patch-pair will be further divided into sub-patches. This procedure is repeated iteratively until each patch-pair meets the stopping criterion. We employ a simple intensity-based homogeneity criterion, where for the patch-pair the split stops if the patch-pair intensity variance is below a specified threshold. An example of the slice partitioning is shown in Fig. 2.

3   Experimental Results

To evaluate the performance of our patch-based resolution enhancement method, we apply our method to a publicly available DIR-lab dataset [11]. Ten cases of 4D-CT were used in this experiment. Each case was acquired at 2.5mm slice spacing with a GE system, and separated into 10 phases. The 4D-CT images cover the entire thorax and upper abdomen. For each case, the in-plane grid size is 256×256 or 512×512, and in-plane voxel dimensions range from (0.97×0.97) to (1.16×1.16) mm^2. We simulated the 4D-CT with 5mm slice thickness by removing one of every two slices from the original 4D-CT with 2.5mm slice thickness. Thus we can quantitatively evaluate the effectiveness of our method in enhancing the resolution from 5mm to 2.5mm. In all experiments, parameter ε is set to 1.2, and parameter λ is set to 0.2. We present both visual and quantitative results to demonstrate the performance of the proposed method, with the comparison to linear interpolation and cubic-spline interpolation.

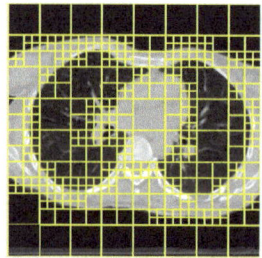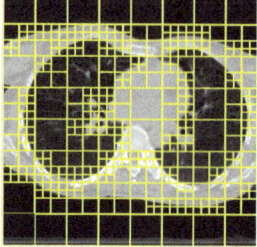

Fig. 2. Quadtree-based adaptive patch partitioning of two consecutive slices

Fig. 3 demonstrates the reconstruction results generated with our method. The top row shows the ground-truth slice together with its respective inferior and superior slices. The bottom row shows the result based on linear interpolation, the reconstructed result based on Equation (1) (the linear interpolation result used as reference for patch distance computation), and the result given by the proposed method (patch distance computed based on Equation (4)). It can be observed that our method provides better reconstruction result that resembles the ground truth more closely. The patch mismatching due to the artifacts in the interpolated patch (see Fig. 3(d)) is avoided effectively.

Fig. 4 shows the results based on the identically sized patches and the quadtree-based adaptively sized patches (described in Section 2.4), respectively. It is clear that the vessels are much clearer with the results given by the adaptively sized patch-based approach.

In Fig. 5, we show typical reconstruction results given by different algorithms. The ground-truth images are shown in the left column. The results given by linear interpolation, cubic spline interpolation, and our method are shown in the 2nd, 3rd, and 4th column, respectively. It is apparent that our proposed method outperforms the conventional interpolation methods, which often cause undesirable artifacts (marked in red squares). Our proposed method makes principled use of information gathered from all other phase images to make up for the missing information and hence expectedly yields better results.

In Fig. 6, we further provide sagittal and coronal views of the same 4D-CT case for further comparison, with similar arrangement as Fig. 5. These results again demonstrate the best performance achieved by our proposed method, as evident from the regions circled in red.

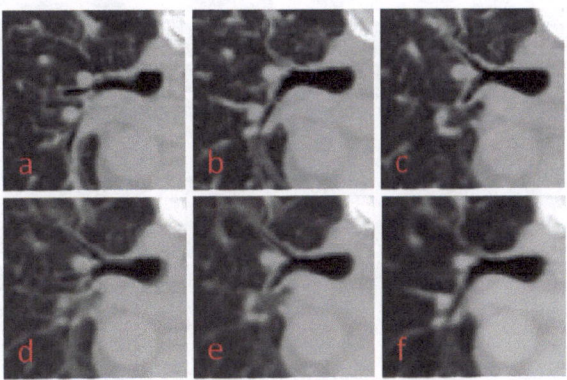

Fig. 3. Reconstructed local patch based on linear interpolation and the proposed method. Top row: (a) inferior slice; (b) ground truth (middle) slice; (c) superior slice. Bottom row: (d) result based on linear interpolation; (e) reconstructed result based on (d); (f) result given by the proposed method.

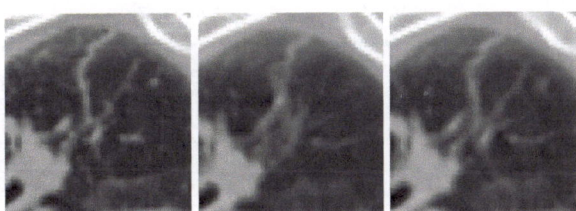

Fig. 4. An example of reconstruction with (middle) identically sized patches and (right) adaptively sized patches. The ground truth is shown on the left.

Finally, in Table 1, we present the mean PSNR (peak signal-to-noise ratio) and SSIM (structural similarity) results for each case. The proposed method again achieves the highest PSNR (usually 3~4dB higher) and SSIM values in all cases.

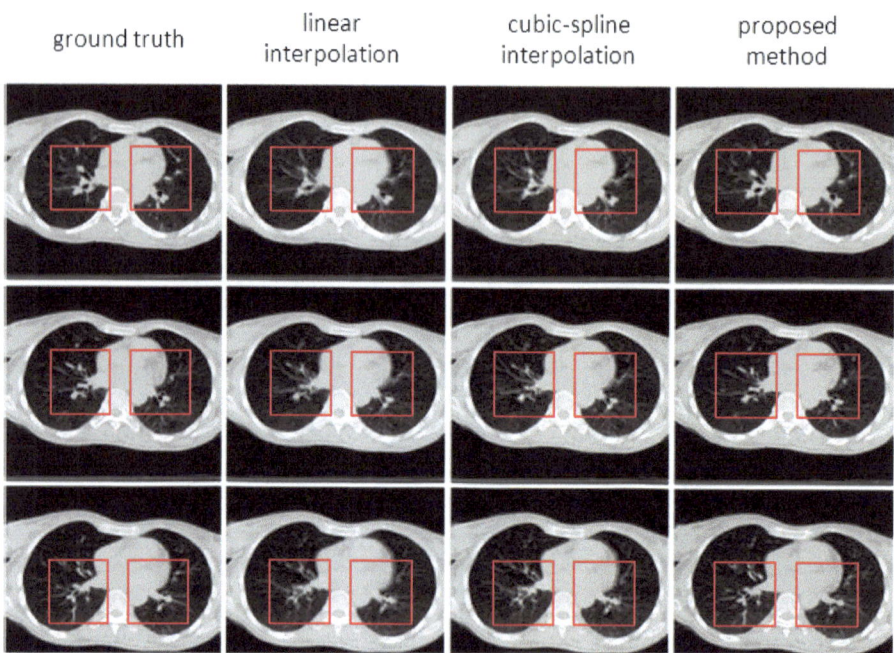

Fig. 5. Reconstruction results for consecutive slices

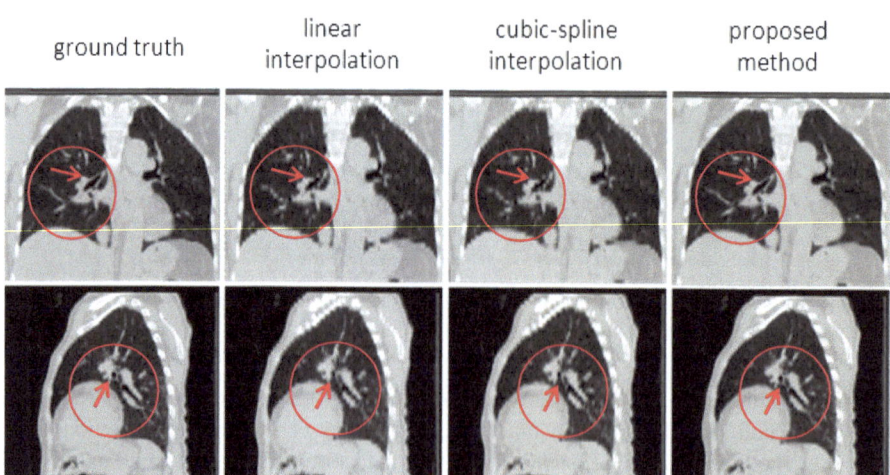

Fig. 6. Sagittal and coronal views of the resolution enhanced images

Table 1. Mean PSNR (top) and SSIM (bottom) for all phases of five 4D-CT cases by linear interpolation, cubic-spline interpolation, and the proposed method

Case	Linear interpolation	Cubic-spline interpolation	Proposed method
Case 1	29.92 0.8861	30.02 0.8849	**33.60** **0.9367**
Case 2	30.02 0.8942	30.22 0.8939	**33.56** **0.9285**
Case 3	30.81 0.9136	31.05 0.9149	**35.30** **0.9579**
Case 4	29.62 0.9187	29.78 0.9202	**33.28** **0.9573**
Case 5	29.85 0.9072	29.91 0.9063	**32.93** **0.9513**
Case 6	28.59 0.8788	28.57 0.8786	**31.14** **0.9219**
Case 7	27.41 0.8515	27.51 0.8520	**31.45** **0.9140**
Case 8	27.16 0.7952	27.23 0.7946	**30.15** **0.8678**
Case 9	29.08 0.9119	29.28 0.9128	**32.76** **0.9454**
Case 10	27.72 0.8569	27.81 0.8579	**30.61** **0.9103**

4   Conclusion

In this paper, we propose a novel lung 4D-CT resolution enhancement algorithm. We take advantage of complementary image information that can be taken from images of different phases captured in 4D-CT, to recover missing structural information. A patch-based non-local strategy, exploiting a new patch distance measure and an adaptively slice-partitioning strategy, is particularly used to achieve the reconstruction. The proposed method demonstrates consistent improvements over all conventional interpolation methods both qualitatively and quantitatively. In the future, detailed aspects of the algorithm, such as parameter optimization, will be studied.

Acknowledgements. This work was supported in part by the Major State Basic Research Development Program of China (No. 2010CB732505), Science and Technology Planning Project of Guangzhou (No. 2010J-E471), and NIH Grant (No. CA140413).

References

1. Khan, F., Bell, G., Antony, J., Palmer, M., Balter, P., Bucci, K., Chapman, M.J.: The use of 4DCT to reduce lung dose: A dosimetric analysis. Medical Dosimetry 34, 273–278 (2009)
2. Freeman, W.T., Jones, T.R., Pasztor, E.C.: Example-based super-resolution. IEEE Computer Graphics and Applications 22, 56–65 (2002)

3. Hong, C., Dit-Yan, Y., Yimin, X.: Super-resolution through neighbor embedding. In: CVPR, pp. 275–282 (2004)
4. Jianchao, Y., Wright, J., Huang, T.S., Yi, M.: Image super-resolution via sparse representation. IEEE Transaction on Image Processing 19, 2861–2873 (2010)
5. Buades, A., Coll, B., Morel, J.M.: A non-local algorithm for image denoising. In: CVPR, vol. 62, pp. 60–65 (2005)
6. Rousseau, F., Habas, P.A., Studholme, C.: A supervised patch-based approach for human brain labeling. IEEE Transactions on Medical Imaging 30, 1852–1862 (2011)
7. Coupé, P., Manjón, J.V., Fonov, V., Pruessner, J., Robles, M., Collins, D.L.: Patch-based segmentation using expert priors: Application to hippocampus and ventricle segmentation. NeuroImage 54, 940–954 (2011)
8. Heinrich, M.P., Jenkinson, M., Bhushan, M., Matin, T., Gleeson, F.V., Brady, J.M., Schnabel, J.A.: Non-local Shape Descriptor: A New Similarity Metric for Deformable Multi-modal Registration. In: Fichtinger, G., Martel, A., Peters, T. (eds.) MICCAI 2011, Part II. LNCS, vol. 6892, pp. 541–548. Springer, Heidelberg (2011)
9. Manjón, J.V., Coupé, P., Buades, A., Fonov, V., Louis Collins, D., Robles, M.: Non-local MRI upsampling. Medical Image Analysis 14, 784–792 (2010)
10. Finkel, R.A., Bentley, J.L.: Quad trees a data structure for retrieval on composite keys. Acta Informatica 4, 1–9 (1974)
11. Castillo, R., Castillo, E., Guerra, R., Johnson, V.E., Mcphail, T., Garg, A.K., Guerrero, T.: A framework for evaluation of deformable image registration spatial accuracy using large landmark point sets. Physics in Medicine and Biology 54, 1849–1870 (2009)

Compressed Sensing Dynamic Reconstruction in Rotational Angiography

Hélène Langet[1,2,3,*], Cyril Riddell[1], Yves Trousset[1], Arthur Tenenhaus[2], Elisabeth Lahalle[2], Gilles Fleury[2], and Nikos Paragios[3,4,5]

[1] GE Healthcare, Interventional Radiology, Buc, France
[2] Supélec, SSE department, Gif-sur-Yvette, France
[3] ECP, Center for Visual Computing, Châtenay-Malabry, France
[4] ENPC, Center for Visual Computing, Champs-sur-Marne, France
[5] INRIA Saclay, GALEN Team, Orsay, France

Abstract. This work tackles three-dimensional reconstruction of tomographic acquisitions in C-arm-based rotational angiography. The relatively slow rotation speed of C-arm systems involves motion artifacts that limit the use of three-dimensional imaging in interventional procedures. The main contribution of this paper is a reconstruction algorithm that deals with the temporal variations due to intra-arterial injections. Based on a compressed-sensing approach, we propose a multiple phase reconstruction with spatio-temporal constraints. The algorithm was evaluated by qualitative and quantitative assessment of image quality on both numerical phantom experiments and clinical data from vascular C-arm systems. In this latter case, motion artifacts reduction was obtained in spite of the cone-beam geometry, the short-scan acquisition, and the truncated and subsampled data.

1 Introduction

Rotational angiography provides three-dimensional (3D) qualitative and quantitative information of high clinical interest as the complexity of minimally invasive procedures increases. However, its spread in the clinical practice is limited by the nature of the measurements: 3D reconstruction of C-arm system data is challenging due to the use of cone-beam (CB) geometry, short-scan orbits, as well as truncated and angularly subsampled data. Besides, physiological times (e.g. heart beat, breathing time) are small compared to the gantry rotation speed of C-arm systems. The resulting temporal variations within a scan are so challenging that they are usually not corrected for in the clinical practice.

Temporal variations are addressed through the decomposition of the dynamic (3D+t) data into phases where the object can be considered "static" so that 3D reconstruction is feasible. Each phase defines a subset of projections that must fully sample the volume at this particular time point [9]. To alleviate

---

* Corresponding author: helene.langet@ge.com. This work was supported in part by ANRT grant number CIFRE-936/2009.

N. Ayache et al. (Eds.): MICCAI 2012, Part I, LNCS 7510, pp. 223–230, 2012.

this sampling requirement, additional a priori information must be integrated. Common approaches rely on modeling the motion (e.g. B-splines or dense vector fields) so that each phase can be deduced from a reference one by the motion model. That is a challenging estimation problem though. Motion of the coronary arteries or of an opaque device can be detected in the projective images [1, 8] while breathing motion can been derived from a previous CT acquisition [10]. Still, even if a perfect knowledge of the motion reduces the number of unknown volumes to just one, it does not guaranty alone that this unique volume is properly sampled; the acquisition itself must be adapted (e.g. ECG-gating, multiple rotations).

These levels of complexity are not adequate for addressing the need for improving standard C-arm imaging marred by accidental motion artifacts or contrast flow variations. Three-dimensional reconstruction based on compressed sensing (CS) is a new alternative that allows for directly reconstructing subsampled data, and that is applicable even in absence of a motion model, yielding a sparse approximation to the solution through spatial constraints (typically wavelets or total variation filtering) and temporal redundancy [2,3,5,7,11]. One particularly seducing approach relies on using a temporal constraint based on a prior image equal to the static reconstruction, so that, schematically, motionless areas are determined from the complete data set, while motion-blurred areas are determined from subsampled reconstruction with a total variation constraint [3]. However, with intra-arterial contrast injection, motion blur is not the only degradation present in the standard Feldkamp (FDK) static reconstruction: any part of the image may be degraded by intense streaks due to the presence of inconsistent high-intensity vessel projections in the data, making the static reconstruction a poor prior image. On the positive side, we have shown in [6] in this same context, that an iterative FDK (iFDK) algorithm combined with a spatial constraint called soft background subtraction (SBS) could mitigate subsampling artifacts while preserving the overall aspect of FDK reconstructions, a point of importance for the clinical practice. However, this strategy is not applicable to removing streaks due to incoherent static data and thus cannot provide an improved prior image. We therefore generalize the approach presented in [6] to the reconstruction of a series of volumes based on combining the SBS spatial constraint to a temporal constraint that enforces the sparsity of the difference between time points. We show how this multiple-phase reconstruction with spatio-temporal constraints can be casted in the same mathematical framework of an iFDK algorithm associated to proximal splitting schemes. It is applied to two types of temporal inconsistencies within injected vessels: small displacements induced by the blood flow pulsatility and contrast flow variability during the scan due to delayed opacification.

2   Dynamic Reconstruction

Let us consider 3D+t data with M phases. We denote f and p the vectors that respectively contain the imaged volume at different time points $f_i = f(t_i)$ and the data, where p_i refers to the 2D projection subset assigned to the volume f_i. R is the block-diagonal matrix that models the rotational CB acquisition process.

$$f = \begin{pmatrix} f_1 = f(t_1) \\ \vdots \\ f_M = f(t_M) \end{pmatrix} \qquad p = \begin{pmatrix} p_1 \\ \vdots \\ p_M \end{pmatrix} \qquad R = \begin{pmatrix} R_1 & & \\ & \ddots & \\ & & R_M \end{pmatrix}$$

The noise-free tomographic problem consists in solving the system of linear equations

$$Rf = p. \tag{1}$$

This problem is underdetermined because the set of measurements p is small with respect to f.

2.1 Compressed Sensing Phase Reconstruction with Spatial Constraint (CS-Ps)

For the case of angiographic data that contain sparse intense vessels over a non-sparse background, we presented in [6] a CS-based reconstruction strategy, here called CS-Ps, that enables the efficient removal of vessel-induced subsampling artifacts. CS-Ps consists in solving a sequence of N ℓ_1-regularized problems indexed by a set of decreasing regularization hyperparameters: $\Lambda_s = \{\lambda_s^{(n)} | n = 1, \cdots, N\}$, such that $\lambda_s^{(1)} \geq \cdots \geq \lambda_s^{(N)}$. Each problem has the form:

$$\underset{f}{\mathrm{argmin}} \left[Q(f) + \chi_{\lambda_s^{(n)}}(f) \right], \tag{2}$$

where $Q(f) = \frac{1}{2}(Rf - p)^T D(Rf - p)$ denotes the ℓ_2-data fitting term, ^{T} the transpose symbol, D the ramp filter that is positive and diagonal in the Fourier domain, and $\chi_{\lambda_s^{(n)}}(f) = \lambda_s^{(n)} \Phi_s(f) = \lambda_s^{(n)} \|f\|_1^+$ the combination of the image ℓ_1-norm with positivity. Problem (2) is solved with proximal operators using a splitting scheme [4]:

$$\begin{cases} f^{(k+\frac{1}{2})} = f^{(k)} - \tau \nabla Q(f^{(k)}) = f^{(k)} + \tau R^T D(p - Rf^{(k)}) \\ f^{(k+1)} = \mathrm{prox}_{\tau \chi_{\lambda_s^{(n)}}} \left(f^{(k+\frac{1}{2})} \right) \equiv \underset{g}{\mathrm{argmin}} \left[\tau \chi_{\lambda_s^{(n)}}(g) + \frac{1}{2} \|g - f^{(k+\frac{1}{2})}\|_2^2 \right] \end{cases}, \tag{3}$$

where τ is a standard gradient descent step. The proximal operator $\mathrm{prox}_{\tau \chi_{\lambda_s^{(n)}}}$ defined in (3) has a direct expression as the SBS operator: it soft-thresholds the positive values by $\tau \lambda_s^{(n)}$ and sets the negative ones to zero. The minimization at $\lambda_s^{(n)}$ identifies a sparse approximation that best fits the data with a level of sparsity that is proportional to $\lambda_s^{(n)}$. It is used as a warm-start to the minimization at $\lambda_s^{(n+1)}$. In practice, iteration (3) results in a standard FDK reconstruction scaled by τ and segmented with threshold $\tau \lambda_s^{(n)}$. Thus, CS-Ps consists in reconstructing high-intensity vessels first, without streaks, while the background is progressively reintroduced as $\lambda_s^{(n)}$ tends to zero. The recent work [12] identifies this process as an approximate homotopy continuation strategy whose convergence is proved given that each problem is solved with sufficient precision and $\lambda_s^{(n)}$ is geometrically decreased. With iterative FDK, we observed convergence when solving each problem with one iteration and using a simple linear decrease.

2.2 Compressed Sensing Phase Reconstruction with Spatio-Temporal Constraint (CS-Pst)

CS-Ps reconstructs each phase independently so that the sampling of the static background structures is significantly reduced. To recover full sampling of the background we have to take inter-phase correlations into account. Since we focus on the vessel temporal variations only, it is relevant to assume sparsity of the difference to the weighted mean $\Phi_t(f) = \sum_{i=1}^{M} \| f_i - \frac{1}{M} \sum_{j=1}^{M} \omega_j f_j \|_1$ where ω_j accounts for the possible difference in the phase subset cardinality. Merging each phase background is relevant only if it does not contain vessel-induced streaks. This suggests extending the sparsity constraint of problem (2) with a temporal constraint Φ_t of hyperparameter λ_t such that:

$$\chi_{\lambda_s^{(n)}}(f) = \lambda_s^{(n)} \Phi_s(f) + \lambda_t \Phi_t(f). \tag{4}$$

Here, hyperparameter λ_s is handled exactly as in CS-Ps because the background is not assumed sparse, while hyperparameter λ_t can be assigned a fixed value without introducing a bias because temporal sparsity can be assumed. We denote CS-Pst this approach. Alternatively, the weighted mean can be replaced by a prior image f_P, leading to $\Phi_t(f) = \sum_{i=1}^{M} \| f_i - f_P \|_1$. We denote CS-Psp this latter constraint (4) with the prior image chosen equal to the static reconstruction as in [3].

Application of $\text{prox}_{\tau \chi_{\lambda_s^{(n)}}}$ means that all constraints are satisfied at once. In absence of a direct expression for $\text{prox}_{\tau \chi_{\lambda_s^{(n)}}}$, we turn to the Dykstra-like proximal algorithm to iteratively compute $\text{prox}_{\tau \chi_{\lambda_s^{(n)}}}(f)$ using $\text{prox}_{\lambda_s^{(n)} \Phi_s}$ and $\text{prox}_{\lambda_t \Phi_t}$. The Dykstra-like scheme is detailed in Sec. 5 of [4] (p.10), and is here nested within scheme (2). The direct expression of $\text{prox}_{\lambda_t \Phi_t}$ is obtained by rewriting the temporal constraint as $\Phi_t(f) = \| H_t(f - f_P) \|_1$, where H_t is an invertible matrix. For the difference to the weighted mean, $f_P = 0$ and H_t transforms the temporal intensity at a given voxel into an average component and differential components that are thresholded. In the case of the prior image, H_t is set equal to the identity matrix.

3   Evaluation

In order to establish the reconstruction performances of CS-Pst and CS-Psp with respect to CS-Ps, we built a numerical phantom with three phases by adding simulated injected arteries (from 1500 to 6000 HU) to a 512×512 abdominal CT cross-section where background structures are valued between 1000 and 2000 HU. Note that we consider positive HU unit, where air is 0 HU and water is 1000 HU. We simulated the acquisition in parallel geometry of data with (a) a pulsatile motion synchronized with an ECG signal, and (b) a motion where each phase is defined by a subset of contiguous projections, resulting in a limited-angle sampling. Acquisition settings were chosen to fit clinical routine, where C-arm systems record projections at 30 frames/s during an approximately 200° rotation at 40°/s delivering about 150 projections in total. Reconstruction settings are as follows: $\tau = 0.9$, N $= 200$ thresholds, $\lambda_s^{(1)} = 3000$ HU and is linearly decreased to $\lambda_s^{(N)} = 0$ HU for CS-Ps, CS-Pst and CS-Psp, and $\lambda_t = 50$ HU for CS-Pst and CS-Psp.

Figure 1 gives comparative assessment of the reconstruction quality. Figure. 1.(a) displays two regions of interest (RoI) of the phantom: with static structures only (top image) and with dynamic injected vessels over static background for two phases (middle and bottom images). CS-Ps reconstruction is shown in Fig. 1.(b) to restore the temporal resolution of the vessels without introducing subsampling streaks, but the background is poorly depicted due to the substantial subsampling of each phase. Comparing to Fig. 1.(c), the prior image constraint of CS-Psp improved the background, while preserving the temporal resolution. A strong streak pattern remains in all RoIs however, that is a slightly attenuated version of the one present in the prior image (image not shown). The best restoration is thus obtained by CS-Pst as shown in Fig. 1.(d). CS-Pst results for the limited-angle case are presented in 1.(e). It outperformed CS-Ps and CS-Psp in the same manner (images not shown). We quantified streak intensity by measuring the maximum intensity which is not a vessel in the RoI with dynamic injected vessels: for the pulsatile case streak intensity decreased from 1872 HU for the prior image to 1636 HU and 1302 HU for CS-Psp and CS-Pst respectively; for the limited-angle case it decreased from 1954 HU to 1629 HU and 1406 HU.

The convergence behavior was monitored at each iteration by the normalized root mean square deviation $d_r = \sqrt{\frac{\sum_{j=1}^{J_r} \left(f_{i,j} - \tilde{f}_{i,j}\right)^2}{\sum_{j=1}^{J_r} \tilde{f}_{i,j}^2}}$ where J_r is the number of pixels in RoI r and $\tilde{f}_i$ is the phantom. Figure 2 contains the plots of $\log d_r$ with respect to the number of iterations for two RoIs: one covering the area with moving vessels displayed in the the middle row of Fig. 1 and shown in graph 2.(a), the other covering the background displayed in the top row of Fig. 1 and shown in graph 2.(b). Discrepancy between the prior image and the reference image over each RoI is shown as a black dashed line. The final deviations of graph 2.(a) reflect the improved recovery of the moving structures with all CS dynamic reconstructions. In graph 2.(b), CS-Ps high deviation reflects poor background recovery. For CS-Psp, background recovery nears the level of the prior image, but cannot improve it by construction. On the contrary, CS-Pst restores the background below the discrepancy level of the prior image.

Results on real data are analyzed in Fig. 3 where standard clinical (i.e. static) reconstruction is compared to CS-Pst. The first dataset is an exam of the renal arteries, in which small displacements of the catheter occur due to the pulsatile blood flow. We manually splitted the scan into four phases, relying on the vertical translation of the tip, that is visible on the 2D projections. The resulting

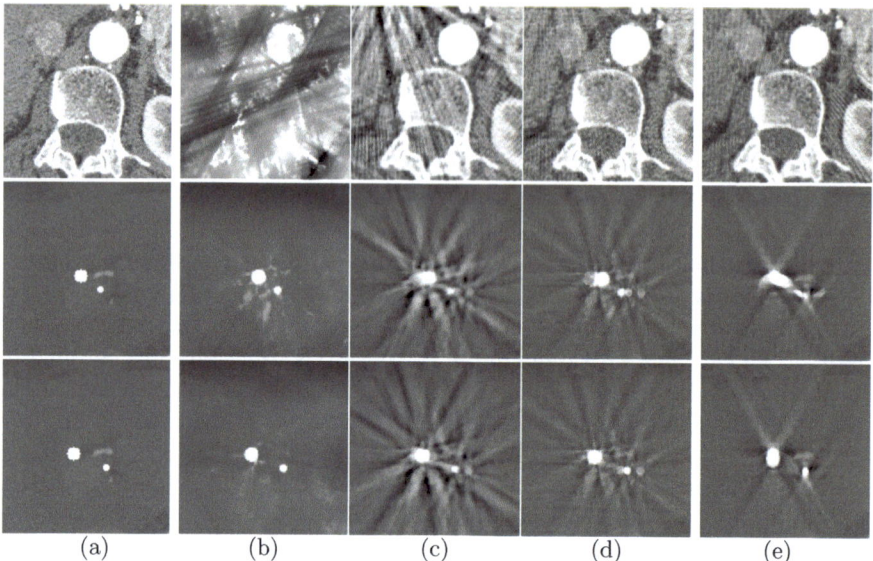

Fig. 1. Simulated data. First row: RoI with static structures - HU display range: 800 to 1400; second and third rows: RoI with dynamic injected vessels over static background for phase 1 and phase 2 respectively - HU display range: 100 to 2800. (a) Ground-truth. Pulsatile case: (b) CS-Ps; (c) CS-Psp; (d) CS-Pst. Limited-angle case: (e) CS-Pst.

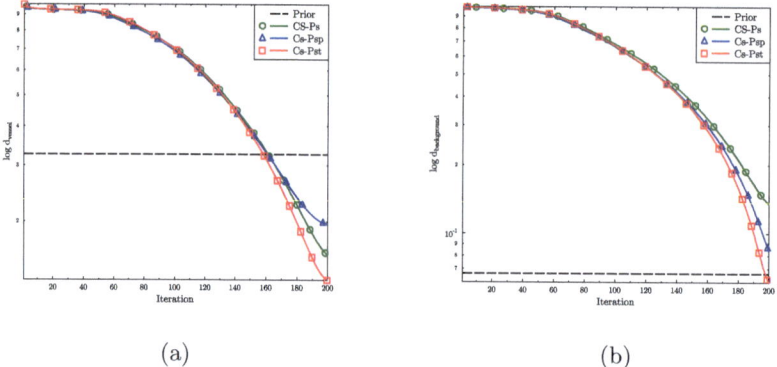

Fig. 2. Convergence curves for the numerical phantom with pulsatile motion: (a) RoI with dynamic injected vessels over static background for phase 1; (b) RoI with static structures

phases contained 33, 36, 40, and 38 projections respectively. The second dataset is an exam of the cerebral vessels. During the first half of the scan the right vertebral artery (RVA, most left vessel in the axial slices in Fig. 3.(2)) did not appear opacified, while the left vertebral artery (LVA, most right vessel) was seen fully opacified during the whole scan. We thus splitted the scan into two phases that contained 72 and 75 projections respectively. Static reconstructions integrate all temporal variations: the position of the tip is blurred in the first exam (Fig. 3.(1a)), while the intensity of the RVA peak is averaged to 9130 HU (Fig. 3.(2a)), that is less than 60% of the LVA peak (15310 HU). In addition, intense streak artifacts degrade the background: the displacements of the catheter yield a rotating pattern of positive and negative streaks in the first case, while the lack of opacification in the lateral projections yields horizontal and vertical negative streaks in the second case. CS-Pst reconstruction recovered some temporal resolution since temporal variations are visible in the reconstructed phases, even though our phase selection was approximate. This is particularly striking when looking at the associated maximum intensity projection (MIP) given in the second row of Fig. 3: the vertical translation of the catheter is well visible (Fig. 3.(1b) and (1c)); the RVA is only visible during phase 2, while the LVA is visible in both phases (Fig. 3.(2b) and (2c)). In terms of quantification the RVA peak was measured to be 1960 HU for phase 1 and 12290 HU for phase 2, while the LVA peak was measured to be around 13600 HU for both phases. As for the background CS-Pst reduced the streaks located close to the catheter tip (Fig. 3.(1b) and (1c)), and nearly eliminated the horizontal and vertical streaks of the RVA (Fig. 3.(2b) and (2c)).

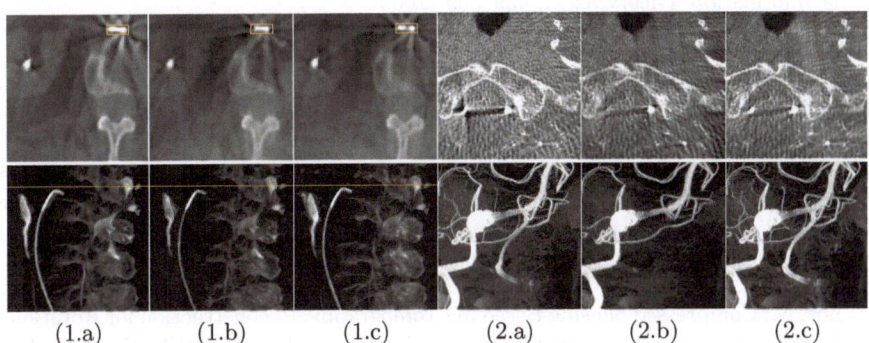

(1.a)   (1.b)   (1.c)   (2.a)   (2.b)   (2.c)

Fig. 3. Clinical data. (1) Pulsatile case; (2) Limited-angle case. First row: axial slice detail - HU display range: (1) 350 to 1550 (2) 0 to 2400. Second row: MIP detail - HU display range: (1) 1100 to 4400 (2) 1000 to 9500. Algorithms: (a) static reconstruction; CS-Pst for (b) phase 1 and (c) phase 2.

4   Conclusion and Discussion

We proposed a 3D+t reconstruction that relies on a CS approach with spatio-temporal constraints. The evaluation of the algorithm with numerical experiments and two typical angiographic datasets demonstrated qualitative and quantitative improvements. These results were obtained in a clinical context with limited assumptions: high-intensity sparse structures but non-sparse background, temporal correlation but no motion modeling, only manual phase selection. For an actual clinical usage, automatic phase selection is a requirement. It is challenging, but to a lesser degree than motion estimation and modeling. Future work will aim at applying the proposed mathematical framework to a larger class of problems because it relies on proximal operators. If applicable, stronger spatial sparsity can be enforced through wavelets or total variation filters, which are proximal operators. Another direction is to strengthen the proposed temporal constraint by computing a mean image that would account for some (i.e. even incomplete) inter-phase registration based upon a priori motion knowledge. This constraint could still be applied through a proximal operator similar to the one presented here. In order to simplify the presentation, the temporal constraint was also set equal for all voxels. This is not a requirement: in the case of a delayed opacification, each voxel could be treated independently, with its own phase selection and associated temporal constraint and proximal operator.

References

1. Blondel, C., Malandain, G., Vaillant, R., Ayache, N.: Reconstruction of coronary arteries from a single rotational X-ray projection sequence. IEEE Transactions on Medical Imaging 25(5), 653–663 (2006)
2. Candès, E., Romberg, J., Tao, T.: Robust Uncertainty Principles: Exact Signal Reconstruction from Highly Incomplete Frequency Information. IEEE Transactions on Information Theory 52(2), 489–509 (2006)
3. Chen, G.H., Tang, J., Leng, S.: Prior Image Constrained Compressed Sensing (PICCS). Medical Physics 35(2), 660–663 (2008)
4. Combettes, P.L., Pesquet, J.C.: Proximal Splitting Methods in Signal Processing. In: Fixed-Point Algorithms for Inverse Problems in Science and Engineering, ch. 10, vol. 49, pp. 185–212 (2011)
5. Jia, X., Lou, Y., Dong, B., Tian, Z., Jiang, S.: 4D Computed Tomography Reconstruction from Few-Projection Data via Temporal Non-local Regularization. In: Jiang, T., Navab, N., Pluim, J.P.W., Viergever, M.A. (eds.) MICCAI 2010, Part I. LNCS, vol. 6361, pp. 143–150. Springer, Heidelberg (2010)
6. Langet, H., Riddell, C., Trousset, Y., Tenenhaus, A., Lahalle, E., Fleury, G., Paragios, N.: Compressed Sensing Based 3D Tomographic Reconstruction for Rotational Angiography. In: Fichtinger, G., Martel, A., Peters, T. (eds.) MICCAI 2011, Part I. LNCS, vol. 6891, pp. 97–104. Springer, Heidelberg (2011)
7. Lustig, M.: Sparse MRI. Ph.D. thesis, Stanford University (September 2008)
8. Perrenot, B., Vaillant, R., Prost, R., Finet, G., Douek, P., Peyrin, F.: Motion correction for coronary stent reconstruction from rotational x-ray projection sequences. IEEE Trans. Med. Imaging 26(10), 1412–1423 (2007)
9. Prümmer, M., Hornegger, J., Lauritsch, G., Wigström, L., Girard-Hughes, E., Fahrig, R.: Cardiac C-Arm CT: A Unified Framework for Motion Estimation and Dynamic CT. IEEE Trans. Med. Imaging 28(11), 1836–1849 (2009)
10. Rit, S., Sarrut, D., Desbat, L.: Comparison of analytic and algebraic methods for motion-compensated cone-beam ct reconstruction of the thorax. IEEE Trans. Med. Imaging 28(10), 1513–1525 (2009)
11. Sidky, E.Y., Duchin, Y., Pan, X., Ullberg, C.: A constrained, total-variation minimization algorithm for low-intensity x-ray CT. Medical Physics 38(S1), S117–S125 (2011)
12. Xiao, L., Zhang, T.: A Proximal-Gradient Homotopy Method for the Sparse Least-Squares Problem. CRR abs/1203.3002 (2012)

Bi-exponential Magnetic Resonance Signal Model for Partial Volume Computation

Quentin Duché[1,2,3,5], Oscar Acosta[1,2], Giulio Gambarota[1,2,3], Isabelle Merlet[1,2], Olivier Salvado[5], and Hervé Saint-Jalmes[1,2,3,4]

[1] Université de Rennes 1, LTSI - Rennes, F-35000, France
[2] INSERM, U1099 - Rennes, F-35000, France
[3] PRISM - Biosit, CNRS UMS 3480 - Biogenouest - Rennes, F-35000, France
[4] CRLCC, Centre Eugène Marquis - Rennes, F-35000, France
[5] CSIRO ICT Centre, The Australian E-Health Research Centre, Brisbane, Australia
quentin.duche@univ-rennes1.fr

Abstract. Accurate quantification of small structures in magnetic resonance (MR) images is often limited by partial volume (PV) effects which arise when more than one tissue type is present in a voxel. PV may be critical when dealing with changes in brain anatomy as the considered structures such as gray matter (GM) are of similar size as the MR spatial resolution. To overcome the limitations imposed by PV effects and achieve subvoxel accuracy different methods have been proposed. Here, we describe a method to compute PV by modeling the MR signal with a biexponential linear combination representing the contribution of at most two tissues in each voxel. In a first step, we estimated the parameters (T1, T2 and proton density) per tissue. Then, based on the bi-exponential formulation one can retrieve fractional contents by solving a linear system of two equations with two unknowns, namely tissue magnetizations. Preliminary tests were conducted on images acquired on a specially designed physical phantom for the study of PV effects. Further, the model was tested on BrainWeb simulated brain images to estimate GM and white matter (WM) PV effects. Root mean squared error was computed between the BrainWeb ground truth and the obtained GM and WM PV maps. The proposed method outperformed traditionally used methods by 33% and 34% in GM and WM, respectively.

Keywords: Bi-exponential model, MR Signal, partial volume correction.

1 Introduction

Magnetic resonance (MR) imaging is a non-invasive imaging modality allowing to detect changes in anatomy and is helpful in diagnosis of several diseases. It is particularly used in brain anatomy as it provides a high-resolution image of the intra cranial structures. Nevertheless, several artifacts arise during the acquisition such as partial volume effects (PVE), bias field and noise that may hamper tissue quantification. PVE may become critical when dealing with small structures like brain cortex where subtle differences in cortical thickness or volume can occur in presence of neurodegenerative diseases such as Alzheimer's disease [1] or focal cortical dysplasia [2], and may yield to significant errors if not taken into account [3,4,5].

N. Ayache et al. (Eds.): MICCAI 2012, Part I, LNCS 7510, pp. 231–238, 2012.

Standard approaches use tissues means and variances within maximum a posteriori classification framework to fit multiple gaussians modeling pure or even mixture of tissues onto the histogram [5,6,7,8,9]. The percentage of each tissue present in each voxel is thus a fractional content of each tissue type modeled by the statistical distributions of pure tissue and mixture voxels in the image.

Other approaches made use of two acquisitions and model the signal intensity of a voxel by two linear combinations of three mean pure tissue values, gray matter (GM), white matter (WM) and cerebrospinal fluid (CSF) [10,11]. However, the mean values estimated in the two images were not computed locally which make the method sensitive to radiofrequency (RF) inhomogeneities. As the authors stated in the paper, "the assumption that a pure tissue will give a constant signal response is a simplification in practice, particularly as field strengths effects can produce position dependent sensitivity" [10].

Here, we describe a model which stands on the physical properties of the signal of the acquisition, namely T1 and T2 relaxation time constants and proton density (PD) of the tissues and the parameters of acquisition TE (Echo Time) and TR (Repetition Time) (and TI -Inversion Time- for inversion recovery -IR- sequences). By using two co-registered images that nowadays may be obtained in a single acquisition such as in the new Fluid Attenuated and White matter Suppression (FLAWS) sequence [12], based on the MP2RAGE [13] technique, a bi-exponential model for MR signal is introduced. This model allows to retrieve the amount of GM, WM and CSF in each voxel of a presegmented intra cranial volume (ICV). We show how this problem leads to a linear system of two equations with two unknowns.

A direct and independent computation of GM/WM and GM/CSF fractional content maps is performed without assumptions about statistical properties of tissue values. This computationally inexpensive method is also robust to RF inhomogeneities as the signal intensities of a voxel in both images are identically biased.

2   Methods

2.1   Bi-exponential Model for MR Signal

We modeled the MR signal with a linear combination of mono-exponentials with weighting as unknowns and representing the magnetizations of the two tissues considered in a voxel. Let's first consider the Spin Echo (SE) signal function for a single tissue as

$$s(\boldsymbol{x}, \boldsymbol{\Phi_{SE}}, \boldsymbol{T}) = M_0 e^{-\frac{TE}{T2}} \left(1 - e^{-\frac{TR}{T1}}\right) \qquad (1)$$

where $\boldsymbol{x} = \{x, y, z\}$, $\boldsymbol{\Phi_{SE}} = \{TE, TR\}$, $\boldsymbol{T} = \{M_0, T1, T2\}$ describe respectively the voxel position, the sequence parameters and tissue properties. M_0 is the longitudinal magnetization in the state of equilibrium and $T1$, $T2$ are respectively the longitudinal and transversal magnetization time constants. If we now consider two magnetic contributions from two different tissues α and β in a single voxel $\boldsymbol{x}$, the acquired signal is written as

$$s(\boldsymbol{x}, \boldsymbol{\Phi_{SE}}, \boldsymbol{T_\alpha}, \boldsymbol{T_\beta}) = M_{0\alpha} e^{-\frac{TE}{T2_\alpha}} \left(1 - e^{-\frac{TR}{T1_\alpha}}\right) + M_{0\beta} e^{-\frac{TE}{T2_\beta}} \left(1 - e^{-\frac{TR}{T1_\beta}}\right) \qquad (2)$$

Here, for a given voxel, $M_{0\alpha}$ and $M_{0\beta}$ are two unkwnowns and $T1$ and $T2$ are either known [14] or experimentally estimated. Thus, two acquisitions with different TE and TR result in a voxel-wise two equation system:

$$(S_{SE}) \Longleftrightarrow \begin{cases} s_1(\boldsymbol{x}) = s(\boldsymbol{x}, \boldsymbol{\Phi_{SE_1}}, \boldsymbol{T_\alpha}, \boldsymbol{T_\beta}) = k_{1\alpha} M_{0\alpha}(\boldsymbol{x}) + k_{1\beta} M_{0\beta}(\boldsymbol{x}) \\ s_2(\boldsymbol{x}) = s(\boldsymbol{x}, \boldsymbol{\Phi_{SE_2}}, \boldsymbol{T_\alpha}, \boldsymbol{T_\beta}) = k_{2\alpha} M_{0\alpha}(\boldsymbol{x}) + k_{2\beta} M_{0\beta}(\boldsymbol{x}) \end{cases}$$

with $k_{i,j} = e^{-\frac{TE_i}{T2_j}} (1 - e^{-\frac{TR_i}{T1_j}})$ where $i = \{1, 2\}$ denotes the acquisition number and $j = \{\alpha, \beta\}$ stands for the tissue. $k_{1\alpha}$, $k_{1\beta}$, $k_{2\alpha}$ and $k_{2\beta}$ are constant values across the image. The solution is:

$$(S_{SE}) \Longleftrightarrow \begin{cases} M_{0\alpha}(\boldsymbol{x}) = \dfrac{k_{2\beta} s_1(\boldsymbol{x}) - k_{1\beta} s_2(\boldsymbol{x})}{k_{2\beta} k_{1\alpha} - k_{2\alpha} k_{1\beta}} \\[3mm] M_{0\beta}(\boldsymbol{x}) = \dfrac{k_{1\alpha} s_2(\boldsymbol{x}) - k_{2\alpha} s_1(\boldsymbol{x})}{k_{2\beta} k_{1\alpha} - k_{2\alpha} k_{1\beta}} \end{cases}$$

This can also be done with an IR sequence of parameters $\boldsymbol{\Phi_{IR}} = \{TR, TE, TI\}$. In this case, although the signal s is slightly different as shown in eq. (3), the bi-exponential model can still be solved as the SE system. Only $k_{1\alpha}$, $k_{1\beta}$, $k_{2\alpha}$ and $k_{2\beta}$ are different.

$$s(\boldsymbol{x}, \boldsymbol{\Phi_{IR}}, \boldsymbol{T}) = M_0 e^{-\frac{TE}{T2}} \left(1 - e^{-\frac{TI}{T1}} (2 - 2e^{-\frac{(TR - \frac{TE}{2})}{T1}} + e^{-\frac{TR}{T1}}) \right) \qquad (3)$$

2.2 Estimation of the Tissue Parameters

Although brain tissue parameters are currently well known [14] a large inter-individual variability may exist and they may need to be consequently estimated. This subsection explains how this information can be retrieved from a pair of acquisitions.

Proton Density. To measure the PD of a tissue relatively to another tissue, one can acquire a sequence with an infinite TR, or at least 5 times the $T1$ of the considered tissues. Then the ratio $\frac{S_{GM}}{S_{WM}}$ (where S_{GM} is the signal of a pure GM tissue) should give the same result as $\frac{PD_{GM}}{PD_{WM}}$.

T1 T1 measurement of a tissue α was made by finding the solution of $g(T1) = \frac{k_{1\alpha}}{k_{2\alpha}} - \frac{\mu_{1\alpha}}{\mu_{2\alpha}} = 0$ where $\mu_{i\alpha} = \frac{1}{|\Omega_\alpha|} \sum\limits_{\boldsymbol{x} \in \Omega_\alpha} s_i(\boldsymbol{x}), i = \{1, 2\}$ is the mean of tissue α in the ith contrast image and Ω_α stands for the domain of pure tissue α.

2.3 Fractional Content Calculation

Signal magnitude M_0 must be positive and hence negative values are set to zero. The preserved M_0 values are subsequently divided by the PD to compensate the difference in water concentration among tissues, the fractional content is eventually computed as :

$$f_{\alpha/\beta}(\boldsymbol{x}) = \frac{M_{0\alpha}(\boldsymbol{x})}{M_{0\alpha}(\boldsymbol{x}) + M_{0\beta}(\boldsymbol{x})} = \frac{k_{2\beta} s_1(\boldsymbol{x}) - k_{1\beta} s_2(\boldsymbol{x})}{s_1(\boldsymbol{x})(k_{2\beta} - k_{2\alpha}) - s_2(\boldsymbol{x})(k_{1\beta} - k_{1\alpha})}$$

$f_{\alpha/\beta}(x)$ thereby represents the percentage of tissue α within the voxel x and it ranges between zero and one. This value is only valid $\forall x \in \Omega_\alpha \cup \Omega_\beta$.

The method computes the fractional content at both boundaries of the GM, namely GM/WM and GM/CSF. To combine the two models, $f_{GM/WM}$ values are computed at the intersection of dilated GM and WM ground truth binary masks (radius 1). The aim of the study is to show the accuracy of the bi-exponential model, thus no segmentation step was included in our work. Likewise on the GM/CSF boundary yielding the $f_{GM/CSF}$ values. Otherwise, the fractional content in the remaining GM is computed as $max(f_{GM/CSF}, f_{GM/WM})$.

3   Experiments

3.1   Physical Phantom

The method was tested on a physical phantom composed of two gel-layers simulating respectively GM and WM tissue relaxation properties. The gels were made of a combination of gadolinium chelate and distilled water (eq. (4)). R_1 and C_{gado} are respectively the relaxivity and the concentration of the contrast agent.

$$T1 = \frac{1}{\frac{1}{T1_{water}} + R_1 C_{gado}} \tag{4}$$

Then, agar (2.5%) was added to the solution and warmed up. While cooling down, the solution jellifies. T2 was fixed as the concentration of agar was the same for the two gels. Thus, a DoubleLayer phantom simulating a flat GM/WM interface was obtained by varying the concentration of gadolinium chelate in the two solutions. SE images were done on a Bruker Biospec 4.7T scanner (Bruker Biospin, Rheinstetten, Germany). The T1 obtained were 903ms for WM and 1130ms for GM. These values are close to the values of brain WM and GM at 3T. Two microtubes as shown in the bottom of Fig. 1(b,c,d) are always present next to the DoubleLayer as a T1 reference.

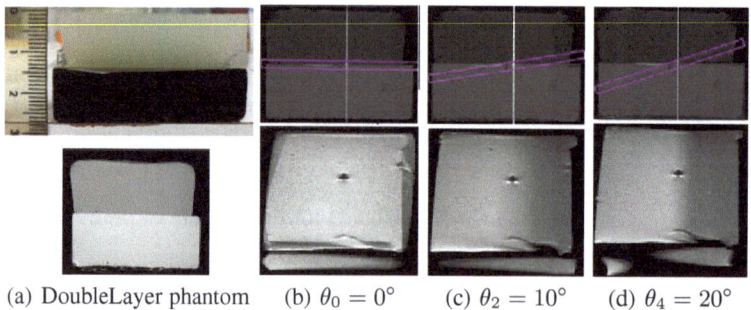

(a) DoubleLayer phantom   (b) $\theta_0 = 0°$ (c) $\theta_2 = 10°$ (d) $\theta_4 = 20°$

Fig. 1. DoubleLayer physical phantom. (a) Picture (*top*) and SE imaging (*bottom*) of the phantom. India ink was added to the GM solution to visually differentiate the two gels. (b,c,d) Acquisition protocol to control partial volume effects. *Top* the tilt, *bottom* the resulting images for different inclination angles (SE, $TR/TE = 800/10ms$, slice thickness $e = 4mm$, FOV = 8cm $*$ 6cm, matrix = 128px $\times$ 128px).

In order to vary the partial volumed zone (PVZ), a first 4mm thick slice was acquired in the middle of the GM/WM interface (Fig. 1(b)). Then, the acquisition was incrementally rotated by a 5° angle, progressively reducing the PVZ with θ, the inclination angle. Each position was acquired twice, the first image with parameters $TR_1/TE_1 = 800/10ms$ and the second image with $TR_2/TE_2 = 3600/10ms$. These parameters were optimized by running Monte Carlo simulations and minimising the error on fractional contents for two tissues.

The actual size d of the PVZ has a theoretical value of $d = \frac{e}{tan(\theta)}$ where e denotes the slice thickness. Then, the PVZ was measured using the resulting GM fractional content map where the values range from zero in the WM to one in the GM as we move from left to right within the image. By denoting n the number of pixels in the slope (*i.e.* $f_{GM/WM} \in]0, 1[$) and r_x (0.625mm/px) the resolution in the x direction, $d_{exp} = nr_x$ gives an experimental value of d. In that way, the fractional content error was estimated.

3.2   Simulated MR Data

We computed the GM and WM fractional content maps for different pairs of noise and field inhomogeneities. Then the root mean squared error (RMSE) was calculated between our maps and the BrainWeb Fuzzy maps for all the experiments. We used the BrainWeb Simulator [16] to build a database of FLAWS-like pairs of IR sequences such as those appearing in Fig. 2 (a,b). Each couple of simulated images was made using the following set of parameters: $TI_1/TR_1/TE_1 = 250/4000/2.3ms$, $TI_2/TR_2/TE_2 = 900/1900/1.6ms$ and flip angle $\alpha = 90°$ for both images. The choice of the parameters was based on the ones provided by the the original FLAWS paper [12]. The method was tested using 0, 3, 5, 7 and 9% as noise values and 0, 20 and 40% as bias field values. T1 and PD parameters were recomputed as section 2.2 describes. We found that the estimated parameters were sligthly different from the ones provided by BrainWeb. While a $\frac{PD_{GM}}{PD_{WM}}$ ratio of 1.04 is given, we estimated it at 1.12. $\frac{PD_{GM}}{PD_{CSF}}$ and $\frac{PD_{WM}}{PD_{CSF}}$ were also different. The T1 obtained were $T1_{GM}/T1_{WM}/T1_{CSF} = 980/556/2947ms$ instead of $833/500/2569ms$.

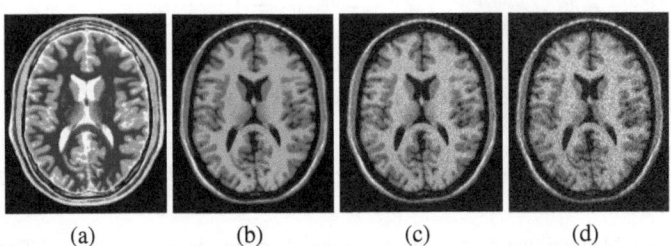

| (a) | (b) | (c) | (d) |

Fig. 2. BrainWeb simulated images. (a,b) No noise and no RF inhomogeneties: example of the two contrasts obtained by simulating the two acquisitions in a typical FLAWS sequence. Next figures show contrast number 2 with 5% of noise, 20% of bias field (c) and 9% of noise, 40% of bias field (d).

4   Results

4.1   Physical Phantom

An example of a bi-exponential response for a voxel shared between GM and WM is shown on Fig. 3, this response is clearly different from a pure GM or WM voxel. Fractional content maps are shown in Fig. 4(a,b,c,d) and must be put in relation with Fig. 1. As it was expected, the greater θ, the smaller the PVZ. The table shown in Fig. 4(e) summarizes these results and shows very good agreement between our measurements and the results from our model. Profiles for the different angles are plotted on Fig. 4(f). The lines intersect in the location $x = x_0 = 70px$ and the fractional content is equal to 0.47, this value is defined by the position of the first slice ($\theta_0 = 0°$).

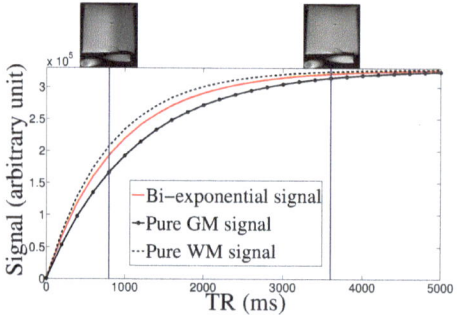

Fig. 3. Graphs of the bi-exponential signal compared to pure GM and WM tissues in a voxel where $f_{GM/WM} = 0.35$. The vertical lines refer to TR_1 and TR_2.

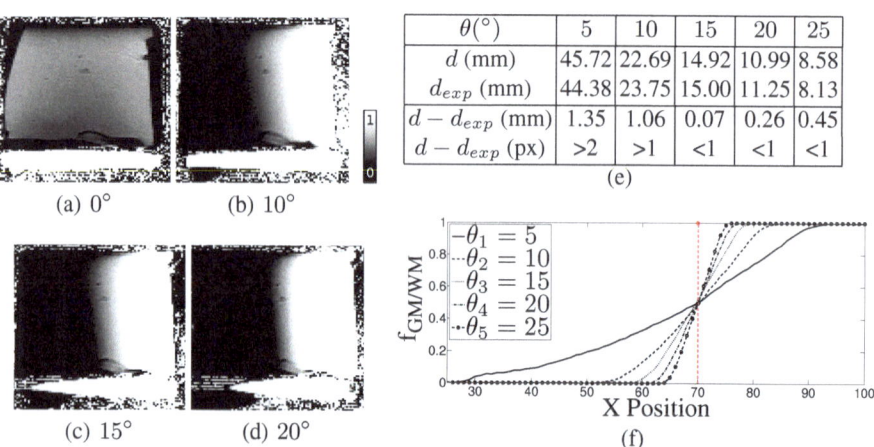

$\theta(°)$	5	10	15	20	25
d (mm)	45.72	22.69	14.92	10.99	8.58
d_{exp} (mm)	44.38	23.75	15.00	11.25	8.13
$d - d_{exp}$ (mm)	1.35	1.06	0.07	0.26	0.45
$d - d_{exp}$ (px)	>2	>1	<1	<1	<1

(e)

(a) $0°$ (b) $10°$

(c) $15°$ (d) $20°$

(f)

Fig. 4. (a,b,c,d) GM fractional content maps on the phantom for four angles. (e) Theoretical and experimental sizes of the PVZ for five angles. (f) Profile of the GM fractional content maps along a few WM-GM lines on the phantom. As expected, all the curves intersect at the same location: the center of rotation of the successive slices.

4.2   BrainWeb MRI Data

GM fractional content maps are shown in Fig. 5, the images show a strong robustness to RF inhomogeneities. As depicted on Fig. 6, our method shows a better RMSE between fractional content maps and BrainWeb references compared to the results reported by Shattuck [5], for instance maximum *a posteriori* (MAP) and maximum likelihood (ML). These results indicate that our method is more robust to RF inhomogeneities than standard methods.

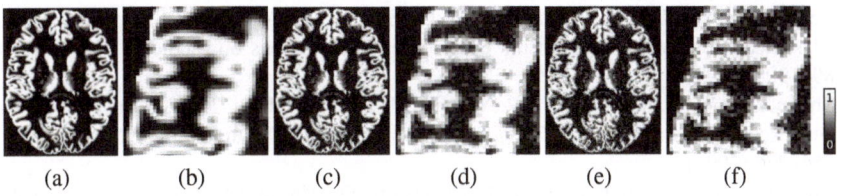

(a)   (b)   (c)   (d)   (e)   (f)

Fig. 5. GM fractional content maps on the BrainWeb phantom. Experiments with 0% noise and 0% RF (a,b), 5% noise and 20% RF (c,d), 9% noise and 40% RF (e,f).

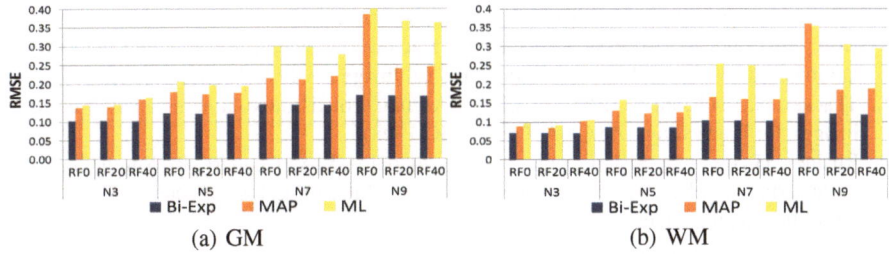

Fig. 6. RMSE obtained on the BrainWeb database for GM and WM, results from [5] are included for comparison. N and RF stand for the percentage of noise and field inhomogeneities, respectively. Our method is robust to RF inhomogeneities as we can observe plateaux when this value increases.

5   Conclusion

We proposed a fast method to accurately estimate fractional content of tissues using a bi-exponential model. It is intrinsically robust to RF inhomogeneities and outperforms already existing and time-consuming approaches. Future work will include evaluation of the current method on actual T1-weighted and T2-weighted images as provided by a standard clinical protocol.

Acknowledgement. This work is partially funded by the "Région Bretagne".

References

1. Acosta, O., Bourgeat, P., Zuluaga, M.A., Fripp, J., Salvado, O., Ourselin, S.: Automated voxel-based 3D cortical thickness measurement in a combined Lagrangian-Eulerian PDE approach using partial volume maps. Medical Image Analysis 13(5), 730–743 (2009)
2. Yang, C.-A., Kaveh, M., Erickson, B.J.: Automated Detection of Focal Cortical Dysplasia Lesions on T1-Weighted MRI using Volume-Based Distributional Features. In: 2011 IEEE International Symposium on Biomedical Imaging: From Nano to Macro, pp. 865–870 (2011)
3. Ballester, A.M., Zisserman, A.P., Brady, M.: Estimation of the partial volume effect in MRI. Medical Image Analysis 6, 389–405 (2002)
4. Leemput, K.V., Maes, F., Vandermeulen, D., Suetens, P.: Automated Model-Based Tissue Classification of MR Images of the Brain. IEEE Transactions on Medical Imaging 18(10), 897–908 (1999)
5. Shattuck, D.W., Sandor-leahy, S.R., Schaper, K.A., Rottenberg, D.A., Leahy, R.M.: Magnetic Resonance Image Tissue Classification Using a Partial Volume Model. NeuroImage 13, 856–876 (2001)
6. Cuadra, M.B., Cammoun, L., Butz, T., Cuisenaire, O., Thiran, J.P.: Comparison and Validation of Tissue Modelization and Statistical Classification Methods in T1-Weighted MR Brain Images. IEEE Transactions on Medical Imaging 24(12), 1548–1565 (2005)
7. Santago, P., Gage, D.: Statistical models of partial volume effect. IEEE Transactions on Image Processing 4, 1531–1540 (1995)
8. Tohka, J., Zijdenbos, A., Evans, A.: Fast and robust parameter estimation for statistical partial volume models in brain MRI. NeuroImage 23, 84–97 (2004)
9. Bricq, S., Collet, C., Armspach, J.: Unifying framework for multimodal brain MRI segmentation based on Hidden Markov Chains. Medical Image Analysis 12, 639–652 (2008)
10. Thacker, N., Jackson, A., Zhu, X., Li, K.: Accuracy of tissue volume estimation in NMR images. In: Proceedings of MIUA, Leeds, UK (1998)
11. Rusinek, H., de Leon, M.J., George, A.E., Stylopoulos, L.A., Chandra, R., Smith, G., Rand, T., Mourino, M., Kowalski, H.: Alzheimer disease: Measuring loss of cerebral Gray Matter with MR imaging. Neuroradiology 178, 109–114 (1991)
12. Tanner, M., Gambarota, G., Kober, T., Krueger, G., Erritzoe, D., Marques, J.P., Newbould, R.: Fluid and white matter suppression with the MP2RAGE sequence. Journal of Magnetic Resonance Imaging 35, 1063–1070 (2011)
13. Marques, J.P., Kober, T., Krueger, G., van der Zwaag, W., de Moortele, P.F.V., Gruetter, R.: MP2RAGE, a self bias-field corrected sequence for improved segmentation and T1-mapping at high field. NeuroImage 49(2), 1271–1281 (2010)
14. Rooney, W.D., Johnson, G., Li, X., Cohen, E.R., Kim, S.G., Ugurbil, K., Springer, C.S.: Magnetic Field and Tissue Dependencies of Human Brain Longitudinal 1H2O Relaxation in Vivo. Magnetic Resonance in Medicine 57, 308–318 (2007)
15. http://www.bic.mni.mcgill.ca/brainweb/
16. Cocosco, C., Kollokian, V., Kwan, R.S., Evans, A.: BrainWeb: Online Interface to a 3D MRI Simulated Brain Database. In: NeuroImage, Proceedings of 3rd International Conference on Functional Mapping of the Human Brain, Copenhagen, vol. 5(4), p. S425 (May 1997)

3D Lung Tumor Motion Model Extraction from 2D Projection Images of Mega-voltage Cone Beam CT via Optimal Graph Search

Mingqing Chen[1,2], Junjie Bai[1], Yefeng Zheng[3], and R. Alfredo C. Siochi[2]

[1] Department of Electrical and Computer Engineering
[2] Department of Radiation Oncology, University of Iowa, Iowa City, IA, USA
[3] Image Analytics and Informatics, Siemens Corporate Research, Princeton, NJ, USA
mingqing-chen@uiowa.com

Abstract. In this paper, we propose a novel method to convert segmentation of objects with quasi-periodic motion in 2D rotational cone beam projection images into an optimal 3D multiple interrelated surface detection problem, which can be solved by a graph search framework. The method is tested on lung tumor segmentation in projection images of mega-voltage cone beam CT (MVCBCT). A 4D directed graph is constructed based on an initialized tumor mesh model, where the cost value for this graph is computed from the point location of a silhouette outline of projected tumor mesh in 2D projection images. The method was first evaluated on four different sized phantom inserts (all above 1.9 cm in diameter) with a predefined motion of 3.0 cm to mimic the imaging of lung tumors. A dice coefficient of 0.87 ± 0.03 and a centroid error of $1.94 \pm 1.31 mm$ were obtained. Results based on 12 MVCBCT scans from 3 patients obtained 0.91 ± 0.03 for dice coefficient and $1.83 \pm 1.31 mm$ for centroid error, compared with a difference between two sets of independent manual contours of 0.89 ± 0.03 and $1.61 \pm 1.19 mm$, respectively.

1 Introduction

The recent advances of mega-voltage cone beam computed tomography (MVCBCT) [1] have enabled the use of linear accelerator (linac) treatment beams for cone beam imaging. This development provides an imaging solution of patient localization to verify the positioning and anatomy information prior to treatment delivery. The 3D volumetric image has potential to improve the accuracy for correcting target misalignments and verifying the treatment plan [2].

However, when the system is used for non-small cell lung cancer (NSCLC) imaging, the existence of respiratory motion during image acquisition causes blurring and streaking artifacts. This motion-blurred 3D volumetric image alone cannot provide much information about tumor size and the motion model, which can change significantly over the full course of a fractionated treatment. It is highly desirable to derive the tumor motion information during the localization scan prior to treatment delivery.

One promising solution is to use cone beam projections to detect tumor motion, since they have high temporal resolution. Previous methods include (1)

N. Ayache et al. (Eds.): MICCAI 2012, Part I, LNCS 7510, pp. 239–246, 2012.

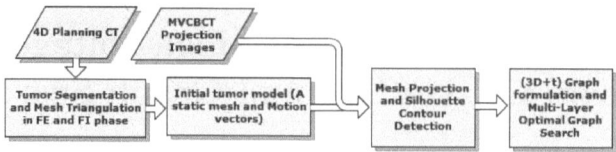

Fig. 1. Flowchart of the proposed approach

monitoring tumor change by projecting a volume of interest for visualization [3], (2) extracting the 2D/3D position of a projected implanted marker [4] or diaphragm edge [5], which can also be used as respiratory signal for gated reconstruction, and (3) registering from 3D image space to projection space for inter-phase motion compensated reconstruction [6]. Direct tumor tracking or detection in 2D images is mainly focused on fluoroscopy [7]. However, few studies have addressed direct tumor detection in MVCBCT projection images, which suffer from relatively poor contrast and the interfering anatomies.

In this study, we present a novel method based on an optimal graph search framework [8] to extract a (3D+t) tumor motion model from 2D projection images. Two major advantages make the method robust in the low-contrast images: (1) The 3D tumor segmentation is based on all the 2D projection images that belong to the corresponding respiratory phase. The detection inaccuracies induced by low contrast and interference of one projection image can thus be reduced. (2) Compared with other 2D-to-3D object shape recovery methods, such as free form deformation [9], B-splines surface model [10] and triangulated mesh pulling [11], our approach incorporates both motion and shape constraints in the segmentation process and obtains a global optimal solution.

2 Method

2.1 General Framework

The main steps of the proposed approach are illustrated in Fig. 1 with the intermediate results shown in Fig. 2. In preparation for the algorithm, the projection images are sorted into several respiratory phase bins according to the 3D anatomical positions of the ipsi-lateral hemi-diaphragm apex (IHDA), which is automatically extracted from projection images based on the dynamic Hough transform [12]. The proposed algorithm starts with an initial 3D static lung tumor mesh model, which reflects the approximate topological structure information of the targeted tumor surface. The initial tumor mesh is projected onto each 2D projection image. The new location of mesh points for all the respiratory bins are determined simultaneously using a multi-surface optimal graph search method [8], which requires computation of the silhouette outline for each projected mesh at first.

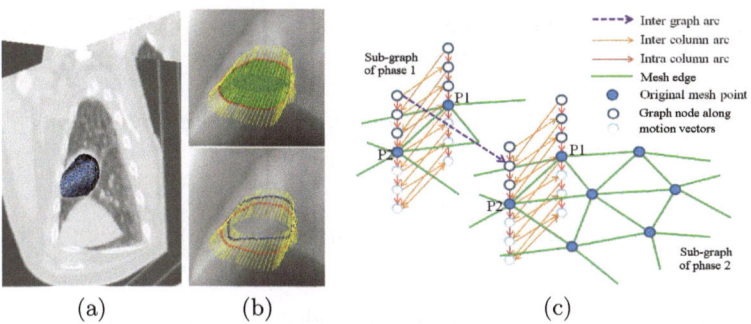

Fig. 2. **(a)** Full exhale phase of 4D diagnostic CT volume overlaid with tumor mesh (blue); **(b)** Projected initial static mesh (green), its silhouette contour (red), motion direction (yellow) and the silhouette contour after the graph search computation (blue); **(c)** A simple illustration of the 4D graph construction

2.2   Model Initialization

The initial static model is the average of the meshes segmented from the full exhale (FE) and full inhale (FI) phases of the 4DCT. For each mesh point, a range of motion is determined using the equation $[P_m + \alpha(P_{fe} - P_m)]$ and $[P_m + \alpha(P_{fi} - P_m)]$, where P_{fe} and P_{fi} is the corresponding positions in the FE and FI phase, respectively, and P_m is the mean position. α is used to control the allowed range, which is typically set between 1.5 and 2. The two meshes are initialized with the same spherical mesh and manually adjusted according to the tumor boundary in the 3D volume using our in-house platform. Thus the correspondence of mesh points is inherently established.

2.3   Silhouette Contour Extraction

The initial mesh, along with pre-defined motion vectors, is projected onto each 2D projection image. In order to move the mesh towards tumor boundary locations in the projection image, the silhouette outline is extracted from each projected mesh by using an efficient algorithm [11]. An example of the detected silhouette outline is shown in Fig. 2.

2.4   Multiple Surface Detection via Optimal Graph Search

A key innovation of the proposed method is converting the segmentation of objects with quasi-periodic motion in 2D rotational cone beam projection images into a 3D multiple interrelated surface detection problem, which can be solved by a graph search framework [8]. The details are presented as follows. A 4D (3D+t) directed graph $G = (V, E)$ is constructed based on the initial tumor mesh. The graph contains T (number of phase bins) subgraphs, where each subgraph corresponds to the tumor surface in one respiratory phase bin. Each subgraph contains $N \times M$ nodes, where N and M are the number of points of the static tumor mesh and the number of sampled points along the pre-defined motion vector. Each combination of $[n, m, t]$ is one unique spatial and temporal location, which represents the mth sampled point in the column defined by mesh point n in phase t. The segmented tumor surfaces are defined by function $\mathcal{N} : (n, t) \rightarrow \mathcal{N}(n, t)$, where $n \in \mathbf{n} = \{0, ..., N - 1\}$, $t \in \mathbf{t} = \{0, ..., T - 1\}$, and $\mathcal{N}(n, t) \in \mathbf{m} = \{0, ..., M - 1\}$.

A cost value is computed for each node $[n, m, t]$, denoted by $c(n, m, t)$, using the following equation:

$$c(n, m, t) = \sum_{p=0}^{P-1} \delta(p, t)\xi(n, p)w(n, m, p), \tag{1}$$

where P and p is the total number and the index of projection images, respectively. The function $\delta(p, t) = 1$ when the pth projection image belongs to the tth bin, otherwise it equals zero. The function $\xi(n, p) = 1$ when the nth point is included in the silhouette contour of the pth projection image, otherwise it equals zero. $w(n, m, p)$ is the cost function of the mth sample point in the nth column in the pth projection image, which is defined as:

$$w(n, m, p) = -\ddot{P}_p(\mathbf{normal}(n)) \cdot \mathbf{grad}(\ddot{P}_p(\mathbf{P}(n, m))), \tag{2}$$

where $\ddot{P}_p$ is the 3D-to-2D projection operation of a vector or point in the pth projection image. $\mathbf{P}(n, m)$ is the location of the mth sample point along the predefined motion vector of the nth mesh point. The operation $\mathbf{normal}(n)$ gives the normal direction of the nth point of the static mesh, while the operation $\mathbf{grad}$ computes the image gradient of a given 2D location. The reason for using the negative dot product between these two vectors is that along the tumor boundary in 2D projection images, the projected normal direction is opposite to the image gradient. Equations (1) and (2) show that the cost for each node in the 4D graph is determined from all the 2D projection images that belong to the corresponding respiratory bin.

Three different types of arcs are added to the graph: (1) **Intra-column arcs** are used to define the graph topology, which connect adjacent nodes that belong to the same column. The arc goes from each node $[n, m, t]$ $(m > 0)$ to the node below $[n, m - 1, t]$. (2) **Inter-column arcs** are used to connect adjacent columns in the same respiratory bin. The arc goes from each node $[n, m, t]$ $(m > \delta_m)$ to $[adj(n), m - \delta_m, t]$, where $adj(n)$ represents adjacent mesh points of n. δ_m is the shape smoothness constraint, which is the maximal allowed difference in m between adjacent columns of one tumor surface. (3) **Inter-phase arcs** are used to connect the same columns in adjacent respiratory bins. The arc goes from each node $[n, m, t]$ $(m > \delta_t)$ to $[n, m - \delta_t, t \pm 1]$. δ_t is the inter-phase constraint, which is the maximal allowed difference in m between adjacent bins of the same column. We define that $[n, m, 0] = [n, m, T]$ to form a closed loop of respiratory bins. Fig. 2c illustrates the main idea for graph construction, where a simple case of $T = 2, M = N = 7, \delta_m = \delta_t = 1$ is shown, where two subgraphs representing the two phases are shown. The forementioned three types of arcs are illustrated. For visualization purposes, only one inter-phase arc is drawn. And only two columns are shown for each subgraph. The subgraph of phase 2 shows all the mesh points, while phase 1 only shows the two points with columns. In our implementation, N

is typically from 1000 to 4000, depending on the tumor size. M is 50, making the step size of the sampled point equal to $1/50$ of the allowed range of motion. T is 20, where larger T makes higher temporal resolution, but reduces the number of projections for each phase bin. The optimal solution can be computed by solving a maximal flow problem in the constructed graph [8]. The running time based on those parameters is about 40s on an Intel Core^{TM} I7 laptop with 4GB RAM.

3   Experiments

3.1   Imaging Data

Our clinic is equipped with a Siemens Oncor MVCBCT system (Siemens Medical Systems, Oncology Care Systems, Concord, CA) with an electrical portal imaging device (EPID) to acquire 2D projection images. Using the standard protocol [1], the 200 EPID projection images are acquired as the gantry rotates clockwise from $-90°$ to $110°$ in about 1 minute.

The proposed approach was first verified on an imaging phantom, which has a predefined motion and size to serve as the ground truth. The phantom consists of a block of basswood and six different sized spherical inserts. The basswood frame has a density of about $0.4g/cc$ to mimic lung tissue, while the six inserts are made of paraffin wax and have 3.81, 3.18, 2.54, 1.91, 0.95, and 0.48 cm in diameter, respectively. Fig. 3 shows a picture of the phantom, a coronal slice of a diagnostic CT and an MVCBCT projection image, respectively. The phantom is placed on a cart attached to the Quasar respiratory motion (QRM) phantom (Modus Medical Devices, INC, London, ON, Canada) to simulate respiratory motion. The QRM phantom is programmed to move only in the superior-inferior (SI) direction, with its position as a function of time t, defined as:

$$z(t) = z_0 + A_0 cos^4(\pi(t + t_0)/\tau), \tag{3}$$

where the motion amplitude A_0 is $30mm$, and the period τ is $4s$ to represent typical breathing. z_0 and t_0 are the DC component of the motion and the starting phase of the phantom motion, which varies among different experiments. The phantom tests were done on two scans, with a dose of 5MU and 10MU, respectively.

The proposed method was also tested on 12 scans from three patients, who have relatively large tumors in the lower lobe of the lung. The patient scans used an imaging dose of 10MU.

3.2   Results

Fig. 4 shows the detection result of the largest insert of the phantom (top) and a real patient whose tumor is right above the diaphragm (bottom). The top-right corner shows the detected 3D mesh in the corresponding respiratory bin. The evaluation is based on 2D contours in projection space. For the phantom images, the detected contour of the inserts is compared with the contour computed from the predefined size and the motion, which is considered ground truth. It can be seen that the insert can be detected robustly in the presence of the interfering superimposed objects,

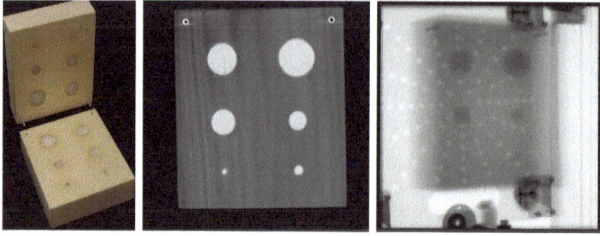

Fig. 3. **Left**: the imaging phantom; **Middle**: a coronal slice of the FE phase of the 4D diagnostic CT; **Right**: one projection image of MVCBCT with a dose of 10MU

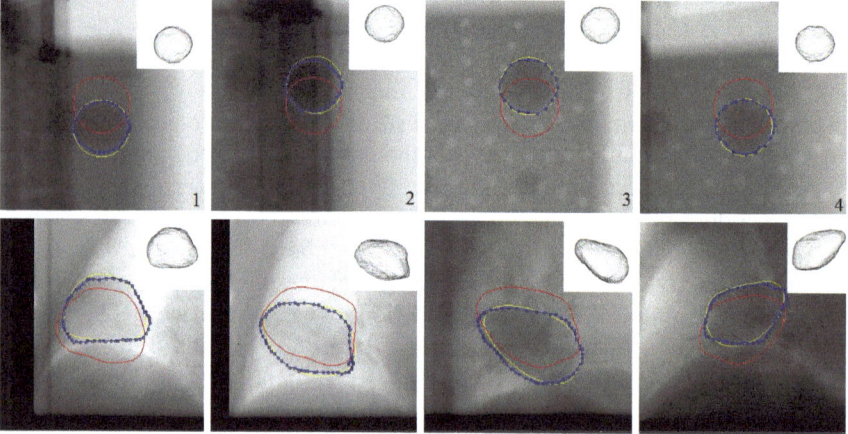

Fig. 4. Detection result on **Top row**: the imaging phantom; **Bottom row**: a patient with tumor above the diaphragm. **Red**: silhouette outline of initial mesh; **blue**: detected tumor contour (deformed silhouette outline); **yellow**: contour of ground truth for phantom images, manually annotated contour for patient images. The detected 3D tumor mesh of the corresponding respiratory bin is displayed on the top-right corner.

such as interfering spheres (Fig. 4.1), the QRM motion phantom (Fig. 4.2) and the holes of the plastic support (small white circles in (Fig. 4.3 & 4)).

The evaluation is based on the four largest inserts, since there is no strong boundary information of the two smaller ones in the projection images (Fig. 3). Two metrics were employed to validate the detection result: the 2D dice coefficient and the difference of centroid positions along the SI direction. Fig. 5 shows the mean and standard deviation values of those metrics over 200 projection images. The dice coefficient decreases slightly when the tumor size goes down, while this phenomenon does not occur in the centroid error. An imaging dose of 10MU obtains better accuracy for centroid and a slight improvement in the dice coefficient. For patient images, the tumor was independently contoured by two clinical experts. The averaged contour was computed to compare with the detection result. The difference between the two manual contours is also quantified. Fig. 6

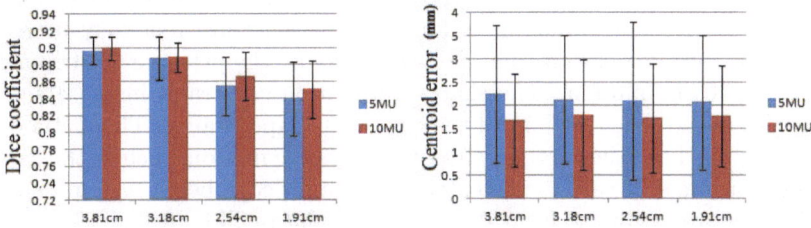

Fig. 5. Mean and standard deviation of **Left**: dice coefficient between detected contour and ground truth; **Right**: centroid difference between detected contour and ground truth over 200 projection images of four spherical inserts

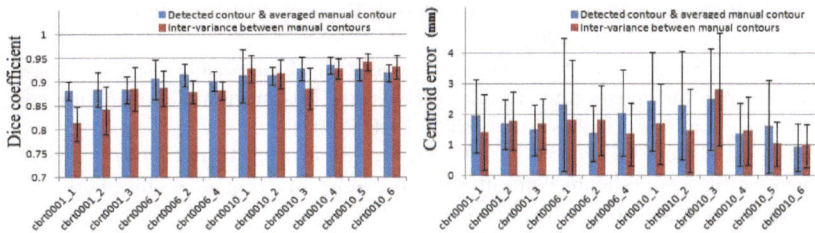

Fig. 6. Mean and standard deviation of **Left**: dice coefficient; **Right**: centroid difference over 200 projection images of 12 patient MVCBCT scans

shows the dice coefficient and centroid difference over 12 MVCBCT scans from 3 patients, where the overall dice coefficient of the proposed method is even better than variations between manual contours. This result is expected, since the segmentation of the 3D shape is based on multiple 2D views, while the manual contour could be confounded by overlapping tissues in one single image. For both phantom and patient studies, the quantified centroid error is clinically acceptable, since a setup error of 5 mm is typically added to the gross tumor volume (GTV) for treatment delivery.

4   Discussion and Conclusion

In this work, we proposed a novel method to extract the 3D tumor motion model from 2D projection images of an MVCBCT system. Experiments based on phantom images show the robustness to detect tumors with diameters larger than $1.9cm$. For patient images, the method can even be used for guidance to assist the clinician for a better visualization of tumor boundaries. The segmentation framework is based on a simple scaling model between the FE and FI phases for each mesh point. Though in reality the motion trajectory is more like an elongated ellipse, the linear scaling model is a good estimation and it has enabled us to derive accurate detection result. It is potentially helpful to use a more complicated model established from multiple phases of 4D CT. However, more computation and complexity will be added to the current framework.

In the patient studies, the shape of the segmentation changes somehow over the respiratory cycle. The tumor mass for those patients are relatively large and they are likely to be deformed in a non-rigid way by the pressure of surrounding tissues and the diaphragm. The shape and motion constraint in the 4D graph can further be adjusted to control the degree of shape change. The method can be easily applied to other organs with quasi-periodic motion, such as the cardiac chambers or lungs. It can also be extended to other cone beam systems, such as the C-arm systems. In the future, more patient data will be tested with various tumor size and shape, imaging dose and breathing pattern.

References

1. Morin, O., Gillis, A., Chen, J., Aubin, M., Bucci, M., Roach III, M., Pouliot, J.: Megavoltage cone-beam CT: system description and clinical applications. Medical Dosimetry 31(1), 51–61 (2006)
2. Jaffray, D., Siewerdsen, J., Wong, J., Martinez, A.: Flat-panel cone-beam computed tomography for image-guided radiation therapy. International Journal of Radiation Oncology Biology Physics 53(5), 1337–1349 (2002)
3. Reitz, B., Gayou, O., Parda, D., Miften, M.: Monitoring tumor motion with on-line mega-voltage cone-beam computed tomography imaging in a cine mode. Physics in Medicine and Biology 53, 823–836 (2008)
4. Li, T., Xing, L., Munro, P., McGuinness, C., Chao, M., Yang, Y., Loo, B., Koong, A.: Four-dimensional cone-beam computed tomography using an on-board imager. Medical Physics 33, 3825–3833 (2006)
5. Siochi, R.: Deriving motion from megavoltage localization cone beam computed tomography scans. Physics in Medicine and Biology 54, 4195–4212 (2009)
6. Li, T., Koong, A., Xing, L.: Enhanced 4D cone-beam CT with inter-phase motion model. Medical Physics 34, 3688–3695 (2007)
7. Shimizu, S., Shirato, H., Ogura, S., Akita-Dosaka, H., Kitamura, K., Nishioka, T., Kagei, K., Nishimura, M., Miyasaka, K.: Detection of lung tumor movement in real-time tumor-tracking radiotherapy. International Journal of Radiation Oncology Biology Physics 51(2), 304–310 (2001)
8. Li, K., Millington, S., Wu, X., Chen, D.Z., Sonka, M.: Simultaneous Segmentation of Multiple Closed Surfaces Using Optimal Graph Searching. In: Christensen, G.E., Sonka, M. (eds.) IPMI 2005. LNCS, vol. 3565, pp. 406–417. Springer, Heidelberg (2005)
9. Lotjonen, J., Magnin, I., Nenonen, J., Katila, T.: Reconstruction of 3-D geometry using 2-D profiles and a geometric prior model. IEEE Trans. Medical Imaging 18(10), 992–1002 (1999)
10. Moriyama, M., Sato, Y., Naito, H., Hanayama, M., Ueguchi, T., Harada, T., Yoshimoto, F., Tamura, S.: Reconstruction of time-varying 3D left ventricular shape from multiview x-ray cineangiocardiograms. IEEE Trans. Medical Imaging, 773–785 (2002)
11. Chen, M., Zheng, Y., Mueller, K., Rohkohl, C., Lauritsch, G., Boese, J., Funka-Lea, G., Hornegger, J., Comaniciu, D.: Automatic Extraction of 3D Dynamic Left Ventricle Model from 2D Rotational Angiocardiogram. In: Fichtinger, G., Martel, A., Peters, T. (eds.) MICCAI 2011, Part III. LNCS, vol. 6893, pp. 471–478. Springer, Heidelberg (2011)
12. Chen, M., Siochi, R.: Diaphragm motion quantification in megavoltage cone-beam CT projection images. Medical Physics 37, 2312–2320 (2010)

Atlas Construction via Dictionary Learning and Group Sparsity

Feng Shi[1], Li Wang[1], Guorong Wu[1], Yu Zhang[1,2],
Manhua Liu[1,3], John H. Gilmore[4], Weili Lin[5], and Dinggang Shen[1]

[1] IDEA Lab.,
University of North Carolina at Chapel Hill, NC, USA
[2] School of Biomedical Engineering, Southern Medical University,
Guangzhou, Guangdong, China
[3] Department of Instrument Science and Technology,
Shanghai Jiao Tong University, Shanghai, China
[4] Department of Psychiatry, University of North Carolina at Chapel Hill, NC, USA
[5] MRI Lab., Department of Radiology and BRIC,
University of North Carolina at Chapel Hill, NC, USA
dgshen@med.unc.edu

Abstract. Atlas construction generally includes first an image registration step to normalize all images into a common space and then an atlas building step to fuse all the aligned images. Although numerous atlas construction studies have been performed to improve the accuracy of image registration step, simple averaging or weighted averaging is often used for the atlas building step. In this paper, we propose a novel patch-based sparse representation method for atlas construction, especially for the atlas building step. By taking advantage of local sparse representation, more distinct anatomical details can be revealed in the built atlas. Also, together with the constraint on group structure of representations and the use of overlapping patches, anatomical consistency between neighboring patches can be ensured. The proposed method has been applied to 73 neonatal MR images with poor spatial resolution and low tissue contrast, for building unbiased neonatal brain atlas. Experimental results demonstrate that the proposed method can enhance the quality of built atlas by discovering more anatomical details especially in cortical regions, and perform better in a neonatal data normalization application, compared to other existing start-of-the-art nonlinear neonatal brain atlases.

1   Introduction

Brain atlases are widely used in the neuroimaging field for disease diagnosis, surgical planning, and educational purpose. Usually, an atlas is created as an average model to represent a population normalized in a common space. Specifically, constructing an atlas needs **1)** an image registration step to normalize all images in the population into a common space and **2)** an atlas building step to fuse all aligned images together. Note that the subject-dependent anatomical details, especially in the cortical regions, may be smoothed out during the image averaging process in the atlas building step.

Many studies have been performed for atlas construction, with main efforts placed on the image registration step. If images in the population can be well aligned, less

N. Ayache et al. (Eds.): MICCAI 2012, Part I, LNCS 7510, pp. 247–255, 2012.

structural discrepancies between aligned images will be obtained and thus the built atlas will keep more anatomical details. Previously, atlas construction is often performed by first choosing one image as a template and then nonlinearly registering all other images to the selected template. This approach could lead to bias in the atlas construction, since the resulting atlas is generally optimized to be similar with the selected template and will has different appearance when different templates are used in registration changes. Thus, groupwise registration is recently proposed to overcome the limitation of template selection, which estimates the geometric mean of the population as the atlas by iteratively performing the step of registering images to the tentatively-estimated atlas and the step of averaging the tentatively-aligned images as new atlas [1]. With the use of groupwise registration, unbiased atlas can be constructed. However, all the aligned images are often simply averaged equally or with some weights for building the atlas. Actually, including all images in the population for building atlas may only marginally improve the details of atlas, but at the risk of introducing more noises and thus making the averaged anatomical structures blurry.

On the other hand, sparse representation has been recently proposed as a powerful tool for robustly representing high-dimensional signals using a small set of basis functions in an over-complete dictionary [2]. This method was developed based on a simple concept that the underlying representations of many real-world images are often sparse, as evidenced by the human biological vision processing system [3]. Sparse representation has several advantages. *First*, the input image can be represented as a linear combination of a small number of basis functions. *Second*, the dictionary with basis functions can be made over-complete to offer a wide range of representing elements. Super-resolution image construction, as a special application of sparse representation, is also an active area of research in computer vision, for recovering a high-resolution image from one or more low-resolution images [4].

In this paper, we propose a novel patch-based sparse representation method for atlas construction, to specially improve the performance of the atlas building step. We hypothesize that, by sparsely representing each patch of the atlas using a small number of image patches, instead of all patches in the whole population, more anatomical details can be revealed and finally an atlas can be obtained. In our implementation, the atlas is constructed locally in a patch-by-patch fashion to ensure the local representativeness, and also the neighboring patches are constrained to have similar representations by using the group sparsity strategy. The overlapping patches are further employed to ensure the structural consistency along the patch boundaries. We apply our proposed method to the neonatal MRI data which often have poor spatial-resolution and low tissue-contrast, thus challenging for building sharp atlas. Experimental results indicate, both qualitatively and quantitatively, that our proposed method can produce much higher quality atlas, compared to the other existing state-of-the-art neonatal atlases.

2   Method

2.1   Overview

In this paper, we consider the atlas construction as image representation problem, with goal of generating representative detailed brain structures from a population of subject images. To do this, we first employ a recently-developed unbiased groupwise registration method to align all subject images onto a common space, and then put our main efforts to introduce our proposed atlas building step. Specifically, for each patch in the to-be-built atlas, a patch dictionary is first adaptively constructed by including the current patch as well as neighboring patches from all aligned subject images. In this way, this dictionary will contain sufficient elements (or local patches) for representation of each atlas patch, under guidance that the reconstructed atlas patch should be similar to the corresponding patches of the subject images distributed near to the population center. By also requiring similar sparse representation for nearby patches in the atlas by using group sparsity, and further making nearby patches to be spatially overlapped, super-resolution brain atlas can be constructed by combining all the reconstructed patches. In the following, details for unbiased groupwise registration, patch-based representation, and group regularization on neighboring patches will be discussed.

2.2   Unbiased Groupwise Registration

This step is to spatially normalize all subject images into a common space, which is a necessary initial step for subsequent atlas building. Unlike the pairwise registration method that needs selection of initial template, groupwise registration is free of template selection and is able to simultaneously register all subject images onto the hidden common space. Although many groupwise registration methods developed in the literature can be employed for our study, we decided to use a state-of-the-art groupwise registration method in [1] for aligning our images, since its software package is freely available at http://www.nitrc.org/projects/glirt. Also, this groupwise registration method used (1) attribute vector as morphological signature of each voxel for guiding accurate correspondence detection among all subject images, and (2) also a hierarchical process for selecting a small number of critical voxels (with distinctive attribute vectors) to guide the whole registration. In this way, the high quality of groupwise registration results can be achieved.

2.3   Patch-Based Representation

We employ a patch-based representation technique for atlas construction, due to its two characteristics. *First*, local anatomical structure could be better captured in a small patch than in a large brain region. *Second*, patch size can be optimized to compromise the local structure representativeness and global structure consistency. We sample local cubic patches to cover the whole brain image. At each point, we can obtain patches $\{p_i | i = 1, ..., N\}$ from all aligned images, where N is the total number of images. Note that each patch is represented with a vector consisting of $M = s \times s \times s$ features (i.e., intensities), where s is the size of patch at each dimension.

We consider all local patches are highly correlated and thus their distribution can be estimated in Euclidean space. The group center of patches is approximated as the group mean of all patches, i.e., $\frac{1}{N}\sum_i^N p_i$. In this feature space, some patches may distribute near the group center, while others may be far away. Generally, patches near the group center have more agreement in representing the population mean, while patches far-away from the group center may introduce anatomical discrepancies and thus make the group mean image or atlas blur. Inspired by this observation, we select K ($< N$) nearest patches to the group center, denoted as $\{y_k | k = 1, ..., K\}$, where the similarity between patches is measured by image correlation coefficient. To formulate the atlas building (or the estimation of group mean image) as a representation problem, for each to-be-estimated patch in the atlas, we require it to represent the common anatomical structure of all K nearest patches simultaneously.

To achieve this, we need to first build a dictionary for each atlas patch under reconstruction. An initial dictionary can include all patches with same location in all aligned images, i.e., $D = [p_1, p_2, ..., p_N]$. To further overcome the possible registration error, the initial dictionary is extended to include more patches from the neighboring locations, thus providing a sufficient number of elements for powerful representation. In this application, we include 26 immediate neighboring locations. Thus, for each aligned image, we will take totally $g = 27$ patches; and from all N aligned images, we will include totally $\bar{N} = g \times N$ patches in the dictionary D.

Then, we can require the reconstructed atlas patch, sparsely represented by the coefficient vector x and the dictionary D, to be similar to all K patches denoted by Y that are closer to the group mean. This problem can be formulated as the following minimization problem:

$$\hat{x} = arg \min_{x>0} \left[\sum_{k=1}^{K} \|Dx - y_k\|_2^2 + \lambda \|x\|_1 \right] \tag{1}$$

where $D \in \mathbb{R}^{M \times \bar{N}}$, $x \in \mathbb{R}^{\bar{N} \times 1}$, $y_k \in \mathbb{R}^{M \times 1}$. The first term measures the discrepancy between observation y_k and the reconstructed atlas patch Dx, and the second term is L_1 regularization of the coefficient vector x (also called LASSO) [5]. Sparsity is encouraged in x under LASSO. $\lambda \geq 0$ is a parameter controlling the influence of the regularization term.

2.4   Group Regularization on Neighboring Patches

Generally, neighboring patches should share similar representations, in order to achieve local structure consistency for the reconstructed atlas. Thus, group sparsity regularization, namely group LASSO [6], is introduced. Specifically, besides solving the representation task for the current patch, we also consider solving the representation tasks in all 26 neighboring patches simultaneously, constraining the coefficients for the whole group.

Denote $g = 27$ as the total number of patches, and let D_{Gj}, and $y_{k,Gj}$, and x_{Gj} denote the respective dictionary, observation variable, and coefficient vector of the j-th patch, respectively, with $j = 1, 2, ..., g$. For simplicity, we use $X = \left[x_{G_1}, x_{G_2}, ..., x_{G_g} \right]$ as a matrix containing all coefficient column vectors. Note that the matrix can also be written in the form of row vectors $X = [u_1; u_2; ...; u_{\bar{N}}]$, where u_i is the i-th row in the matrix X. Then, we reformulate the Eq. (1) into a group LASSO problem as below:

$$\hat{x} = arg \min_{x>0} \left[\sum_{j=1}^{g} \sum_{k=1}^{K} \left\| D_{G_j} x_{G_j} - y_{k,G_j} \right\|_2^2 + \lambda \|X\|_{2,1} \right] \tag{2}$$

where $\|X\|_{2,1} = \sum_{i=1}^{\bar{N}} \|u_i\|_2$. The first term is a multi-task least square minimizer for all the g groups. The second term is for regularization. The $\|X\|_{2,1}$ is a combination of both L_2 and L_1 norms, in which the L_2 norm is imposed to each row of the matrix X (i.e., u_i) to make the neighboring patches have similar representations while the L_1 norm is imposed to the results of L_2 norm to ensure the sparsity of the representation by the respective dictionary (reflected by the sum of $\|u_i\|_2$). In this way, the nearby patches share the same sparsity pattern in finding their representations. The group LASSO in Eq. (2) can be solved efficiently by using algorithm in [6].

Using non-overlapping patches could result in steep gradient changes along patch boundaries and also inconsistent structures across patches. Thus, to alleviate this problem, overlapping patches are used here by taking average from multiple results for each voxel. Specifically, we sample patches in the whole brain by moving the current patch point for half patch size at each time. By doing so, each voxel is now included by 8 patches. Then, by combining all overlapping patches together, the atlas can be finally obtained.

3   Experiments

3.1   Data Specification

Data for Atlas Construction. Neonatal data generally has low spatial resolution and insufficient tissue contrast, and would considerably benefit from the proposed method for building an atlas. Specifically, 73 healthy neonatal subjects (42 males/31 females) were recruited, and their MR images were scanned at 33-42 gestational weeks. MR images were acquired on a Siemens head-only 3T scanner with a circular polarized head coil. T2-weighted images were obtained with 70 transverse slices using turbo spin-echo (TSE) sequences: TR=7380 ms, TE=119 ms, Flip Angle=150°, and resolution=1.25×1.25×1.95 mm^3. The study has been proved by IRB and the written informed consent forms were also obtained from all parents. All the 73 neonatal images were resampled into 1×1×1 mm^3, bias corrected, skull stripped [7], and tissue segmented [8].

Data for Normalization Evaluation. We evaluate the performance of proposed atlas with other state-of-the-art neonatal atlases by measuring how well they are able to spatially normalize a neonatal population. MR images of 20 healthy neonatal subjects (10 males/10 females) were obtained at 40±1 (37-41) gestational weeks, using TSE sequences with parameters: TR=6200 ms, TE=116 ms, Flip Angle=150°, and resolution=1.25×1.25×1.95 mm^3. All the images were resampled into 1×1×1 mm^3, bias corrected, skull stripped [7], and tissue segmented [8].

3.2   Parameter Settings

Fig. 1 shows our constructed atlases as functions of patch size and the number of nearest subjects to the group mean image. Generally, larger patch size will affect the ability of local representation and make the atlas more blur. In our experiments, we use 6×6×6 patches with overlap of 3 voxels between adjacent patches. We choose $K = 10$ center subjects, as observed from experiments that, if K is too large, the resulting atlas will appear blur, while if K is too small, e.g., $K = 2$, the resulting atlas can be easily affected by noises. Regularization parameter was set as $\lambda = 0.01$, since too high regularization values will reduce the number of non-zero coefficients in patch representation and thus become unstable.

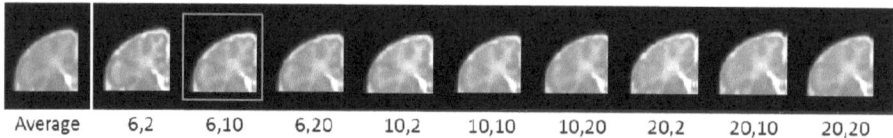

| Average | 6,2 | 6,10 | 6,20 | 10,2 | 10,10 | 10,20 | 20,2 | 20,10 | 20,20 |

Fig. 1. Close-up views of our constructed atlases. The number (d,K) in this figure represents patch size and the number of center subjects, with (6,10) chosen in this paper. Average of all aligned images is also shown in the left panel for comparison.

3.3   Experimental Results

Fig. 2 compare results obtained with different atlas construction methods. Top row shows the axial views of the constructed atlases, and bottom row shows the close-up views of the top-left part of brain region. Patch size is set as 6×6×6 with 3 voxels overlap between patches. As we can see, the result obtained from the average of 10 center images (adaptive at each local patch) (Fig. 2b) shows higher level of details than the result from the average of all images (Fig. 2a), while it still suffers from steep gradient changes along patch boundaries (or boundary effect) and inconsistent intensities between neighboring patches. Better structural consistency is observed in the result by sparse representation (Fig. 2c), and further enhanced in the result by using group sparsity (Fig. 2d).

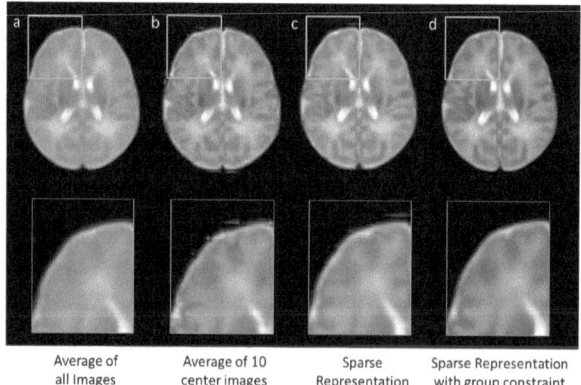

| Average of all Images | Average of 10 center images | Sparse Representation | Sparse Representation with group constraint |

Fig. 2. Comparison of atlases built by different construction methods. Note that the atlases in (b-d) are constructed in a patch-by-patch fashion.

Comparison with Other State-of-the-Art Neonatal Atlases. The proposed atlas is further compared with other state-of-the-art neonatal atlases constructed by nonlinear registration techniques. Typical views of atlases are shown in Fig. 3. Kuklisova-Murgasova *et al* [9] created a 4D atlas using 142 neonatal subjects between 29 and 44 gestational weeks, in which the atlas for 41 weeks was used and referred here to as Atlas-A. Oishi *et al* [10] constructed atlas using 25 brain images from neonates of 38-41 post-conceptional weeks, here referred to as Atlas-B. Serag *et al* [11] also made a 4D atlas using 204 premature neonates between 26.7 to 44.3 gestational weeks, in which the atlas for 41 weeks was used and referred here to as Atlas-C. Average atlas of our 73 aligned neonate images is also provided by simply averaging them. Our proposed atlas, constructed from 73 neonates using sparse representation with group constraints, establishes the highest level of details than any other neonatal atlases.

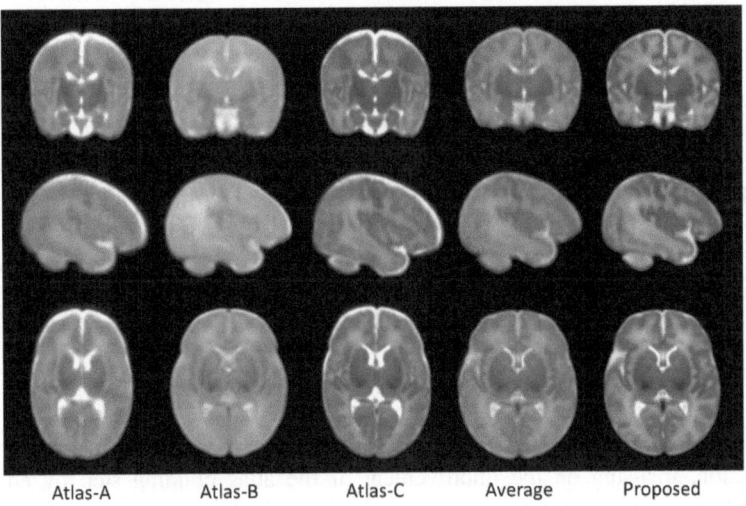

Atlas-A   Atlas-B   Atlas-C   Average   Proposed

Fig. 3. Comparison of nonlinear neonatal atlases among the results from Kuklisova-Murgasova *et al* (2010) (Atlas-A), Oishi *et al* (2011) (Atlas-B), Serag *et al* (2012) (Atlas-C), equal averaging of 73 aligned images (Average), and our proposed method (Proposed). Similar slices were selected directly from these 5 atlases for easy comparison.

Evaluation of Atlas Quality through Image Registration. To quantitatively evaluate the quality of our atlas, we also design an experiment to spatially normalize a population of neonatal images separately by using the 5 atlases shown in Fig. 3 as templates. In this experiment, we use 20 neonates as detailed in Data subsection which are independent of the data used for atlas construction. All images were aligned to the 5 atlases using a nonlinear registration method, Diffeomorphic Demons [12], respectively. Registration parameters were conservatively set as $5 \times 5 \times 5$ iterations and 3 smoothing sigma for the deformation field. Brain tissues, i.e., gray matter (GM), white matter (WM), and ventricular cerebrospinal fluid (CSF) in segmented images, were also aligned to the common space by using the deformation fields. Since the ground truth for normalization is not available, we generate a mean image representing the common structures of population by using voxel-wise majority voting on the 20 aligned segmented images. Brain tissues of each warped image were then compared with the mean image, and the structural agreement was assessed by the Dice coefficient.

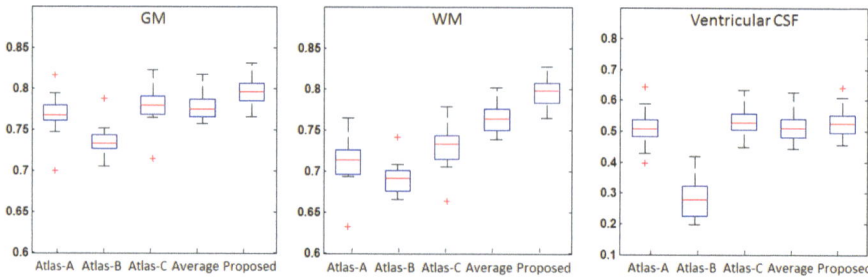

Fig. 4. Dice coefficients of structural consistency between the warped images and their respective mean image for each of 5 atlases, respectively

Results are shown in Fig. 4. The performance of our proposed atlas outperforms other 4 atlases for GM and WM (p<0.05), while no difference for CSF when compared to Atlas-A, Atlas-B, and Average atlas. Average atlas has similar performance with Atlas-A and Atlas-C for GM and CSF, while superior for WM consistency.

4   Conclusion and Future Work

We have presented a novel patch-based sparse representation method for atlas construction, focusing on the improvement of the atlas building step by employing sparse representation and group sparsity techniques. To the best of our knowledge, the present paper is the first work of exploiting sparse representation for building atlases. Experimental results have shown that the local sparse representation method can improve the anatomical details in the constructed neonatal atlas. Our method is flexible enough to be incorporated into any registration algorithms to further improve the atlas quality. Note that a potential limitation of experiment is that the testing data has similar imaging protocol with the data used for our atlas construction, and thus may favor the proposed atlas. In the future work, we would run evaluations on more datasets.

References

1. Wu, G., Wang, Q., Jia, H., Shen, D.: Feature-based groupwise registration by hierarchical anatomical correspondence detection. Human Brain Mapping 33, 253–271 (2012)
2. Zhang, S., Zhan, Y., Dewan, M., Huang, J., Metaxas, D.N., Zhou, X.S.: Towards robust and effective shape modeling: sparse shape composition. Med. Image Anal. 16, 265–277 (2012)

3. Vinje, W.E., Gallant, J.L.: Sparse coding and decorrelation in primary visual cortex during natural vision. Science 287, 1273–1276 (2000)
4. Yang, J., Wright, J., Huang, T.S., Ma, Y.: Image super-resolution via sparse representation. IEEE Transactions on Image Processing 19, 2861–2873 (2010)
5. Tibshirani, R.: Regression shrinkage and selection via the lasso. Journal of the Royal Statistical Society 58, 267–288 (1996)
6. Liu, J., Ji, S., Ye, J.: Multi-task feature learning via efficient l2,1-norm minimization. Uncertainty in Artificial Intelligence (UAI), 339–348 (2009)
7. Shi, F., Wang, L., Dai, Y., Gilmore, J.H., Lin, W., Shen, D.: LABEL: Pediatric Brain Extraction using Learning-based Meta-algorithm. NeuroImage (in press, 2012)
8. Wang, L., Shi, F., Lin, W., Gilmore, J.H., Shen, D.: Automatic Segmentation of Neonatal Images Using Convex Optimization and Coupled Level Sets. NeuroImage 58, 805–817 (2011)
9. Kuklisova-Murgasova, M., Aljabar, P., Srinivasan, L., Counsell, S., Doria, V., Serag, A., Gousias, I., Boardman, J., Rutherford, M., Edwards, A.: A dynamic 4D probabilistic atlas of the developing brain. NeuroImage 54, 2750–2763 (2010)
10. Oishi, K., Mori, S., Donohue, P.K., Ernst, T., Anderson, L., Buchthal, S., Faria, A., Jiang, H., Li, X., Miller, M.I.: Multi-contrast human neonatal brain atlas: application to normal neonate development analysis. NeuroImage 56, 8–20 (2011)
11. Serag, A., Aljabar, P., Ball, G., Counsell, S.J., Boardman, J.P., Rutherford, M.A., Edwards, A.D., Hajnal, J.V., Rueckert, D.: Construction of a consistent high-definition spatio-temporal atlas of the developing brain using adaptive kernel regression. NeuroImage 59, 2255–2265 (2012)
12. Vercauteren, T., Pennec, X., Perchant, A., Ayache, N.: Diffeomorphic demons: Efficient non-parametric image registration. NeuroImage 45, S61–S72 (2009)

Dictionary Learning and Time Sparsity in Dynamic MRI

Jose Caballero[1], Daniel Rueckert[1], and Joseph V. Hajnal[2]

[1] Department of Computing, Imperial College London, UK
[2] Institute of Clinical Sciences, Imperial College London and MRC Clinical Sciences Centre, Hammersmith Hospital, London, UK
{jose.caballero06,d.rueckert,jo.hajnal}@imperial.ac.uk

Abstract. Sparse representation methods have been shown to tackle adequately the inherent speed limits of magnetic resonance imaging (MRI) acquisition. Recently, learning-based techniques have been used to further accelerate the acquisition of 2D MRI. The extension of such algorithms to dynamic MRI (dMRI) requires careful examination of the signal sparsity distribution among the different dimensions of the data. Notably, the potential of temporal gradient (TG) sparsity in dMRI has not yet been explored. In this paper, a novel method for the acceleration of cardiac dMRI is presented which investigates the potential benefits of enforcing sparsity constraints on patch-based learned dictionaries and TG at the same time. We show that an algorithm exploiting sparsity on these two domains can outperform previous sparse reconstruction techniques.

1 Introduction

Medical research and diagnosis rely heavily on magnetic resonance imaging (MRI) for the visualisation of anatomical structures and physiological function. This technology is non-invasive, non-ionizing and offers an unmatched quality in soft tissues contrast. However, physical and physiological limits on scanning speed make this an inherently slow process. Sampling constraints are particularly challenging for dynamic MRI (dMRI). The use of compressed sensing (CS) theory [1,2] has been shown repeatedly to be successful at reducing acquisition time. The philosophy behind CS is that if a signal is known a-priori to be sparse in some transform domain, much fewer samples are needed for its acquisition than those dictated by the Nyquist rate.

Spatio-temporal correlations were early on exploited for MRI acceleration by k-t BLAST/SENSE [3], but with the introduction of Lustig's developments [4] they could be linked to CS theory under a more general framework named k-t FOCUSS [5,6]. Structural dMRI such as cardiac cine, has mainly exploited sparsity in the x-f space, which is obtained through a Fourier transform of the data along time [7,8]. The wavelet domain has also been proposed for the sparse representation of spatial information [9]. However, fixed basis transforms such as the aforementioned have recently been outperformed by adaptive transforms

N. Ayache et al. (Eds.): MICCAI 2012, Part I, LNCS 7510, pp. 256–263, 2012.

resulting from dictionary learning (DL) [10] for the case of 2D structural MRI reconstruction [11,12]. Also, dMRI objects are known to vary through time at a few constrained locations, e.g. edges of a heart, and Fourier transforms along time are not able to capture information about the location of temporal changes.

In this paper, a novel algorithm is proposed for the acceleration of cardiac dMRI acquisition. The contribution is two-fold: First, DL is extended to the dynamic case for the first time through the use of 3D dictionaries as an attempt at finding a better sparsifying domain than those obtained with fixed basis. Secondly, sparsity is additionally enforced on the temporal gradient (TG) of the reconstruction. This simple transform has not received much attention in previous techniques although it can greatly improve the reconstruction performance by capturing very sparse constrained spatio-temporal changes.

The paper is organised as follows: Section 2 introduces the theory behind the compressed sensing MRI (CSMRI) problem and the sparsifying transforms exploited in the method proposed. Our algorithm is described in section 3 and its performance is evaluated and compared with the k-t FOCUSS algorithm [5] in section 4. We summarise the characteristics of the novel technique and future work in section 5.

2 Compressed Sensing in Dynamic MRI

2.1 The CSMRI Problem

Assuming a desired cardiac sequence to be represented as a 3D volume of size $P = P_x \times P_y \times P_t$, time being the third dimension, the column vector $\mathbf{x}_d \in \mathbb{R}^P$ can be built as a concatenation of its columns. Denote $\hat{\mathbf{x}}_d$ as the Fourier transform of $\mathbf{x}_d$ such that $\mathcal{F}\{\mathbf{x}_d\} = \hat{\mathbf{x}}_d$. The acquisition of MR data takes place in the frequency domain, referred to as k-space. To accelerate the process, only $m << P$ k-space samples are acquired according to the sampling subset Ω, which are represented by $\hat{\mathbf{x}}_u \in \mathbb{C}^m$. If the sampling process is assumed to be corrupted by additive white Gaussian noise (AWGN) $\mathbf{n} \in \mathbb{C}^m$, then we can write $\hat{\mathbf{x}}_u = \mathcal{F}_u\{\mathbf{x}_d\} + \mathbf{n}$, where $\mathcal{F}_u\{.\}$ is the undersampling Fourier operator. Given that there exists a sparsifying transform $\mathcal{S}\{.\}$ such that $\|\mathcal{S}\{\mathbf{x}_d\}\|_0 << P$, the problem of recovering $\mathbf{x}_d$ from $\hat{\mathbf{x}}_u$ reduces to solving

$$\min_{\mathbf{x}} \|\mathcal{S}\{\mathbf{x}\}\|_0 \quad s.t. \quad \|\mathcal{F}_u\{\mathbf{x}\} - \hat{\mathbf{x}}_u\|_2^2 < \epsilon, \tag{1}$$

where ϵ is a small constant accounting for sampling noise in k-space. In general both k-space data and the resulting image space are complex, although it is common to reconstruct magnitude images. In this paper fully sampled magnitude images have been used as gold standard input data, implying pure real objects.

Three requirements ensure that the underdetermined system of equations (1) has a unique and attainable solution [1]: (a) $\|\mathcal{S}\{\mathbf{x}_d\}\|_0$ must be sparse or compressible, (b) aliasing has to be incoherent in the transform domain and (c) there must be a non-linear reconstruction process able to enforce sparsity and data-consistency at the same time. The latter two conditions are easily met in

MRI with the use of random undersampling masks [4] and a variety of optimisation algorithms [13]. The success of a CSMRI method therefore relies heavily on the choice of the transform $\mathcal{S}\{.\}$, which should sparsify information as much as possible.

2.2   Sparsifying Transforms in Dynamic MRI

Local Learned Sparsity. An alternative to fixed compression transforms are learned dictionaries. These are constructed through a training process based on example patches extracted from one or multiple signals sharing similar features with the target $\mathbf{x}_d$. Because they are adaptive and more flexible, they can provide sparser representations by discarding redundancies specific to a signal [10], therefore enhancing the potential of the CSMRI framework.

The learning of a dictionary is an optimisation problem in which a dictionary containing N patches of n pixels as columns in a matrix $\mathbf{D} \in \mathbb{R}^{n \times N}$ is tailored to sparsely represent $M > N$ training patches. Available algorithms such as the K-SVD [10] can perform this for 3D training patches and dictionary atoms, suitable for the coding of image sequences. Learning bases for natural video has been successfully tested [14], but the complexity involved can scale very fast if objects in the sequence are rapidly changing because at each time instance the dictionary must be relearned. This disadvantage, however, does not apply to dMRI where the signal's characteristics undergo minimal and locally constrained changes through time and a fixed dictionary is enough for the coding of an entire sequence.

Global Temporal Gradient Sparsity. Total variation (TV) sparsity has been exploited for dMRI reconstruction [15] and is generally included as an extra constraint in sparse reconstructions under the assumption that medical images are piecewise smooth. Nevertheless, the analysis of finite-difference sparsity along the three dimensions of a typical cardiac sequence reveals that temporal finite-differences, which approximate TG, are sparser than any other transform based on spatio-temporal finite-differences.

We empirically compared the sparsity of TV and finite-differences along the three dimensions from a cardiac sequence $\mathbf{x}_d$ of size $128 \times 128 \times 30$ that will be used in experiments of section 4. The l_1 norm, a usual sparsity metric, for these transforms was $\|TV\{\mathbf{x}_d\}\|_1 = 2.9 \times 10^4$, $\|\nabla_x\{\mathbf{x}_d\}\|_1 = 1.7 \times 10^4$, $\|\nabla_y\{\mathbf{x}_d\}\|_1 = 1.8 \times 10^4$ and $\|\nabla_t\{\mathbf{x}_d\}\|_1 = 6.2 \times 10^3$, where $\nabla_f\{.\}$ is the finite-difference operator along dimension f and $TV\{\mathbf{x}\} = \sqrt{\nabla_x\{\mathbf{x}\}^2 + \nabla_y\{\mathbf{x}\}^2 + \nabla_t\{\mathbf{x}\}^2}$.

3   Proposed Method

The method suggested for undersampled dMRI reconstruction consists in an iterative refinement of the zero-filled sequenced $\mathbf{x}_{zf} \in \mathbb{R}^P$ until sparsity constraints under a learned dictionary and TG are simultaneously met. An additional step ensures k-space samples of the solution in the sampling subset Ω are consistent with acquired samples in $\hat{\mathbf{x}}_{zf}$. The method, referred to as dictionary learning temporal gradient (DLTG), is broken down into three main blocks, in which an approximate generic solution $\mathbf{y} \in \mathbb{R}^P$ is refined towards a better solution $\mathbf{x} \in \mathbb{R}^P$. Algorithm 1 summarises the solution proposed.

– **Subproblem 1:** Local patch sparse coding

$$\min_{\boldsymbol{\Gamma}} \|\boldsymbol{\gamma}_j\|_0 \quad s.t. \quad \|\mathbf{R}_j\mathbf{y} - \mathbf{D}\boldsymbol{\gamma}_j\|_2^2 < \epsilon, \forall j \tag{2}$$

Assuming a dictionary $\mathbf{D}$ is trained on $\mathbf{y}$, this step will approximate $\mathbf{y}$ with a sparse representation under $\mathbf{D}$ up to a small error ϵ. A patch $\mathbf{R}_j\mathbf{y}$ is extracted with the matrix operator $\mathbf{R}_j$ and coded in $\boldsymbol{\gamma}_j$ for each pixel of $\mathbf{y}$. Patches wrap around sequence edges, meaning each pixel is contained by a total of n patches. Problem (2) can be efficiently solved through orthogonal matching pursuit [16].

Once a sparse coding is obtained for all pixels in $\mathbf{y}$, the output sequence is recovered through

$$\mathbf{x} = \frac{\sum_{j=1}^{P} \mathbf{R}_j^T \mathbf{D}\boldsymbol{\gamma}_j}{n}, \tag{3}$$

which numerically is interpreted as the superposition of all coded patches according to their spatial correspondence within $\mathbf{x}$, and the averaging of their contribution at each pixel position.

– **Subproblem 2:** Global TG sparse coding

$$\min_{\mathbf{x}} \lambda \|\nabla_t\{\mathbf{x}\}\|_1 + \frac{1}{2}\|\mathbf{y} - \mathbf{x}\|_2^2 \tag{4}$$

The solution of (4) will be close to $\mathbf{y}$ in the least squares sense and will have sparse TG. This can be solved using an interior-point method with an empirical complexity of $O(P^{1.2})$ [17]. To solve equation (4) we operate on $\nabla_t\{\mathbf{x}\}$ directly and update $\mathbf{x}$ for the second term using forward cumulative sums of the TG. This requires the DC level to be set in an independent step. Further details are excluded here due to space restrictions.

– **Subproblem 3:** Data consistency in k-space

$$\hat{\mathbf{x}}(\mathbf{k}) = \begin{cases} \hat{\mathbf{y}}(\mathbf{k}) & , \mathbf{k} \notin \Omega \\ \frac{\hat{\mathbf{y}}(\mathbf{k}) + \nu\hat{\mathbf{x}}_{zf}(\mathbf{k})}{1+\nu} & , \mathbf{k} \in \Omega \end{cases} \tag{5}$$

The entire process relies on acquired k-space samples $\mathbf{k} = (k_x, k_y, t) \in \Omega$, which are non-zero samples in $\hat{\mathbf{x}}_{zf}$. Hence, the k-space representation $\hat{\mathbf{x}}$ of the solution will have to be consistent with these. A weighting factor $\nu = q/\sigma$ determines how much these samples are trusted considering noise power σ in k-space.

Algorithm 1. DLTG

Input: Undersampled zero-filled k-space data - $\hat{\mathbf{x}}_{zf}$
Output: Reconstructed MR sequence - $\mathbf{x}_{I_1, I_2}$
Initialise: $\mathbf{x}_{0,0} = \mathbf{x}_{zf} = \mathcal{F}^{-1}\{\hat{\mathbf{x}}_{zf}\}$
for $k = 0$ **to** $I_1 - 1$ **do**
    1. Train $\mathbf{D}$ using patches from $\mathbf{x}_{k,0}$
    2. Obtain local patch sparse coding $\boldsymbol{\Gamma}$ of $\mathbf{x}_{k,0}$ under $\mathbf{D}$ by solving (2)
    3. Update $\mathbf{x}_{k,0}$ based on $\boldsymbol{\Gamma}$ through (3)
    4. Enforce data consistency on $\mathbf{x}_{k,0}$ by (5)
    for $i = 0$ **to** $I_2 - 1$ **do**
        5. Enforce global TG sparsity on $\mathbf{x}_{k,i}$ solving (4)
        6. Enforce data consistency on $\mathbf{x}_{k,i}$ by (5) and store result in $\mathbf{x}_{k,i+1}$
    end
    7. Update reconstruction: $\mathbf{x}_{k+1,0} \leftarrow \mathbf{x}_{k,I_2}$
end

Many of the parameters do not require very precise settings and can be chosen from a reasonably large spectrum without excessively affecting the end result [11]. This is the case for patch sizes n, the number of dictionary atoms N, the number of training patches M and the scaling factor q. Stopping criteria are chosen as maximum number of iterations I_1 and I_2, although convergence to stable solutions is also a valid condition. Variables ϵ and λ set a compromise on the performance and speed of the algorithm. The smaller they are, the better the result but the slower the convergence rate. Ideally, a regularisation path would optimally initialise them with large values and decrease them at each iteration. For the production of results in section 4, they were sequentially updated such that at outer iteration k, $\epsilon_k = \sqrt{mse_{k,0} \times n}$, and at inner iteration i, $\lambda_{k,i} = \sqrt{mse_{k,i}}/2$, where $mse_{k,i} = \mathbb{E}\{\|\mathbf{x}_{k,i} - \mathbf{x}_d\|_2^2\}$ and $\mathbb{E}\{.\}$ is the expectation operator. The use of the gold standard $\mathbf{x}_d$ is exclusive for demonstration purposes. Fixed parameters ϵ and λ have been tested to provide the same results simply slower.

4   Experimental Results

In the following experiments, a cardiac sequence of size $128 \times 128 \times 30$ with normalised intensity is artificially corrupted by multiplying its k-space representation with a binary undersampling mask and by adding complex AWGN of power σ. Assuming a Cartesian trajectory sampling, acquisitions of the mask are randomly drawn from a 1D Gaussian distribution prioritising the rejection of high frequency components and are independent realisations for each frame.

Results are all drawn using a dictionary of $N = 300$ cubic atoms of size $n = 125$ trained from $M = 5000$ patches. The noise regularisation factor is chosen to be $q = 150$ from empirical observation, but results were found to be reasonably stable (less than 0.5 PSNR variation) for a range between 60 and 200. The algorithm is run using $I_1 = 20$ and $I_2 = 10$ iterations, and its performance is evaluated in terms of its Peak Signal-to-Noise Ratio (PSNR). The result from

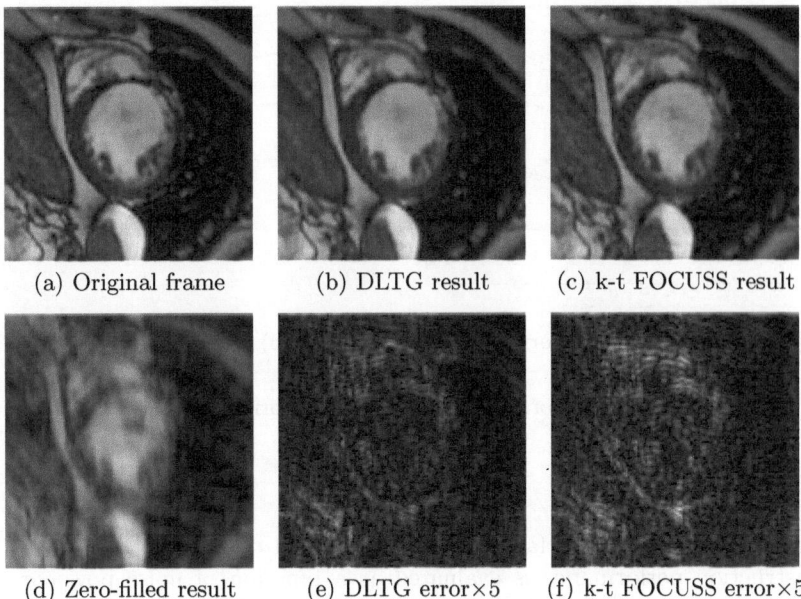

(a) Original frame   (b) DLTG result   (c) k-t FOCUSS result

(d) Zero-filled result   (e) DLTG error×5   (f) k-t FOCUSS error×5

Fig. 1. One frame in a reconstruction of a sequence acquired at a 0.15 sampling factor

k-t FOCUSS [5] is provided as a reference x-f based method and an algorithm exploiting only DL sparsity (ignoring steps 5 and 6 in algorithm 1) is assessed in order to understand the benefits of imposing TG sparsity on the solution.

4.1 Visual Appearance

A frame from the reconstructed sequence is shown in figure 1. The sampling factor used in this example was $m/P = 0.15$ and a noise-free acquisition was assumed. Amplified error images are also shown. The DLTG method is able to recover the sequence with PSNR = 31.6dB from the original PSNR = 23.7dB of the zero-filled sequence compared to the PSNR = 29.7dB of k-t FOCUSS.

4.2 Noiseless Case

Figure 2(a) shows the performance of the proposed method assuming $\sigma = 0$ for different sampling factors. For very high ones (above 0.5), the reconstruction power is completely attributed to the enforcement of sparsity under the learned dictionary. As the sampling is reduced, more aliasing is introduced in $\mathbf{x}_{zf}$ and the dictionary starts incorporating it as part of the sequence features to be learned, therefore lowering the performance of DL. The aliasing reproduced, however, prevents the reconstruction from meeting the sparsity requirement in the TG domain, which is why enforcing it is beneficial for the end result. The algorithm is shown to be superior to k-t FOCUSS for all sampling factors and the same was observed for 20 different short axis data as well as on long axis examples.

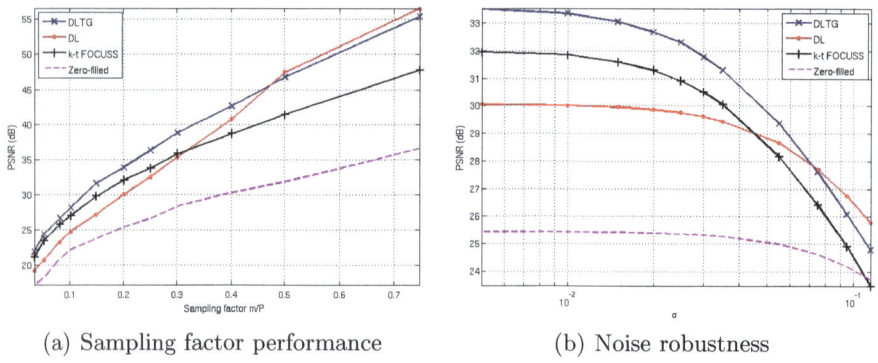

(a) Sampling factor performance   (b) Noise robustness

Fig. 2. Compared performance of the DLTG algorithm and k-t FOCUSS

4.3   Noisy Case

In figure 2(b), a sampling factor of 0.2 is imposed on the acquisition and the reconstruction performance is evaluated as a function of noise power σ. The spectrum covered is SNR = 34.5dB ($\sigma = 0.005$) up to SNR = 7.2dB ($\sigma = 0.115$) and the DLTG method is consistently superior to k-t FOCUSS. Also, it can be observed that the gain obtained from the TG constraint becomes smaller as noise is increased and its enforcement can be detrimental for high levels of noise.

5   Conclusion and Future Work

A novel reconstruction method for the acceleration of dMRI acquisition called DLTG has been proposed which, for the first time, adapts DL to dMRI data and introduces the TG transform as a suitable sparsifying transform. A dictionary learned from the acquired k-space data provides a sparse representation that can outperform methods based on fixed basis transforms. Sparsity enforced on TG is seen as the best performing one out of those exploiting spatio-temporal finite-differences and effectively reduces aliasing further whenever the DL constraint alone is not sufficient. On top of being reasonably robust to noise, results show that the method provides better results than the k-t FOCUSS method.

One important improvement of the DLTG method needs to explore the reconstruction of complex data. All the results were based on the assumption that the target sequence was real, but information such as blood flow in cardiac dMRI is encoded in complex format. Also, a more efficient way to combine DL and TG sparsity will be imperative to widen the algorithm's applicability. The DLTG algorithm is nevertheless an encouraging first attempt at using learned bases for dMRI and sets path for the extension of learned sparsity to other MRI modalities such as functional or parallel MRI, with the expectation of experiencing the same benefits previously observed in 2D MRI and confirmed here for structural dMRI.

References

1. Candes, E.J., Romberg, J., Tao, T.: Robust uncertainty principles: Exact signal reconstruction from highly incomplete frequency information. IEEE Transactions on Information Theory 52(2), 489–509 (2006)
2. Donoho, D.: Compressed sensing. IEEE Transactions on Information Theory 52(4), 1289–1306 (2006)
3. Tsao, J., Boesiger, P., Pruessmann, K.P.: k-t BLAST and k-t SENSE: Dynamic MRI with high frame rate exploiting spatiotemporal correlations. Magnetic Resonance in Medicine 50(5), 1031–1042 (2003)
4. Lustig, M., Donoho, D., Pauly, J.M.: Sparse MRI: The application of compressed sensing for rapid MR imaging. Magnetic Resonance in Medicine 58(6), 1182–1195 (2007)
5. Jung, H., Ye, J.C., Kim, E.Y.: Improved k-t BLAST and k-t SENSE using FOCUSS. Physics in Medicine and Biology 52(11), 3201–3226 (2007)
6. Jung, H., Sung, K., Nayak, K.S., Kim, E.Y., Ye, J.C.: k-t FOCUSS: A general compressed sensing framework for high resolution dynamic MRI. Magnetic Resonance in Medicine 61(1), 103–116 (2009)
7. Gamper, U., Boesiger, P., Kozerke, S.: Compressed sensing in dynamic MRI. Magnetic Resonance in Medicine 59(2), 365–373 (2008)
8. Usman, M., Prieto, C., Schaeffter, T., Batchelor, P.G.: k-t group sparse: A method for accelerating dynamic MRI. Magnetic Resonance in Medicine 66(4), 1163–1176 (2011)
9. Lustig, M., Santos, J.M., Donoho, D.L., Pauly, J.M.: k-t SPARSE: High frame rate dynamic MRI exploiting spatio-temporal sparsity. In: Proc. of the 13th Annual Meeting of ISMRM, Seattle, vol. 50(5), p. 2420 (2006)
10. Aharon, M., Elad, M., Bruckstein, A.: K-SVD: Design of dictionaries for sparse representation. In: Proc. of SPARS, vol. 5, pp. 9–12 (2005)
11. Ravishankar, S., Bresler, Y.: MR image reconstruction from highly undersampled k-space data by dictionary learning. IEEE TMI 30(5), 1028–1041 (2011)
12. Chen, Y., Ye, X., Huang, F.: A novel method and fast algorithm for MR image reconstruction with significantly under-sampled data. Inverse Problems and Imaging 4(2), 223–240 (2010)
13. Tropp, J.A., Wright, S.J.: Computational methods for sparse solution of linear inverse problems. Proc. of the IEEE 98(6), 948–958 (2010)
14. Protter, M., Elad, M.: Image sequence denoising via sparse and redundant representations. IEEE Transactions on Image Processing 18(1), 27–35 (2009)
15. Montefusco, L.B., Lazzaro, D., Papi, S., Guerrini, C.: A fast compressed sensing approach to 3D MR image reconstruction. IEEE TMI 30(5), 1067–1075 (2011)
16. Pati, Y., Rezaiifar, R., Krishnaprasad, P.: Orthogonal matching pursuit: Recursive function approximation with applications to wavelet decomposition. In: Proc. of 27th Asilomar Conference on Signals, Systems and Computers, vol. 1, pp. 40–44 (2011)
17. Kim, S.J., Koh, K., Lustig, M., Boyd, S., Gorinevsky, D.: An interior-point method for large-scale l1-regularized least squares. IEEE Journal of Selected Topics in Signal Processing 1(4), 606–617 (2007)

Joint Reconstruction of Image and Motion in MRI: Implicit Regularization Using an Adaptive 3D Mesh

Anne Menini[1,2], Pierre-André Vuissoz[1,2],
Jacques Felblinger[1,2], and Freddy Odille[2]

[1] IADI, Université de Lorraine, Nancy, France
[2] U947, INSERM, Nancy, France
{a.menini,pa.vuissoz,j.felblinger}@chu-nancy.fr, freddy.odille@inserm.fr

Abstract. Magnetic resonance images are affected by motion artefacts due to breathing and cardiac beating that occur during the acquisition. Methods for joint reconstruction of image and motion have been proposed recently. Such optimization problems are ill-conditioned, therefore regularization methods are required such as motion smoothness constraints using the Tikhonov method. However with Tikhonov methods the solution often relies on a good choice of the regularization parameter μ, especially in large parameter search spaces (e.g. in 3D reconstructions). In this paper, we propose an adaptive, implicit regularization method which results in subject-specific, spatially varying smoothness constraints on the motion model. It is based on the idea of solving for motion only in certain key points that form a mesh. A practical algorithm is proposed for generating this mesh automatically. The proposed method is shown to have a better convergence rate than the Tikhonov method, both in silico and in vivo. The accuracy of the reconstructed image and motion is also improved.

Keywords: Magnetic Resonance Imaging, reconstruction, non-rigid motion, regularization, mesh, inverse problem.

1 Introduction

A magnetic resonance imaging (MRI) acquisition is a sequential process and therefore often exceeds tolerable breath hold time. Thus, respiratory motion and heart beating can occur during the acquisition. Since data are acquired in the Fourier domain, such non-rigid motions lead to complex artefacts that affect the whole image. These cannot be fixed using entirely image post-processing methods such as registration. Solutions cannot be found among acquisition strategies either. Indeed, despite effective acceleration methods [1], motion correction remains a challenge because of the growing interest in 3D and 4D (3D + time), high resolution imaging and quantitative MRI which take minutes to acquire.

Reconstruction methods have been proposed based on the joint optimization of image and motion [2, 3]. The two unknowns obtained in this way are an

N. Ayache et al. (Eds.): MICCAI 2012, Part I, LNCS 7510, pp. 264–271, 2012.
© Springer-Verlag Berlin Heidelberg 2012

artefact-free image and a non-rigid motion model that describes the displacements of each voxel during the acquisition. This leads to a non-linear optimization which is generally ill-conditioned. Therefore, a regularization is applied to constrain the solution. A typical constraint consists of picking up the solution whose motion field is smoothest, as defined by the gradient $\mathcal{L}_2$ norm, which is one kind of Tikhonov regularization.

Such Tikhonov methods have several drawbacks : i) the weight of the smoothness constraint, as expressed by a regularization parameter called μ in the remainder of the paper, is generally adjusted empirically (optimizing μ itself would necessitate a considerable increase in reconstruction time) ; ii) such regularizers may not depict certain classes of motion, e.g. shearing or piecewise smooth motion ; iii) when the dimensionality of the problem is increased (e.g. from 2D to 3D), the conditioning of the problem decreases and thus leads to a higher sensitivity of the solution to μ, both in terms of accuracy and convergence rate.

In this paper, we propose an alternative regularization method intended to avoid these drawbacks. Instead of dealing with a large amount of unknowns and imposing a strong constraint, here we solve the problem only for a small subset of unknowns that can be thought of as describing the principal components of motion. The method proceeds by generating an adaptive mesh which inherently contains local smoothness information. Once integrated into the joint reconstruction process, it allows voxels with similar displacements to be grouped and thereby provides an implicit regularization for the optimization of the motion model, meaning the explicit regularization term is no longer necessary.

The proposed method, the adaptive regularization (AR), was compared with a classical Tikhonov regularization (TR), both in silico and in vivo. Results were assessed in term of convergence rate, image similarity and motion recovery.

2   Joint Reconstruction of Image and Motion

2.1   Inverse Problem

We are interested in reconstructing a volume (or an image) ρ_0 that was acquired while an unknown non-rigid motion occurs. This can be described by a set of images $(\rho_t)_{t=1..N_t}$ at several physiological states,

$$\rho_t = W_t(u_t)\rho_0 \tag{1}$$

where W_t is an image transformation matrix that depends on an unknown displacement u_t. The displacement u_t can be parametrized, e.g. using physiological signals $(S_k)_{k=1..N_k}$ from motion sensor that are temporally correlated with physiological movements (e.g. abdominal or thoracic breathing, heart beating). Then the displacement can be approximated by a linear combination

$$u_t(r) = \sum_{k=1}^{N_k} \alpha_k(r)S_k(t) \tag{2}$$

where $(\alpha_k)_{k=1..N_k}$ are unknown motion models coefficients. The warping of the image is rewritten as a function of the unknown motion parameters.

$$\rho_t = W_t(\alpha)\rho_0 \tag{3}$$

The acquisition process can be expressed by a linear forward projection operator P. Then, the raw data s acquired by the scanner are given by an encoding operator $E(\alpha)$ affected by noise ν.

$$s = \sum_{t=1}^{N_t} P_t W_t(\alpha)\rho_0 + \nu = E(\alpha)\rho_0 + \nu \tag{4}$$

Eventually, the joint reconstruction problem consists in solving the inverse problem of (4). Generally, it is done by minimizing the negative log likelihood of:

$$L(\rho_0, \alpha) = \|s - E(\alpha)\rho_0\|^2 \ . \tag{5}$$

2.2   Joint Optimization with Explicit Regularization

While the problem of reconstructing ρ_0 for a fixed motion model α reduces to a well conditioned least squares problem, the problem of recovering both ρ_0 and α is ill-posed. This is because several motion models can lead to the same warped image ρ_t. A regularization is applied to constrain the solution, for example to be smooth or to have a low energy. It is achieved by adding a regularization operator.

$$(\tilde{\rho}_0, \tilde{\alpha}) = \underset{\rho_0, \alpha}{\operatorname{argmin}} \{L(\rho_0, \alpha) + \Psi(\alpha)\} \tag{6}$$

With a Tikhonov regularization, we can write $\Psi(\alpha) = \mu\|\nabla\alpha\|_2^2$. Equation (6) can be solved by alternating optimization with respect to ρ_0 and α. Two linearised problems are solved alternately using standard iterative linear system solvers. A multi-resolution scheme can also be used as no initial guess of the motion model α is available in general.

We consider an acquisition with N_k motion models like in (2). In 2D, the displacements can only be described in-plane (2 directions), so we obtain $N_{\alpha,2D}$ unknowns for the motion with $N_{\alpha,2D} = 2 \times N_k \times N_x \times N_y$ and $N_{s,2D}$ data acquired with $N_{s,2D} = N_x \times N_y$. Then in 3D, we obtain $N_{\alpha,3D} = 3 \times N_k \times N_x \times N_y \times N_z$ and $N_{s,3D} = N_x \times N_y \times N_z$. The amount of unknowns raises $3/2$ times more than the amount of data. Consequently, the inverse problem is much more ill-conditioned in 3D. To tackle that issue the constraint should have a stronger weight, however this can result in excessive smoothing.

3   Implicit Regularization

3.1   Assumptions about Motion

Regularizations are often based on the assumption that motion is relatively smooth. While this is a reasonable assumption within a single tissue, it is invalidated at the interface between different tissues moving in independent directions (e.g. shearing between liver and ribs).

Then, it would be more efficient to allow local variations of the constraint rather than applying the same constraint to the whole image. This can be achieved by varying the density of points where the motion is described (referred as key points). By doing so, motion is constrained to be smooth only where the density of key points is low (Fig. 1). Furthermore, it reduces drastically the number of unknowns which makes the optimization task more tractable.

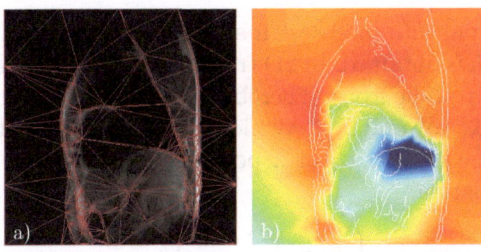

Fig. 1. Example of a 2D mesh adapted for a short axis MRI acquisition (a). The motion model reconstructed is smooth where the density of the mesh is low (b)

3.2   Mesh Generation

We suppose that we have a first estimate of the image ρ and the motion α. These can be provided by a previous iteration of the joint reconstruction algorithm. We propose the algorithm 1 to select the set of points Ω where the motion should be solved for.

Algorithm 1. Building of the key points set Ω

1: $\Omega \leftarrow \emptyset$
2: $\delta\rho \leftarrow \|\nabla\rho\|_2$
3: $\delta\alpha \leftarrow \|\nabla\alpha\|_2$
4: **for** voxel x_i s.t. $\delta\rho_i = \delta\rho_{\max}$ **to** $\delta\rho_i = \delta\rho_{\min}$ **do**
5:     $r \leftarrow \lambda(\delta\alpha_i - \delta\alpha_{\max})/(\delta\alpha_{\min} - \delta\alpha_{\max})$ ▷ λ is a characteristic length of the structures on the image (it does not have to be tuned).
6:     **if** $\Omega \cap \{$voxel x_j s.t. $\|x_i - x_j\|_2 < r\} = \emptyset$ **then**
7:         $\Omega \leftarrow \Omega \cup x_i$
8:     **end if**
9: **end for**

This mesh generation algorithm results in selecting with higher priority points that lie at the interfaces between different tissues (corresponding to large image gradients). Moreover, the density of points is proportional to the complexity of the motion (reflected in the motion model gradients). To initialize the algorithm when no motion model estimate is available, vertices are simply spread along the image gradients. With this point set, voxels with similar displacements are automatically grouped which has the effect of a spatially varying regularization. In addition, we avoid the pitfalls of classical regularizations. More particularly, the selection of the key point set is automatic (no parameter tuning). The mesh generation should be relatively fast for the joint reconstruction algorithm to benefit from it. Hence this direct method is preferable to iterative ones.

3.3 Mesh Integration

The image can be split into pieces with a Delaunay tesselation of the key points set [4]. Thus, a mesh is obtained. In 2D (resp. 3D), each point P_i in space belongs a triangle T_i (resp. tetrahedron). Thereby, its motion depends on the unknown motion $(\hat{\alpha}_{T_i,j})_{j=1..N_V}$ of only N_V vertices $(V_{T_i,j})_{j=1..N_V}$ with $N_V = 3$ (resp. $N_V = 4$). Then, the motion α_i of a point P_i in space can be obtained by a barycentric interpolation.

$$\begin{cases} P_i = \sum_{j=1}^{N_V} \beta_{ij} V_{T_i,j} \\ \alpha_i = \sum_{j=1}^{N_V} \beta_{ij} \hat{\alpha}_{T_i,j} \end{cases} \tag{7}$$

As a consequence of using a mesh, there is no need to compute the motion explicitly in every point to warp an image. Indeed, we can compute a texture mapping based on the mesh. It can be achieved with a piece-wise affine interpolation (Algo. 2 and Fig. 2).

Algorithm 2. Image warping

1: **for** voxel $x_i^t \in \rho_t$ **do**
2:    Find T_i^t s.t. $x_i^t \in T_i^t$
3:    Compute $(\beta_{i,j})_{j=1..N_V}$ s.t. (7)
4:    Compute x_i^0 using $(\beta_{i,j})_{j=1..N_V}$
5:    $\rho_i^t \leftarrow$ nearest neighbourhood interpolation of ρ_0 around x_i^0
6: **end for**

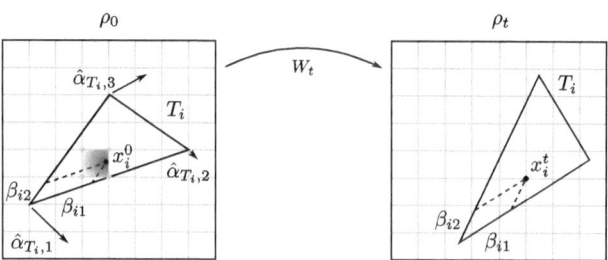

Fig. 2. Image warping with a piece-wise affine interpolation

The mesh could be updated each time the image or motion parameters are updated. Here, in a multiresolution reconstruction, we suggest to update the mesh only once at the beginning of each resolution loop.

4   Validation

4.1   In Silico

A 3D MRI acquisition was simulated from a synthetic image (Fig. 3 (a)), a predefined motion model (Fig. 3 (b, c, d)) and real physiological signals according to (2, 4). This data set simulate a sagittal view of a liver through a 3D MRI sequence with parallel imaging. Two joint reconstructions of the image and the motion models were performed with a fixed-point multi-resolution scheme [2], one with the classical Tikhonov method and the other with our adaptive method to regularize the motion optimization. Several reconstructions were tested with the Tikhonov method in order to find a fair regularization parameter ($\mu = 0.01$).

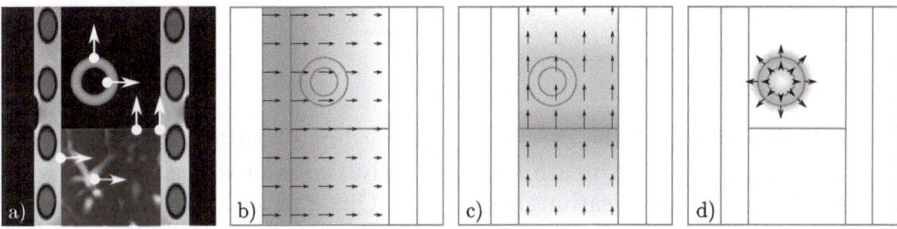

Fig. 3. Synthetic image with locations where the motion accuracy was assessed (a), and motion models used to simulate the data: thoracic breathing (b), abdominal breathing (c) and cardiac beating (d)

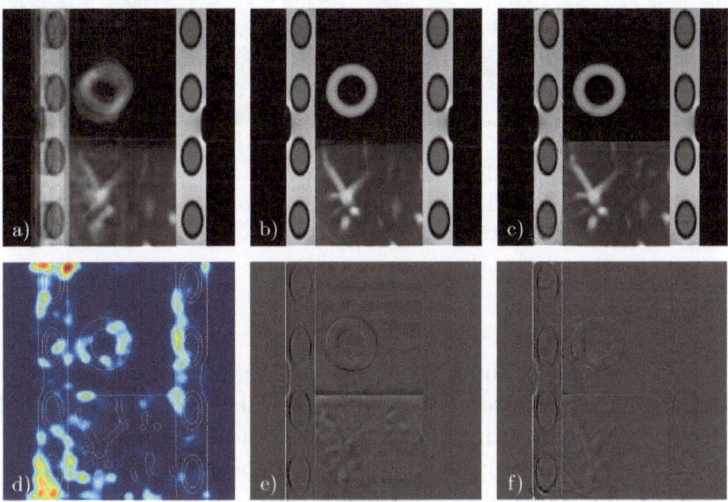

Fig. 4. Reconstructions of the synthetic data set: without motion correction (a), with the motion correction using TR (b), using AR (c). Point density of the adaptive mesh (d). Error with TR (e) and error with AR (f).

The image obtained with the naive Fourier reconstruction presents motion artefacts as expected (Fig. 4 (a)). Both regularizations have successfully solved for the thoracic breathing and the cardiac beating (Fig. 4 (b, c)). However, motion artefacts from abdominal breathing remain with the classical regularization. Since the latter motion model includes abrupt variations unlike the other ones, it points out the limitation of a homogeneous smoothing constraint. The NRMSE computed on the image reaches 5.3 % with the classical method, against 4.7 % with the adaptive one (Fig. 4 (e, f)). Similarly, the NRMSE computed on 6 specific locations of the motion reaches 69.5 %, against 22.3 % (Fig. 3 (a)). The amount of unknowns for the motion was divided by 100 with the adaptive method. At last, for each resolution level, the number of iterations n required for the optimization to converge to the same given tolerance systematically reached the maximum number allowed ($n_{max} = 8$) with the Tikhonov regularization whereas it reached 3.3 in average with our method.

4.2   In Vivo

3D MRI acquisitions[1] of the liver were performed in a healthy volunteer during free breathing and during breath hold. Similarly, two joint reconstructions were performed from the free breathing acquisitions. Qualitatively, both regularization methods resulted in a drastic improvement of the image compared to uncorrected images, and were similar to the breath hold acquisition (Fig. 5). The convergence behaviour was better for the adaptive method like in silico ($n = 3$ against 8).

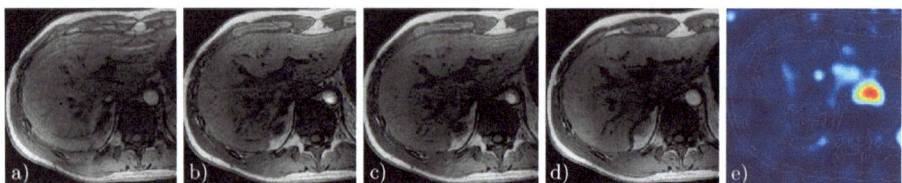

Fig. 5. Reconstructions of the liver on a healthy volunteer (zoom): free breathing acquisition without motion correction (a), with the motion correction using TR (b), using AR (c) and acquisition in breath hold (d). Point density of the adaptive mesh (e).

5   Discussion

Finally, our method makes the regularization of highly ill-conditioned problems more tractable. Therefore, compared with the Tikhonov method, it improves the accuracy of the joint optimization solutions and in addition, speeds up the convergence rate and reduces the number of unknowns by 100.

Here we chose to report the convergence rate (number of iteration), rather than the effective computation time. Indeed, our new method involves several

---

[1] LAVA, $TE/TR = 1.82/3.92$ ms, matrix size: $320 \times 288 \times 60$, asset factor $= 2$, 3T SIGNA HDxt, GE Healthcare, Milwaukee, WI.

time consuming algorithms (e.g. Delaunay tesselation, search for the triangle containing some point, interpolation), which have not been optimized yet in our current implementation. Till then, these loss in computation time are compensated by the drop-off of iterations required. A GPU implementation of these steps should improve the computation time as well.

Alternative regularizers have been proposed in the literature to address the limitations of Tikhonov regularizers. In particular, total variation regularization [5] allows discontinuities to be preserved. However this is at the cost of an increased complexity of the optimization leading to increased computation time.

Finite element approaches are often used [6]; however these are not always adaptive. Others have proposed adaptive meshes [7]. Their adaptation consists of an iterative refinement based on residual errors at the previous iteration. In our case, the construction is direct when we have a motion estimate, which is available after only one iteration. These adaptive techniques could be combined.

The adaptive mesh-based implicit regularization is not limited to free-breathing MRI reconstruction. Image registration techniques [8] might also apply.

References

[1] Tsao, J.: Ultrafast imaging: Principles, pitfalls, solutions, and applications. Journal of Magnetic Resonance Imaging 32(2), 252–266 (2010)

[2] Odille, F., Vuissoz, P., Marie, P., Felblinger, J.: Generalized reconstruction by inversion of coupled systems (GRICS) applied to free-breathing MRI. Magnetic Resonance in Medicine 60(1), 146–157 (2008)

[3] Jacobson, M.W., Fessler, J.A.: Joint estimation of image and deformation parameters in motion-corrected PET. In: 2003 IEEE Nuclear Science Symposium Conference Record, vol. 5, pp. 3290–3294. IEEE (October 2003)

[4] Barber, C.B., Dobkin, D.P., Huhdanpaa, H.: The quickhull algorithm for convex hulls. ACM Transaction on Mathematical Software 22(4), 469–483 (1996)

[5] Rudin, L.I., Osher, S., Fatemi, E.: Nonlinear total variation based noise removal algorithms. Physica D: Nonlinear Phenomena 60(14), 259–268 (1992)

[6] Arridge, S.R., Schweiger, M., Hiraoka, M., Delpy, D.T., et al.: A finite element approach for modeling photon transport in tissue. Medical Physics-Lancaster PA 20, 299–299 (1993)

[7] Joshi, A., Bangerth, W., Sevick-Muraca, E.: Adaptive finite element based tomography for fluorescence optical imaging in tissue. Optics Express 12(22), 5402–5417 (2004)

[8] Rueckert, D., Sonoda, L.I., Hayes, C., Hill, D.L., Leach, M.O., Hawkes, D.J.: Non-rigid registration using free-form deformations: application to breast MR images. IEEE Transactions on Medical Imaging 18(8), 712–721 (1999)

Sparsity-Based Deconvolution
of Low-Dose Perfusion CT Using Learned Dictionaries

Ruogu Fang[1], Tsuhan Chen[1], and Pina C. Sanelli[2]

[1] Department of Electrical and Computer Engineering, Cornell University, Ithaca, NY, USA
[2] Department of Radiology, Weill Cornell Medical College, NYC, NY, USA

Abstract. Computational tomography perfusion (CTP) is an important functional imaging modality in the evaluation of cerebrovascular diseases, such as stroke and vasospasm. However, the post-processed parametric maps of blood flow tend to be noisy, especially in low-dose CTP, due to the noisy contrast enhancement profile and the oscillatory nature of the results generated by the current computational methods. In this paper, we propose a novel sparsity-base deconvolution method to estimate cerebral blood flow in CTP performed at low-dose. We first built an overcomplete dictionary from high-dose perfusion maps and then performed deconvolution-based hemodynamic parameters estimation on the low-dose CTP data. Our method is validated on a clinical dataset of ischemic patients. The results show that we achieve superior performance than existing methods, and potentially improve the differentiation between normal and ischemic tissue in the brain.

1   Introduction

Stroke is the third-leading cause of death in the United States after heart disease and cancer. Early and rapid diagnosis of stroke can save critical time for thrombolytic therapy. Cerebral perfusion imaging via computed tomography perfusion (CTP) has become more commonly used in clinical practice for the evaluation of patients with acute stroke and vasospasm. Various mathematical models have been used to process the acquired temporal data to ascertain quantitative information, such as cerebral blood flow (CBF), cerebral blood volume (CBV) and mean transit time (MTT) [1-3]. However recent reports on over-exposure of radiation in CTP have brought the dosage problem to the limelight because many patients reported biologic effects from radiation exposure, including hair loss and skin burns. A key challenge in CTP is to obtain a high-quality CBF image from a low-dose perfusion scan.

The most commonly used deconvolution method to quantify the perfusion parameters in CTP is truncated singular value decomposition (TSVD) and its variants, such as circular TSVD (cTSVD) [2]. The oscillatory nature [4] of the TSVD-based method has initiated research that incorporates different regularization methods to stabilize the deconvolution, and have shown varying degrees of success in recovering the residue function or the perfusion parameters [3][5-8]. However, prior studies have focused exclusively on imposing regularizations on the noisy low-dose CTP, without considering the corpus of high-dose CTP data.

N. Ayache et al. (Eds.): MICCAI 2012, Part I, LNCS 7510, pp. 272–280, 2012.
© Springer-Verlag Berlin Heidelberg 2012

In this paper, we propose a new sparsity-based deconvolution method to estimate cerebral blood flow in CTP at low-dose. We first learned a dictionary of CBF maps from a corpus of high-dose CTP data and then performed deconvolution-based hemo-dynamic parameter estimation of the low-dose CTP. This method produces perfusion parameter maps with better signal-to-noise characteristics.

Our major contribution in this work is two-fold: First, we propose to train a dictionary of perfusion parameter maps from the high-dose CT data to improve the quantification of low-dose CT perfusion. Second, we use local sparsity and redundancy in a global spatial Bayesian objective combined with the temporal convolution model. Then on the in vivo brain ischemic stroke CTP data, we demonstrate that our estimated CBF values lead to better separation between ischemic tissue—which by its angiogenic nature tends to have less blood flow—and normal tissue.

2   A Dictionary Approach to Deconvolution

In this section, we present the new sparsity based deconvolution framework for CTP quantification. The framework is comprised of two steps: dictionary learning and sparse coding.

2.1   Perfusion Parameter Model

Based on the theoretical model provided in [1], in CTP, the amount of contrast in the region is characterized by

$$C_v(t) = CBF \int_0^t C_a(\tau)R(t-\tau)d\tau \tag{1}$$

where $C_v(t)$ is the tissue enhancement curve (TEC) of tracer at the venous output in the volume of interest (VOI), CBF is the cerebral blood flow, $C_a(t)$ is an arterial input function (AIF) and $R(t)$ is the tissue impulse residue function (IRF), which measures the mass of contrast media remaining in the given vascular network over time. To discretize the computation, we assume that $C_a(t)$ and $C(t)$ are measured with N equally spaced time points $t_1, t_2, \ldots, t_N$, with time increment Δt. The convolution is discretized

$$C = CBF \cdot \Delta t \cdot C_a \cdot R \tag{2}$$

where

$$C = \begin{pmatrix} C(t_1) \\ C(t_2) \\ \vdots \\ C(t_N) \end{pmatrix} \quad R = \begin{pmatrix} R(t_1) \\ R(t_2) \\ \vdots \\ R(t_N) \end{pmatrix} \quad C_a = \begin{pmatrix} C_a(t_1) & 0 & \cdots & 0 \\ C_a(t_2) & C_a(t_1) & \cdots & 0 \\ \vdots & \vdots & \ddots & \vdots \\ C_a(t_N) & C_a(t_{N-1}) & \cdots & C_a(t_1) \end{pmatrix}$$

When $R(t)$ is estimated from Equation (2), CBF can be computed from

$$CBF = R(t = 0) \tag{3}$$

since from the definition of the residue function $R(t)$, $R(t = 0) = 1$.

2.2   Proposed Dictionary Learning Approach to Deconvolution

Sparse representations over trained dictionaries for perfusion parameter maps restoration rest on the assumption that the image priors in the perfusion maps can be learned from images, rather than choosing a prior based on some simplifying assumptions, such as spatial smoothness, non-local similarity, or sparsity in the transformed domain. Since the low dose CTP have high noise level in TEC, it is important to learn the dictionaries from the high-dose (thus low noise level) CTP. Therefore, we implement the sparse and redundant representation in the spirit of Sparseland [9]. In our model, we estimate perfusion parameters by considering both temporal correlations and example-based restoration based on dictionaries learned from high-dose data.

Problem Formulation: Suppose $C(x,y,z,t) \in \mathbb{R}^{N \times T}$ is TEC in VOI $[x,y,z]^T$ from a spatial-temporal patch of size $\sqrt{N} \times \sqrt{N} \times 1$ pixels and T time points. $R(x,y,z,t) \in \mathbb{R}^{N \times T}$ represent the remaining tracer concentration (RIF) of the voxel $[x,y,z]$ at a given time point t, where x, y and z are the respective row, column and slice coordinates of the spatial-temporal data. The least-square form of (2) is

$$J_{ls} = \|C - C_a R\|_2^2 \tag{4}$$

Due to the noise in the low-dose CTP data, the solution of (4) may be severely distorted. In the spirit of Sparseland model, we incorporate *a prior* of not only temporal correlation but also sparse representation from the learned dictionaries of the parameter map patches through the inclusion of two constraints to the original least-square cost function. This results in the new cost function

$$J = \mu_1 \|C - C_a R\|_2^2 + \|x - D\alpha\|_2^2 + \mu_2 \|\alpha\|_0 \tag{5}$$

where $x \in \mathbb{R}^N$ is the CBF perfusion map we want to estimate for the VOI at $[x,y,z]$, $D \in \mathbb{R}^{N \times K}$ is the learned dictionary of CBF perfusion map patches that consists of K key patches from the training data. $\alpha \in \mathbb{R}^K$ represents a sparse vector so that $D\alpha$ can approximate x with certain error tolerance. From the definition of the residue function, we can get $x = R(t = 0)$. The choice of two parameters μ_1 and μ_2 dictate how important the temporal correlation term (the first term) and the sparsity term (the third term) should be weighted.

Dictionary Learning: To solve D, we use the recently developed K-SVD algorithm [10] which solves (5) by iterating exact K times of Singular Value Decomposition (SVD). We first learn a dictionary by using randomly sampled patches from the CBF perfusion maps estimated from the high-dose CTP data. Given a set of image patches $Z = \{z_j\}_{j=1}^M$, each of $\sqrt{N} \times \sqrt{N} \times 1$. We seek the dictionary D that minimizes

$$\min_{D,A} \sum_{j=1}^M \|\alpha_j\|_0, \text{ subject to} \|z_j - D\alpha_j\|_2 \le \epsilon, i = 1, \dots, N \tag{6}$$

where $\epsilon > 0$ is the prescribed error tolerance of representation error.

To solve (6), we start from an initial dictionary (i.e. the overcomplete DCT dictionary), and an initial estimation of the CBF parameter map (i.e. CBF map from cTSVD algorithm). Then K-SVD algorithm approaches the solution of (6) by alternating the following two steps: the minimization with respect to α with D fixed using orthogonal matching pursuit (OMP), and the update of atoms in D using the current A. The update stage modifies the atoms in D one by one to better represent the data Z. For each column $k = 1,2,...,K$, we find the index set $I_k = \{i: \alpha_{ki} \neq 0\}$, which is the set of indices of z_j's who used d_k in representation in the sparse coding step. Then we set error matrix $E_k = Z_k - D_k A_k$, where D_k is D with d_k replaced by 0. Z_k and A_k collect the columns with indices in I_k from Z and A. Finally, we apply SVD decomposition $E_k = U \Lambda V^T$. Update d_k in D with the first column of U, and the coefficients in α_j with the entries in V multiplied by $\Lambda(1,1)$. Theoretically K-SVD solver may not produce stable results, while in this specific application and in all experimental the solver works very well and yields stable reconstructed images.

Sparse Perfusion Deconvolution (SPD): When the dictionary D is known, the CBF perfusion parametric map from the low-dose CTP data can be estimated using our sparse perfusion deconvolution method by minimizing (5) in an iterative fashion. Our SPD method also consists of *iterating* the following two steps: minimization with respect to α with x fixed, and update of x with α fixed.

The first step is sparse coding, which is formulated a

$$\text{Min}_\alpha \|\alpha\|_0, \quad \text{subject to} \quad \|x - D\alpha\|_2 \leq \epsilon \tag{7}$$

where the value of ϵ implies specific value for μ_2. Equation (7) can be solved by any matching pursuit algorithm. Here we use orthogonal matching pursuit (OMP).

The second step is to minimize

$$\min_x \mu_1 \|C - C_a R\|_2^2 + \|x - D\alpha\|_2^2 \tag{8}$$

Because $x = R(t = 0)$, (8) can be rewritten as

$$\min_x \mu_1 \|C - C_a \hat{R} \cdot diag(x)\|_2^2 + \|x - D\alpha\|_2^2 \tag{9}$$

where $\hat{R}$ is the residue functions normalized by x so that $\hat{R}(t = 0) = 1$. (9) is a quadratic term that has a closed-form solution.

If vec(B) denotes the vector formed by the entries of a matrix B in column major order, and define $P = C_a \hat{R}$, then

$$\text{vec}\left(C - C_a \hat{R} \cdot diag(x)\right) = \text{vec}\left(C - P \cdot diag(x)\right) = \text{vec}(C) - Mx \tag{10}$$

where M is a $TN \times N$ matrix in form of

$$M = \begin{pmatrix} P_{,1} & 0 & \cdots & 0 \\ 0 & P_{,2} & \cdots & 0 \\ \vdots & \vdots & \ddots & \vdots \\ 0 & 0 & \cdots & P_{,N} \end{pmatrix}$$

where $P_{.i}$. dictates the ith column of matrix P in its column vector form. Equation (9) can be transformed into the conventional least square problem

$$\min_x \|(I_n; M)x - [D\alpha; \text{vec}(C)\|_2^2 \tag{11}$$

Let $A = (I_n; M)$. and $B = (D\alpha; \text{vec}(C))$, we get

$$x = A^+ B \tag{12}$$

where A^+. is the pseudo-inverse of matrix A, $(.;,)$ denotes a vector or matrix by stacking the arguments vertically.

To address the global CBF deconvolution problem, we use a sliding window of size $\sqrt{N} \times \sqrt{N}$ on the specific slice and overlaps the windows by step size of 1. The final global CBF parametric map is generated by averaging the areas that the windows overlap.

3   Experiments

In this section, we describe the results from comparing our approach with cTSVD on two clinical subjects with ischemia related to vasospasm. The presence and location of the perfusion deficits were identified by board-certified radiologists with subspecialty training in neuroradiology.

3.1   Data Acquisition

CTP was performed during the typical time-period for vasospasm in aneurysmal subarachnoid hemorrhage, between days 6-8 in asymptomatic patients and on the same day clinical deterioration occurred in symptomatic patients. There is a standard scanning protocol for CTP at our institution using GE Lightspeed or Pro-16 scanners (General Electric Medical Systems, Milwaukee, WI) with cine 4i scanning mode and 45 second acquisition at 1 rotation per second using 80 kVp and 190 mA.

3.2   Experimental Results

For cTSVD, a threshold of 6% of the maximum singular value is used, in accordance with parameter tuning in our experiments. For all experiments, the dictionary used are of size 64×256, designed to handle perfusion image patches of 8×8 pixels. In all experiments, the denoising process uses a sparse coding of each patch of size 8×8 pixels from noisy image. The parameters are chosen empirically and the experimental results are not sensitive to the parameters. Repetitive scanning of the same patient at different radiation doses is unethical and a physiological phantom which can uptake contrast agent is currently not available. Thereby, low-dose CTP data is simulated following the practice in [11], where Gaussian noise $\varepsilon \sim N(0, \sigma^2)$ is added to the high-dose CTP data. In the following, peak signal-to-noise ratio (PSNR) is calculated by dividing the peak value of the tissue time-enhancement curve by the noise standard deviation σ.

1) *Learned Dictionaries:* Figure 1 shows the redundant DCT dictionary on the left, with each atom of an 8×8 pixel image. This dictionary was used as the initialization for the training. The globally trained dictionary is shown on the right side of Fig. 1. This dictionary was trained on a data-set of 10,000 8×8 patches of high-dose CBF perfusion maps.

2) *LACA Estimation:* Figure 2 shows CBF maps and the zoomed-in regions of a normal clinical subject. The zoomed-in region of the left anterior cerebral artery (LACA) territory (in X-ray image left and right are opposite) of the CBF map using TSVD in high-dose (190mA), low-dose   (PSNR=20) and using SPD in low-dose (PSNR=20) are shown on the right. The vascular region supplied by the LACA has increased noise in the CBF map using TSVD.

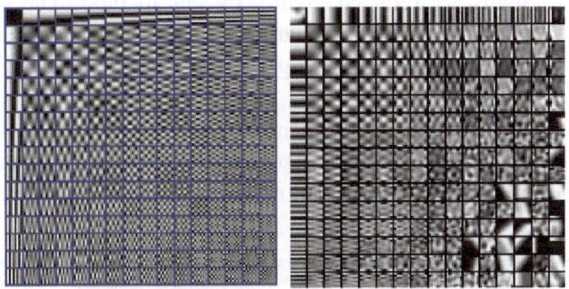

Fig. 1. Left: DCT dictionary. Right: Globally trained dictionary using high-dose CBF maps.

In comparison, significantly improved spatial smoothness in the vascular region and higher color contrast between the artery region and the vascular region can be observed from the CBF map computed using our proposed method. The standard deviation the LACA region computed using TSVD and SPD under different PSNR are shown in Table 1.

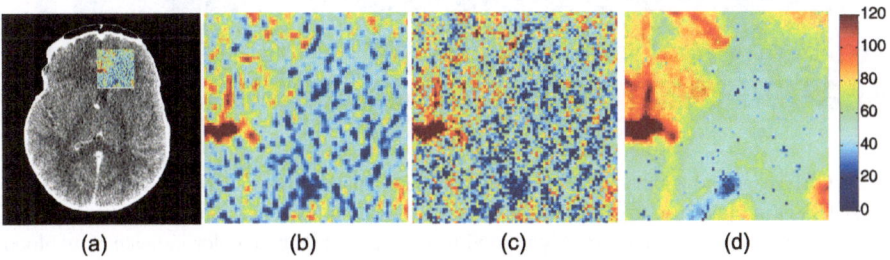

(a)   (b)   (c)   (d)

Fig. 2. (a) An acquired CT image from a CTP exam in a normal subject. (b) Left anterior cerebral artery (LACA) territory using cTSVD in high-dose (190mA) (c) cTSVD in low-dose (PSNR=20) (d) our proposed SPD in low-dose (PSNR=20) data.

Table 1. Standard deviation of the LACA region on a patient with normal blood flow under different PSNR using TSVD and our SPD method

PSNR	20	40	60	80
TSVD	56.09	47.11	23.14	22.98
SPD	41.94	42.12	16.44	16.47

3) Ischemic Comparison: We also show the CBF maps processed for patients with ischemic deficits (Figure 3) using TSVD and our proposed SPD on high-dose and low-dose CTP data. On the left, the low value of CBF in the ischemic patient becomes more evident while the vascular regions become smoother and variations in the estimated blood flow maps are reduced greatly by our method. The difference of the blood flows between the vascular and the artery regions were significantly enlarged.

4) Ischemic Voxels Clustering: By aggregating all voxels (within the VOI) from the normal patient data sets into a single "normal" group with n_1 samples, and the ischemia patient data sets into an "abnormal" group with n_2 samples. In our case, $n_1=1000$ and $n_2=1000$. To quantify the separability between normal and ischemic CBF values, we define the distance between these two clusters as:

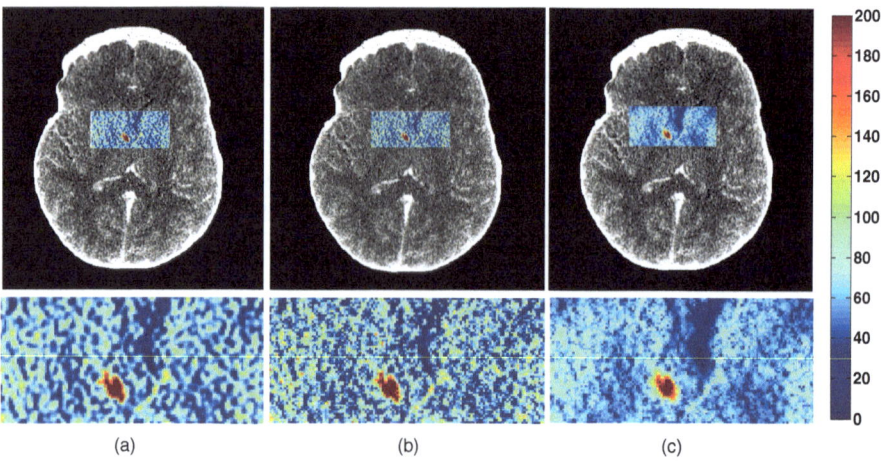

(a)   (b)   (c)

Fig. 3. CBF maps and zoomed-in regions in an ischemic patient with a RMCA deficit estimated by (a) TSVD in high-dose (b) TSVD in low-dose (c) SPD in low-dose. Low blood flow is delineated in blue. Red color indicates high blood flow value, while blue color indicates low blood flow value.

$$d = \frac{\mu_1 - \mu_2}{\sqrt{\sigma_1^2 / n_1 + \sigma_2^2 / n_2}} \tag{13}$$

where μ_1, μ_2 are the means, and σ_1, σ_2 are the standard deviations of CBF in the normal and ischemic clusters respectively. We expect our SPD algorithm to produce larger distance d as defined in Eq. (13), that is, to more definitely differentiate between normal and ischemic regions in the brain. Fig.4 show scatter plots of normal vs. ischemic clusters. It is apparent that the two clusters are more separable in data processed via SPD than TSVD.

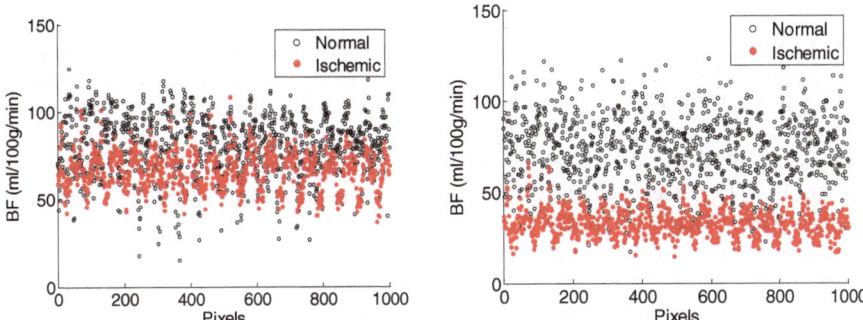

Fig. 4. (a) Two clusters of normal vs. ischemic regions in the brain generated by TSVD method. The distance d between two clusters is 22.67. (b) Two clusters of normal vs. ischemic regions by our sparse perfusion deconvolution method. The distance d between two clusters is 63.79.

4   Conclusion

In this paper, we introduced a novel sparsity-based deconvolution algorithm to estimate cerebral blood flow in low-dose CTP. We trained a dictionary using CBF maps computed from high-dose CTP and then performed deconvolution-based hemodynamic parameter estimation of the low-dose CTP data. The experimental results indicated that our algorithm not only outperforms TSVD algorithm but also may significantly improve the diagnostic performance of ischemia related to vasospasm in aneurysmal subarachnoid hemorrhage patients.

Acknowledgement. The authors would like to thank Prof. David Bindel for his valuable comments on matrix computation and Prof. Krishna Juluru for making the phantom data of the noise model available.

References

1. Østergaard, L., Weisskoff, R.M., Chesler, D.A., Gyldensted, C., Rosen, B.R.: High Resolution Measurement of Cerebral Blood Flow Using Intravascular Tracer Bolus Passages. Part I: Mathematical Approach and Statistical Analysis. Magn. Reson. Med. 36, 715–725 (1996)
2. Wittsack, H.J., Wohlschlager, A., Ritzl, E., Kleiser, R., Cohnen, M., Seitz, R., Moder, U.: CT-Perfusion Imaging Of The Human Brain: Advanced Deconvolution Analysis Using Circulant Singular Value Decomposition. Computerized Med. Imag. Graphics 32, 67–77 (2008)

3. He, L., Orten, B., Do, S., Karl, W.C., Kambadakone, A., Sahani, D.V., Pien, H.: A Spatio-Temporal Deconvolution Method To Improve Perfusion CT Quantification. IEEE Transactions on Medical Imaging 29(5), 1182–1191 (2010)
4. Mouridsen, K., Friston, K., Hjort, N., Gyldensted, L., Ostergaard, L., Kiebel, S.: Bayesian estimation of cerebral perfusion using a physiological model of microvasculature. Neuro Image 33, 570–579 (2006)
5. Pack, N., DiBella, E., Rust, T., Kadrmas, D., McGann, C., Butterfield, R., Christian, P., Hoffman, J.: Estimating Myocardial Perfusion From Dynamic Contrast-Enhanced CMR With A Model-Independent Deconvoution Method. J. Cardiovas. Magn. Reson. 10, 52 (2008)
6. Wong, K., Tam, C., Ng, M., Wong, S., Young, G.: Improved Residue Function and Reduced Flow Dependence In MR Perfusion Using Least-Absolute-Deviation Regularization. Magn. Reson. Med. 61, 418–428 (2009)
7. Fang, R., Chen, T., Sanelli, P.C.: Sparsity-Based Deconvolution of Low-dose Brain Perfusion CT in Subarachnoid Hemorrhage Patients. In: IEEE Proceedings of the Ninth International Symposium on Biomedical Imaging (2012)
8. Fang, R., Raj, A., Chen, T., Sanelli, P.C.: Radiation Dose Reduction In Computed Tomography Perfusion Using Spatial-Temporal Bayesian Methods. In: Pelc, N.J., Nishikawa, R.M., Whiting, B.R. (eds.) Medical Imaging. SPIE, vol. 8313, pp. 45–53 (2012)
9. Elad, M., Aharon, M.: Image Denoising Via Sparse and Redundant Representations Over Learned Dictionaries. IEEE Transactions on Image Processing 15(12) (2006)
10. Aharon, M., Elad, M., Bruckstein, A., Katz, Y.: K-SVD: An Algorithm for Designing of Overcomplete Dictionaries for Sparse Representation. IEEE Transactions on Signal Processing 54, 4311–4322 (2006)
11. Britten, A., Crotty, M., Kiremidjian, H., Grundy, A., Adam, E.: The Addition of Computer Simulated Noise to Investigate Radiation Dose and Image Quality in Images with Spatial Correlation of Statistical Noise: An Example Application to X-Ray CT of the Brain. British Journal of Radiology 77(916), 323 (2004)

Fast Multi-contrast MRI Reconstruction

Junzhou Huang[1], Chen Chen[1], and Leon Axel[2]

[1] Department of Computer Science and Engineering, University of Texas at
Arlington, TX, USA 76019
[2] Department of Radiology, New York University, New York, NY 10016

Abstract. This paper proposes an efficient algorithm to simultaneously
reconstruct multiple T1/T2-weighted images of the same anatomical
cross section from partially sampled k-space data. The simultaneous reconstruction problem is formulated as minimizing a linear combination
of three terms corresponding to a least square data fitting, joint total-
variation (TV) and group wavelet-sparsity regularization. It is rooted in
two observations: 1) the variance of image gradients should be similar for
the same spatial position across multiple contrasts; 2) the wavelet coefficients of all images from the same anatomical cross section should have
similar sparse modes. To efficiently solve this formulation, we decompose
it into group sparsity and joint TV regularization subproblems, respectively. Finally, the reconstructed image is obtained from the weighted
average of solutions from two subproblems in an iterative framework.
We compare the proposed algorithm with previous methods on SRT24
multi-channel Brain Atlas Data. Experiments demonstrate its superior
performance for multi-contrast MR image reconstruction.

1 Introduction

Magnetic Resonance Imaging (MRI) has been widely used to image the same
anatomical cross section under multiple contrast settings, since the multi-contrast
MRI can achieve superior power for clinical diagnosis over individual T1, T2 or
proton-density weighted images.

Recent developments in compressive sensing (CS) theory [1] show that accurate MRI reconstruction can be achieved from highly undersampled k-space
data. Motivated by the CS theory, Lustig et al. [2] proposed their pioneering
work SparseMRI for CS-MRI. They showed that the combination of gradient
and wavelet sparsity is far better than each of them separately in CS-MRI.
However, their method based on conjugate gradient (CG) is not fast enough for
practical MR images. Operator-splitting (TVCMRI [3]) and variable splitting
(RecPF [4]) techniques were proposed then to accelerate this problem. Both
of them gain time savings over the SparseMRI [2]. Recently, a composite splitting algorithm (FCSA [5] [6]) further accelerated this problem with convergence
guarantee $\mathcal{O}(1/\sqrt{\varepsilon})$), where ε is the accuracy. It was the best algorithm among
ones that were tested.

All above introduced methods are designed for individual MR image reconstruction. When they are directly applied to each of multi-contrast MR

N. Ayache et al. (Eds.): MICCAI 2012, Part I, LNCS 7510, pp. 281–288, 2012.

images, the CS theory guides us that the necessary measurement number is $\mathcal{O}(TK + TKlog(n/K))$ [1], where T is the contrast number, K is the sparsity number and n is the pixel number. However, the multi-contrast MR images are not independent but highly correlated. If one of them has smaller values in wavelet or gradient domain in a spatial position, all of them should likely have smaller values in wavelet or gradient domain for the same position. So, they should be group sparse on wavelet or gradient domain, not only standard sparse. According to the group sparsity theory for CS [7], the necessary measurement number can be reduced to $\mathcal{O}(TK + Klog(n/K))$ instead of $\mathcal{O}(TK + TKlog(n/K))$.

Unfortunately, no work has fully utilized these benefits so far. In [8], group sparsity is exploited on wavelet coefficients of multi-contrast MR images to achieve better results than standard sparsity. However, they did not consider the group sparsity on gradients. In [9], group sparsity on gradients of multi-contrast MRI is exploited under a multi-task Bayesian framework [10]. However, it is unknown how to couple group wavelet-sparsity into their method. Intuitively, better performance can be achieved by fully exploiting group sparsity on both wavelet and gradient domains for multi-contrast MRI.

This paper proposes an efficient algorithm to further accelerate multi-contrast MRI by fully exploiting the group sparsity on both wavelet and gradient domain over multi-contrast. The reconstruction problem is formulated as minimizing a linear combination of three terms corresponding to a least square data fitting, joint total-variation (TV) and group wavelet-sparsity regularization. A novel algorithm FCSA-MT is developed to efficiently solve this problem. It can obtain an ϵ-optimal solution in $\mathcal{O}(1/\sqrt{\epsilon})$ iterations. Extensive experiments on Multi-contrast Brain MRI data demonstrate its superior performance over all previous methods in term of the reconstruction accuracy and computational complexity.

2   Related Work

2.1   Compressed Sensing MRI

The CS MRI [2][3][4][5] can be formulated as follows:

$$\hat{x} = \arg\min_x \{\frac{1}{2}\|Rx - b\|^2 + \alpha\|x\|_{TV} + \beta\|\Phi x\|_1\} \tag{1}$$

where α and β are two positive parameters, b is the undersampled measurements of k-space data, R is a partial Fourier transform, Φ is a wavelet transform and x denotes the MR image. The TV was defined discretely as $\|x\|_{TV} = \sum_{i=1}^{n}\sqrt{((\nabla_1 x_i)^2 + (\nabla_2 x_i)^2)}$ where ∇_1 and ∇_2 denote the forward finite difference operators on the first and second coordinates, respectively. Several classic methods have been proposed to attack this problem, including CG [2], TVCMRI [3], RecPF [4] and FCSA [5]. As far as we know, the FCSA is the best in terms of both reconstruction accuracy and computational complexity.

The FCSA [5] solves the problem :$\min_x\{F(x) \equiv f(x) + g_1(x) + g_2(x), x \in \mathbf{R}^n\}$, where f is a smooth convex function with Lipschitz constant L_f, and $g_{i=1,2}$ are

Algorithm 1 FCSA [5]	**Algorithm 2** Proposed FCSA-MT
Input: $\rho = \frac{1}{L_f}$, α, β, $t^1 = 1$ $z = x^0$	**Input:** $\rho = \frac{1}{L_f}$, α, β, $t^1 = 1$ $z_s = x^0$
for $k = 1$ **to** N **do**	**for** $k = 1$ **to** N **do**
$\quad y = z - \rho \nabla f(z)$	$\quad Y(:,s) = z_s - \rho \nabla f_s(z_s)$, $s = 1, \ldots, T$
$\quad x_1 = \arg\min_x \{\frac{1}{4\rho}\|x-y\|^2 + \alpha\|x\|_{TV}\}$	$\quad X_1 = \arg\min_X \{\frac{1}{4\rho}\|X-Y\|^2 + \alpha\|X\|_{JTV}\}$
$\quad x_2 = \arg\min_x \{\frac{1}{4\rho}\|x-y\|^2 + \beta\|\Phi x\|_1\}$	$\quad X_2 = \arg\min_X \{\frac{1}{4\rho}\|X-Y\|^2 + \beta\|\Phi X\|_{2,1}\}$
$\quad x^k = \frac{x_1+x_2}{2}$; $t^{k+1} = \frac{1+\sqrt{1+4(t^k)^2}}{2}$	$\quad X^k = \frac{X_1+X_2}{2}$; $t^{k+1} = \frac{1+\sqrt{1+4(t^k)^2}}{2}$
$\quad z = x^k + \frac{t^k-1}{t^{k+1}}[x^k - x^{k-1}]$	$\quad z_s = X^k(:,s) + \frac{t^k-1}{t^{k+1}}[X^k(:,s) - X^{k-1}(:,s)]$
end for	**end for**

convex functions. $\nabla f(x)$ denotes the gradient of the function f at the point x. $x \in \mathbf{R}^n$ is called an ϵ-optimal solution to the problem if $F(x) - F(x^*) \leq \epsilon$ holds.

In the problem of CS-MRI, $f(x) = \frac{1}{2}\|Rx - b\|^2$, $g_1(x) = \alpha\|x\|_{TV}$ and $g_2(x) = \beta\|\Phi x\|_1$. Algorithm 1 outlines the FCSA. It can obtain an ϵ-optimal solution in $\mathcal{O}(1/\sqrt{\epsilon})$ iterations. Moreover, the cost of each iteration is $\mathcal{O}(n\log(n))$ in FCSA for problem (1).

2.2   Multi-contrast Reconstruction

Multi-contrast MRI reconstruction means the simultaneous reconstruction of multiple T1/T2-weighted MR images $\{x_s\}_{s=1}^T \in \mathbf{R}^n$ for the same anatomical cross section from partially sampled k-space data $\{b_s\}_{s=1}^T$. In [8], group sparsity is exploited on wavelet coefficients of multi-contrast MR images instead of standard sparsity. Its formulation is as follows:

$$\hat{X} = \arg\min_X \|\Phi X\|_{2,1}; \sum_{s=1}^T \|R_s X(:,s) - b_s\|^2 \leq \sigma^2 \qquad (2)$$

where $X = [x_1, ..., x_T] \in \mathbf{R}^{n \times T}$ are multi-contrast images, and R_s is the measurement matrix of $m_s \times n$ for x_s. The L21 norm term was defined as $\|\Phi X\|_{2,1} = \sum_{i=1}^n (\sqrt{\sum_{s=1}^T (\Phi X_{is})^2})$. Then, the SPGL1 [11] is directly used to solve it. However, they did not consider the group sparsity on gradients (unknown how to add it into their framework).

In [9], group sparsity on gradients of multi-contrast MRI is exploited under a multi-task Bayesian framework [10]. In their work, the gradients of images are reconstructed from their measurements in k-space under a Bayesian framework. Their experiments show the advantage of group sparsity on gradients over conventional sparsity. However, due to the inherent shortcoming of Bayesian frameworks, their method is very slow. It is also unknown how to couple group wavelet-sparsity into their method.

Algorithm 3 Proposed FJGP for Joint Total Variation

Input: ρ,α, Y, $(R_s, S_s) = (P_s, Q_s) = (\mathbf{0}_{(n_1-1) \times n_2}, \mathbf{0}_{n_1 \times (n_2-1)})$
for $k = 1$ **to** N **do**
   $t^{k+1} = \frac{1+\sqrt{1+4(t^k)^2}}{2}$
   for $s = 1$ **to** T **do**
     $(P_s^k, Q_s^k) = \mathbb{P}_p[(R_s, S_s) + \frac{1}{16\rho\alpha}\mathcal{L}^T\mathbb{P}_C[Y(:, s) - 2\rho\alpha\mathcal{L}(R_s, S_s)]]$
     $(R_s, S_s) = (P_s^k, Q_s^k) + \frac{t^k-1}{t^{k+1}}(P_s^k - P_s^{k-1}, Q_s^k - Q_s^{k-1})$
   end for
end for
$X(:, s) = \mathbb{P}_C[Y(:, s) - 2\rho\alpha\mathcal{L}(P_s^K, Q_s^K)]$ for $i = 1, ..., T$

---

3   Fast Multi-contrast Reconstruction

3.1   Formulation and Algorithm

In the multi-contrast setting, the MR images denote MRI scans with different image weights. We have two observations about them: 1) the variance of image gradients should be similar for the same spatial position across multiple contrasts; 2) the wavelet coefficients of all MR images from the same spatial positions have similar sparse modes. Intuitively, better performance can be achieved by fully exploiting group sparsity on both wavelet and gradient domains for multi-contrast MRI. Motivated by these, the simultaneous reconstruction problem can be formulated as follows:

$$\hat{X} = \arg\min_{X}\{\frac{1}{2}\sum_{s=1}^{T}\|R_sX(:, s) - b_s\|^2 + \alpha\|X\|_{JTV} + \beta\|\Phi X\|_{2,1}\} \qquad (3)$$

where α and β are two positive parameters, b_s is the undersampled measurements of k-space data for the s-th MR image $x_s = X(:, s)$, R_s is a partial Fourier transform for x_s and Φ is a wavelet transform. The JTV was defined discretely as $\|X\|_{JTV} = \sum_{i=1}^{n}\sqrt{\sum_{s=1}^{T}((\nabla_1 X_{is})^2 + (\nabla_2 X_{is})^2)}$. Algorithm 2 outlines the proposed algorithm for the multi-contrast reconstruction. Its efficiency is highly dependent on how quickly we can solve the second step and third step in each iteration. They correspond to two subproblems: JTV and group wavelet sparsity problem.

3.2   Group Wavelet Sparsity

The step 3 in Algorithm 2 is to solve the group wavelet sparsity problem:

$$\hat{X} = \arg\min_{X}\{\frac{1}{4\rho}\|X - Y\|^2 + \beta\|\Phi X\|_{2,1}\} \qquad (4)$$

It has a closed form solution by the soft thresholding:

$$(\Phi\hat{X})_i = max(1 - \frac{2\rho\beta}{\|(\Phi Y)_i\|_2}, 0)(\Phi Y)_i \tag{5}$$

where $(\cdot)_i$ denotes the i-th row of the matrix for $i = 1, ..., n$.

3.3   Joint Total Variation

The step 2 in Algorithm 2 is to solve the JTV denoising problem:

$$X_1 = \arg\min_{X}\{\frac{1}{4\rho}\|X - Y\|^2 + \alpha\|X\|_{JTV}\} \tag{6}$$

As far as we know, there is no closed form solution for it. The Fast Gradient Projection (FGP) algorithm for TV [12] can not directly solve it, due to the different formulation. Fortunately, we can develop a new method, called Fast Joint-Gradient Projection (FJGP) algorithm, for this JTV problem by modifying the FGP algorithm in [12].

Algorithm 3 outlines the proposed FJGP. Due to page limitation, we follow the notations in FGP [12]. Please refer FGP [12] for more details. n_1 and n_2 denote the width and height of an image with $n_1 * n_2 = n$, $\mathcal{L}(P, Q)_{i,j,s} = P_{i,j,s} - P_{i-1,j,s} + Q_{i,j,s} - Q_{i,j-1,s}$ for $i \in [1, n_1]$, $j \in [1, n_2]$, $s \in [1, T]$. The $\mathcal{L}^T$ is defined as $\mathcal{L}^T(X) = (P, Q)$, where $P \in \mathbf{R}^{(n_1-1)\times n_2 \times T}$ and $Q \in \mathbf{R}^{n_1 \times (n_2-1) \times T}$. The $\mathbb{P}_p$ is a projection operator used to ensure that $\sum_{s=1}^{T}(P_{i,j,s}^2 + Q_{i,j,s}^2) \leq 1$, $|P_{i,n_2,s}| \leq 1$ and $|Q_{n_1,j,s}| \leq 1$. The $\mathbb{P}_C$ is a projection operator to ensure the reconstructed X stay in the constrained set C. The proposed FJGP algorithm has fast convergence performance, borrowed from the FGP [12]. It converges in $\mathcal{O}(1/\sqrt{\epsilon})$ iterations. The computation cost is $\mathcal{O}(Tn)$ in each iteration.

3.4   Convergence and Complexity

The proposed FCSA-MT algorithm has fast convergence performance, borrowed from the FCSA [5]. It can obtain an ϵ-optimal solution in $\mathcal{O}(1/\sqrt{\epsilon})$ iterations. The cost of each iteration in the proposed algorithm is $\mathcal{O}(Tn \log(n))$, as confirmed by the following observations. The steps 4 and 5 only involve adding vectors or scalars, and thus cost only $\mathcal{O}(Tn)$ or $\mathcal{O}(1)$. In step 1, $\nabla f_s(z_s) = R_s^T(R_s z_s - b_s)$, since $f_s(z_s) = \frac{1}{2}\|R_s z_s - b_s\|^2$ in this case. Thus, this step only costs $\mathcal{O}(Tn \log(n))$. The second step (JTV) can be quickly solved by the proposed FJGP with cost $\mathcal{O}(Tn)$; the third step (group wavelet sparsity) has a closed form solution and can be computed with cost $\mathcal{O}(Tn \log(n))$.

4   Experiments

4.1   Experiment Setup

Our experiments were conducted on the multi-contrast data extracted from the SRI24 Multi-Channel Brain Atlas Data [13]. The MR images were acquired

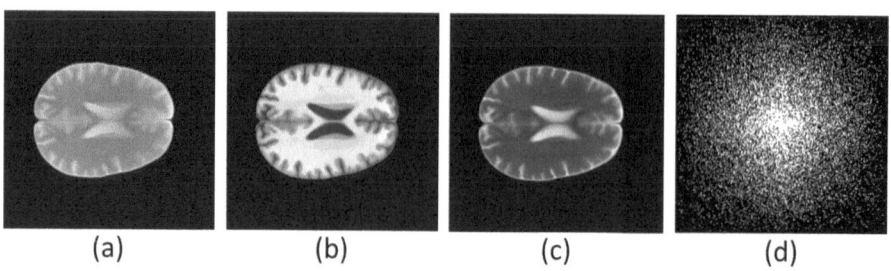

(a)   (b)   (c)   (d)

Fig. 1. SRI24 Multi-Channel Brain Atlas Data [13]: a) Proton density-weighted image; (b) T1-weighted image; (c) T2-weighted image and (d) Sampling mask

with three different contrast settings at 3T: 1) Proton density-weighted images: they were acquired with a 2D axial dual-echo fast spin echo (FSE) sequence (TR=10,000 ms, TE=14 ms); 2) T1-weighted images: they were acquired with a 3D axial IR-prep Spoiled Gradient Recalled (SPGR) sequence, where TR=6.5 ms and TE=1.54 ms; and 3) T2-weighted images: they were acquired with the same sequence as the proton density-weighted scan. However, TE equals 98 ms in this case. The data includes 620 MR images with size 256×256 covering a 24-cm field-of-view.

The partial Fourier transform R_s in problem (3) consists of m_s rows of a $n \times n$ matrix corresponding to the full 2D discrete Fourier transform. The m_s selected rows correspond to the acquired b_s. The sampling ratio is defined as m_s/n. To randomly select rows in k-space, we randomly obtained more samples at low frequencies and less samples at higher frequencies. This sampling scheme is the same as those in [2][3][4][5] and has been widely used in CS-MRI. Figure 1 shows example images and the sampling mask.

All experiments were conducted on a 2.2GHz PC in Matlab environment. We compared the proposed FCSA-MT [1] with conventional CS-MRI methods (CG [2], TVCMRI [3], RecPF [4] and FCSA[5]) and two recent multi-contrast reconstruction methods (SPGL1 [8] and Bayesian [9]). For fair comparisons, the codes were obtained by downloading them from their websites or asking for them from the authors. We carefully followed their experiment setup. The regularization parameters α and β were set as 0.001 and 0.035.

4.2   Numerical Results

We first compared the proposed method with conventional CS-MRI methods on all images. The sample ratio was set to be approximately 25%. To perform fair comparisons, all methods ran 50 iterations, except that the CG ran only 8 iterations due to its higher complexity. To reduce the randomness, each experiment ran 100 times. Figure 2(a) gives the performance comparisons between different methods in terms of the CPU time over SNR. The proposed algorithm

---

[1] Code available in http://ranger.uta.edu/~huang/R_CSMRI.htm

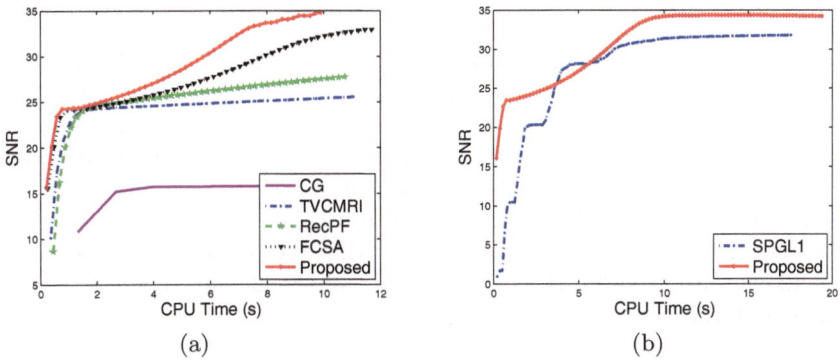

Fig. 2. Performance comparisons (CPU-Time vs. SNR): a) Conventional CS-MRI, CG [2], TVCMRI [3],RecPF [4] and FCSA [5]; b) Multi-contrast CS-MRI:SPGL1 [8] vs. Proposed

Table 1. Bayesian [9] vs. Proposed for Multi-contrast CS-MRI

	BAYESIAN [9]					PROPOSED				
ITERATIONS	1000	1500	2000	2500	3000	10	15	20	25	30
TIME (S)	144	305	516	829	1199	0.4	0.5	0.7	0.9	1.1
SNR (DB)	24.9	25.2	27.9	28.3	29.1	25.4	29.7	30.9	31.1	31.2
MSSIM (%)	97.75	98.62	99.05	99.30	99.47	93.32	98.75	99.25	99.44	99.63

is always the best, by achieving the highest SNR in less CPU time. The FCSA is always inferior to the proposed FCSA-MT, which shows the effectiveness of simultaneous reconstruction for multi-contrast MRI.

We then compared the proposed method with two multi-contrast reconstruction methods (SPGL1 [8] and Bayesian [9]) on all images. The sample ratio was set to be approximately 25%. To reduce the randomness, each experiment ran 100 times for each parameter setting of each method. Figure 2(b) gives the performance comparisons between the proposed method and SPGL1 [8] in terms of the CPU time vs. SNR. The proposed algorithm is always better, by achieving the higher SNR in less CPU time. As the Bayesian method is too slow, we resized the images to 128 × 128. Table 1 tabulates the comparison between the Bayesian method [9] and the proposed method on all images. Besides SNR, mean Structural Similarity (MSSIM) [14] is also considered for result evaluation. The proposed method is always best, in terms of both reconstruction accuracy and computational complexity. These results are reasonable, as we consider group sparsity on both wavelet domain and gradient domain while others only exploit one of them. This clearly demonstrates its effectiveness and efficiency for multi-contrast reconstruction.

5   Conclusion

We have proposed an efficient algorithm for multi-contrast CS-MRI. The contributions of our work are as follows. First, the proposed FCSA-MT achieves the best reconstruction performance over all previous methods. Second, the computational cost of the proposed method is only $\mathcal{O}(Tn\log(n))$ in each iteration. It can obtain an ϵ-optimal solution in $\mathcal{O}(1/\sqrt{\epsilon})$ iterations. These properties make real-time multi-contrast CS-MRI much more feasible than before. Finally, numerous experiments were conducted to show that the proposed method outperforms all conventional CS-MRI methods and two recent multi-contrast CS-MRI methods in terms of accuracy and complexity.

References

1. Donoho, D.: Compressed sensing. IEEE Transactions on Information Theory 52(4), 1289–1306 (2006)
2. Lustig, M., Donoho, D., Pauly, J.: Sparse MRI: The application of compressed sensing for rapid MR imaging. Magnetic Resonance in Medicine 58, 1182–1195 (2007)
3. Ma, S., Yin, W., Zhang, Y., Chakraborty, A.: An efficient algorithm for compressed MR imaging using total variation and wavelets. In: Proceedings of CVPR (2008)
4. Yang, J., Zhang, Y., Yin, W.: A fast alternating direction method for TVL1-L2 signal reconstruction from partial fourier data. IEEE Journal of Selected Topics in Signal Processing, Special Issue on Compressive Sensing 4(2) (2010)
5. Huang, J., Zhang, S., Metaxas, D.: Efficient MR Image Reconstruction for Compressed MR Imaging. In: Jiang, T., Navab, N., Pluim, J.P.W., Viergever, M.A. (eds.) MICCAI 2010, Part I. LNCS, vol. 6361, pp. 135–142. Springer, Heidelberg (2010)
6. Huang, J., Zhang, S., Metaxas, D.: Efficient MR image reconstruction for compressed MR imaging. Medical Image Analysis 15, 670–679 (2011)
7. Huang, J., Zhang, T.: The benefit of group sparsity. Annals of Statistics 38, 1978–2004 (2010)
8. Majumdar, A., Ward, R.: Joint reconstruction of multiecho MR images using correlated sparsity. Magnetic Resonance Imaging 29, 899–906 (2011)
9. Bilgic, B., Goyal, V., Adalsteinsson, E.: Multi-contrast reconstruction with bayesian compressed sensing. Magnetic Resonance Medicine 66, 1601–1615 (2011)
10. Ji, S., Dunson, D., Carin, L.: Multitask compressive sensing. IEEE Transactions on Signal Processing 57, 92–106 (2009)
11. Berg, E., Friedlander, M.: Probing the pareto frontier for basis pursuit solutions. SIAM Journal on Scientific Computing 31, 890–912 (2008)
12. Beck, A., Teboulle, M.: Fast gradient-based algorithms for constrained total variation image denoising and deblurring problems. IEEE Transaction on Image Processing 18(113), 2419–2434 (2009)
13. Rohlfing, T., Zahr, N.M., Sullivan, E., Pfefferbaum, A.: The sri24 multichannel atlas of normal adult human brain structure. Human Brain Mapping 31, 798–819 (2010)
14. Wang, Z., Bovik, A.C., Sheikh, H.R., Simoncelli, E.P.: Image quality assessment: From error measurement to structural similarit. IEEE Transactions on Image Processing 13(4), 600–612 (2004)

Steady-State Model
of the Radio-Pharmaceutical Uptake
for MR-PET

Stefano Pedemonte[1], M. Jorge Cardoso[1], Simon Arridge[1],
Brian F. Hutton[2], and Sebastien Ourselin[1]

[1] The Centre for Medial Image Computing, UCL, London, United Kingdom
[2] Institute of Nuclear Medicine, UCL Hospitals NHS Trust, London, United Kingdom

Abstract. This work explores a fully-automated algorithm for estimation of the uptake of radio-pharmaceutical in brain MR-PET imaging. The algorithm is based on a model of the pharmaceutical uptake coupled with probabilistic models of the PET and MR acquisition systems. In contrast to algorithms that attempt to correct for the Partial Volume Effect (PVE), the problem is tackled here in the reconstruction by means of a probabilistic model of the pharmaceutical uptake. We make use of Hybrid Bayesian Networks to describe the joint probabilistic model and to obtain an efficient optimisation algorithm. We describe solutions adopted in order to mitigate the effect of local maxima and to reduce the sensitivity to the initialisation of the parameters, rendering the algorithm fully automatic. The algorithm is evaluated on simulated MR-PET data and on the reconstruction of clinical PET FDG acquisitions.

1   Introduction

Uncertainty in Emission Tomography is dominated by photon count statistics. It is therefore essential to adopt a probabilistic model of the emission and interaction of the Gamma photons in order to use optimally the information at hand for the quantification of the uptake of the radio-pharmaceutical. Given a generative probabilistic model of the emission imaging system (outlined here in Sec. 2.1), the spatial density of radio pharmaceutical can be estimated by Maximum Likelihood (ML) [1]. However, due to the acquisition being photon-limited, the information about the pharmaceutical density is scarce, thus determining an infinity of equally likely solutions (ill-posedness). Furthermore, optimisation of the likelihood can only be treated currently with greedy optimisation algorithms because of the high dimensionality of the unknown pharmaceutical density, and yet the unknowns (pharmaceutical density in each voxel) are strongly correlated due to the measurement of line integrals by the emission imaging system. For these reasons, algorithms for the optimisation of the likelihood present slow convergence rates, practically never reaching convergence, posing the unsolved problem of establishing a stopping criterion [2]. A smoothing prior is typically adopted in order to obtain a convergent algorithm; PET images obtained under

N. Ayache et al. (Eds.): MICCAI 2012, Part I, LNCS 7510, pp. 289–297, 2012.
© Springer-Verlag Berlin Heidelberg 2012

the assumption of smoothness, however, when overlaid on an intra-subject MR image, present the problem of *partial volume* or *spill out* effect: an observer can distinguish certain regions in common between the two images, but the PET image is smoother than the MR image, giving the observer the impression of spill out of the pharmaceutical. The partial volume effect, which is nothing else but the *bias* of the estimate of the pharmaceutical density, highlights how it is problematic to quantify the uptake of pharmaceutical in a region of interest obtained by segmentation of the MR image. Partial volume *correction* algorithms attempt to deconvolve the PET image in order to estimate the dose in one or more regions of interest by introducing certain assumptions about uniformity of the uptake in each region. However, since partial volume is due to the photon count statistics, the problem cannot be solved in the domain of the PET image for the reason that the PET reconstruction is a point estimate of the high dimensional likelihood function that describes the uncertainty of the measurement (and the photon counting process does not admit *sufficient statistics*). Though a number of partial volume *correction* algorithms have been proposed and are sometimes considered state of the art, concerns about the efficacy of such algorithms are starting to be raised [3].

In this paper we extend the work proposed by [4], which replaces the assumption of smoothness with a parametric model of the pharmaceutical uptake. Here we extend and improve on both the stability and convergence of the pharmaceutical uptake model of [4], making it suitable for clinical usage. Full automation is obtained by means of integration of population-based prior information, by the use of a local contextual model and by improving the robustness to intensity inhomogeneity of the MR image. To the best of our knowledge, this paper presents the first algorithm that combines models of the MRI and PET acquisition systems, pharmaceutical uptake, MRI intensity inhomogeneity correction and local contextual information in a unified framework.

2   Generative Model of the Pharmaceutical Uptake in Brain Tissue

This section will first introduce the Poisson model of the PET acquisition system (Sec. 2.1), followed by the hidden-state model of the pharmaceutical uptake (Sec. 2.2) and the hidden-state model of the MR acquisition system (Sec. 2.3). Sec. 2.4 will describe the joint model and Sec. 2.5 the algorithm for optimisation of the joint probability distribution.

2.1   Model of the PET Acquisition System

The rate of emission of Gamma rays is a continuous function over the spatial domain of the patient's body and proportional to the local density of radiopharmaceutical. Assuming that photon counts z_d for the lines of response (LOR) indexed by $d = 1, \ldots, N_d$, are caused only by the radiation emitted by the radio pharmaceutical and approximating the continuous emission rate by a discrete set

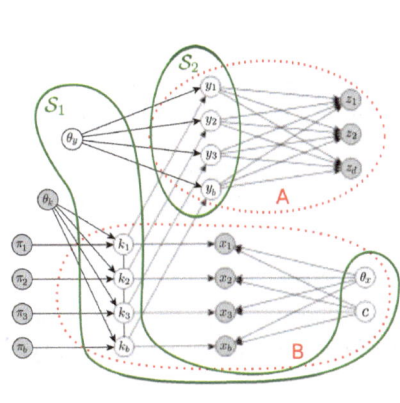

MR image:
$x = \{x_b\};\quad b = 1, \ldots, N_b;\quad x_b \in \mathbb{R}^+$
Pharmaceutical density:
$y = \{y_b\};\quad b = 1, \ldots, N_b;\quad y_b \in \mathbb{R}^+$
Photon counts:
$z = \{z_d\};\quad d = 1, \ldots, N_d;\quad z_d \in \mathbb{N}$
Hidden states:
$k = \{k_b\};\quad b = 1, \ldots, N_b;\quad k_b \in \{e_1, .., e_N\}$
Tissue-specific parameters of MR image:
$\theta_x = \{\mu_{x_n}, \sigma_{x_n}\};\quad n = 1, \ldots, N;\quad \mu_{x_n}, \sigma_{x_n} \in \mathbb{R}^+$
Parameters of the pharmaceutical uptake model:
$\theta_y = \{\mu_{y_n}, \sigma_{y_n}\};\quad n = 1, \ldots, N;\quad \mu_{y_n}, \sigma_{y_n} \in \mathbb{R}^+$
Coeff. of the polynomials for bias field correction:
$c = \{c_j\};\quad j = 1, \ldots, J;\quad c_j \in \mathbb{R}$
Parameters of the spatial dependence of k:
$\theta_k = G_i;\quad i = 1, \ldots, N^2;\quad g_i \in \mathbb{R}$
Population-based multinomial prior distrib. of k:
$\pi = \pi_{bn};\quad n = 1, \ldots, N;\quad \pi_{bn} \in (0, 1);\quad \sum_n \pi_{bn} = 1$
N_b: num. of voxels; N_d: num. of lines of response; N: num. of classes; J: num. of basis functions; e_n: unit vector of length N, n-th element is 1.

Fig. 1. Hybrid Bayesian Network model of the pharmaceutical uptake for the MR-PET imaging system. Observed and assumed quantities are shaded. The MR image intensity x_b and the pharmaceutical density y_b are assumed to be independent conditionally to the hidden tissue state k_b. Hidden states are drawn from a MRF with first order neighbourhood structure and have a spatially dependent multinomial prior probability distribution π_b, obtained from population data. A: PET acquisition system; B: MR imaging system. The optimisation algorithm iteratively updates variables $\mathcal{S}_1$ and $\mathcal{S}_2$.

of point sources $y = y_b, b \in \{1, \ldots, N_b\}$ displaced on a regular grid of voxels, the model of the imaging system is expressed graphically by Fig. 1-A. Letting p_{bd} be the probability that a photon emitted in b is detected in d, by the sum and thinning properties of the Poisson distribution, denoted by $\mathcal{P}$, and observing (from the d-separation property of the graph) that $z_{d'} \perp z_d | y, \forall\, d' \neq d$, the probability to observe photon counts z when activity is y, is expressed by (see [1]):

$$p(z|y) = \prod_{d=1}^{N_d} \mathcal{P}\left(\sum_{b=1}^{N_b} p_{bd} y_b, z_d\right) \tag{1}$$

The system matrix p_{bd} encompasses the characteristics of the imaging system (location, size, sensitivity, spatial resolution of the Gamma detectors, eventual collimators) and the attenuation of Gamma radiation through the patient, which can be approximated with a simple generic phantom of the brain or estimated from the MR image for the patient under examination Patient specific estimation of the attenuation coefficients from the MR image, however, is out of the scope of this paper.

2.2 Steady-State Model of the Pharmaceutical Uptake

It is assumed that there exist a finite number of tissue types and that, in a given type of tissue, the pharmaceutical uptake is to some extent predictable. The expectation and the extent of variation of the uptake within each type of tissue are captured by a parametric finite mixture model.

The hidden tissue states $k = \{k_1, \ldots, k_{N_b}\}$ are modelled as the realisation of a random process with parametric probability distribution $p(k|\theta_k)$, where $k_b = e_n$ for some value $n, 1 \leq n \leq N$, with N being the number of tissue types and e_n a unit vector of length N with n-th component equal to 1. The density of radio-pharmaceutical y_b in a voxel b belonging to class n is assumed to be normally distributed around a certain mean μ_{y_n}, with variance $\sigma_{y_n}^2$, grouped in $\theta_{y_n} = \{\mu_{y_n}, \sigma_{y_n}^2\}$:

$$p(y_b|k_b = e_n) = \mathcal{G}\left(y_b; \mu_{y_n}, \sigma_{y_n}\right) \tag{2}$$

$\theta_y = \{\theta_{y_1}, \ldots, \theta_{y_N}\}$ are the parameters of the pharmaceutical uptake model, describing the expectation and the extent of variation of the uptake in each type of tissue.

2.3 Model of the MR Acquisition System

The MR imaging system is described by a parametric voxel-based finite mixture model commonly employed for classification of tissue types by means of MR images [5]. It relates the observed image intensities to the underlying finite hidden tissue states. The log intensity x_b of a voxel b that belongs to class n is assumed to be normally distributed around a certain mean μ_{x_n}, with variance $\sigma_{x_n}^2$. The smoothly varying bias due to inhomogeneity of the magnetic field is modelled by a linear combination of J polynomial basis functions $\phi_j(X)$, where X denotes the 3D coordinates. Intensity is *log* transformed, as suggested in [5], in order to treat the bias field, which multiplicates the intensity, as an additive term:

$$p(x_b|k_b = e_n) = \mathcal{G}\left(x_b - \sum_{j=1}^{J} c_j \phi_j(X_b); \mu_{x_n}, \sigma_{x_n}\right) \tag{3}$$

where X_b are the coordinates of the voxels b. The model of the MR imaging system (3) is represented by the Bayesian Network in Fig. 1-B. The set of parameters are the bias field coefficients $c = \{c_1, \ldots, c_J\}$ and the mean and spread of the (log) intensity for each class, grouped in $\theta_x = \{\mu_{x_n}, \sigma_{x_n}^2\}, n = 1, \ldots, N$.

2.4 Joint Model

The hidden tissue states are considered the unique underlying cause of mutual dependence of the two images (as expressed by the arrows of the graph in Fig. 1). The hidden state in each voxel is related to the intensity of the MR image and to the pharmaceutical density (which is also a hidden variable) by the parametric models of Sec. 2.2 and Sec. 2.3. Such models are local, expressing the probability of the hidden state in voxel b only as a function of the MR intensity and pharmaceutical uptake in the voxel. The model is made more robust by adding contextual information in the form of spatial dependence of the hidden labels. Not only k_b depends on x_b and y_b, but on $k_{b'}, b' \neq b$ elsewhere. For computational convenience, the spatial dependence of k is modelled with a joint distribution of the variables k_b which factorises on the first order neighbourhood structure of the image lattice (Markov Random Field - MRF): k_b is assumed to be conditionally independent from all other states if its 6 nearest neighbours are known. The dependence of state k_b upon its neighbours $\mathcal{N}_b$ is expressed by the following Potts model $p(k_b|\mathcal{N}_b, \theta_k)$, parametrised by θ_k, which corresponds (Markov-Gibbs equivalence) to the joint density of the hidden states $p(k|\theta_k)$:

$$p(k_b|\mathcal{N}_b, \theta_k) = \frac{e^{-k_b^T G_{\theta_k} g_b}}{\sum_n^N e^{-k_b^T G_{\theta_k} g_b}} \qquad p(k|\theta_k) = \frac{e^{-\sum_b^{N_b} -k_b^T G_{\theta_k} g_b}}{Z} \qquad (4)$$

where g_b counts the labels of each class between the neighbours, G_{θ_k} is a $[N \times N]$ matrix of parameters of the Potts model that expresses the affinity of all pairs of states and Z is the partition function, not involved in the maximisation of the joint probability.

Finally, the probability of voxel b being in state n depends a priori on the location of b. Such prior distribution is expressed by a multinomial probability distribution π_{bn}, $\sum_n^N \pi_{bn} = 1$. The use of the spatially varying multinomial prior probability of the hidden states is key to automating the algorithm, as otherwise the parameters of the mixture models converge to different tissue classes non predictably.

2.5   Greedy Optimisation Algorithm

The joint probability distribution is optimised with the Iterated Conditional Modes (ICM) optimisation algorithm, consisting of iterating the optimisation of two subsets of the unknowns: $\mathcal{S}_1$ and $\mathcal{S}_2$ in Fig. 1. Iteratively, the algorithm computes $\mathcal{S}_1$ that increases the conditional probability distribution $p(\mathcal{S}_1|\mathcal{S}_2)$, given the provisional estimate of $\mathcal{S}_2$, then it computes a new value of $\mathcal{S}_2$ that increases $p(\mathcal{S}_2|\mathcal{S}_1)$. The choice of the two subsets corresponds to the existence of Generalised Expectation Maximisation (GEM) formulations for the optimisation of $p(\mathcal{S}_1|\mathcal{S}_2)$ and $p(\mathcal{S}_2|\mathcal{S}_1)$. The GEM algorithm to update $\mathcal{S}_1$ involves 4 steps (i.i, i.ii, i.iii, i.iv); while the One Step Late EM algorithm to update $\mathcal{S}_2$, involves a single step: ii. Derivation of the update formulae for the subsets $\mathcal{S}_1$ and $\mathcal{S}_2$ is described in [4] and [5], whose notation we maintain here; we report in the following the algorithm, which consists in iterating in order i.i, i.ii, i.iii, i.iv, ii:

i.i Estimate the probability p_{bn} that tissue state in voxel b is n. This step is necessary for the successive steps and arises from the GEM formulation [5].

$$p_{bn}^{(m+1)} \equiv \frac{p(y_b|k_b = e_n; \theta_y^{(m)})p(x_b|k_b = e_n; \theta_x^{(m)})p(k_b = e_n|p_{\mathcal{N}_b}^{(m)}; \theta_k)\pi_{bn}}{\sum_{n=1}^N p(y_b|k_b = e_n; \theta_y^{(m)})p(x_b|k_b = e_n; \theta_x^{(m)})p(k_b = e_n|p_{\mathcal{N}_b}^{(m)}; \theta_k)\pi_{bn}} \qquad (5)$$

where the spatial dependence term $p(k_b = e_n|p_{\mathcal{N}_b}^{(m)}; \theta_k)$ is approximated from the previous estimate of p_{bn} by the Mean Field approximation [5]:

$$p(k_b = e_n | p_{N_b}^{(m)}; \theta_k) = \frac{e^{-U_{\theta_k}(e_n | p_{N_b}^{(m)})}}{\sum_{n'=1}^{N} e^{-U_{\theta_k}(e_{n'} | p_{N_b}^{(m)})}} \qquad U_{\theta_k}(e_n | p_{N_b}^{(m)}) = k_b^T \, G_{\theta_k} \, g_b^{(m)}$$

(6)

$g_b^{(m)}$ being the vector of length N with elements $g_{bn}^{(m)} = \sum_{N_b} p_{bn}^{(m)}$. **i.ii** Update the tissue-specific parameters of the MR imaging system:

$$\mu_{x_n}^{(m+1)} = \frac{1}{N_b} \frac{\sum_{b=1}^{N_b} p_{bn}^{(m+1)} x_b}{\pi_{bn}} \qquad \sigma_{x_n}^{2(m+1)} = \frac{1}{N_b} \frac{\sum_{b=1}^{N_b} p_{bn}^{(m+1)} (\mu_{x_n}^{(m+1)} - x_b)^2}{\pi_{bn}} \quad (7)$$

i.iii Update the parameters of the pharmaceutical uptake model:

$$\mu_{y_n}^{(m+1)} = \frac{1}{N_b} \frac{\sum_{b=1}^{N_b} p_{bn}^{(m+1)} y_b}{\pi_{bn}} \qquad \sigma_{y_n}^{2(m+1)} = \frac{1}{N_b} \frac{\sum_{b=1}^{N_b} p_{bn}^{(m+1)} (\mu_{y_n}^{(m+1)} - y_b)^2}{\pi_{bn}} \quad (8)$$

i.iv Update the bias field parameters:

$$\begin{bmatrix} c_1^{(m+1)} \\ c_2^{(m+1)} \\ \cdots \end{bmatrix} = \left(A^T \, diag \, w_b^{(m+1)} \, A \right)^{-1} A^T \, diag \, w_b^{(m+1)} \begin{bmatrix} x_1 - \tilde{x}_1^{(m+1)} \\ x_2 - \tilde{x}_2^{(m+1)} \\ \cdots \end{bmatrix} \quad (9)$$

where A is the geometrical matrix of the bias field model, each of its columns evaluating the polynomial basis function ϕ_j at voxel coordinates X_b and

$$w_b^{(m+1)} = \sum_{n=1}^{N} w_{bn}^{(m+1)} \qquad w_{bn}^{(m+1)} = \frac{p_{bn}^{(m+1)}}{\sigma_{x_n}^{2(m+1)}} \qquad \tilde{x}_b^{(m+1)} = \frac{\sum_{n=1}^{N} w_{bn}^{(m+1)} \mu_{x_n}^{(m+1)}}{\sum_{n=1}^{N} w_{bn}^{(m+1)}}$$

ii Update the estimate of the pharmaceutical density (One Step Late EM algorithm for the Poisson model - see [1]):

$$y_b^{(m+1)} = y_b^{(m)} \frac{1}{\sum_{d=1}^{N_d} p_{bd} + \sum_{n=1}^{N} p_{bn}^{(m+1)} \frac{y_b^{(m)} - \mu_n^{(m+1)}}{\sigma_{x_n}^2}} \sum_{d=1}^{N_d} \frac{p_{bd} \, z_d}{\sum_{b'=1}^{N_b} p_{b'd} \, y_{b'}^{(m)}} \quad (10)$$

3   Results

Synthetic MR-PET FDG: Uptake of FDG was simulated by assigning typical average values observed in PET FDG scans to the BrainWeb (http://mouldy.bic.mni.mcgill.ca/brainweb/) ground truth tissue model: 4 parts uptake in the gray matter, 1 part in white matter, 0 in CSF. One hot and one cold spherical lesions of 14 mm diameter were simulated by augmenting the activity by 30% in the hot lesion and reducing it by 50% in the cold lesion. 30 PET scans with $150M$ counts were simulated with the PET-Sorteo simulator

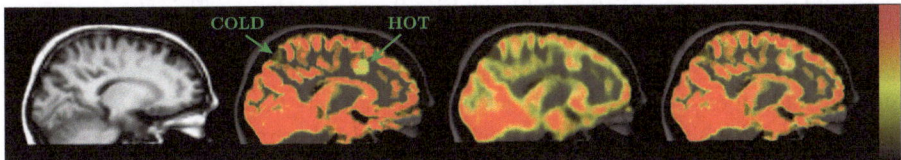

		White Matter	Internal Gray Matter	External Gray Matter	External CSF	Internal CSF	Hot Lesion	Cold Lesion
MLEM	COR	0.53	0.84	0.87	0.42	0.50	0.14	0.21
	SNR	10.21	7.78	17.67	7.59	3.65	1.13	1.01
UPTAKE MODEL	COR	0.86	0.95	0.95	0.81	0.84	0.14	0.20
	SNR	11.98	10.85	30.00	11.65	2.10	1.58	1.01

Fig. 2. Synthetic MR-PET FDG imaging data (see-through volume-rendering of 5 mm-thick sagittal slices). From left to right: T1-weighted MR image, activity phantom, MLEM reconstruction, reconstruction with the proposed pharmaceutical uptake model using 6 classes from the MNI-152 brain statistical atlas.

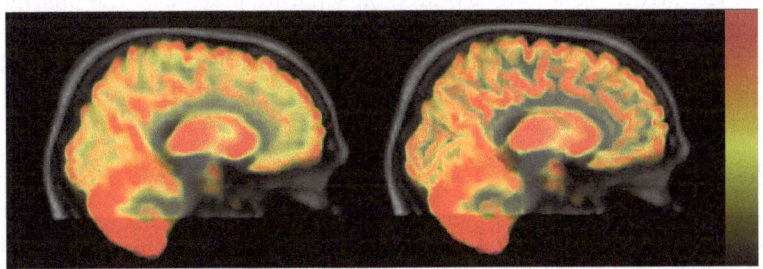

Fig. 3. PET FDG reconstructions obtained with MLEM (left) and with the proposed pharmaceutical uptake model (right) using 6 classes from the MNI-152 brain statistical atlas. See-through volume-rendering of 5 mm-thick sagittal slices.

and adding Poisson noise. The attenuation map was simulated by aligning non-rigidly a clinical CT-derived attenuation image to the Brainweb MR image with Normalised Mutual Information cost function. The 30 sinograms were then pre-corrected for scatter by energy thresholding and reconstructed with MLEM [1] and with the proposed algorithm. The number of classes N was set to 6: White Matter, Internal Gray Matter, External Gray Matter, External CSF, Internal CSF, everything else. The statistical atlas for the 6 classes was obtained from the MNI-152 atlas by splitting manually internal and external regions for the Gray Matter and CSF classes and aligning rigidly the MNI-152 T1-weighted MR template to the MR image with NMI cost function. The off-diagonal elements of the $N \times N$ parameter matrix θ_k were set to 0.1 and the diagonal elements to 0, penalising equally all transitions except for the transition to the identical class (more sophisticated parameter selection criteria are reported in [5]). The order of the polynomial for bias field correction J was set to 4. For simplicity both MLEM (non-convergent) and the proposed (convergent) algorithm were terminated after 50 iterations. Fig. 2 reports a sagittal slice of the reconstructions obtained for one of the 30 noise instances. The table in Fig. 2 reports the coefficient of recovery (COR) and signal to noise ratio (SNR) of the mean uptake in 8 regions of interest including the two lesions. The results highlight that the pharmaceutical uptake model yields measurements with less noise and less bias when the uptake is consistent with the model, producing remarkably truthful estimates. It is also remarkable that the lesions are well reconstructed even though they are outliers of the model (there isn't a class that captures the lesions), presenting overall improved SNR. This fact can be explained with the strong inter-correlation of the unknowns in emission imaging due to the line-integral measurements: improving the estimate everywhere outside of the lesion already improves the estimate in the lesion. Execution time on a Xeon E5430 equipped with NVidia GTX285 GPU is approximately 3 minutes for MLEM and 12 min for the Bayesian uptake model.

Clinical Data: The algorithm has been applied to clinical PET FDG using the same 6 classes that were employed in the synthetic PET FDG study. The emission data and the MR images were acquired on separate machines: the pharmaceutical density was estimated initially with MLEM, aligned with the MR image by rigid registration with NMI cost function and reconstructed again with the uptake model. Reconstructions are reported in Fig. 3.

4   Conclusion

In this paper we have extended the pharmaceutical uptake model presented by [4], making it fully automated. Robust estimation is achieved by 1) adopting a population-based statistical atlas to initialise and drive the optimisation of the parameters of the pharmaceutical uptake model and of the MR acquisition system model; 2) adding contextual information in the form of a Markov Random Field over the hidden tissue labels; 3) capturing the MR image bias field. We have evaluated the algorithm in a synthetic study, showing that it improves the quantification of the pharmaceutical uptake when the simulated data reflects the assumptions of the model and, remarkably, that the uptake estimate may improve also in regions that do not obey to the model. Validation with real data remains an open problem as it would require large sets of imaging data, possibly labelled with long term clinical outcome for specific imaging tasks. To this extent, automation of the reconstruction algorithm is crucial.

Source code of the synthetic experiment: http://niftyrec.sourceforge.net

Acknowledgement. This work has been supported by the EPSRC under Grant EP/G026483/1.

References

1. Green, P.G.: Bayesian Reconstructions From Emission Tomography Data Using a Modified EM Algorithm. IEEE Trans. on Med. Imag. 9(1), 84–93 (1990)
2. Nuyts, J., Baete, K., Bequ, D., Dupont, P.: Comparison between MAP and post-processed ML for image reconstruction in emission tomography when anatomical knowledge is available. IEEE Trans. on Med. Imag. 24(5), 667–675 (2005)
3. Moghbel, M.C., Saboury, B., Basu, S., Metzler, S.D., Torigian, D.A., Langstrom, B., Alavi, A.: Amyloid-β imaging with PET in Alzheimers disease: is it feasible with current radiotracers and technologies? E. J. of Nuc. Med. and Mol. Im. 39(2) (2012)
4. Pedemonte, S., Bousse, A., Hutton, B.F., Arridge, S., Ourselin, S.: 4-D Generative Model for PET/MRI Reconstruction. In: Fichtinger, G., Martel, A., Peters, T. (eds.) MICCAI 2011, Part I. LNCS, vol. 6891, pp. 581–588. Springer, Heidelberg (2011)
5. Van Leemput, K., Maes, F., Vandermeulen, D., Suetens, P.: Automated Model-Based Bias Field Correction of MR Images of the Brain. IEEE Trans. on Med. Imag. 18(10), 885–896 (1999)

Oriented Pattern Analysis
for Streak Detection in Dermoscopy Images

Maryam Sadeghi[1,2,3], Tim K. Lee[1,2,3], David McLean[2],
Harvey Lui[2], and M. Stella Atkins[1,2]

[1] School of Computing Science, Simon Fraser University, Canada
msa68@sfu.ca
[2] Department of Dermatology and Skin Science, University of British Columbia, Canada
[3] Cancer Control Research Program, BC Cancer Research Center, Canada

Abstract. There is an increasing demand for automated detection and analysis of dermoscopy structures and malignancy clues such as streaks in dermoscopy images, for computer-aided early diagnosis of deadly melanoma. This paper presents a novel approach for streak detection and visualization on dermoscopic images. We tackle the detection of streaks by means of ridge and valley estimation. Orientation estimation and correction is applied to detect low contrast and fuzzy streaks lines, and candidate streaks are used to classify dermoscopy images into streaks *Absent* or *Present* with the AUC of 90.5% on 300 dermoscopy images. Our approach can also detect starburst pattern of regular streaks using detected linear structures with accuracy of 81.5% and AUC of 87.7%.

1 Introduction

Melanoma is the most deadly form of skin cancer, yet treatable via excision if detected early. There is, therefore, a demand to develop computer-aided diagnostic systems to facilitate the early detection of melanoma. Dermoscopy, also known as epiluminescence microscopy (ELM), is an in-vivo noninvasive skin imaging method useful for the early recognition of malignant melanoma. For melanoma detection, in almost all of the dermoscopy methods, evaluation of dermoscopic structures focuses on structural features such as pigment network, streaks, dots, and globules [1].

Clinical Definition: Streaks is a term used interchangeably with radial streaming or pseudopods. Radial streaming is a linear extension of pigment at the periphery of a lesion radially arranged linear structures in the growth direction, and pseudopods represent finger-like projections of dark pigment (brown to black) at the periphery of the lesion. In order to ensure accurate recognition, streaks are numerated only when at least 3 near linear and parallel structures are clearly visible [1]. Streaks are *local* dermoscopy features of skin lesions, however they can correlate with a *global* pattern of skin lesions called a starburst pattern if symmetrically arranged over the entire lesion.

Mathematical Definition: The above clinical definition is translated to mathematical concepts with justified parameters to be captured by image processing techniques: 1) Streaks are 3 or more linear structures co-radially oriented in the boundary which is a contour with the thickness equal to $1/3$ of the minor axis of the lesion. 2) Streaks are

N. Ayache et al. (Eds.): MICCAI 2012, Part I, LNCS 7510, pp. 298–306, 2012.
© Springer-Verlag Berlin Heidelberg 2012

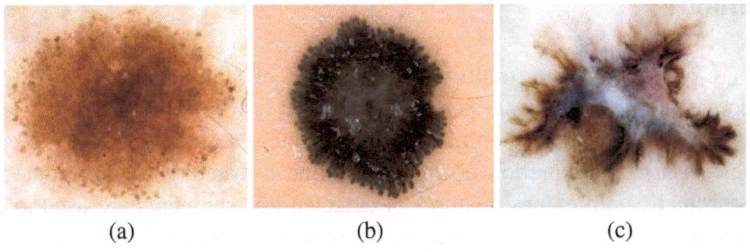

(a)   (b)   (c)

Fig. 1. Examples of absent, regular and irregular streaks. (a) shows a lesion without streaks (*Absent*). (b) illustrates a lesion with a complete symmetric regular streaks pattern called *starburst* (*Present*), and in (c), a melanoma lesion with irregular streaks is shown (*Present*).

darker than their neighborhood. 3) Streaks are shorter than the $1/3$ of the minor axis of the lesion and they should be longer than one percent of the major axis. 4) Streaks do not branch and their curvature is smaller than one.

Figure 1 shows examples of lesions with no streaks (*Absent*), regular (*Present*), and irregular (*Present*) streaks. Figure 1-a shows *Absent, 1-b* shows a starburst pattern, and Figure 1-c shows a lesion with irregular streaks and partial pattern.

Diagnostic Importance: Streaks are important morphologic expressions of malignant melanoma, specifically melanoma in the radial growth phase [2]. Irregular streaks is one of the most critical features (included in almost all of dermoscopy procedures) that shows the high association with melanoma. Also Menzies et al. [2] found pseudopods to be one of the most specific features of superficial spreading melanoma which is a subset of malignant melanoma. In addition, symmetric streaks (starburst pattern) is one of the specific dermoscopic criteria to differentiate usually benign Spitz nevi (a dark nevus common in children) from melanoma, thus increasing diagnostic accuracy for pigmented Spitz nevus. However, all lesions in adults exhibiting a starburst pattern should be excised for histopathological evaluation [2]. Therefore detection of streaks can be a significant step towards computer-aided diagnosis of skin lesions and melanoma detection.

As a fundamental step towards computer-aided diagnosis of skin cancers, automatic detection of many of these dermoscopic structures have been recently addressed in the literature [3,4]. However, the automatic detection of streaks has only recently been investigated [5,6]. Streaks on dermoscopy images usually are difficult to detect since they are not perfect linear structures, but often fuzzy and low-contrast oriented intensities. Furthermore, streaks may have unpredictable spatial distribution (partial pattern) with just a few streaks lines in a small region of a lesion. Therefore, it is not easy to detect them using general oriented pattern analysis. Mirzaalian et al. [6] have used a machine-learning approach for classifying streaks in dermoscopic images. Although the methodology is interesting, it, unfortunately, has been tested on a small number (99) of dermoscopic images with wide exclusion criteria. It is not clear how the method generalizes to all conditions of dermoscopic images captured in a dermatologist clinic.

This paper presents a novel method to estimate, enhance, detect and visualize streaks.

2 Method

After a pre-processing step, multi-scale Laplacian of Gaussian is applied to detect dermoscopy structures with Gaussian cross-sectional profile. After finding linear structures, the orientation flow of the image is analyzed to determine the orientation of detected objects in the orientation flow to select linear structures of candidate streaks. Finally, chromatic and textural features of detected line segments are used to classify the lesions into *Absent* or *Present* images. These steps are shown in Figure 2.

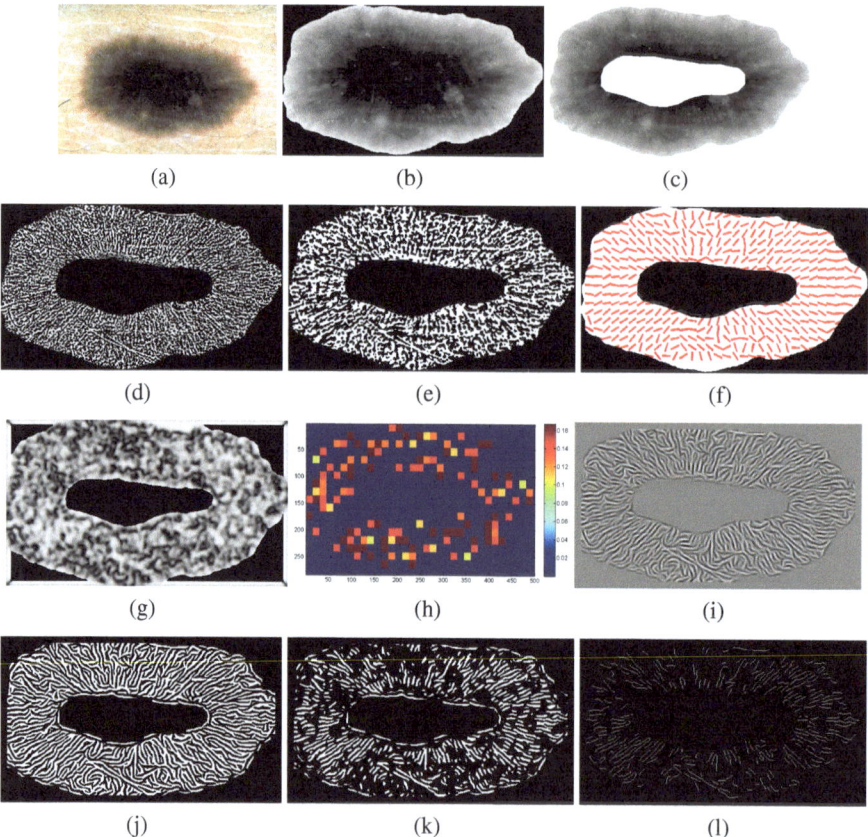

Fig. 2. The overview of the method. (a) shows a lesion with regular streaks and (b) illustrates the result of segmentation re-orientated and sharpening in the L* channel. (c) illustrates the region of interest that will be processed to find streaks. (d), and (e) show the LOG filter responses in the two scales $hsize_k = 3, 9$ respectively. In (f), the directional flow is plotted with red lines for $hsize_k = 9$, and (g) shows the reliability of estimation. The median frequency of the parallel pattern, illustrated in (h), is used in Gabor filters applied to enhance the estimated orientation shown in (i). (j) shows the binary image of the enhanced orientation with 1 for ridges and 0 for valleys. (k) is created from (g) and (j) by removing pixels with $reliability \leq 50\%$ and skeleton of the result is shown in (l) as detected candidate streaks structures.

2.1   Preprocessing

First the lesion is segmented using Wighton et al.'s method [7] and the orientation of the lesion is found, and the image is rotated to align the major axis horizontally since the major axis represents the lesion growth direction. Then, to have a relatively uniform image size, the lesion is re-sized so that its major axis occupies 500 pixels. Finally, the image is enhanced using a simple 3x3 high pass filter that removes the low frequency noise [3]. To get a single plane luminance image, the given RGB image is converted to the L*a*b color-space and L*, is used for the rest of our analysis (Figure 2-b).

2.2   Identifying Linear Structures after Enhancing Orientation

The region of interest (the boundary of the lesion) is found by computing the distance transform of the lesion mask. $1/3$ of the length of the lesion's minor-axis is used to compute the boundary area. Figure 2-c shows the region of interest to find streaks.

Blob Detection Using LOG: Since streaks are linear structures with Gaussian cross-sectional profiles, we detect them using Laplacian of Gaussian (LOG). To capture objects of different sizes a multi-scale approach is necessary. Thus, an input image $f(x, y)$ is filtered by rotationally symmetric LOG filters of size $hsize = 3, 5, 7, 9$ with a small value of 0.1 assigned to the standard deviation in order to achieve high sensitivity even to a small changes in intensity. At the end, we will union results of the four scales to form a multi-scale result. Figure 2-d and 2-e show the LOG responses at two different scales of $hsize_k = 3, 9$ respectively.

Estimating Orientation: After finding linear structures by LOG, the orientation estimation is performed using the Averaged Squared Gradient Flow (ASGF) algorithm [8]. The reason for using squared gradient instead of the elementary gradient is that after computing the local orientation for a pixel, the estimation will be averaged over a block of 16*16. Since a ridge line has two edges, the gradient vectors at both sides of a ridge are opposite to each other. Therefore, gradients cannot directly be averaged since opposite vectors will cancel each other, although they indicate the same ridge-valley orientation. Therefore, by applying ASGF that doubles the angles of the gradient vectors before averaging, opposite gradient vectors will point in the same direction and will reinforce each other. Also, the length of the gradient vectors is squared, as if the gradient vectors are considered as complex numbers that are squared. Thus, strong orientations have a higher vote in the average orientation than weaker orientations.

The qualitative analysis that was given above is made quantitative here. The algorithm starts by computing the gradients $G_x(i, j)$ and $G_y(i, j)$ at each pixel (i, j) in image I. For doubling the angle and squaring the length in ASGF, the gradient vector is converted to *polar* coordinates, in which it is given by $[G_\rho, G_\theta]$:

$$G_\rho = \sqrt{G_y^2 + G_x^2}, \qquad G_\theta = tan^{-1}(G_y, G_x) \qquad (1)$$

$$G_x = G_\rho * cos(G_\theta), \qquad G_y = G_\rho * sin(G_\theta) \qquad (2)$$

$$\begin{bmatrix} G_{s,x} \\ G_{s,y} \end{bmatrix} = \begin{bmatrix} G_\rho{}^2 cos(2G_\theta) \\ G_\rho{}^2 sin(2G_\theta) \end{bmatrix} = \begin{bmatrix} G_\rho^2(cos^2(G_\theta) - sin^2(G_\theta)) \\ G_\rho^2(2sin(G_\theta)cos(G_\theta)) \end{bmatrix} = \begin{bmatrix} G_x^2 - G_y^2 \\ 2G_x G_y \end{bmatrix} \qquad (3)$$

$$DF = \frac{1}{2} tan^{-1} \begin{bmatrix} \frac{2G_x G_y}{G_x^2 - G_y^2} \end{bmatrix} \qquad (4)$$

where $\begin{bmatrix} G_{s,x} \\ G_{s,y} \end{bmatrix}$ is the squared gradient and DF is the directional flow of image I.

The image is divided into blocks of size W=16. For each block, the local orientation centered at pixel (i, j) is estimated and averaged using DF as follows:

$$\begin{bmatrix} \overline{G_{s,x}} \\ \overline{G_{s,y}} \end{bmatrix} = \frac{1}{|W|} \begin{bmatrix} \sum_W G_x^2 - G_y^2 \\ \sum_W 2G_x G_y \end{bmatrix} \qquad (5)$$

To reduce the effect of noise on the estimated orientation, a low-pass filter (Gaussian) is used to modify the local ridge orientation. In order to apply the Gaussian filter, the orientation image is converted back to a continuous vector as follows:

$$\Phi_x(i,j) = cos(2G_\theta(i,j)), \qquad \Phi_y(i,j) = sin(2G_\theta(i,j)) \qquad (6)$$

$$\Phi'_x(i,j) = \sum_W F(i,j)\Phi_x(i,j), \qquad \Phi'_y(i,j) = \sum_W F(i,j)\Phi_y(i,j) \qquad (7)$$

where F is the Gaussian filter with unit integral and specified size $w_\Phi = 5$. Now, the local orientation and its reliability (the coherence of the squared gradients given by [8]) can be computed at pixel (i, j) using the following equation:

$$O(i,j) = \frac{1}{2} tan^{-1} \left(\frac{\Phi'_y(i,j)}{\Phi'_x(i,j)} \right), \qquad Reliability = \frac{|\sum_W (G_{s,x}, G_{s,y})|}{\sum_W |(G_{s,x}, G_{s,y})|}. \qquad (8)$$

which means if all squared gradient vectors are pointing in exactly the same direction, the sum of the vectors equals the modulus of the sum of the vectors, resulting in a coherence value of 1. On the other hand, if the gradient vectors are random in all directions, the sum of them will be 0, resulting in a coherence equal to 0. This algorithm results in a smooth intensity flow orientation over the image (shown in Figure 2-f), and Figure 2-g shows the reliability map of the orientation estimation in the example image.

Estimating Ridge Frequency: After finding the local orientation and averaging for image blocks, the local ridge frequency is estimated by rotating the block so that the ridges are vertical. Then, the columns are projected down to find peaks. The frequency of ridges can be calculated by dividing the distance between the first and last peaks by (number of peaks -1), and finally the median frequency is computed over all the blocks in the image. Figure 3-a shows an example block the image given in Figure 3-a. The result of rotating the block with the average block orientation to make it vertical is

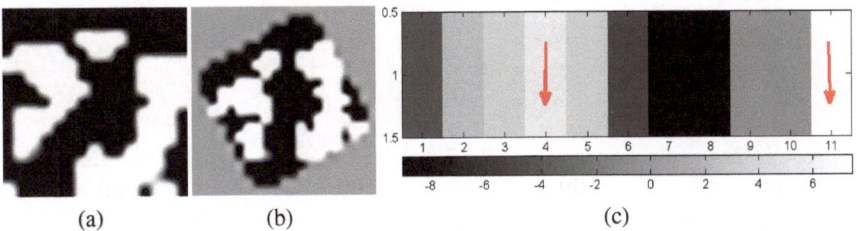

Fig. 3. Ridge frequency estimation. (a) shows an example block magnified for illustration (b) illustrates the result of rotation with average block orientation which is 30 degree for this block. (c) shows the projection result with red arrows pointing the peaks. The wavelength of this block is 11-4=7 that results in frequency of $1/7 = 0.14$.

shown in Figure 3-b, and the projection step is shown in 3-c. Now peaks of the block can be easily found using the histogram of projection. The frequency can be found using these peaks and their wavelength. The final result of frequency estimation for all blocks of our example image (2-d) is shown in Figure 2-h.

Enhancing Orientation Image: From [9], a Gabor filter with tuned ridge frequency and orientation, can remove the noise efficiently while preserving true ridges and valleys. The even-symmetric Gabor filter has the general form of $g(x, y; f, \theta, \sigma) = \exp\left(-\frac{x'^2+y'^2}{2\sigma^2}\right)\cos(2\pi f x')$, $x' = x\cos\theta + y\sin\theta$, and $y' = -x\sin\theta + y\cos\theta$, where σ is the sigma of the Gaussian kernel in the filter, and f and θ are the corresponding median ridge frequency over the image and local orientation respectively. The result of this step is shown in Figure 2-i. Figure 2-j shows the binary image of the enhanced orientation created by thresholding (1 for ridges and 0 for valleys), and Figure 2-k is created from (j) and (g) by removing pixels with $reliability \leq 50\%$. The skeleton of the result is shown in (l) as detected linear structures in the image. These line segments will be used for feature extraction in the next step.

Figure 4 demonstrates our streak detection method qualitatively. Figures 4-a, and 4-c illustrate *absent* images and their results are shown in 4-b and 4-d. In the second row, Figure 4-e and 4-g, shows two starburst lesions (*regular* streaks) with their streaks detected in Figure 4-f and 4-h respectively. Two melanomas with *irregular* streaks are shown in the third row with their corresponding results.

2.3   Feature Extraction and Classification

Based on our mathematical definitions of streaks, we propose a new set of 12 features called *STR* which includes three structural, six chromatic, and 3 textural characteristics of candidate streaks. In *STR*, **Structural** set includes the number of candidate streaks in the image, average number of pixels of candidate streaks, and the ratio of the streaks size to the lesion size in pixels; **Chromatic** set consists of the mean, standard deviation and reciprocal of coefficient of variation (mean/stdev) of candidate streaks in L* and S, and std of H; and **Textural** features are energy, contrast, and homogeneity of candidate streaks. We have also used common color and texture features [4] of the lesion itself

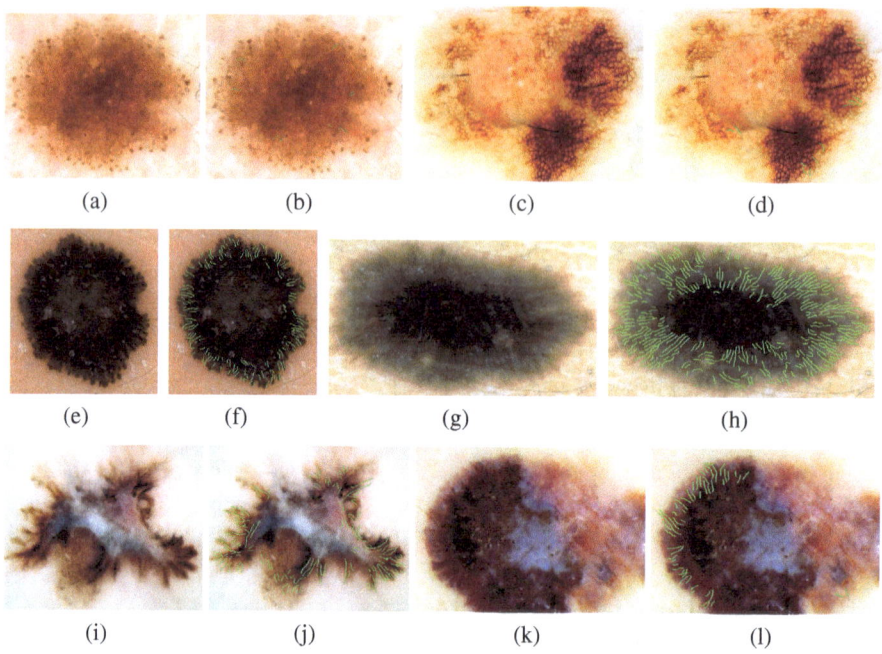

Fig. 4. Qualitative results. (a), and (c) illustrate *absent* lesions with their results in (b) and (d). (e) and (g) are starburst lesions. Their *regular* streaks are shown in (f) and (h). Two melanomas with *irregular* streaks are shown in the third row, (i) and (k), with their results in (j) and (l).

(called *LCT*). *LCT* includes the following 13 features: The mean, standard deviation and reciprocal of coefficient of variation (mean/stdev) of values in H, S, and V from HSV and L* of L*a*b*, and four of the classical Gray-level co-occurrence matrix based texture measures; energy, contrast, correlation, and homogeneity [4]. Finally, these 25 features are fed into the SimpleLogistic classifier implemented in Weka.

3   Results

Using ten-fold cross-validation, we evaluated our proposed approach on streak detection on a set of 300 dermoscopy images, including 105 *absent* and 195 *present*. 250 images are chosen randomly from two atlases of dermoscopy [10,1], and 50 images are taken from experts' archives with permission. Corrupted images due to the acquisition parameters such as lighting and magnification, partial lesions (entire lesion was not visible), or lesions occluded with an unreasonable amount of either oil or hair are excluded. Using the L channel of the L*a*b* colour channel as the luminance image for streak detection, we obtained the best performance for both data sets. For 300 images, accuracy of *Absent/Present* classification using L* is 85%, with AUC of 90.5%. In the second experiment, 200 images (100 *starburst*, and 100 *non-starburst*) are used to evaluate the performance of our method on starburst detection. We achieved the accuracy

Table 1. This table shows results of *LCT* (first row) and *STR* (second row) separately and combined (third row) for the multi-scale analysis on the L* on classifying N lesions with (*Present*) and without (*Absent*) streaks. The last row shows the evaluation on another set ($N = 200$) for finding starburst pattern. The last column (AUC) shows the Area Under ROC curve.

Experiment	N	Features	Prec.	Recall	FMeasure	Acc.	AUC
Abs/Pres	300	LCT	0.712	0.722	0.713	0.722	0.779
		STR	0.835	0.837	0.835	0.837	0.901
		LCT+STR	**0.85**	**0.87**	**0.86**	**0.85**	**0.905**
Starburst	200	**LCT+STR**	**0.815**	**0.815**	**0.815**		**0.815**	**0.877**

of 81.5% and AUC of 87.7% using 10-fold cross validation. Table 1 reports the details. Assuming the difficulty level of the images in [6] is similar to those of one of our data sets, our approach achieves an AUC of 90.5% comparing to 80% reported in [6].

4   Conclusion

We have presented an automatic approach for detection of radially oriented streaks on 300 real dermoscopic images, using techniques based on ridge and valley detection used in fingerprint image recognition. We demonstrated that the proposed approach can detect streaks in dermoscopy images and visualize them. Furthermore, with locating streaks and providing a qualitative analysis, it can be used to highlight suspicious areas for experts diagnosis and for visualization and training purposes.

Acknowledgments. This work was funded by the Canadian NSERC, CIHR-Skin Research Training Center and a grant from the Canadian Health Research Project (CHRP).

References

1. Soyer, H., Argenziano, G., et al.: Dermoscopy of pigmented skin lesions. An atlas based on the Consensus Net Meeting on Dermoscopy 2000. Edra, Milan (2001)
2. Menzies, S., Ingvar, C., McCarthy, W.: A sensitivity and specificity analysis of the surface microscopy features of invasive melanoma. Melanoma Research 6(1), 55–62 (1996)
3. Sadeghi, M., Razmara, M., Lee, T., Atkins, M.: A novel method for detection of pigment network in dermoscopic images using graphs. Computerized Medical Imaging and Graphics 35(2), 137–143 (2011)
4. Sadeghi, M., Razmara, M., Wighton, P., Lee, T.K., Atkins, M.S.: Modeling the Dermoscopic Structure Pigment Network Using a Clinically Inspired Feature Set. In: Liao, H., Eddie Edwards, P.J., Pan, X., Fan, Y., Yang, G.Z. (eds.) MIAR 2010. LNCS, vol. 6326, pp. 467–474. Springer, Heidelberg (2010)
5. Betta, G., Di Leo, G., et al.: Automated application of the 7-point checklist diagnosis method for skin lesions: Estimation of chromatic and shape parameters. In: Proceedings of the IEEE Instrumentation and Measurement Technology Conference, pp. 1818–1822 (2005)

6. Mirzaalian, H., Lee, T., Hamarneh, G.: Learning features for streak detection in dermoscopic color images using localized radial flux of principal intensity curvature. In: IEEE Workshop on Mathematical Methods for Biomedical Image Analysis, pp. 97–101 (2012)

7. Wighton, P., Sadeghi, M., Lee, T.K., Atkins, M.S.: A Fully Automatic Random Walker Segmentation for Skin Lesions in a Supervised Setting. In: Yang, G.-Z., Hawkes, D., Rueckert, D., Noble, A., Taylor, C. (eds.) MICCAI 2009, Part II. LNCS, vol. 5762, pp. 1108–1115. Springer, Heidelberg (2009)

8. Kass, M., Witkin, A.: Analyzing oriented patterns. Computer Vision, Graphics, and Image Processing 37(3), 362–385 (1987)

9. Hong, L., Wan, Y., Jain, A.: Fingerprint image enhancement: Algorithm and performance evaluation. IEEE Trans. on Pattern Anal and Machine Intelligence 20, 777–789 (1998)

10. Argenziano, G., Soyer, H., et al.: Interactive Atlas of Dermoscopy (Book and CD-ROM). Edra Medical Publishing and New Media (2000)

Automated Foveola Localization in Retinal 3D-OCT Images Using Structural Support Vector Machine Prediction

Yu-Ying Liu[1], Hiroshi Ishikawa[2,3], Mei Chen[4], Gadi Wollstein[2],
Joel S. Schuman[2,3], and James M. Rehg[1]

[1] College of Computing, Georgia Institute of Technology, Atlanta, GA
[2] UPMC Eye Center, University of Pittsburgh School of Medicine, Pittsburgh, PA
[3] Department of Bioengineering, University of Pittsburgh, Pittsburgh, PA
[4] Intel Science and Technology Center on Embedded Computing, Pittsburgh, PA

Abstract. We develop an automated method to determine the foveola location in macular 3D-OCT images in either healthy or pathological conditions. Structural Support Vector Machine (S-SVM) is trained to directly predict the location of the foveola, such that the score at the ground truth position is higher than that at any other position by a margin scaling with the associated localization loss. This S-SVM formulation directly minimizes the empirical risk of localization error, and makes efficient use of all available training data. It deals with the localization problem in a more principled way compared to the conventional binary classifier learning that uses zero-one loss and random sampling of negative examples. A total of 170 scans were collected for the experiment. Our method localized 95.1% of testing scans within the anatomical area of the foveola. Our experimental results show that the proposed method can effectively identify the location of the foveola, facilitating diagnosis around this important landmark.

1 Introduction

The foveola is an important anatomical landmark for retinal image analysis [1]. It is located in the center of the macula, responsible for sharp central vision. Several clinically-relevant indices are measured with respect to the foveola location, such as the retina's average thickness, or drusen size within concentric circles around the foveola [1, 2]. In addition, many macular diseases are best observed around the foveola, such as macular hole, and age-related macular degeneration [3]. Therefore, the localization of the foveola in retinal images is an important first step for diagnosis and longitudinal data analysis.

There has been extensive work in determining the foveola location in 2D color fundus images [1, 4]. However, there has been *no published work on automated foveola localization in retinal 3D-OCT images*. Researchers in ophthalmology typically need to determine this landmark in 3D-OCT images manually [2, 3].

Examples of the foveola location in 3D-OCT images are illustrated in Fig. 1, where the *OCT en-face* is a 2D image generated by projecting the 3D-OCT volume along the z (depth) axis, a x-y plane analogous to the *fundus* image.

N. Ayache et al. (Eds.): MICCAI 2012, Part I, LNCS 7510, pp. 307–314, 2012.
© Springer-Verlag Berlin Heidelberg 2012

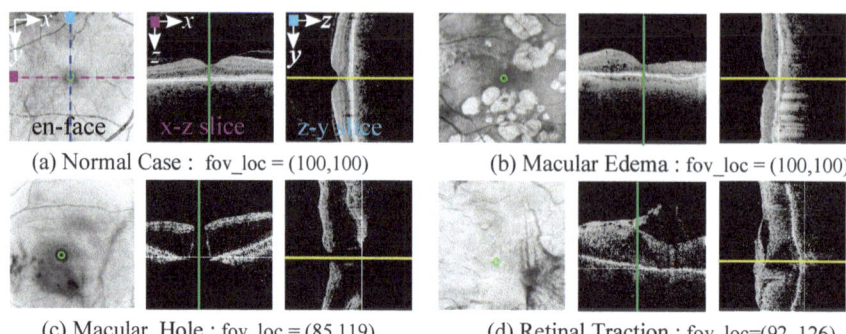

(a) Normal Case : fov_loc = (100,100)   (b) Macular Edema : fov_loc = (100,100)

(c) Macular Hole : fov_loc = (85,119)   (d) Retinal Traction : fov_loc=(92, 126)

Fig. 1. Examples of the foveola's (x,y) location in normal and diseased cases. On the en-face image, the (x, y) location is marked by a *green* circle, while in the corresponding x-z (horizontal) and z-y (vertical) slice, the x and y location is shown in *green* and *yellow* line, respectively. (The 3D scan is normalized to 200x200x200 dimension.)

From Fig. 1, we can see that the localization task is not trivial, since the foveola can have significant appearance changes due to various ocular diseases.

In the literature, an object localization or detection task is usually formulated as a discriminative binary classification problem [5–7], where *zero-one* loss term is employed. In training, the annotated ground truth locations form the positive set, while a number of negative examples are typically randomly-sampled. Each negative example is treated *equally negative*, regardless of its distance or area of overlap to the ground truth. Thus, the loss function used in training may not be the same as the one utilized in performance evaluation in testing (e.g. the Euclidean distance). This scheme has been applied to localizing organs in whole-body scans [5] and detection of liver tumors [6].

Recently Blaschko et. al [8] proposed to pose the object localization task as a *structural prediction* problem. Specifically, they adopted Structural Support Vector Machine (S-SVM) formulation [9, 10] to directly predict the coordinates of the target object's bounding box in a 2D image. S-SVM learns to predict outputs that can be a multivariate structure. The relationship between a possible output and the ground truth is explicitly modeled by a desired *loss* function. During training, the constraints state that the score at the ground truth should be higher than that of any other output by a required margin set to the loss term [9]. This formulation considers all possible output locations during training, and directly minimizes the empirical risk of localization. They have shown that the S-SVM outperforms binary classification for object localization in several 2D image datasets. However, *S-SVM has not yet been applied to medical image analysis.*

In the context of our task, the output space is the space of possible locations of the foveola in the 3D-OCT scan, which makes this problem a multivariate structural prediction problem. We adopt S-SVM framework to directly minimize the localization risk during training. A coarse-to-fine sliding window search approach is proposed to efficiently find the most-violated constraint in S-SVM's cutting-plane training and in prediction. In feature construction, multi-scale spatially-distributed texture features are designed to encode the appearance in the neighborhood of any candidate 3D position. We conducted experiments to compare S-SVM's performance with a human expert, and with the binary SVM classifier to validate our approach.

This paper makes three main contributions: (1) Introduce a formulation of the foveola localization problem in 3D-OCT as structured output prediction, which can be solved using S-SVM method. (2) Propose a coarse-to-fine sliding window-based approach to identify the most-violated constraint during S-SVM training. (3) Demonstrate high prediction accuracy using a dataset of 170 scans.

2   Approach

2.1   Formulation of Structural SVM in Foveola Localization Task

For our task, the optimization problem is formulated as follows: given a set of training scans $(a_1, ..., a_n) \subset A$ and the annotated foveola locations $(b_1, ..., b_n) \subset B$, the goal is to learn a function $g : A \mapsto B$ with which we can automatically label novel images. Note that since there is no consensus in defining the z (depth) location of the foveola in ophthalmology, we consider the output space B consisting of only the (x, y) labels. The extent of the retina in z direction can be estimated by a separate heuristic procedure and serves as an input for feature extraction (explained in Section 2.3).

The mapping g is learned by using the structured learning formula [9] as

$$g(a) = \text{argmax}_b \ f(a, b) = \text{argmax}_b \ \langle w, \phi(a, b) \rangle \tag{1}$$

where $f(a, b) = \langle w, \phi(a, b) \rangle$ is a linear discriminant function that should give a large score to pair (a, b) if they are well-matched, $\phi(a, b)$ is a feature vector associating input a and output b, and w is the weight vector to be learned. To learn w, we use the following *1-slack margin-rescaling* formulation of S-SVM [9],

$$\min_{w, \xi \geq 0} \ \frac{1}{2} w^T w + C\xi \tag{2}$$

$$s.t. \ \forall (\bar{b}_1, ..., \bar{b}_n) \in B^n : \frac{1}{n} \sum_{i=1}^{n} [\langle w, \phi(a_i, b_i) \rangle - \langle w, \phi(a_i, \bar{b}_i) \rangle] \geq \frac{1}{n} \sum_{i=1}^{n} \Delta(b_i, \bar{b}_i) - \xi \tag{3}$$

where $\Delta(b_i, \bar{b}_i)$ is the loss function relating the two outputs, and is set to $\|b_i - \bar{b}_i\|_2$ representing their Euclidean distance, ξ is the slack variable, and C is a free parameter that controls the tradeoff between the slack and model complexity.

The constraints state that for each training pair (a_i, b_i), the score $\langle w, \phi(a_i, b_i) \rangle$ for the correct output b_i should be greater than the score of *all* other outputs $\bar{b}_i$ by a required margin $\Delta(b_i, \bar{b}_i)$. If the margin is violated, the slack variable ξ becomes non-zero. In fact, ξ is the upper bound of the empirical risk on the training set [9], and is directly minimized in the objective function.

Algorithm 1. S-SVM training with margin-rescaling and 1-slack [9]

Input: Examples $S = \{(a_1, b_1), ..., (a_n, b_n)\}$, C, ϵ; **Init**: Constraints $W \leftarrow \emptyset$
Do
  $(w, \xi) \leftarrow \text{argmin}_{w, \xi \geq 0} \; \frac{1}{2} w^T w + C\xi$
  $s.t. \; \forall (\bar{b}_1, ..., \bar{b}_n) \in W : \frac{1}{n} \sum_{i=1}^{n} w^T [(\phi(a_i, b_i) - \phi(a_i, \bar{b}_i)] \geq \frac{1}{n} \sum_{i=1}^{n} \Delta(b_i, \bar{b}_i) - \xi$
  For $i = 1, ..., n$
    $\bar{b}_i = \text{argmax}_b \; [w^T \phi(a_i, b) + \Delta(b_i, b)]$
  End for
  $W \leftarrow W \cup \{(\bar{b}_1, ..., \bar{b}_n)\}$
Until $\frac{1}{n} \sum_{i=1}^{n} w^T [\phi(a_i, b_i) - \phi(a_i, \bar{b}_i)] \geq \frac{1}{n} \sum_{i=1}^{n} \Delta(b_i, \bar{b}_i) - \xi - \epsilon$
Return (w, ξ)

Note that the number of constraints in Eq. (3) is intractable, with the total number of constraints in $O(|B|^n)$. By using the *cutting-plane* training algorithm [9] (presented in Algo. 1 for completeness) that employs constraint-generation techniques, this large-scale optimization problem can be solved efficiently. Briefly, the weight vector w is estimated using a working set of constraints W which is set to *empty* initially, and new constraints are then added by finding the $\bar{b}_i$ for each a_i that violates the constraint the most (i.e., has the highest sum of the score function and the loss term). These two steps are alternated until no constraint can be found that is violated by more than the desired *precision* ϵ. This generally ends with a small set of active constraints [9]. Note that when the algorithm terminates, *all* constraints in B^n are satisfied within precision ϵ.

2.2   Finding the Most-Violated Constraint and Prediction

Note that in Algo. 1, we need an efficient method to find $\bar{b}_i = \text{argmax}_b \; [w^T \phi(a_i, b) + \Delta(b_i, b)]$ for each a_i, so as to construct the next constraint. Similarly, in prediction, it is desirable to efficiently derive $\hat{b} = \text{argmax}_b$ $\langle w, \phi(a, b)\rangle$ for a novel input a. Previous work [8] addressed the above problems using a branch-and-bound procedure which exploited a bag-of-words feature model. Unfortunately such a technique cannot be easily adapted for the dense feature vectors (Section 2.3) needed for OCT image analysis. As an alternative, we propose to use a *coarse-to-fine sliding window search* approach to approximately obtain the desired result. Specifically, we first search the entire output range (x=[1 200], y=[1 200]) with 16-pixel spacing in both x and y, to identify the coarse position with the maximum score. The subsequent search ranges are $\pm 48, \pm 8, \pm 4$ in both x and y, with the sliding window centered around the previously found best location, at 4, 2, and 1 pixel spacing, respectively. A similar search strategy has been used for object detection [7] with a conventional classifier for improving the search speed.

2.3   Image Pre-processing and Feature Construction

We now describe the construction of our feature vector $\phi(a, b)$. First, before we can reliably extract features from a raw scan, a necessary pre-processing is

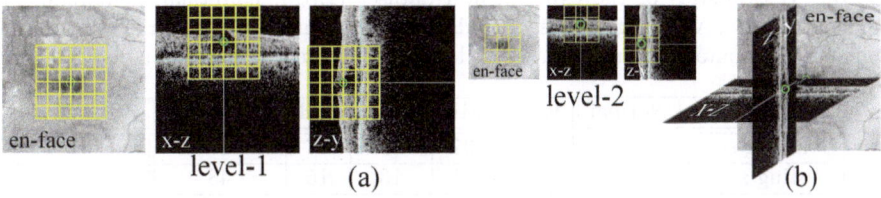

Fig. 2. (a) Illustration of our multi-scale spatially-distributed feature encoding for a given position (x, y, z). A 6x6 and 3x3 spatial grid is centered at the corresponding position on the en-face image, x-z slice and z-y slice for image scale level-1 and level-2, respectively. Appearance features are computed for each spatial cell. The automatically identified z position of the RPE layer is shown as a *light blue* line. (b) 3D presentation of the three orthogonal images (en-face, x-z slice, z-y slice) for a given 3D position.

to conduct eye-motion correction for restoring the 3D integrity of the volume. We apply Xu's [11] method to correct the eye motion artifacts, which usually produces a corrected volume with a roughly *flattened* retinal pigment epithelium (RPE) layer (the bottom retinal layer that shows high intensity in OCT images). This effect largely reduces the appearance variations across scans caused by different retinal curvatures or imagining deviation.

Before we can extract a volumetric feature vector centered at a candidate foveola location (x,y), we need to decide the retina's spatial extent in z. We now describe an empirical procedure to identify the maximum z value, $\hat{z}$, for analysis. We begin by estimating an average z position of the RPE layer in the volume. For each x-z slice, we find one row z that has the maximum average energy in the slice. This is usually located at the bottom RPE layer, but could sometimes map to the top nerve fiber layer. Then, the maximum z value among all x-z slices is found, and only the z within a specified distance to this maximum are retained, in order to exclude outliers. The z location of the RPE layer is estimated by taking the average of these retained z values. We found that this procedure can robustly derive the desired results (*light blue* line in Fig. 2(a)). We then set $\hat{z} = (z\_RPE + \frac{1}{10} dim\_z)$ as the largest z position for further analysis.

In constructing the feature $\phi(a, b)$ for a candidate output $b = (x, y)$, we compute features within the neighborhood centered at (x, y, z), where $z = (\hat{z} - \frac{1}{4} dim\_z)$. Specifically, we calculate features in the *three orthogonal context windows* (in en-face, x-z slice, and z-y slice) centered at (x, y, z). The window width/height is set to be $\frac{1}{2} dim\_size$ for each dimension. For each window, we divide it into 6x6 spatial cells, and compute intensity mean and gradient orientation histogram [12] with 16 angular bins for each cell. The same feature types are also computed for the down-scaled volume with 3x3 spatial grids. An example is shown in Fig. 2. To reduce the boundary effect, we also include the 5x5 and 2x2 central overlapped cells in the two scales, respectively. These measurements are concatenated to form an overall appearance descriptor. Also, since the relative location to the scan center is also a useful cue, we include $(dx, dy) = (\frac{|x - scan\_center\_x|}{dim\_x}, \frac{|y - scan\_center\_y|}{dim\_y})$ in our overall descriptor.

Table 1. Statistics of the experimental dataset (ERM: epiretinal membrane, ME: macular edema, AMD: age-related macular degeneration, MH: macular hole). Note that one eye can contain several diseases and may be counted in more than one category.

Num. of Eyes	Normal	ERM	ME	AMD	MH	All diseased	Total Eyes
Training set	30	28	37	16	17	59	89
Testing set	33	19	31	13	15	48	81

Table 2. The localization distance (in pixels) of all methods

Results	Normal (33 cases)		Diseased (48 cases)		Overall (81 cases)	
	mean	median	mean	median	mean	median
Second Expert	1.78±1.37	1.56	1.84±1.42	1.75	1.82±1.39	1.61
S-SVM	2.87±1.45	2.73	3.14±1.96	2.78	3.03±1.77	2.73
B-SVM	3.57±1.94	3.16	3.98±2.15	3.80	3.81±2.06	3.61

Table 3. Percentage of testing scans within various localization distances (in pixels)

Percentage	≤ 2	≤ 4	≤ 6	≤ 8	≤ 10	≤ 12
Second Expert	67.9%	91.4%	98.8%	100%	100%	100%
S-SVM	30.9%	77.8%	95.1%	97.5%	98.8%	100%
B-SVM	18.5%	55.6%	87.7%	97.5%	98.8%	100%

3   Experimental Results

We collected a large sample of 3D SD-OCT macular scans (200x200x1024 or 512x128x1024 protocol, 6x6x2 mm; Cirrus HD-OCT; Carl Zeiss Meditec). Each scan is then normalized to be 200x200x200 in x, y, z. For each scan, two ophthalmologists labeled the (x, y) location of the foveola independently. We then included a total of 170 scans from 170 eyes/126 subjects in which all scans have good expert labeling agreement (distance ≤ 8 pixels). One expert's labeling was adopted as the ground truth while the other was used to assess the inter-expert variability. We split the dataset to a training and a testing set such that they have similar disease distributions, and eyes from the same subject were assigned to the same set. The statistics of our dataset is detailed in Table 1.

We conducted experiments to compare the performance of the proposed S-SVM with binary SVM (B-SVM), both using linear kernel for localization efficiency. We used *SVMStruct* package [13] and *SVMLight* [14] for S-SVM and B-SVM, respectively. The precision ϵ is set to 0.1 and the parameter C is set by performing 2-fold cross validation on the training set. In B-SVM training, for each training scan, we sampled k locations which are at least 8 pixels away from the ground truth as negative examples. We tested for $k = 1, \cdots, 5, 10, 25, 50$. The best result of B-SVM was reported for comparison to S-SVM.

The mean and median localization distance of the S-SVM, B-SVM (best $k = 1$), and the second human expert are detailed in Table 2. The results for the percentage of scans within various precision are shown in Table 3. From Table 2,

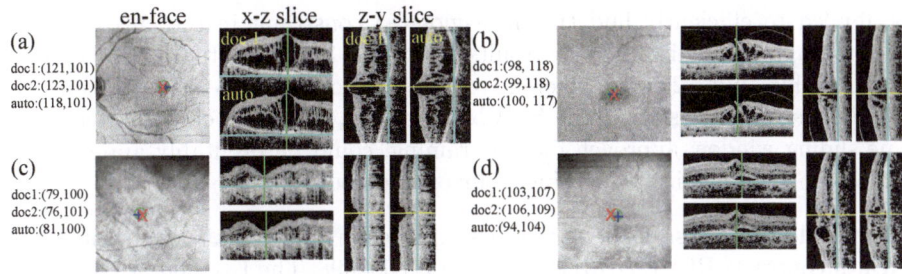

Fig. 3. (a)-(d): example results of the proposed method (auto) compared to the ground truth (doc 1). In the en-face, the labeling of *auto* is marked as "red x", *doc 1* as "green o", and the second expert (doc 2) as "blue +". The slices that cross the foveola defined by *doc 1* and *auto* are shown, where the x, y, z (at RPE layer) position are illustrated in *green*, *yellow*, and *light blue* line. (d): An example of larger error in *auto*.

the performance of the second expert is the best, followed by S-SVM, and then B-SVM. The labeling difference between S-SVM and the second expert is only 1.25 pixels on average, though this is statistically significant (t-$test$, $p \ll 0.001$). From Table 3, our S-SVM can localize 95.1% of scans within 6 pixels, well within the foveola's diameter (12 pixels). Example outputs of S-SVM are in Fig. 3.

In comparison to B-SVM, S-SVM achieved smaller median, mean and standard deviation in all cases as shown in Table 2, and their performance difference is statistically significant (t-$test$, $p = 0.004$). From Table 3, S-SVM also shows larger percentage of scans within anatomical foveola area (95% vs. 87%). S-SVM's better performance is intuitively due to its direct minimization of the localization risk, and its efficient use of all negative locations (the final constraint size $|W| = 22$). In addition, we observed that when using B-SVM, sampling more negative examples (≥ 3 per scan) in training doesn't give us higher performance (some scans have ≥ 20 pixel errors). This is likely due to the higher imbalanced sample number between the two classes that can result in classifier degeneration. Our results demonstrate the value of the proposed S-SVM approach.

The running time of the training of our S-SVM is about 5 hours while for a B-SVM is 1 hour (with 2.67GHz CPU, Matlab+SVM software). Both methods gave the prediction result in 1 minute for each scan. This running time can be improved by parallelizing the score evaluations in sliding window search for both methods, and the loop in finding the most-violated constraint in S-SVM training.

4   Conclusion

In this paper, we propose an effective approach to determine the location of the fovea in retinal 3D-OCT images. Structural SVM is learned to directly predict the foveola location, such that the score at the ground truth position is higher than that of any other position by a margin set to the localization loss. This S-SVM formulation directly minimizes the empirical risk of localization, naturally fitting the localization problem. A coarse-to-fine sliding window search approach is applied to efficiently find the most-violated constraint in the cutting-plane training and in prediction. Our results show that S-SVM outperforms B-SVM, and is within only 1.25 pixel difference on average compared to the second expert.

Our results suggest that the S-SVM paradigm, using the efficient coarse-to-fine sliding window approach during training, could be profitably applied in a broad range of localization problems involving medical image datasets.

Acknowledgments. This research is supported in part by National Institutes of Health contracts R01-EY013178 and P30-EY008098, The Eye and Ear Foundation (Pittsburgh, PA), unrestricted grants from Research to Prevent Blindness, Inc. (New York, NY), and grants from Intel Labs Pittsburgh (Pittsburgh, PA).

References

1. Abramoff, M.D., Garvin, M.K., Sonka, M.: Retinal imaging and image analysis. IEEE Reviews in Biomedical Engineering 3, 169–208 (2010)
2. Yehoshua, Z., Wang, F., Rosenfeld, P.J., Penha, F.M., Feuer, W.J., Gregori, G.: Natural history of drusen morphology in age-related macular degeneration using spectral domain optical coherence tomography. American Academy of Ophthalmology 118(12), 2434–2441 (2011)
3. Liu, Y.Y., Chen, M., Ishikawa, H., Wollstein, G., Schuman, J., Rehg, J.M.: Automated macular pathology diagnosis in retinal OCT images using multi-scale spatial pyramid and local binary patterns in texture and shape encoding. Medical Image Analysis 15, 748–759 (2011)
4. Niemeijer, M., Abramoff, M.D., van Ginneken, B.: Fast detection of the optic disc and fovea in color fundus photographs. Medical Image Analysis (13), 859–870 (2009)
5. Zhan, Y., Zhou, X.S., Peng, Z., Krishnan, A.: Active Scheduling of Organ Detection and Segmentation in Whole-Body Medical Images. In: Metaxas, D., Axel, L., Fichtinger, G., Székely, G. (eds.) MICCAI 2008, Part I. LNCS, vol. 5241, pp. 313–321. Springer, Heidelberg (2008)
6. Pescia, D., Paragios, N., Chemouny, S.: Automatic detection of liver tumors. In: IEEE Intl. Symposium on Biomedical Imaging (2008)
7. Pedersoli, M., Gonzàlez, J., Bagdanov, A.D., Villanueva, J.J.: Recursive Coarse-to-Fine Localization for Fast Object Detection. In: Daniilidis, K., Maragos, P., Paragios, N. (eds.) ECCV 2010, Part VI. LNCS, vol. 6316, pp. 280–293. Springer, Heidelberg (2010)
8. Blaschko, M.B., Lampert, C.H.: Learning to Localize Objects with Structured Output Regression. In: Forsyth, D., Torr, P., Zisserman, A. (eds.) ECCV 2008, Part I. LNCS, vol. 5302, pp. 2–15. Springer, Heidelberg (2008)
9. Joachims, T., Finley, T., Yu, C.N.J.: Cutting-plane training of strucural SVMs. Journal of Machine Learning (2009)
10. Tsochantaridis, I., Hofmann, T., Joachims, T., Altun, Y.: Support vector learning for interdependent and structured output spaces. In: ICML (2004)
11. Xu, J., Ishikawa, H., Wollstein, G., Schuman, J.S.: 3D OCT eye movement correction based on particle filtering. In: EMBS, pp. 53–56 (2010)
12. Freeman, W.T., Roth, M.: Orientation histogram for hand gesture recognition. In: Intl. Workshop on Automatic Face and Gesture Recognition, pp. 296–301 (1994)
13. Joachims, T.: Support vector machine for complex outputs, software http://svmlight.joachims.org/svm_struct.html
14. Joachims, T.: SVMLight support vector machine, software http://svmlight.joachims.org/

Intrinsic Melanin and Hemoglobin Colour Components for Skin Lesion Malignancy Detection

Ali Madooei, Mark S. Drew, Maryam Sadeghi, and M. Stella Atkins

School of Computing Science
Simon Fraser University
amadooei@cs.sfu.ca
http://www.cs.sfu.ca/~amadooei

Abstract. In this paper we propose a new log-chromaticity 2-D colour space, an extension of previous approaches, which succeeds in removing confounding factors from dermoscopic images: (i) the effects of the particular camera characteristics for the camera system used in forming RGB images; (ii) the colour of the light used in the dermoscope; (iii) shading induced by imaging non-flat skin surfaces; (iv) and light intensity, removing the effect of light-intensity falloff toward the edges of the dermoscopic image. In the context of a blind source separation of the underlying colour, we arrive at intrinsic melanin and hemoglobin images, whose properties are then used in supervised learning to achieve excellent malignant vs. benign skin lesion classification. In addition, we propose using the geometric-mean of colour for skin lesion segmentation based on simple grey-level thresholding, with results outperforming the state of the art.

1 Introduction

The three most common malignant skin cancers are basal cell carcinoma (BCC), squamous cell carcinoma (SCC), and melanoma, among which melanoma is the most deadly with a high increasing rate in most parts of the world. Melanoma is often treatable if detected in the early stage, particularly before the metastasis phase. Therefore, there is an increasing demand for computer-aided diagnostic systems to catch early melanomas.

Colour has played a crucial role in the diagnosis of skin lesions by experts in most clinical methods (see e.g. [1]). For instance, the presence of multiple colours with an irregular distribution can signal malignancy.

Few studies have investigated the use of colour features representing biological properties of skin lesions. In particular, the work of Claridge et al. has figured prominently, with emphasis on the use of intermediate multispectral modelling to generate images disambiguating dermal and epidermal melanin, thickness of collagen, and blood [2]. At the same time, another stream of work has focused on using Independent Component Analysis (ICA) [3] in the context of 3-channel RGB images with no intermediate spectral-space model, aimed both at non-medical images and dermoscopic images of skin [4].

Here we concentrate on the latter, simpler, approach to utilizing colour and consider only RGB, not multispectral image modelling. We show that, combined with texture features, one can successfully carry out classification, disambiguating Malignant vs. Benign; Melanoma vs. Benign; and Melanoma vs. Spitz Nevus.

N. Ayache et al. (Eds.): MICCAI 2012, Part I, LNCS 7510, pp. 315–322, 2012.
© Springer-Verlag Berlin Heidelberg 2012

2   Method

We first adopt the ICA-based idea [4] in spirit and show that, in a particular novel colour space, pixel triples live on a plane, with (non-orthogonal) basis vectors assumed attributable to melanin and hemoglobin only.

Here, in an innovative step, we introduce a new colour 2-D chromaticity which removes (i) the effects of the particular camera characteristics for the camera system used in forming RGB images; (ii) the colour of the light used in the dermoscope; (iii) shading induced by imaging non-flat skin surfaces; (iv) and also light intensity, removing the effect of light-intensity falloff toward the edges of the image. The output from this colour processing is a set of two 1-D-colour chromaticity images, one for melanin content and one for hemoglobin content.

Together with the above colour space features, we also employ greyscale and texture features, including all features in a final 25-D feature-space vector. Such vectors are then amenable to machine learning techniques for effective skin lesion classification. In this paper we achieve comparable to state of the art results for distinguishing malignant from benign lesions.

2.1   Colour Space Image Formulation

Tsumura et al. first suggested using a simple Lambert-Beer type of law for radiance from a multilayer skin surface, resulting from illumination by polarized light [5]. That is, employing a model similar to a simple logarithm model based on optical densities for accounting for light passing for example through multilayer slide film. The transmittance through each colour layer is proportional to the exponential of the negative optical density for that layer. Such a simple model stands in contradistinction to a considerably more complex model based on Kubelka-Monk (KM) theory such as used in [2]. In the latter, full modelling of interreflection inside each layer is used to set up equations detailing light transport. This uses estimates of the absorption K and scattering S in each layer to predict overall transmittance and reflection [6]. KM theory has been found to be useful in tasks such as visualizing different components including surface and deep melanin etc. [2]. Here, we are simply focused on the classification task, and make use of the simpler model.

In the simpler approach, then, we utilize the model developed by Hiraoka et al. [7], which formulates a generalization of the Lambert-Beer law. In [7], the spectral reflection of skin (under polarized light) at pixel indexed by (x, y) is given by

$$S(x, y, \lambda) = \exp\{-\rho_m(x,y)\alpha_m(\lambda)l_m(\lambda) - \rho_h(x,y)\alpha_h(\lambda)l_h(\lambda) - \zeta(\lambda)\} \quad (1)$$

where $\rho_{m,h}$ are densities of melanin and hemoglobin respectively (cm^{-3}), and are assumed to be independent of each other. The cross sectional areas for scattering absorption of melanin and hemoglobin are denoted $\alpha_{m,h}$ (cm^2) and $l_{m,h}$ are the mean pathlength for photons in epidermis and dermis layers, which are used as the depth of the medium in this modified Lambert-Beer law. These quantities are used as well in [4]. Finally, we also extend the model by including a term ζ standing for scattering loss and any other factors which contribute to skin appearance such as absorbency of other chromophores (e.g. β-carotene) and thickness of the subcutis. The reason we can extend the model will become clear below, when we form logarithms of ratios in a novel step.

In keeping with [8] we adopt a standard model in computer vision for colour image formation. Suppose the illuminant spectral power distribution is $E(\lambda)$ and, in any reflective case, the spectral reflectance function at pixel (x, y) is $S(x, y, \lambda)$, e.g. as given in eq. (1) above. Then measured RGB values are given by

$$R_k(x, y) = \omega(x, y) \int E(x, y, \lambda_k) S(x, y, \lambda_k) Q_k(\lambda) d\lambda, \ k = 1..3 \qquad (2)$$

where ω denotes shading variation (e.g., Lambertian shading is surface normal dotted into light direction, although we do not assume Lambertian surfaces here); and $Q_k(\lambda)$ is the camera sensor sensitivity functions in the R,G,B channels.

Following [8] we adopt a simple model for the illuminant: we assume the light can be written as a Planckian radiator (in Wien's approximation):

$$E(x, y, \lambda, T) \simeq I(x, y) k_1 \lambda^{-5} exp\left(-k_2/(T\lambda)\right) \qquad (3)$$

where k_1 and k_2 are constants, T is the correlated colour temperature characterizing the light spectrum, and I is the lighting intensity at pixel (x, y), allowing for a possible rolloff in intensity towards the periphery of the dermoscopic image. We assume light temperature T is constant across the image (but is, in general, unknown).

Finally, with [8] we assume camera sensors are narrowband or can be made narrowband via a spectral sharpening operation [9]. In this approximation. sensor curve $Q_k(\lambda)$ is simply assumed to be a delta function: $Q_k(\lambda) = q_k \delta(\lambda - \lambda_k)$, where specific wavelengths λ_k and sensor-curve heights q_k are properties of the camera used. Simplifying by taking logs (cf. [4]), we arrive at a model for pixel log-RGB as follows:

$$\log R_k(x, y) = -\rho_m(x, y)\sigma_m(\lambda_k) - \rho_h(x, y)\sigma_h(\lambda_k) - \zeta(\lambda_k) \\ + \log(k_1 I(x, y)\omega(x, y)) + \left[\log(1/\lambda_k^5) - k_2/(\lambda_k T)\right] \qquad (4)$$

where we have lumped terms $\sigma_m(\lambda_k) = \alpha_m(\lambda_k) l_m(\lambda_k)$, $\sigma_h(\lambda_k) = \alpha_h(\lambda_k) l_h(\lambda_k)$. For notational convenience, denote $u_k = \log(1/\lambda_k^5)$, $e_k = -k_2/\lambda_k$, $m_k = \sigma_m(\lambda_k)$, $h_k = \sigma_h(\lambda_k)$, $\zeta_k = \zeta(\lambda_k)$.

Now let us move forward from [4] by making the novel observation that the same type of chromaticity analysis as appears in [8] can be brought to bear here for the skin-reflectance model (4) [but N.B., [8] does not use the density model (1)]. Chromaticity is colour without intensity, e.g. an L_1-norm based chromaticity is $\{r, g, b\} = \{R, G, B\}/(R + G + B)$. Here, suppose we instead form a band-ratio chromaticity by dividing by one colour-channel R_p, e.g. Green for $p = 2$. [In practice, we shall instead follow [8] and divide by the geometric-mean colour, $\mu = \sqrt[3]{R \cdot G \cdot B}$, so as not to favour one particular colour-channel, but dividing by R_p is clearer in exposition.] Notice that dividing removes the effect of shading ω and light-intensity field I.

Defining a log-chromaticity $\chi(x, y)$ as the log of the ratio of colour component R_k over R_p, we then have

$$\chi_k(x, y) = \log\left(R_k(x, y)/R_p(x, y)\right) \\ = -\rho_m(x, y)(m_k - m_p) - \rho_h(x, y)(h_k - h_p) + w_k - (e_k - e_p)(1/T) \qquad (5)$$

with $w_k \equiv (u_k - u_p) - (\zeta_k - \zeta_p)$. The meaning of this equation is that, if we were to vary the lighting (in this simplified model) then the chromaticity χ would follow a straight line as temperature T changes. In fact, this linear behaviour is also obeyed by the mean $\bar{\chi}$ over the image of this new chromaticity quantity:

$$\bar{\chi}_k = -\bar{\rho}_m(m_k - m_p) - \bar{\rho}_h(h_k - h_p) + w_k - (e_k - e_p)(1/T) \tag{6}$$

Now we notice that we can remove all terms in the camera-offset term w_k and the illuminant-colour term T by subtracting the mean from χ. Let χ^0 be the mean-subtracted vector $\chi_k^0(x, y) = \chi_k(x, y) - \bar{\chi}_k$. We then arrive at a feature which depends only on melanin m and hemoglobin h:

$$\chi_k^0(x, y) = -(\rho_m(x, y) - \bar{\rho}_m)(m_k - m_p) - (\rho_h(x, y) - \bar{\rho}_h)(h_k - h_p) \tag{7}$$

If we apply the assumption that m and h terms can be disambiguated using ICA, then from the new feature χ^0 we can extract the melanin and hemoglobin content in dermoscopic images, where we take vectors $(m_k - m_p)$ and $(h_k - h_p)$ as constant vectors in each image. The log-subtraction step removes intensity and shading, and the mean-subtraction removes camera-offset and light colour, as opposed to [4] where one must attempt to recover approximations of these quantities.

As an example, consider Fig. 1(a) showing a Melanoma lesion, and the ρ_m and ρ_h components in Figs.(b,c). Below, we show how these two new image features, $\rho_m^0(x, y) = (\rho_m(x, y) - \bar{\rho}_m)$ and $\rho_h^0(x, y) = (\rho_h(x, y) - \bar{\rho}_h)$, can be used in lesion classification. In computer vision, images with lighting removed are denoted "intrinsic images", and thus our two new features are indeed intrinsic.

Geometric Mean Chromaticity. To not rely on any particular colour channel, we divide not by R_p but by the geometric mean μ at each pixel, for which the invariance properties above persist: $\psi_k(x, y) \equiv \log[R_k(x, y)/\mu(x, y)]$. Then ψ is a 3-vector; it is orthogonal to $(1, 1, 1)$. Therefore instead of 3-vectors one can easily treat these as 2-vector values, lying in the plane orthogonal to $(1, 1, 1)$: if the 3×3 projector onto that 2-D subspace is P, then the singular value decomposition of $P = UU^T$, where U is a 3×2 matrix. We project onto 2-D vectors ϕ in the plane coordinate system via U^T:

$$\psi_k(x, y) = \log[R_k(x, y)/\mu(x, y)]; \quad \phi = U^T \psi \tag{8}$$

where ϕ is 2-D. The mean-subtraction above still holds in projected colour, and we therefore here propose carrying out ICA in the plane: *feature* $= \eta = ICA(\phi - \bar{\phi})$.

2.2 Texture and Colour Feature Vectors

So far, we have discarded the luminance (intensity) part of the input image, focusing on intrinsic colour. However, we can go on to include the greyscale geometric-mean image (Fig. 1(d)) information μ as well. Thus, we extract features for each of $\{\mu, \eta_1, \eta_2\}$.

As colour features, we generate mean; standard deviation; the ratio of these; and entropy of each channel, in addition to $|var(\eta_1) - var(\eta_2)|$, adding up to a 13-D colour feature vector. Further, we add texture features to our colour feature-vectors, in a similar fashion as in [10]: four of the classical statistical texture measures of [11] (contrast, correlation, homogeneity and energy) are derived from the grey level co-occurrence matrix (GLCM) of each channel. This is an additional 12-D texture feature vector; thus we arrive at a 25-D feature vector.

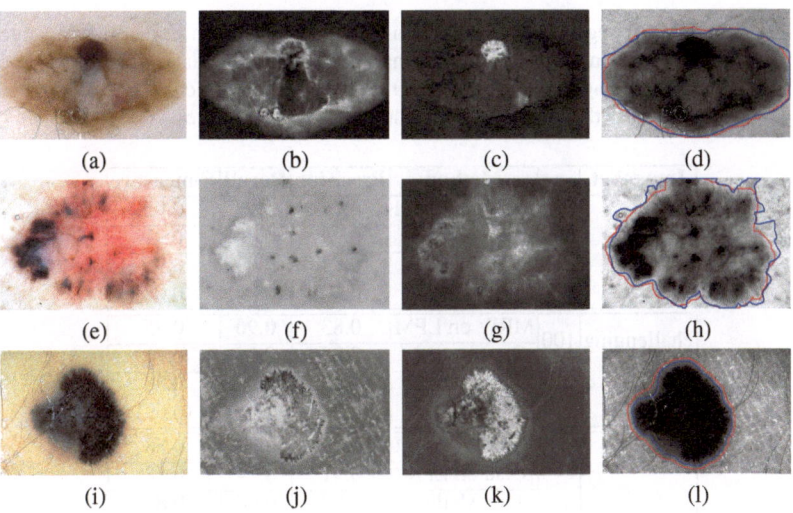

Fig. 1. (a): Input image (Melanoma); (b): melanin component; (c): hemoglobin component; (d): greyscale geometric mean. Blue border: expert segmentation, Red border: our segmentation. (e-h): BCC. (i-l): Spitz Nevus.

3   Image Masks

Each of the features calculated above is applied only within a mask surrounding the lesion, normalized accordingly. For automatic segmentation of lesions, we found that using the geometric-mean μ is as good as or better than the state of the art [12] for these dermoscopic images, in a much simpler algorithm. Here we simply apply Otsu's method [13] for selecting a grey-level threshold. Note that Otsu's method (and also most commercially available automated systems) fail in segmenting low contrast lesions. However our approach achieved very high precision and recall, since we discovered that geometric-mean greyscale highlights the lesion from its surrounding.

We tested our method on a dataset of images used by Wighton et al. [12]. They presented a modified random walker (MRW) segmentation where seed points were set automatically based on a lesion probability map (LPM). The LPM was created through a supervised learning procedure using colour/texture properties. Table 1 shows results for our method compared to results in [12]. While our method for segmentation uses a much simpler algorithm and does not require learning, it achieves competitive results. It is worth mentioning [12] also applied Otsu's method on their lesion probability maps. Their result included in Table 1 under 'Otsu on LPM', with results not nearly as good as ours. In another test on **944 test images**, we achieved precision 0.86, recall 0.95, and f-measure 0.88 (with STD 0.19, 0.08 and 0.15 respectively) compared to expert segmentations.

4   Experiments

We applied a Logistic classifier to a set of 500 images, with two classes consisting of malignant (melanoma and BCC) vs. all benign lesions (congenital, compound, dermal,

Table 1. Comparing our segmentation method to the modified random walker (MRW) algorithm and Otsu's thresholding, on lesion probability map (LPM)[12]. The dataset is divided into a set of 20 easy-to-segment images, and another 100 images that pose a challenge to segmentation methods. Note that our method consistently produces higher f-measures.

ImageSet	n	Method	Precision	Recall	F-measure
simple	20	MRW on LPM	0.96	0.95	0.95
		Otsu on LPM	**0.99**	0.86	0.91
		Our Method	0.94	**0.97**	**0.95**
		(STD)	(0.04)	(0.04)	(0.02)
challenging	100	MRW on LPM	0.83	**0.90**	0.85
		Otsu on LPM	0.88	0.68	0.71
		Our Method	**0.88**	0.90	**0.88**
		(STD)	(0.15)	(0.1)	(0.09)
whole	120	MRW on LPM	0.87	**0.92**	0.88
		Otsu on LPM	**0.91**	0.74	0.78
		Our Method	0.89	0.90	**0.89**
		(STD)	(0.13)	(0.09)	(0.09)

Table 2. Results of classifying the dataset using different colour spaces. MHG is our proposed colour space; We win and improve the f-measure somewhat, but the AUC is substantially boosted. Since our dataset is unbalanced, a classifier trained on e.g. RGB achieved high score while assigned benign label to most malignant instances. We on the other hand produced equally high and steady results for both classes; improving e.g. recall for malignant cases up to 23%. Since same feature-set & classifier is used, the improvement is the result of using our proposed colour-space.

Colour Space	Class	n	Precision	Recall	F-measure	AUC
MHG	Malignant	135	0.806	**0.8**	**0.803**	
	Benign	365	**0.926**	0.929	**0.927**	**0.953**
	Weighted Avr.	500	**0.894**	**0.894**	**0.894**	
RGB	Malignant	135	**0.895**	0.57	0.697	
	Benign	365	0.86	**0.975**	0.914	0.773
	Weighted Avr.	500	0.869	0.866	0.855	
HSV	Malignant	135	0.807	0.652	0.721	
	Benign	365	0.88	0.942	0.91	0.797
	Weighted Avr.	500	0.86	0.864	0.859	
LAB	Malignant	135	0.837	0.57	0.678	
	Benign	365	0.858	0.959	0.906	0.765
	Weighted Avr.	500	0.852	0.854	0.844	

Clark, Spitz and blue nevus; dermatofibroma; and seborrheic keratosis). Table 2 results are averaged over 10-fold cross-validation. We achieve **f-measure: 89.4%** and **AUC: 0.953**, an excellent performance. For comparison, we compare using our feature set on RGB, HSV, and CIELAB colour spaces. We see that our proposed colour space, $\{\eta_1, \eta_2, \mu\}$ (denoted MHG for melanin, hemoglobin and geometric-mean), improves accuracy (f-measure) as well as the performance (AUC) of classification, particularly formative for malignant lesions, where the results show significantly higher precision and recall for our method.

Table 3. Results of classifying the dataset using different subsets of our feature-set (colour/texture), and different channels of our proposed colour space MHG

Description	n	Precision	Recall	F-measure	AUC
Colour Features Only on MHG		0.728	0.754	0.72	0.731
Texture Features only on MHG		0.855	0.854	0.842	0.858
Colour+Texture on Melanin only	500	0.783	0.794	0.786	0.831
Colour+Texture on Hemoglobin only		0.765	0.78	0.766	0.829
Colour+Texture on Geo-mean only		0.817	0.824	0.817	0.877
Colour+Texture on MHG		**0.894**	**0.894**	**0.894**	**0.953**

Table 4. Classification results for skin cancer categories using our proposed feature space

Classification Task	n	Precision	Recall	F-measure	AUC
Malignant vs. Benign	500	0.894	0.894	0.894	0.953
Melanoma vs. Benign	486	0.897	0.899	0.897	0.946
Melanoma vs. Spitz Nevus	167	0.915	0.916	0.916	0.96

To judge the effect of colour vs. texture and the different channels of our proposed colour space MHG, Table 3 shows that 1)texture features have higher impact than colour features; 2)the three channels of MHG contribute more than each individually; best overall is from combining all.

To further analyze the robustness and effectiveness of our method, we tried different classifiers using Weka [14]. On the main classification task of malignant vs. benign, Logistic Regression produced the highest result (Table 4) whereas e.g. using support vector machine (SVM) we attained precision 0.872, recall 0.87, f-measure 0.871 and AUC 0.828; sequential minimal optimization (SMO) produced 0.892, 0.891, 0.888, 0.883 respectively. Table 4 shows results for classifying melanoma vs. benign and melanoma vs. Spitz nevus, as well as malignant vs. benign, with excellent results for these difficult problems. Spitz nevus is a challenging classification, to the extent that expert dermatologists usually have to take into consideration other criteria such as patient's age.

5 Conclusion

We have proposed a new colour-feature η which is aimed at apprehending underlying melanin and hemoglobin biological components of dermoscopy images of skin lesions. The advantage of the new feature, in addition to its biological underpinnings, lies in removing the effects of confounding factors such as light colour; intensity falloff; shading; and camera characteristics. The new colour-feature vectors $\{\eta_1, \eta_2\}$ combined with geometric-mean vector, μ, is proposed as a new colour-space MHG (abbreviation of melanin, hemoglobin and geometric-mean). In our experiments, MHG is shown to produce excellent results for classification of Malignant vs. Benign; Melanoma vs. Benign; and Melanoma vs. Spitz Nevus. Moreover, in the lesion segmentation task, μ is shown to improve accuracy of segmentation. Future work will include i) Exploration of effects and contributions of other colour and texture features, combined with those reported here. ii) Experimenting with different learning algorithms and strategies, in particular the possibility of multi-class classification. iii) Examination of the extracted melanin and hemoglobin colour components as a set of two full-colour images, since the equations leading to (8) are in fact invertible for each component separately. As 3-D colour features these will support descriptors such as colour histograms and correlograms, which may lead to even more improvement.

References

1. Henning, J.S., Dusza, S.W., Wang, S.Q., Marghoob, A.A., Rabinovitz, H.S., Polsky, D., Kopf, A.W.: The CASH (color, architecture, symmetry, and homogeneity) algorithm for dermoscopy. J. of the Amer. Acad. of Dermatology 56, 45–52 (2007)
2. Claridge, E., Cotton, S., Hall, P., Moncrieff, M.: From colour to tissue histology: Physics-based interpretation of images of pigmented skin lesions. Med. Im. Anal. 7, 489–502 (2003)
3. Hyvärinen, A., Karhunen, J., Oja, E.: Independent Component Analysis. John Wiley and Sons, Inc., New York (2001)
4. Tsumura, N., Ojima, N., Sato, K., Shiraishi, M., Shimizu, H., Nabeshima, H., Akazaki, S., Hori, K., Miyake, Y.: Image-based skin color and texture analysis/synthesis by extracting hemoglobin and melanin information in the skin. ACM Trans. Graph. 22, 770–779 (2003)
5. Tsumura, N., Haneishi, H., Miyake, Y.: Independent-component analysis of skin color image. J. of the Optical Soc. of Amer. A 16, 2169–2176 (1999)
6. Kang, H.R.: Color technology for electronic imaging systems. SPIE Optical Eng. Press (1997)
7. Hiraoka, M., Firbank, M., Essenpreis, M., Cope, M., Arrige, S.R., Zee, P.V.D., Delpy, D.T.: A Monte Carlo investigation of optical pathlength in inhomogeneous tissue and its application to near-infrared spectroscopy. Phys. Med. Biol. 38, 1859–1876 (1993)
8. Finlayson, G.D., Drew, M.S., Lu, C.: Intrinsic Images by Entropy Minimization. In: Pajdla, T., Matas, J(G.) (eds.) ECCV 2004, Part III. LNCS, vol. 3023, pp. 582–595. Springer, Heidelberg (2004)
9. Finlayson, G.D., Drew, M.S., Funt, B.V.: Spectral sharpening: sensor transformations for improved color constancy. J. Opt. Soc. Am. A 11(5), 1553–1563 (1994)
10. Sadeghi, M., Razmara, M., Wighton, P., Lee, T., Atkins, M.: Modeling the Dermoscopic Structure Pigment Network Using a Clinically Inspired Feature Set. In: Liao, H., Eddie Edwards, P.J., Pan, X., Fan, Y., Yang, G.-Z. (eds.) MIAR 2010. LNCS, vol. 6326, pp. 467–474. Springer, Heidelberg (2010)
11. Haralick, R.M., Shapiro, L.G.: Computer and Robot Vision, vol. 1, p. 459. Addison-Wesley, New York (1992)
12. Wighton, P., Sadeghi, M., Lee, T.K., Atkins, M.S.: A Fully Automatic Random Walker Segmentation for Skin Lesions in a Supervised Setting. In: Yang, G.-Z., Hawkes, D., Rueckert, D., Noble, A., Taylor, C. (eds.) MICCAI 2009, Part II. LNCS, vol. 5762, pp. 1108–1115. Springer, Heidelberg (2009)
13. Otsu, N.: A threshold selection method from gray-level histograms. IEEE Trans. on Systems, Man and Cybernetics 9(1), 62–66 (1979)
14. Hall, M., Frank, E., Holmes, G., Pfahringer, B., Reutemann, P., Witten, I.H.: WEKA data mining software (2001), http://www.cs.waikato.ac.nz/ml/weka/

Anisotropic ssTEM Image Segmentation Using Dense Correspondence across Sections

Dmitry Laptev, Alexander Vezhnevets,
Sarvesh Dwivedi, and Joachim M. Buhmann

Department of Computer Science, ETH Zurich, Switzerland
{dlaptev,alexander.vezhnevets,sdwivedi,jbuhmann}@inf.ethz.ch

Abstract. Connectomics based on high resolution ssTEM imagery requires reconstruction of the neuron geometry from histological slides. We present an approach for the automatic membrane segmentation in anisotropic stacks of electron microscopy brain tissue sections. The ambiguities in neuronal segmentation of a section are resolved by using the context from the neighboring sections. We find the global dense correspondence between the sections by SIFT Flow algorithm, evaluate the features of the corresponding pixels and use them to perform the segmentation. Our method is 3.6 and 6.4% more accurate in two different accuracy metrics than the algorithm with no context from other sections.

Keywords: Membrane Segmentation, Anisotropic Data, Dense Correspondence, SIFT Flow.

1 Introduction

Neuroanatomists face the challenging task of reconstructing neuronal structure with synaptic resolution in order to gain insights into the functional connectivity of brain. Performing this geometry extraction manually has been demonstrated to be tedious, error prone and requires an impractical amount of time. Therefore, accurate algorithms for automatic neuronal segmentation are indispensable for large scale geometric reconstruction of densely interconnected neuronal tissue. In this paper we focus on the segmentation problem, i.e., to annotate neuronal structures in tissue as either membranes or the inside volume of neurons.

Currently serial section transmission electron microscopy (ssTEM) [5] is the only available technique which can provide sufficient resolution. ssTEM data depicts the observed volume as a stack of images (sections). This imaging technique visualizes the resulting volumes in a highly "anisotropic" way, i.e., the x- and y-directions[1] have a high resolution, whereas the z-direction has a low resolution, primarily dependent on the precision of serial cutting.

Local appearance around the pixel in a section may be insufficient to discriminate between the membrane or the inner area of a neuron. This ambiguity arises

---

[1] Here, x and y coordinates correspond to the dimensions of a section, and z corresponds to the vertical dimension of the stack.

N. Ayache et al. (Eds.): MICCAI 2012, Part I, LNCS 7510, pp. 323–330, 2012.

from the fact that electron microscopy produces the images as a projection of the whole section, so some of the membranes that are not orthogonal to a cutting plane can appear very blurred.

To allow automatic methods to exploit information from neighboring sections we have to resolve the correspondence problem - finding a mapping from a neighboring section to the current one. We propose to solve this problem by finding global dense correspondence with SIFT flow algorithm [10] and to use the features from different sections to perform segmentation.

1.1 Related Work

There are three general approaches for anisotropic data segmentation. The first approach focuses on the detection of neuron membranes in each section independently [7]. The software package Fiji [1] implements this approach: first, in every pixel the vector of features is evaluted, and then this vectors are used to train Random Forest classifier. We use this package for feature extraction, described in details in Section 2.3.

The second approach incorporates context from different sections without correspondence alignment. In [8] the authors propose two terms for graph cut segmentation, one of them incorporates context from neighboring sections. In contrast to our algorithm, this term depends only on the feature vector evaluated in the pixel in a direct z-neighborhood, with no correspondence alignment. As the difference between the sections is usually quite significant, incorporating of this term doesn't lead to significant improvements.

The third approach [15] generates many, possibly contradictory, segmentation hypotheses in individual sections and combine them in order to optimize the global agreement functional defined on the whole stack. In contrast to this approach, we are not dealing with given segmentation hypotheses, but incorporate the context from neighboring sections to improve the segmentation of every single section.

The novel contribution describes how to exploit context from neighboring sections by solving the correspondence problem. We present it in the following sections.

2   Proposed Method

Let $\tau = \left\{ I^k, Y^k \right\}_{k=1}^K$ be a training set, consisting of K images with a given labeling. Here $I^k = \{x_p^k\}_{p=1}^N$ respresents an input image of section k, x_p^k corresponds to a pixel in section k. $Y^k = \{y_p^k\}_{p=1}^N$ represents the labels of the corresponding pixels p for a section k. y_p^k equals 1 for the class "membrane" and 0 otherwise. Let $\varphi(x_p^k)$ be a feature vector for the pixel x_p^k. Our goal is to build a segmentation algorithm that would automatically label new sets of images.

The proposed method constructs a dense correspondence between the neighboring sections and it uses features that are evaluated in all the corresponding pixels for classification. Our workflow is illustrated in Figure 1. For a given section I^k we first find warpings from the neighboring sections I^{k+1} and I^{k-1}: $F_{k+1,k}$ and $F_{k-1,k}$. Then, for every pixel x_p^k we find the corresponding pixels $\hat{x}_p^k$ and $\check{x}_p^k$. Next, we calculate features in all three pixels $\varphi(\hat{x}_p^k)$, $\varphi(x_p^k)$, $\varphi(\check{x}_p^k)$, concatenate the feature vectors and use this extended feature vector as input to a Random Forest (RF) classifier. Finally, we use the probabilities returned by the RF for Graph Cut segmentation.

2.1   Framework

Suppose we are given a non-linear warping $F_{k-1,k}$ that establishes the correspondence between the pixels in the image I^{k-1} and I^k. We discuss a method to obtain it in Section 2.2. We introduce two more images to the dataset: $I^0 \equiv I^1$ and $I^{K+1} \equiv I^K$ both for training and test sets, so that now there are two neighbors for every section from 1 to K. Every pixel x_p^k is then assigned to the corresponding pixels in the neighboring sections:

$$\hat{x}_p^k = F_{k-1,k}(x_p^k), \quad \check{x}_p^k = F_{k+1,k}(x_p^k). \tag{1}$$

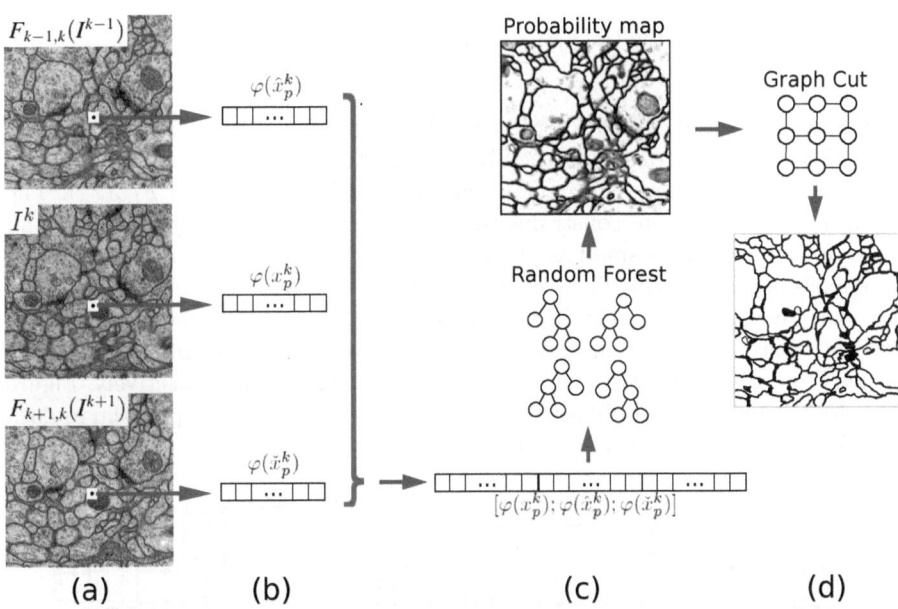

(a)   (b)   (c)   (d)

Fig. 1. Based on the non-linear correspondings $F_{k-1,k}$ and $F_{k+1,k}$ the algorithm evaluates the warped images $F_{k-1,k}(I^{k-1})$ and $F_{k+1,k}(I^{k+1})$ (a). Then, feature vectors in the corresponding pixels are evaluated: $\varphi(\hat{x}_p^k)$, $\varphi(x_p^k)$, $\varphi(\check{x}_p^k)$ (b). After that the method concatenates them and passes the concatenated feature vector to a RF (c). RF returns a probability map that is segmented by Graph Cut algorithm (d).

To incorporate the context from neighboring sections, an extended feature vector has to capture the contextual feature information associated with the pixel x_p^k itself, as well as with the pixels $\hat{x}_p^k$ and $\check{x}_p^k$. The extended feature vectors form a training set for a RF classifier [4].

$$\tau = \left\{ [\varphi(x_p^k); \varphi(\hat{x}_p^k); \varphi(\check{x}_p^k)], y_p^k, \ 1 \le p \le N, 1 \le k \le K \right\}. \tag{2}$$

A trained RF returns the probability of every pixel of the image to belong to a membrane, i.e., a probability map. Afterwords, graph cut segmentation [3] with the probability map as unary potentials partitions the image into semantically meaningful segments.

2.2   Dense Correspondence

To find a dense correspondence between the sections we use the recently proposed method "SIFT Flow" [10]. SIFT Flow finds the non-linear warping $F_{1,2}$ on the pixel grid x_p^1 between the images I^1 and I^2 by minimizing the following energy:

$$E(F_{1,2}) = \sum_{p=1}^{N} \min \left(\|s(x_p^2) - s(F_{1,2}(x_p^1))\|, t \right) + \sum_{p=1}^{N} \gamma D(x_p^1, F_{1,2}(x_p^1)) +$$
$$\sum_{(p,q)\in\epsilon} \min \left(\alpha D(F_{1,2}(x_p^1), F_{1,2}(x_q^1)), d \right). \tag{3}$$

$E(F_{1,2})$ is comprised of a data term, a small displacement term and a smoothness term. The first term constrains the SIFT descriptors $s(x_p^2)$ [11] evaluated in pixel x_p^2 to be matched along with the descriptors evaluated in pixel $F_{1,2}(x_p^1)$. The small displacement term constrains the changes between the original image and a wrapped one to be as small as possible. D is equal to the distance between the two pixels in a pixel grid. The smoothness term constrains the transformation of adjacent pixels to be similar. In this objective function, truncated L_1 norms are used in both the data term and the smoothness term to account for matching outliers and discontinuities, with t and d as the threshold, respectively. Figure 2 shows the results of applying SIFT Flow algorithm to a drosophila larva data set. For further information we refer to [10].

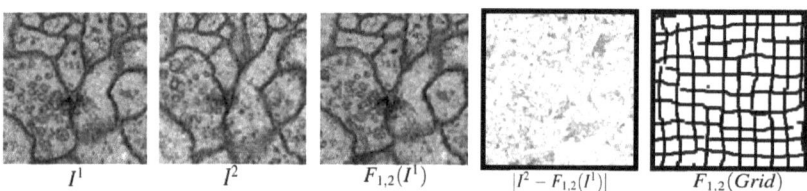

$$I^1 \qquad\qquad I^2 \qquad\qquad F_{1,2}(I^1) \qquad |I^2 - F_{1,2}(I^1)| \qquad F_{1,2}(Grid)$$

Fig. 2. An example of non-linear warping between images I^1 and I^2 found by SIFT Flow. Image $F_{1,2}(I^1)$ shows the warping applied to image I^1 and image $F_{1,2}(Grid)$ shows the warping applied to a grid image.

2.3   Features

We use 626 pixel features. When we incorporate the features from the neighboring section this number increases to 1878. RF performs well even in presence of lots of noisy features [4], therefore we need no feature selection procedure.

The whole set of features provided by [1] is used in this study: Gaussian blur, Sobel filter, Hessian, Difference of gaussians, Membrane projections, Variance, Mean, Minimum, Maximum, Median, Anisotropic diffusion, Bilateral, Lipschitz, Kuwahara, Gabor, Laplacian, Structure, Derivatives. Additionally, we incorporate newly developed features that proved to be informative for neuronal reconstruction: radon-like features [9], ray features [12] and line filter transform [13]. Also we use all the components of SIFT histogram [11] in the pixel.

2.4   Graph Cut Segmentation

We use graph cut segmentation to take into account the fact that the labels of the neighboring pixels are more likely to have the same label. For simplicity we drop the upper index in the following equations, as graph cut algorithm deals with one section at a time: $y_p = y_p^k$.

The segmentation task is formulated as an energy minimization problem $\hat{Y} = \arg\min_Y E(Y)$, where

$$E(Y) = \sum_{p=1}^{N} E_u(y_p) + \lambda_s \sum_{(p,q)\in\epsilon} E_s(y_p, y_q) + \lambda_{gf} \sum_{p=1}^{N} E_{gf}(y_p) + \lambda_{gc} \sum_{(p,q)\in\epsilon} E_{gc}(y_p, y_q). \tag{4}$$

Here the first term is a unary potential that equals to the negative log probabilities given by the RF in every pixel. Let $i(x_p)$ be an intensity of the image in pixel x_p. Then the second term is a smoothness term:

$$E_s(y_p, y_q) = \exp\left(-\frac{(i(x_p) - i(x_q))^2}{2\sigma_s^2}\right) \frac{\delta(y_p, y_q)}{D(x_p, x_q)}, \tag{5}$$

where $\delta(y_p, y_q)$ is a Kronecker function that equals 0 if $y_p = y_q$ and 1 otherwise.
The gradient flux term [14] is defined as follows:

$$E_{gf}(y_p) = \begin{cases} \max(0, F(x_p)) & \text{if } y_p = 1 \\ -\min(0, F(x_p)) & \text{if } y_p = 0, \end{cases} \tag{6}$$

where $F(x_p)$ denotes a gradient flux, $F(x_p) = \sum_{x_q:(x_p,x_q)\in\epsilon} < u_{x_p,x_q}, v_{x_p} >$, u_{x_p,x_q} represents a unit vector pointing from pixel x_p to the neighboring pixel x_q and vector v_{x_p} corresponds to the gradient vector at pixel x_p.
The good-continuation term [8] is defined as follows:

$$E_{gc}(y_p, y_q) = |< v_{x_p}, u_{x_p,x_q} >| \exp\left(-\frac{(i(x_p) - i_m)^2}{2\sigma_{gc}^2}\right) \frac{\delta_\rightarrow(y_p, y_q)}{D(x_p, x_q)}, \tag{7}$$

The variable i_m encodes the average gray value of membrane pixels and σ_{gc} is estimated as the variance of these gray values. The factor $\delta_{\rightarrow}(y_p, y_q) = 1$ for $y_p = 1$, $y_q = 0$ and equals 0 for all other cases.

The minimum of $E(Y)$ is computed by max-flow/min-cut computation [3]. The cross-validation procedure determines the unknown parameters λ_s, λ_{gf}, λ_{gc} such that the results generalize in an optimal way.

As a post-processing procedure two steps are performed iteratively: region removing and line filter transform [13]. Region removing is performed by a series of thresholding operations based on region properties such as Area, Solidity, Euler Number and Eccentricity.

3   Experiments

Data. Our experiments are performed with the data provided for the ISBI 2012 challenge "Segmentation of neuronal structures in EM stacks" [2]. The dataset [5] is comprised of a training and a test set. Each set consists of 30 sections from a ssTEM of the Drosophila first instar larva ventral nerve cord (VNC), imaged at a resolution of 4x4x50 nm/pixel and cover a 2x2x1.5 micron cube of neural tissue. Training and test sets are taken from different volumes of the same VNC.

Error Metrics. There are two metrics used for the task of membrane segmentation: *Pixel error* and *Splits and Mergers Warping error*. Given the estimated labeling $\hat{Y}$ and ground truth $Y^\star$, the pixel error is defined as the Hamming distance between the two labelings $\sum_p \delta(\hat{Y}_p, Y_p^\star)$.

Splits and Mergers Warping error is a segmentation metric that penalizes topological disagreements between the two labelings [6]. The warping error is the squared Euclidean distance between $Y^\star$ and the "best warping" L of $\hat{Y}$ onto $Y^\star$ such that the warping L is from the class Λ that preserve topological structure: $\min_{L \in \Lambda} \sum_p \delta(L(\hat{Y})_p, Y_p^\star)$.

Both types of errors are evaluated automatically on the test set when the results are submitted to the testing server. The challenge also provides the error value caused by discrepancy in human labeling.

3.1   Results

Our experiments are conducted with the default parameters of the SIFT flow algorithm: $\gamma = 0.05$, $t = 0.1$, $\alpha = 2$, $d = 40$. We compare the results of three different versions of our algorithm: with no context from neighboring sections (*one slice*), with direct correspondence (we incorporate the context from the pixels being a direct z-neighbors, with no warping procedure), and with dense correspondence found by SIFT flow algorithm.

Results are presented in Table 1. Some examples of the resulting images are presented in Figure 3. Incorporating the context from the neighboring sections with direct correspondence leads to improvement in terms of pixel error, but it performs worse in terms of warping error. On the other hand, using dense

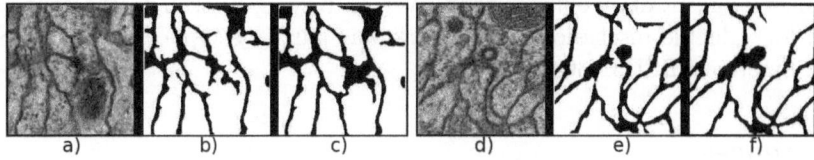

Fig. 3. Original images: (a, d), one slice results: (b, e), dense correspondense: (c, f)

Table 1. Comparison of error results on a testing set for different versions of the algorithm and the results of other teams. **Human** denotes the error of human annotators.

Method	Pixel error	Warping error	Method	Pixel error	Warping error
Human	$6.7 * 10^{-2}$	$3.4 * 10^{-4}$	*IDSIA*	$6.0 * 10^{-2}$	$4.3 * 10^{-4}$
Dense *ETH*	$7.9 * 10^{-2}$	$6.2 * 10^{-4}$	*CSIRO*	$8.7 * 10^{-2}$	$6.8 * 10^{-4}$
Direct *ETH*	$8.0 * 10^{-2}$	$6.5 * 10^{-4}$	*Utah*	$1.3 * 10^{-1}$	$1.6 * 10^{-2}$
One slice *ETH*	$8.5 * 10^{-2}$	$6.4 * 10^{-4}$	*NIST*	$1.5 * 10^{-1}$	$1.6 * 10^{-2}$

correspondence leads to improvement in both objectives: 3.6% improvement in warping error and 6.4% for pixel error.

Most of other algorithms applied in the ISBI challenge exploited the context of only one single slice. S. Iftikhar & A. Godil (NIST) and X. Tan & C. Sun of CSIRO Enquiries employed Support Vector Machine (SVM) as a classifier. A team from Scientific Computing and Imaging Institute, University of Utah[2] designed Series of Classifiers and Watershed Tree. The Swiss AI Lab IDSIA team[3] trained Deep Neural Networks which appeared to be competitive to ours and their solution was slightly better in quantitative terms. This approach, however, requires almost a week of training time with specialized hardware, and it is therefore much more difficult to apply in real-world scenarios.

4   Conclusion

This paper addresses the problem of automatic membrane segmentation in stacks of electron microscopy brain tissue sections. Since the image stacks in our applications are anisotropic, we are not able to exploit information from neighboring sections by exploring direct z-neighborhood. This paper demonstrates, for the first time, how to exploit context information from neighboring sections by robustly solving the correspondence problem.

We show that this problem can be effectively solved with the SIFT Flow algorithm. Our method calculates features in all the corresponding pixels, concatenates their feature vectors and uses this extended feature vector for a RF classifier. Finally Graph Cut segmentation is performed. The proposed method is 3.6% more accurate for warping error, and 6.4% for pixel error.

---

[2] T. Liu, M. Seyedhosseini, E. Jurrus, & T. Tasdizen.

[3] D. Ciresan, A. Giusti, L. Gambardella, & J. Schmidhuber.

Acknowledgement. We like to thank Verena Kaynig-Fittkau, GVI Group Harvard, for valuable discussions. This work was partially supported by the SNF grant Sinergia CRSII3_130470/1.

References

1. Advanced Weka Segmentation (Fiji), http://bit.ly/MdCr0v
2. ISBI 2012 challenge, http://bit.ly/riGDUm
3. Boykov, Y., Kolmogorov, V.: An experimental comparison of min-cut/max-flow algorithms for energy minimization in vision. Trans. Pattern Anal. Mach. Intell. 26, 1124–1137 (2004)
4. Breiman, L.: Random forests. Machine Learning 45(1), 5–32 (2001)
5. Cardona, A., Saalfeld, S., Preibisch, S., Schmid, B., Pulokas, A.C.J., Tomancak, P., Hartenstein, V.: An integrated micro- and macroarchitectural analysis of the drosophila brain by computer-assisted serial section electron microscopy. PLoS Biol. 10 (2010)
6. Jain, V., Bollmann, B., Richardson, M., Berger, D.R., Helmstaedter, M., Briggman, K.L., Denk, W., Bowden, J.B., Mendenhall, J.M., Abraham, W.C., Harris, K.M., Kasthuri, N., Hayworth, K.J., Schalek, R., Tapia, J.C., Lichtman, J.W., Seung, H.S.: Boundary learning by optimization with topological constraints. In: CVPR, pp. 2488–2495 (2010)
7. Kaynig, V., Fuchs, T.J., Buhmann, J.M.: Geometrical Consistent 3D Tracing of Neuronal Processes in ssTEM Data. In: Jiang, T., Navab, N., Pluim, J.P.W., Viergever, M.A. (eds.) MICCAI 2010, Part II. LNCS, vol. 6362, pp. 209–216. Springer, Heidelberg (2010)
8. Kaynig, V., Fuchs, T.J., Buhmann, J.M.: Neuron geometry extraction by perceptual grouping in sstem images. In: CVPR, pp. 2902–2909. IEEE (2010)
9. Kumar, R., Reina, A.V., Pfister, H.: Radon-like features and their application to connectomics. In: MMBIA. IEEE (2010)
10. Liu, C., Yuen, J., Torralba, A.: Sift flow: Dense correspondence across scenes and its applications. Trans. Pattern Anal. Mach. Intell. 33(5), 978–994 (2011)
11. Lowe, D.G.: Object recognition from local scale-invariant features. In: ICCV, p. 1150. IEEE (1999)
12. Lucchi, A., Smith, K., Achanta, R., Lepetit, V., Fua, P.: A Fully Automated Approach to Segmentation of Irregularly Shaped Cellular Structures in EM Images. In: Jiang, T., Navab, N., Pluim, J.P.W., Viergever, M.A. (eds.) MICCAI 2010, Part II. LNCS, vol. 6362, pp. 463–471. Springer, Heidelberg (2010)
13. Sandberg, K., Brega, M.: Segmentation of thin structures in electron micrographs using orientation fields. Journal of Structural Biology 157(2), 403–415 (2007)
14. Vasilevskiy, A., Siddiqi, K.: Flux maximizing geometric flows. Trans. Pattern Anal. Mach. Intell. 24, 1565–1578 (2001)
15. Vazquez-Reina, A., Huang, D., Gelbart, M., Lichtman, J., Miller, E., Pfister, H.: Segmentation fusion for connectomics. In: ICCV. IEEE (2011)

Apoptosis Detection for Adherent Cell Populations in Time-Lapse Phase-Contrast Microscopy Images

Seungil Huh[1], Dai Fei Elmer Ker[2], Hang Su[1], and Takeo Kanade[1]

[1] Robotics Institute, Carnegie Mellon University
{seungilh,hangs,tk}@cs.cmu.edu
[2] Department of Orthopedic Surgery, Stanford University
elmerker@stanford.edu

Abstract. The detection of apoptosis, or programmed cell death, is important to understand the underlying mechanism of cell development. At present, apoptosis detection resorts to fluorescence or colorimetric assays, which may affect cell behavior and thus not allow long-term monitoring of intact cells. In this work, we present an image analysis method to detect apoptosis in time-lapse phase-contrast microscopy, which is non-destructive imaging. The method first detects candidates for apoptotic cells based on the optical principle of phase-contrast microscopy in connection with the properties of apoptotic cells. The temporal behavior of each candidate is then examined in its neighboring frames in order to determine if the candidate is indeed an apoptotic cell. When applied to three C2C12 myoblastic stem cell populations, which contain more than 1000 apoptosis, the method achieved around 90% accuracy in terms of average precision and recall.

Keywords: Apoptosis detection, Time-lapse phase-contrast microscopy, Microscopy image restoration, Event detection in videos.

1 Introduction

The detection of apoptosis, or programmed cell death, is critical for furthering our understanding in biology as apoptosis plays a significant role in both normal tissue development and disease progression, e.g., proper organ development, stress-induced neurodegeneration, and cancer cell development. In addition, apoptosis detection is often used for toxicity screening of compounds, such as pharmacological reagents and biomaterials, as well as drug discovery and subsequent dosage optimization of chemotherapeutic agents.

Apoptosis occurs in an orderly, step-wise manner starting with a series of biochemical events that lead to characteristic changes in the cell prior to its death. The process of apoptosis includes cell shrinking, membrane blebbing, DNA degradation, and the formation of apoptotic bodies that serve to minimize spillage of the internal contents of a dying cell to its surroundings [1].

N. Ayache et al. (Eds.): MICCAI 2012, Part I, LNCS 7510, pp. 331–339, 2012.

Presently, apoptosis is detected using a variety of assays, which include absorbance measurements and fluorescence or colorimetric stains, to measure the levels and activity of apoptotic molecules. These procedures often require a sample to be harvested for each time-point measurement; thus, long-term cell monitoring is not feasible and multiple samples may be required. On the other hand, image analysis of cells using non-destructive imaging such as phase-contrast microscopy offers a way to monitor and detect apoptosis in a population of cells over time without adversely affecting cell behavior or requiring additional samples.

In this work, we present a method to detect apoptosis in time-lapse phase-contrast microscopy, particularly for adherent cells, which involves changes in cell morphology and image intensity during apoptosis. The method first detects the cells that shrink and become bright as candidates for apoptotic cells in order to reduce the search space. For this candidate detection, we propose a computational model of phase-contrast microscopy that can be used to detect both bright and dark cells. Each candidate is examined to determine if apoptosis indeed occurs based on changes in image intensity and texture over the neighboring frames. The proposed method was tested on three time-lapse microscopy image sequences of C2C12 myoblastic stem cells.

1.1 Related Work

There have been little-to-no reports of apoptosis detection in phase-contrast microscopy. To the best of our knowledge, cell death event detection has only been implicitly performed as a byproduct of cell tracking; i.e., if the trajectory of a cell terminates during cell tracking, the cell is considered dead. However, this simple heuristic often yields poor results because many cell trajectories terminate due to failures in cell tracking as opposed to actual cell death.

One may think that apoptosis detection can be performed by the methods for mitosis (cell division) detection, such as the method in [2]. However, such methods are not effective because mitosis detection depends on a unique visual presentation lasting only a short time, namely a figure eight shape, while apoptosis does not involve such a distinctive visual hallmark. In addition, after cells die through apoptosis, the dead cells often form a cluster with other living or dead cells, which makes apoptosis detection more difficult than mitosis detection.

2 Method

To narrow down the locations where apoptosis begins, we first locate bright cells whose formation is followed by size shrinkage and brightness increase. Each candidate is then validated based on temporal changes in brightness and texture.

2.1 Cell Region Detection

To detect apoptosis candidates, we detect both bright and dark cell areas using a computational model for the optical principle of phase-contrast microscopy.

According to [3], phase-contrast imaging can be modeled by two waves: the unaltered surround wave $\tilde{l}_S(x)$ and the diffracted wave $\tilde{l}_D(x)$, computed as

$$\tilde{l}_S(x) = i\zeta_p A e^{i\beta} \tag{1}$$

$$\tilde{l}_D(x) = \zeta_c A e^{i(\beta+f(x))} + (i\zeta_p - 1)\zeta_c A e^{i(\beta+f(x))} * airy(r) \tag{2}$$

where $i^2 = -1$; A and β are the illuminating wave's amplitude and phase before hitting the specimen plate, respectively; ζ_p and ζ_c are the amplitude attenuation factors by the phase ring and the specimen, respectively; $f(x)$ is the phase shift caused by the specimen at location x; and, $airy(r)$ is an obscured Airy pattern.

The intensity of the final observed image $g(x)$ is then computed as

$$g(x) = |\tilde{l}_S(x) + \tilde{l}_D(x)|^2 \tag{3}$$

$$= |i\zeta_p A e^{i\beta} + \zeta_c A e^{i(\beta+f(x))} + (i\zeta_p - 1)\zeta_c A e^{i(\beta+f(x))} * airy(r)|^2 \tag{4}$$

$$\approx 2\zeta_c\zeta_p(1+\zeta_c)A^2\left(\frac{\zeta_p(1+\zeta_c)}{2\zeta_c} + f(x) - f(x)*airy(r)\right) \tag{5}$$

$$\propto f(x) * (\delta(r) - airy(r)) + C \tag{6}$$

where $C = \frac{\zeta_p(1+\zeta_c)}{2\zeta_c}$ is a constant. Based on this approximate linear relation between $f(x)$ and $g(x)$ in Eq. (6), $f(x)$ can be reconstructed from $g(x)$. Since $f(x)$ is the phase shift caused by the specimen, thresholding $f(x)$ results in the detection of cell areas [3].

Note that in order to obtain Eq. (5) from Eq. (4), it is assumed that $f(x)$ is close to zero, based on which following three approximations are applied:

$$e^{if(x)} \approx 1 + if(x), \quad f(x)^2 \approx 0, \quad (f(x)*airy(r))^2 \approx 0. \tag{7}$$

However, these approximations are not valid particularly for bright cells, which cause greater phase retardations than dark cells[1]. As a result, the method has difficulty in detecting mitotic or apoptotic cells, which appear bright due to their increased thickness.

To detect bright cells (and also dark cells more properly), we generalize the model by assuming that $f(x)$ is close to a certain phase θ, which is not necessarily zero. More formally, $f(x)$ is replaced with $\theta + \tilde{f}(x)$, where θ is a constant and $\tilde{f}(x)$ is close to zero. Based on this relaxed assumption, $g(x)$ is computed as

$$g(x) = |i\zeta_p A e^{i\beta} + \zeta_c A e^{i(\beta+\theta+\tilde{f}(x))} + (i\zeta_p - 1)\zeta_c A e^{i(\beta+\theta+\tilde{f}(x))} * airy(r)|^2 \tag{8}$$

to which we apply the following approximations

$$e^{i\tilde{f}(x)} \approx 1 + i\tilde{f}(x), \quad \tilde{f}(x)^2 \approx 0, \quad (\tilde{f}(x)*airy(r))^2 \approx 0, \tag{9}$$

---

[1] Even for the detection of dark cells, the assumption $f(x) \approx 0$ is not quite valid because the diffracted wave is retarded in phase by approximately 90 degrees through interaction with the specimen [4].

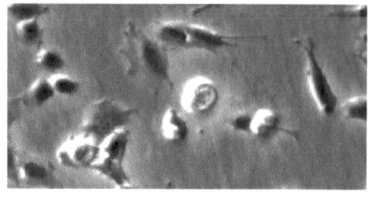 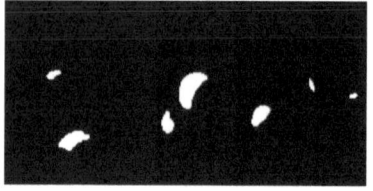

Fig. 1. A sample image and bright cell areas on it detected by the proposed model

(a) 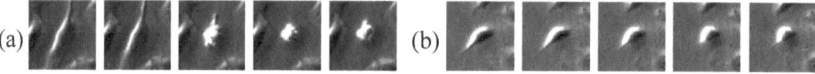 (b)

Fig. 2. Apoptosis processes in consecutive frames. An apoptotic cell shrinks and its brightness increases (a) abruptly for a short time period (less than five minutes) or (b) gradually for a long time period (tens of minutes or a few hours).

resulting in

$$g(x) \approx 2\zeta_c\zeta_p(\cos\theta + \zeta_c)A^2$$
$$\times \left(\frac{\zeta_p(1 + \zeta_c^2 + 2\zeta_c\cos\theta)}{2\zeta_c(\cos\theta + \zeta_c)} + \tilde{f}(x) - \frac{\cos\theta + \zeta_c + \zeta_p\sin\theta}{\cos\theta + \zeta_c}\tilde{f}(x) * airy(r)\right) \quad (10)$$
$$\propto \tilde{f}(x) * (\delta(r) - B \cdot airy(r)) + C' \quad (11)$$

where $B = \frac{\cos\theta + \zeta_c + \zeta_p\sin\theta}{\cos\theta + \zeta_c}$ and $C' = \frac{\zeta_p(1 + \zeta_c^2 + 2\zeta_c\cos\theta)}{2\zeta_c(\cos\theta + \zeta_c)}$. Note that, if $\theta = 0$, then $\tilde{f}(x) = f(x)$, $B = 1$, and $C' = C$; thus, Eq (11) reduces to Eq (6). Since this is also a linear relation between $\tilde{f}(x)$ and $g(x)$, $\tilde{f}(x)$ can be reconstructed from $g(x)$ and cell areas can be detected by thresholding $\tilde{f}(x)$.

Using this model, we detect bright and dark cell areas, separately with two different parameters: θ_b and θ_d. For the parameter setting, we tested several values $(0, \pi/6, \cdots, 11\pi/6)$ and selected the best ones based on apoptosis detection accuracy on the training set. (This can also be conducted by visual examination on a first few images.) The proposed model can detect bright cells as well as dark cells, unlike the previous model. Fig. 1 shows bright cell areas detected by our model, where bright halos are undetected or weakly detected.

2.2   Apoptosis Candidate Detection

To detect the cells that undergo the beginning of an apoptotic process, we examine each bright cell area to determine if its formation is followed by the decrease of dark area and/or the increase of bright area, which represent cell shrinkage and brightness increase, respectively. If the change is not trivial, the bright cell area is considered a candidate for an apoptotic cell; otherwise, it is regarded an already dead cell or a bright halo, and thus is not further taken into account.

Algorithm 1. Apoptosis candidate detection at frame t

Input:
$\{B^{(s)}, D^{(s)}$: binary images indicating bright/dark cell areas at frame $s\}$,
K: maximum number of frames investigated prior to the frame t,
R: radius of the neighboring region, th: threshold for bright/dark area change.
Output:
$\{(cx, cy)\}$: a set of (x,y) positions of candidate apoptotic cells.

1: // Compute dark/bright area change over consecutive frames prior to frame t
2: **for** $k = 1 \rightarrow K$ **do**
3:     $\Delta B_k \leftarrow (B^{(t-k+1)} - B^{(t-k)})$ filtered by the average disk filter with radius R.
4:     $\Delta D_k \leftarrow (D^{(t-k)} - D^{(t-k+1)})$ filtered by the average disk filter with radius R.
5: **end for**
6: // Examine bright/dark area change.
7: $\{C_i\} \leftarrow$ a set of bright cell areas (lists of positions) at frame t, obtained from $B^{(t)}$.
8: **for each** $C_i = \{(x_j, y_j)\}$ **do**
9:     $found \leftarrow false, k \leftarrow 0$
10:    **while** not $found$ and $k < K$ **do**
11:       $k \leftarrow k + 1$
12:       **if** $\exists (x, y) \in C_i$ s.t. $\forall j \in \{1, \cdots, k\}, \Delta B_j(x, y) > th/k$ or $\Delta D_j(x, y) > th/k$ **then**
13:          $found \leftarrow true$
14:       **end if**
15:    **end while**
16:    **if** $found$ **then**
17:       // Keep the point that shows the most brightness change over the k frames.
18:       $\{(cx, cy)\} \leftarrow \{(cx, cy)\} \cup \arg\max_{(x,y) \in C_i} \sum_{k'=1}^{k} \Delta B_{k'}(x, y)$
19:    **end if**
20: **end for**

More formally, for each bright cell area at frame t, we examine its neighboring region over consecutive frames prior to the frame t. If the proportion of the bright area expanded or dark area shrunk in the region to the region's area is greater than a certain threshold, then the bright cell area is considered a candidate for an apoptotic cell. As the duration of cell shrinking and brightness change varies (See Fig. 2.) and the image acquisition interval can also be different among experiments, we investigate different numbers of frames (up to K frames) prior to frame t. More specifically, if the change between every two consecutive frames among the $k + 1$ preceding frames is greater than the reduced threshold th/k for any $k \in \{1, \cdots, K\}$, then the bright cell area is considered a candidate for an apoptotic cell. The detailed procedure of apoptosis candidate detection is described in Algorithm 1.

The neighboring region is set to be a circle with radius R. Hence, this scheme involves three parameters: K, R, and th. We set these parameters to achieve at least a certain high level of recall (e.g., 99%) and as high a precision as possible in candidate detection among the training data (Note that as th decreases, recall increases while precision decreases.). K and R can also be determined based on

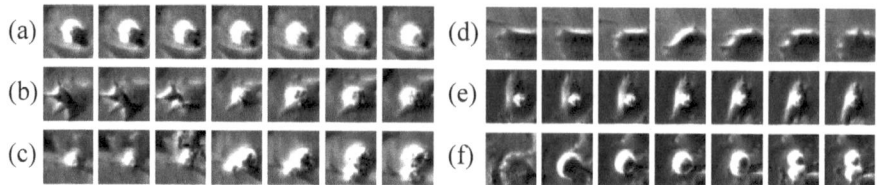

Fig. 3. Candidate patch sequences containing apoptosis (left) and non-apoptosis (right): (a-c) apoptotic cells in contact with none, a living cell, and a (or a group of) dead cell(s); (d-f) a change of halo, a (or a group of) dead cell(s), and mitosis

the observation of apoptosis duration and cell size/movement, respectively. In our experiments, K, R, and th were set to be 5, 10, and 0.25, respectively.

2.3   Feature Extraction

Each candidate is tracked in the neighboring frames in order to incorporate temporal information by using a standard correlation tracking method, resulting in candidate patch sequences as shown in Fig. 3. Investigating temporal information helps to avoid detecting mitosis, which shows similar visual change to apoptosis at the beginning, as well as bright halos and dead cells. This step involves two parameters, the size of patch and the number of frames tracked on one side (preceding or following a candidate), which can be set by a typical validation scheme. In our experiments, they were set to be 50 pixels and 3 patches. From each patch in a patch sequence, we extract the following features:

- Brightness change histogram binning to 16 bins,
- Rotation invariant uniform local binary pattern (LBP^{riu2}) [5].

The former, which is computed on the difference between a patch and its previous patch, captures brightness change over time, the major cue for apoptosis detection, more precisely and in more detail than the candidate detection step. The latter captures the texture property of apoptotic cells, which is quite different from that of non-apoptotic cells as apoptosis involves membrane blebbing and the formation of apoptotic bodies. It is worth mentioning that these features are robust to global illumination change due to experimental setting.

2.4   Candidate Validation

We applied a linear Support Vector Machine (SVM) to classify candidate patch sequences. We tested several other classifiers used for mitosis detection, Hidden Conditional Random Field (HCRF) [6] and its variations [2,7]. All these classifiers as well as an RBF kernel SVM did not outperform a linear SVM despite their higher computational cost, presumably because visual features of apoptosis are less informative and more noisy in the sense that apoptosis does not

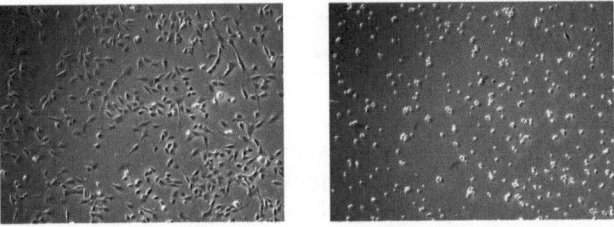

Fig. 4. The first (left) and last (right) frames of the data

involve distinctive morphological features, such as a figure eight shape during mitosis. Under such a circumstance, a max-margin classifier with a simple decision boundary might be more effective to eliminate outliers or meaningless patterns. After classification, the post-processing in [7] is conducted to prevent one apoptosis from being detected multiple times.

3   Experiments

We introduce the experimental setup and results with discussions.

3.1   Image and Ground Truth Acquisition

After C2C12 myoblastic stem cells were cultured for one day, Mitomycin C was added to induce apoptosis. Afterward, three populations were imaged every 5 minutes over 45 hours, resulting in three sets of 540 image frames. As shown in Fig. 4, most of cells were dead at the last frame. We manually annotated apoptosis by marking the center of each apoptotic cell after it shrinks and becomes bright, obtaining 1154 cases in total. The image sequences and ground truths are available on the first author's web page (www.cs.cmu.edu/∼seungilh).

3.2   Evaluation

A detection is considered a true positive if an apoptotic cell is detected within spatially 30 pixels and temporally 3 frames from an annotated location. If an apoptotic cell is detected more than once, the only one that temporally the closest to the ground truth was considered true positive, the others false positives.

We used one sequence as a training set and another one as a test set, testing all six training-testing set pairs. We set all the parameters including the SVM parameter through a four-fold cross validation on the training set.

3.3   Results and Discussions

Our method achieved an average precision of 93.0%±1.1% and an average recall of 89.8%±1.4% for apoptosis detection. False positives mostly happened due to

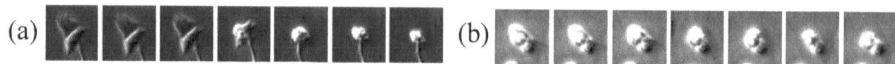

Fig. 5. Examples of undetected apoptosis after candidate validation. (a) As two cells in contact with each other undergo apoptosis simultaneously, only one apoptosis is detected. (b) An apoptotic cell is barely observable as it is covered with two dead cells.

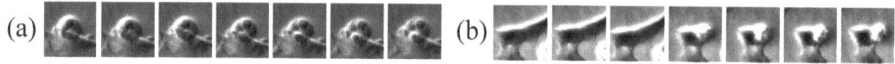

Fig. 6. Examples of undetected apoptosis at the candidate detection step. (a) Apoptosis occurs without brightness change. (b) As a small apoptotic cell is located in contact with a compact and dark cell, the bright apoptotic cell is considered the bright halo of the dark cell and thus not detected at the bright cell area detection step.

rapidly changing halos and moving dead cells attached to living cells. Duplicate detection sometimes occurred as apoptotic cells abruptly and considerably move while they shrink or when cell internal contents spill out. False negatives mostly happened when cells form a cluster in which multiple apoptosis simultaneously occur or apoptotics cells are occluded by other cells, as shown in Fig. 5.

In the candidate detection step, our method detected almost all apoptosis except a few cases (See Fig. 6.). The number of candidates were approximately three times as many as the number of apoptosis.

Our model-based cell area detection is effective, particularly when cell density is high and thus cells are in contact with one another and halos appear among them. The scheme outperformed a cell area detection scheme based on intensity thresholding by 3.3% and 10.3% in terms of average apoptosis detection precision and recall, respectively, on the last 100 frames of the three sequences.

4   Conclusion

We have presented an apoptosis detection method for adherent cells that detects apoptosis candidates and then validates them. For the candidate detection, we proposed a cell area detection method based on the optical principle of phase-contrast microscopy. When applied to three cell populations, our method achieved around 90% accuracy in terms of average precision and recall.

References

1. Fuchs, Y., Steller, H.: Programmed cell death in animal development and disease. Cell 147(4), 742–758 (2011)
2. Huh, S., et al.: Automated mitosis detection of stem cell populations in phase-contrast microscopy images. IEEE Trans. Med. Imaging 30(3), 586–596 (2011)

3. Yin, Z., Kanade, T., Chen, M.: Understanding the phase contrast optics to restore artifact-free microscopy images for segmentation. Med. Image Anal. 16(5), 1047–1062 (2012)
4. http://www.microscopyu.com/articles/phasecontrast/phasemicroscopy.html
5. Ojala, T., Pietikäinen, M., Mäenpää, T.T.: Multiresolution gray-scale and rotation invariant texture classification with local binary pattern. IEEE Trans. Pattern. Anal. Mach. Intell. 24(7), 971–987 (2002)
6. Quattoni, A., Wang, S., Morency, L., Collins, M., Darrell, T.: Hidden conditional random fields. IEEE Trans. Pattern Anal. Mach. Intell. 29(10), 1848–1853 (2007)
7. Huh, S., Chen, M.: Detection of mitosis within a stem cell population of high cell confluence in phase-contrast microscopy images. In: IEEE CVPR, pp. 1033–1040 (2011)

Modeling Dynamic Cellular Morphology
in Images

Xing An[1,2,*], Zhiwen Liu[1], Yonggang Shi[1], Ning Li[3],
Yalin Wang[2], and Shantanu H. Joshi[4]

[1] School of Information and Electronics, Beijing Inst. of Tech., Beijing, China
[2] School of Computer Sci. and Engineering, Arizona State University, Tempe, USA
[3] Department of General Surgery, Beijing You'An Hospital, Beijing, China
[4] Laboratory of Neuro Imaging, UCLA School of Medicine, Los Angeles, CA, USA

Abstract. This paper presents a geometric method for modeling dynamic features of cells in image sequences. The morphological changes in cellular membrane boundaries are represented as sequences of parameterized contours. These sequences are analyzed as paths on a shape space equipped with an invariant metric, and matched using dynamic time warping. Experimental results show high sensitivity of the proposed dynamic features to the morphological changes observed in lymphocytes of healthy mice after undergoing skin transplantation when compared with standard representation methods and shape features.

1 Introduction

Morphological analysis of cells features prominently in a wide range of applications including digital pathology and is essential for improving our understanding of the basic physiological processes of organisms. Although the underlying cellular structure is $3D$, a $2D$ morphological analysis can still be conclusive and effective for several applications [1]. Accordingly, advanced image processing techniques involving tasks such as cell tracking, extraction, cell shape representation and analysis [1–3] have enabled accurate analysis of $2D$ static cell images. However, these static analyses do not provide information about the dynamic cellular activity. To date, an increasing number of studies are using live-cell $(2D + t)$ imaging to provide insight into the nature of cellular functions [4]. The task of cell shape analysis in image sequences $(2D + t)$ is challenging due to the following reasons: i) it is difficult to compactly reduce and represent the high dimensional geometric data from information-rich image sequences for accurately capturing the biologically relevant phenomena under investigation, ii) live cells are non-rigid bodies, and thus classical methods optimized for rigid transformations are unsuitable for their analysis, and finally, iii) the geometric information from the cell shapes needs to be appropriately isolated from the pose in an invariant manner.

---

* This work is sponsored by the National Natural Science Foundation of China (60971133) and the China Scholarship Council. anxing@bit.edu.cn

N. Ayache et al. (Eds.): MICCAI 2012, Part I, LNCS 7510, pp. 340–347, 2012.

In this paper we propose a dynamic framework for quantitative analysis of lymphocyte morphological changes in $2D + t$ image sequences. We represent cell shape boundaries by continuous, closed, parameterized curves, and analyze them dynamically on the shape space of such representations. Our framework conveniently lends itself to i) the interpolation of intermediate shapes in a sequence, ii) the invariant and symmetrical matching of different cell shape sequences, and iii) statistical analysis of dynamic cell morphology. We test our method on a collection of 42 lymphocyte sequences and present results on i) discrimination of normal and abnormal cellular morphology, ii) local statistical differences between abnormal and normal shape sequences, and iii) classification of shape sequences based on the dynamic cellular shape changes from one time point to another.

2 Dynamic Cellular Morphometry

2.1 Shape Analysis of Static Cellular Boundaries

While normal morphological changes in cells show subtle changes in shape, abnormal cells exhibit structural irregularities due to various disease processes or disruptions in cellular mechanisms caused by isolated cellular activity. It is critical that the shape representation be sensitive to pathological changes as well as regular normative variation. In this section, we briefly describe the representation, invariances, and matching framework for static cell shape analysis.

Shape Representation: We represent the segmented cell boundary by $2D$ closed, continuously parameterized curve [5–7] $c \subset \mathbb{R}^2$ given by $c(s) : [0, 2\pi) \rightarrow \mathbb{R}^2$. In order to analyze the geometry of them exclusively without the confounding effects of global location and scale, we represent the translation invariant geometric shape of this curve using the parameterized function given by

$$q(s) = \frac{\dot{c}(s)}{\sqrt{||\dot{c}(s)||}} \in \mathbb{R}^2, s \in [0, 2\pi]. \tag{1}$$

Here $||\cdot|| \equiv \sqrt{(\cdot, \cdot)_{\mathbb{R}^2}}$, and $(\cdot, \cdot)_{\mathbb{R}^2}$ is the standard Euclidean inner product in $\mathbb{R}^2$.

Shape Invariances: The representation is automatically invariant to translation. To make that invariant to scale, we divide the q function by its magnitude $\sqrt{\int_0^{2\pi} (q(s), q(s))_{\mathbb{R}^2}}$. A rigid rotation of a curve is a shape-preserving operation and is defined as $O \cdot q(s) = Oq(s)$, where $O \in \mathrm{SO}(2)$. Additionally the cell shape distances should also be independent of the origin of the curve. The choice of the origin is modeled as a shift operation by $r \in \mathbb{S}^1$, $r \cdot q(s) = q((s - r)_{\mathrm{mod}\ 2\pi})$. Lastly, the variable speed reparameterizations of the curve are modeled as diffeomorphic group actions of $\gamma : [0, 2\pi) \rightarrow [0, 2\pi)$ on the curve and given as $q \cdot \gamma = \sqrt{\dot{\gamma}}\ (q \circ \gamma)$. Of these, the contribution due to the starting point, rotation, and the reparameterization are removed during the next shape matching stage.

Shape Matching: Since a cell boundary necessarily corresponds to a closed curve, we define the space of all translation and scale invariant closed curves

as $\mathcal{C} \equiv \{q|q(s) : [0, 2\pi] \to \mathbb{R}^2| \int_0^{2\pi} (q(s), q(s))_{\mathbb{R}^2} ds = 1, \int_0^{2\pi} q(s) \ ||q(s)||ds = 0\}$.
Owing to the conditions of scale invariance, translation invariance, and closure, the space $\mathcal{C}$ becomes a subset of a spherical Hilbert space. For the purpose of discriminating between cell boundaries, we need a computable metric on the space of cellular shapes. We define a $\mathbb{L}^2$ inner product on the ambient Hilbert space given by $\langle u, v \rangle = \int_0^{2\pi} (u(s), v(s))_{\mathbb{R}^2} ds$, and induce it on $\mathcal{C}$. This inner product is analogous to the vector form of the Euclidean inner product and measures infinitesimal perturbations of shapes. The advantage of the ambient spherical Hilbert space is that geodesics are specified analytically. The geodesic as a function of time τ, between two cell shapes q_1 and q_2 on the sphere is given by $\chi_\tau(q_1, q_2) = \cos\left(\tau \cos^{-1}\langle q_1, q_2 \rangle\right) q_1 + \sin\left(\tau \cos^{-1}\langle q_1, q_2 \rangle\right) f$, where $f = q_2 - \langle q_1, q_2 \rangle q_1$. Then the scale and translation invariant distance between the two cell shapes is given by $d(q_1, q_2) = \int_0^{2\pi} \sqrt{\langle \dot{\chi}_\tau, \dot{\chi}_\tau \rangle} d\tau$. Thus we need to enable fully pose, and initial-point invariant, as well as elastic mappings between cell shapes. This is achieved as follows. Rotational invariance is achieved by finding the optimal distance over all rotations $O \in SO(2)$, and the invariance to starting point is obtained by searching over all starting points $r \in \mathbb{S}^1$. It is easier to implement in the discrete setting. For obtaining an elastic mapping, we optimize over all reparameterizations of the curve given by $q \cdot \gamma$. Thus the fully pose and scale invariant, elastic shape distance between two cell boundaries is given by

$$d_e(q_1, q_2) = \underset{r, O \in SO(2), \gamma}{\text{argmin}} \frac{1}{2} \left[d(q_1, r \cdot O(q_2 \cdot \gamma)) + d(q_2, r \cdot O(q_1 \cdot \gamma^{-1})) \right]. \quad (2)$$

After solving Eqn. 2 using a combination of dynamic programming (for initialization) and gradient descent, we not only get a distance between the shapes q_1 and q_2, but also get a geodesic path χ_τ between them. The distance obtained by solving Eqn. 2 is a shape distance between two static cell boundaries.

2.2   Dynamic Shape Analysis of Cell Sequences

Since our goal is to model the dynamic nature of the cell behaviors by analyzing the spatial as well as temporal changes, we now propose a general framework for representation, matching, and statistical analysis of dynamic cell shape sequences. In this paper, we assume that the cell motion for all populations is captured in a fixed time interval, $t \in [0, T]$. Fig. 1 (A) provides an overview of the acquisition of the cell shape sequences from phase contrast microscopy images as well as two representative sequences of abnormal (Fig. 1 (B)) and normal (Fig. 1 (C)) lymphocyte morphology.

We denote $X(t)$ as a time-valued sequence of cell shapes for a given observation, where $X(t) \subset \mathbb{R}^2|X(t, s) : [0, 2\pi] \times [0, T] \to \mathbb{R}^2$. We represent the time sequence $X(t)$ as $X(t) \equiv \{q_t^X\}, t \in [0, T]$, where q_t^X is the observed shape in sequence X at time t. The quantity $X(t)$ can be thought of as a path of a collection of shapes exhibiting infinitesimal changes on the shape space. Now given two such shape sequences, $X(t)$, and $Y(t)$, we are interested in finding an optimal correspondence between them, that takes the temporal variation in the

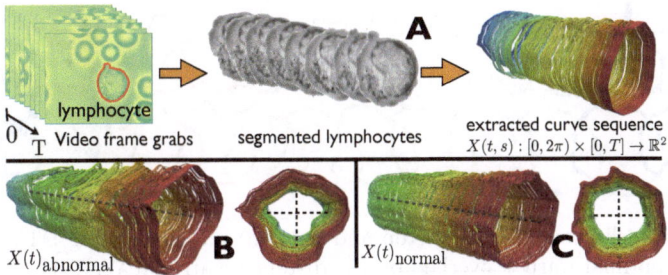

Fig. 1. (A) Lymphocyte shape sequence extraction workflow. Lateral and cross-sectional views of cell sequences belonging to the (B) abnormal category and the (C) normal category.

sequences into account. Dynamic time warping (DTW) [8] has been originally used for aligning different speech time series for speech recognition, and subsequently used to compare human gait [9, 10]. Matching cellular forms is more challenging than comparing human silhouettes, since cellular shapes lack well defined structure. In this work, we extend and adapt the dynamic time warping algorithm for comparing dynamic sequences on the shape space of elastically parameterized cell boundaries.

Cell Sequence Matching. Given two shape sequences X_1 and X_2, we want to find a distance between them that takes into account i) the changes between individual shapes along the temporal direction, and ii) the differences between individual shapes within the two sequences. Myers et al. [8] have used a square root weighting function compensated by the time rate change between two time sequences for speech recognition. Following the same principle, we define an invariant, symmetrical distance between the two shape sequences X_1 and X_2 as

$$d_s(X_1, X_2) = \min_{\psi} \int_0^T d_e \left(q_t^{X_1}, q_{\psi(t)}^{X_2} \right)^2 \{1 + \dot{\psi}(t)\} dt, \qquad (3)$$

with the optimal time warp $\hat{\psi}$ given by the minimizer of Eqn. 3. This function is a weighted Euclidean distance between the two shape sequences compensated by a non-linear weighting function that adjusts the time rate change of the two sequences. Furthermore, this distance is invariant to the rate change by time t, and symmetrical with respect to the two shape sequences. For the purpose of computer implementation, Eqn. 3 is discretized by considering finite samples from the shape sequences, and solved using dynamic programming. Fig. 2 shows an example of a dynamic alignment between two lymphocyte sequences along with the optimal warping function $\hat{\psi}$ overlaid on the discrete distance matrix given by $d(X_1, X_2)$.

Statistics of Dynamic Shape Sequences. In order to find statistical differences between two populations of cell shape sequences, we establish the notion

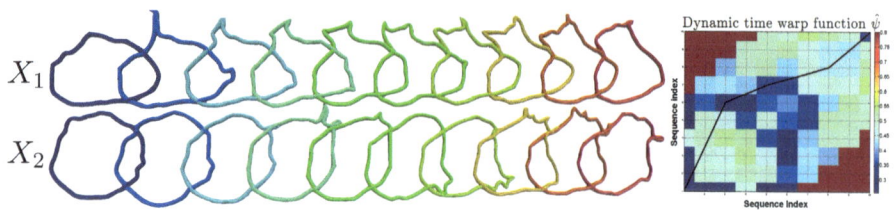

Fig. 2. Left: Cell shape sequence (top and bottom) matching using DTW in Eqn. 3. Right: The optimal warp $\hat{\psi}$ overlaid on the distance matrix $d(X_1, X_2)$.

of an average dynamic shape sequence. The average shape sequence is the local minimizer of the variance of a collection of shape sequences. We define the dynamic shape variance as $X_\sigma^2 = \frac{1}{N-1} \sum_{i=1}^{N} d_s(X_i, X)^2$. Then using Eqn. 2 and 3, the dynamic shape average becomes

$$X_\mu = \underset{X}{\text{argmin}} \frac{1}{N-1} \left[\sum_{i=1}^{N} \left\{ \underset{\psi}{\text{argmin}} \int_0^T d_e\left(q_t^{X_i}, q_{\psi(t)}^X\right)^2 \{1 + \dot{\psi}(t)\} dt \right\}^2 \right]. \quad (4)$$

Specifically X_μ is a sequence of shapes denoted by $X_\mu \equiv \{q_t^{X_\mu}\}, t \in [0, T]$. In practice, the mean shape sequence is computed by performing the dynamic time warping of the shape sequences and then computing the Karcher mean [11] shapes of all the corresponding shapes. The Karcher mean is an intrinsic mean on the space of shapes and is computed iteratively by minimizing the sum-squared geodesic distances between all the shapes in the population.

Shape Discrimination between Cell Morphologies. Since our main goal is to differentiate the shape variation between the dynamic behavior of normal and abnormal lymphocytes, we derive a discrete shape-sequence feature vector which can used to classify different sequences of lymphocytes. This feature vector should ideally be efficient to compute as well as capture the relevant shape dynamics along the sequence. For a given sequence $X(t)$, we first sample N shapes uniformly along the time interval $t \in [0, T]$ as $\{q_i^X\}, i = 1, \ldots, N$. We then compute $N - 1$ piecewise geodesics between the adjacent shapes of the sequence and denote the respective geodesic paths by χ . We then construct a parameter vector by taking the magnitude of the velocity vector given by

$$f_i = \int_0^1 \sqrt{\langle \dot{\chi}_t(q_i^X, q_{i+1}^X), \dot{\chi}_t(q_i^X, q_{i+1}^X) \rangle} dt, i = 0, \ldots, N - 2. \quad (5)$$

The adjacent velocity vectors $\dot{\chi}_\tau$ are analogous to the approximation of the difference operators in the well-known ARIMA model, although we do not impose any such parametric constraints in our work. This $N - 1$ dimensional parameter vector is can now be used as the input feature for classification of dynamic lymphocyte shape changes in image sequences.

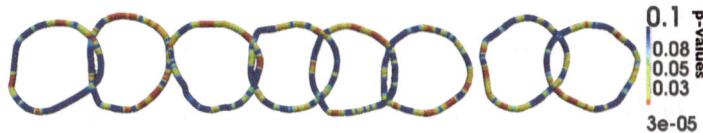

Fig. 3. Average for all the 42 lymphocyte sequences. The overlaid p-values (FDR-corrected) on the shapes denote significant differences of the invariant shape deformation fields between the abnormal and normal classes.

3 Experimental Design and Results

3.1 Data

Our data consists of 42 lymphocyte image sequences (20~30 seconds) of mice undergoing back skin transplantation (age: 6-8 weeks, weight 20-22 g) observed with phase contrast microscopy (Olympus BX51, 0.3 μ resolution, 16 × 1000 magnification). The first group consisted of 21 healthy Balb/C mice as hosts and 21 healthy Balb/C mice as donors, whereas the second group consisted of 21 healthy Balb/C mice as hosts and 21 healthy C57BL/6 mice as donors. The lymphocytes were obtained from the blood samples of the 42 hosts collected from the tail 7 days after the skin transplant. Lymphocytes in the second group showed irregular dynamic behavior such as cell elongation from different angles and a temporary projection at the border, and were characterized as abnormal, while the lymphocytes in the first group were characterized as normal.

3.2 Dynamic Shape Differences between Lymphocytes

To find differences in changes of shape across the entire population, we computed an average shape sequence for all the 42 lymphocytes using Eqn. 4. For efficiency, we sampled each sequence into 8 shapes per sequence, aligned all the sequences to this average sequence using dynamic time warping, and measured the magnitude of the velocity vectors along the geodesics between the corresponding shapes in the sequence. Since the velocity vectors are invariant to pose, we denoted this measure as the magnitude of the element wise shape deformation between the two sequences. We then performed a t-test comparing the magnitude of the velocity vector across the abnormal and normal groups. Fig. 3 shows the mean shape sequence for all the 42 lymphocyte sequences computed using Eqn. 4 with color-code false-discovery rate (FDR) corrected p-values ($p_{FDR} < 0.0059$)) denoting the differences in shape. It is observed that there are significant localized statistical differences in shape across the normal and abnormal populations.

Next, we test the discriminative properties of the shape-sequence distance by computing $42 \times \frac{41}{2} = 861$ pairwise shape distances for all the 42 sequences. The shape sequence distances were visualized by projecting the distance matrix into two dimensions using multidimensional scaling (MDS). To test the improvement due to dynamic time warping, we also computed 861 pairwise distances without DTW ($\psi(t) = t$). Fig. 4 shows a comparison of the MDS projections of the pairwise distances between all 42 (21 abnormal (denoted by A_n), and 21 normal (denoted by N_n) shape sequences. It is observed that pairwise distances using DTW exhibit a better separation of the sequences compared to shape matching using a linear time correspondence. Additionally, Fig. 4 also shows possible outlier sequences for abnormal cases A_1, A_5, A_8, and A_{21}.

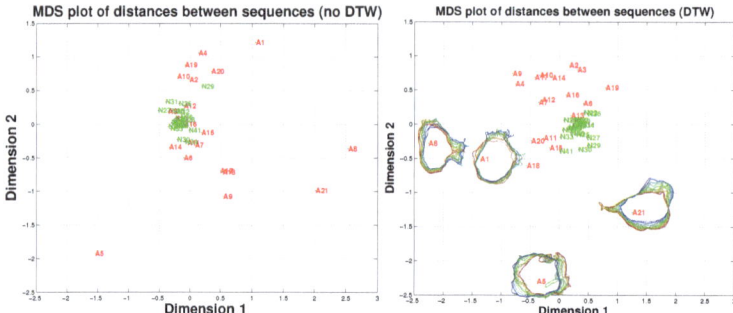

Fig. 4. MDS projections of the pairwise distances between all 42 sequences without (left) DTW ($\psi(t) = t$), and with DTW (right) along with outlier sequences. The abnormal and normal samples are plotted in red and green respectively.

3.3   Classification of Dynamic Lymphocyte Cell Morphology

Finally we present results of the classification of lymphocyte cell sequences using the feature vector defined in Eqn. 5. We sampled $N = 7$ cell shapes from each image sequences and computed 42 6-dimensional feature vectors for the population. Learning Vector Quantization (LVQ) was then used to classify these two categories with 10-fold cross-validation. We compared our results with standard cell shape features such as area, elongation, and Fourier descriptors coefficients ($n = 360$) of cell shapes [1]. Each of these features were represented by a 6-parameter vector using the same 7 images used for the geodesic feature vectors, except computing Euclidean norms instead of geodesic distances. This ensured that the comparisons were consistent across different methodologies. All the classification experiments were randomly repeated for 100 times, trained with one prototype for each class, and the performance was evaluated over the other disjoint members of the set. Table 1 shows the comparison results of mean recognition accuracy of training (TrAc), testing (TeAc), sensitivity (TrSe) and specificity (TrSp) of training, and sensitivity (TeSe), and specificity (TeSp) of testing for these features. As seen in Table 1, our method shows a good performance in terms of recognition rate and stability. Although specificity for some features was better than ours, the balance of sensitivity and specificity for the geodesic-based features was superior. Statistically, our geodesic-based feature vector method showed significant ($p < 1e - 6$) improvement in the total recognition accuracy over the Fourier descriptor-based method.

Table 1. Classification Results of Lymphocyte Cell Sequences using LVQ

Feature	TrAc(%)	TeAc(%)	TrSe(%)	TrSp(%)	TeSe(%)	TeSp(%)
Area	86.44	68.50	86.78	86.11	56.67	80.33
Elongation	95.06	84.50	90.56	99.56	79.00	90.00
Fourier	92.58	92.33	85.17	100.00	84.67	100.00
Geodesic	**95.22**	**94.33**	**95.44**	**95.00**	**92.00**	**96.67**

4   Discussion

We have presented a morphometry method for analyzing dynamic cell boundaries, and it showed improved discriminative properties over linear time matching. The performance was visually verified by projecting the data into its MDS coordinates, as well as detailed classification comparisons using LVQ. The proposed method required minimal manual intervention, thus offering a significant advantage for analyzing large scale time-lapsed cellular imaging data.

References

1. Pincus, Z., Theriot, J.A.: Comparison of quantitative methods for cell-shape analysis. Journal of Microscopy 227(2), 140–156 (2007)
2. Ali, S., Veltri, R., Epstein, J., Christudass, C., Madabhushi, A.: Adaptive Energy Selective Active Contour with Shape Priors for Nuclear Segmentation and Gleason Grading of Prostate Cancer. In: Fichtinger, G., Martel, A., Peters, T. (eds.) MICCAI 2011, Part I. LNCS, vol. 6891, pp. 661–669. Springer, Heidelberg (2011)
3. Meijering, E., Smal, I., Danuser, G.: Tracking in Molecular Bioimaging. IEEE Signal Processing Magazine 23(3), 46–53 (2006)
4. Terryn, C., Bonnomet, A., Cutrona, J., Coraux, C., Tournier, J., Nawrocki-Raby, B., Polette, M., Birembaut, P., Zahm, J.: Video-microscopic imaging of cell spatio-temporal dispersion and migration. Critical Reviews in Oncology/Hematology 69(2), 144–152 (2009)
5. Joshi, S.H., Klassen, E., Srivastava, A., Jermyn, I.: Removing Shape-Preserving Transformations in Square-Root Elastic (SRE) Framework for Shape Analysis of Curves. In: Yuille, A.L., Zhu, S.-C., Cremers, D., Wang, Y. (eds.) EMMCVPR 2007. LNCS, vol. 4679, pp. 387–398. Springer, Heidelberg (2007)
6. Joshi, S.H., Klassen, E., Srivastava, A., Jermyn, I.: A novel representation for Riemannian analysis of elastic curves in Rn. In: IEEE CVPR, pp. 1–7 (2007)
7. Srivastava, A., Klassen, E., Joshi, S.H., Jermyn, I.: Shape analysis of elastic curves in euclidean spaces. IEEE Trans. PAMI 33(7), 1415–1428 (2011)
8. Myers, C., Rabiner, L.: A level building dynamic time warping algorithm for connected word recognition. IEEE Trans. ASSP 29(2), 284–297 (1981)
9. Veeraraghavan, A., Chowdhury, A., Chellappa, R.: Role of shape and kinematics in human movement analysis. In: IEEE CVPR, vol. 1, pp. 1–6 (2004)
10. Kaziska, D., Srivastava, A.: Gait-based human recognition by classification of cyclostationary processes on nonlinear shape manifolds. Journal of the American Statistical Association 102(480), 1114–1124 (2007)
11. Le, H.: Locating Fréchet means with application to shape spaces. Advances in Applied Probability 33(2), 324–338 (2001)

Learning to Detect Cells
Using Non-overlapping Extremal Regions

Carlos Arteta[1], Victor Lempitsky[2], J. Alison Noble[1], and Andrew Zisserman[1]

[1] Department of Engineering Science, University of Oxford, U.K.
[2] Yandex, Moscow, Russia

Abstract. Cell detection in microscopy images is an important step in the automation of cell based-experiments. We propose a machine learning-based cell detection method applicable to different modalities. The method consists of three steps: first, a set of candidate cell-like regions is identified. Then, each candidate region is evaluated using a statistical model of the cell appearance. Finally, dynamic programming picks a set of non-overlapping regions that match the model. The cell model requires few images with simple dot annotation for training and can be learned within a structured SVM framework. In the reported experiments, state-of-the-art cell detection accuracy is achieved for H&E-stained histology, fluorescence, and phase-contrast images.

1 Introduction

Automatic cell detection is a subject of interest in a wide range of cell-based studies, as it is the basis of many automatic methods for cell counting, segmentation and tracking. The broad diversity of cell lines and microscopy imaging techniques require that cell detection algorithms adapt well to different scenarios. The difficulty of the problem also increases when the cell density of the sample is high, as in this case the cell size can vary and cell clumping is usual. Moreover, in some applications different cell types or other similar structures can be present in the same image, and in this case the algorithm is required to detect only the cells of interest, posing a barrier hard to overcome with classical image processing techniques.

In this paper we propose a learning-based method that is general enough to perform well across different microscopy modalities. Rather than invoking computationally-intensive segmentation frameworks [1,9], or classifying all image patches in a sliding-window manner [15], it uses a highly-efficient MSER region detector [8] to find a broad number of candidate regions to be scored with a learning-based measure. The non-overlapping subset of those regions with high similarity to the class of interest can then be selected via dynamic programming, while the learning can be done within the structured output framework [12].

The new method is evaluated on three data sets (Figure 1), which are annotated with dots; a dot is placed inside each cell. Given only this minimalistic annotation, the method is able to learn a model that achieves state-of-the-art detection accuracy, in our evaluation, despite all the variation between the data sets.

N. Ayache et al. (Eds.): MICCAI 2012, Part I, LNCS 7510, pp. 348–356, 2012.
© Springer-Verlag Berlin Heidelberg 2012

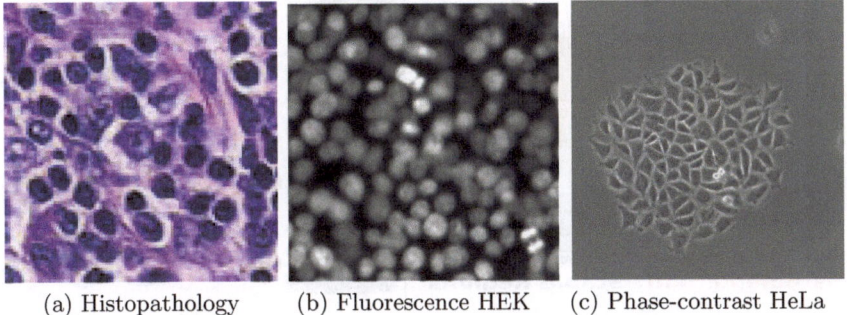

(a) Histopathology   (b) Fluorescence HEK   (c) Phase-contrast HeLa

Fig. 1. Example images from the data sets used for cell detection. (a) Histopathology image of breast cancer tissue, which is stained to highlight lymphocyte nuclei (100×100 pix.; cell size 6–8 pix.) (b) Fluorescence microscopy image of human embryonic kidney cells (190×190 pix.; cell size 10–20 pix.) (c) Phase-contrast image of cervical cancer cells of the HeLa cell line (400×400 pix.; cell size 10–40 pix.).

2   Learning Non-overlapping Extremal Regions

The model operates by first producing a set of candidate *extremal regions*, and then picking a subset of those regions based on a learned classifier score and subject to a *non-overlap constraint*. We discuss the components of the method, namely the detection of candidate regions, the inference, and the structured learning, next.

Extremal Regions of the grey-value image $\mathcal{I}$ are defined as connected components of a thresholded image $\mathcal{I}_{>t} = \{\mathcal{I} > t\}$ for some t. In other words, a region is extremal if the image intensity everywhere inside of it is higher than the image intensity at its boundary. Our approach thus builds on the fact that in many microscopy modalities, cells show up as bright or dark blobs in one of the intensity channels, and therefore can be closely approximated by extremal regions of this intensity channel. An important property of extremal regions is their *nestedness*, i.e. the fact that for the same image $\mathcal{I}$ two extremal regions R and S can be either nested or non-overlapping ($R \subset S$ or $R \supset S$ or $R \cap S = \emptyset$. See Figure 2).

The number of extremal regions can be combinatorial, so in practice we consider only regions that are *maximally stable* in the sense of [8], i.e. the speed of their area variation w.r.t. changing threshold t is a local minimum and is below a separate *stability threshold*. We thus use a popular and efficient maximally stable extremal region detector (MSER) [8] to find a representative subset of all extremal regions. To boost the recall for cell detection, we set the stability threshold to a very high value, so that the MSER-detector produces a manageable but very large (thousands) number of candidate regions. Our inference procedure then determines which of those candidates correspond to cells.

Inference under the Non-overlap Constraint. Let $R_1, R_2, \ldots R_N$ be the candidate set of N extremal regions detected in an image. Let us assume that

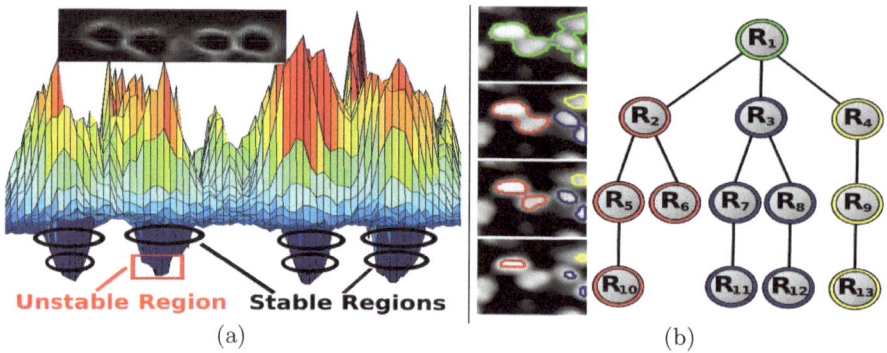

Fig. 2. (a) Example of the intensity profile of an image region containing cells. The MSER algorithm detects extremal regions that are stable in area growth while varying an intensity threshold. Typically, many extremal regions are nested within and between cells (especially when there is cell clumping) forming a tree structure. For example, (b) the boundaries of several MSERs that appear in the close-up of a cell image are shown, which can be represented by the tree structure. The parent-child relationships in the tree correspond to the nestedness of the regions. The tree structure is utilized by the inference algorithm.

each region R_i is assigned a value V_i, which is produced by a classifier and indicates the appropriateness score of this region to the class of cells we want to detect. Our method then picks a subset of extremal regions so that the sum of scores of the picked regions is maximized, while the picked regions do not overlap (the non-overlap constraint).

To formalize this task, we define a set of binary indicator variables $\mathbf{y} = \{y_1, y_2, \ldots y_N\}$ so that $y_i = 1$ implies the region R_i being picked. Let $\mathcal{Y}$ be a set of those region subsets that do not have region overlap, that is, $\mathcal{Y} = \{\mathbf{y} \,|\, \forall i, j : (i \neq j) \wedge (y_i = 1) \wedge (y_j = 1) \Rightarrow R_i \cap R_j = \emptyset\}$. Then, the optimization task faced by the model is:

$$F(\mathbf{y}) = \max_{\mathbf{y} \in \mathcal{Y}} \sum_{i=1}^{N} y_i \, V_i \ . \tag{1}$$

For an arbitrary set of regions, maximizing (1) over $\mathbf{y} \in \mathcal{Y}$ is NP-hard (equivalent to *submodular maximization*). Fortunately, the nestedness property of extremal regions permits fast and exact maximization of (1). The idea is to organize the extremal regions into trees according to the nestedness property, so that each tree corresponds to a set of overlapping extremal regions (Figure 2b). The exact solution of (1) can then be obtained via dynamic programming on those trees [11] after an appropriate variable substitution (see implementation details).

Learning Formulation. As discussed above, our method relies on machine learning to score each region for the detection task. A suitable scoring can be learned in a principled fashion from the dot-annotated training data as follows. Assume a set of M training images $\mathcal{I}^1, \mathcal{I}^2, \ldots \mathcal{I}^M$, where each training image

$\mathcal{I}^j$ has a set of N^j MSER regions $R_1^j, R_2^j, \ldots R_{N^j}^j$. For each of these regions R_i^j a feature vector $\mathbf{f}_i^j$ is computed (the feature vector choice is described in the implementation details). Finally, assume that the images are annotated, so that n_i^j denotes the number of user-placed dots (annotations) inside the region R_i^j.

To obtain the score for each region, we use a linear classifier so that the value V_i^j for the region R_i^j is computed as a scalar product $(\mathbf{w} \cdot \mathbf{f}_i^j)$ with the *weight vector* $\mathbf{w}$. The goal of learning is then to find a weight vector so that the inference procedure tends to pick regions with $n_i^j = 1$, and also to ensure that for each dot a region is picked that contains it. In this way, the produced set of regions tends to be in a one-to-one correspondence with the user-placed dots.

Learning via Binary Classification. The simplest way to learn $\mathbf{w}$, and one that already produces competitive results in our comparisons, is to learn a binary classifier. For this, all regions in the training images are considered, and those with $n_i^j = 1$ are assigned to the positive class while all others are assigned to the negative class. Training any linear classifier, e.g. via a support vector machine algorithm, then produces a desired $\mathbf{w}$.

Structured Learning. Learning via binary classification does not take into account the non-overlap constraint. A more principled approach is to use a structured SVM [12] that directly optimizes the performance of the inference procedure on the training set. Consider the configuration $\mathbf{y}^j \in \mathcal{Y}^j$ defining the set of non-overlapping regions for the image $\mathcal{I}^j$. It is natural to define an error measure (the *loss*) associated with $\mathbf{y}^j$ as the deviation from the one-to-one correspondence between the user-placed dots and the picked regions:

$$L(\mathbf{y}^j) = \sum_{i=1}^{N^j} y_i^j \, |n_i^j - 1| + U^j(\mathbf{y}^j) \tag{2}$$

$U^j(\mathbf{y}^j)$ denotes the number of user-placed dots that are not covered by any region R_i^j with $y_i^j = 1$ (i.e. have no correspondence).

To perform the learning, the "ground truth" configuration $\bar{\mathbf{y}}^j = \{\bar{y}_1^j, \bar{y}_2^j, \ldots \bar{y}_{N^j}^j\} \in \mathcal{Y}$ is defined for each training image by assigning a unique extremal region to each dot (see implementation details). The structured SVM method [12] then finds the optimal weight vector $\mathbf{w}$ by minimizing the following convex objective:

$$\mathcal{L}(\mathbf{w}) = \frac{1}{2}||\mathbf{w}||^2 + \frac{C}{M} \sum_{j=1}^{M} \max_{\mathbf{y}^j \in \mathcal{Y}^j} \left(\sum_{i=1}^{N^j} (\mathbf{w} \cdot \mathbf{f}_i^j) \, y_i^j - \sum_{i=1}^{N^j} (\mathbf{w} \cdot \mathbf{f}_i^j) \, \bar{y}_i^j + L(\mathbf{y}^j) \right) \tag{3}$$

where the first term is a regularization on $\mathbf{w}$, C is a scalar regularization parameter, and the maximum inside the sum represents a convex (in $\mathbf{w}$) upper bound on the loss (2), that the inference (1) incurs on the jth training image [12].

The objective (3) can be optimized with a standard cutting-plane algorithm [12] provided that it is possible to perform the *loss-augmented inference*, which corresponds to finding maxima inside the second term of (3) for a fixed $\mathbf{w}$. Thus, one needs to solve:

$$
\max_{\mathbf{y}^j \in \mathcal{Y}^j} \left(\sum_{i=1}^{N^j} (\mathbf{w} \cdot \mathbf{f}_i^j)\, y_i^j - \sum_{i=1}^{N^j} (\mathbf{w} \cdot \mathbf{f}_i^j)\, \bar{y}_i^j \; + \; \sum_{i=1}^{N^j} y_i^j \, |n_i^j - 1| + U^j(\mathbf{y}^j) \right) \tag{4}
$$

We then note that under the non-overlap constraint, the number of un-matched dots $U^j(\mathbf{y}^j)$ can be rewritten as $D^j - \sum_{i=1}^{N^j} y_i^j n_i^j$, where D^j is the total number of dots in the jth training image. After substituting $U(\mathbf{y}^j)$ and omitting the terms independent of $\mathbf{y}^j$, an equivalent optimization problem is obtained:

$$
\max_{\mathbf{y}^j \in \mathcal{Y}^j} \sum_{i=1}^{N^j} \left((\mathbf{w} \cdot \mathbf{f}_i^j) + |n_i^j - 1| - n_i^j \right) y_i^j \tag{5}
$$

which has exactly the same form as (1) with $V_i = (\mathbf{w} \cdot \mathbf{f}_i^j) + |n_i^j - 1| - n_i^j = (\mathbf{w} \cdot \mathbf{f}_i^j) - [n_i^j \geq 0]$. Thus, we can perform loss-augmented inference exactly via dynamic programming on trees, and get an optimal $\mathbf{w}$ through the cutting-plane procedure [12].

Implementation Details. We use the MSER implementation from [14]. The feature vector for each region in a grayscale image is 92-dimensional, and consists of several concatenated histograms: (a) a 10-dimensional histogram of intensities within the region (separate histograms are computed for color images), (b) two 6-dimensional histograms of differences in intensities between the region border and a dilation of it for two different dilation radii (these histograms capture the spatial context of the region), (c) a shape descriptor represented by a 60-dimensional histogram of the distribution of the boundary of the region on a size-normalized polar coordinate system, and, finally, (d) the area A of the region represented by a 10-dimensional binary vector with the entry $\lceil \log A \rceil$ set to 1.

To generate the ground truth configuration for the structured learning, we first score all regions using the weight vector w_{bin} learned through a binary SVM. Then, for each dot, we include into the ground truth configuration the region that contains only this dot and has the highest score.

The dynamic programming within the inference (1) can be implemented via the following variable substitution: each $\mathbf{y}$ is mapped to a new set of binary variables $\mathbf{z} = \{z_1, z_2, \ldots, z_N\}$, so that $z_i = 1$ iff the y-variable for either the ith node or any of its ancestors in the MSER-tree is 1. The tree-structured graphical model on z-variables is defined for each region tree. For the root node i, the cost for $z_i = 1$ is set to V_i. For every edge in the tree connecting nodes i (parent) and j (child), the cost for $z_i = 0$ and $z_j = 1$ is set to V_j, while the cost for $z_i = 1$ and $z_j = 0$ is set to $-\infty$. The latter restricts inference to only those z-configurations that correspond to $\mathbf{y} \in \mathcal{Y}$. All other costs within pairwise and unary terms are set to 0. A standard max-product algorithm is run in each tree and the optimal z-variables are mapped back to y-variables.

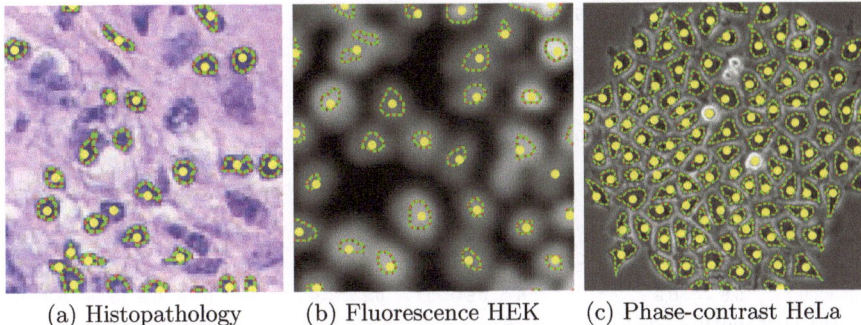

(a) Histopathology	(b) Fluorescence HEK	(c) Phase-contrast HeLa

Fig. 3. Example results on each of the data sets. The boundaries of the detected MSER regions are shown in dashed green/red over the test images with yellow dots indicating the ground truth annotations. Note, the features are computed over a support region that is larger than the MSER region.

The learning is done via the SVM^{struct} code [5, 13]. In general, detecting cells on a 400-by-400 pixel HeLa image takes 30 seconds on an i7 CPU (dominated by our unoptimized MATLAB code for feature computation).

3   Experiments

Evaluating the Model. Although the algorithm produces a set of regions, our aim is to optimize the detection accuracy (and not the segmentation) w.r.t. the ground truth provided in the form of dots. Therefore, we evaluate the output of our method based on the position of the region centroids. A centroid is considered a true positive (TP) if it is within a radius ρ of the ground truth dot. In our experiments, ρ is set to the radius of the smallest cell in the data set. Thus, only centroids that lie inside cells are considered correct. Centroids further than ρ from ground truth dots are considered false positives (FP). Finally, missed ground truth dots are counted as false negatives (FN). The results are reported in terms of Precision=TP/(TP + FP) and Recall=TP/(TP + FN).

Three data sets for cell detection have been used to validate the method (Figure 1). Firstly, the ICPR 2010 Histopathology Images contest [4], which consists of 20 images of stained breast cancer tissue. It is required to detect lymphocyte nuclei, while discriminating them from breast cancer nuclei having very similar appearance. The second data set comes from [1] and contains 12 fluorescence microscopy images of human embryonic kidney (HEK) cells, where the detection task is challenging due to the significant intensity variation between cells across the image, fading boundaries, and frequent cell clumping. The third data set contains 22 phase-contrast images of cervical cancer cell colonies of the HeLa cell line, which presents a high variability in cell shapes and sizes.

Three variations of our method are evaluated: (I) *direct classification (DC)*, which evaluates all MSERs with a **w** vector learned via a binary classifier and chooses the region with the highest score in every set of overlapping regions with positive scores, (II) *binary SVM + inference (B+I)*, which does the full

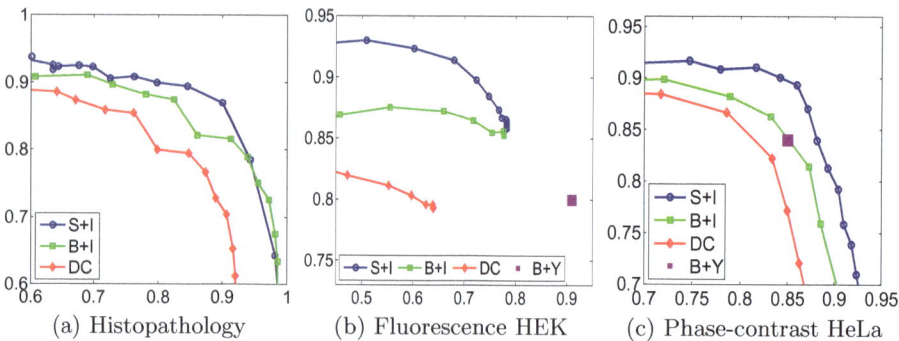

Fig. 4. Precision (vertical) vs Recall (horizontal) curves for the three datasets for the three variations of our approach and [1] (denoted as B+Y, where available). Significant improvements brought by the non-overlap constraint (B+I) and the structured SVM (S+I) can be observed.

Table 1. Results for the data set of the ICPR 2010 Pattern Recognition in Histopathological Images contest [4]. Seven measures are reported: precision, recall and F1-score (when available), where higher numbers are better, and the four measures used in the evaluation of the ICPR contest, where lower numbers are better. The contest criteria consisted of the mean and standard deviation of two measurements: the Euclidean distance between detected dots and ground truth dots (**d**), and the absolute difference between the number of cells found and the ground truth number of cells (**n**).

Method	Prec.	Rec.	F_1-score	$\mu_d \pm \sigma_d$	$\mu_n \pm \sigma_n$
Our method	**86.99**	**90.03**	**88.48**	**1.68** $\pm$ **2.55**	**2.90** $\pm$ **2.13**
LIPSyM [6]	70.21	70.08	69.84	3.14 $\pm$ 0.93	4.30 $\pm$ 3.09
Bernadis et al. [1]	-	-	-	3.13 $\pm$ 3.08	12.7 $\pm$ 8.70
Kuse et al. [7]	65.23	69.99	67.29	3.04 $\pm$ 3.40	14.01 $\pm$ 4.40
Cheng et al. [2]	-	-	-	8.10 $\pm$ 6.98	6.98 $\pm$ 12.5
Graf et al. [3]	-	-	-	7.60 $\pm$ 6.30	24.5 $\pm$ 16.2
Panagiotakis et al. [10]	-	-	-	2.87 $\pm$ 3.80	14.23 $\pm$ 6.30

inference (1) based on the weight vector learned through binary classification, and (III) *structured SVM + inference (S+I)*, which uses inference with the weight vector learned by the structured SVM (3). The histopathology and the HeLa datasets were split into halves for training and testing, whereas the HEK data was evaluated in a leave-one-out fashion in order to test on the entire set and be able to fully compare results with [1].

Figure 4 shows the precision-recall curves for the three variations of our method. The curves were obtained by varying a constant τ added to the score of each region. It can be seen that enforcing the non-overlap constraint increases the accuracy of the method considerably, especially when **w** is learned within the structured SVM framework.

Comparison with State of the Art. Table 1 compares our experimental results (S+I method) on the histopathology data set to the methods presented in the ICPR 2010 contest, and to [6] and [1], published since then. The overall comparison is favourable to our method, with a considerable improvement on precision and recall over all other methods.

Figure 4 includes the results of the method [1] on the HEK and HeLA data sets, kindly provided by its authors. Overall, on the HeLa data set our method was uniformly better (Figure 4(c)) (despite [1] requiring masking out the homogeneous areas of the images to remove the phantom detections), and achieves higher precision but lower recall on the HEK data set.

4 Summary

We have presented a method for cell detection in microscopy images that is able to achieve state-of-the-art performance across different scenarios. It is tolerant to changes in image intensities, cell densities and cell sizes, whilst being specific to the structures of interest. The in-built non-overlap constraint, which is taken into account during learning, allows the method to perform well even in the presence of cell clumping.

Acknowledgements. We are grateful to Dr. N. Rajpoot, Dr. E. Bernadis, Dr. B. Vojnovic and Dr. G. Flaccavento for providing cell data sets. Financial support was provided by the RCUK Centre for Doctoral Training in Healthcare Innovation (EP/G036861/1) and ERC grant VisRec no. 228180.

References

1. Bernardis, E., Yu, S.X.: Pop out many small structures from a very large microscopic image. Med. Image Anal. 15(5), 690–707 (2011)
2. Cheng, J., Veronika, M., Rajapakse, J.: Identifying Cells in Histopathological Images. In: Ünay, D., Çataltepe, Z., Aksoy, S. (eds.) ICPR 2010. LNCS, vol. 6388, pp. 244–252. Springer, Heidelberg (2010)
3. Graf, F., Grzegorzek, M., Paulus, D.: Counting Lymphocytes in Histopathology Images Using Connected Components. In: Ünay, D., Çataltepe, Z., Aksoy, S. (eds.) ICPR 2010. LNCS, vol. 6388, pp. 263–269. Springer, Heidelberg (2010)
4. Gurcan, M.N., Madabhushi, A., Rajpoot, N.: Pattern Recognition in Histopathological Images: An ICPR 2010 Contest. In: Ünay, D., Çataltepe, Z., Aksoy, S. (eds.) ICPR 2010. LNCS, vol. 6388, pp. 226–234. Springer, Heidelberg (2010)
5. Joachims, T., Finley, T., Yu, C.N.: Cutting-plane training of structural SVMs. Mach. Learn. 77, 27–59 (2009)
6. Kuse, M., Khan, M., Rajpoot, N., Kalasannavar, V., Wang, Y.F.: Local isotropic phase symmetry measure for detection of beta cells and lymphocytes. J. Pathol. Inform. 2(2), 2 (2011)
7. Kuse, M., Sharma, T., Gupta, S.: A Classification Scheme for Lymphocyte Segmentation in H&E Stained Histology Images. In: Ünay, D., Çataltepe, Z., Aksoy, S. (eds.) ICPR 2010. LNCS, vol. 6388, pp. 235–243. Springer, Heidelberg (2010)
8. Matas, J., Chum, O., Urban, M., Pajdla, T.: Robust wide-baseline stereo from maximally stable extremal regions. Image Vision Comput. 22(10), 761–767 (2004)

9. Nath, S., Palaniappan, K., Bunyak, F.: Cell Segmentation Using Coupled Level Sets and Graph-Vertex Coloring. In: Larsen, R., Nielsen, M., Sporring, J. (eds.) MICCAI 2006, Part I. LNCS, vol. 4190, pp. 101–108. Springer, Heidelberg (2006)
10. Panagiotakis, C., Ramasso, E., Tziritas, G.: Lymphocyte Segmentation Using the Transferable Belief Model. In: Ünay, D., Çataltepe, Z., Aksoy, S. (eds.) ICPR 2010. LNCS, vol. 6388, pp. 253–262. Springer, Heidelberg (2010)
11. Pearl, J.: Probabilistic reasoning in intelligent systems. Morgan Kaufmann (1988)
12. Tsochantaridis, I., Hofmann, T., Joachims, T., Altun, Y.: Support vector machine learning for interdependent and structured output spaces. In: ICML 2004, p. 104. ACM (2004)
13. Vedaldi, A.: A MATLAB wrapper of SVM^{struct} (2011), http://www.vlfeat.org/~vedaldi/code/svm-struct-matlab.html
14. Vedaldi, A., Fulkerson, B.: VLFeat (2010), http://www.vlfeat.org/
15. Yin, Z., Bise, R., Chen, M., Kanade, T.: Cell segmentation in microscopy imagery using a bag of local Bayesian classifiers. In: ISBI 2010, pp. 125–128 (2010)

Application of the IMM-JPDA Filter
to Multiple Target Tracking in Total Internal
Reflection Fluorescence Microscopy Images

Seyed Hamid Rezatofighi[1,2], Stephen Gould[1], Richard Hartley[1,3],
Katarina Mele[2], and William E. Hughes[4,5]

[1] College of Engineering & Computer Sci., Australian National University, ACT, AU
[2] Quantitative Imaging Group, CSIRO Math., Informatics & Statistics, NSW, AU
[3] National ICT (NICTA), AU
[4] The Garvan Institute of Medical Research, NSW, AU
[5] Department of Medicine, St. Vincent's Hospital, NSW, AU
hamid.rezatofighi@anu.edu.au

Abstract. We propose a multi-target tracking method using an Interacting Multiple Model Joint Probabilistic Data Association (IMM-JPDA) filter for tracking vesicles in Total Internal Reflection Fluorescence Microscopy (TIRFM) sequences. We enhance the accuracy and reliability of the algorithm by tailoring an appropriate framework to this application. Evaluation of our algorithm is performed on both realistic synthetic data and real TIRFM data. Our results are compared against related methods and a commercial tracking software.

Keywords: Multi-Target tracking, Bayesian tracking, IMM Filter, Data association, JPDA filter, Total internal reflection fluorescence microscopy.

1 Introduction

Many biological mechanisms such as intracellular trafficking involve the interaction of diverse subcellular components moving between different intracellular locations and cellular membrane [1]. Analyzing these movements is an essential preliminary step in understanding many biological processes. This spatiotemporal analysis has become feasible using recent developments in time-lapse fluorescence imaging, such as total internal reflection fluorescence microscopy (TIRFM). However, manual scrutiny of hundreds of moving subcellular structures over numerous sequences is painstakingly slow and suffers from poor accuracy and repeatability. Therefore, the development of a reliable automated tracking algorithm is required for better biological exploration. However, many challenging difficulties such as high levels of noise, high object densities and intricate motion patterns confront the development of reliable automated tracking algorithms. Moreover, the subcellular structures generally have complex interactions while entering, exiting or temporarily disappearing from the frame [2].

Bayesian tracking approaches are a class of tracking algorithm that have became popular for cell tracking applications in recent years [2–8]. These tracking

N. Ayache et al. (Eds.): MICCAI 2012, Part I, LNCS 7510, pp. 357–364, 2012.

methods can properly deal with the interaction between the targets and long disappearance intervals by incorporating prior knowledge of object dynamics and measurement models. Particle filtering (PF) methods are a type of Bayesian tracking technique well suited to nonlinear models. Therefore, they have been applied in many biological applications [3, 5]. However, the main weakness of these methods is their high computation cost [3]. For this reason, Kalman filtering based methods, such as the interacting multiple model (IMM) filter, which are computationally effective, are still a popular alternative for biological applications [2, 4, 6]. In order to solve the measurement-to-target assignment problem, accurate multi-target tracking also requires robust data association. Some examples of these algorithms used in cell tracking applications include multiple hypothesis tracking (MHT) [7] and joint probabilistic data association (JPDA) [8]. MHT is a preferred technique for solving the data association problem due to considering all possible measurement-to-track assignments for a number of successive frames. However, it is computationally intensive, especially in the regions with high target density [9]. JPDA is a special case of MHT and considers all possible measurement-to-target assignments in each frame separately. In diverse applications, this data association technique provides acceptable performance whilst having significantly less processing time compared to the MHT algorithm. Moreover, it has been shown that for tracking highly maneuvering targets in the presence of clutter, the PDA-based filter in conjunction with the IMM filter yields one of the best solutions and has comparable performance to MHT [9].

Since in our application the objects of interest embody nonlinear dynamics we propose a combination of the IMM and the JPDA filters. The combination of these filters, the so called IMM-JPDA filter, was first introduced by Bar-Shalom *et al.* [10] and has been used in various applications such as radar [11] and robotics [12]. However, to our knowledge, this is the first application of the IMM-JPDA filter to biological imaging. As the main contribution of this paper we tailor a framework for tracking vesicles in TIRFM images. We evaluate the performance of our algorithm on realistic synthetic sequences as well as a real TIRFM data set. In addition, our results are compared with those of related methods and one popular commercial software package. The results show that our algorithm is robust enough to track different vesicle dynamics whilst maintaining tracks after their temporary disappearance.

2   Background

In this section, we briefly review the IMM and JPDA filters. For a complete treatment see Blackman and Popoli [13]. The IMM filter is a Bayesian state estimation algorithm which models nonlinear dynamic and measurement equations using multiple switching linear models. For each model k, the posterior density $p(x_t|z_t, k_t = k)$, where x_t is the system state vector and z_t is the measurement vector at time t, evolves based on the Kalman filter equations [13]. The switching between models is regulated by a transition probability matrix. To this end, IMM switching weights, so called IMM model probabilities λ_t^k, are calculated and updated at each time index t using this matrix. Next, these weights are used for mixing the posterior densities of each model $p(x_t|z_t, k_t)$ and calculating the final posterior density $p(x_t|z_t)$.

The JPDA filter is a method of associating the detected measurements in the current frame with existing targets using a joint probabilistic score. This score is calculated based on the set of all valid joint associations, Θ_{ji}, which assign measurement j to target i. Here, a set of all possible measurement-to-track hypotheses are first generated such that each detected measurement is uniquely chosen by one track in each hypothesis. A null assignment $\emptyset$, representing the assignment of no observation to a given track, is also considered. Next, the probability $P(\theta|z_t)$ corresponding to each hypothesis, θ, is calculated. In the case of linear Gaussian models, this probability can be calculated as $P(\theta|z_t) \propto \prod_{(i,j)\in\theta} g_{ij}$, where g_{ij} is a likelihood function,

$$g_{ij} = \begin{cases} 1 - P(D) & \text{if } j = \emptyset, \\ \dfrac{\exp(-d_{ij}^2/2)}{(2\pi)^{M/2}\sqrt{|S|}} & \text{otherwise,} \end{cases} \tag{1}$$

where $P(D)$ is the probability of detection, M is dimension of the measurement, and S is innovation covariance matrix of the Kalman filter. Here d_{ij} is the normalized statistical distance between track i and measurement j using the innovation covariance matrix S.

Consequently, the joint probabilistic score, β_{ji}, that measurement j was generated by track i is obtained by $\sum_{\theta\in\Theta_{ji}} P(\theta|z_t)$. Finally, tracks are updated with a weighted sum of measurements where the weights are the score probabilities.

3 Method

An accurate multiple target tracking algorithm requires robust detection for track initialization, initiation, and termination. To this end, we use the maximum possible h-dome (MPHD) method [14]. This detection method is accurate enough to detect most of targets with a low false detection rate. The output of the algorithm is a set of detected positions and an estimated background $\mathbf{B}_t$ in frame t (see Rezatofighi et al. [14] for details). Then, we use an enhanced IMM-JPDA filter along with a track management procedure as follows.

3.1 An Enhanced IMM-JPDA Filter

Since the data in our case consists of two dimensional sequences, the state vector and the measurement vector are typically defined as $x_t = (x_t, \dot{x}_t, y_t, \dot{y}_t)$, including positions $\acute{x}_t = (x_t, y_t)$ and velocities $\dot{x}_t = (\dot{x}_t, \dot{y}_t)$, and $z_t = (\hat{x}_t, \hat{y}_t)$ respectively. In the IMM-JPDA filter, the prediction density of the state $x_t \in \mathbb{R}^4$ in each model is first estimated based on each linear dynamic model of the IMM filter. Next, each density is updated by the JPDA filter. Last, the posterior density $p(x_t|z_t)$ is calculated based on a weighted combination of posterior densities $p(x_t|z_t, k_t)$ using the IMM model probabilities. To improve the performance of this filter in TIRFM sequences, we tailor the framework as described below.

IMM with a State Dependent Transition Probability Matrix. To deal with nonlinear dynamics of the biological structures, different numbers of linear dynamic models have been proposed in the literature [3, 4, 6]. Although, a large number of linear dynamics [4, 6] may result a better estimation of these non-linear dynamics, they are more computationally demanding. In addition, more dynamic models increase the uncertainty of the estimated state; because in the IMM filter, a mixture of weighted Gaussian posterior densities results in higher variance. For these reasons, we use the two dynamic models defined by Smal *et al.* [3] including random walk and nearly constant velocity motion with small accelerations. These two types of dynamics properly model the nonlinear motion of the vesicles in TIRFM sequences. The random walk and constant velocity models resemble vesicle motion patterns described as tethering and docking, and linear movements, respectively [1]. Also for abrupt changes in direction, the random walk model operates as the transition state between two linear movements.

Traditionally, the elements of the transition probability matrix (TPM) are almost always considered as constant and chosen empirically. In Li *et al.* [4], these values are adaptively improved using an online minimum mean-square error estimation. However, it is still a shared matrix for all targets and requires an assumed distribution for probabilities of TPM. In contrast, we use an adaptive transition probability matrix which evolves based on the state of each target in the previous frame. Biologically, a vesicle can occasionally switch between these two states based on its kinetic energy. In other words, a vesicle with low velocity is more likely to either remain in the first model (docking and tethering dynamics) ($k_t = k_{t-1} = 1$) or switch from the linear movement model ($k_{t-1} = 2$) to the first model. The transition probability for the above states can be modeled by a decreasing function of the velocity of each target in the previous frame $\dot{X}_{t-1}$. Here, we define this function by a Gaussian-like probability function as

$$P(k_t|k_{t-1} = k, \dot{X}_{t-1}) = \begin{cases} \mathcal{S}^k \exp(-\frac{1}{2}\dot{X}_{t-1}\left(\mathcal{A}^k\right)^{-1}\dot{X}_{t-1}), & k_t = 1, \\ 1 - \mathcal{S}^k \exp(-\frac{1}{2}\dot{X}_{t-1}\left(\mathcal{A}^k\right)^{-1}\dot{X}_{t-1}), & k_t = 2, \end{cases} \quad (2)$$

where $\mathcal{S}^k$ is the maximum switching probability from model k_{t-1} to model k_t and $\mathcal{A}^k$ is a user specified positive semi-definite matrix. In our work, we set $\mathcal{A}^k = \sigma^k \mathbf{I}$, where $\mathbf{I}$ is the identity matrix. These parameters are fixed for each model based on prior knowledge. Finally, the elements of the transition probability matrix can be obtained by marginalization over $\dot{X}_{t-1}$:

$$P(k_t|k_{t-1}, Z_{t-1}) = \int P(k_t|k_{t-1}, \dot{X}_{t-1})p(\dot{X}_{t-1}|Z_{t-1}, k_{t-1})d_{\dot{X}_{t-1}}. \quad (3)$$

Since $p(\dot{X}_{t-1}|Z_{t-1}, k_{t-1} = k)$ is a Gaussian with mean $\dot{\mu}^k_{t-1}$ and covariance $\dot{\Sigma}^k_{t-1}$, $P(k_t|k_{t-1} = k, Z_{t-1})$ can be written in a closed form as

$$\mathcal{S}^k \sqrt{\frac{|\mathcal{A}^k|}{|\dot{\Sigma}^k_{t-1} + \mathcal{A}^k|}} \exp(-\frac{1}{2}(\dot{\mu}^k_{t-1})^T(\dot{\Sigma}^k_{t-1} + \mathcal{A}^k)^{-1}(\dot{\mu}^k_{t-1})), \quad \text{for } k_t = 1. \quad (4)$$

For the case $k_t = 2$, this probability is simply one minus the above.

An Enhanced JPDA for Vesicle Tracking. The performance of the JPDA algorithm is enhanced if the probability of detection in Equation 1 is a function of the position of each target. The detection of each target directly depends on the performance of the detection algorithm. In MPHD, a missed detection is more likely to occur at the edge of background structures. Therefore, the distribution of this probability can be modeled as a function of the background $\mathbf{B}_t$ estimated by the MPHD method. In this paper, we define this probability as $P(D|\acute{x}_{t|t-1}^k) = 1 - \Omega(\|\nabla \mathbf{B}_t(\acute{x})\|)_{\acute{x}=\acute{x}_{t|t-1}^k}$, where $\|\nabla.\|$ is the gradient magnitude operator and $\Omega(\cdot)$ is a function that normalizes its argument to the interval $[0,1]$. Because a closed form for the probability of detection by marginalization over $\acute{x}_{t|t-1}^k$ can not be calculated, we approximate it by the point estimate $P(D|\acute{\mu}_{t|t-1}^k)$.

In the 2D TIRFM imaging system, the emitting intensity of each fluorescence object is a nonlinear function of its depth as $z_t - z_0 = \zeta \log(I_0/I_t)$, where ζ is a decaying factor and z_0 and I_0 are a known depth and its equivalent intensity, respectively. Therefore, we can use the relative changes in the target's depth movement to better assign each measurement to its corresponding targets. To this end, we assume that the maximum intensity (I_{max}) corresponds to $z_0 = 0$. By extending the state vector to $x_t = (x_t, \dot{x}_t, y_t, \dot{y}_t, z_t, \dot{z}_t)$ and the measurement vector to $z_t = (\hat{x}_t, \hat{y}_t, \hat{z}_t = \zeta \log(I_{max}/I_t))$, the performance of the JPDA algorithm is enhanced.

3.2   Track Management

Initialization and Track Initiation. In order to initialize the trajectories, we apply the MPHD method for the first two consecutive sequences. The positions are initialized with the output of this method for the first frame. The initial velocities are estimated as the difference between the detected positions in the first frame and the nearest corresponding detected positions in the second frame. For track initiation of newly appearing targets, we use the joint probabilistic score described in §2. To this end, a total joint probabilistic score $\beta_{ji}^{\mathcal{K}}$ is first calculated as $\sum_{k=1}^{2} \lambda_t^k \beta_{ji}^k$, where β_{ji}^k is the joint probabilistic score of each model and λ_t^k are the IMM weights. Next, the detected measurements in frame t with the highest total score are considered as the most plausible measurements for the existing targets in this frame. The remaining detected measurements are initiated as new born targets.

Temporary Target Disappearance and Track Termination. Due to the depth movements of the targets in TIRFM sequences, they can temporarily disappear for several sequential frames. In this situation, the first element of the total joint probabilistic score ($\beta_{0i}^{\mathcal{K}}$) representing the missed detection probability is maximum in the frames where a target has either disappeared or was not detected. To deal with this temporary disappearance, our algorithm is allowed to continue tracking missed detections for up to N consecutive frames. Otherwise, the track is terminated from the last frame where the maximum score is not allotted to the $\beta_{0i}^{\mathcal{K}}$.

4   Experimental Results

The proposed tracking algorithm was evaluated using synthetic data (with ground truth) and also real TIRFM sequences. To show the efficacy of the combination of IMM and JPDA filters, we compared the performance of the proposed method (IMM-JPDA) with those of two related methods including the JPDA filter with a small acceleration dynamic model [8] and IMM filter along with a data association technique using the innovation matrix [6]. We also validate our experiments against a state-of-the-art commercial tracking software package (ImarisTrack).

In the first experiment, the tracking methods were tested using realistic synthetic sequences. The synthetic data consists of 80 targets moving through 40 frames inside a 450×450 pixel region. The spatial intensity profile of the targets were modeled by a 2D Gaussian distribution and were generated in different sizes similar to the size of the vesicles in the real TIRFM. Furthermore, due to the 3-D dimensional motion of the targets, their intensity is modulated according to their depth (see §3.1). To add an appropriate background, the background of a real TIRFM image estimated using the MPHD method [14], was added to the generated synthetic sequences. Next, the sequences were contaminated with Poisson noise. The dynamics of the targets were modeled using two aforementioned models. Also, targets can switch between these two dynamics (Fig. 1).

In order to quantitatively assess the performance of the tracking methods, we need an appropriate measure to characterize different aspects of tracking performance such as track accuracy, track truncation, data association and missed or false tracks. Metrics used in previous works [2–8] can not properly represent the performance of a multi-target tracking algorithm. Recently, a metric based on optimal subpattern assignment (OSPA) has been introduced by Risitc *et al.* [15] that captures the aforementioned aspects by a single value. This value can be seen as the sum of two errors including cardinality and location errors. The cardinality error can be interpreted as errors related to missed or false tracks while location error shows track accuracy error and labeling error. In other words, the accuracy of a tracking filter in tracking of a target and the performance of its data association technique are better shown by location error. On the other hand, a truncated track increases both cardinality and location errors because of missed tracks in the gaps and labeling error of truncated tracks.

In Table 1, the performance of the IMM, JPDA, IMM-JPDA and ImarisTrack for realistic synthetic data is compared using OSPA metric. For the first three methods, same detection scheme (MPHD) was used. As a result, they track similar false targets and have similar cardinality error. Differences in this error are due to their performance in filling the gaps between two tracks (missed track error). This error is noticeably higher for the ImarisTrack software because of its different detection scheme. The location error in this table demonstrates the performance of both the tracking filter and data association technique. As expected, selection of the JPDA filter as data association technique enhances the performance of the tracking system. However, the JPDA filter can not track nonlinear dynamics as well as the IMM-JPDA filter. Fig. 1 (b)-(e) shows results from the IMM-JPDA method for some complex situations.

Table 1. Comparison of the performance of the IMM, JPDA, IMM-JPDA and Imaris-Track for realistic synthetic data using OSPA metric (lower value is better)

Methods	IMM [6]	JPDA [8]	IMM-JPDA	ImarisTrack
OSPA [15]	7.81	5.78	**5.45**	13.61
Cardinality error	2.68	2.65	**2.36**	6.75
Location error	5.13	3.13	**3.09**	6.86

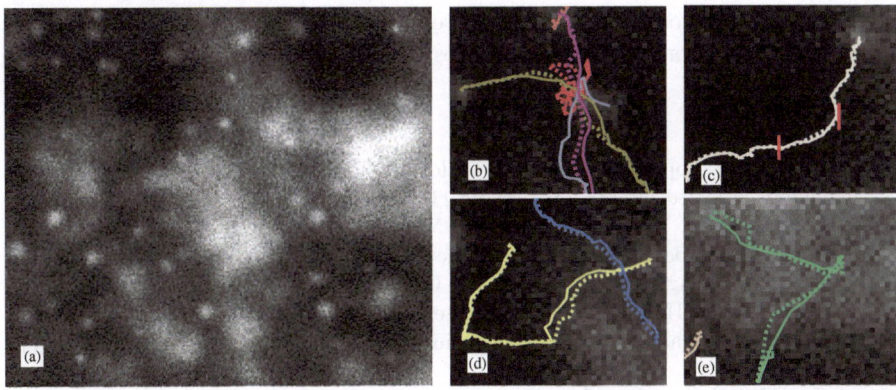

Fig. 1. (a) A part of the realistic synthetic data with locally varying SNR= $2 - 6$. (b)-(e) The result of tracking using the proposed algorithm (dashed line) and the ground truth (solid line): (b) a complex assignment, (c) a temporary disappearance (between two red lines), (d) a maneuvering motion, and (e) a switching dynamics

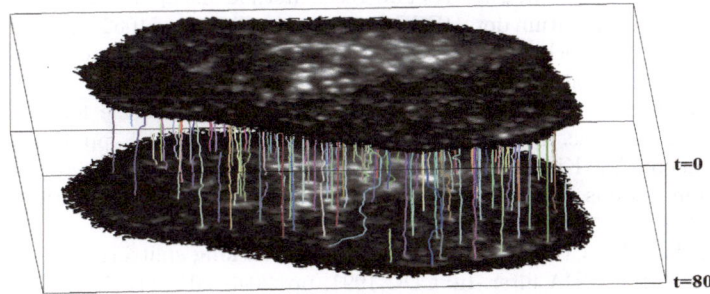

Fig. 2. Tracking result of the proposed method for 80 real TIRFM sequences

The described tracking methods were also tested on real TIRFM sequences (Fig. 2). Since the ground truth was not available for these real data, the results of the tracking were only visually evaluated by expert biologist. Our method in many cases such as temporary disappearance of the targets and their maneuvering or switching dynamics outperforms the other methods.

5   Conclusion

Due to complex interaction of subcellular structures, the performance of tracking systems can be noticeably affected by their method for data association. Our results show that the combination of IMM with JPDA can be effective in both tracking nonlinear dynamics and solving the complex measurement-to-track assignment problem. Moreover, our method has significantly lower processing time with comparable performance to particle filter based approaches. Specifically, it takes only few minutes to track hundreds of targets using our method. This suggests that our method can be used as a reliable algorithm for tracking hundreds moving targets in long TIRFM sequences.

References

1. Burchfield, J., Lopez, J., Mele, K., Vallotton, P., Hughes, W.: Exocytotic vesicle behaviour assessed by TIRFM. Traffic 11, 429–439 (2010)
2. Feng, L., Xu, Y., Yang, Y., Zheng, X.: Multi. Dense particle tracking in fluoresc. microsc. images based on MAP. J. Struct. Biol. 173(2), 219–228 (2011)
3. Smal, I., Meijering, E., Draegestein, K., Galjart, N., Grigoriev, I., Akhmanova, A., Van Royen, M., Houtsmuller, A., Niessen, W.: Multi. object tracking in molecular bioimag. by rao-blackwellized marginal PF. Med. Image Anal. 12(6), 764–777 (2008)
4. Li, K., Miller, E., Chen, M., Kanade, T., Weiss, L., Campbell, P.: Cell population tracking and lineage construction with spatiotemporal context. Med. Image Anal. 12(5), 546–566 (2008)
5. Smal, I., Draegestein, K., Galjart, N., Niessen, W., Meijering, E.: PF for multi. object tracking in dynamic fluoresc. microsc. images: Application to microtubule growth analysis. IEEE Trans. Med. Imag. 27(6), 789–804 (2008)
6. Genovesio, A., Liedl, T., Emiliani, V., Parak, W., Coppey-Moisan, M., Olivo-Marin, J.: Multi. particle tracking in 3-D+t microsc.: Method and application to the tracking of endocytosed quantum dots. IEEE Trans. Image Process., 1062–1070 (2006)
7. Chenouard, N., Bloch, I., Olivo-Marin, J.: MHT in microsc. images. In: ISBI 2009, pp. 1346–1349 (2009)
8. Smal, I., Niessen, W., Meijering, E.: A new detection scheme for multi. object tracking in fluoresc. microsc. by JPDA filtering. In: ISBI 2008, pp. 264–267 (2008)
9. Bar-Shalom, Y., Kirubarajan, T., Lin, X.: PDA techniques for target tracking with applications to sonar, radar and EO sensors. IEEE Aerosp. Electron. Syst. Mag. 20(8), 37–56 (2005)
10. Bar-Shalom, Y., Chang, K.C., Blom, H.A.P.: Tracking splitting targets in clutter using an IMM JPDA filter. In: CDC 1991, pp. 2043–2048 (1991)
11. Chen, B., Tugnait, J.K.: Tracking of multi. maneuvering targets in clutter using IMM/JPDA filtering and fixed-lag smoothing. Automatica 37(2), 239–249 (2001)
12. Hoffmann, C., Dang, T.: Cheap joint probabilistic data association filters in an interacting multiple model design. Robot. Auton. Syst. 57(3), 268–278 (2009)
13. Blackman, S., Popoli, R.: Design and analysis of modern tracking systems, vol. 685. Artech House, Norwood (1999)
14. Rezatofighi, S.H., Hartley, R., Hughes, W.E.: A new approach for spot detection in TIRFM. In: ISBI 2012, pp. 860–863 (2012)
15. Ristic, B., Vo, B., Clark, D., Vo, B.: A metric for performance evaluation of multitarget tracking algorithms. IEEE Trans. Signal Process. 59(7), 3452–3457 (2011)

Image Segmentation with Implicit Color Standardization Using Spatially Constrained Expectation Maximization: Detection of Nuclei

James Monaco[1], J. Hipp[2], D. Lucas[2], S. Smith[2],
U. Balis[2], and Anant Madabhushi[1,*]

[1] Department of Biomedical Engineering, Rutgers University, USA
[2] Department of Pathology, University of Michigan, USA

Abstract. Color nonstandardness — the propensity for similar objects to exhibit different color properties across images — poses a significant problem in the computerized analysis of histopathology. Though many papers propose means for improving color constancy, the vast majority assume image formation via reflective light instead of light transmission as in microscopy, and thus are inappropriate for histological analysis. Previously, we presented a novel Bayesian color segmentation algorithm for histological images that is highly robust to color nonstandardness; this algorithm employed the expectation maximization (EM) algorithm to dynamically estimate — for each individual image — the probability density functions that describe the colors of salient objects. However, our approach, like most EM-based algorithms, ignored important spatial constraints, such as those modeled by Markov random field (MRFs). Addressing this deficiency, we now present spatially-constrained EM (SCEM), a novel approach for incorporating Markov priors into the EM framework. With respect to our segmentation system, we replace EM with SCEM and then assess its improved ability to segment nuclei in H&E stained histopathology. Segmentation performance is evaluated over seven (nearly) identical sections of gastrointestinal tissue stained using different protocols (simulating severe color nonstandardness). Over this dataset, our system identifies nuclear regions with an area under the receiver operator characteristic curve (AUC) of 0.838. If we disregard spatial constraints, the AUC drops to 0.748.

1 Introduction

Color nonstandardness, the propensity for similar objects (e.g. cells) to exhibit different color properties across images, poses a significant challenge in the analysis of histopathology images. This nonstandardness typically results from variations in tissue fixation, staining, and digitization. Though methods have been proposed for improving color constancy in images formed via reflective light

* This work was made possible through funding from the NCI (R01CA136535-01, R01CA140772-01A1, R03CA128081-01) and the Burroughs Wellcome Fund.

N. Ayache et al. (Eds.): MICCAI 2012, Part I, LNCS 7510, pp. 365–372, 2012.

(see [1] for a review) and for mitigating the analogous intensity drift in grayscale images (e.g. MRI [2]), these methods are not extensible to color images formed via light transmission as in microscopy, and thus are inappropriate for histological analysis.

We previously presented a novel Bayesian color segmentation algorithm for histological images that is highly robust to color nonstandardness [3]. With respect to Bayesian classification, color nonstandardness manifests as inter-image changes in the probability densities that describe the colors of salient objects. To account for such changes, we estimated the requisite distributions in each image individually using expectation maximization (EM). However, our methodology did not account for spatial coherency among pixels.

Within a Bayesian framework, spatial dependencies are modeled as Markov random fields. Unfortunately, using EM to estimate Markov priors is notoriously complex: the EM equations become intractable. In an effort to maintain tractability, authors have invoked simplifying assumptions; unfortunately, these assumptions tended to reduce the generality of the solutions. For example, Comer and Delp [4] demanded that the Markov prior remain constant during the EM iteration; Nikou *et al.* [5] imposed Gaussianity constraints; Marroquin [6] tied the implementation to a predetermined cost function, thus linking estimation (i.e. model fitting) and classification.

In this work, we introduce spatially-constrained EM (SCEM), a novel approach for incorporating Markov priors into the EM framework. This approach 1) employs the pseudo-likelihood [7] to simplify the EM equations without incurring any loss of generality and 2) leverages our recently presented Markov chain Monte Carlo (MCMC) method [8] to estimate the resulting complex marginal distributions. As we will discuss later, previous MCMC methods [9] are ill-equipped to perform this estimation.

We validate SCEM by integrating it into our computerized system to segment nuclei in H&E stained histopathology. To test our system, we cut seven consecutive slices from a block of paraffin embedded gastrointestinal (GI) tissue, H&E stain the slices using different protocols (to simulate the gamut of color nonstandardness), digitized the sections, and then use our algorithm to segment the nuclear regions from the background. We then compare the resulting performance to that of our previous approach, which ignored spatial constraints.

2   Spatially Constrained Expectation Maximization

2.1   Definitions and Terminology

Let $R = \{1, 2, \ldots, |R|\}$ reference $|R|$ sites to be classified. Each site $r \in R$ has two associated random variables: $X_r \in \Lambda \equiv \{1, 2, \ldots, |\Lambda|\}$ indicating its class and $Y_r \in \mathbb{R}^D$ representing its D-dimensional feature vector. Let $\mathbf{X} = \{X_r : r \in R\}$ and $\mathbf{Y} = \{Y_r : r \in R\}$ refer to all X_r and Y_r in aggregate. The state spaces of $\mathbf{X}$ and $\mathbf{Y}$ are the Cartesian products $\Omega = \Lambda^{|R|}$ and $\mathbb{R}^{D \times |R|}$. Instances of random variables are denoted by their associated lowercase letters, e.g. $P(\mathbf{X} = \mathbf{x})$.

The random field $\mathbf{X}$ is a Markov random field if its local conditional probability density functions satisfy the Markov property: $P(X_r = x_r | \mathbf{X}_{-r} = \mathbf{x}_{-r}) = P(X_r = x_r | \mathbf{X}_{\eta_r} = \mathbf{x}_{\eta_r})$, where $\mathbf{x}_{-r} = \{x_s : s \in R, s \neq r\}$ and $\eta_r \subseteq R$ is the set of sites that neighbor r. Note that where it does not cause ambiguity, we will henceforth simplify probabilistic notations by omitting the random variables, e.g. $P(\mathbf{x}) \equiv P(\mathbf{X} = \mathbf{x})$. The joint probability distribution describing $\mathbf{X}$ and $\mathbf{Y}$ is as follows: $P(\mathbf{y}, \mathbf{x} | \boldsymbol{\theta}) = P(\mathbf{y} | \mathbf{x}, \boldsymbol{\theta}) P(\mathbf{x} | \boldsymbol{\theta})$, where $P(\mathbf{y} | \mathbf{x}, \boldsymbol{\theta})$ is the conditional distribution, $P(\mathbf{x} | \boldsymbol{\theta})$ is the Markov prior, and $\boldsymbol{\theta}$ is the vector of free parameters.

2.2 Derivation of Spatially Constrained Expectation Maximization

Typically, we infer $\boldsymbol{\theta}$ from the observations $\mathbf{y}$. The most common method of inference is maximum likelihood estimation (MLE). In an unsupervised context, EM provides an effective method for performing MLE. In brief, the EM algorithm employs the following iterative approach: at each step t, EM selects $\boldsymbol{\theta}^{t+1}$ such that $Q(\boldsymbol{\theta}^{t+1} | \boldsymbol{\theta}^t) > Q(\boldsymbol{\theta}^t | \boldsymbol{\theta}^t)$, where $Q(\boldsymbol{\theta} | \boldsymbol{\theta}^t) = \sum_{\mathbf{x}} P(\mathbf{x} | \mathbf{y}, \boldsymbol{\theta}^t) \ln P(\mathbf{y}, \mathbf{x}, \boldsymbol{\theta})$. Typically, $\boldsymbol{\theta}^{t+1}$ is set to the $\boldsymbol{\theta}$ that maximizes $Q(\boldsymbol{\theta} | \boldsymbol{\theta}^t)$ [10].

Unfortunately, the above form of Q is not amenable to implementation. To construct a more tractable form, we present the following derivation:

$$Q(\boldsymbol{\theta} | \boldsymbol{\theta}^t) = \sum_{\mathbf{x}} P(\mathbf{x} | \mathbf{y}, \boldsymbol{\theta}^t) \left[\ln P(\mathbf{y} | \mathbf{x}, \boldsymbol{\theta}) + \ln P(\mathbf{x} | \boldsymbol{\theta}) \right]$$

$$\approx \sum_{\mathbf{x}} P(\mathbf{x} | \mathbf{y}, \boldsymbol{\theta}^t) \sum_{r \in R} \left[\ln P(y_r | x_r, \boldsymbol{\theta}) + \ln P(x_r | \mathbf{x}_{\eta_r}, \boldsymbol{\theta}) \right] \quad (1)$$

$$= \sum_{r \in R} \sum_{x_r} P(x_r | \mathbf{y}, \boldsymbol{\theta}^t) \ln P(y_r | x_r, \boldsymbol{\theta}) +$$

$$\sum_{r \in R} \sum_{\mathbf{x}_{r \cup \eta_r}} P(\mathbf{x}_{r \cup \eta_r} | \mathbf{y}, \boldsymbol{\theta}^t) \ln P(x_r | \mathbf{x}_{\eta_r}, \boldsymbol{\theta}) \quad (2)$$

Equation (1) results from 1) making the common assumption that each observation Y_r is conditionally independent given its associated state X_r, i.e. $P(\mathbf{y} | \mathbf{x}) = \prod_{r \in R} P(y_r | x_r)$ and 2) replacing the Markov prior with its pseudo-likelihood representation [7]: $P(\mathbf{x} | \boldsymbol{\theta}) \approx \prod_{r \in R} P(x_r | \mathbf{x}_{\eta_r}, \boldsymbol{\theta})$. Equation (2) follows from changing the order of summation and then summing out the superfluous variables. Note that the first term in (2) is the formulation proposed by Comer and Delp [4]. It is the second term that allows us to estimate the MRF parameters during the SCEM iteration.

In summary, the expectation step in SCEM requires estimating the marginal probabilities $P(\mathbf{x} | \mathbf{y}, \boldsymbol{\theta}^t)$ and $P(\mathbf{x}_{r \cup \eta_r} | \mathbf{y}, \boldsymbol{\theta}^t)$ using the current estimate $\boldsymbol{\theta}^t$. The maximization step involves determining the $\boldsymbol{\theta}^{t+1}$ that maximizes (2). The difficultly lies in estimating the marginals needed for the expectation step.

2.3 Estimating the Marginals Densities

The (large) range Ω of $\mathbf{X}$ precludes determining $P(x_r | \mathbf{y}, \boldsymbol{\theta})$ and $P(\mathbf{x}_{r \cup \eta_r} | \mathbf{y}, \boldsymbol{\theta})$ via the direct marginalization of $P(\mathbf{x} | \mathbf{y}, \boldsymbol{\theta})$. However, it is possible to use the Gibbs sampler [11] (or the Metropolis-Hastings algorithm) to generate a Markov chain $(\mathbf{X}^0, \mathbf{X}^1, \mathbf{X}^2, \ldots | \mathbf{y}, \boldsymbol{\theta})$ whose elements are random samples of $P(\mathbf{x} | \mathbf{y}, \boldsymbol{\theta})$ — and consequently, samples of $P(x_r | \mathbf{y}, \boldsymbol{\theta})$ and $P(\mathbf{x}_{r \cup \eta_r} | \mathbf{y}, \boldsymbol{\theta})$. Using these samples, a Monte Carlo procedure can then estimate the requisite marginals. Unfortunately, previous MCMC approaches, which employed a histogramming strategy for density estimation [9], are ill-equipped to estimate distributions for which the sample space is large, such as $P(\mathbf{x}_{r \cup \eta_r} | \mathbf{y}, \boldsymbol{\theta})$.

We recently presented a more effective Rao-Blackwellized MCMC density estimator [8]. Consider the general marginal $P(\mathbf{x}_{\widetilde{R}})$, where $\mathbf{x}_{\widetilde{R}} = \{x_r : r \in \widetilde{R} \subseteq R\}$. Our estimator is as follows:

$$\widehat{P}\left(\mathbf{X}_{\widetilde{R}} = \boldsymbol{\lambda} | \mathbf{y}\right) = \frac{1}{c \cdot m} \sum_{j=1}^{c} \sum_{k=b+1}^{b+m} P(\mathbf{X}_{\widetilde{R}} = \boldsymbol{\lambda} | \mathbf{x}_{\eta_{\widetilde{R}}}^{j,k}, \mathbf{y}), \tag{3}$$

where $\boldsymbol{\lambda} \in \Lambda^{|\widetilde{R}|}$, c is the number of Markov chains, b is the number of iterations needed for the Markov chain to reach equilibrium, m is the number of iterations past equilibrium required to accurately estimate $P(\mathbf{x}_{\widetilde{R}})$, and $\mathbf{x}_{\eta_{\widetilde{R}}}^{j,k}$ is the states of all sites that neighbor $\widetilde{R}$ in Markov chain j at iteration k.

By averaging over the functional forms $P(\mathbf{x}_{\widetilde{R}} | \mathbf{x}_{\eta_{\widetilde{R}}}, \mathbf{y})$ — instead of the samples themselves as with typical histogramming [9] — each "sample" in (3) updates $\widehat{P}(\mathbf{x}_{\widetilde{R}} | \mathbf{y})$ for all $\mathbf{x}_{\widetilde{R}} \in \Lambda^{|\widetilde{R}|}$, greatly decreasing the number of samples needed for an accurate estimate. Furthermore, using multiple Markov chains (instead of the typical one [9]) improves robustness to the presence of multiple modes in $P(\mathbf{x}_{\widetilde{R}})$, each of which can trap the Markov chain.

3   Segmenting Nuclei on H&E Stained GI Tissue

We begin with an overview of the algorithm. Step 1) SCEM adapts the parameterized distributions to model the color — hue in HSV color-space — and spatial properties of nuclear and stromal pixels. Step 2) Using the MCMC estimator in (3), we calculate the probability that a given pixel is nuclei or stroma. Step 3) We threshold the pixel-wise probabilities to create hard classifications.

3.1   Color and Spatial Distributions of Nuclear and Stromal Pixel

First, we restate the segmentation problem using the nomenclature presented in Section 2.1. Let the set $R = \{1, 2, \ldots, |R|\}$ reference the $|R|$ pixels in an image. Each pixel $r \in R$ has two associated random variables: $X_r \in \Lambda \equiv \{1, 2\}$ indicating its class as either nuclei $\{1\}$ or stroma $\{2\}$ and $Y_r \in [0, 2\pi]$ representing its hue (color) in HSV space. We assume all X_r are identically distributed; we assume all Y_r are conditionally independent given X_r and identically distributed.

Conditional Distribution. The conditional distribution models the color properties of nuclear and stromal pixels. Since these biological structures stain differently (blue and red, respectively), their hue in HSV color-space provides a

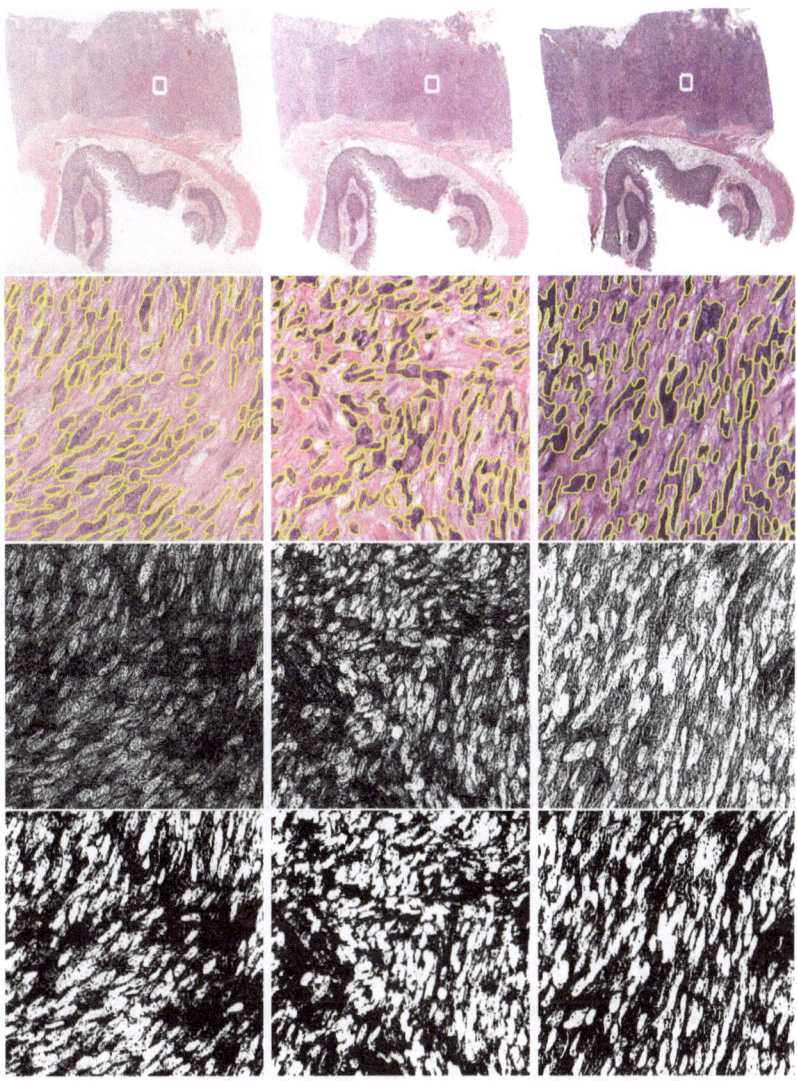

Fig. 1. Row 1) H&E stained GI specimens: (left to right) under-stained in both H and E ($\downarrow$H$\downarrow$E), normal (HE), and over-stained with both H and E ($\uparrow$H$\uparrow$E). Row 2) Magnified view of white boxes in the first row (boxes in Row 1 shown at 5x size to ensure visibility); yellow lines indicate manually delineated nuclear boundaries used as ground-truth. Row 3) Probability maps: $P(X_r = 1|y_r, \boldsymbol{\theta}_{hue})$. Row 4) Probability maps: $P(X_r = 1|\mathbf{y}, \boldsymbol{\theta})$.

reasonably discriminative feature. To model hue, an angular variable, we select the von Mises density. This leads to the following conditional distribution:

$$P(\mathbf{y}|\mathbf{x}, \boldsymbol{\theta}) = \prod_{r \in R} P(y_r|x_r, \boldsymbol{\theta}) = \prod_{r \in R} \exp\{\kappa_{x_r} \cos(y_r - \mu_{x_r})\}/[2\pi I_0(\kappa_{x_r})] \qquad (4)$$

where μ_{x_r} is the mean, κ_{x_r} is the concentration (i.e. shape), and I_0 is the modified Bessel function; the subscript x_r indicates that the means and concentrations are functions of the class x_r.

Prior Distribution. The Markov prior models spatial coherency. We establish this prior by defining its local conditional probability density functions, electing to use the Ising formulation:

$$P(x_r|\mathbf{x}_{\eta_r}) = \frac{1}{Z(\eta_r, \beta)} \exp\left\{\beta \sum_{s \in \eta_r} \delta(x_r - x_s)\right\}, \tag{5}$$

where $\beta \in \mathbb{R}$ and $Z(\eta_r, \beta) = \sum_{x_r} \exp\left\{\beta \sum_{s \in \eta_r} \delta(x_r - x_s)\right\}$ is the normalizing constant. The neighborhood η_r is the typical 4-connected region.

3.2 Parameter Estimation Using SCEM

The parameter vector for the MRF model is $\boldsymbol{\theta} = [\boldsymbol{\theta}_{hue}\ \boldsymbol{\theta}_{mrf}]^\mathsf{T} = [\mu_1\ \kappa_1\ \mu_2\ \kappa_2\ \beta]^\mathsf{T}$. Due to variabilities in staining, these parameters will vary from image to image. Consequently, we use SCEM to estimate $\boldsymbol{\theta}$ for each image. Inserting (4) and (5) into (2) yields the following EM equations:

$$Q(\boldsymbol{\theta}|\boldsymbol{\theta}^t) = \sum_{r \in R} P(X_r{=}1|\mathbf{y}, \boldsymbol{\theta}^t)\left[\kappa_1 \cos(y_r - \mu_1) - \ln I_0(\kappa_1) - \ln 2\pi\right] +$$

$$\sum_{r \in R} P(X_r{=}2|\mathbf{y}, \boldsymbol{\theta}^t)\left[\kappa_2 \cos(y_r - \mu_2) - \ln I_0(\kappa_2) - \ln 2\pi\right] +$$

$$\sum_{r \in R}\sum_{\mathbf{x}_{r \cup \eta_r}} P(\mathbf{x}_{r \cup \eta_r}|\mathbf{y}, \boldsymbol{\theta}^t)\left[-\ln Z(\eta_r, \beta) + \beta \sum_{s \in \eta_r} \delta(x_s - x_r)\right] \tag{6}$$

Notice that each of the three terms in the sum can be maximized independently. The first two yield analytical solutions. The final requires a numerical method; we employed the Nelder-Mead simplex. (Note that the initial conditions were chosen empirically, and remain fixed across all images.)

3.3 Pixel-Wise Classification

Having determined $\boldsymbol{\theta}$ with SCEM, classification becomes straightforward. We simply estimate $P(x_r|\mathbf{y}, \boldsymbol{\theta})$ with (3). Employing $P(x_r|\mathbf{y}, \boldsymbol{\theta})$ for classification is called maximum posterior marginal (MPM) estimation. Instead of MPM, we could have chosen maximum *a posteriori* (MAP) estimation, implementing it with iterated conditional modes [7] or simulated annealing [11]. However, MPM is the natural choice since $P(x_r|\mathbf{y}, \boldsymbol{\theta})$ is already calculated during the SCEM iteration. As a final step, the probabilities are converted to hard classifications via thresholding.

Table 1. Comparison of AUC values for both algorithms across sub-images; comparison of SCEM-estimated beta $\widehat{\beta}$ with β derived from ground-truth

	Area Under the ROC Curve		Markov Parameter		
Stain	$P(X_r=1\|y_r,\boldsymbol{\theta}_{hue})$	$P(X_r=1\|\mathbf{y},\boldsymbol{\theta})$	β	$\widehat{\beta}$	$\|\beta-\widehat{\beta}\|/\beta$
HE	0.761	**0.823**	2.826	2.936	0.0391
H↓E	0.787	**0.860**	3.149	2.936	0.0677
H↑E	0.735	**0.823**	3.111	2.845	0.0853
↓HE	0.638	**0.781**	2.976	2.741	0.0789
↓H↓E	0.717	**0.834**	2.765	2.867	0.0367
↑HE	0.803	**0.867**	2.978	2.823	0.0520
↑H↑E	0.814	**0.881**	3.102	2.845	0.0829
Mean	0.748	**0.838**	2.987	2.856	0.0632

4 Results of Nuclear Segmentation

4.1 Dataset

We cut seven consecutive sections from a block of paraffin embedded GI tissue. To simulate the common variability resulting from differing staining protocols, we dyed the specimens as follows: HE, H↓E, H↑E, ↓HE, ↓H↓E, ↑HE, and ↑H↑E, where ↑ and ↓ indicate over- and under-staining of the specified dye. Each slide was then digitized using an Aperio whole-slide scanner at 40x apparent magnification (0.25 μm per pixel). From each image, we extracted the same 768x793 sub-image for which we manually delineated the nuclear regions, establishing the "ground-truth" (Figure 1). We used these seven sub-images and their associated ground-truths to evaluate our algorithm.

4.2 Results

For each sub-image, we perform the segmentation algorithm described in the previous section. For comparison, we also apply an additional algorithm, identical to the first with the exception that it ignores spatial information. That is, $P(x_r|\mathbf{x}_{\eta_r},\boldsymbol{\theta})=P(x_r|\boldsymbol{\theta})$. In this instance, SCEM devolves into standard EM and $P(x_r|\mathbf{y},\boldsymbol{\theta})$ reduces to $P(x_r|y_r,\boldsymbol{\theta}_{hue})$.

Both of these algorithms create a probability map (either $P(X_r=1|y_r,\boldsymbol{\theta}_{hue})$ or $P(X_r=1|\mathbf{y},\boldsymbol{\theta})$) for each image. Please see Figure 1 for illustrations. Using each map, we generate a single receiver operator characteristic (ROC) curve and then measure the area under the curve (AUC). The resulting AUC values are listed in Table 1. Both algorithms perform consistently across all images, validating their robustness to color nonstandardness. However, including spatial constraints increases AUC performance substantially. Table 1 also reports our SCEM estimates of β along with the values obtained from the ground-truth (estimated using pseudo-likelihood). The relative difference between the two estimates never exceeds 9%. (Note that for MCMC estimation, we use $b=5$, $m=15$, and $c=4$; all values were chosen empirically.)

5   Conclusion

Color nonstandardness poses a significant problem in the computerized analysis of histopathology. In this work, we presented a novel Bayesian color segmentation algorithm that is highly robust to such nonstandardness; this algorithm employed a novel spatially-constrained extension of the EM algorithm, called spatially-constrained EM (SCEM), to dynamically estimate the probability density functions that describe the color and spatial properties of salient objects. Evaluating this algorithm over a dataset consisting of sections of gastrointestinal tissue stained using different protocols (to simulate severe color nonstandardness) we found that 1) the algorithm performed consistently across images and 2) the inclusion of spatial constraints increased AUC performance by over 12%.

An important goal of this paper was to introduce the SCEM algorithm. Unlike previous approaches for incorporating Markov priors into the EM framework, SCEM does not limit the type of Markov model (as in [5]) nor the parameters that can be estimated (as in [4]). On a final note, we should mention that SCEM is not specific to nuclear segmentation, or even image segmentation, but instead is applicable to any task requiring the unsupervised estimation of MRF models.

References

1. Finlayson, G., et al.: Color by correlation: A simple, unifying framework for color constancy. IEEE Trans. on Patt. Anal. and Mach. Intel. 23, 1209–1221 (2001)
2. Madabhushi, A., Udupa, J.: New methods of mr image intensity standardization via generalized scale. Medical Physics 33(9), 3426–3434 (2006)
3. Monaco, J., et al.: Image segmentation with implicit color standardization using cascaded em: Detection of myelodysplastic syndromes. In: ISBI (2012)
4. Comer, M.L., Delp, E.J.: The em/mpm algorithm for segmentation of textured images: analysis and further experimental results. IEEE Trans. Imag. Proc. 9(10), 1731–1744 (2000)
5. Nikou, C., et al.: A class-adaptive spatially variant mixture model for image segmentation. IEEE Trans. on Imag. Proc. 16(4), 1121–1130 (2007)
6. Marroquin, J.L., Vemuri, B.C., Botello, S., Calderon, F., Fernandez-Bouzas, A.: An accurate and efficient bayesian method for automatic segmentation of brain mri. IEEE Trans. on Med. Imag. 21(8), 934–945 (2002)
7. Besag, J.: On the statistical analysis of dirty pictures. J. of the Roy. Stat. Soc. Series B (Methodological) 48(3), 259–302 (1986)
8. Monaco, J., Madabhushi, A.: Weighted maximum posterior marginals for random fields using an ensemble of conditional densities from multiple markov chain monte carlo simulations. IEEE Trans. on Med. Imag. 30, 1352–1364 (2011)
9. Marroquin, J., Mitter, S., Poggio, T.: Probabilistic solution of ill-posed problems in computational vision. J. of the Amer. Stat. Assoc. 82(397), 76–89 (1987)
10. Dempster, A., Laird, N., Rubin, D.: Maximum likelihood from incomplete data via the em algorithm. J. of the Roy. Stat. Soc. Series B 39(1), 1–38 (1977)
11. Geman, S., Geman, D.: Stochastic relaxation, gibbs distribution, and the bayesian restoration of images. IEEE Transactions on Pattern Recognition and Machine Intelligence 6, 721–741 (1984)

Detecting and Tracking Motion
of *Myxococcus xanthus* Bacteria in Swarms*

Xiaomin Liu[1], Cameron W. Harvey[2], Haitao Wang[1],
Mark S. Alber[2], and Danny Z. Chen[1]

[1] Department of Computer Science & Engineering, University of Notre Dame, USA
[2] Department of Applied and Computational Mathematics and Statistics,
University of Notre Dame, USA

Abstract. Automatically detecting and tracking the motion of *Myxococcus xanthus* bacteria provide essential information for studying bacterial cell motility mechanisms and collective behaviors. However, this problem is difficult due to the low contrast of microscopy images, cell clustering and colliding behaviors, etc. To overcome these difficulties, our approach starts with a level set based pre-segmentation of cell clusters, followed by an enhancement of the rod-like cell features and detection of individual bacterium within each cluster. A novel method based on "spikes" of the outer medial axis is applied to divide touching (colliding) cells. The tracking of cell motion is accomplished by a non-crossing bipartite graph matching scheme that matches not only individual cells but also the neighboring structures around each cell. Our approach was evaluated on image sequences of moving *M. xanthus* bacteria close to the edge of their swarms, achieving high accuracy on the test data sets.

1   Introduction

Myxococcus xanthus is a rod-shaped, Gram-negative soil bacterium that has become a model organism for the study of multicellular development because of the coordinated collective motion that the bacterial cells exhibit when moving on surfaces [1]. Understanding the biomechanical interactions of bacterial cells during movement, such as collisions and cells moving within clusters, will shed light on the collective motion of cells and ultimately on both the processes of swarming and multicellular-structure formation. An important step towards achieving this goal is to track the cell movement and interactions. However, accurate quantification of cell motion faces a number of challenges, including low image contrast, intra- or inter-frame intensity variations, and the frequent clustering and colliding behaviors of multiple cells.

The current cell tracking methods mainly fall into two basic categories: segmentation-based methods and model-based methods. Model-based algorithms such as the geodesic active contour method [2] have gained popularity in recent

---

* This work was supported in part by NSF under grant CCF-0916606 and by NIH under grants R01GM095959 and R01GM100470.

N. Ayache et al. (Eds.): MICCAI 2012, Part I, LNCS 7510, pp. 373–380, 2012.

years due to their flexibility in capturing topological changes such as mitosis. However, such methods cannot avoid merging multiple touching cells, which occur quite frequently in our images. Segmentation-based methods consist of two steps: segmenting individual cells in each image frame and mapping segmented cells between consecutive frames. Once segmented cells are obtained in different frames, the remaining task in fact becomes a certain matching problem that could be solved globally by methods such as optimal bipartite graph matching [3], Softassign Procrustes algorithm [4], etc. But, these matching methods utilize only information of independent cells (e.g., their appearances) as matching criteria, and do not consider relations among different cells, such as the spatial distribution of cells in a neighborhood. Indeed, the relative positions of moving cells and their local structures keep changing from frame to frame, which may not be captured directly by simple graph matching methods (e.g., [5]).

We observed that in image sequences of moving *M. xanthus* cells, the changes of relative cell positions are quite moderate, and thus the spatial structures of cells between consecutive image frames remain relatively similar. Based on this observation, we propose a new tracking algorithm that considers the neighboring cells of every target cell in consecutive frames, and captures their similarity despite of certain changes caused by the cell movement.

In this paper, we present a new method that combines cell shape segmentation and optimal graph matching to overcome the difficulties of tracking *M. xanthus* bacteria. First, cell clusters are identified using a level set method. Then individual cells within clusters are segmented by enhancing the cells' rod-like shape features with the eigenvalues of Hessian matrices. Next, false merging of neighboring cells is separated by an approach based on the structures of the outer medial axis of the cells. Finally, a non-crossing maximum bipartite graph matching scheme is applied to compare cell neighboring structures in consecutive frames, producing the frame-to-frame correspondence in image sequences. Based on the tracking results, we can quantitatively study cell motility mechanisms such as the reversal behavior of the bacteria and how they avoid blocking in cell motions.

2   Method

2.1   Segmentation of Cell Clusters

The regions of cell clusters in each image frame are first identified by a gradient based level set approach [6] that maintains the regularity during the level set evolution (see Fig. 1). To speed up the process, we assign the initial level set function as a binary image generated as follows. (1) Obtain the shadow area surrounding each bacterium by the method introduced in Sec. 2.2; (2) apply the morphological dilation method to the binary image obtained in Step (1) to cover the entire regions of cells. As shown in Sec. 2.2, the segmentation of cell clusters helps eliminate false positive cell segmentation errors near the cell clusters.

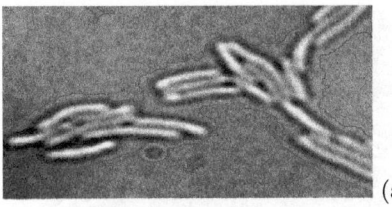 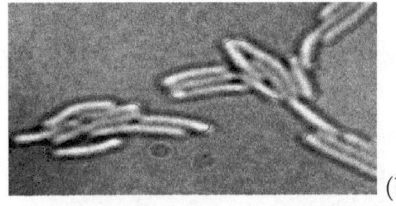

(a)   (b)

Fig. 1. An example for the level set segmentation of the cell clusters: (a) The initialization of the level set function (in red); (b) the final segmentation

2.2 Segmentation of Individual Cells

The appearance of an *M. xanthus* bacterium in our images is like a bright rod-shaped object surrounded by dark shadow area. We propose a method based on the eigenvalues of the Hessian matrix to detect such distinct shape features of each individual cell, which are insensitive to inter- and intra-frame intensity changes. For a 2D image I of bacterial cells, let $I(x, y)$ denote the intensity value at a pixel of coordinates (x, y). We first obtain a smoothed image $L(x, y; \sigma)$ by convolving $I(x, y)$ with a Gaussian kernel $G(x, y; \sigma)$, where σ is a scale parameter corresponding to the size of the target object [7]. Then the Hessian matrix of a pixel at (x, y) is composed of the second order derivatives of L: $H(x, y) = \begin{bmatrix} L_{xx} & L_{xy} \\ L_{xy} & L_{yy} \end{bmatrix}$. We can learn the second order local intensity changes by computing the eigenvalues λ_1 and λ_2 of $H(x, y)$: $\lambda_{1,2} = \frac{L_{xx} + L_{yy} \pm \sqrt{(L_{xx} - L_{yy})^2 + 4L_{xy}^2}}{2}$.

If one of the two eigenvalues is close to zero and the other exhibits a high negative or positive value, then it corresponds to a ridge-like local structure. Let λ_S and λ_L denote the two eigenvalues such that $|\lambda_S| < |\lambda_L|$, and let $\lambda = \lambda_S - \lambda_L$. In our approach, we enhance the image for each pixel that has a high positive λ value in the rod-like cell regions and a high (absolute) negative λ value in the surrounding shadow regions. Those regions are then segmented by thresholding. As shown in Fig. 2(b), a narrow band around each cell cluster also presents high positive λ values in the enhanced image, which can be eliminated by the accurate segmentation of the cell cluster boundaries (see Fig. 2(d)). The scale space based image segmentation algorithm may cause over-partitioning due to intensity changes inside the cells. These cases, which occurred rather infrequently in our images, are mostly near the ends of the cells.

2.3 Separation of Touching Cells

The moving bacterial cells frequently touch each other while exhibiting no significant intensity changes around the cell boundaries at the touching areas. The watershed method is commonly used for segmenting touching cells [8]. However, for objects with elongated shapes such as *M. xanthus* bacteria, the watershed method tends to under-segment cell regions and produce too many small fragments. To capture the concavity of the boundary locations where two cells touch,

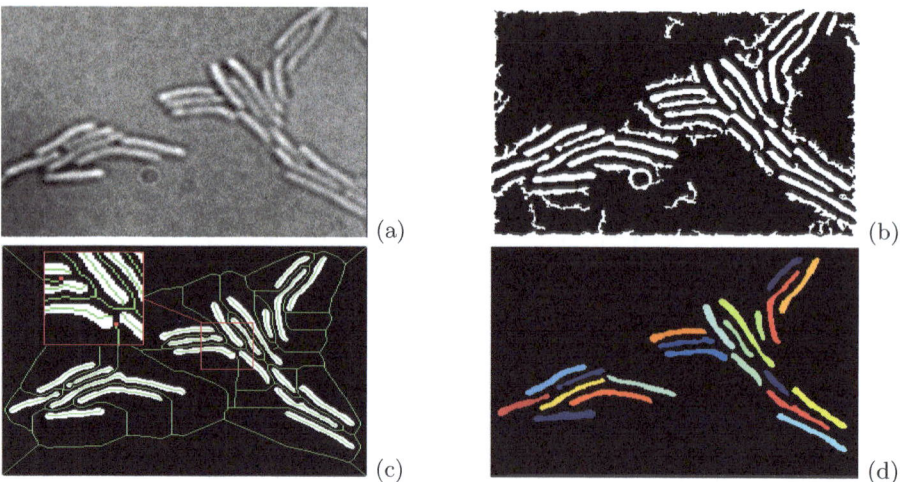

Fig. 2. Illustrating the cell segmentation approach: (a) An original image; (b) cell regions segmented by using the eigenvalues of the Hessian matrix (in Sec. 2.2); (c) cell regions after removing the false positives outside the clusters and separating touching cells based on the outer medial axis (the outer medial axis is in green and the endpoints of the outer medial axis spikes in a boxed area are in red); (d) the final segmentation

a method based on the "spikes" of the outer medial axis of the cell regions is applied to detect the locations of the touching areas [9]. As shown in Fig. 2(c), the outer medial axis of well separated bacteria is similar to their Voronoi diagram. The "spikes" are the segments of the outer medial axis with one disjoint endpoint, which are associated with the boundary concavity between touching cells and actually point at the locations where cell touching occurs.

Fig. 3 illustrates several typical touching cases involving two or more cells (more complex cases can be viewed as combinations of these basic cases). In our settings, almost all touching locations are at the ends of the rod-shaped cells: either two cells merge at two end positions (Fig. 3(a), (c), (d)) or one cell's end touches another cell's body (Fig. 3(b)). After computing the outer medial axis by an iterative thinning method [10], we prune away the false "spikes" that are caused by noisy cell boundaries instead of by true cell touching [9]. Then the endpoints of the remaining spikes are identified and extended along the centerline directions of the spikes to divide the touching cells. An extension line stops if it crosses a neighboring extension line (Fig. 3(b), (c)). If it does not cross any neighboring extension line, then it divides the cell region by itself (Fig. 3(a)).

2.4   Tracking Cells Based on Non-crossing Maximum Matching of Neighborhood Structures

Once individual cells are segmented, we map cells in consecutive frames and establish their correspondence throughout an image sequence. For each cell C

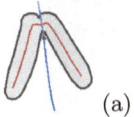 (a)   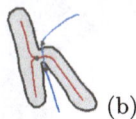 (b)   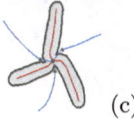 (c)   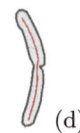 (d)

Fig. 3. Examples of separating touching cells based on the outer medial axis: (a) End-to-end touching of two cells; (b) end-to-body touching of two cells; (c) end-to-end touching of multiple cells; (d) a difficult case of end-to-end touching with no spikes presented on the outer medial axis. The outer medial axis is marked in blue and the arrow markers correspond to the endpoints of spikes of the outer medial axis.

in a frame I_t, we find its corresponding cell C' in frame I_{t+1} by comparing the neighboring cells of C in frame I_t with those of C' in frame I_{t+1}, which we model as a bipartite matching problem based on their order around C (and C'). The neighbors of a cell C in a frame are those bacteria whose Voronoi regions share a common edge with the Voronoi region of C. Note that since moving cells may enter or leave the neighborhood (i.e., the set of neighbors) of a cell C in consecutive frames, C's neighborhood in I_t may be somewhat different from C's neighborhood in I_{t+1}. For a cell C_i in I_t and a candidate cell C_j of C_i in I_{t+1}, let N_i and N_j denote their neighborhoods in I_t and I_{t+1} in (say) clockwise cyclic order around C_i and C_j, respectively. We build a bipartite graph $G = (U, V, E)$ with weighted edges, where $U = \{u_1, u_2, \ldots, u_{n_i}\}$ is for N_i and $V = \{v_1, v_2, \ldots, v_{n_j}\}$ is for N_j. To capture the similarity between N_i and N_j that may contain some common cells, we apply a non-crossing bipartite matching algorithm [11] that aims to preserve the order of the neighboring cells while finding a matching with the maximum total edge weight. A *non-crossing matching* in the graph $G = \{U, V, E\}$ is a subset of edges $M \subseteq E$ such that for any two edges (u_a, v_b) and (u_c, v_d) in M, either ($a < c$ and $b < d$) or ($c < a$ and $d < b$) holds. In our problem, it is crucial to obtain a non-crossing maximum matching (instead of just a maximum matching) because an edge crossing corresponds to a wrong order of the matched neighbors which may not reflect the correct neighboring structures. The algorithm in [11] takes $O(m \log n)$ time, where $n = |U| + |V|$ and $m = |E|$.

Our cell mapping algorithm for an image sequence takes the following steps:

1. For the cells in every binary image frame, compute their outer medial axis [10] and associate each cell with its corresponding Voronoi region.
2. In every frame I_t, for each cell C_i, identify its neighborhood $N_i = \{C_i^1, C_i^2, \ldots, C_i^{n_i}\}$ in clockwise cyclic order around C_i (the Voronoi region of every C_i^k shares a common edge with that of C_i). For a candidate cell C_j of C_i in frame I_{t+1}, let its neighborhood $N_j = \{C_j^1, C_j^2, \ldots, C_j^{n_j}\}$ (see Fig. 4).
3. For each pair (C_i^k, C_j^l) of C_i and C_j, build a bipartite graph $G_{kl} = \{U, V, E\}$, with $U = \{C_i^k, C_i^{k+1}, \ldots, C_i^{n_i}, C_i^1, \ldots, C_i^{k-1}\}$ (when $k = 1$, $U = \{C_i^1, C_i^2, \ldots, C_i^{n_i}\}$), and $V = \{C_j^l, C_j^{l+1}, \ldots, C_j^{n_j}, C_j^1, \ldots, C_j^{l-1}\}$ (when $l = 1$, $U = \{C_j^1, C_j^2, \ldots, C_j^{n_j}\}$). An edge in E connects two vertices $u \in U$ and $v \in V$ if the two corresponding cells satisfy some constraints on their relative distance, their

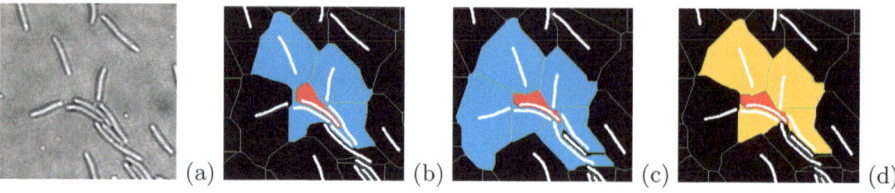

Fig. 4. Illustrating the non-crossing maximum matching between two sets of neighboring cells: (a) An original image; (b)(c) segmented cell regions and their outer medial axes (in green) in frames I_t and I_{t+1}, with the center cell in the red region and the neighboring cells in the blue regions; (d) the cells in the non-crossing maximum matching of the two neighboring sets (in the yellow regions)

length difference, and their orientation difference with respect to C_i and C_j; its edge weight $w(u, v)$ is defined by the similarity between the two cells of u and v, $w(u, v) = (c - MHD(u, v))/c$, where $MHD(u, v)$ is the modified Hausdorff distance between the two cells of u and v, and c is a constant that is two times the maximum cell width. Then we compute the non-crossing maximum weight matching M_{kl}^* in G_{kl} using the algorithm in [11]. Find the matching M^* with the largest weight among all such graphs G_{kl} for C_i and C_j. Add the similarity value $w(C_i, C_j)$ for the cells C_i and C_j to the weight of M^*, which is the "best" match weight $W(C_i, C_j)$ for C_i and C_j. If $W(C_i, C_j)$ is smaller than a threshold, then ignore the pair (C_i, C_j).

4. Repeat Step 3 for every possible candidate cell C_j of C_i in frame I_{t+1}.
5. For every two frames I_t and I_{t+1}, sort the remaining "best" match pairs (C_i, C_j) based on their "best" match weights $W(C_i, C_j)$. Scan the sorted list of "best" match pairs starting from the largest one. Assign correspondence between the paired cells (C_i, C_j) in frames I_t and I_{t+1}. Once a cell C_i (C_j) for I_t (I_{t+1}) is assigned a matched cell, all other pairs containing C_i (C_j) in I_t and I_{t+1} are removed from the list. After the scan, all unmatched cells are viewed as "single" cells (e.g., new cells entering the frames).

3   Experimental Results

Swarms of M. xanthus are made on agar plates as detailed in [12]. Time-lapse microscopy is performed either on the swarm plates or on specially designed imaging chambers that are similar to the submerged agar chambers (SAC) described in [13]. The image size is 512 by 512. The pixel size is 0.14*0.07 μm. The cells move approximately 10-25 pixels in two consecutive frames. The time interval between two consecutive image frames is 15 seconds.

The experiments were performed on 4 image sequences containing 384 cells in total. Cells were visually tracked in the sequences and compared with the output of our algorithm. The tracking result of one moving cell is considered as correct if the cell is segmented correctly in each frame and the correspondence throughout the entire image sequence is correctly maintained. Incomplete trajectories and

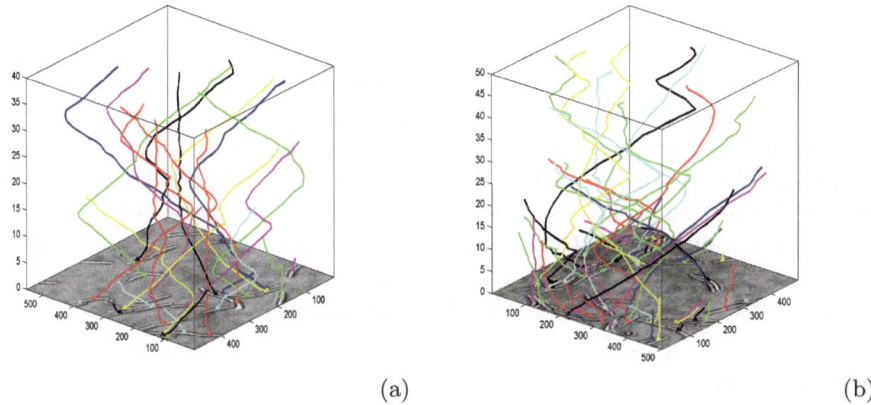

(a)   (b)

Fig. 5. Two examples of tracked trajectories of cell centroids in frame stacks, with frame 1 positioned at the $z = 0$ plane. Different cells are distinguished by colors.

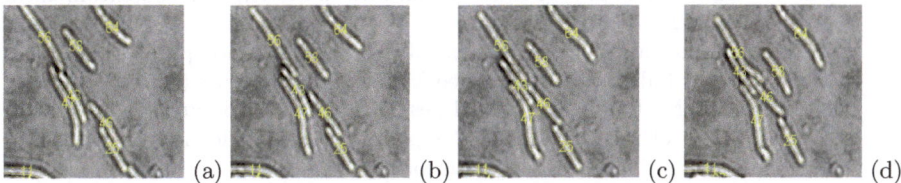

(a)   (b)   (c)   (d)

Fig. 6. Consecutive frames of tracking results

Table 1. The tracking accuracy of cell trajectories

	Independent tracking	With neighborhood	Number of cells
Seq1	76.9%	89.2%	65
Seq2	71.7%	87.1%	124
Seq3	77.7%	92.2%	103
Seq4	78.3%	89.1%	92

wrong trajectories are all considered as errors. Fig. 5 shows two examples of tracked cell traces in 3D spatio-temporal space. Fig. 6 is another example of the frame-by-frame correspondence in a magnified region. The tracking errors are mostly due to incorrect segmentation in regions that are blurred when the focal plane of the microscope is being adjusted. Table 1 lists the accuracy of cell trajectories measured in the 4 sequences. It shows our method achieved higher accuracy comparing to the method without utilizing the neighboring structures, which has met the requirement of the current biological application.

4   Conclusions

We present new algorithms for segmenting and tracking *M. xanthus* bacteria that are moving and closely interacting. One of our major contributions is a non-crossing maximum matching method to track moving cells based on their neighborhood structures. The experiments showed high accuracy of tracking cell trajectories by our algorithm. Our approach is applicable to other tracking problems with the assumption that the cell movement is moderate between consecutive image frames, so that the neighboring structure around each cell does not change too substantially from frame to frame (otherwise, it may be meaningless to incorporate the neighboring cell information into the tracking process).

References

1. Dworkin, M.: Recent advances in the social and developmental biology of the myxobacteria. Microbiological Reviews 60, 70–102 (1996)
2. Li, K., Miller, E.D., Chen, M., Kanade, T., Weiss, L.E., Campbell, P.G.: Cell population tracking and lineage construction with spatiotemporal context. Medical Image Analysis 12, 546–566 (2008)
3. Munkres, J.: Algorithms for the assignment and transportation problems. Journal of the Society for Industrial and Applied Mathematics 5, 32–38 (1957)
4. Gor, V., Elowitz, M., Bacarian, T., Mjolsness, E.: Tracking cell signals in fluorescent images. In: Proc. of the 2005 IEEE Computer Society Conference on Computer Vision and Pattern Recognition - Workshops, p. 142 (2005)
5. Liu, M., Roy-Chowdhury, A.K., Reddy, G.V.: Robust estimation of stem cell lineages using local graph matching. In: IEEE Computer Society Conference on Computer Vision and Pattern Recognition Workshops, pp. 194–201 (2009)
6. Li, C., Xu, C., Gui, C., Fox, M.D.: Distance regularized level set evolution and its application to image segmentation. IEEE Trans. Image Processing 19, 3243–3254 (2010)
7. Lindeberg, T.: Scale-space theory in computer vision. Kluwer Academic Publishers (1994)
8. Vincent, L., Soille, P.: Watersheds in digital spaces: An efficient algorithm based on immersion simulations. IEEE Transactions on Pattern Analysis and Machine Intelligence 13, 583–598 (1991)
9. Liu, X., Setiadi, A.F., Alber, M.S., Lee, P.P., Chen, D.Z.: Identification and classification of cells in multi-spectral microscopy images of lymph node. In: Proceedings of SPIE Medical Imaging: Image Processing, vol. 7962, p. 79620J (2011)
10. Lam, L., Lee, S.W., Suen, C.Y.: Thinning methodologies – A comprehensive survey. IEEE Trans. on Pattern Analysis and Machine Intelligence 14, 869–885 (1992)
11. Malucelli, F., Ottmann, T., Pretolani, D.: Efficient labelling algorithms for the maximum non crossing matching problem. Discrete Applied Mathematics 47, 1–4 (1993)
12. Harvey, C., Morcos, F., Sweet, C.R., Kaiser, K., Chatterjee, S., Liu, X., Chen, D.Z., Alber, M.: Study of elastic collisions of myxococcus xanthus in swarms. Physical Biology 8, 026016 (2011)
13. Welch, R., Kaiser, D.: Cell behavior in traveling wave patterns of myxobacteria. Proc. Natl. Acad. Sci. USA 98, 14907–14912 (2001)

Signal and Noise Modeling in Confocal Laser Scanning Fluorescence Microscopy

Gerlind Herberich[1], Reinhard Windoffer[2,*],
Rudolf E. Leube[2,*], and Til Aach[1,*,**]

[1] Institute of Imaging and Computer Vision, RWTH Aachen University, Germany
[2] Institute of Molecular and Cellular Anatomy, RWTH Aachen University, Germany

Abstract. Fluorescence confocal laser scanning microscopy (CLSM) has revolutionized imaging of subcellular structures in biomedical research by enabling the acquisition of 3D time-series of fluorescently-tagged proteins in living cells, hence forming the basis for an automated quantification of their morphological and dynamic characteristics. Due to the inherently weak fluorescence, CLSM images exhibit a low SNR. We present a novel model for the transfer of signal and noise in CLSM that is both theoretically sound as well as corroborated by a rigorous analysis of the pixel intensity statistics via measurement of the 3D noise power spectra, signal-dependence and distribution. Our model provides a better fit to the data than previously proposed models. Further, it forms the basis for (i) the simulation of the CLSM imaging process indispensable for the quantitative evaluation of CLSM image analysis algorithms, (ii) the application of Poisson denoising algorithms and (iii) the reconstruction of the fluorescence signal.

Keywords: Fluorescence microscopy, Confocal laser scanning microscopy, Model, Noise, Pixel intensity statistics.

1 Introduction

4D (3D+time) live cell fluorescence imaging by means of CLSM has become a widely used tool in cell biology for the analysis of the dynamics of subcellular structures. To avoid phototoxicity, the excitation laser power has to be kept in a low range. In consequence, the fluorescence signal is very weak and the SNR is low. Fig. 1b shows a typical CLSM slice image, depicting fluorescently-labeled keratin intermediate filaments, which are subcellular protein fibers that build an essential part of the cytoskeleton in epithelial cells, illustrating how much CLSM images are corrupted by noise.

Noise reduction is therefore a crucial preprocessing step to be applied before the image analysis. To perform a sound denoising a noise model is needed. An extended model describing signal and noise transfer in CLSM which does not only

---

* The authors gratefully acknowledge funding by the German Research Council (DFG, AA5/5-1, LE566/18-1, WI1731/8-1).

** Deceased 16.01.2012.

N. Ayache et al. (Eds.): MICCAI 2012, Part I, LNCS 7510, pp. 381–388, 2012.

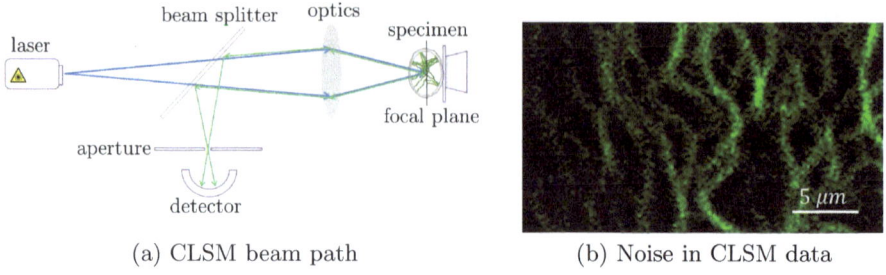

(a) CLSM beam path   (b) Noise in CLSM data

Fig. 1. CLSM imaging: (a) Scheme of the beam path in a confocal laser scanning microscope and (b) Noise in CLSM images: Image section showing fluorescently-labeled keratin intermediate filaments, subcellular protein fibers, that appear in the image as curvilinear structures. Their granular appearance is due to noise.

account for the system noise but also for the randomness of the fluorescence input signal further enables the simulation of CLSM imaging so that synthetic images may be generated for the quantitative evaluation of image analysis algorithms for CLSM. Furthermore, such an extended model can serve for the reconstruction of the fluorescence input signal. The latter is related to the concentration of fluorescently-labeled proteins such that quantitative spatiotemporal analyses of the protein-of-interest can be performed.

Few models have been proposed for the noise in CLSM images as well as for the pixel intensity statistics. It is often assumed, that due to the photon-counting process in CLSM, the noise follows a Poisson distribution [1]. Denoising methods for CLSM that rely on this assumption have been designed [2] [3]. For the pixel intensity statistics in CLSM images, a mixture model [4] has been proposed recently, claiming that the pixel intensity statistics follow a linear mixture of a discrete normal distribution and a negative binomial distribution. The discrete normal distribution serves as a model for additive electronic noise while the negative binomial distribution, also known as Gamma-Poisson distribution, accounts for the fact that the photon-counting process at the detector described by the Poisson model depends itself on a random variable – namely the random fluorescence field after smoothing by the CLSM point-spread-function (PSF). The distribution of the latter is approximated by a Gamma distribution by simulation [4]. Further related work on pixel intensity statistics includes a Poisson approximation to the noise of the integrating detectors [5] where the pixel intensity statistics are modeled as two cascaded Poisson processes and a linear mapping which accounts for the offset and gain of the analog-to-digital conversion.

We found that all of the above models did not fit well to our data (Fig. 5). Instead of performing a simulation of the input such as is done in [4], we provide a theoretically derived model which is substantiated by measurements of signal-dependence, spatial-frequency-dependence and distribution of the pixel intensity statistics.

2   Image Formation

In fluorescence CLSM, subcellular structures are labeled with fluorescent dyes called fluorochromes. The structure to be imaged can thus be considered as a spatial fluorochrome distribution. A 3D image of such a specimen is acquired as follows (Fig. 1a): A laser is focused by the optics onto a point within the specimen (excitation beam path). Any fluorochromes present at that position randomly emit photons in all directions. As the fluorescence emitted by an excited fluorochrome has a longer wavelength than the excitation light (Stokes' law) the fluorescence photons are deflected at the dichroic beam splitter towards the detector, a photomultiplier tube (PMT). To mask fluorescence that originates from structures that are out-of-focus, an aperture is placed in front of the detector (detection beam path). By moving the focal point, the whole focal plane is scanned point-wise yielding a 2D image which represents a section of the specimen. This process is repeated at different depths of the 3D specimen such that it is imaged in a stack of 2D slices forming a 3D image.

For a better understanding of the way the fluorescence signal and the noise are transferred through the microscope system, in the following, we detail the single pixel acquisition process, i.e. the detection beam path, as illustrated in Fig. 2. Note that throughout the description the wavelength-dependency of the quantities involved is not mentioned explicitly for reasons of simplicity.

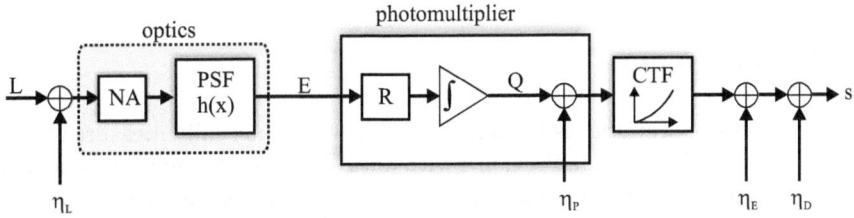

Fig. 2. Block diagram of the single pixel acquisition process in a confocal laser scanning microscope: See main text for explanation

The emission photon flux from a single fluorescent molecule depends on the excitation photon flux, the quantum yield of the fluorochrome and its molecular cross-section. It gives the number of photons emitted per unit time. However, not only a single fluorescent molecule contributes to the signal formation of one pixel, but rather all fluorescent molecules contained in the sensing volume form the input to the detection beam path, the radiant flux L. The number of fluorescent molecules in the sensing volume is determined by the fluorochrome concentration. The sensing volume is defined by the effective support of the PSF of the excitation beam path: It is the small volume within the specimen, that is illuminated by the laser during the pixel time.

Due to the quantum nature of light and electric charge, the emission of particles such as photons or electrons is associated with an uncertainty referred to as shot noise. According to this random process, photons are emitted in all spatial directions. Only a small fraction - the effective fraction - of them are collected by the microscope objective. Its numerical aperture NA is a measure for its acceptance cone. An objective with NA = 1.4 will capture about 30% of all photons. These photons pass the optics. The resulting radiant flux or radiant power E specifies the number of photons per unit time arriving at the detector where they are integrated over the pixel dwell time dt. The detector responsivity $R \in [0, 1]$ describes its quantum efficiency, i.e. how efficient incident photons cause photoelectrons to emit from the photocathode as a consequence of the photoelectric effect. Because of the quantum nature of electric charge, this process is subject to shot noise η_P. The electric field between photocathode and anode in the PMT accelerates the photoelectrons on their way to the anode while striking several dynodes where further electrons are emitted due to secondary emission. In this way, the number of electrons is multiplied and the accumulation of charge at the anode forms the detected signal which is largely amplified compared to the weak fluorescence radiant power arriving at the detector. The signal then passes an analog-to-digital converter (ADC), defining the final dynamic range of the output signal. It is sampled and quantized such that electronic noise η_E and quantization noise η_D are added to the signal. PMT gain, ADC offset, ADC gain and possible non-linearities in e.g. the electronics or nonlinear quantum efficiencies are summarized in the camera transfer function (CTF)[6]. The resulting noisy pixel intensity is called s.

3   Measurements

The pixel intensity statistics is the only quantity we can actually measure to corroborate our model derived in Section 4 with data. To measure signal-dependence, spatial-frequency-dependence and distribution of the pixel intensity statistics, under the assumption that all noise processes in the imaging chain are ergodic, we have sought specimens with a spatially homogeneous fluorochrome distribution to obtain a homogeneous input to the imaging chain. To this end, we prepared sodium fluorescein dilution series with known concentrations ranging from $5\mu g/ml$ to $200\mu g/ml$. Sodium fluorescein is a water soluble fluorochrome that has been proposed for fluorescence calibration [7]. Following [7] we stabilized the pH at 9.5 using borate buffer. Each specimen then yields a homogeneous fluorochrome distribution with a radiant power depending on the fluorescein concentration. At room temperature, from each specimen, we acquired a 16-bit 3D image stack using a Zeiss LSM710 with the following parameters: Excitation laser from the Argon line (wavelength of emission maximum: $488\,nm$), lateral voxel size $dx = dy = 24\,nm$, interslice distance $dz = 11nm$, 63× oil-immersion objective with numerical aperture NA = 1.4, pixel dwell time $dt = 1.58\,\mu s$, pinhole diameter $49\,\mu m$, PMT gain 911, ADC gain $K_d = 1$, ADC offset $K_0 = 0$.

To investigate whether the pixel intensity variance is signal-dependent, we measured sample variance and sample mean slicewise (Fig. 3a) over $1.8 \cdot 10^8$ samples from concentrations which spanned a range from 20 to $200\mu g/ml$ at

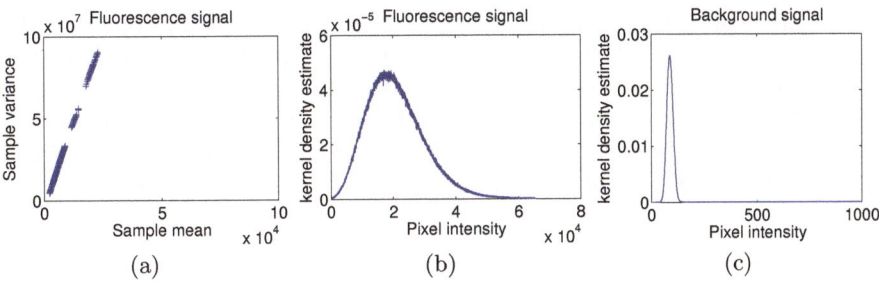

Fig. 3. Fluorescence signal: (a) signal-dependence of variance and (b) kernel density estimate of pixel intensity distribution. Background signal: (c) kernel density estimate of intensity distribution. Note that the gaps in plot (a) are due to a limited number of fluorescein concentrations used for the analysis.

$20\mu g/ml$ increments and from $5\mu g/ml$ and $10\mu g/ml$. Note that the slope is not equal to one as would be the case for samples of a Poisson distribution where the variance equals the expected value.

As estimate of the intensity distribution, for each fluorescein image, we computed a kernel density estimate from the pixel intensities. We used the Epanechnikov kernel with a width of 10. Fig. 3b shows a kernel density estimate of $2 \cdot 10^6$ samples drawn from a 3D image of a $180\mu g/ml$-concentration specimen and Fig. 3c a density estimate from $8 \cdot 10^5$ samples of a 3D image acquired without a specimen to measure the electronic noise.

We have estimated the 3D noise power spectrum (NPS) by periodogram averaging (Bartlett method). Fig. 4 shows the results of averaging over 700 xy- and xz-slices of size 100×100 respectively.

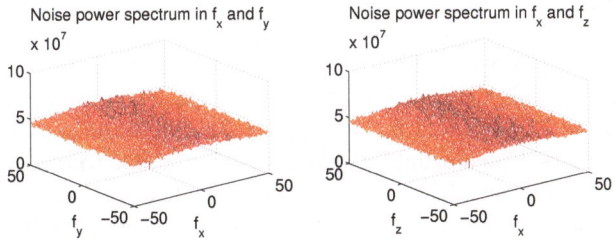

Fig. 4. NPS estimates in x, y and z: White spectrum in f_y and f_z and a slight increase in low spatial frequencies in f_x due to linewise scanning. (The sharp negative peak at $\mathbf{f} = 0$ is due to subtraction of the sample mean prior to periodogram averaging.).

We can draw the following conclusions: As expected, the electronic noise η_E can be modeled as additive Gaussian noise and is of negligible amplitude. Quantization noise η_D may be neglected as it exhibits an amplitude smaller than half a quantization level. Obviously, the dominating noise sources are the fluorescence noise η_L and/or the PMT noise η_P. This conclusion is confirmed by the measurement of the signal-dependence which indicates by its slope that the noise samples have largely been amplified. The 3D NPS further indicates that the power of η_P must be superior to that of the fraction of η_L that arrives at the detector: White noise η_L passing through optics becomes colored noise with an NPS shaped by the squared magnitude of the Fourier transform of the PSF. As the measured NPS is not colored, the power of η_P must be larger.

4   Model

The random fluorescence signal is the input to the imaging system. In the case of weak signals, the law of rare events holds and the uncertainty of the fluorescence photon emission can be modeled by a Poisson distribution describing the probability to find k successes (i.e. photon emissions) in a given time interval. Let X_L be a discrete random variable, $X_L \sim \mathcal{P}(L)$ with probability mass function (pmf) $P_{X_L}(k) = \frac{L^k e^{-L}}{k!}$, $k \in \mathbb{N}$, $L \in \mathbb{R}^{>0}$. Recall that for a Poisson distribution, the variance equals the expected value: $Var(X_L) = L$. Hence, to model this as additive noise, we rewrite $\eta_L = k - L$ as depicted in Fig. 2.

In the following, we describe step by step how the random fluorescence signal is transferred through each of the blocks in the diagram Fig. 2 and where it is corrupted by noise.

1) NA: From k emitted photons, only a small fraction l are collected by the microscope objective: The random variates k become new random variates $l = f_1(k)$ of the discrete random variable X_{NA}, according to $f_1(x) = a_1 x$, $a_1 \in [0, 1]$. $Var(X_{\text{NA}}) = a_1^2 Var(X_f)$.

2) PSF: The l collected photons are then filtered by the PSF which corresponds to a convolution of the effective fraction of the spatial fluorochrome distribution with the PSF $h(\mathbf{x})$ of the microscope, $\mathbf{x} = (x, y, z)^T$ being the spatial coordinates. Estimating the PSF using the fluorescein images in a similar fashion as in [8] is not possible because of the PMT noise η_P. We thus base our modeling upon a PSF description by a linear shift-invariant (LSI) lowpass. As an example, the 3D anisotropic Gaussian approximation [9] leads to Gaussian parameters $\sigma_x = \sigma_y = 78.5\,nm$ and $\sigma_z = 294\,nm$ for the paraxial model given our imaging parameters. Calculating how the pmf changes due to transfer of the random variates through an LSI-system is a nontrivial task. We approximate this by considering how the linear and quadratic mean change: The linear mean becomes $E(X_E) = H(0)E(X_{\text{NA}})$, $H(\mathbf{f})$ being the Fourier transform of $h(\mathbf{x})$ and $\mathbf{f} = (f_x, f_y, f_z)^T$ being the spatial frequencies. The variance of zero-mean white noise after filtering is $Var(X_E) = Var(X_{\text{NA}}) \sum_{\mathbf{i}} h^2(\mathbf{i})$. In consequence, for an LSI-lowpass PSF model, the mean remains unchanged by filtering and the variance is highly reduced. Hence, we approximate the pmf after filtering by a mapping of the input pmf that leaves the mean unchanged while decreasing the variance. This yields new variates $m = f_2(l)$ with $f_2(x) = a_2(x - E(X_{\text{NA}})) + E(X_{\text{NA}})$, $a_2^2 = \sum_{\mathbf{i}} h^2(\mathbf{i})$.

3) R: The detector responsivity R leads to new random variates $n = f_3(m)$ of the random variable X_R, $f_3(x) = a_3 x$, $a_3 \in [0, 1]$ and $Var(X_R) = a_3^2 Var(X_E)$.

To summarize the mappings above, $n = f(k)$ according to $f(x) = y = a_2 a_3 (a_1 x - E(X_{\text{NA}}) + \frac{E(X_{\text{NA}})}{a_2})$. The variance has become

$$Var(X_R) = a_3^2 \sum_i h^2(\mathbf{i}) a_1^2 L = a_1^2 a_2^2 a_3^2 L = cL \tag{1}$$

and $c \ll 1$ because a_1, describing the acceptance cone of the optics, is very small and $a_2^2 \ll 1$ for the Gaussian PSF model introduced above. Hence, even for ideal detector responsivity $R = 1$, $c \ll 1$ and $Var(X_R)$ becomes negligible as L decreases or rather is in the low signal range. Note that this assessment is in accordance with our NPS measurement Fig. 4. The conclusion we can draw is that Q can be approximated as deterministic signal $Q = a_1 a_3 L$.

4) PMT: The PMT shot noise can be modeled by a Poisson distribution: $X_Q \sim \mathcal{P}(Q)$ according to the pmf $P_{X_Q}(k_q) = \frac{Q^{k_q} e^{-Q}}{k_q!}$.

5) CTF: The CTF accounts for the signal amplification in the PMT, the rescaling in the ADC, the ADC offset, dark current and possible non-linearities in the imaging chain. We model it using a gamma curve to obtain a simple model of possible non-linearities which still contains a linear transform as special case. The random variates k_q are transformed into new samples $k_s = f_{CTF}(k_q)$ according to $y = f_{CTF}(x) = \alpha + \beta x^\gamma$, $\alpha \geq 0$. The substitution $f_{CTF}^{-1}(y) = \varphi(y) = \left(\frac{y-\alpha}{\beta}\right)^{1/\gamma}$ with the continuously differentiable function $\varphi(y)$ gives the new pmf

$$P_{X_s}(k_s) = \frac{d\varphi}{dy} P_{X_Q}(k_q) = \frac{Q^{\left(\frac{k_s-\alpha}{\beta}\right)^{1/\gamma}} e^{-Q}}{\left(\left(\frac{k_s-\alpha}{\beta}\right)^{1/\gamma}\right)!} \frac{1}{\gamma \beta} \left(\left(\frac{k_s-\alpha}{\beta}\right)^{\frac{1}{\gamma}-1}\right). \tag{2}$$

As η_E and η_D are negligible, the noisy signal $s = k_s$ and the pixel intensity statistics follow $P_{X_s}(k_s)$.

To fit this model to our data, we used the Stirling approximation for factorial computation. Fig. 5 shows the estimated CTF with the parameters $\alpha = 58.5$, $\beta = 3028$ and $\gamma = 1.08$ as fitting result. Fig. 5 shows two example distributions illustrating that our model provides a very accurate description of the data.

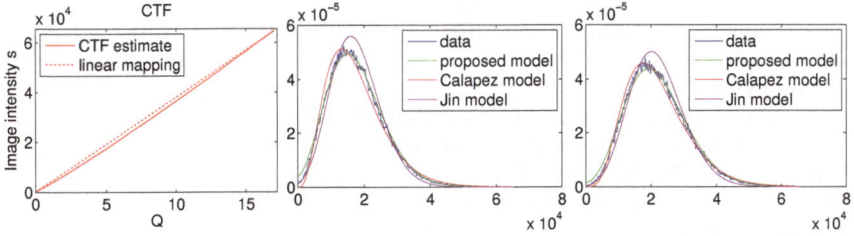

Fig. 5. Model fit. Left: Estimated CTF showing that the imaging system exhibits a slight non-linearity. A linear mapping is shown for comparison. Center and Right: The proposed model is plotted over the kernel density estimate. The Calapez model fit [4] and the Jin model fit [5] are shown for comparison.

The Calapez model [4] and the Jin model [5] are shown for comparison. The mean absolute fitting error (MAE) over $2 \cdot 10^6$ samples confirms this result. The MAE of the proposed model is $8.04 \cdot 10^{-7}$ while the MAE of the Calapez model is $1.23 \cdot 10^{-6}$ and that of Jin model fit is $1.96 \cdot 10^{-6}$. Note that as η_E is negligible, the Jin model fit corresponds to the fit of our model for $\gamma = 1$ which equals a fit of the standard model of a linearly-scaled Poisson.

5   Summary and Conclusions

In the present work, we have a proposed a novel model for signal and noise transfer in CLSM. We have acquired homogeneous exposures from sodium fluorescein dilution series. These images served as basis for a rigorous analysis of the pixel intensity statistics via assessment of their distribution, signal-dependence and spatial frequency-dependence. These measurements illuminated the understanding of the imaging process and substantiate our new model which gives a description of the pixel intensity statistics derived from a Poisson process whose variates are mapped to the pixel intensity via the camera transfer function accounting for possible non-linearities in the system. It enables simulation of the CLSM image formation so that CLSM image analysis algorithms can quantitatively be evaluated. After inverse CTF, established Poisson denoising methods can be applied. Finally it forms the basis for a reconstruction of the input fluorescence signal. As the model fit is performed with data acquired from sodium fluorescein concentration series, the procedure can easily be repeated to determine the model parameters for other microscopes.

References

1. Sheppard, C.J.R., Gan, X., Gu, M., Roy, M.: Signal-To-Noise Ratio in Confocal Microscopes. In: Pawley, J.B. (ed.) Handbook of Biological Confocal Microscopy, 3rd edn. ch. 22, pp. 442–452. Springer (2006)
2. Rodrigues, I., Sanches, J.: Convex total variation denoising of poisson fluorescence confocal images with anisotropic filtering. IEEE TIP 20(1), 146–160 (2011)
3. Kervrann, C., Trubuil, A.: An adaptive window approach for poisson noise reduction and structure preserving in confocal microscopy. In: Proc. ISBI, pp. 788–791 (2004)
4. Calapez, A., Rosa, A.: A statistical pixel intensity model for segmentation of confocal laser scanning microscopy images. IEEE TIP 19(9), 2408–2418 (2010)
5. Jin, X.: Poisson approximation to image sensor noise. Master's thesis, University of Dayton, Ohio (2010)
6. Bell, A.A., Brauers, J., Kaftan, J.N., Meyer-Ebrecht, D., Böcking, A., Aach, T.: High dynamic range microscopy for cytopathological cancer diagnosis. IEEE JSTSP (Special Issue: Dig. Im. Proc. Techniques for Oncology) 3(1), 170–184 (2009)
7. Marti, G.E., et al.: Fluorescence calibration and quantitative measurement of fluorescence intensity; approved guideline. NCCLS 24(26) (2004)
8. Brauers, J., Aach, T.: Direct PSF estimation using a random noise target. In: IS&T/SPIE Electronic Imaging. SPIE-IST, vol. 7537 (2010)
9. Zhang, B., Zerubia, J., Olivo-Marin, J.C.: Gaussian approximations of fluorescence microscope point-spread function models. App. Opt. 46(10), 1819–1829 (2007)

Hierarchical Partial Matching
and Segmentation of Interacting Cells

Zheng Wu[1], Danna Gurari[1], Joyce Y. Wong[2], and Margrit Betke[1]

[1] Department of Computer Science, Boston University, Boston, MA 02215, USA
[2] Department of Biomedical Engineering, Boston University, Boston, MA 02215, USA

Abstract. We propose a method that automatically tracks and segments living cells in phase-contrast image sequences, especially for cells that deform and interact with each other or clutter. We formulate the problem as a many-to-one elastic partial matching problem between closed curves. We introduce Double Cyclic Dynamic Time Warping for the scenario where a collision event yields a single boundary that encloses multiple touching cells and that needs to be cut into separate cell boundaries. The resulting individual boundaries may consist of segments to be connected to produce closed curves that match well with the individual cell boundaries before the collision event. We show how to convert this partial-curve matching problem into a shortest path problem that we then solve efficiently by reusing the computed shortest path tree. We also use our shortest path algorithm to fill the gaps between the segments of the target curves. Quantitative results demonstrate the benefit of our method by showing maintained accurate recognition of individual cell boundaries across 8068 images containing multiple cell interactions.

1 Introduction

Cell morphology and behavior analysis has an important role for studying biological processes, developing biomaterials, and diagnosing and fighting diseases. Reliable automated analysis of cell morphology and behavior depends on accurately finding the contours of each cell in every image. This is challenging because many cells undergo significant appearance variation in short periods of time. Amplifying the difficulty of maintaining shape recognition is the fact that cells frequently approach or touch other cells and clutter for a variety of reasons, including dense clustering of cells on the substrate, imperfect segmentation of the cell boundaries, and insufficient image resolution. The key computer vision challenge addressed in this paper is how to obtain cell shape information as cells deform during interactions with multiple other cells.

General segmentation algorithms that address cell deformation were summarized thoroughly by Rittscher [1]. They are limited to scenarios without apparent cell-to-cell or cell-to-clutter contacts or collisions. When a contact event occurs, the image of the shared boundary typically does not have a sufficiently strong intensity gradient, as in Fig. 1. This makes it difficult to detect the boundary where cells are touching. Segmentation methods that distinguish between cells

N. Ayache et al. (Eds.): MICCAI 2012, Part I, LNCS 7510, pp. 389–396, 2012.

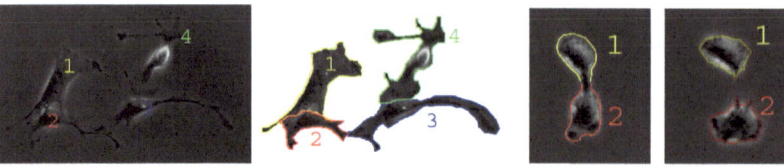

Fig. 1. Matching cell boundaries through time-lapse sequences are challenging tasks for these cases of colliding, dividing, and otherwise interacting cells

within a cluster of cells include static image-based and temporal-based methods. Nath et al. [2] added constraints to the level set method using the assumption that cells in the image share similar characteristics. Liu and Sclaroff [3] noted segmentation success in the presence of small amounts of cell overlap. Heuristics about expected intensity changes along boundaries between cells, or cells and clutter, have also been adopted [4]. These static image-based methods limit the generalizabilty across imaging modalities, degree of overlap, or cell type. Object boundaries have been propagated between successive frames such that each pixel on the merged boundary is associated to a pixel on one of the cell boundaries in the previous frame [5]. However, to avoid the high computational cost associated with this partial matching problem, heuristics were adopted which limit segmentation accuracy. The heuristics also make it difficult to increase the scale of the proposed method and apply it successfully to scenarios where multiple cells are involved in an interaction.

In this paper, we treat the segmentation of interacting cells as a partial matching problem between cell boundaries obtained from consecutive frames. Methods addressing the issue of *partial* matching were either applied to rigid transformations only [6] or chose distance measures such as the *edit distance* [7] that are not suitable for modeling the effects of stretching and shrinking. To the best of our knowledge, we are not aware of any competing method that can be applied directly to our elastic partial matching problem. Our contributions are: 1) A general framework to address the task of many-to-one partial matching, as opposed to the traditional tasks of one-to-one or two-to-one matching; 2) A new Double Cyclic Dynamic Time Warping procedure with a mechanism that reuses shortest path trees to speed up computation; 3) A tracking system embedded with the matching scheme that achieves high segmentation accuracy for varying numbers of deforming cells over long durations of interactions.

2   Method

Our segmentation method is embedded in a tracking system, which performs initial segmentation, frame-by-frame data association, partial or complete boundary matching, and curve gap completion. During the preprocessing step, we followed the work by Theriault et al. [8] to obtain the initial segmentation. The Hungarian algorithm is adopted to solve the frame-by-frame data association problem and identify merging and splitting events. Based on the relative positions of cells, the number and the order of cells involved in partial matching could be determined. In the following, the main effort is to address the problems of many-to-one partial matching and gap completion.

2.1   Partial Matching with Hierarchical Dynamic Programming

The shape of a deformable object is represented by its closed boundary curve c of length L_c. The curve is re-parameterized as a function $C\colon s \to \mathbf{f}$, where $s \in [0, L]$ is the arc length and $\mathbf{f}$ is a d-dimensional local feature descriptor. A matching or alignment between curves C and C' is a monotonic mapping function $g : [0, L] \to [0, L'], g(s) = s'$. Given a set of K candidate curves $\{C_k\}$ representing individual cells and a target curve C_t extracted from a merged cluster, where every segment of the target curve must be uniquely matched to a segment of one of the candidate curves, our goal is to minimize the following functional:

$$E(g_1, g_2, ..., g_K, l_1, l_2, ..., l_{K+1}) = \sum_{k=1}^{K} \int_{l_k}^{l_{k+1}} \|C_k(g_k(s)) - C_t(s)\|^2 \, ds \quad (1)$$

Particularly, we set $l_1 = 0, l_{K+1} = L$ so that the target curve C_t will be *completely* matched, while each segment of C_t will be *partially* matched to the candidate curve C_k. The search space of this functional includes all possible matching functions $\{g_k\}$ and cutting points $\{l_k\}$ along the target curve C_t. Note that, when $K = 1$, Eq. 1 is reduced to the functional commonly used for the *complete* alignment between two curves [9,10].

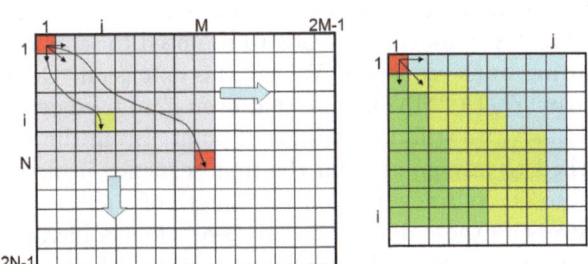

Fig. 2. Extended dynamic programming table for Double Cyclic Dynamic Time Warping. Left: Every $M{\times}N$ block has to be computed to find the optimal alignment starting at pair (i, j) to any ending pair up to $(i{+}N, j{+}M)$. Shortest paths computed from adjacent blocks can be reused to speed up the computation. Right: After a block $[1{:}i, 1{:}j]$ has been computed, all shortest paths going through $(2,1)$ (green) remain the same in block $[2{:}i{+}1, 1{:}j]$; Similarly, those going through $(1,2)$ (blue) can be reused in block $[1{:}i, 2{:}j{+}1]$; those going through $(2,2)$ (yellow) can be reused in block $[2{:}i{+}1, 2{:}j{+}1]$.

We chose Dynamic Time Warping (DTW) to search for the matching function g. DTW allows us to capture the significant stretching and shrinking effects of the boundary of moving fibroblast cells. Given two sequences of *ordered* data points, the best alignment is computed with the following subproblem structure:

$$d(i, j) = c(i, j) + \min\{d(i-1, j) + w_i, d(i, j-1) + w_j, d(i-1, j-1) + w_{ij}\} \quad (2)$$

where $c(i, j)$ measures the dissimilarity between data point i from one of the sequences and data point j from the other sequence and w_i, w_j, w_{ij} are penalty terms for different types of pairings. $d(i, j)$ is the accumulated matching cost up to pair (i, j). The whole process can be visualized by a dynamic programming (DP) table, as in Fig. 2. If the lengths of two sequences are M and N respectively, it takes $O(MN)$ steps to compute the global optimal alignment for the *complete* matching, which corresponds to the shortest path from entry $(1, 1)$ to entry (N, M) in the DP table. As a byproduct, every entry (i, j) in the DP table encodes the alignment from the pair $(1, 1)$ to the pair (i, j).

If a matching of *closed* curves is desired, as in our case, it is also required to search for the start pair. This has been accomplished with Cyclic Dynamic Time Warping (CDTW) [10]. For the problem of matching *complete* curves, only one of the two sequences has to be cyclically shifted in order to search for the correct start pair. A straightforward implementation of CDTW leads to $O(MN \min(M, N))$ computations while the fastest algorithm known for this task can compute the optimal alignment of *complete* curves in $O(MN \log \min(M, N))$ steps, which is based on the key observation that the optimally aligned curves corresponding to different start pairs cannot intersect in the DP table [10].

Standard DTW/CDTW methods have been mostly applied to solve the *complete matching problem*. They are essentially used to search for the alignment function g only in Eq. 1. The complexity of the *partial matching problem* comes from the need to search for "cutting points" of the target curve in the functional in Eq. 1. Such complexity inevitably leads to the need to search for a start pair by cyclically shifting **both** sequences. We call this extension "Double Cyclic Dynamic Time Warping" (DCDTW). Note that even if we tried every possible pair (n, j), for $n = 1, ..., N$, we still do not know if point j from the second sequence should be matched to any point from the first sequence in first place. At the same time, we also do not know the optimal length of a subsequence we should look for. To address all these difficulties, we here adopt a hierarchical dynamic programming approach to solve the partial matching problem optimally.

At the first stage of our proposed algorithm, we need to compute the optimal alignment for pairs (s_k, s_t) and (s'_k, s'_t), where $s_k, s'_k \in \{1, 2, ...N_k\}$ are the start and end points from the candidate curve C_k and, similarly, $s_t, s'_t \in \{1, 2, ...M\}$ are the start and end points from the target curve C_t. To search for the start pair, we extend the DP table to size $(2N_k - 1) \times (2M - 1)$ as shown in Fig. 2. In the extended table, the shortest path from cell (s_k, s_m) to cell (s'_k, s'_t) (such that $|s_k - s'_k| \leq N, |s_t - s'_t| \leq M$) gives the optimal alignment between curve segment $C_k^{s_k \to s'_k}$ and $C_t^{s_t \to s'_t}$. To compute all such shortest paths, we can apply DTW for every $N \times M$ block from the extended DP table, which requires $O(N^2 M^2)$

steps. However, the following proposition shows that approximately at least one third of this computation is not necessary.

Proposition 1. *When applying the standard DTW $N \times M$ times for every $N \times M$ block of the extended DP table, $\frac{1}{3}O(M^2N^2)$ of the computation is redundant.*

The proposition uses the observation that the DP table for one block can be reused for the adjacent blocks because of the non-intersect property of shortest path. We find such reduction is usually much higher in practice.

We denote all shortest paths from DCDTW as the set of matching functions G with the matching cost $\{c_{s_t \to s'_t}^{s_k \to s'_k}\}$. Given a segment of the target curve $C_t^{l_k \to l'_k}$ such that $1 \leq l_k \leq l'_k \leq M$, the optimal partial matching with the candidate curve C_k is chosen to be $g_k^{k'} = \arg\min_{g \in G} c_{l_k \to l'_k}^{s_k \to s'_k}$ and the corresponding minimum cost is denoted as $c_{l_k}^{l'_k}$. There will be $K \times M \times M$ matching functions selected, each of which represents the best alignment if we want to match one segment cut from the target curve to one of the candidate curves (possibly partially).

Multiple candidate curves compete for the matching points on the target curve, because every data point on the target curve can only be matched exactly once to one of the candidate curves. We find the best cutting points $\{l_k\}$ on the target curve through the iterative steps:

$$\gamma(k,m) = \begin{cases} c_1^m, & \text{if } k = 1 \\ \min_{1 \leq l \leq m} \gamma(k-1,l) + c_l^m + w_m, & \text{otherwise.} \end{cases} \quad (3)$$

where $\gamma(k,m)$ is the compositional cost for matching segment $C_t^{1 \to m}$ to k candidate curves and w_m is the penalty for choosing point m as the cutting point. We here assume the relative order of candidate curves is known (through tracking) but the first curve to be matched has to be searched. The above computation takes $O(KM^2)$ steps, and $\gamma(K,M)$ is the minimum matching cost corresponding to the global minimum of the functional in Eq. 1. After the global minimum is found at $\gamma(K,M)$, the best cutting points can be traced back and the best alignment with each individual cell can be recovered from its corresponding matching function $g_k^{k'}$. We want to emphasize that there could be repetition in the K candidate curves in order to handle the situation where more than one segment from the target curve is matched to the same individual curve, as shown in Fig. 3.

2.2   Gap Completion with Shortest Path

To obtain a complete segmentation of interacting cells, we need to fill in the gaps between disconnected pieces of the boundaries of touching cells (Fig. 3). Similar to the path tracing for actin filament segmentation [11], we close the boundary by dynamic programming. For each gap, we create a directed graph that connects two points, the sink and source nodes, that delineate the gap. The pixels of the image patch between these points become nodes in the graph. Two nodes are connected if the corresponding pixels are neighboring pixels. A cost

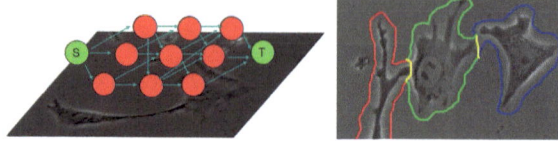

Fig. 3. Left: To fill the gap between boundary pixels represented by S and T, the shortest path through a graph, which models the image properties of the gap, is computed, Right: Output result. Given the input of a single combined outline, our method cuts it into the separate boundaries of three cells (red, green, blue) and fills boundary gaps (yellow) where the cells touch.

is associated with each node that captures the preference of attraction/repelling when a node is visited. In our application, we use as the node cost the minimum Euclidean distance to the predicted location of the boundary of the cell obtained via tracking. A transition cost is associated with each edge that penalizes moving into the interior of the cell, which is chosen to be the intensity gradient. Once the graph is constructed, the goal is to find the shortest path traveling from the source node to the sink node with minimum accumulated cost. Since the cost along a path is additive, it favors paths with short lengths and avoids crossing high gradient regions. The shortest path can be computed efficiently, again, by using dynamic programming.

3   Experiments and Results

We collected a dataset including phase-contrast images of fibroblast cells of the Balb/c 3T3 mouse strain cultured at $37°C$ in 5% CO_2 observed with a Zeiss Axiovert S100 microscope. A library of merge events was extracted, which consisted of cell-to-cell/clutter interactions, mitosis, and apparent collisions due to over-segmentation. We collected 41 merge subsequences with 7052 images showing 2-to-1 merging and 975 frames showing 3-1 merging as exemplified in Fig. 5.

We used the precision measure to evaluate the initial outline of a segmented merged object. Given the ground truth A and segmentation result B, precision calculates the average overlap between the two regions as $\frac{|A \cap B|}{|A \cup B|}$. As a baseline, the average annotator agreement using this criterion is 0.58, which indicates the challenge of obtaining a reliable ground truth due to inter-annotator disagreement. The precision of the segmentation algorithm over 100 non-merged cells was 0.408 which is close to the agreement between annotators. The error is attributed in part to the algorithm incorporating the halos surrounding cells while annotators did not include halos in the cell boundaries when annotating.

To evaluate the performance of separating merged objects, we modified the accuracy measure [12]. Given the ground truth region A and the segmentation region result B, accuracy calculates the fraction of the true cell region captured by the segmented region as $\frac{|A \cap B|}{|A|}$. To capture the fact that one segmentation result may be better at the expense of another when separating merged objects,

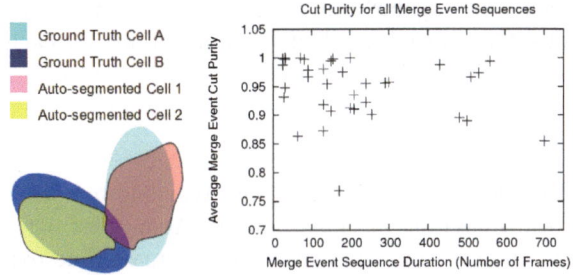

Fig. 4. Performance of Boundary Cutting Algorithm. Left: the accuracy is the area of intersection between the ground truth and auto-segmented region normalized by the area of the ground truth. The cut purity is computed as the average of accuracy of all merged objects. Right: Each tick mark on the x-axis represents the number of frames in a unique merge-event subsequence. The mean values shown are measured using the scores from all cells observed across all images in the subsequence. Higher values indicate stronger results.

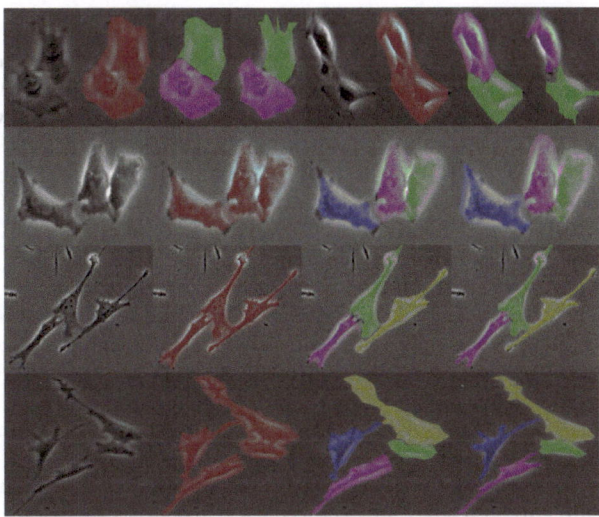

Fig. 5. Qualitative result of interacting cells. Four images for each merging event are shown, which are (from left to right) the original image, the initial segmentation, the final output and the manual segmentation.

we report a single score we call "cut purity" to indicate the average accuracy score for all objects involved in the merge event. The cut purity measure limits obtaining a good score to the situation when all cells in the merge event are accurately segmented. Fig. 4 shows results for all image sequences with each point indicating an average cut purity score across all images in the merge event. As is shown, our method remains strong for both short and long duration merge events as fibroblast cells regularly undergo significant amounts of deformation during interactions. Our Matlab implementation can process each merging event in 5 secs on a Intel Xeon(R) 3.20GHz PC.

4   Conclusions

We introduced Double Cyclic Dynamic Time Warping to solve the problem of many-to-one partial matching of closed curves. A shortest path was chosen to fill the gaps between the segments of the target curve. The experiments show that our methods produce accurate cell boundaries by appropriately cutting the combined outline of touching cells. In future work, we plan to apply our methods to other types of cells with additional imaging modalities.

Acknowledgement. This work is supported by NSF grant 0910908. We thank Matthew Walker, Diane Theriault, Gordon Towne and Quan Fang for data collection.

References

1. Rittscher, J.: Characterization of biological processes through automated image analysis. Annual Review of Biomedical Engineering 12, 315–344 (2010)
2. Nath, S.K., Palaniappan, K., Bunyak, F.: Cell Segmentation Using Coupled Level Sets and Graph-Vertex Coloring. In: Larsen, R., Nielsen, M., Sporring, J. (eds.) MICCAI 2006, Part I. LNCS, vol. 4190, pp. 101–108. Springer, Heidelberg (2006)
3. Liu, L., Sclaroff, S.: Medical image segmentation and retrieval via deformable models. In: Proc. of Intl. Conf. on Image Processing (ICIP), pp. 1071–1074 (2001)
4. Pan, J., Kanade, T., Chen, M.: Learning to detect different types of cells under phase contrast microscopy. In: Proc. of MIAAB, pp. 49–52 (2009)
5. Bise, R., Li, K., Eom, S., Kanade, T.: Reliably tracking partially overlapping neural stem cells in dic microscopy image sequences. In: MICCAI Workshop on Optical Tissue Image Analysis in Microscopy, Histopathology and Endoscopy, OPTMHisE (2009)
6. Bruckstein, A., Katzir, N., Lindenbaum, M., Porat, M.: Similarity-invariant signatures for partially occluded planar shapes. Int. J. Comp. Vis. 7, 271–285 (1992)
7. Chen, L., Feris, R.S., Turk, M.: Efficient partial shape matching using smithwaterman algorithm. In: NORDIA, pp. 1–6 (2008)
8. Theriault, D., Walker, M., Wong, J., Betke, M.: Cell morphology classification and clutter mitigation in phase-contrast microscopy images using machine learning. In: Machine Vision and Applications (2011)
9. Sebastian, T.B., Klein, P.N., Kimia, B.B.: On aligning curves. IEEE Trans. Pattern Anal. Mach. Intell. 25(1), 116–125 (2003)
10. Schmidt, F.R., Farin, D., Cremers, D.: Fast matching of planar shapes in sub-cubic runtime. In: Proc. of Intl. Conf. on Computer Vision (ICCV), pp. 1–6 (2007)
11. Li, H., Shen, T., Huang, X.: Actin Filament Segmentation Using Dynamic Programming. In: Székely, G., Hahn, H.K. (eds.) IPMI 2011. LNCS, vol. 6801, pp. 411–423. Springer, Heidelberg (2011)
12. Udupa, J.K., LeBlanc, V.R., Zhuge, Y., Imielinska, C., Schmidt, H., Currie, L.M., Hirsch, B.E., Woodburn, J.: A framework for evaluating image segmentation algorithms. Comput. Med. Imaging Graph 30(2), 75–87 (2006)

Hybrid Tracking and Mosaicking for Information Augmentation in Retinal Surgery

Rogério Richa, Balázs Vágvölgyi, Marcin Balicki,
Gregory D. Hager, and Russell H. Taylor

Johns Hopkins University
rogerio.richa@jhu.edu

Abstract. Current technical limitations in retinal surgery hinder the ability of surgeons to identify and localize surgical targets, increasing operating times and risks of surgical error. In this paper we present a hybrid tracking and mosaicking method for augmented reality in retinal surgery. The system is a combination of direct and feature-based tracking methods. A novel extension for direct visual tracking using a robust image similarity measure in color images is also proposed. Several experiments conducted on phantom, *in vivo* rabbit and human images attest the ability of the method to cope with the challenging retinal surgery scenario. Applications of the proposed method for tele-mentoring and intra-operative guidance are demonstrated.

Keywords: tracking, mosaicking, information augmentation, retinal surgery.

1 Introduction

Retinal surgery is considered one of the most demanding types of surgical intervention. Difficulties related to this type of surgery arise from several factors such as the difficult visualization of surgical targets, poor ergonomics, lack of tactile feedback, complex anatomy and high accuracy requirements. Specifically regarding intra-operative visualization, surgeons face limitations in field and clarity of view, depth perception and illumination which hinder their ability to identify and localize surgical targets. These limitations result in long operating times and risks of surgical error.

A number of solutions for aiding surgeons during retinal surgery including robotic assistants for improving surgical accuracy and mitigating the impact of physiological hand tremor [1], micro-robots for drug delivery [2] and sensing instruments for intra-operative data acquisition [3] have been proposed. Addressing the limitations in visualization, systems for intra-operative view expansion and information overlay have been developed in [4,5]. In such systems, a mosaic of the retina is created intra-operatively and pre-operative surgical planning and data (e.g. fundus images) are displayed during surgery for improved guidance.

Although several solutions have been proposed in the field of minimally invasive surgery and functional imaging [6,7], retinal surgery imposes additional

N. Ayache et al. (Eds.): MICCAI 2012, Part I, LNCS 7510, pp. 397–404, 2012.

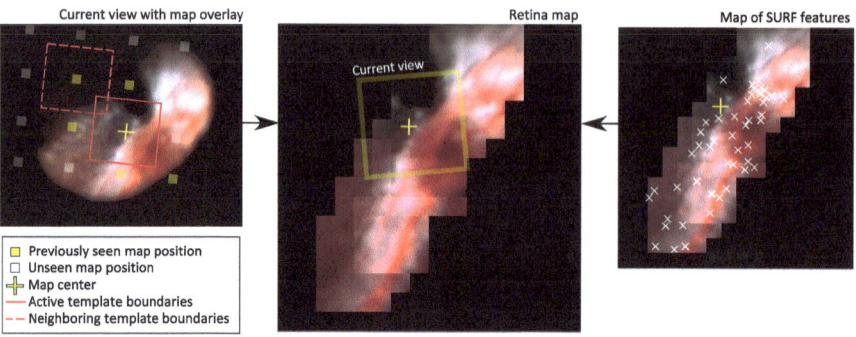

Fig. 1. The proposed hybrid tracking and mosaicking method. A direct visual tracking method (left) is combined with a SURF feature map (right) for coping with full occlusions. The result is the intra-operative retina map shown in the middle. Notice the retina map displayed above is a simple overlay of the templates associated with each map position.

challenges such as highly variable illumination (the illumination source is manually manipulated inside the eye), partial and full occlusions, focus blur due to narrow depth of field and distortions caused by the eye lens. Although the systems proposed in [4,5] suggest potential improvements in surgical guidance, they lack robustness to such disturbances. Furthermore, tracking and mapping in such conditions is much harder compared to non-invasive retinal interventions such as laser photocoagulation [8].

In this paper we present a hybrid tracking and mosaicking method designed for the challenging conditions in retinal surgery. The method is a combination of both direct and feature-based tracking methods. Similar to [5] and [9], a two dimensional map of the retina is build on-the-fly using a direct tracking method based on a robust similarity measure called Sum of Conditional Variance (SCV) [10]. In parallel, a map of SURF features is built and updated as the map expands, enabling tracking to be reinitialized in case of full occlusions. The method has been tested on a database of phantom, rabbit and human surgeries, with successful results.

This paper is organized as follows. In the next section, we describe the components of the proposed hybrid tracking and mosaicking method. In section 3, we describe the experimental analysis conducted on *in vivo* data. In section 4, we demonstrate potential applications of the proposed system in intra-operative navigation and tele-mentoring systems. We conclude the paper in section 5.

2   Methods

A schematic overview of the proposed hybrid tracking and mosaicking method is given in Figure 1. A combination of feature-based and direct based methods was necessary due to the specific nature of the retina images, where low frequency texture information is predominant. As explained in details in section 3, a purely feature-based tracking and mosaicking method could not produce the same results as the proposed method in the *in vivo* human datasets shown in Figure 3 due to the lack of salient features in certain areas of the retina.

During surgery, only a small portion of the retina is visible. For initializing the tracking and mosaicking method, an initial reference image of the retina is selected. The center of the initial reference image represents the origin of a retina map. As the surgeon explores the retina, additional templates are incorporated to the map, as the distance to the map origin increases. New templates are recorded at even spaces, as illustrated in Figure 1(left) (notice that regions of adjacent templates overlap). At a given moment, the template closest to the current view of the retina is tracked using the direct tracking method detailed next.

2.1   Direct Visual Tracking Using a Robust Similarity Measure

As explained in the introduction, tracking must cope with disturbances such as illumination variations, partial occlusions (e.g. due to particles floating in the vitreous), distortions, etc. To this end, we tested several robust image similarity measures from the medical image registration domain such as Mutual Information (MI), Cross Cumulative Residual Entropy (CCRE), Normalized Cross Correlation (NCC) and the Sum of Conditional Variance (SCV) (see [10] for more information). Among these measures, the SCV has shown the best trade-off between robustness and convergence radius. In addition, efficient optimization schemes can be derived for the SCV, which is not the case for NCC, MI or CCRE.

Tracking can be formulated as an optimization problem, where we seek to find at every image the parameters $\mathbf{p}$ of the transformation function $w(\mathbf{x}, \mathbf{p})$ that minimize the SCV between the template and current images T and $I(w(\mathbf{x}, \mathbf{p}))$:

$$\mathcal{SCV}(\mathbf{p}) = \sum_{\mathbf{x}} \left(I(w(\mathbf{x}, \mathbf{p})) - \hat{T}_{(i,j)}(\mathbf{x})\right)^2, \text{ with } \hat{T}(\mathbf{x}) = \mathcal{E}(I(w(\mathbf{x}, \mathbf{p}))|T_{(i,j)}(\mathbf{x}))$$

(1)

where $\mathcal{E}(.)$ is the expectation operator. The indexes (i, j) represent the row and column of the template position in the retinal map shown in Figure 1. The transformation function $w(.)$ is chosen to be a similarity transformation (4 DOFs, accounting for scaling, rotation and translation). Notice that more complex models such as the quadratic model [11] can be employed for mapping with higher accuracy.

In the medical imaging domain, images T and I are usually intensity images. Initial tests of retina tracking in gray-scale images yielded poor tracking performance due to the lack of image texture in certain parts of the retina. This motivated the extension of the original formulation in equation (1) to tracking in color images for increased robustness:

$$\mathcal{SCV}^*(\mathbf{p}) = \sum_{c} \sum_{\mathbf{x}} \left(^c I(w(\mathbf{x}, \mathbf{p})) - {}^c \hat{T}_{(i,j)}(\mathbf{x})\right)^2$$

(2)

In the specific context of retinal images, the blue channel could be ignored as it is not a strong color component. Hence, tracking is performed using red and

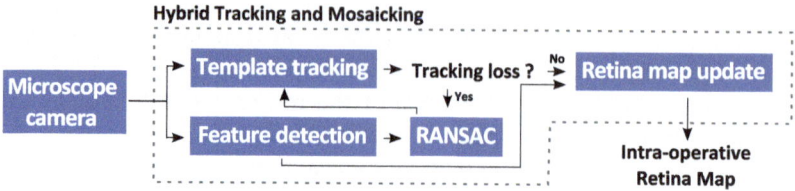

Fig. 2. Schematic overview of the proposed tracking system

green channels. For finding the transformation parameters **p** that minimize equation (2), the Efficient Second-Order Minimization (ESM) strategy is adopted [9]. Finally, it is important to highlight the fact that new templates are only incorporated to the retina map when tracking confidence is high (*i.e.* over an empirically defined threshold ϵ). Once a given template is incorporated to the map, it is no longer updated. Tracking confidence is measured as the average NCC between $^c\hat{T}$ and $^cI(w(\mathbf{x}, \mathbf{p}))$ over red and green color channels c. Notice this specific NCC is a bounded measure derived directly from the SCV coefficient (the expected $^c\hat{T}$ is used instead of ^cT).

2.2   Creating a Feature Map

For recovering tracking in case of full occlusions, a map of SURF features on the retina is also created. For every new template incorporated in the map, the set of SURF features within the new template is included in the feature map. Due to the overlap between templates, new features are matched against the existing features in the map and if the distance (in pixels) between old and new features on the map is small, two features are merged by taking the average of their positions and descriptor vectors.

If the template tracking confidence drops below a pre-defined threshold λ, tracking is deemed unreliable and is suspended. For re-establishing tracking, RANSAC is employed for matching features from the feature map to those on the current image from the surgery. In practice, due to the poor visualization conditions in retinal surgery, the SURF Hessian thresholds are set very low. This creates a large number of false matches, which consequently requires a large number of RANSAC iterations. A schematic diagram of the hybrid tracking and mosaicking method is shown in Figure 2.

3   Experiments

For acquiring phantom and *in vivo* rabbit images, we use a FireWire Point Grey camera acquiring 800x600 pixel color images at 25 fps. For the *in vivo* human sequences, a standard NTSC camera acquiring 640x480 color images was used. The method was implemented using OpenCV on a Xeon 2.10GHz machine. The direct tracking branch (see Figure 2) runs at frame-rate while the feature detection and RANSAC branch runs at ≈ 6 fps (depending on the

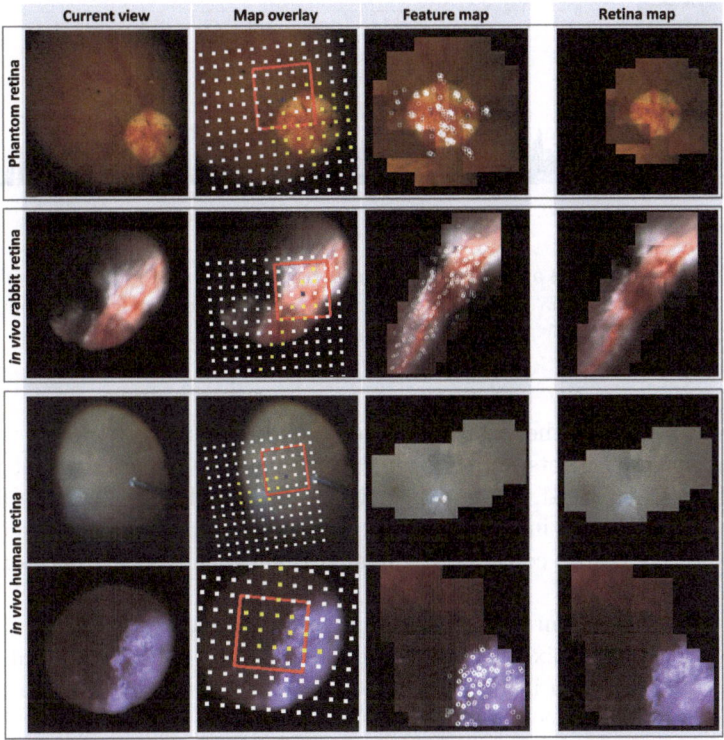

Fig. 3. Examples of intra-operative retina maps obtained using the proposed hybrid tracking and mosaicking method

number of detected features). Although the two branches already run in parallel, considerable speed gains can be achieved with further code optimization.

3.1 Reconstructed Retina Maps

Figure 3 shows examples of retina maps obtained using the proposed method. In addition, an example of an on-line map reconstruction can be found in the supplementary videos. For all sequences, we set the template size for each map position to 90x90 pixels. Map positions are evenly spaced by 30 pixels. Due to differences in the acquisition setup (zoom level, pupil dilation, etc), the field of view may vary between sequences. The rabbit image dataset consists of two sequences of 15s and 20s and the human image datasets consist of two sequences of 46s and 39s (lines 3 and 4 in Figure 3, respectively). The tracking confidence threshold ϵ for incorporating new templates and the threshold λ for detecting tracking failure were empirically set to 0.95 and 0.6, respectively, for all experiments. In addition, the number of RANSAC iterations was set to 1000.

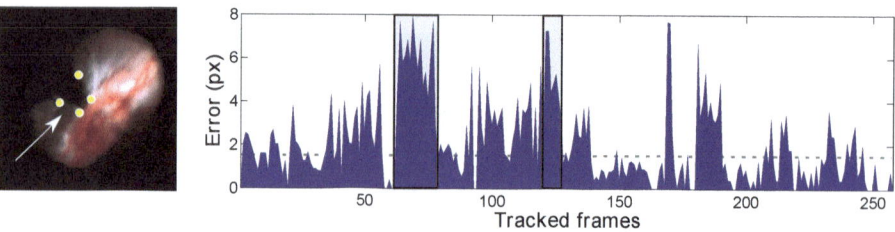

Fig. 4. For a quantitative analysis, the average tracking error of four points arbitrarily chosen on the rabbit retina is manually measured. Slight tracking drifts are highlighted in the plot.

The advantages of the proposed extension to tracking in color are clearly shown in the experiments with human *in vivo* images. In these specific images, much information is lost in the convertion to gray-scale, reducing the tracking convergence radius and increasing chances of tracking failure. Consequently, the estimated retina map is considerably smaller than when tracking in color images (see example in 5(a)).

For a quantitative analysis of the proposed method, we manually measured the tracking error (in pixels) of four points arbitrarily chosen on 500 images of the rabbit retina shown in Figure 4. The error is only measured when tracking is active (*i.e.* tracking confidence above ϵ). In average, tracking error is below 1.60 ± 3.1 pixels, which is close the manual labeling accuracy (estimated to be ≈ 1 pixel). Using the surgical tool shaft as reference in this specific image sequence, the ratio between pixels and millimeters is approximately 20 px/mm. From the plot, slight tracking drifts can be detected (from frame intervals [60,74] and [119,129] highlighted in the plot), as well as error spikes caused by image distortions. Overall, even though tracking accuracy is too large for applications such as robotic assisted vein cannulation, it is sufficient for consistent video overlay.

3.2   Current Limitations

A visual inspection of Figure 3 suggests a correlation between SURF features and blood vessels on the retina. In fact, few features are available where blood vessels are not clearly visible or in regions distant from the nerve bundle. In the proposed method, a minimum number of feature matches is necessary to recover from full occlusions. A possible solution to circumvent this issue is the use of additional feature detection methods adapted to retinal images.

The proposed tracking and mosaicking method strongly relies on the NCC coefficient as a measure of tracking quality. However, the NCC does not provide reliable results when tracking images with little texture information. Since the transformation model is not constrained, tracking errors result in the incorporation of falsetemplates to the map (see Figure 5(b)). As an alternative to

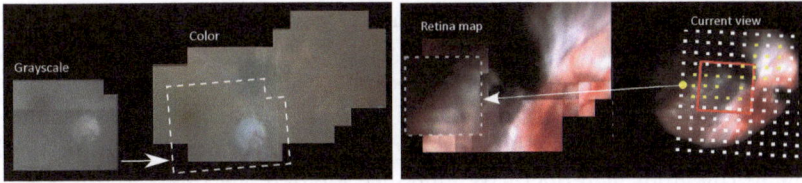

Fig. 5. (left) A considerably smaller retina map is obtained when tracking in gray-scale images. (right) Poor tracking quality measurements lead to the incorporation of wrong templates to the map in areas with little texture.

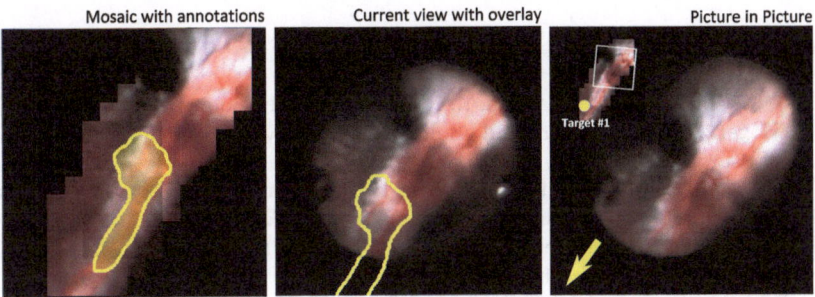

Fig. 6. Annotations created by a mentor on the intra-operative mosaic can be overlayed on the novice surgeon view for assistance and guidance during surgery. The mosaic could also be displayed to the surgeon for facilitating the localization of surgical targets.

circumvent this problem, consistency checks can be implemented for verifying the similarity between a given patch and its surrounding neighbors.

4   Applications

The proposed hybrid tracking and mosaicking method can be applied in a variety of scenarios. The most natural extension would be the creation of a photo realistic retina mosaic, taking advantage of the overlap between stored templates. The proposed system could also be used in an augmented reality scenario for tele-mentoring. Through intra-operative video overlay, a mentor could guide a novice surgeon by indicating points of interest on the retina, demonstrate surgical gestures or even create virtual fixtures in a robotic assisted scenario (see Figure 6(left-middle)). Similar to [4], the proposed tracking and mosaicking method can also be used for intra-operative guidance, facilitating the localization and identification of surgical targets as illustrated in Figure 6 (right). Videos illustrating these capabilities can be found in the supplementary materials.

5   Conclusion

In this paper we propose a hybrid tracking and mosaicking method for view expansion and surgical guidance during retinal surgery. The system is a combination of direct and feature-based tracking methods. A novel extension for direct visual tracking using a robust similarity measure named SCV in color images is proposed. Several experiments conducted on phantom, *in vivo* rabbit and human images illustrate the ability of the method to cope with the challenging retinal surgery scenario. Furthermore, applications of the proposed method for tele-mentoring and intra-operative guidance are demonstrated.

Acknowledgements. This research was supported in part by NIH BRP grant 1 R01 EB 007969 and in part by Johns Hopkins University internal funds. Other equipment and systems infrastructure support were developed within the CISST ERC under NSF grant EEC9731748.

References

1. Mitchell, B., Koo, J., Iordachita, I., Kazanzides, P., Kapoor, A., Handa, J., Taylor, R., Hager, G.: Development and application of a new steady-hand manipulator for retinal surgery. In: ICRA, Rome, Italy, pp. 623–629 (2007)
2. Bergeles, C., Kummer, M.P., Kratochvil, B.E., Framme, C., Nelson, B.J.: Steerable Intravitreal Inserts for Drug Delivery: *In Vitro* and *Ex Vivo* Mobility Experiments. In: Fichtinger, G., Martel, A., Peters, T. (eds.) MICCAI 2011, Part I. LNCS, vol. 6891, pp. 33–40. Springer, Heidelberg (2011)
3. Balicki, M., Han, J., Iordachita, I., Gehlbach, P., Handa, J., Taylor, R., Kang, J.: Single Fiber Optical Coherence Tomography Microsurgical Instruments for Computer and Robot-Assisted Retinal Surgery. In: Yang, G.-Z., Hawkes, D., Rueckert, D., Noble, A., Taylor, C. (eds.) MICCAI 2009, Part I. LNCS, vol. 5761, pp. 108–115. Springer, Heidelberg (2009)
4. Fleming, I., Voros, S., Vagvolgyi, B., Pezzementi, Z., Handa, J., Taylor, R., Hager, G.: Intraoperative visualization of anatomical targets in retinal surgery. In: IEEE Workshop on Applications of Computer Vision (WACV 2008), pp. 1–6 (2008)
5. Seshamani, S., Lau, W., Hager, G.: Real-Time Endoscopic Mosaicking. In: Larsen, R., Nielsen, M., Sporring, J. (eds.) MICCAI 2006, Part I. LNCS, vol. 4190, pp. 355–363. Springer, Heidelberg (2006)
6. Totz, J., Mountney, P., Stoyanov, D., Yang, G.-Z.: Dense Surface Reconstruction for Enhanced Navigation in MIS. In: Fichtinger, G., Martel, A., Peters, T. (eds.) MICCAI 2011, Part I. LNCS, vol. 6891, pp. 89–96. Springer, Heidelberg (2011)
7. Hu, M., Penney, G., Rueckert, D., Edwards, P., Bello, F., Figl, M., Casula, R., Cen, Y., Liu, J., Miao, Z., Hawkes, D.: A Robust Mosaicing Method with Super-Resolution for Optical Medical Images. In: Liao, H., Eddie Edwards, P.J., Pan, X., Fan, Y., Yang, G.-Z. (eds.) MIAR 2010. LNCS, vol. 6326, pp. 373–382. Springer, Heidelberg (2010)
8. Broehan, A.M., Rudolph, T., Amstutz, C., Kowal, J.: Real-time multimodal retinal image registration for computed-assisted laser photocoagulation system. IEEE Transactions on Biomedical Engineering (TBME) 58(10), 2816–2824 (2011)
9. Silveira, G., Malis, E., Rives, P.: An efficient direct approach to visual SLAM. IEEE Transactions on Robotics 24(5), 969–979 (2008)
10. Richa, R., Sznitman, R., Taylor, R., Hager, G.: Visual tracking using the sum of conditional variance. In: IROS, San Francisco, USA, pp. 2953–2958 (2011)
11. Stewart, C., Tsai, L., Roysam, B.: The dual-bootstrap iterative closest point algorithm with application to retinal image registration. IEEE Transactions on Pattern Analysis and Machine Intelligence (PAMI) 22(1), 1379–1394 (2003)

Real Time Assistance for Stent Positioning and Assessment by Self-initialized Tracking

Terrence Chen[1], Yu Wang[3,*], Peter Durlak[2], and Dorin Comaniciu[1]

[1] Siemens Corporation, Corporate Research & Technology, Princeton, NJ, USA
[2] Siemens Healthcare, Forchheim, Germany
[3] Riverain Technologies, Miamisburg, OH, USA

Abstract. Detailed visualization of stents during their positioning and deployment is critical for the success of an interventional procedure. This paper presents a novel method that relies on balloon markers to enable real-time enhanced visualization and assessment of the stent positioning and expansion, together with the blood flow over the lesion area. The key novelty is an automatic tracking framework that includes a self-initialization phase based on the Viterbi algorithm and an online tracking phase implementing the Bayesian fusion of multiple cues. The resulting motion compensation stabilizes the image of the stent and by compounding multiple frames we obtain a much better stent contrast. Robust results are obtained from more than 350 clinical data sets.

Keywords: percutaneous coronary interventions, stent positioning, stent enhancement.

1 Introduction

Stent thrombosis and restenosis are associated with stent under-expansion, which has been shown as a major risk factor for patients undergoing percutaneous coronary intervention (PCI) [4]. This procedure is monitored by X-ray fluoroscopy where the guidewire, markers, or stent visibility are often quite low. Two of the major risk factors concern with the success rate of this procedure are: 1. Whether the stent is implanted precisely at the desired location. 2. Whether the stent is expanded properly against the vessel wall. Due to poor contrast, clinical preference, and rapid motion of the coronaries, physicians often have difficulty making a precise judgement from live fluoroscopic images.

To overcome the problem where the low visibility of stent undermines the assessment of the stent implantation outcome, image processing techniques have been proposed to improve the image quality for better stent visibility. Most of the algorithms applied a motion-compensated noise reduction via landmark-based registration of multiple images [1,3,6]. Interested readers may refer to [2] for a comprehensive study of existing work.

---

* Contributions from Yu Wang are results from his internship at Siemens Corporation, Corporate Research and Technology.

N. Ayache et al. (Eds.): MICCAI 2012, Part I, LNCS 7510, pp. 405–413, 2012.
© Springer-Verlag Berlin Heidelberg 2012

Existing solutions are mostly offline where the physician can only observe the enhanced stent from one static image. We propose a method to assist the physician in visualizing the stent during live monitoring. It is achieved by robust tracking of the balloon marker pair in an online manner such that real time guidance can be provided throughout the procedure. Physician can directly assess the stent expansion and the blood flow over the lesion area after stent implantation. It can also be applied to facilitating stent positioning. To achieve this goal, a robust self-initialized tracking framework is proposed. It can be directly applied to automation of other device tracking problems and potentially makes the image-based tracking techniques more practical in clinical applications.

Our work is essentially different from existing industrial solutions. Comparing to StentViz [11], Stentboost [9], ClearStent [8], and StentOptimizer [10], which apply post-processing to a short fluoroscopic acquisition to present an image of enhanced stent in relation to the vessel, our work has the following advantages: 1. Our work presents the enhanced stent in real time during acquisition. 2. The enhancement is visualized in every frame. On the other hand, comparing to Sync-RX [12], which also provides real-time solutions, our work has the following advantages: 1. We propose a global optimization framework to use a few frames in the beginning for self-initialization. This improves the robustness of the tracking significantly (about 15%). 2. The quality of our real time stent enhancement is much higher even for cases with low-dose radiation since we do not achieve the enhancement only by anchoring the original scene with the balloon marker locations. At last, our work provides one unique advantage, which is to allow the physician visualize the stent clearly in its original context. No information is lost or distorted in the whole scene. To the best of our knowledge, this is the first work to provide a clear stent in its original context. Our work is validated through a quantitative evaluation over more than 350+ clinical scenes, a scale which is previously unreported.

2   The Self-initialization Tracking Framework

Our tracking framework is illustrated in figure 1 (A), which consists of three phases - the self-initialization phase (I), the computation phase (II), and the online tracking phase (III). For a specific tracking target (in our applications, the balloon marker pair), we assume an offline detector D is trained. It can be applied to an image and output multiple candidates of the target object with confidence scores. In our work, a probabilistic boosting tree [7] is used as the classifier to train the offline detector D. In phase I, we collect n frames ($n = 10$ by default), apply D to all images, and then localize the target pattern, balloon marker pair, in every frame by the spatial-temporal cues. A few frames (4 to 5 frames in our cases) may be skipped during computation of phase I, which is named the computation phase (II) in this paper. Once the computation is done, real time tracking can be performed to track the target pattern online.

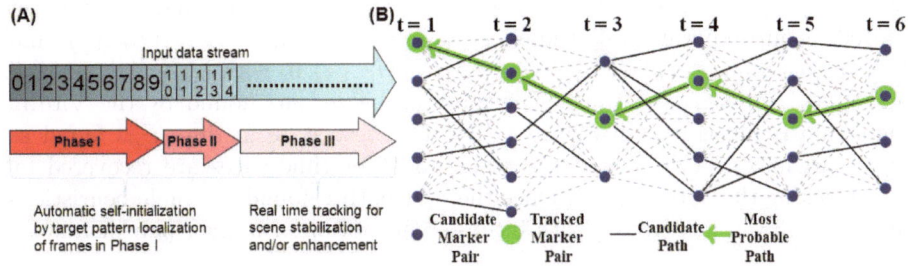

Fig. 1. (A) The proposed tracking framework (B) The trellis graph of the Viterbi algorithm. Each node represents a marker pair. The bold green path is the most probable path/viterbi path.

2.1 Automatic Self-initialization

To automatically initialize the tracking process, we take the first n frames ($n = 10$) from the live fluoroscopic stream and apply a novel offline tracking method based on the Viterbi algorithm to find the marker pair sequence in a globally optimal manner. In addition, results in phase I are used to create an adaptive joint marker pair template **T** and statistical models that can robustify the online tracking phase. Specifically, after obtaining detection results by applying **D** to the first 10 frames, the goal is to find the best sequence of the marker pairs that maximizes the following posterior probability:

$$\hat{X} = \arg\max_X P(X|\mathbf{Y}), \tag{1}$$

where $X = \{x_1, ..., x_{T=10}\}$ is the state sequence, and $x_{t,k} = (b_{t,k}, e_{t,k})$ is the kth state of the marker pair $b_{t,k}$ and $e_{t,k}$ at time t. $\mathbf{Y} = \{I_1, ..., I_{T=10}\}$ are the images. This problem is solved by the Viterbi algorithm which recursively finds the weight of the most likely state sequence ending with each $x_{t,k}$ ($V_{t,k}$) at t:

$$V_{1,k} = P(I_1|x_{1,k})P(x_{1,k}); \tag{2}$$
$$V_{t,k} = P(I_t|x_{t,k}) \max_j (P(x_{t,k}|x_{t-1,j})V_{t-1,j}), \tag{3}$$

where, $P(x_{1,k})$ represents the prior probability of the kth marker pair at the first frame and is set to 1. $P(I_t|x_{t,k})$ represents the observation probability defined as the sum of the detection confidences of both markers:

$$P(I_t|x_{t,k}) \propto P(I_t|b_{t,k}) + P(I_t|e_{t,k}), \tag{4}$$

$P(x_{t,k}|x_{t-1,j})$ represents the transition probability from the jth state of time $t-1$ to the kth state of time t and is defined as a combination of length and direction consistencies, and the movement probability:

$$P(x_{t,k}|x_{t-1,j}) \propto U_{motion} * U_{length} * U_{dir}, \tag{5}$$

where $U_{motion} = exp(-(||b_{t,k} - b_{t-1,j}|| + ||e_{t,k} - e_{t-1,j}||)/\sigma)$ and the σ is set to 100 in our experimental studies, $U_{length} = exp(-|l_{t,k} - l_{t-1,j}|/l_{t-1,j})$, and $U_{dir} = max((b_{t,k} - e_{t,k}) \cdot (b_{t-1,j} - e_{t-1,j})/(l_{t,k} \cdot l_{t-1,j}), 0)$ with $l_{t,k} = ||b_{t,k} - e_{t,k}||$ and $l_{t-1,j} = ||b_{t-1,j} - e_{t-1,j}||$. The most probable path found by the Viterbi algorithm is illustrated in Figure 1 (B). The best state in time T is found as $\hat{x}_T = \arg\max_{x_{T,k}}(V_{T,k})$, and the states in other time slices are recovered by backtracking the Viterbi path. Once the best path is found, a simple heuristic is applied to invalidate frames with inconsistent motion or marker pair distance.

2.2   Online Tracking

Tracking by Detection. In the online tracking phase, **D** is also applied to generate marker pair candidates with confidence scores at each frame. A Bayesian inferencing framework to maximize the posterior probability of the balloon marker pair model x_t at time t is formulated as:

$$\hat{x}_t = \arg\max_{x_t} P(x_t|I_{1...t}), \tag{6}$$

where $I_{1...t}$ is image observation from 1 to t-th frame. By assuming a Markovian representation of the stent motion the above formula can be expanded as:

$$\hat{x}_t = \arg\max_{x_t} P(I_t|x_t) \int_{x_{t-1}} P(x_t|x_{t-1})P(x_{t-1}|I_{1...t-1})dx_{t-1}. \tag{7}$$

Eq. (7) essentially combines two parts: the likelihood term, $P(I_t|x_t)$, and the prediction term, $P(x_t|x_{t-1})$. The likelihood term $P(I_t|x_t)$ is estimated by combining the detection score from **D** and the template matching as follows:

$$P(I_t|x_t) = P(Z_t|x_t) \cdot P(C_t|x_t) \tag{8}$$

where $P(Z_t|x_t)$ is probability measure of the marker pair at the t-th frame and is obtained directly by **D**. $P(C_t|x_t)$ is obtained by the cross-correlation between a local patch defined by the current evaluating marker pair at frame t and the same-sized patch defined by the marker pair in the adaptive joint template **T** generated from the initialization phase.

   The motion smoothness term $P(x_t|x_{t-1})$ in (7) is formulated as a combination of translation, orientation, and shape consistencies of the joint marker pair at time t compared to the joint marker pair at time $t-1$. The translation and shape consistencies are defined based on the Gaussian models ($l \sim \mathcal{N}(u_{length}, \sigma_{length})$, $w \sim \mathcal{N}(u_{width}, \sigma_{width})$, $h \sim \mathcal{N}(u_{height}, \sigma_{height})$, $m \sim \mathcal{N}(u_{motion}, \sigma_{motion})))$ generated in initialization phase to model the lengths, widths and heights (the bounding box of the marker pair), and movements of the marker pair, respectively. In the online tracking phase, the parameters of the marker pair length model are updated with the length of the tracked marker pair ($\hat{l}_t$) as follows:

$$u_{length}^t = (1 - \lambda)u_{length}^{t-1} + \lambda \hat{l}_t \tag{9}$$

$$(\sigma_{length}^t)^2 = (1 - \lambda)(\sigma_{length}^{t-1})^2 + \lambda(\hat{l}_t - u_{length}^t)^2 \tag{10}$$

where λ is the learning rate and is set as 0.1 in our studies. The other Gaussian models are updated in the same manner in the online tracking phase.

The joint template $\mathbf{T}$ is also updated online during the online tracking phase with new template $\mathbf{T}_t$ using the following equation:

$$\mathbf{T} = (1 - \lambda)\mathbf{T} + \lambda \mathbf{T}_t, \tag{11}$$

To reduce the false detection, top 5 candidates are sorted based on their scores and fed into a tracking validation process. The first valid marker pair is output as the final result. Our approach of validating the maker pair candidate online is based on the Gaussian models of lengths ($\mathcal{N}(u_{length}, \sigma_{length})$) and movements ($\mathcal{N}(u_{motion}, \sigma_{motion})$), a Gaussian model ($\mathcal{N}(u_{tmp}^{joint}, \sigma_{tmp}^{joint})$) of the matching scores (cross-correlation) between the joint template $\mathbf{T}$ and the template of one frame , and another Gaussian model ($\mathcal{N}(u_{tmp}^{prev}, \sigma_{tmp}^{prev})$) for the matching scores between templates at one frame and its previous frame . As a result, the marker pair is invalid if the length is abnormal (less than $u_{length} - \sigma_{length}$ or larger than $u_{length} + \sigma_{length}$) or the motion is too large (larger than $u_{motion} + \sigma_{motion}$). The marker pair is also invalid if either one of the matching scores is too small (less than $u_{tmp}^{joint} - \sigma_{tmp}^{joint}$ or $u_{tmp}^{prev} - \sigma_{tmp}^{prev}$).

3 Stent Positioning

The first application we present using the proposed tracking framework is to facilitate stent positioning during PCI, where the main difficulty for physicians is to observe the balloon markers in relation with the lesion and vessels. This is sometimes quite challenging due to the rapid motion of coronaries during live monitoring. This procedure could be improved if a scene can be stabilized by the location of the balloon markers. For this purpose, we track the balloon marker pair in streaming data, transform the image such that the balloon marker pair is always aligned at exactly the same coordinates, and then display the transformed image to the physician. In our framework, $n = 10$ is set in phase I. In a typical 15 fps acquisition rate, phase I takes 0.67 seconds, phase II takes 0.27 seconds, and followed by the real time online tracking. Once the online tracking starts, the new coming scene is stabilized by the coordinates of the balloon marker pair. Physician can inject contrast and observe the relation between the marker pair (undeployed stent) and the lesion area.

Real-time stent positining has been studied and is not a new application [12]. Nevertheless, by the proposed framework of using a few frames for self-initialization, it improves the robustness significantly. Applying a well-trained detector to any single image results in a detection accuracy of about 82% (c.f. Table 1 Part B. Accuracy of $\mathbf{D}$). With the proposed framework, the initialization successful rate is validated to be improved to 97% (c.f. Table 1 the 3rd row).

4   Stent Assessment

In this section, we present a new way to assist physicians in assessing the stent expansion in real time by the same framework, which is the main application of the proposed paper. One additional step implemented here is that once the marker pairs are all localized in phase I, a motion-compensated based stent enhancement [6] is applied to obtain a stent enhancement image (*SEI*). To make sure *SEI* with good quality, $n = 25$ is set in phase I. After the online tracking phase starts, a compound of *SEI* and the streaming data is output as the visual result to the physician.

Specifically, let $f_1, ..., f_t$ be the t frames of the input data stream, *SEI* is obtained by $\{f_1, ..., f_{25}\}$. Once *SEI* is obtained, a guidewire localization [6] technique is applied to *SEI* to obtain the guidewire τ which passes through the two markers. A weighting field $\mathbf{W}$ is then generated by applying a Gaussian kernel to the guidewire location on *SEI*. Once phase III starts, which normally begins with f_{40} to f_{45}, the *SEI* is rigidly transformed to $\hat{SEI}$ such that marker pair of $\hat{SEI}$ is aligned with the marker pair in the current frame f_i. The output image $\hat{f}_i$ is then obtained by compounding the $\hat{SEI}$ and f_i with $\mathbf{W}$:

$$\hat{f}_i = \mathbf{W} \times \hat{SEI} + (1 - \mathbf{W}) \times f_i, \tag{12}$$

where i is the frame index, which normally begins with 40 to 45. In other words, the computation time for the *SEI* is up to 3 seconds in a 15 fps acquisition. Figure 2 shows an example of the stent assessment results.

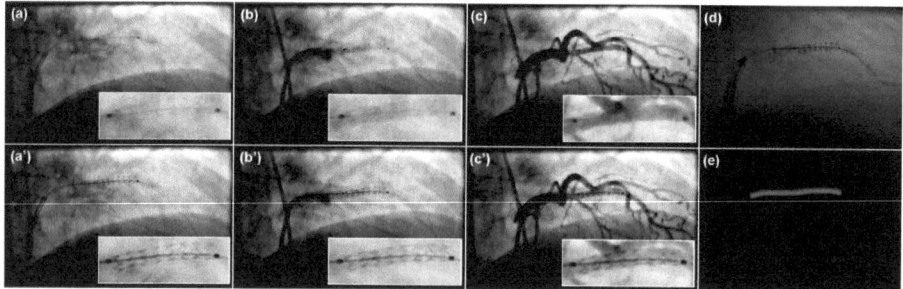

Fig. 2. (a)(b)(c): Three frames of the original scene; (a')(b')(c'): Corresponding frames of the output enhanced scene. Bottom right windows are zoom-in views of the stent; (d):Stent Enhancement Image (*SEI*) from the first 25 frames;(e): Weighting field ($\mathbf{W}$)

Two notable comments we would like to address here are: 1. If a live acquisition is followed by a playback, the same enhancement can be applied to frames in phase I and II as well. That is, during playback mode, stent is enhanced in every frame ($\{f_1, ..., f_t\}$) 2. Based on the clinical preference, during stent enhancement and assessment, scene stabilization based on the balloon markers can also be provided just like what we do during stent positioning.

5   Results

356 clinical sequences with a total of 17234 frames are collected in PCI procedures from clinical sites in US, Europe, and Asia. They are either collected
during stent positioning or after stent implantation, when the balloon is still in
place. All the evaluated sequences have at least 20 frames, and 145 sequences
have more than 50 frames. Image size ranges from 720 × 720 to 1024 × 1024. We
evaluated the performance by a Intel Xeon PC (2.2 GHz) in an online manner
- the testing program sends one frame at a time by the speed of 15 fps. (Real
time in this paper is defined as 15 fps as this is the most common setting in
real world clinics. Nevertheless, the online tracking of our algorithm performs
far beyond this speed.) Both the results and processing time are monitored. In
our evaluation, error is defined as the average displacement between the two
markers to their ground truth positions. If the error is less than 1.5 mm, it is
regarded as correct. 1.5 mm is used to tolerate the manual annotation errors for
small markers. The tracking accuracy after validation drops slightly from 98.5%
to 97.7% if the error threshold is set as 0.6mm (c.f. Table 1 Part B. the last row).

We first compared the robustness of the proposed Viterbi algorithm for the
self-initialization phase (I). Two measures are used for this evaluation - *Success*
is defined by if all returned marker pairs are correct in phase I. *Recall* is defined
by the number of marker pairs that are localized and returned in phase I. Table
1 Part A shows the results. **D** denotes the method if we directly apply **D** and
use the top candidate as the marker pair. We also compared the method by Lu
et al. [6]. It can be shown that the proposed method has the highest *Success*
rate and can localize much more marker pairs than [6]. Please note that the
evaluation were conducted for both stent positioning (POS) with 356 sequences
and stent assessment (ASM) with 145 sequences.

Table 1. Part A. Evaluation and comparison for the self-initialization phase. Part B.
Evaluation and comparison for phase III.

Part A.	POS.Success	POS. Recall	ASM. Success	ASM. Recall
D	0.68(285/356)	100%	0.52 (75/145)	100%
Lu et al. [6]	0.96 (342/356)	78.9%	0.95 (138/145)	79.2%
Proposed	0.97(345/356)	88.9%	0.97(140/145)	90.3%

Part B.	Accuracy	Accuracy after validation	FPS
D	81.93%(11203/13674)	N/A	35.54
Online Boosting	53.00%(7247/13674)	N/A	9.08
Proposed method	96.50%(13195/13674)	98.50%(12651/12844)	29.04

Next, we evaluated our tracking method in phase III. For this experiment, we
also compared with the online boosting (OB) detector [5]. In the experiments
with the online boosting detector, we initialized two online boosting detectors
that track the markers independently. 50 base classifiers are used in each detector

and the Haar features are employed. At each frame, the online boosting detector is updated with the tracking result (20×20 window centering at the tracked marker) as the positive sample and randomly sampled windows in the neighboring region as the negative samples. We evaluated the tracking by number of correctly tracked frames. Since there are more frames (13674) used in the stent positioning procedure, the evaluation was conducted by this procedure only. For fair comparison, the same initialization was applied for all methods. As shown in Table 1 Part B, the proposed online tracking method outperformed the other two tacking methods and reached 96.5% accuracy and an average speed of 29.04 FPS. After applying the validation approach the accuracy is boosted to 98.5%.

We report the running time of the entire workflow below. In the stent positioning procedure, the self-initialization of 10 frames takes an average of 0.27 seconds after phase I, which means 4 to 5 frames are needed for phase II. For the stent assessment procedure, the self-initialization of 25 frames takes an average of 0.36 seconds after phase I. The registration of all frames and generation of the *SEI* takes about additional 0.82 seconds. In total, a 1.18 second is needed for phase II, which is about 15 to 20 frames. Online stent enhancement can start to be displayed after about 40 to 45 frames.

In summary, main advantages of the proposed tracking framework include: 1. It is more efficient and accurat than manual initialization, and it is more robust than a single frame initialization. 2. Results obtained at phase I can be used to learn the scene specific statistics and provide an appearance template to improve the tracking robustness in phase III. This is another key factor how we achieve such robust tracking performance.

6   Conclusion

We present a framework to assist stent positioning and post implantation assessment, which provides physicians a clearly observable stent in real time fluoroscopy. The proposed framework can be potentially applied to other interventional applications to streamline the workflow and improve the results.

References

1. Bismuth, V., Vaillant., R.: Elastic registration for stent enhancement in X-ray image sequences. ICIP (2008)
2. Bismuth, V., Vaillant., R., Funck, F., Guillard, N., Najman., L.: A comprehensive study of stent visualization enhancement in X-ray images by image processing means. In: Prince, J. L., Pham, D. L., Myers, K. J. (eds.) Medical Image Analysis, vol. 15, No. 4:565-76, Springer (2011)
3. Florent, R., Nosjean, L., Lelong, P., Rongen, P.M.J.: Medical viewing system and method for enhancing structures in noisy images. US Patent 7415169.

4. Fujii, K., Carlier, S.G., Mintz, G.S., Yang, Y.M., Moussa, I., Weisz, G., Dangas, G., Mehran, R., Lansky, A.J., Kreps, E.M., Collins, M., Stone, G.W., Moses, J.W., Leon., M.B.: Stent underexpansion and residual reference segment stenosis are related to stent thrombosis after sirolimus-eluting stent implantation: An intravascular ultrasound study. Journal of the American College of Cardiology. 45:995-998 (2005)
5. Grabner, H., Bischof, H.: On-line Boosting and Vision. CVPR (2006)
6. Lu, X., Chen, T., Comaniciu, D.: Robust Discriminative Wire Structure Modeling with Application to Stent Enhancement in Fluoroscopy. CVPR (2011)
7. Tu, Z.: Probabilistic boosting-tree: Learning discriminative models for classification, recognition, and clustering. ICCV (2005)
8. ClearStent, http://www.swe.siemens.com/france/web/fr/med/produits/angio/solutions/applications_cliniques/Pages/IC-stent.aspx
9. StentBoost, http://www.gehealthcare.com/euen/interventional_xray/clinical_cases/bifurcation_lesion.html
10. StentOptimizer, http://www.paieon.com/Products.asp?Par=9.27&id=75
11. StentViz, http://www.genewscenter.com/content/detail.aspx?ReleaseID=8465&NewsAreaID=2
12. Sync-RX, http://www.sync-rx.com/EN/contents/page.aspx?contentPageID=13

Marker-Less Reconstruction of Dense 4-D Surface Motion Fields Using Active Laser Triangulation for Respiratory Motion Management

Sebastian Bauer[1], Benjamin Berkels[3], Svenja Ettl[2], Oliver Arold[2],
Joachim Hornegger[1], and Martin Rumpf[4]

[1] Pattern Recognition Lab, Dept. of Computer Science
[2] Institute of Optics, Information and Photonics
Friedrich-Alexander-Universität Erlangen-Nürnberg, Erlangen, Germany
sebastian.bauer@cs.fau.de
[3] Interdisciplinary Mathematics Institute,
University of South Carolina, Columbia, SC, USA
[4] Institute for Numerical Simulation,
Rheinische Friedrich-Wilhelms-Universität Bonn, Bonn, Germany

Abstract. To manage respiratory motion in image-guided interventions a novel sparse-to-dense registration approach is presented. We apply an emerging laser-based active triangulation (AT) sensor that delivers sparse but highly accurate 3-D measurements in real-time. These sparse position measurements are registered with a dense reference surface extracted from planning data. Thereby a dense displacement field is reconstructed which describes the 4-D deformation of the complete patient body surface and recovers a multi-dimensional respiratory signal for application in respiratory motion management. The method is validated on real data from an AT prototype and synthetic data sampled from dense surface scans acquired with a structured light scanner. In a study on 16 subjects, the proposed algorithm achieved a mean reconstruction accuracy of ± 0.22 mm w.r.t. ground truth data.

1 Introduction

Respiration-synchronized image-guided radiation therapy (IGRT) techniques aim at tracking the tumor location and reposition the beam dynamically. To reduce additional radiation exposure, recent hybrid tumor-tracking techniques combine episodic radiographic imaging with continuous monitoring of external breathing surrogates based on the premise that the internal tumor position can be accurately predicted from external motion. The underlying correlation model can be established from a series of simultaneously acquired external-internal position measurements [1] or 4-D CT planning data [2]. Clinically available solutions for hybrid tumor-tracking [1,3] measure external motion using a single or a few passive markers on the patient's chest as a low-dimensional surrogate. Thus, these techniques are incapable of depicting the full complexity of respiratory motion, they involve extensive patient preparation, and require reproducible

N. Ayache et al. (Eds.): MICCAI 2012, Part I, LNCS 7510, pp. 414–421, 2012.
© Springer-Verlag Berlin Heidelberg 2012

marker placement with a substantial impact on model accuracy. Modern IGRT solutions that allow to monitor the motion of the complete external patient surface help to reduce correlation model uncertainties. In particular, range imaging (RI) technologies can acquire a dense 3-D surface model of the patient [4,5,6]. Based on the estimation of a dense displacement field representing the deformation of the instantaneous torso surface w.r.t. a reference surface (either from RI or planning CT data), a highly accurate correlation model can be established [7,8]. The deformation estimation from dense surface scans for application in RT has been investigated recently [8,9]. Available RI-based IGRT solutions are capable of delivering dense surface information in a marker-less manner but focus on patient positioning, do not support dense sampling in real-time [4,5] or at the cost of a limited field of view [6], often imply high costs in terms of hardware and are subject to measurement uncertainties due to the sampling principles e.g. active stereo [6] or swept lasers [4,5]. The temporal resolution of these solutions may be insufficient to characterize respiratory motion. In this paper, we propose a marker-less system based on a non-moving active laser triangulation (AT) sensor that delivers sparse but accurate measurements in real-time (30 Hz). Using prior patient shape knowledge from planning data, a variational model is proposed to recover a dense and accurate displacement field and to reconstruct a complete and reliable patient surface model at the instantaneous respiration phase. Estimating the dense deformation is combined with recovering a sparse displacement field from AT measurements to planning data, thus the approach is closely related to the field of inverse-consistent registration [10,11]. The variational model is discretized using Finite Elements, the optimization is guided by a step-size controlled gradient flow to guarantee fast and smooth relaxation.

2   Method

In this section, we derive the variational model for the reconstruction of a dense displacement field from sparse measurements. Given is a reference shape $\mathcal{G} \subset \mathbb{R}^3$ extracted from planning data and the instantaneous body surface $\mathcal{M}$ represented by a sparse sampling Y. For instance, let us assume that the AT sensor acquires a set of n measurements $Y = \{y_1, \ldots, y_n\}$, $y_i \in \mathbb{R}^3$, arranged in a grid-like structure (Fig. 1). We assume that $\mathcal{G}$ is given as a graph, i.e. there is a domain $\Omega \subset \mathbb{R}^2$ usually associated with the plane of the patient table and a function $g : \Omega \to \mathbb{R}$ such that $\mathcal{G} = \{(\zeta, g(\zeta)) \in \mathbb{R}^3 : \zeta \in \Omega\}$. Due to respiration, the intra-fractional sampling Y is not aligned with $\mathcal{G}$. Now, the goal is to estimate the unknown, non-rigid, dense deformation ϕ of $\mathcal{G}$ with $Y \subset \phi(\mathcal{G})$. For this purpose, in a joint manner, we estimate ϕ together with an inverse deformation ψ matching Y and $\mathcal{G}$ in the sense that $\psi(Y) \subset \mathcal{G}$. When registering Y onto $\mathcal{G}$ we solely deal with a sparse displacement field $(\psi(y_i))_{i=1,\ldots,n}$ on the n positions measured by the AT sensor. A geometric sketch of the registration configuration is depicted in Fig. 1. Estimating ψ allows us to establish a correspondence between the AT measurements and the reference patient surface, whereas the dense deformation ϕ enables the reconstruction of the complete instantaneous patient surface. We represent

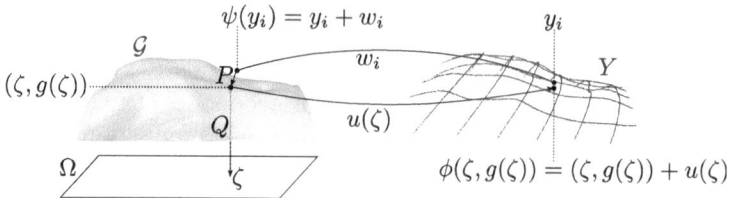

Fig. 1. Geometric configuration for reconstructing the dense deformation ϕ with $\phi(\zeta, g(\zeta)) = (\zeta, g(\zeta)) + u(\zeta)$ from sparse sampling data $Y = \{y_1, \ldots, y_n\}$ and the approximate sparse inverse ψ with $\psi(y_i) = y_i + w_i$ (for a better visibility $\mathcal{G}$ and Y have been pulled apart). Furthermore, the projection P onto $\mathcal{G}$ and the orthogonal projection Q from the graph $\mathcal{G}$ onto the parameter domain Ω are sketched.

ψ by a vector of displacements $W = \{w_1, \ldots, w_n\}$ with $\psi(y_i) = y_i + w_i$. Furthermore, the deformation ϕ is represented by a displacement $u : \Omega \to \mathbb{R}^3$ defined on the parameter domain Ω of the graph $\mathcal{G}$ with $\phi(\zeta, g(\zeta)) = (\zeta, g(\zeta)) + u(\zeta)$. To quantify the matching of $\psi(Y)$ onto $\mathcal{G}$ let us assume that the signed distance function d with respect to $\mathcal{G}$ is precomputed in a sufficiently large neighborhood in $\mathbb{R}^3$. We set $d(x) := \pm\text{dist}(x, \mathcal{G})$, where the sign is positive outside the body, i. e. above the graph, and negative inside. Then $\nabla d(x)$ is the outward pointing normal on $\mathcal{G}$ and $|\nabla d(x)| = 1$. Based on this signed distance map d we can define the projection $P(x) := x - d(x)\nabla d(x)$ of a point $x \in \mathbb{R}^3$ in a neighborhood of $\mathcal{G}$ onto the closest point on $\mathcal{G}$ and compute the mismatch of $\psi(Y)$ and $\mathcal{G}$ pointwise via $|P(\psi(y_i)) - \psi(y_i)| = |d(y_i + w_i)|$. Let us emphasize that we do not expect ψ to be equal to the projection P. Indeed, the computational results discussed below underline that it is the prior in the deformation ϕ which leads to general matching correspondences for a minimizer of our variational approach.

2.1   Definition of the Registration Energy

Now, we define a functional $\mathcal{E}$ on dense displacement fields u and sparse vectors of displacements W such that a minimizer represents a suitable matching of the planning data and AT measurements:

$$\mathcal{E}[u, W] := \mathcal{E}_{\text{match}}[W] + \kappa\,\mathcal{E}_{\text{con}}[u, W] + \lambda\,\mathcal{E}_{\text{reg}}[u] \tag{1}$$

where κ and λ are nonnegative constants controlling the contributions of the individual terms. $\mathcal{E}_{\text{match}}$ denotes a term measuring closeness of $\psi(Y)$ to $\mathcal{G}$. The consistency functional $\mathcal{E}_{\text{con}}$ is responsible for establishing the relation between both displacement fields. Finally, $\mathcal{E}_{\text{reg}}$ ensures a regularization of the dense displacement u. The detailed definitions of these functionals are as follows.

Matching Energy. In order to measure closeness of $\psi(Y)$ to $\mathcal{G}$, we use the pointwise mismatch measure discussed above and define

$$\mathcal{E}_{\text{match}}[W] := \frac{1}{2n} \sum_{i=1}^{n} |d(y_i + w_i)|^2 . \tag{2}$$

Consistency Energy. For a known instantaneous deformation ϕ of the patient surface $\mathcal{G}$ and an exact deformation correspondence $\psi(Y) \subset \mathcal{G}$ of the AT measurement Y the identity $\phi(\psi(Y)) = Y$ holds. But for an arbitrary deformation ψ described by some vector of displacements W in general $\psi(Y) \not\subset \mathcal{G}$. To relate ϕ and ψ in this case we have to incorporate the projection P because ϕ is only defined on $\mathcal{G}$. In fact, to ensure that $(\phi \circ P \circ \psi)(W) \approx W$ for a minimizer of the total energy we introduce the consistency energy

$$\mathcal{E}_{\text{con}}[u, W] := \frac{1}{2n} \sum_{i=1}^{n} |P(y_i + w_i) + u(Q\, P(y_i + w_i)) - y_i|^2 , \qquad (3)$$

where $Q \in \mathbb{R}^{2 \times 3}$ denotes the orthographic projection matrix with $Q(\zeta, g(\zeta)) = \zeta$. Here, we have used that $\phi(P(\psi(y_i))) = P(y_i + w_i) + u(Q\, P(y_i + w_i))$. Indeed, this definition of the consistency energy allows us to compute a dense smooth displacement of the patient planning surface even though only a sparse set of measurements is available.

Prior for the Displacement. To ensure smoothness of the deformation ϕ on $\mathcal{G}$ we incorporate a thin plate spline type regularization of the corresponding displacement u [12] and define

$$\mathcal{E}_{\text{reg}}[u] := \frac{1}{2} \int_{\Omega} |\triangle u|^2 \, dx , \qquad (4)$$

where $\triangle u = (\triangle u_1, \triangle u_2, \triangle u_3)$ and thus $|\triangle u|^2 = \sum_{k=1}^{3} (\triangle u_k)^2$. Indeed, since our input data Y only implicitly provide information for ϕ on a sparse set, a first order regularizer is inadequate to ensure sufficient regularity for the deformation. Let us emphasize that (discrete) smoothness of the approximate inverse deformation ψ is implicitly controlled by the regularization of ϕ.

2.2   Numerical Optimization

To minimize the functional $\mathcal{E}$ (Eq. 1), we apply a Finite Element approximation and optimize the functional using a gradient descent scheme. In particular, after an appropriate scaling of $\mathcal{G}$ we choose $\Omega = [0, 1]^2$ and consider a piecewise bilinear, continuous Finite Element approximation on a uniform rectangular mesh covering Ω. In the experiments we used a 129×129 grid. Furthermore, the signed distance function d is precomputed using a fast marching method on a uniform rectangular 3-D grid covering the unit cube $[0, 1]^3$ and stored on the nodes of this grid. In the algorithm d and ∇d are evaluated using trilinear interpolation of nodal values. For the gradient descent, derivatives of the energy have to be computed numerically. The derivatives of $\mathcal{E}_{\text{match}}$ and $\mathcal{E}_{\text{con}}$ w.r.t. w_j are given as:

$$\partial_{w_j} \mathcal{E}_{\text{match}}[W] = \frac{1}{n} d(y_j + w_j) \nabla d(y_j + w_j)$$

$$\partial_{w_j} \mathcal{E}_{\text{con}}[u, W] = \frac{1}{n} \left(P(y_j + w_j) + u(Q\, P(y_j + w_j)) - y_j \right)^T$$
$$\left(D P(y_j + w_j) + \nabla u(Q\, P(y_j + w_j)) Q\, D P(y_j + w_j) \right)$$

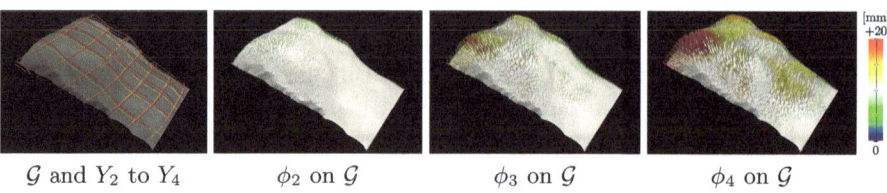

$\mathcal{G}$ and Y_2 to Y_4 ϕ_2 on $\mathcal{G}$ ϕ_3 on $\mathcal{G}$ ϕ_4 on $\mathcal{G}$

Fig. 2. Validation on real AT data. Estimation of ϕ_p transforming $\mathcal{G}$ into $\mathcal{M}_p$, from AT sampling data Y_p. For the glyph visualization of ϕ_p on $\mathcal{G}$, $|u(\varsigma)|$ is color coded [mm].

where DP denotes the Jacobian of the projection P. The variations of $\mathcal{E}_{\text{con}}$ and $\mathcal{E}_{\text{reg}}$ w.r.t. u in a direction $\vartheta : \Omega \to \mathbb{R}^3$ are given by:

$$\langle \partial_u \mathcal{E}_{\text{con}}[u, W], \vartheta \rangle = \frac{1}{n} \sum_{i=1}^{n} \left(P(y_i + w_i) + u(Q\, P(y_i + w_i)) - y_i \right) \vartheta(Q\, P(y_i + w_i))$$

$$\langle \partial_u \mathcal{E}_{\text{reg}}[u], \vartheta \rangle = \sum_{k=1}^{3} \int_{\Omega} \triangle u_k \triangle \vartheta_k \, \mathrm{d}x$$

The evaluation of DP involves the Hessian $D^2 d(x)$ of the distance function. One can either compute $D^2 d(x)$ based on second order finite differences or - as actually implemented here - replace the projection direction in P by the already computed direction from the last update. Furthermore, the Laplacian of a Finite Element function is evaluated by the discrete Finite Element Laplacian. In the gradient descent scheme we stop iterating as soon as the energy decay is smaller than a threshold value ϵ, $\epsilon = 10^{-4}$ proved to be sufficient to achieve the accuracy reported below. For the first frame of the respiratory motion we initialize $u = 0$ and $w_j = P(y_j) - y_j$ leading to approx. 60 gradient descent steps on average. For all subsequent frames we take u from the previous step and $w_j = P(y_j) - y_j$ as initial data resulting in approx. 45 descent steps on average.

3   Experiments and Results

Experimental Setup. For validation of the method, we have used an eye-safe AT prototype that acquires a sparse grid of 11×10 accurate 3-D sampling lines in real-time (30 Hz), using two perpendicular laser line pattern projection systems and a 1024×768 px resolution CCD chip [13]. Within the measurement volume, the mean AT measurement uncertainty is $\sigma = 0.39$ mm. The evaluation dataset is composed of 32 datasets from 16 subjects, each performing abdominal and thoracic breathing, respectively. Per subject, we synchronously acquired both real AT data and surface data using a moderately accurate but rather dense structured light (SL) system with a resolution of 320×240 px. Both sensors were mounted at a height of 1.2 m above the patient table, at a viewing angle of $30°$. AT and SL data were aligned using calibration. From each dataset, we extracted sparse AT measurements Y_p and dense SL meshes $\mathcal{M}_p$ for 8 phases within one

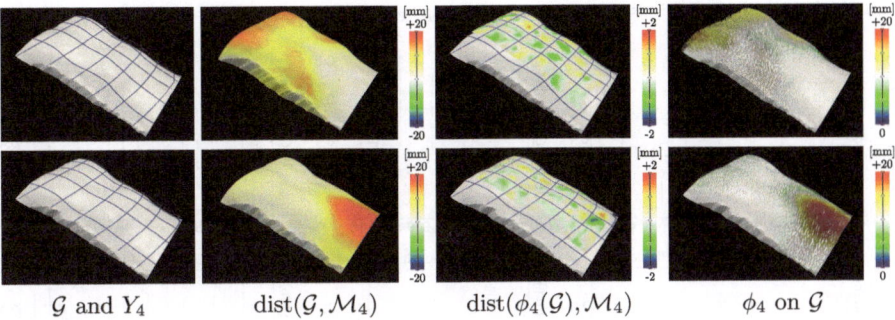

$\mathcal{G}$ and Y_4 dist$(\mathcal{G}, \mathcal{M}_4)$ dist$(\phi_4(\mathcal{G}), \mathcal{M}_4)$ ϕ_4 on $\mathcal{G}$

Fig. 3. Estimation of ϕ_p transforming $\mathcal{G}$ into $\mathcal{M}_p$ from realistic AT sampling data Y_p, for thoracic (top row) and abdominal respiration (bottom row). $p = 4$ represents the respiration state of fully inhale, roughly. For the glyph visualization of ϕ on $\mathcal{G}$, $|u(\zeta)|$ is color coded [mm]. Please note that the color coding differs by a factor of 10.

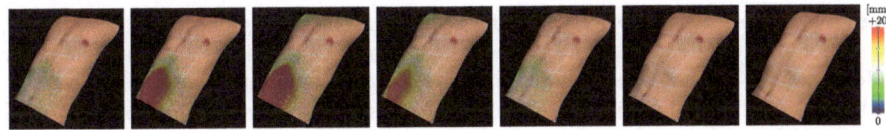

Fig. 4. Glyph visualization of ϕ_2 to ϕ_8 on $\mathcal{G}$ for an abdominal respiration cycle

respiration cycle, the index p denotes the phase. In the experiments below, the subject's body surface at full expiration $\mathcal{M}_1$ is considered as the given planning data $\mathcal{G}$. The model parameters were empirically set to $\kappa = 8 \cdot 10^{-1}$, $\lambda = 4 \cdot 10^{-8}$.

Validation on Real AT Data. Results for the reconstruction of ϕ_p for phase p on real AT data are given in Fig. 2. A quantitative evaluation on real AT and aligned SL data was unfeasible, as the SL camera exhibited local sampling artifacts due to the underlying measurement principle and interferences between the laser grid (AT) and speckle pattern projections (SL) of the synchronously used modalities, which cause local deviations in the scale of several millimeters.

Quantitative Evaluation on Realistic AT Data. For quantitative evaluation, we developed a simulator for the generation of realistic AT sampling data from dense SL surfaces. For this purpose, the noise characteristics of our AT sensor prototype were measured in an optics lab and used to augment the synthetic sampling, providing realistic AT data. We considered the reconstruction of the displacement field ϕ_p from realistic AT data Y_p, $p = \{2, \ldots, 8\}$, sampled from $\mathcal{M}_p$. An evaluation is given in Fig. 3 and the displacements for a full respiration cycle are shown in Fig. 4. The accuracy of the deformation estimation is assessed by the absolute error $|\text{dist}(\phi_p(\mathcal{G}), \mathcal{M}_p)|$ in Fig. 5 representing the mismatch between the transformed reference surface and the ground truth surface. To discard boundary effects, the evaluation is performed within the central surface of interest covering the torso. Over all subjects and phases, the mean

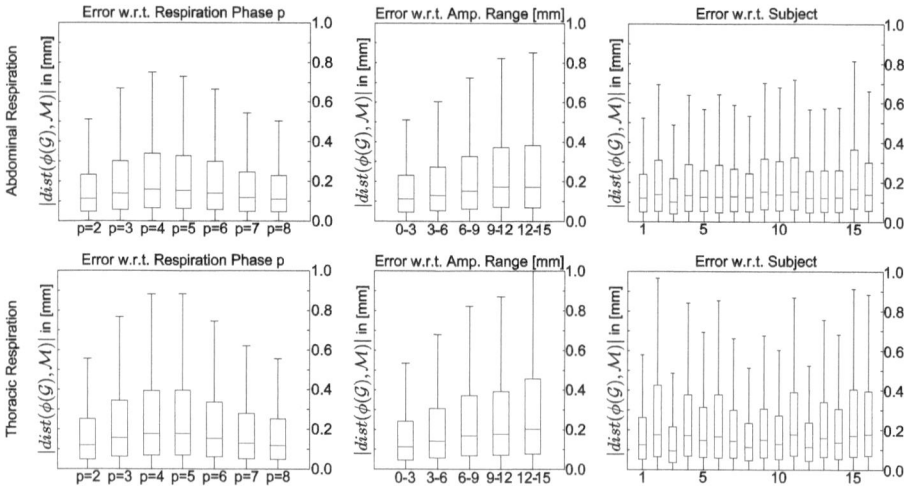

Fig. 5. Box plots of $|\text{dist}(\phi_p(\mathcal{G}), \mathcal{M}_p)|$ for realistic AT sampling data from 16 subjects, for abdominal (top row) and thoracic (bottom row) respiration. Given are plots for different phases of the respiration cycle (left), w.r.t. the respiration amplitude (center), and for the individual subjects (right). The reconstruction error scales approximately linearly with the respiration amplitude observing a peak at the respiration state of fully inhale (phase 4/5). The whiskers indicate that >99% of the residual error is <1 mm.

reconstruction error was 0.22 mm w.r.t. ground truth dense SL data. This indicates that the method can reliably recover the dense displacement field from a sparse sampling of the instantaneous patient state using prior shape knowledge.

Performance. With our proof of concept implementation, a single gradient descent step on a single core of a Xeon X5550 2.67GHz CPU takes $\approx$ 60 ms. Over all subjects, we achieved total runtimes of 2.6±0.7 s, thus significantly outperforming related work on dense-to-dense surface registration [8] with runtimes in the scale of minutes (25 iterations, 11.9 s per iteration on comparable CPU and for a surface mesh with a comparable number of vertices).

4   Conclusions and Outlook

In this paper, a variational approach to marker-less reconstruction of dense non-rigid 4-D surface motion fields from sparse but accurate AT sampling data has been introduced. The algorithm can precisely reconstruct the dense respiratory displacement field using prior shape knowledge from planning data. The implications for RT motion management are manifold. The motion fields can be used as multi-dimensional respiration surrogates, as input for accurate external-internal motion correlation models, and to reconstruct the body shape for patient positioning. Beyond its application in RT, the approach holds potential for motion-compensated tomographic reconstruction and image-guided interventions.

Acknowledgments. S. Bauer acknowledges support by the European Regional Development Fund & the Bayerisches Staatsministerium für Wirtschaft, Infrastruktur, Verkehr und Technologie under Grant IUK338/001, and by the Graduate School of Information Science in Health (GSISH) & TUM Graduate School.

References

1. Hoogeman, M., Prvost, J.B., Nuyttens, J., Pll, J., Levendag, P., Heijmen, B.: Clinical accuracy of the respiratory tumor tracking system of the Cyberknife: assessment by analysis of log files. Int. J. Radiat. Oncol. Biol. Phys. 74(1), 297–303 (2009)
2. Verellen, D., Depuydt, T., Gevaert, T., Linthout, N., Tournel, K., Duchateau, M., Reynders, T., Storme, G., Ridder, M.D.: Gating and tracking, 4D in thoracic tumours. Cancer Radiother. 14(67), 446–454 (2010)
3. Willoughby, T.R., Forbes, A.R., Buchholz, D., Langen, K.M., Wagner, T.H., Zeidan, O.A., Kupelian, P.A., Meeks, S.L.: Evaluation of an infrared camera and X-ray system using implanted fiducials in patients with lung tumors for gated radiation therapy. Int. J. Radiat. Oncol. Biol. Phys. 66(2), 568–575 (2006)
4. Brahme, A., Nyman, P., Skatt, B.: 4D laser camera for accurate patient positioning, collision avoidance, image fusion and adaptive approaches during diagnostic and therapeutic procedures. Med. Phys. 35(5), 1670–1681 (2008)
5. Moser, T., Fleischhacker, S., Schubert, K., Sroka-Perez, G., Karger, C.P.: Technical performance of a commercial laser surface scanning system for patient setup correction in radiotherapy. Phys. Med. 27(4), 224–232 (2011)
6. Peng, J.L., Kahler, D., Li, J.G., Samant, S., Yan, G., Amdur, R., Liu, C.: Characterization of a real-time surface image-guided stereotactic positioning system. Med. Phys. 37(10), 5421–5433 (2010)
7. Fayad, H., Pan, T., Clement, J.F., Visvikis, D.: Correlation of respiratory motion between external patient surface and internal anatomical landmarks. Med. Phys. 38(6), 3157–3164 (2011)
8. Schaerer, J., Fassi, A., Riboldi, M., Cerveri, P., Baroni, G., Sarrut, D.: Multidimensional respiratory motion tracking from markerless optical surface imaging based on deformable mesh registration. Phys. Med. Biol. 57(2), 357–373 (2012)
9. Bauer, S., Berkels, B., Hornegger, J., Rumpf, M.: Joint ToF Image Denoising and Registration with a CT Surface in Radiation Therapy. In: Bruckstein, A.M., ter Haar Romeny, B.M., Bronstein, A.M., Bronstein, M.M. (eds.) SSVM 2011. LNCS, vol. 6667, pp. 98–109. Springer, Heidelberg (2012)
10. Cachier, P., Rey, D.: Symmetrization of the Non-rigid Registration Problem Using Inversion-Invariant Energies: Application to Multiple Sclerosis. In: Delp, S.L., DiGoia, A.M., Jaramaz, B. (eds.) MICCAI 2000. LNCS, vol. 1935, pp. 472–481. Springer, Heidelberg (2000)
11. Christensen, G., Johnson, H.: Consistent image registration. IEEE Trans. Med. Imaging 20(7), 568–582 (2001)
12. Modersitzki, J., Fischer, B.: Curvature based image registration. Journal of Mathematical Imaging and Vision 18(1), 81–85 (2003)
13. Ettl, S., Arold, O., Yang, Z., Häusler, G.: Flying triangulation–an optical 3D sensor for the motion-robust acquisition of complex objects. Appl. Opt. 51(2), 281–289 (2012)

Modeling of Multi-View 3D Freehand Radio Frequency Ultrasound

T. Klein[1,*], M. Hansson[2,**], and Nassir Navab[1]

[1] Computer Aided Medical Procedures (CAMP), TU München, Germany
[2] Malmö University, School of Technology, Sweden

Abstract. Nowadays ultrasound (US) examinations are typically performed with conventional machines providing two dimensional imagery. However, there exist a multitude of applications where doctors could benefit from three dimensional ultrasound providing better judgment, due to the extended spatial view. 3D freehand US allows acquisition of images by means of a tracking device attached to the ultrasound transducer. Unfortunately, view dependency makes the 3D representation of ultrasound a non-trivial task. To address this we model speckle statistics, in envelope-detected radio frequency (RF) data, using a finite mixture model (FMM), assuming a parametric representation of data, in which the multiple views are treated as components of the FMM. The proposed model is show-cased with registration, using an ultrasound specific distribution based pseudo-distance, and reconstruction tasks, performed on the manifold of Gamma model parameters. Example field of application is neurology using transcranial US, as this domain requires high accuracy and data systematically features low SNR, making intensity based registration difficult. In particular, 3D US can be specifically used to improve differential diagnosis of Parkinson's disease (PD) compared to conventional approaches and is therefore of high relevance for future application.

Keywords: Envelope-Detected RF, Ultrasound, Registration, 3D Reconstruction, Finite mixture, Nakagami, View-dependent.

1 Introduction

Ultrasonography is often the modality of choice in terms of e.g. intra-operative and screening applications due to its safety, mobility and inexpensiveness compared to other imaging techniques. This together with the steady increase in image quality has made it a widely used diagnostic method in various medical disciplines in recent years. However, the interpretation of US imagery is typically not straightforward and of quite subjective nature and therefore highly dependent on the expertise of its users. This largely stems from the inherent process of US imaging, which is above all view-dependent, as well as subject to noise and

---

* This work was partially sponsored by EU grant FP7-ICT-2009-6-270460.
** This work was partially sponsored by The Royal Physiographic Society in Lund.

N. Ayache et al. (Eds.): MICCAI 2012, Part I, LNCS 7510, pp. 422–429, 2012.
© Springer-Verlag Berlin Heidelberg 2012

prone to containing various types of artifacts. The characteristic speckle noise, dependent on factors such as spatial arrangement and size of scatterers, forms patterns, which are largely characteristic for various types of tissue. Different statistical models have been proposed to model speckle, including the Rician, generalized K, homodyned K, Rayleigh and Nakagami distribution [1]. Specifically in [2], Shankar showed that the envelope detected RF signal follows the Nakagami distribution [3], which serves as a very general model for a multitude of speckle scenarios.

In this paper we extend classical US RF envelope modeling by employing a Nakagami FMM-based approach for 3D US freehand data. This allows us to embed the view-dependent property of US in a statistical formulation. FMMs have already been successfully applied to US data for segmentation of the carotid artery [4]. However, our target applications for this model are registration and reconstruction. To our knowledge we are the first to apply a statistical parametric approach in conjunction with similarity measures (in our case the J-divergence distance metric) to registration of 3D US data. Previous works [5] have applied similarity metrics, e.g Kullback-Leibler (KL), Hellinger and Bhattacharyaa, directly without any parametric distributional assumptions on the data.

Performance and use is show-cased on transcranial US (TCUS) brain data, where 3D freehand image sequences are taken through a narrow bone window at the temporal lobe. The domain of neuro-US is quite relevant for the proposed approach. This is because of the need of high registration accuracy for brain data for applications such as electrode implantation in the brain. Also, TCUS has been recently shown to be appropriate for early diagnosis of PD [6]. This illness is related to degeneration of the substantia nigra (SN). The process is associated with the agglomeration of ferrite deposits, which form hyperechogenic areas in the SN [7] that are visible in US. In this regard, generating 3D data from 2D images by means of a tracked transducer can help in reducing subjectivity in diagnosis [8]. Furthermore, accurate registration of 3D data is required to perform continuous staging of hyperechogenic SN regions.

2   Method

2.1   Freehand 3D RF Data

Due to the spatial relationship of the data, the RF image requires disintegration into individual scanlines such that the reconstruction process, following [9], becomes ray-based - see Fig. 1. Beside the intensity data we also record geometric information such as view point and direction. This additional data is used in a follow-up processing step. The distribution of the envelope of the RF signal, resulting from backscattered tissue echo, has been shown to be modeled, in a simple and versatile way, by the Nakagami distribution [2]. Thus we assume all intensities in the RF envelope image to follow a Nakagami distribution

$$\mathcal{N}(x|\mu,\omega) = \frac{2\mu^\mu x^{2\mu-1}}{\Gamma(\mu)\omega^\mu} \exp\left(-\frac{\mu}{\omega}x^2\right) \quad \text{s.t.} \quad \forall x \in \mathbb{R}_+ \,, \tag{1}$$

with μ, ω denoting the shape and scale parameters, respectively.

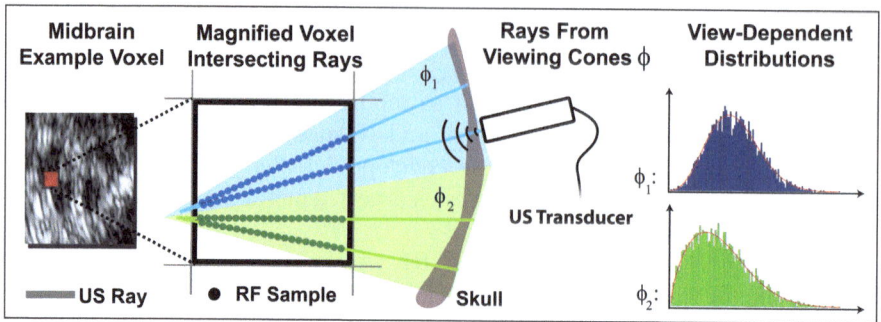

Fig. 1. Distributional change for cones ϕ_1 and ϕ_2 within a single view of midbrain

2.2   Mixture Model Motivation

Since ultrasound is highly view-dependent [10], it is desirable to incorporate this property when modeling back-scatter. However, we are not interested in the individual backscatter intensities, but in the distribution within a small finite volumetric element (voxel) w.r.t views of a data point x, i.e.

$$p(x) = \int_{\mathcal{D}(x)} p(x|\phi)p(\phi)d\phi \,, \tag{2}$$

where $\mathcal{D}(x)$ is the set of all possible viewing cones ϕ of x. The distribution $p(x)$ is approximated by a FMM of K Nakagami densities [4],

$$p(x) \approx \sum_{k=1}^{K} p(\phi_k)p(x|\phi_k) = \sum_{k=1}^{K} w_k \mathcal{N}(x|\mu_k, \omega_k) \quad \text{s.t.} \quad \sum_{k=1}^{K} w_k = 1 \,, \tag{3}$$

where the distribution $p(\phi_k)$ of the kth cone is represented by a mixture weight. The K viewing cones are assumed approx. evenly spaced around the object of interest. See Fig. 1 for illustration of viewing cones of the midbrain with beams originating at different skull positions. A popular choice for FMM estimation is the Expectation-Maximization (EM) algorithm [11]. However, as the EM algorithm can potentially overfit the data and is also quite flexible in component modeling, we do not instantiate it on the pooled data from all views. Rather, we instantiate individual mixture estimations within geometrical subspaces obtained from each view (each containing viewing cones) that were recorded during the acquisition process. Altogether this yields robust component estimation, s.t.

$$p(x) = \sum_{i=1}^{N} \sum_{k=1}^{K_i} w_k p(x|\phi_{i,k}) = \sum_{i=1}^{N} \sum_{k=1}^{K_i} w_k \mathcal{N}(x|\mu_{i,k}, \omega_{i,k}) \,. \tag{4}$$

Specifically, within each view $i \in N$ we determine the number of components $K \leq K_{max}$, following the approach of Frayley and Raftery [12]. Here the Asymptotic Minimum Description Length (AMDL / BIC) principle selects the FMM with d free parameters, which minimizes the quantity $-2 \log \mathcal{L} + d \log n$, where $\mathcal{L}$ is the likelihood of data given model parameters and n the number of observations. This estimation process is performed voxelwise in the entire volume, yielding a mixture model representation for each voxel, where the number of components naturally varies from voxel to voxel.

2.3 Registration

For registration, we perform a voxel-wise distribution matching employing J-divergence in conjunction with a data fidelity term. This provides higher robustness compared to a pure intensity-based model, as was also observed in [5]. Considering a fixed volume (A) and moving volume (B), we seek the rigid transformation $\hat{T}$ that yields optimal alignment between the two, s.t. $\hat{T} = \arg \min_T D_{\text{PJD}}(A, T(B))$ for the pseudo-distance

$$
D_{\text{PJD}}(C, D) = \arg \min_{i,j} \sum_{k=1}^{Z} \mathcal{J}(f^i_{C_k}, f^j_{D_k}) \cdot e^{\left(\lambda \cdot ((1 - w^i_{C_k}) + (1 - w^j_{D_k}))\right)} . \tag{5}
$$

We refer to this pseudo-distance as *Pseudo-J-Divergence*. For each voxel $k \in Z$ it takes the mixture components pair $f^i_{C_k}$ and $f^j_{D_k}$ from the two volumes C and D, resp., to be registered with least J-divergence[13] times the exponentially scaled sum of corresp. mixture weights $w^i_{C_k}, w^j_{D_k} \geq \tau$, where τ is the min. weight. Lastly, λ is a parameter. The pseudo-distance D_{PJD} does not satisfy the triangle inequality, but inherits symmetricity and uniqueness from the J-divergence $\mathcal{J}(f, g)$. The exponential weight in (5) punishes distances formed from components with low mixture weights, since these components are assumed to be less descriptive of the underlying distribution. The J-divergence between two Gamma distributions $f, g \in \mathcal{GA}$, is the sum of two non-symmetric KL distances with switched arguments, s.t.

$$
\mathcal{J}(f, g) = \int \log \frac{f(x)}{g(x)} (f(x) - g(x)) dx = (\mu_a - 1)\Psi(\mu_a) - \log \omega_a - \mu_a
$$
$$
- \log \frac{\Gamma(\mu_a)}{\Gamma(\mu_b)} + \mu_b \log \omega_b - (\mu_b - 1)(\Psi(\mu_a) + \log \omega_a) + \frac{\omega_a \mu_a}{\omega_b} . \tag{6}
$$

Although the data follows Nakagami distribution, the Gamma distribution may be used instead, as they are related by a simple transformation, given by $Y \sim \mathcal{GA}(x \mid \mu_{gam}, \omega_{gam}), X \sim \mathcal{N}(x \mid \mu_{nak}, \omega_{nak}) \Rightarrow \sqrt{X} = Y(\mu_{nak}, \omega_{nak}/\mu_{nak})$.

2.4 Reconstruction

Given the voxel FMM representation we can perform a novel type of reconstruction. Therefore a reference component is chosen from the mixture for each

---

[1] Jeffreys (J) divergence is also known as symmetric KL distance.

voxel, on basis of maximum mean intensity, although other approaches are conceivable. However, this criterion guarantees that no high intensity backscatter is missed during reconstruction. Note that artifacts, such as shadows, might require specific treatment, which is beyond the scope of this work. By optimizing the reference component parameters, i.e. minimizing the sum of geodesic distances to neighbours component parameters, on the manifold $\mathcal{G}$ of Gamma model parameters, smoothness of the reconstructed volume is achieved. Thus, given a point $\theta_a = (\mu_a, \omega_a) \in \mathcal{G}$, the geodesic distance D_{geo} to a locally neighbouring point $\theta_b = (\mu_b, \omega_b) \in \mathcal{G}$ is bounded s.t.

$$D_{geo}(\theta_a, \theta_b) \leq \left| \frac{d^2 \log \Gamma}{d\mu^2}(\mu_b) - \frac{d^2 \log \Gamma}{d\mu^2}(\mu_a) \right| + \left| \mu_a \cdot \log \frac{\mu_a \omega_a}{\mu_b \omega_b} \right| , \qquad (7)$$

cf. Ch. 7, [14] and [15]. Applying (7), the reference distribution θ_{ref} is optimized by minimizing the sum of geodesic distances to all of its neighbors s.t.

$$\hat{\theta}_{\mathrm{ref}} = \underset{\theta_{\mathrm{ref}}}{\mathrm{argmin}} \sum_{k \in N_{\mathrm{ref}}} D_{geo}(\theta_{\mathrm{ref}}, \theta_k) , \qquad (8)$$

keeping the neighbours $\theta_k \in N_{\mathrm{ref}}$ fixed, where N_{ref} defines the neighborhood of a reference voxel. This yields a spatially consistent image without over-smoothing or loss of detail in terms of highlights. Typically a few optimization steps are sufficient and allow for a fast reconstruction.

For data reconstruction within a voxel we apply a Gaussian-weighted (GW) [9] reconstruction scheme in order to increase homogeneity,

$$y_j = \frac{1}{Z} \sum_{i=1}^{N} x_i e^{-d_i^2/\sigma^2} \quad \mathrm{s.t.} \quad Z = \sum_{i=1}^{N} e^{-d_i^2/\sigma^2} , \qquad (9)$$

yielding the reconstructed intensity y_j at voxel position j. Here the intensities x_i are sampled from the reference distribution, where d_i are the distances from the voxel centroid that can be obtained by regression from the measured data.

3   Results

Registration. The 3D US RF freehand data used is obtained using the optical tracking system NDI Spectra in conjunction with an Ultrasonix MDP US machine. For testing the registration performance multiple transcranial 3D volumes for several patients were acquired. An acquisition consisted of bilateral scans; in doing so various sweeps from numerous possible views were obtained. Furthermore, each patient was recorded with a reference target rigidly attached to the head, which allows establishment of groundtruth position between numerous volumes. The three-dimensional RF datasets were acquired using a phased-array probe with a frequency of 3.3 MHz and depth 14 cm. RF data is sampled at 40 MHz. Each 3D RF data set is built from approximately 4000 2D RF images (2000 images from each side of the skull), each having a resolution of 3648 x 96 pixels.

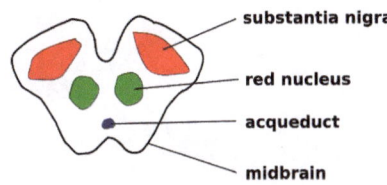

Fig. 2. Schematic illustration of midbrain and structures within

Table 1. Median errors (mm) and std. dev. of registration study

Dataset	SSD	NCC	PJD
#1	3.2 ± 1.3	3.0 ± 1.3	$\mathbf{2.7 \pm 1.1}$
#2	2.7 ± 1.3	2.7 ± 1.2	$\mathbf{2.4 \pm 1.2}$
#3	3.2 ± 1.2	3.3 ± 1.1	$\mathbf{2.9 \pm 1.1}$
#4	3.7 ± 1.1	3.4 ± 1.1	$\mathbf{3.0 \pm 1.1}$
#5	3.4 ± 1.1	3.2 ± 1.1	$\mathbf{2.9 \pm 1.1}$
#6	3.3 ± 1.2	3.4 ± 1.2	$\mathbf{2.9 \pm 1.1}$

Acquisition time is 2-4 min (1800 images/min unilateral scan). Volumes were reconstructed with isotropic voxel size of 0.65 mm (mean 1400 samples/voxel). For the mixture modeling we assumed $N = 2$ views (bilateral) as well as $K_{max} = 2$. This yielded a maximum of four mixture components per voxel and sufficiently modeled the data while avoiding overfits.

For evaluating the quality of the proposed approach, we performed registration by block matching, which is commonly used for US [16,17]. For each patient two multi-view volumes are constructed for distinct US data. These two distinct volumes are then rigidly registered by taking 27 equally distributed blocks (each of size $6 \times 6 \times 6$ voxels) for matching, within each multi-view volume. For each of 10 runs we randomly displace, with initial deviation of ±6 cm, the moving subvolume/block from the ground truth position (obtained via head target), in each spatial direction from its ground truth position. This is followed by registration by block-matching at each position using state of the art similarity metrics for US, aligning the moving and the fixed volume. In the case of global registration, the result from each block is accumulated. Parameters for our distance metric were set to $\lambda = 2$ and $\tau = 0.3$. In spite of rigidity, registration of transcranial brain US brain data is quite challenging due to the relative low SNR as a result of variable transmission through skull bone and the low transducer frequency required. Nevertheless, the proposed pseudo-J-Divergence (PJD) yields up to 15% better registration results compared to Normalized Cross-Correlation (NCC) and Sum of Squared Differences (SSD) [16,17], as can be seen in Tab. 1. Intensity volumes were created using GW [9]. The difference in median between methods is statistically significant. The Hodges-Lehmann 95% confidence interval for the difference in median error between PJD and NCC is (-0.25,-0.08), and (-0.3,-0.12) for PJD and SSD. The corresp. Mann-Whitney U-test yields p-values $0.14 \cdot 10^{-3}$ and $0.2 \cdot 10^{-6}$, resp. Obtained results are quite close to technical possible limits due to the errors that are propagated through the processing chain. In this respect, US calibration affects the accuracy significantly, depending largely on the approach used. In our setup, calibration was performed using a single wall phantom, yielding an error between 1-2 mm [18,19].

Reconstruction. As reconstruction methods are difficult to compare due to the highly subjective nature of US image analysis, we will elaborate on the obvious differences between a state of the art method (GW - increased smoothness

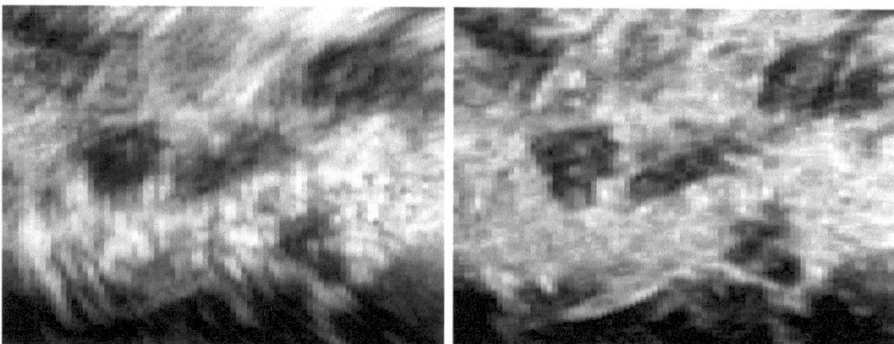

Fig. 3. TCUS reconstruction. Butterfly-shaped region in the image center corresponds to the midbrain. Left: Gaussian-weighted Right: Geodesic.

favourable for segmentation and registration [9]) and our approach as well as discuss the potential implications. Reconstructions following the geodesic approach yield more coherent and homogeneous images - see Fig. 3. Note that for Gaussian reconstruction we chose $\sigma = 1$ in all cases. Checker-board and radial artifacts disappear, which are visible in the GW approach due to the multi-view mixture nature of the signal. Additionally, the mid-brain area exhibits sharper edges using the proposed approach. Regions that are clinically relevant for classification such as the SN, where the level of hyperechogenicity is a risk-assessment criterion for PD [6], are more pronounced and less blurred (see Fig. 2 for a schematic illustration of the midbrain and structures within). The clinical benefit for applications such as classification, however, remains to be evaluated.

4   Conclusion

We have presented a FMM representation of 3D RF data exploiting its view-dependent statistical properties. Making use of view-dependency has potential to facilitate several applications; specifically, results from a block-matching based rigid registration study suggest improvements in terms of accuracy compared to conventional similarity metrics. Moreover, image reconstruction promises to be an interesting domain of application. Further applications will be studied e.g. multi-view bone imaging where, as a result of varying reflectance properties of bone, muscle, and ligaments, different backscatter scenarios are encountered.

References

1. Destrempes, F., Cloutier, G.: A Critical Review and Uniformized Representation of Statistical Distributions Modeling the Ultrasound Echo Envelope. Ultrasound Med. Biol. 36(7), 1037–1051 (2010)
2. Shankar, P.M.: A General Statistical Model for Ultrasonic Scattering from Tissues. IEEE Trans. Ultrason. Ferroelectr. Freq. Control 47(3), 339–343 (2000)

3. Nakagami, N.: The m-distribution, a General Formula for Intensity Distribution of Rapid Fadings. In: Hoffman, W.G. (ed.) Statistical Methods in Radio Wave Propagation, pp. 3–36. Pergamon, Oxford (1960)

4. Destrempes, F., Meunier, J., Giroux, M.F., Soulez, G., Cloutier, G.: Segmentation in Ultrasonic B-Mode Images of Healthy Carotid Arteries Using Mixtures of Nakagami Distributions and Stochastic Optimization. IEEE Trans. Med. Imag. 28(2), 215–229 (2009)

5. Ijaz, U.Z., Prager, R.W., Gee, A.H., Treece, G.M.: A Study of Similarity Measures for In Vivo 3D Ultrasound Volume Registration Acoustical Imaging. Acoustical Imaging, vol. 30, pp. 315–323. Springer, Netherlands (2011)

6. Walter, U., Dressler, D., Probst, T., Wolters, A., Abu-Mugheisib, M., Wittstock, M., Benecke, R.: Transcranial Brain Sonography Findings in Discriminating Between Parkinsonism and Idiopathic Parkinson Disease. Arch. Neurol. 64(11), 1635–1640 (2007)

7. Becker, G., Seufert, J., Bogdahn, U., Reichmann, H., Reiners, K.: Degeneration of Substantia Nigra in Chronic Parkinson's Disease Visualized by Transcranial Color-coded Real-time Sonography. Neurology 45(1), 182–184 (1995)

8. Plate, A., Ahmadi, S.-A., Klein, T., Navab, N., Weisse, J., Mehrkens, J.H., Boetzel, K.: Towards a More Objective Visualization of the Midbrain and its Surroundings Using 3D Transcranial Ultrasound. In: Deutschen Gesellschaft für Klinische Neurophysiologie und Funktionelle Bildgebung (DGKN), Halle, Germany (2010)

9. Wein, W., Pache, F., Röper, B., Navab, N.: Backward-Warping Ultrasound Reconstruction for Improving Diagnostic Value and Registration. In: Larsen, R., Nielsen, M., Sporring, J. (eds.) MICCAI 2006, Part II. LNCS, vol. 4191, pp. 750–757. Springer, Heidelberg (2006)

10. Hedrick, W.R., Hykes, D.L., Starchman, D.E.: Ultrasound Physics and Instrumentation. Mosby (2004)

11. Dempster, A.P., Laird, N.M., Rubin, D.B.: Maximum Likelihood for Incomplete Data via the EM Algorithm. J. Roy. Statist. Soc. Ser. B 39, 1–38 (1977)

12. Fraley, C., Raftery, A.E.: Model-based Clustering, Discriminant Analysis, and Density Estimation. J. Amer. Statist. Assoc. 97(458), 611–631 (2002)

13. Jeffreys, H.: An Invariant Form for the Prior Probability in Estimation Problems. Proc. R. Soc. A. Series A, Mathematical and Physical Sciences 186, 453–461 (1946)

14. Arwini, K., Dodson, C., Doig, A., Sampson, W., Scharcanski, J., Felipussi, S.: Information Geometry: Near Randomness and Near Independence. Lect Notes Math. Springer, Heidelberg (2008)

15. Dodson, C., Matsuzoe., H.: An Affine Embedding of the Gamma Manifold. Inter-Stat, 1–6 (2002)

16. Poon, T.C., Rohling, R.N.: Three-dimensional Extended Field-of-view Ultrasound. Ultrasound Med. Biol. 32(3), 357–369 (2006)

17. Krucker, J.F., LeCarpentier, G.L., Fowlkes, J.B., Carson, P.L.: Rapid Elastic Image Registration for 3-d Ultrasound. IEEE Trans. Med. Imag. 21(11), 1384–1394 (2002)

18. Hsu, P.W., Prager, R.W., Gee, A.H., Treece, G.M.: Freehand 3D Ultrasound Calibration: A Review (2007)

19. Mercier, L., Lango, T., Lindseth, F., Collins, D.: A Review of Calibration Techniques for Freehand 3-d Ultrasound Systems. Ultrasound Med. Biol. 31(4) (2005)

Towards Intra-operative PET for Head and Neck Cancer: Lymph Node Localization Using High-Energy Probes

Dzhoshkun I. Shakir[1,2], Aslı Okur[1,2], Alexander Hartl[1,2], Philipp Matthies[1],
Sibylle I. Ziegler[2], Markus Essler[2], Tobias Lasser[1,3], and Nassir Navab[1]

[1] Computer Aided Medical Procedures (CAMP),
Technische Universität München, Germany
[2] Department of Nuclear Medicine, Klinikum rechts der Isar,
Technische Universität München, Germany
[3] Institute of Biomathematics and Biometry, HelmholtzZentrum München, Germany

Abstract. We present a novel approach for intra-operative localization
of lymph nodes and metastases in the head and neck region using the
radio-tracer [18F]FDG. By combining an optical tracking system with
a high-energy gamma probe to detect 511keV annihilation gammas, we
enable intra-operative PET to visualize activity distributions. Detection
of these gammas is modeled ad-hoc analytically, taking into account several factors affecting the detection process. This allows us to iteratively
reconstruct the radio-tracer distribution within a localized volume of interest. As a feasibility study we analyze clinical data of 7 patients with
tumors in the head and neck region, and derive a realistic neck phantom
configuration with [18F]FDG-filled lesions mimicking tumors and lymph
nodes. We demonstrate the capabilities and limitations of our approach
using that neck phantom. We also outline possible improvements to make
our method clinically viable towards less invasive surgeries.

1 Introduction

Head and neck squamous (epithelial) cell carcinoma (HNSCC) is diagnosed in
500,000 patients each year. HNSCC primarily affects the oropharynx, oral cavity
hypopharynx and larynx [1], but has a risk of metastasizing into the cervical
lymph nodes (LNs). It is therefore important for prognosis to assess the status
of LNs in this region and remove the ones containing metastases. In the current
clinical workflow, sonography, MRI, Computed tomography (CT) or [18F]FDG–
Positron-Emission-Tomography ([18F]FDG-PET – referred to as simply *PET*
from this point on) are used for pre-operative LN staging in HNSCC patients.
Compared to others, PET was found to detect cervical LN metastases with
the highest sensitivity and specificity [2]. The aim of surgical treatment is to
completely resect the tumor and all LN metastases. However, the intra-operative
localization of metastatic LNs only is difficult, so in practice all LNs in the
vicinity of the suspicious one(s) are resected by a neck dissection procedure. On
the other hand, the high post-operative morbidity risk due to the presence of

N. Ayache et al. (Eds.): MICCAI 2012, Part I, LNCS 7510, pp. 430–437, 2012.

vital anatomic structures is an indication for minimizing invasiveness in head and neck (HN) interventions. Aesthetic motivations are also obvious. Thus it is of high clinical relevance to intra-operatively guide the surgeon to selectively resect the few PET-positive metastatic LNs, especially when critical structures such as nerves or vessels make resection difficult.

In this work we describe freehand PET (fhPET), a novel system for the intra-operative detection of metastatic LNs with an increased glucose metabolism. fhPET allows to intra-operatively image the region containing the PET-positive LNs. Our system combines a high-energy gamma probe (HE probe) (that can detect the 511 keV gammas released upon the annihilation of the positrons emitted by [^{18}F]FDG with electrons) with a 3D optical tracking system, similar to the freehand SPECT (fhSPECT) system mentioned in [3,4]. The detection physics are modeled with an analytical ad-hoc model that allows for iterative reconstruction of the 3D radio-tracer distribution within the volume of interest (VOI). In contrast to freehand SPECT, this technique has to deal with high-energy (511 keV) gamma rays (compared to the 140 keV gamma rays of ^{99m}Tc).

Most related work uses HE probes without tracking and navigation support; for instance in HNSCC [5] and thyroid cancer applications [6]. There is work on dedicated intra-operative PET scanners [7,8], combined intra-operative PET and trans-rectal ultrasound [9], or handheld PET imaging probes with an external detector ring for full tomographic data [10]. A more suitable approach for the operating room (OR) is outlined in [11,12].

2   Materials and Methods

2.1   High-Energy Gamma Probes (HE Probes)

A HE probe is a pen-sized, hand-held device, typically with a big shielding head around the detector (see fig. 1(a)), that can detect annihilation gamma rays. The annihilation takes place within a very limited distance from the emitting atom (typically below 2 mm [13]) and results in two 511 keV gamma rays in opposite directions to each other. PET systems are based on hardware that can detect such simultaneous gamma rays (*coincidences*). A HE probe does not detect coincidences, but only single 511 keV gamma rays.

2.2   Tomographic Imaging with 1D HE Probes

To generate tomographic images from the HE probe data we need to combine it with a spatial localization system, such that the VOI can be scanned with the probe while the probe signals are recorded synchronously to the probe positions with respect to the VOI. This VOI is discretized into voxels and we decompose each measurement m_j into a linear combination of the contributions a_{ij} of the unknown activity values x_i in all voxels:

$$m_j = \sum_i a_{ij} x_i \tag{1}$$

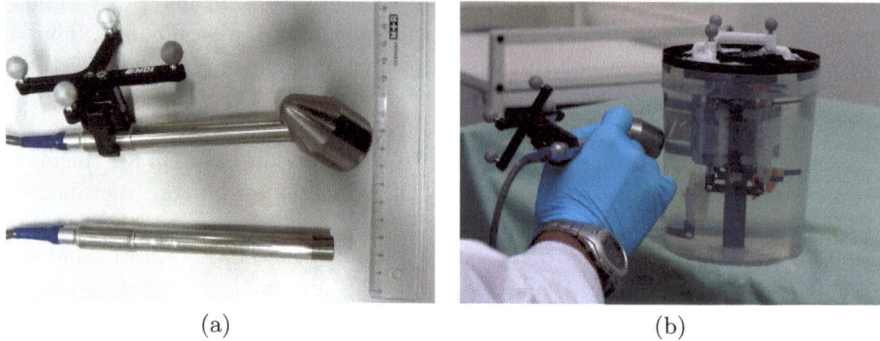

(a)   (b)

Fig. 1. (a) *top:* HE probe, *bottom:* low-energy gamma probe. (b) Neck phantom.

Using this decomposition, all the measurements within a scan can be stacked into a system of linear equations: $m = Ax$. By inverting this system we can retrieve the activity distribution in our VOI using a solver like MLEM (Maximum Likelihood Expectation Maximization) [3]. However, for the inversion, the system matrix A with the contributions a_{ij} is needed. As we do not have a fixed acquisition geometry we need to compute the contributions on the fly using an ad-hoc model of the detection physics of our probe.

2.3   Ad-Hoc Model of Detection Physics

We model the physical factors affecting the detection of gamma rays analytically, based on the known geometric properties of our HE probe. This is our *ad-hoc model* of detection physics.

First of all, our model computes the geometric attenuation, which determines the portion of the initial radiation that should in the ideal case reach the detector due to the isotropy of radiation. This is computed with the solid angle Ω subtended by the detector of the probe on a point source.

In the next step, the effects of the shielding and the absorption in the detector of the probe are computed using the mean lengths that gamma rays will traverse through the shielding and the detector. These lengths are obtained by dividing the space around the probe into partitions in each of which these lengths can be computed with a unique formula. Due to symmetry the computations can be reduced to a profile slice through the probe. In this slice we consider the four rays that reach the four corners of the detector and for each of these rays we compute the length of interaction l_i that the ray traverses through the detector (see fig. 2(a)). The probability of an interaction in the detector along this ray can be computed using the formula $p = 1 - e^{\mu l_i}$, with μ being a material coefficient (detector: BGO, shielding: tungsten [14]). Using this probability function we can now compute the mean probability $\bar{p}$ of an interaction between two successive rays by integrating over the probability function with the two rays as boundaries and then dividing by the difference in the length of interaction of both rays:

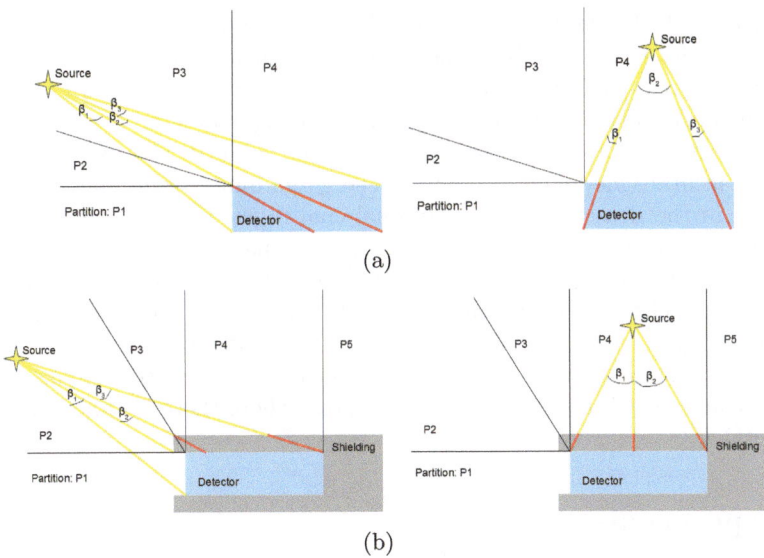

Fig. 2. The length rays take through the detector (a) and through the shielding (b) are computed depending on the partition (P1,P2...) in which the source lies. This is done by using several example rays between which this length *(red)* changes smoothly. For these rays the probability of an interaction is computed and by integrating between two successive rays. This is then weighted with the angle β_i between the two rays divided by the sum of all angles, so we get the mean probability for an interaction in the detector/shielding from a specific source position.

$$\overline{p} = \frac{\int_{l_{in}}^{l_{in+1}} \left[1 - e^{\mu l_i}\right] dl_i}{|l_{in} - l_{in+1}|} = \frac{1 - \left|e^{\mu l_{in+1}} - e^{\mu l_{in}}\right|}{|l_{in} - l_{in+1}|} \tag{2}$$

By weighting these probabilities with the angle β_i between these rays and dividing by the total angle between the two outer rays we get the mean probability for an interaction of a gamma ray emitted by a point source on a specific position relative to the probe. Absorption in the shielding is computed in a similar way (see fig. 2(b)).

The mean probability for an absorption in the shielding $\overline{p_s}$ and in the detector $\overline{p_d}$ are then used to compute the amount of radiation that is detected:

$$a = (1 - \overline{p_s} * \overline{p_d} * \frac{\Omega}{4\pi}) \tag{3}$$

2.4   System Setup and Challenges

Our system combines a 1D HE probe (NodeSeeker 800, Intra Medical Imaging LLC, CA, USA) with a 3D (6DOF) optical tracking system (Polaris Vicra, Northern Digital Incorporated, ON, Canada). The combined data gets synchronized by the software running on the application workstation (CSS300, SurgicEye

GmbH, Munich, Germany). We tuned the software on this workstation to accommodate the described ad-hoc model. Data acquisition and reconstruction are performed in real-time using the workstation (about 5min for data acquisition and 1min for reconstruction). It also provides an augmented-reality visualization.

Our system is similar in terms of hardware to the fhSPECT technology. However, the accurate modeling of the high–energy gamma rays in matter and their detection in the detector poses additional challenges. One big problem is that due to their high energy levels, these 511 keV gamma rays can penetrate through matter more than e.g. the 140 keV gamma rays of ^{99m}Tc. Thus, HE probes require much thicker shielding, which can still not stop all the gammas. Another problem is the background radiation due to the partially unspecific [^{18}F]FDG uptake (e.g. muscle activity, inflammation - see fig. 3(a)), contrary to e.g. ^{99m}Tc– marked tracers used in sentinel LN procedures, where there is almost no unspecific uptake.

3   Experiments

We conducted three different sets of experiments to evaluate fhPET for the localization of tumors and LNs/metastases in HNSCC. For these, we prepared a phantom simulating a tumor mass and a LN in the neck region, using a plastic box and three plastic lab reservoirs (2 ml each) (see fig. 1(b)). The reservoirs were attached rigidly and reproducibly to the construction. For the first set of experiments, we evaluated PET/CT images from 7 HNSCC patients (mean age: 53 year, 6 m/1 f). Each patient had one or two PET-positive LNs. Following the surgical resection, the LNs were histologically examined for metastases and 5 cases were positive. Using these data sets, we calculated the values seen in table 1 we used for injecting [^{18}F]FDG into the reservoirs (simulating the tumor and the LN). The rest of the phantom was filled with water and with background (BG) activity respectively (simulating cases with no BG and unspecific BG).

Table 1. The geometrical and activity-related parameters obtained from patient data

tumor depth from the surface:	5.3 ± 1.06 cm
lymph node depth from the surface:	2.6 ± 0.99 cm
tumor-to-background (T/BG) uptake ratio:	3.3 ± 1.17
tumor-to-lymph node (T/LN) uptake ratio:	1.5 ± 0.97
tumor uptake:	23.8 ± 9.41 kBq/ml
lymph node uptake:	21.3 ± 12.75 kBq/ml

In the second set of experiments, we used higher activity, which we also varied, in order to be able to assess the boundary conditions of our system, i.e. from which activity level on we can actually see the tumor and the LN.

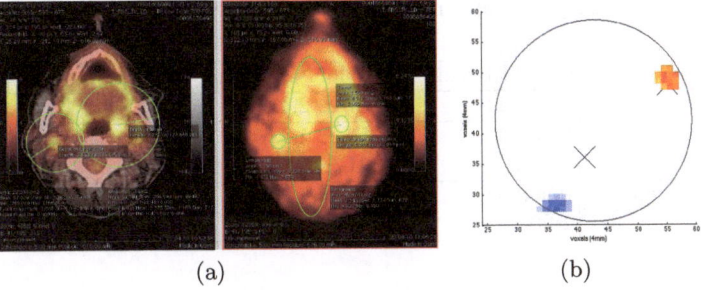

(a)   (b)

Fig. 3. (a) The tumor and LN locations, as well as depths, were identified in the over-laid PET/CT images (left). The corresponding average activity values were obtained from PET images (right). In addition, the unspecific background radiation values were calculated (in this case the large elliptic region).(b) A transverse slice of one recon-structed image. Blue blob: reconstructed tumor (the cross nearby showing the tumor location in the ground truth). Red figure: reconstructed LN (the cross within showing the LN location in the ground truth). Circle: an outline of the phantom.

In the third set of experiments, we used the same activity ratios as in the second set, but this time we used ^{99m}Tc. Our aim here was to compare the images obtained with the fhSPECT system and our fhPET system, in the light of the discussion about the additional challenges of fhPET within sec. 2.4.

Two operators scanned each phantom configuration two or three times respec-tively, each time covering about 120 degrees around the phantom, and obtaining 3000 measurement points. In each case the resulting system of linear equations was inverted using MLEM with 20 iterations. The obtained reconstruction was smoothed using a 4 or 6 mm Gaussian filter to reduce reconstruction noise due to the highly under-sampled acquisition with insufficient statistics.

4 Evaluation and Results

For qualitative evaluation, we checked the visibility of the tumor and the LN in the reconstructions. Within the first set of scans (realistic activity concentra-tions) we were able to identify the LN in 3 (none with BG activity) of the 7 reconstructions. We could identify the tumor in none of the 7 reconstructions, as it was seated much deeper than the LN.

In the second set of experiments we were able to identify the LN in all of the 17 reconstructions. Moreover, we were able to see the tumor in 6 (3 of those with BG activity) reconstructions (for example see fig. 3(b)). In one of these we could even distinguish the two reservoirs next to each other, simulating the tumor.

We further obtained a CT image of our phantom to serve as a ground truth. Using the phantom tracking target seen in fig. 1(b) (already visible in the CT), we registered the CT image to the fhPET images. In the CT images, we manu-ally selected the midpoint of the LN and the tumor. Using the registration, we computed the distance between the centroid of the LN in the fhPET images and

Table 2. Different phantom configurations and accuracies achieved with fhPET

Experiment setup	BG:T:L	Lymph node loc. error (mm)	Tumor loc. error (mm)
1. [18F]FDG low	0:17:10	12.67 ± 2.48	NA
2. [18F]FDG high	0:20:20	13.57 ± 4.22	34.79 ± 6.20
	1:20:20	14.41 ± 5.75	47.39 ± 22.28
3. 99mTc high	0:20:20	11.35 ± 4.26	39.39 ± 10.60
	1:20:20	10.85 ± 4.07	20.42 ± 2.55

its midpoint in the CT. We did the same for the tumor as well, for the cases where the tumor was visible in the fhPET images.

5   Discussion and Conclusion

The results show the ability to reconstruct the mock LN in all cases, with a localization error between 12.7 to 14.4mm (see table 2). While deviations of 10mm are typically considered acceptable in a surgical setting, our error is a bit higher. Also, the tumor site was not detectable at realistic activity concentrations, while at higher activities it was visible with high localization errors. The errors are due to several reasons. Sub-optimal collimation in hand-held devices at high energies contributes to a decrease in accuracy. A remedy for this is to detect coincidences, which requires placing a detector block under the patient. On the other hand our system does not need such a complicated setup, and is thus a more feasible solution if it can meet the OR accuracy requirements. Although positron range in general affects PET image resolution [15], we do not think that it has a major effect on our system currently, due to the differences in the resolution range.

Some factors, however, can still be improved, like a better physical model of the detection process, taking also into account attenuation correction and scatter effects. The best solution to improve image quality would be to include registered prior PET/CT data, providing attenuation correction information as well as the possibility of guiding the scanning procedure and constraining the reconstruction process using priors. The combination with intra-operative ultrasound could for example yield the basis for registration of the prior data.

In summary, we have shown first results demonstrating feasibility of PET-like intra-operative imaging using HE probes within certain constraints with phantoms. In addition we have outlined the improvements to our method required for making it viable for clinical applications.

Acknowledgments. This research was funded/supported by the Graduate School of Information Science in Health (GSISH), the TUM Graduate School (Munich, Germany) and SFB 824 (DFG, Germany).

References

1. Haddad, R.I., Shin, D.M.: Recent advances in head and neck cancer. The New England Journal of Medicine 359(11), 1143–1154 (2008)
2. Adams, S., Baum, R.P., Stuckensen, T., Bitter, K., Hör, G.: Prospective comparison of 18F-FDG PET with conventional imaging modalities (CT, MRI, US) in lymph node staging of head and neck cancer. Eur. J. Nucl. Med. 25(9), 1255–1260 (1998)
3. Wendler, T., Feuerstein, M., Traub, J., Lasser, T., Vogel, J., Daghighian, F., Ziegler, S.I., Navab, N.: Real-Time Fusion of Ultrasound and Gamma Probe for Navigated Localization of Liver Metastases. In: Ayache, N., Ourselin, S., Maeder, A. (eds.) MICCAI 2007, Part II. LNCS, vol. 4792, pp. 252–260. Springer, Heidelberg (2007)
4. Wendler, T., Herrmann, K., Schnelzer, A., Lasser, T., Traub, J., Kutter, O., Ehlerding, A., Scheidhauer, K., Schuster, T., Kiechle, M., Schwaiger, M., Navab, N., Ziegler, S.I., Buck, A.K.: First demonstration of 3-D lymphatic mapping in breast cancer using freehand SPECT. Eur. J. Nucl. Med. 37(8), 1452–1461 (2010)
5. Meller, B., Sommer, K., Gerl, J., von Hof, K., Surowiec, A., Richter, E., Wollenberg, B., Baehre, M.: High energy probe for detecting lymph node metastases with 18F-FDG in patients with head and neck cancer. Nuklearmedizin 45(4), 153–159 (2006)
6. Kim, W.W., Kim, J.S., Hur, S.M., Kim, S.H., Lee, S., Choi, J.H., Kim, S., Choi, J.Y., Lee, J.E., Kim, J., Nam, S.J., Yang, J., Choe, J.: Radioguided surgery using an intraoperative PET probe for tumor localization and verification of complete resection in differentiated thyroid cancer: a pilot study. Surgery 149(3), 416–424 (2011)
7. Stolin, A.V., Majewski, S., Raylman, R.R., Martone, P.: Hand-Held SiPM-Based PET imagers for surgical applications. In: Proceedings of IEEE Nuclear Science Symposium and Medical Imaging Conference (IEEE NSS-MIC), Valencia, Spain (October 2011)
8. Majewski, S., Stolin, A., Martone, P., Raylman, R.: Dedicated mobile pet prostate imager. J. Nucl. Med. Meeting Abstracts 52(1), 1945 (2011)
9. Huber, J., Moses, W., Pouliot, J., Hsu, I.: Dual-Modality PET/Ultrasound imaging of the prostate, vol. 4, pp. 2187–2190. IEEE (October 2005)
10. Huh, S.S., Rogers, W.L., Clinthorne, N.H.: An investigation of an Intra-Operative PET imaging probe. In: Nuclear Science Symposium Conference Record, NSS 2007, pp. 552–555. IEEE (October 2007)
11. Huh, S.S., Rogers, W.L., Clinthorne, N.H.: On-line sliding-window list-mode PET image reconstruction for a surgical PET imaging probe. In: Nuclear Science Symposium Conference Record, NSS 2008, pp. 5479–5484. IEEE (October 2008)
12. Huh, S., Han, L., Rogers, W., Clinthorne, N.: Real time image reconstruction using GPUs for a surgical PET imaging probe system. In: Nuclear Science Symposium Conference Record, NSS 2009, pp. 4148–4153. IEEE (October 2009)
13. Cho, Z.H., Chan, J.K., Ericksson, L., Singh, M., Graham, S., MacDonald, N.S., Yano, Y.: Positron ranges obtained from biomedically important positron-emitting radionuclides. J. Nucl. Med. 16(12), 1174–1176 (1975)
14. National Institute of Standards and Technology, Physical Measurements Laboratory, http://physics.nist.gov/PhysRefData/Xcom/html/xcom1.html
15. Levin, C.S., Hoffman, E.J.: Calculation of positron range and its effect on the fundamental limit of positron emission tomography system spatial resolution. Physics in Medicine and Biology 44(3), 781–799 (1999)

Data-Driven Breast Decompression and Lesion Mapping from Digital Breast Tomosynthesis

Michael Wels[1], B.M. Kelm[1], M. Hammon[2], Anna Jerebko[3],
M. Sühling[1], and Dorin Comaniciu[4]

[1] Siemens AG, Corporate Technology, Erlangen, Germany
[2] University Hospital Erlangen, Department of Radiology, Germany
[3] Siemens AG, Healthcare, Erlangen, Germany
[4] Siemens Corporation, Corporate Research and Technology, Princeton, NJ, USA

Abstract. Digital Breast Tomosynthesis (DBT) emerges as a new 3D modality for breast cancer screening and diagnosis. Like in conventional 2D mammography the breast is scanned in a compressed state. For orientation during surgical planning, e.g., during presurgical ultrasound-guided anchor-wire marking, as well as for improving communication between radiologists and surgeons it is desirable to estimate an uncompressed model of the acquired breast along with a spatial mapping that allows localizing lesions marked in DBT in the uncompressed model. We therefore propose a method for 3D breast decompression and associated lesion mapping from 3D DBT data. The method is entirely data-driven and employs machine learning methods to predict the shape of the uncompressed breast from a DBT input volume. For this purpose a shape space has been constructed from manually annotated uncompressed breast surfaces and shape parameters are predicted by multiple multi-variate Random Forest regression. By exploiting point correspondences between the compressed and uncompressed breasts, lesions identified in DBT can be mapped to approximately corresponding locations in the uncompressed breast model. To this end, a thin-plate spline mapping is employed. Our method features a novel completely data-driven approach to breast shape prediction that does not necessitate prior knowledge about biomechanical properties and parameters of the breast tissue. Instead, a particular deformation behavior (decompression) is learned from annotated shape pairs, compressed and uncompressed, which are obtained from DBT and magnetic resonance image volumes, respectively. On average, shape prediction takes 26 s and achieves a surface distance of 15.80±4.70 mm. The mean localization error for lesion mapping is 22.48±8.67 mm.

1 Introduction

According to the World Cancer Report 2008 (globocan.iarc.fr, 2012/01/23) breast cancer is the most frequent cancer diagnosis in women among all specifiable kinds of cancer. Early detection is assumed to significantly improve outcomes. That is why breast cancer screening is recommended by many national organizations for most older women, e.g., the American Cancer Society (www.cancer.org,

N. Ayache et al. (Eds.): MICCAI 2012, Part I, LNCS 7510, pp. 438–446, 2012.

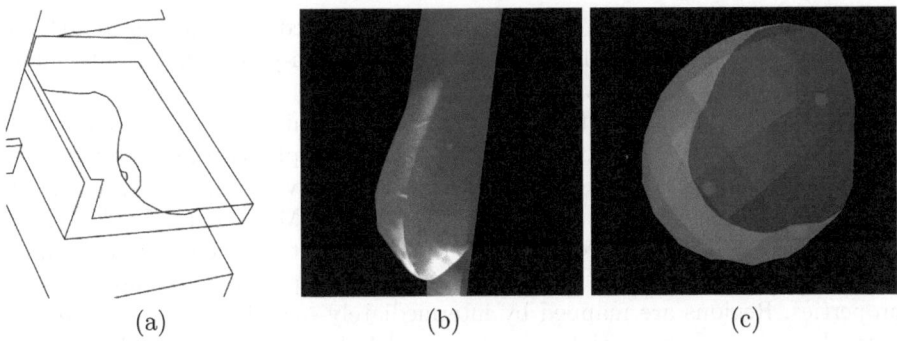

(a)   (b)   (c)

Fig. 1. The MLO image acquisition (a), a 3D DBT scan (b), and a 3D rendering of an uncompressed breast with mapped lesions (c). Radiographic image with courtesy of University Hospital Erlangen.

2012/05/31) recommends yearly screening mammography for women aged 40 and above as long as they are in good health.

Recently, Digital Breast Tomosynthesis (DBT) increasingly replaces common 2D mammography for differential diagnosis and is in discussion for screening [1]. It provides 3D image volumes of the compressed breast (see Fig. 1 (b)) that are reconstructed from multiple 2D projections acquired at varying angles. Being a 3D imaging modality DBT naturally allows superior spatial localization of suspicious lesions. For a mediolateral-oplique (MLO) scan the breast is compressed as sketched in Fig. 1 (a). Typically, a second scan is acquired in craniocaudal (CC) direction during an examination. For surgical planning it is common clinical practice to mark the lesions in the scans and to communicate the rough localization of suspicious findings in the uncompressed breast via schematic 2D drawings. The latter naturally suffers from inaccuracies and can often only be dissolved by additional, potentially ionizing and costly, imaging. Providing more accurate lesion localization in the uncompressed breast, e.g., in terms of a 3D rendering view (see Fig. 1 (c)), without additional imaging has the potential to facilitate surgical planning and related procedures, e.g., placing pre-operative markers, at low cost.

We therefore propose a method for estimating uncompressed 3D breast shapes from 3D DBT MLO scans. The reconstructed uncompressed shape and the original compressed shape depicted in the DBT scan establish a reference frame that can be used to map lesions found in the image of the compressed breast to the corresponding location in the uncompressed breast. Essentially, our method consists of two major steps: shape prediction and lesion mapping. For shape prediction the input data is transformed to a representation suitable for multiple multi-variate regression. This is done by fully-automatically detecting the nipple (or papilla) from the DBT images, segmenting the breast area, extracting the breast surface, and canonically re-sampling it. For lesion mapping we make use of the point correspondences established by applying the same canonical re-sampling to the uncompressed shapes used for predictor training and shape model construction. This allows us to compute a thin-plate spline (TPS) interpolation for lesion mapping.

Despite the huge body of literature on biomechanical breast modeling [2,3] and its applications in the context of 2D mammography [4] there are few publications dealing with DBT. As a notable exception van Schie et al. [5] match corresponding regions from ipsilateral DBT views (MLO and CC). Unlike in our case, the behavior of breasts—that are assumed to be hemispheres—under compression/decompression is explicitly modeled by approximating breast tissue properties. Regions are mapped by intermediately mapping them to a decompressed version of the initial geometric model that has been matched to the compressed breast before. The matching region in the ipsilateral view is finally found after rotation and repeated compression. This is different from our approach as we predict the shape of the uncompressed breast directly without intermediate steps and without explicitly modeling tissue behavior. We rather rely on a purely data-driven approach inherently capturing tissue behavior as it is present in the available training data.

2   Methods

2.1   Input Data and Feature Extraction

For shape prediction feature vectors $x \in \mathbb{R}^K$ of uniform length K have to be extracted from the 3D DBT image volumes. For this we first segment the breast tissue area by thresholding and region growing, then extract the breast surface using Marching Cubes [6], and canonically re-sample it starting from the nipple to a fixed number of surface points. This re-sampling scheme is also relevant to lesion mapping, which will be discussed in more detail later. Finally, a high-dimensional feature vector suitable for machine learning-based shape prediction is obtained by composing the distances between every individual surface point and the nipple. Here, the nipple position is automatically determined by a machine learning-based landmark detection algorithm using 3D Haar-like features [7,8]. It has been rapidly prototyped using an Integrated Detection Network (IDN) [9]. Note that, for processing, any breast is treated as a left breast, i.e., right breast images are mirrored.

2.2   Target Shape Model and 3D Shape Reconstruction

For the purpose of shape prediction we construct a statistical shape model [10] of the target shapes, i.e., the uncompressed breasts, from real patient data for the following two reasons. First, we are interested in a realistic but smooth estimate of the uncompressed breast shape omitting artefactual shape variations of individual examples. Second, the statistical shape model significantly reduces the number of shape parameters to be estimated (see below). From a statistical point of view, this simplifies the prediction problem, allowing successful training with less training data. Thus we strive for capturing as much shape information as possible in as few parameters as possible.

Here, we employ a simple linear shape model [10]: a shape $s = (x_n, y_n, z_n)_{n=1,\ldots,N}$ consisting of N points is described as linear combination $s = \bar{s} + Py$ where P is a matrix formed by base vectors of the shape space, $\bar{s}$ is the mean shape, and $y = (y_1, \ldots, y_L)$ are the shape parameters. The base vectors are found by Principal Component Analysis (see reference [10]). The amount of variation captured by the model is determined by the number of principal components L included in the model. Here, it turns out

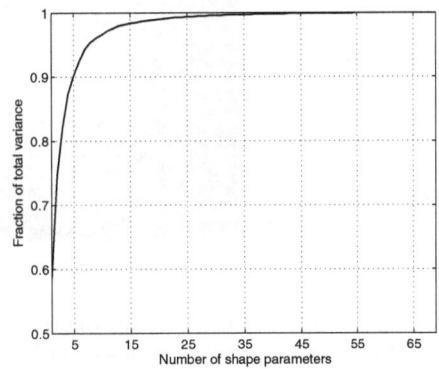

Fig. 2. The fraction of total shape variance plotted against the number of used shape parameters

that only $L = 5$ shape parameters are sufficient for preserving 90% of the total variance in a sample of 74 breasts (see Fig. 2). After verifying the shape space projections of these 74 breasts and given our training base for shape prediction we consider 5 shape parameters to be sufficient for our current system. This restriction also leverages the problem of the imperfect ground-truth at hand, i.e., larger uncompressed breasts within our data collection are occasionally deformed by the coils used for MR scanning as depicted in Fig. 4 (c). Note that in order to align the model shapes and establish point correspondence we re-sample relative to the same anatomical entities as for the compressed DBT shapes.

2.3 3D Shape Prediction by Multiple Multi-variate Random Forest Regression

Predicting $L = 5$ real-valued shape coefficients from a K-dimensional feature vector can be cast as the multiple multi-variate regression problem $f : \mathcal{X} \to \mathcal{Y}$ with $y = f(x)$, $x \in \mathcal{X} = \mathbb{R}^K$, $y \in \mathcal{Y} = \mathbb{R}^L$.

Here, we have chosen to use a Random Forest (RF) regressor [11] since it can capture linear as well as nonlinear dependencies and is known to achieve good generalization performance in general. While the more popular RF classifier employs randomized *decision* trees, RF regression uses an ensemble of M randomized *regression* trees. Like classification trees, regression trees partition the domain $\mathcal{Y}$ of response variables y into J regions $\mathcal{R} = \{\mathcal{R}_j | j = 1, \ldots, J\}$ with $\mathcal{Y} = \bigcup_{j=1}^{J} \mathcal{R}_j$ and $\bigcap_{j=1}^{J} \mathcal{R}_j = \emptyset$. Unlike classification trees, regression trees model the distribution of response variables for any region R_j as a joint normal distribution with constant mean μ_j and covariance Σ_j. Since the response variables y are the shape parameters of a linear statistical shape model here, they are uncorrelated by construction [10]. Hence, we assume that $\Sigma_j = \text{diag}(\sigma_{j_1}^2, \sigma_{j_2}^2, \ldots, \sigma_{j_L}^2)$

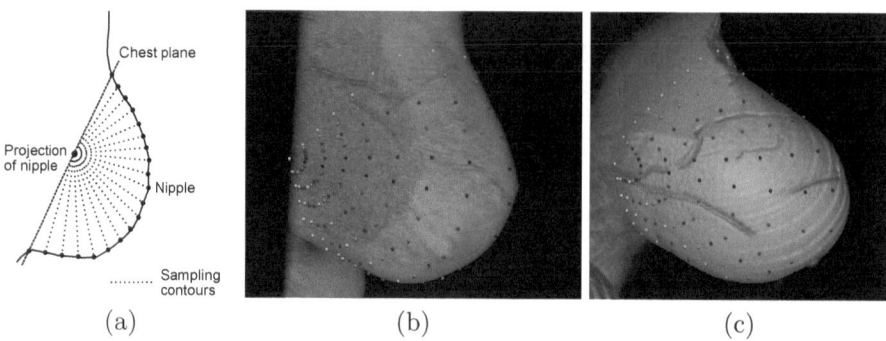

(a)   (b)   (c)

Fig. 3. The anatomical entities and the contours of the surface re-sampling planes in the MLO plane (a), and the canonical surface re-sampling scheme applied to a DBT scan (b) and an MR scan (c) of a compressed and uncompressed breast, respectively. Radiographic images with courtesy of University Hospital Erlangen.

is a diagonal matrix with determinant $|\boldsymbol{\Sigma}_j| = \prod_{l=1}^{L} \sigma_{j_l}^2$. Randomized regression tree induction can be summarized as follows: given a training sample $\mathcal{T} = \{(\boldsymbol{x}_i, \boldsymbol{y}_i)|i = 1, \ldots, I\} \subset \mathcal{X} \times \mathcal{Y}$ with cardinality T, regions $\mathcal{R}_\nu$ are recursively split into $\mathcal{R}_\nu = \mathcal{R}_{\nu_1} \cup \mathcal{R}_{\nu_2}$ with $\mathcal{R}_{\nu_1} \cap \mathcal{R}_{\nu_2} = \emptyset$, where each region $\mathcal{R}_\nu$ is associated with a node ν of a binary tree and a subset $\mathcal{T}_\nu \subset \mathcal{T}$ of the training sample with cardinality T_ν. Each split is defined by a threshold t and an index m to one of the features. It partitions $\mathcal{T}_\nu$ into subsets $\mathcal{T}_{\nu_1} = \{(\boldsymbol{x}_i, \boldsymbol{y}_i) \in \mathcal{T}_\nu | x_{i_m} \leq t\}$ and $\mathcal{T}_{\nu_2} = \{(\boldsymbol{x}_i, \boldsymbol{y}_i) \in \mathcal{T}_\nu | x_{i_m} > t\}$. The optimal split is chosen among randomly selected features as to maximize the decrease in sample entropy

$$\triangle i(\nu) = T_\nu \cdot \ln |\boldsymbol{\Sigma}_\nu| - (T_{\nu_1} \cdot \ln |\boldsymbol{\Sigma}_{\nu_1}| + T_{\nu_2} \cdot \ln |\boldsymbol{\Sigma}_{\nu_2}|).$$

During application, i.e., shape prediction, a feature vector $\boldsymbol{x}$ is passed to appropriate tree leaf nodes ν_m according to the induced feature thresholds for each regression tree $m \in \{1, \ldots, M\}$. Finally, the mean values $\boldsymbol{\mu}_j = \boldsymbol{\mu}_{\nu_m} \in \mathcal{Y}$ from the leaf nodes (corresponding to a region R_j) are averaged for prediction.

2.4   Thin-Plate Spline-Based Lesion Mapping from Corresponding Surface Points

A TPS mapping [12], which is computed based on two input shapes $\boldsymbol{s}$ and $\boldsymbol{s}'$, is a function $f_{TPS} : \mathbb{R}^3 \rightarrow \mathbb{R}^3$ that maps each point of the input shape to its corresponding point in the target shape, i.e., $f_{TPS}(x_n, y_n, z_n) = (x'_n, y'_n, z'_n)$. Its parameters are based on closed-form solutions minimizing the integral quadratic variation for each coordinate axis. Being a continuous mapping it interpolates between the known data points and can therefore be used for mapping lesions $\boldsymbol{p} = (x, y, z)^T$ from within the compressed breast $\boldsymbol{s}$ to within the predicted uncompressed breast $\boldsymbol{s}' = \bar{\boldsymbol{s}} + \boldsymbol{P}\boldsymbol{y}$.

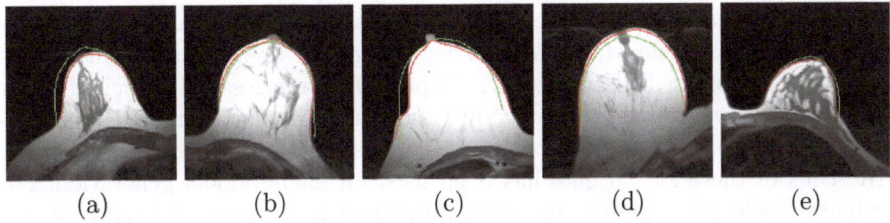

Fig. 4. Exemplary results for shape prediction on unseen data (a–e). The contour of the predicted shape is depicted in green, the one of the ground-truth annotation in red. Radiographic images with courtesy of University Hospital Erlangen.

For that reason we establish point correspondences between compressed and uncompressed shapes s and s'. Both the source shapes and the target shapes are parameterized relative to common anatomical entities that are identifiable in both cases. Figure 3 (a) summarizes the scheme with respect to an MLO scan.

- The first entity used is the nipple. It is automatically detected in the DBT images and has been manually annotated in the uncompressed breast shapes.
- The second entity is the chest plane, which we define as the plane orthogonal to the MLO plane intersecting with the inframammary fold and its counterpart at the top of the DBT MLO scan. Both points are detected in the image slice aligning with the MLO plane and going through the nipple of the 3D MLO scan by analyzing the surface contour for curvature characteristics. In the uncompressed breast shapes these points have been manually annotated.
- The rotation axis for surface re-sampling is the axis orthogonal to the MLO plane intersecting with the nipple's projection onto the chest plane.
- Further surface points within the MLO plane through the nipple are equidistantly sampled between the nipple and the inframammary fold and between the nipple and the top delineation of the breast. Then, intersection contours between the surface and the planes rotated around the rotation axis defined before and passing through the re-sampled points in the MLO plane are extracted. Equidistant re-sampling of these contours yields the remaining points of the re-sampled surface. This is done the same way for surfaces originating from DBT scans as well as uncompressed breast surfaces.

Figure 3 (b+c) shows a compressed/uncompressed breast pair where the described canonical re-sampling scheme has been applied.

3   Experimental Setting and Results

Nipple detection has been trained and evaluated on 122 annotated training data sets, i.e., DBT scans. The 8-fold cross-validated mean position error is $5.89\pm6.56\,\mathrm{mm}$, which reflects the annotation uncertainty.

The shape model has been computed from a population of 74 surface breast shapes. They all have been manually annotated in MR data showing hanging breasts as the patients all lay prone at the time of image acquisition. Evaluation of shape prediction has been carried out on 24 breast shape pairs (compressed/uncompressed). For these 24 shapes, DBT images and associate input shapes as well as ground-truth uncompressed target shapes from MR are available as the patients underwent both types of examination. However, none of the MR scans of these 24 patients has been used for shape model generation. For evaluation of lesion mapping, an expert radiologist has annotated 49 corresponding points inside the breast both in the DBT scan and in the accompanying MR scan. These expert annotations are used to assess accuracy of lesion mapping.

The projection of the original breast shapes into the 5-dimensional shape space yields nice and smooth shapes but also a mean average surface distance of already 10.57±4.36 mm. Using fully-automatic nipple detection and the proposed regression approach, the mean average surface distance slightly increases to 15.80±4.70 mm (result from 8-fold cross-validation). Exemplary results are depicted in Fig. 4, which also demonstrates the desired smoothing behavior of our method (see Fig. 4(c)). The

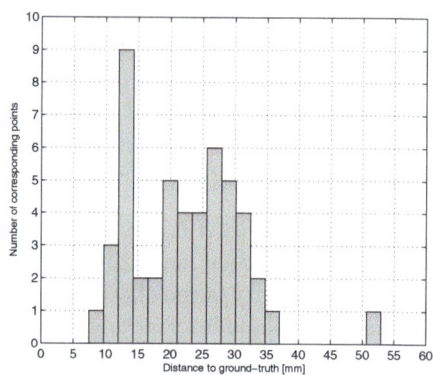

Fig. 5. The histogram of localization errors achieved for lesion mapping

evaluation of the final lesion mapping step yields a mean localization error of 22.48±8.67 mm (see Figs. 5 and 6). Note, however, that this error also includes the intentional discrepancy between the smoothed breast surface after shape space projection and the annotated breast surface in MR. Thus, it cannot be compared with accuracies obtained by methods that have access to the exact target shape. Feature extraction takes 26 s on average where 86% of the time is spent detecting the nipple. Shape prediction takes 36 ms. Comparison of our results to existing methods for lesion mapping is difficult due to the lack of

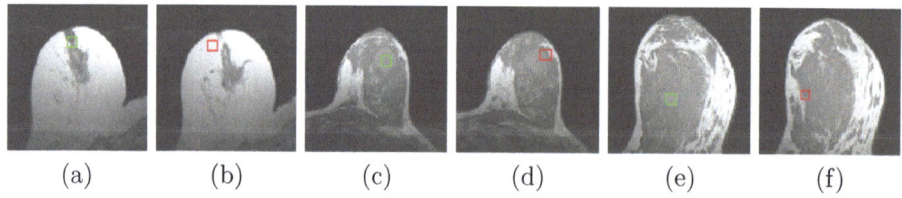

| (a) | (b) | (c) | (d) | (e) | (f) |

Fig. 6. Lesion mapping results. The images show ground-truth annotations (a, c, and e) and associated locations estimated by our method (b, d, and f). Radiographic images with courtesy of University Hospital Erlangen.

competing methods addressing exactly the same problem. In spite of this, van Schie et al. [5] report position errors for lesion mapping between ipsilateral DBT scans in a comparable range, which they consider reasonably accurate. Further improvement is certainly desirable for clinical application of our method.

4   Conclusions

In this paper we have presented a novel method for uncompressed breast shape prediction from 3D DBT image volumes. As a core contribution, the method does not involve any explicit biomechanical modeling of deformations, e.g., induced by gravity or compression. Instead, we make use of data-driven multiple multivariate RF regression to immediately predict uncompressed target shapes in terms of their shape parameters describing them in a statistical shape space. We apply a TPS mapping to map lesions identified in the input data to the corresponding location in the predicted uncompressed breast. For that, breast surface point correspondences have been defined relative to anatomical entities that are identifiable both in the compressed and in the uncompressed breast. These entities are fully-automatically detected in the DBT scans. Processing one data set takes less than half a minute where most of the time is due to feature extraction. The achieved lesion mapping accuracy is encouraging and supports further refinement of the proposed data-driven approach.

References

1. Gilbert, F.J., Young, K.C., Astley, S.M., Whelehan, P., Gillan, M.G.C.: Digital Breast Tomosynthesis. NHS Cancer Screening Programmes, Sheffield (2010)
2. Tanner, C., White, M., Guarino, S., Hall-Craggs, M.A., Douek, M., Hawkes, D.J.: Large breast compressions: Observations and evaluation of simulations. Med. Phys. 38(2), 682–690 (2011)
3. Samani, A., Bishop, J., Yaffe, M.J., Plewes, D.B.: Biomechanical 3-D finite element modeling of the human breast using MRI data. IEEE Trans. Med. Imag. 20(4), 271–279 (2001)
4. Zhang, Y., Qiu, Y., Goldgof, D.B., Sarkar, S., Li, L.: 3D finite element modeling of nonrigid breast deformation for feature registration in X-ray and MR images. In: IEEE Workshop Appl. Comp. Vis., Austin, TX, USA, p. 38 (2007)
5. van Schie, G., Tanner, C., Snoeren, P., Samulski, M., Leifland, K., Wallis, M.G., Karssemeijer, N.: Correlating locations in ipsilateral breast tomosynthesis views using an analytical hemispherical compression model. Phys. Med. Biol. 56(15), 4715–4730 (2011)
6. Lorensen, W.E., Cline, H.E.: Marching cubes: A high resolution 3D surface construction algorithm. Comput. Graph. 21(4), 163–169 (1987)
7. Zheng, Y., Barbu, A., Georgescu, B., Scheuering, M., Comaniciu, D.: Four-chamber heart modeling and automatic segmentation for 3D cardiac CT volumes using Marginal Space Learning and steerable features. IEEE Trans. Med. Imag. 27(11), 1668–1681 (2008)

8. Wels, M., Zheng, Y., Carneiro, G., Huber, M., Hornegger, J., Comaniciu, D.: Fast and Robust 3-D MRI Brain Structure Segmentation. In: Yang, G.-Z., Hawkes, D., Rueckert, D., Noble, A., Taylor, C. (eds.) MICCAI 2009, Part II. LNCS, vol. 5762, pp. 575–583. Springer, Heidelberg (2009)
9. Sofka, M., Ralovich, K., Zhang, N.B.J., Zhou, S.K.: Integrated Detection Network (IDN) for pose and boundary estimation in medical images. In: IEEE Int. Symp. Biomed. Imag.: Nano To Macro, Chicago, IL, USA, pp. 294–299 (2011)
10. Cootes, T.F., Taylor, C.J., Cooper, D.H., Graham, J.: Active Shape Models—their training and application. Comput. Vis. Image Understand. 61(1), 38–59 (1995)
11. Breiman, L.: Random Forests. Mach. Learn. 45(1), 5–32 (2001)
12. Bookstein, F.L.: Principal warps: Thin-plate splines and the decomposition of deformations. IEEE Trans. Pattern Anal. Mach. Intell. 11(6), 567–585 (1989)

Real Time Image-Based Tracking
of 4D Ultrasound Data

Ola Kristoffer Øye[1,2], Wolfgang Wein[3],
Dag Magne Ulvang[2], Knut Matre[4], and Ivan Viola[1]

[1] Department of Informatics, University of Bergen, Norway
[2] Christian Michelsen Research, Bergen, Norway
olak@cmr.no
[3] Chair for Computer Aided Medical Procedures (CAMP),
Technische Universität München, Germany
[4] Institute of Medicine, University of Bergen, Norway

Abstract. We propose a methodology to perform real time image-based tracking on streaming 4D ultrasound data, using image registration to deduce the positioning of each ultrasound frame in a global coordinate system. Our method provides an alternative approach to traditional external tracking devices used for tracking probe movements. We compare the performance of our method against magnetic tracking on phantom and liver data, and show that our method is able to provide results in agreement with magnetic tracking.

Keywords: Ultrasound, image registration, real time image processing.

1 Introduction

Medical ultrasound is a flexible, non-invasive, hand-held imaging modality used in a wide range of clinical applications. There is increased interest to assign precise 3D location information to ultrasound data, in order to enable reproducible results and diagnostic processes similar to how e.g. CT and MRI data are used. Such approaches often suffer from motion of the examined subject due to body movement, respiration and heart beat. Navigation in neurosurgical treatments is utilizing high-precision optical tracking systems by fixing optical markers to the cranium, surgical instrument, and ultrasound probe so that their mutual positions are known and involuntary movements are avoided. In the scenario of abdominal ultrasound, large organs in general do not fit into a single scan sector and they exhibit significant shifts due to respiration movements. In this scenario, external positional magnetic tracking is employed to measure position and rotation of the US probe in 3D space. This does not require line-of-sight, but suffers from other severe drawbacks. Most importantly, it tracks the position of the probe and not of the subject of examination, therefore assumptions have to be made that neither the magnetic transmitter nor the subject did move. This assumption is carried out by asking the patient to perform shallow breathing, or to stop breathing for a limited time period within the same phase of

N. Ayache et al. (Eds.): MICCAI 2012, Part I, LNCS 7510, pp. 447–454, 2012.
© Springer-Verlag Berlin Heidelberg 2012

a respiration cycle. These workarounds reduce to some degree positioning errors, but are sensitive to patient movement and unreliable when high precision is needed. Also, any presence of ferromagnetic objects deforms the magnetic field and makes the measurements imprecise. Thus, reliable positioning technology is urgently needed for abdominal US examinations. Our concept addresses exactly this challenge. First, we propose a novel tracking approach, where the positioning information is obtained internally, as a result of image registration of streaming US 3D data. Without an external reference, systematic errors such as drift influence the precision. As a second contribution, we therefore present effective strategies to minimize the drift. Third, registration as a tracking concept is carried out as a fast GPU implementation that converges sufficiently fast so that the probe can be tracked in real-time.

Related Work: A method for intensity-based registration of 3D US of the prostate is presented in [1]. In [2], a variational method is proposed to register a single pair of 3D US volumes of the liver while considering soft tissue deformations. [3] develops strategies for the mosaicing of multiple US volumes, including the use of multi-variate similarity measures. Designated similarity measures to deal with ultrasonic noise statistics have been developed as well, see e.g. [4]. All those works have however focused on the methodology as opposed to real-time computation. Work in [5] presents a fast GPU implementation and adds the registration to CT as a global map guiding the local US volumes. In [6], real-time 2D US with magnetic tracking is used to establish abdominal 4D US covering respiratory motion. Our new contribution is a designated approach for fully replacing an external tracking system using real-time registration of 4D US.

2   Methodology

Our image based tracking consists of two main steps (Fig. 1). First, a sweep over the organ of interest is performed. Using *dead reckoning tracking*, the individual frames from the sweep are mosaiced into a larger *compound volume*. Second, the compound volume is used as the reference for tracking streaming US data, using *reference volume tracking*. We have developed a solution that streams data real time from a GE Vivid E9 scanner over ethernet to any computer running our software, providing the registration framework with a stream of US volumes.

"Dead Reckoning" Image Based Tracking: In order to build the compound volume from streaming US data without an external tracking reference, we deduce the position of the current image from the position of the previous images, a principle known as "dead reckoning" from navigation. The most basic approach would be to use pairwise (PW) image registration to find the relative transformation T between the current image and the previous image in the stream. For each new image, we could use the product of all previous Ts to find the position of this image in a common coordinate system. This will however propagate the error from every PW registration to all following frames, leading to a significant drift over time. We therefore extend the classical PW image registration to multi-frame registration: Instead of registering a moving image to a single

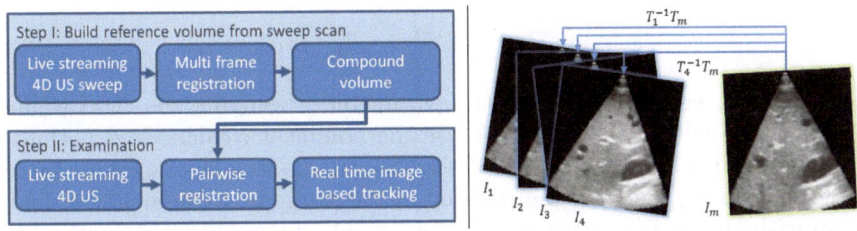

Fig. 1. Image based tracking workflow (left) and multiframe registration (right)

fixed image, we register our image to n fixed images in a global coordinate system (Fig. 1). For the live streaming case, we use the n most recent images. We use the sum of squared differences (SSD) as our image similarity measure. Specific US similarity measures have been developed [4], but their practical advantage has never been conclusively shown for clinical applications. Besides, the image noise statistics assumed for such methods are generally manipulated further down in the US processing chain (i.e. time-gain compensation, log-compression, scan-conversion etc.). Since we are registering neighbouring frames, we can assume that the anatomical regions have echoes of similar intensity due to only small changes in probe orientation. Given a linear transformation T, a fixed image I_f and a moving image I_m, we define the similarity between two images as

$$d(I_f, I_m; T) = \frac{\sum_x [I_f(x) - I_m(Tx)]^2}{N} + \begin{cases} 0 & \text{if } N \geq N_0 \\ \beta(1 - N/N_0) & \text{if } N < N_0 \end{cases} \tag{1}$$

where the sum is taken over all voxels x in the image and N is the number of overlapping voxels. The last term is a penalty function to avoid artificial low overlap minima, added for overlaps less than N_0 (typically 20% of total number of voxels). β is a constant penalty weight. Only voxels with an intensity over a certain threshold are included in the SSD calculation to avoid taking shadow regions into account. Based on (1), we construct a similarity measure D for a moving image vs. any number of fixed images in a common frame of reference:

$$D(\mathbf{I}^{(n)}, \mathbf{T}^{(n)}, I_m, T_m) = \sum_{i=0}^{n} \alpha_i [d(I_i, I_m, T_i^{-1} T_m)] \tag{2}$$

where $\mathbf{I}$ and $\mathbf{T}$ are vectors of size n containing the set of fixed images and their respective global transformations. The factor α_i is the fraction of total overlap for frame i, giving more overlapping frames stronger contribution. For $n = 1$, the equation reduces to PW image similarity. We allow for two types of linear transformations: rigid transformation with 6 degrees of freedom (DOF) and affine transformation without scaling with 9 DOF. We use the rigid transformation for dead reckoning tracking for compounding, assuming that the object does not deform under the compound sweep. The registration problem can be stated as:

$$\min_{x} D(\mathbf{I}^{(n)}, \mathbf{T}^{(n)}, I_m, T_m(x)) \tag{3}$$

where x is the vector containing the parameters specifying the rigid (affine) transformation with 6 (9) DOF. We use the nonlinear Nelder-Mead optimizer to minimize Eq. (3). The outcome of the registration of image I_m is the global transformation T_m, defining the position of the image in a common coordinate system with all previous registered frames, essentially providing the path of the ultrasound scan relative to the scanned object.

Compound Reference Volume Construction: Using the dead reckoning tracking, we can resample each frame with its T_m into a larger compound volume. The value of each individual voxel of the compound volume is updated for each new resampled frame by averaging over the current and all previous contributions to each particular voxel, as described in [7], appendix B.

Reference Volume Image Based Tracking: We can now use the compound volume as a fixed image, and streamed volumes as moving images to track probe movement, avoiding accumulated drift. This is the tracking mode that is to be used in an examination phase. We use our registration approach with $n = 1$ and with affine transformation. This is to allow for some deformation due to breathing and patient movement. Since we track wrt. a reference anatomical map instead of an external reference, the method is independent of patient movement and up to a certain level organ deformations. When starting the registration, an initial search for a good fit is performed using a large step size in the optimizer. Once a good fit is found, for each new frame, we seed the registration with the position of the previous frame. If the tracking fails, the user reinitializes the tracking.

Implementation: For real time performance, we implement registration and compounding on the GPU using OpenCL. The pipeline starts with the streaming providing the most recent US volume in GPU memory. The similarity (1) is computed on the GPU: given T, I_f and I_m, the calculation of a squared difference image (SDI) is fully parallizable. A parallel sum reduction is performed on the SDI, producing the scalar SSD, which is transferred to the CPU where the optimizer is running. For the compounding, we use a kernel that given T resamples the streaming volume to the compound volume for each voxel in parallel.

3   Results

We evaluate the performance of our proposed method on phantom and liver scans, using a GE Vivid E9 scanner with a 4V matrix array 3D probe with a typical framerate of 10 FPS. We compare image based tracking to magnetic tracking by attaching a magnetic tracker sensor (Flock of Birds) to the probe. This system is today used in commercial systems for compounding and landmark positioning ('GPS'). As the magnetic sensor can not be placed exactly on the transducer element, we need to calibrate the offset T_C between the magnetic sensor and the image coordinate system. We use the procedure in [7], appendix

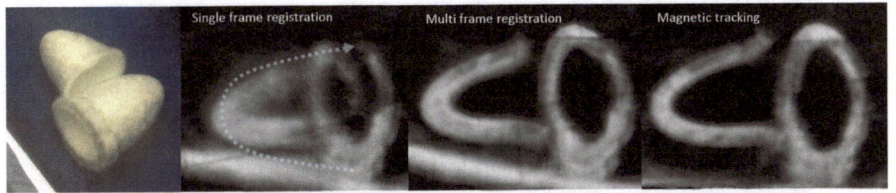

Fig. 2. Phantom used for evaluation (left). Compound volumes produced from image based tracking and magnetic tracking (top view).

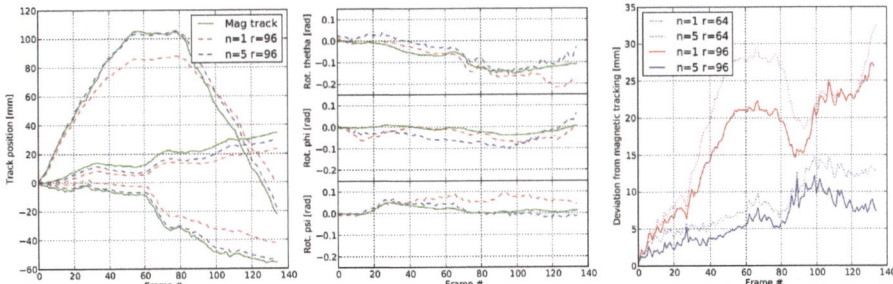

Fig. 3. Comparison of magnetic and image based tracking for sweep over phantom. Left: Tracked position of a point at the centre of the US volume, shown for all three coordinate components individually. Mid: Rotational components. Right: Discrepancy between magnetic and image based tracking for a point in the centre of the US volume.

B: Three volumes are acquired with external tracking (T_1, T_2, T_3). The relative Ts between the volumes are found using image registration. Using optimization, we find the rigid tracker offset T_C that minimizes the difference in relative movement as measured by the magnetic tracker and by the image registration.

Evaluation on Phantom: For our evaluation we use two heart phantoms in a water tank (Fig. 2). We calibrate T_C using the phantom, and from the variation of T_C over multiple calibrations, we find that the calibration has an error of the order of mms and a few degrees of rotation. The error is a combination of the magnetic tracking positioning error and the error in the image registration.

We start by performing a sweep over the phantom to build a compound volume. Fig. 3 shows the reconstructed probe path and the discrepancy between the calibrated magnetic tracking and our image based tracking for $n=1,5$ and volume number of voxels $r=64^3$, 96^3 (in our streaming we can vary the resolution of the scan converted US volume). The path of the sweep is indicated by the dotted arrow in Fig. 2. We see that for $n = 1$ (PW registration), there is a quite large drift between the image based and the magnetic tracking for both resolutions. By increasing n, we see that the discrepancy is significantly reduced. Further increases in n or r did not improve the results further. Using the tracking information, we build compound volumes for each of the cases. Slices from

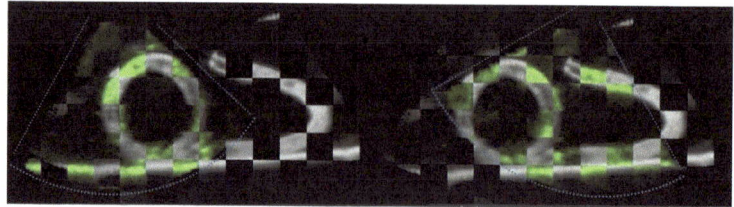

Fig. 4. Slice view of two time steps of image based tracking using compound volume as tracking reference. Streaming data in green, field of view indicated by dotted lines.

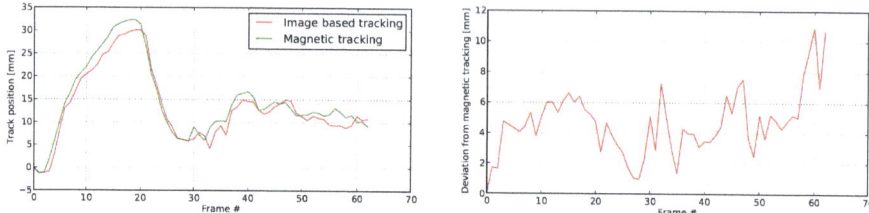

Fig. 5. Image based tracking for phantom scan using compound volume reference

the resulting volumes are shown in Fig. 2. We see that the PW registration has a quite large error as expected from Fig. 3, leading to a fuzzy and misaligned compound image. For the $n = 5$ case however, we see that we produce a compound volume with no visible drift. We actually get a better result than for the magnetic tracking, where we see that there is a shift in the right part of the image towards the end of the sweep. This can be explained by imperfections in the magnetic tracking calibration, and shows that magnetic tracking does not provide an absolute ground truth in our case. We then evaluate the *reference volume tracking* using the $n=5$ compound volume as a fixed image. To test the robustness of the method, we use a different probe path and a different FOV on the scanner from what was used when building the compound volume. Results are shown in Fig. 4, and we see that there is a good match between the compound volume and the streamed data. In Fig. 5 left, we compare with the magnetic tracking, plotting the distance between the centre of the tracked current frame and the initial frame. The right plot shows the distance between the centre point as tracked by magnetic and image based tracking. We see a discrepancy of the same magnitude as seen in Fig. 3. This is as expected, since we are using the compound volume from this scan as our tracking reference. We are also able to make a visual qualitative assessment that the image based tracking is able to follow the "anatomical" features of the phantom in the reference volume. As the $n=5$ compound volume was of higher quality than the one produced using magnetic tracking, this indicates that the image based tracking in this case provides a tracking of higher *anatomical* precision than the magnetic tracking.

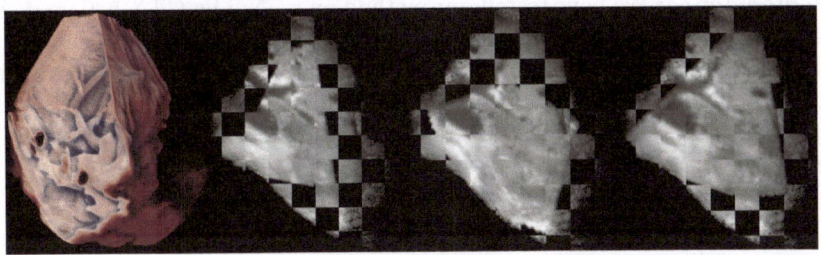

Fig. 6. Volume rendering of compound liver volume (left), three examples of streaming data with varying field-of-view registered to a reference compound volume for tracking

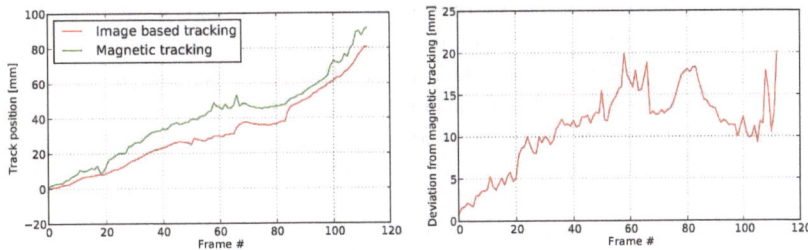

Fig. 7. Comparison of image based and magnetic tracking for a liver scan

Evaluation on Liver Scans: Having seen that we are able to build a compound volume and perform image based tracking on a phantom, we move to liver scans of a healthy volunteer (HV). We perform a sweep scan to build a compound volume while the HV is performing a deep breath hold. We avoid putting heavy pressure on the probe to minimize organ deformation. The subject is then allowed to breathe freely for a while, and then asked to perform a breath hold again. A new scan is then tracked wrt. to the compound volume, and we see from Fig. 6 that we are able to track the image in the anatomical reference of the compound volume using affine registration. We are using a FOV different from what was used for building the compound volume. Fig. 7 shows a comparison of the path reconstructed from the image based and magnetic tracking. They follow the same shape, but some discrepancy is expected due to the fact that the image based tracking registers into the anatomical reference, thus following an *anatomical path*, while the magnetic tracking simply follows the spatial path of the sensor. Since the HV had a period of breathing between the scans, there will inevitably be some movement and deformation of the liver compared to the initial sweep. Using affine registration, we are however able to handle this. This is an important point, since anatomical markers such as "GPS points" placed using magnetic tracking will be invalidated after patient movement, while our method is not affected by global patient movement, and able to handle some organ deformation.

Performance: We have tested our method on an Nvidia GTX 580, and show framerates for image based tracking for varying n and r in the table below. We are using $(1, 64)$ for the reference volume tracking results shown. We have also compared our results with a corresponding CPU based setup using C++ ITK. We find that PW reg. at $r = 64(96)$ takes ~10 (35)s per frame on an Intel i5 2.5 GHz, making our GPU implementation faster by two orders of magnitude.

(n, r)	$(1, 64)$	$(5, 64)$	$(1, 96)$	$(5, 96)$
FPS	8.2	2.5	4.5	1.2

4 Conclusion

We have presented an approach for real time image based tracking, and shown that we achieve results that are in agreement with magnetic tracking, currently the industry standard for tracking in abdominal US. The major advantage of our method is that we are tracking the location of the probe wrt. anatomy instead of an external tracking reference. This means that the tracking precision of our method is not affected by global patient movement. We are able to track the probe relative to the organ also under some deformation, in contrast to magnetic tracking which assumes an entirely static organ. For further work on evaluation, optical tracking or a phantom with fiducial features should be used. We also intend to improve our algorithms for deformable abdominal motion, which may eventually be used to create large-scale 4D US over the entire respiratory cycle.

References

1. Baumann, M., Mozer, P., Daanen, V., Troccaz, J.: Towards 3D Ultrasound Image Based Soft Tissue Tracking: A Transrectal Ultrasound Prostate Image Alignment System. In: Ayache, N., Ourselin, S., Maeder, A. (eds.) MICCAI 2007, Part II. LNCS, vol. 4792, pp. 26–33. Springer, Heidelberg (2007)
2. Zikic, D., Wein, W., Khamene, A., Clevert, D.-A., Navab, N.: Fast Deformable Registration of 3D-Ultrasound Data Using a Variational Approach. In: Larsen, R., Nielsen, M., Sporring, J. (eds.) MICCAI 2006, Part I. LNCS, vol. 4190, pp. 915–923. Springer, Heidelberg (2006)
3. Wachinger, C., Wein, W., Navab, N.: Three-Dimensional Ultrasound Mosaicing. In: Ayache, N., Ourselin, S., Maeder, A. (eds.) MICCAI 2007, Part II. LNCS, vol. 4792, pp. 327–335. Springer, Heidelberg (2007)
4. Wachinger, C., Navab, N.: Ultrasound Specific Similarity Measures for Three-Dimensional Mosaicing. In: Proc. SPIE Medical Imaging 2008, San Diego, USA (2008)
5. Kutter, O., Wein, W., Navab, N.: Multi-modal Registration Based Ultrasound Mosaicing. In: Yang, G.-Z., Hawkes, D., Rueckert, D., Noble, A., Taylor, C. (eds.) MICCAI 2009, Part I. LNCS, vol. 5761, pp. 763–770. Springer, Heidelberg (2009)
6. Nakamoto, M., et al.: Recovery of respiratory motion and deformation of the liver using laparoscopic freehand 3D ultrasound system. Medical Image Analysis 11(5), 429–442 (2007)
7. Wein, W.: Multimodal Integration of Medical Ultrasound for Treatment Planning and Interventions. PhD dissertation, Fakultät fur Informatik, Technische Universität München (2007), http://mediatum2.ub.tum.de/doc/620979/620979.pdf

Development of an MRI-Compatible Device for Prostate Focal Therapy

Jeremy Cepek[1], Blaine Chronik[1], Uri Lindner[2],
John Trachtenberg[2], and Aaron Fenster[1]

[1]Robarts Research Institute, Western University, London, Canada
{jcepek,afenster}@robarts.ca, bchronik@uwo.ca
[2]Department of Surgical Oncology, Division of Urology,
University Health Network, Toronto, Canada
lindneruri@gmail.com, john.trachtenberg@uhn.ca

Abstract. We present a device that has been developed for delivering prostate focal thermal therapy under magnetic resonance imaging (MRI) guidance. Unlike most existing devices, ours is capable of delivering needles to targets in the prostate without removing the patient from the scanner. This feature greatly reduces procedure time and increases accuracy. The device consists of a mechanical linkage encoded with optical incremental encoders, and is manually actuated. A custom magnetic resonance (MR) compatible alignment interface allows the user to manually align the device to its target with high accuracy in-bore in very short time. The use of manual actuation over motors greatly reduces the complexity and bulk of the system, making it much more compact and portable. This is important when dealing with such tight space constraints. Needle targeting experiments in gel phantoms have demonstrated the device's ability to deliver needles with an accuracy of 2.1 +/- 1.3 mm.

Keywords: MRI-compatible device, prostate cancer, focal thermal therapy.

1 Introduction

1.1 Background

It is estimated that over 240,000 men will be diagnosed with prostate cancer (PCa) in the United States in 2012, and over 28,000 men will die from it [1]. While treatments of the disease can be very effective if caught in the early stages, there is a growing belief among many clinicians that PCa is being over-treated with radical approaches. As a result, patients are being subjected to unnecessary morbidity, particularly those with low-risk disease. For patients in the low-risk category, disease management options range from radical prostatectomy to active surveillance (AS). AS has proven to reduce over-treatment [2], but the dropout rate is about 20%, as the disease either progresses or the patient makes the decision to request definitive therapy [3]. In some of these cases complete radical resection may be "therapeutic overkill", and leave the patient with reduced sexual, urinary and bowel functions. Alternatively, properly

N. Ayache et al. (Eds.): MICCAI 2012, Part I, LNCS 7510, pp. 455–462, 2012.

executed selective focal ablative therapy could provide an effective option for definitive disease management with minimal treatment-related morbidity. Thus, there is a need for an accurate method of delivering focal prostate therapies.

One of the most common methods of delivering needles to the prostate for biopsy or therapy is with the aid of transrectal ultrasound (TRUS) imaging. While TRUS does provide real-time visualization of needles during insertion, it is not capable of accurately locating tumours or clearly visualizing the peripheral zone; the site of ~80% of prostate cancers [4]. Magnetic resonance imaging (MRI) has the ability to image tumours, delineate the peripheral zone, and display tissue temperature for thermal ablative procedures [4]. MRI is therefore a very promising imaging modality for guiding focal thermal ablation therapies, since it can provide accurate target localization, real-time needle trajectory and depth tracking, and monitoring of the ablative procedure, all in the same session.

1.2   Previous Work

Various authors have reported the development of devices for the delivery of needles to the prostate under MRI guidance [5,6,7,8]. Most of these devices use either pneumatic or ultrasonic motors to align a needle with a target, and require removal of the patient from the scanner for manual needle insertion. Verification of needle placement is then made by placing the patient back into the scanner and re-imaging [5,6]. This approach increases procedure time considerably, and reduces the potential needle placement accuracy due to increased patient motion. Other authors report fully automated devices [7,8]. With these devices, needle insertion is motorized, and patient safety is compromised, since there is no haptic feedback provided to the physician. In an attempt to overcome these issues, we have developed an MRI-compatible needle trajectory alignment device that is manually actuated, and allows for adjustment of the needle trajectory and manual needle insertion with the patient in-bore. It is hypothesized that this system will allow for accurate delivery of prostate focal thermal therapy with minimal procedure time, while maintaining patient safety. The target accuracy to be achieved is +/- 2.5 mm, based on the finding that tumours of clinically significant size are at least ~10 mm in diameter [9].

2   Methods and Materials

2.1   Device Design

We present a device that allows a physician to precisely align a needle guide with an intended target in the prostate under MRI guidance. This is achieved through the use of four linear motion stages attached to an arm that holds needle templates. Movement of the arm is achieved manually by the physician. Two locking handles allow the needle insertion point and trajectory to be independently adjusted using the alignment handle. This approach removes the complexity and bulk that would be added by using motors for positioning, and still allows accurate targeting in less than 40 s with the patient in-bore. The two rear templates allow the physician to insert needles without moving the patient out of the bore of the scanner by extending the point of needle insertion within reach. The vertical slides are supported by spring counterbalances and ensure the device's position is maintained when the handle is released. An MR-visible fiducial arrangement is used to register the device's initial position in the scanner, and subsequent movements are tracked with optical linear encoders. The device is shown in Figure 1.

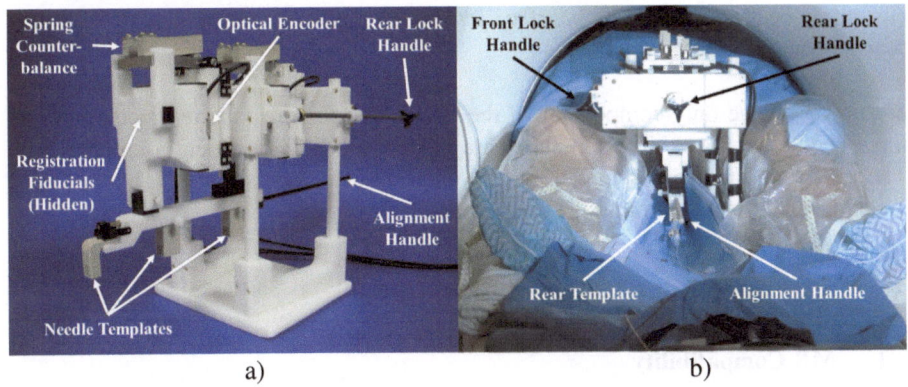

Fig. 1. a) Device components, b) device in position with a patient

The patient is positioned head first supine in the scanner, and needles are inserted through the perineum. The needle is imaged as it is inserted, providing direct comparison between its position and the patient's anatomy. The templates allow for large tumours to be treated with multiple needles simultaneously.

User Interface. MR images are transferred from the scanner to a custom graphical user interface on a laptop via FTP. This interface allows the user to localize the device's registration fiducials and targets (tumours). The registration and target data is sent to a custom embedded electronics system that decodes linear position from the encoders and computes kinematics solutions. The kinematics solutions are used to send data to a custom MR-compatible visual alignment interface, placed immediately outside of the MRI bore. The interface indicates which direction the handle must be moved to reach the given target. Once the device has been aligned to the target within a given level of precision, only the middle LED in the grid will be displayed. Figure 2 shows this interface.

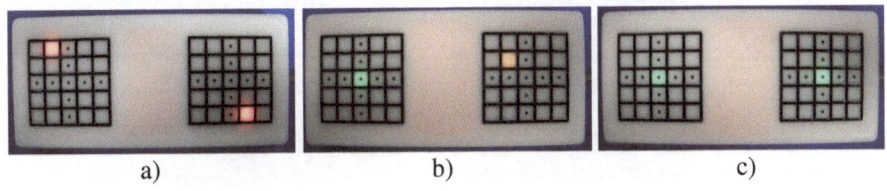

Fig. 2. Alignment interface: a) not aligned, b) front stages aligned, rear stages within 3 mm in both directions, c) all stages within 0.25 mm of target

Materials & Components. All major components of the device are constructed of either Delrin or fiberglass. The linear ball slide bearings in the linear stages consist of stainless steel (grade 303) rods and titanium races with ceramic balls. All fasteners are either brass or plastic. Aluminum was used for various small components. Linear position encoding is achieved with non-magnetic incremental encoders (LIA-20, Numerik Jena, Jena, Germany). The encoders output a sine-cosine signal in the kHz range and do not interfere with the MRI's RF system. The encoders are connected to a custom embedded electronics interface inside the console room via RF filters in the scanner room's penetration panel.

Sterilization. The only components of the device that require full sterilization are the three needle templates. The templates are made from PEEK, which is autoclavable. The rest of the device is completely enclosed in a sterile plastic bag. The templates are attached to device through the plastic bag.

3   Experimental Methods and Results

3.1   MR Compatibility

It is important for the device to not interfere with the scanner's ability to produce high-quality images, and for the scanner to not interfere with the device's ability to accurately target tumours. Specifically, the presence of the device must not produce any distortion or reduction in signal-to-noise ratio (SNR) in the images, and the scanner must not interfere with the device's operation by introducing significant force, torque, vibration, or heating, or affect the operation of the encoders.

The distortion and SNR tests were based on the relevant ASTM and NEMA standards, respectively. Accordingly, these effects were evaluated by imaging a grid phantom located superior to the device for each of the following cases: 1) device not present (baseline), 2) device in position, not connected, 3) device in position, cables connected, not powered, 4) device in position, cables connected, powered. Since the device will not be moved during imaging, this case was not considered. The experimental setup is shown in Figure 3.

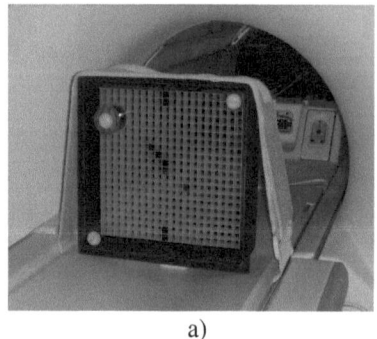
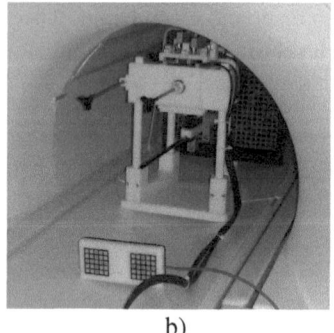

a)   b)

Fig. 3. Setup for MR-compatibility tests: a) the grid phantom used, b) device positioning

The device was positioned so the distance from the template to the center of the phantom was equivalent to the average distance to the center of a patient's prostate (~10 cm), with the center of the phantom at the isocenter. Axial gradient echo images were acquired on a 3 T scanner (MR750, GE Healthcare, Milwaukee, WI) with the parameters: field of view (FOV): 400 mm x 400 mm, matrix: 256 x 256, TR = 270 ms, TE = 4 ms, flip angle: 25°. Each set of images was acquired with bandwidths of both 195 and 977 Hz/pixel. The low bandwidth image set was used to evaluate image distortion, while the higher bandwidth set was used for SNR calculations. This presents an overestimate of the effect of the device on the images. There was negligible distortion in all cases. SNR was calculated using a mean signal in a 30 x 60 voxel region near the middle of the FOV, and the standard deviation of the signal in a region of the same size outside the phantom. The SNR was calculated in image slices that contained only fluid. SNR was found to decrease by no more than 6% from its value in case 1 in all other cases. MR thermometry images have also been acquired with the device present, and no significant interference was detected.

Effects of the scanner on the device were minimized by using non-magnetic materials for all major components. Non-magnetic metals were used only for small components, and did not cause any significant force, torque, heating or vibration effects. Fidelity of the encoder operation is ensured by rechecking that the encoder counts are zero each time an index pulse is received.

3.2   Calibration

Open-Air Calibration. An experiment was performed to quantify the device's ability to place a needle at a target in open air. The experiment involved fitting the manipulator arm with two steel tooling balls, and measuring their positions over the device's full range of motion using a coordinate measuring machine (CMM). The CMM has a total volumetric accuracy of 5.2 μm. Error in position of the furthest tooling ball (representative of the placement of a needle tip at the base of the prostate) was found to be 0.29 +/- 0.11 mm.

MRI Calibration. Calibration of the device within the MRI workspace requires careful consideration of the sources of geometric errors present in MR images. Figure 4 shows a breakdown of the major sources of error that contribute to the total error in needle targeting.

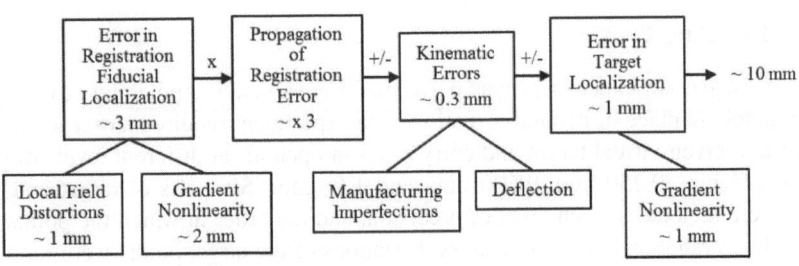

Fig. 3. Sources of needle targeting error

Errors from local field distortions mainly result in errors in the image readout direction. For calibration purposes, minimization of this error can be achieved by acquiring two sets of fiducial images, with the readout direction swapped, and only measuring coordinates in the phase encode direction [10]. Gradient field nonlinearity results in both in-plane geometric errors and slice select errors [11]. These errors are specific to the MR system and are corrected for using image warping algorithms applied by the scanner software after image acquisition. Distortion correction algorithms generally do not correct the slice select errors; furthermore, residual in-plane errors remain due to truncation of the spherical harmonic expansion terms [11].

The propagation error exists because the distance from the registration fiducial arrangement to the prostate is much larger than the distance between the fiducials. This source of error is fixed by the device geometry. The kinematic errors result from imperfections in manufacturing of the device, and deflection of materials. As found in the open air calibration experiment, these errors are relatively small (~ 0.3 mm), and are considered insignificant. Before calibration, the total error in targeting a point within the MRI is estimated to be as much as ~ 10 mm.

A simple calibration method has been applied, whereby the MRI image space in the region of the prostate is registered to the device space with a rigid transformation. Registration was performed using Procrustes analysis. Justification for the effectiveness of this method is based on the observations:

1. The main source of error is gradient field nonlinearity (assumes a good shim over the target volume).
2. The gradient field nonlinearity error is a function of position in the scanner and varies only a small amount over small distances (i.e. over the size of a prostate and the registration fiducial arrangement).
3. The patient and device will always be placed in approximately the same position.

The calibration procedure was performed by fitting the device's manipulator arm with an arrangement of two MR-visible spheres. These spheres were positioned over a region the size of a typical prostate and imaged. A 3D rigid transformation was computed between the positions of the fiducials in the images and their supposed locations from the kinematics solution. Before correction, the maximum error in fiducial position was greater than 5 mm. Calibration reduced this to less than 1 mm. This transformation was then applied to subsequent targeting sessions.

3.3   Targeting Tests

Time to Target. An experiment was performed to evaluate the potential advantage of using motors in place of manual actuation. The experiment required a user to align the device to a given virtual target and entry point in open-air at different levels of precision: 0.125 mm, 0.250 mm, 0.500 mm, and 1.00 mm. Six pairs of target and entry points were targeted at each level of precision, and the order in which the points were targeted was randomized for four users. Locations of the target points were representative of targets in each sextant of the prostate. Table 1 shows the time to successfully target the device (and lock it in position) at various levels of precision.

Table 1. Time to target at various precision levels

	0.125 mm	0.250 mm	0.500 mm	1.00 mm
Mean Time (s)	38	21	15	11
Standard Deviation (s)	11	6	4	2

The results show that targeting was possible in less than 40 s, even at a higher precision level than device's accuracy in open air. Since each therapy session requires insertion of no more than 3 or 4 needles, it is reasoned that motorized positioning could save no more than a few minutes in a procedure that lasts about 2 hours. Thus, we conclude that the addition of motorized trajectory alignment is not justified.

Needle Targeting Accuracy. After calibration, as described in section 2.3, the device was used to deliver needles to targets in a 3T scanner (MR750, GE Healthcare, Milwaukee, WI). The targets consisted of 10 mm spheres of gelatin, doped with gadolinium (Magnevist, 0.005 mmol/ml). Nine such spheres were embedded in a rectangular alginate phantom, as alginate has mechanical properties similar to that of pelvis connective tissue [12]. The spheres were arranged in an approximate grid pattern of size ~ 65 mm x 65 mm, at a depth of ~ 85 mm under the surface of the alginate. This arrangement is representative of typical locations of tumours in a prostate relative to the device. The experimental setup is shown in Figure 5a (needles were inserted with the phantom at the isocenter). Figure 5b shows the needles inserted to their targets (axial slices). Note that this is a concatenation of images from needle insertions into each of the nine spheres. The needles appear as bright dots within the gel spheres.

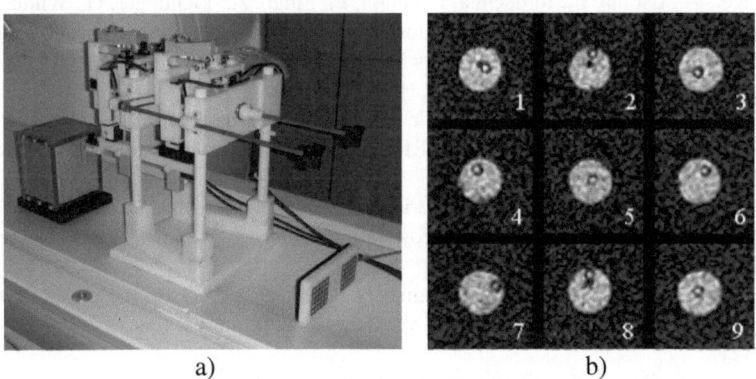

a)   b)

Fig. 5. Needle targeting test: a) setup, b) axial slices showing needles inserted into gel spheres

Positioning error was calculated as the distance between the centroid of the needles after each insertion and the centroid of the gel spheres before needle insertion. The mean error was found to be 2.1 +/- 1.3 mm. These results show that the device is capable of accurately delivering needles to tumours of the smallest clinically significant size.

4   Summary

We have presented a system for the delivery of MR-guided prostate focal therapies. Targeting tests showed that the device can be aligned to targets in less than 40 seconds with a precision that is greater than its accuracy in open air, validating the use of a manual actuation method. A needle insertion experiment in a gel phantom has shown the device to be capable of delivering needles to targets with an average error of 2.1 mm. Results from initial clinical testing will be presented at the conference.

References

1. Siegel, R., Naishadham, D., Jemal, A.: Cancer statistics. Cancer J. Clin. 62(1), 10–29 (2012)
2. Klotz, L., Zhang, L., Lam, A., Nam, R., Mamedov, A., Loblaw, A.: Clinical Results of Long-Term Follow-Up of a Large, Active Surveillance Cohort With Localized Prostate Cancer. J. Clin. Oncol. 28(1), 126–131 (2010)
3. Ercole, B., Marietti, S., Fine, J., Albertsen, P.: Outcomes Following Active Surveillance of Men With Localized Prostate Cancer Diagnosed in the Prostate Specific Antigen Era. J. Urology 180(4), 1336–1341 (2008)
4. Haider, M., van der Kwast, T., Tanguay, J., Evans, A., Hashmi, A.-T., Lockwood, G., Trachtenberg, J.: Combined T2-Weighted and Diffusion-Weighted MRI for Localization of Prostate Cancer. Am. J. Roentgenol. 189(2), 323–328 (2007)
5. Schouten, M., Ansems, J., Renema, W.K.J., Bosboom, D., Scheenen, T., Futterer, J.: The accuracy and safety aspects of a novel robotic needle guide manipulator to perform trans-rectal prostate biopsies. Med. Phys. 37(9), 4744–4750 (2010)
6. Krieger, A., Csoma, C., Iordachita, I., Guion, P., Singh, A., Fichtinger, G., Whitcomb, L.: Design and Preliminary Accuracy Studies of an MRI-Guided Transrectal Prostate Intervention System. In: Ayache, N., Ourselin, S., Maeder, A. (eds.) MICCAI 2007, Part II. LNCS, vol. 4792, pp. 59–67. Springer, Heidelberg (2007)
7. Goldenberg, A., Trachtenberg, J., Yi, Y., Weersink, R., Sussman, M., Haider, M., Ma, L., Kucharczyk, W.: Robot-assisted MRI-guided prostatic interventions. Robotica 28(2), 215–234 (2010)
8. Stoianovici, D., Song, D., Petrisor, D., Ursu, D., Mazilu, D., Mutener, M., Schar, M., Patriciu, A.: "MRI Stealth" robot for prostate interventions. Minimal. Invasiv. Ther. 16(4), 241–248 (2007)
9. Villers, A., McNeal, J., Freiha, F., Stamey, T.: Multiple cancers in the prostate. Morphologic features of clinically recognized versus incidental tumors. Cancer 70(9), 2313–2318 (1992)
10. Haacke, M., Brown, R., Thompson, M., Venkatesan, R.: Magnetic Resonance Imaging: Physical Principles and Sequence Design. J. Wiley-Liss, New York (1999)
11. Wang, D., Strugnell, W., Cowin, G., Doddrell, D., Slaughter, R.: Geometric distortion in clinical MRI systems. Part I: evaluation using a 3D phantom. Magn. Reson. Imaging 22(9), 1211–1221 (2004)
12. Lindner, U., Lawrentschuk, N., Weersink, R., Raz, O., Hlasny, E., Sussman, M., Davidson, S., Gertner, M., Trachtenberg, J.: Construction and Evaluation of an Anatomically Correct Multi-Image Modality Compatible Phantom for Prostate Cancer Focal Ablation. J. Urology 184(1), 352–357 (2010)

Intraoperative Ultrasound Guidance
for Transanal Endoscopic Microsurgery

Philip Pratt, Aimee Di Marco, Christopher Payne, Ara Darzi, and Guang-Zhong Yang

Hamlyn Centre for Robotic Surgery
Imperial College of Science, Technology and Medicine
London SW7 2AZ, UK
{p.pratt,a.di-marco,cjp04,a.darzi,g.z.yang}@imperial.ac.uk

Abstract. Local excision of rectal cancer with transanal endoscopic microsurgery has proved to be a viable alternative to conventional, more radical techniques, but the reduced sensory experience presents significant challenges for the surgeon. Accurate identification and complete removal of lesions and subsurface targets is currently a difficult task, often exacerbated by intraoperative tissue deformation. This work describes novel ultrasound calibration and effective visualisation methods designed to meet these requirements, relying solely on optical measurements and pattern tracking. Detailed quantitative phantom and porcine validation experiments confirm that the technique is both practical and an accurate means for assessing lesion thickness intraoperatively, leading directly to human clinical trials.

1 Introduction

Rectal carcinoma accounts for a significant number of cancer-related deaths in the developed world. Transanal endoscopic microsurgery [1] was introduced as an alternative to conventional, more radical resection techniques for the treatment of early-stage lesions, with the goal of reducing the relatively high mortality and morbidity, including functional impairment and stoma. Indeed, the recent prevalence of cancer screening programmes demands the more widespread use of an effective minimally invasive technique, capable of proportionately safe and accurate resection. The goal of this work is to provide real-time, intraoperative ultrasound guidance using a small microsurgery transducer, such that its images are correctly registered to and fused with endoscopic views of the surgical scene. Moreover, by addressing some of the remaining barriers that typically impede use in human subjects, the quantitative phantom and porcine study presented here suggests a rapid path for clinical translation.

Safety and convenience, combined with recent advances in image quality, have made ultrasound images an attractive candidate for use in augmented reality systems designed for diagnosis and intervention. This is particularly true in the context of minimally invasive, including robotic, surgical procedures where the reduced sensory experience presents the surgeon with significant challenges. Notable advances in this area include the 'sonic flashlight' of Stetten *et al.* [2], the 'DaVinci Canvas' developed by Leven *et al.* [3], the technique for freehand 3D ultrasound described by Ali and Logeswaran [4],

N. Ayache et al. (Eds.): MICCAI 2012, Part I, LNCS 7510, pp. 463–470, 2012.

and applications during laparoscopic partial nephrectomy and bronchoscopy introduced by Cheung *et al.* [5] and Dressel *et al.* [6], respectively. Langø *et al.* [7] provide an extensive review of navigated laparoscopic ultrasound and describe their own experiences of optimal resection planning during adrenalectomy in a porcine model. In addition, Schneider *et al.* [8] have performed a feasibility study for 'pick-up' ultrasound, using the renal vasculature to perform registration to preoperative CT images.

However, the relatively small scale afforded by the transanal approach and transducer size dictates that the localisation techniques employed to date in the most relevant studies, namely exogenous electromagnetic or optical tracking, robot kinematic feedback, either individually or in combination, are not sufficiently accurate or practical for the intended application. Indeed, the difficulties associated with performing precise hand-eye and probe calibrations, typically required in a contemporaneous manner, present important barriers to successful clinical translation.

During surgery, the radial extent of lesions is significantly easier to assess than the depth of penetration through the mucosal and sub-mucosal layers of the rectum wall. This can lead to excisions being too deep, resulting in perforation, or too shallow, leading to incomplete margins. The paucity of depth information is apparent in Fig. 1 (left), which shows a typical endoscopic view during a human case immediately prior to resection. Adopting lesion thickness measurement as an exemplar application, this work therefore describes a novel use for ultrasound overlay, based on optical pattern tracking alone, using a new dual pattern calibration method. An efficient tracking algorithm, driven by topological relationships between features, and visualisation methods is described. Phantom and porcine validation experiments are performed to measure overlay accuracy and gauge suitability for clinical translation.

2   Materials and Methods

2.1   Microsurgery Probe Calibration

The ultrasound transducer used in this study is a UST-533 multi-frequency linear array microsurgery probe (Hitachi Aloka Medical Ltd., Tokyo, Japan), driven by a ProSound ALPHA 10 cart. As illustrated in Fig. 1 (centre), its small dimensions and associated field of view (approximately 60mm) make it an ideal choice given the limited workspace imposed by the transanal endoscopic approach and the intended targets. By selecting a relatively high zoom factor on the cart (1 pixel ~ 50μm), the appropriate balance between level of detail and depth of tissue penetration is struck.

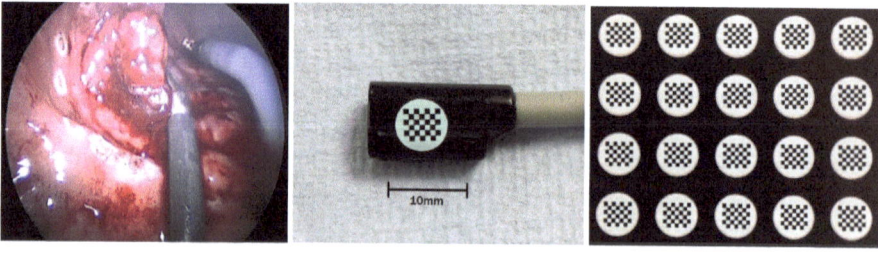

Fig. 1. Endoscopic view prior to resection, microsurgery probe and KeySurgical marker dots

The probe calibration process seeks to determine the static spatial transformation from the ultrasound image frame to the transducer frame. The latter is defined by a semi-permanently attached *KeyDot*® marker (KeySurgical Inc., Eden Prairie, MN, USA). Fig. 1 (right) illustrates the design, where non-symmetrical chessboard patterns are laser-engraved on 6.35mm diameter, 76.2µm thickness destructible acrylate discs. Overcoming another important translational barrier, the markers and adhesive are approved for human use and can withstand harsh environments and temperatures, including repeated sterilisation cycles. Further promoting longevity, the radial design ensures that there are no corners to lift. Once calibrated, the relationship between image and transducer frames remains fixed until the marker is replaced.

The spatial transformation, represented as an image scaling followed by a 6 DOF translation and rotation, is estimated by scanning a calibration object of known geometry and associating image points and their corresponding spatial positions. Following Chen *et al.* [9] and other studies, a multiple Z-wire arrangement is employed, where the scan images are manually segmented. The main challenge here is in the accurate manufacture of the phantom at a necessarily small scale. To this end, the calibration phantom is printed using an *Objet260 Connex* rapid prototype 3D printer (Objet Ltd., Rehovot, Israel). Typical build accuracies are in the range 20-85µm.

Fig. 2 (left) shows a cross-section through the phantom design, revealing conical guide holes and the boss on which a calibration pattern is mounted. Chosen for their very high straightness tolerance, Micron Hard high speed steel wires (Nachi-Fujikoshi Corp., Tokyo, Japan), of nominal diameter 250µm, are threaded through 300µm diameter holes in the opposing phantom walls. The complete device is shown in Fig. 2 (centre), together with a typical ultrasound scan image (right), the well having been filled with water at a temperature of approximately 38°C.

Images are captured using a 5mm diameter mono laparoscope (Karl Storz GmbH, Tuttlingen, Germany), forming part of the standard equipment inventory. Intrinsic camera parameters and distortion coefficients are estimated using an implementation of Zhang's calibration method [10, 12], using at least twenty phantom pattern images at different distances and orientations. This study employs the novel method of capturing both the phantom and transducer patterns in the same image (Fig. 3, left). By recovering the extrinsic parameters comprising the transformations between the patterns and their projections in that image, through the minimisation of reprojection error [12], it is possible to estimate the relationship between the phantom and transducer coordinate systems.

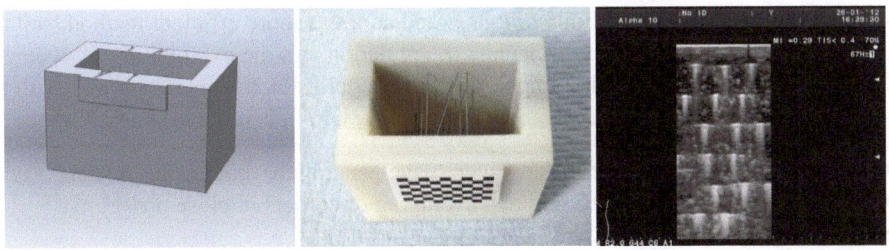

Fig. 2. Calibration phantom section, internal Z-wire pattern and microsurgery probe image

Specifically, Fig. 3 (centre) illustrates the coordinate frames involved during the calibration procedure: the calibration phantom frame **P**, the ultrasound image frame **U** and the transducer frame **T**. The camera coordinate frame is not shown. Given 2D points $\mathbf{p}_i$ in the ultrasound image frame and corresponding 3D locations $\mathbf{q}_i$ in the calibration phantom frame, the desired scale factor s and transformation $\mathbf{M}_{UT}$, mapping from the ultrasound image frame to the transducer frame, are found by minimisation of the following expression.

$$\sum_i \| \mathbf{M}_{UT}.s.\mathbf{p}_i - \mathbf{E}_T^{-1}\mathbf{E}_P.\mathbf{q}_i \|^2 \tag{1}$$

The matrices $\mathbf{E}_T$ and $\mathbf{E}_P$ represent the transducer and phantom extrinsics, respectively. Formulated as an absolute orientation problem [11], the solution can be found in closed form. The scale factor s is determined as the ratio of the root mean-squared deviations of the coordinates from their respective centroids. For comparison, the expression is also minimised in a more general form where the X and Y image scale factors are allowed to vary independently. Since the image-to-probe transformation is independent of the camera and associated video hardware, probe calibrations performed at different resolutions are, in principle, interchangeable once an appropriate ultrasound image scaling and translation has been applied. In this study, calibrations are performed at both SD (720×576i) and HD (1920×1080i) resolution to determine whether any improvement in accuracy using the latter is sufficient to warrant the inevitable decrease in processing performance.

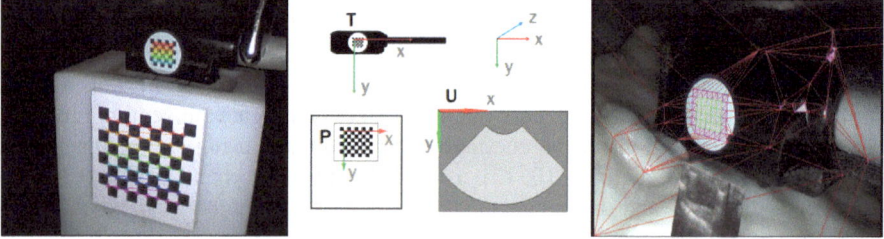

Fig. 3. Dual chessboard pattern recovery, coordinate frames and pattern tracking with overlay

2.2   Real-Time Pattern Tracking

While contour-based approaches to chessboard tracking [12] are typically robust, this study builds on the work of Shu *et al.* [13] and adopts a more efficient method, suitable for real-time use, based on Delaunay triangulation and the exploitation of geometric and topological constraints imposed by the pattern. Each frame, captured with a Quadro SDI card (NVIDIA Corp., Santa Clara, CA, USA), is processed as follows:

- feature selection (i.e. Sobel filter, Eigenimage generation, thresholding) [12]
- sub-pixel corner refinement [12] and averaging of corners in close proximity
- Delaunay triangulation [12]
- elimination of triangles with edge length greater than specified threshold
- elimination of triangles where edge ratio metric is greater than specified limit
- elimination of triangles that do not have three neighbours

- conversion to quadrilaterals by comparison and pairing of longest edges
- vertex orientation using cross products
- recursive flood-fill to determine relationships between quadrilaterals
- trim quadrilaterals that have fewer than two neighbours
- select largest group of connected quadrilaterals then locate 'top left' corner
- check width and height of connected quadrilateral pattern
- determine pattern orientation by comparing pixel averages in opposing corners.

The optimal tracking parameters (e.g. corner quality threshold) are determined by empirical optimisation over archetypal footage. In the event of a recognition failure, the last good pattern is used for up to a maximum of eight frames. Fig. 3 (right) shows the triangulation and quadrilaterals comprising a successful recognition.

2.3 Visualisation

Once a valid pattern has been identified, the corners and prevailing camera parameters are used to find the optimal extrinsic transformation [12]. Concatenated with the calibrated transformation M_{UT} this is used subsequently to project and render the ultrasound image texture in the correct location. The texture is blended with the underlying scene, using an adjustable alpha coefficient. The user may move the crop boundaries applied to the image texture, and also enable a measurement grid overlay with 1mm and 5mm graduations (Fig. 4, left). Textures and extrinsics are stored in a GPU ring buffer, such that 3D freehand reconstructions from multiple slices can be made at any time (Fig. 4, centre). Furthermore, a custom pixel shader is used to pass the ultrasound image through a 1D transfer function performing histogram equalisation on-the-fly. This markedly improves image contrast and thus interpretation of structure.

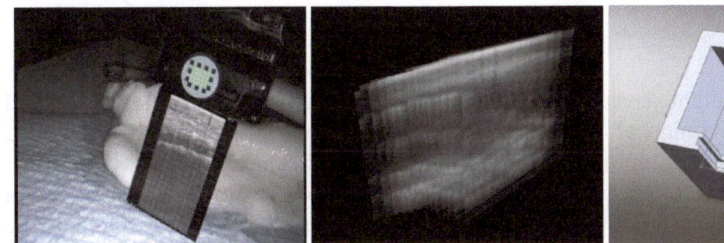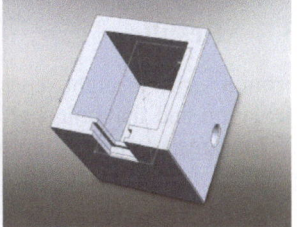

Fig. 4. Overlay ruler markings, freehand 3D reconstruction and validation phantom design

2.4 Validation

The first validation stage aims to measure ultrasound overlay accuracy and the extent of the operational envelope defined by probe angle of incidence and laparoscope proximity. The original calibration phantom was modified to support a single cross-wire feature (Fig. 4, right). Direct line of sight was achieved by sliding out its removable door and removing the plug, thereby draining the water bath. Once the two image features representing the wires are made coincident in the ultrasound scan, overlay accuracy can be assessed by superimposing the overlay and undistorted direct view of the wire crossing point (Fig. 5, left).

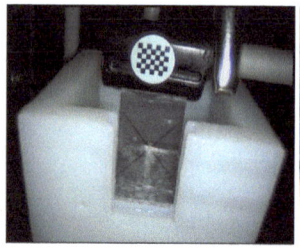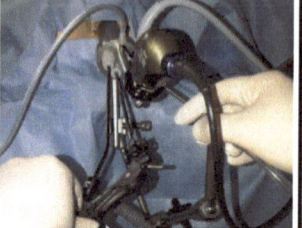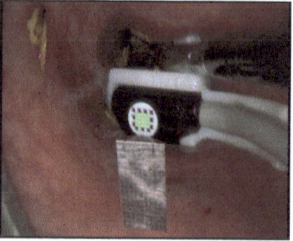

Fig. 5. Validation phantom superimposition, equipment setup and *in vivo* porcine study

Thereafter, intact *ex vivo* porcine rectum samples were used to assess the accuracy of lesion thickness measurement. The microsurgery probe was mounted in a custom-designed holder and wire guide, with exposed foot to facilitate secure mating with the grasping instrument. In each sample, six simulated silicone lesions of varying thicknesses (from 1.5mm to 4mm) were inserted between tissue layers. This material was chosen as it exhibits imaging responses similar to those observed during preoperative examination. Six subjects (five surgeons, one engineer) were recruited to the study and asked to estimate lesion thickness using ultrasound overlay. Thickness estimates were compared against subsequent caliper measurements.

Finally, an *in vivo* porcine trial was conducted to confirm that the system as a whole is sufficiently practical and robust in a live theatre environment. Following proctoscope and instrument insertion (Fig. 5, centre), pneumorectum was established. Although there was no specific pathology to investigate, surveys of rectum wall thickness were made with a view, in practice, of reducing the chance of perforation. This is of relevance to any lesion above the peritoneal reflection, and is of particular importance in human female subjects with lesions situated in the anterior wall, where accidental creation of a rectovaginal fistula must be avoided.

3   Results

From a series of eight separate calibration runs at SD resolution, the mean, standard deviation and maximum of the residual errors were found to be 206μm, 53μm and 277μm, respectively. Employing the most accurate of these calibrations, the corresponding results for ultrasound image and direct sight superimposition, gathered over a range of eight different camera poses and transducer positions, were found to be 669μm, 255μm and 961μm. The calibrations performed at HD resolution did not result in a significant residual error improvement. Similarly, the use of a general transformation (i.e. separate scaling in the X and Y directions) resulted in only a 23μm improvement in residual error. The relative size of the validation error in comparison to the residuals can be attributed to the difficulty in achieving an accurate cross-wire image feature alignment when configuring the phantom and probe.

Table 1. Probe tracking operational envelope

	range	min	max
rotate X	97°	-44°	53°
rotate Y	102°	-54°	48°
translate Z	42mm	22mm	64mm

Table 1 shows a typical measurement of the probe tracking algorithm's operational envelope, i.e. the range of probe positions resulting in consistently successful pattern recognitions, where a perpendicular arrangement of probe and endoscope defines the rotation origins, and the Z translation is measured from endoscope tip to pattern centre. It can be seen that there is a relatively wide operating envelope, although at high illumination levels, performance was observed to deteriorate in a region close to the rotational origins. This is due to the intensity of reflections and blooming in the camera sensor. The design of the probe mounting's angled foot ensures that this region is avoided in practice, while offering significant help in maintaining wide overlay areas.

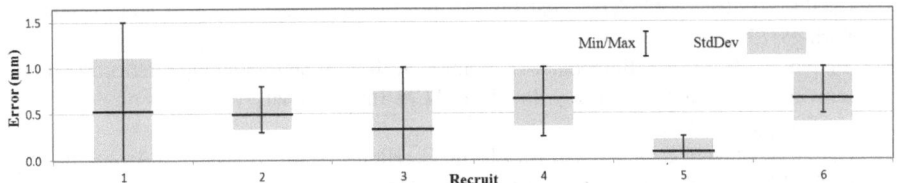

Fig. 6. Mean *ex vivo* lesion thickness measurement errors

Mean lesion thickness measurement errors for each recruit assessed on the *ex vivo* model are shown in Fig. 6. The overall mean error is 0.46mm, showing an admissible result given typical sizes (9-40mm) of transanally resected lesions. Median responses to the study questionnaire indicate that integrated ultrasound image overlay makes depth measurement much easier and convenient than use of the cart separately, that it helps convey a relative sense of scale, and that the inevitable small video delay is not noticeable. Fig. 5 (right) shows a typical snapshot from the *in vivo* porcine trial. This exercise highlighted the importance of selecting optimal illumination levels.

4   Discussion and Conclusion

In common with most camera-based systems, this work has the limitation that it cannot automatically adjust to changes in zoom or focus position. Although, crucially, no probe re-calibration is required in this event, the current setup still demands a repeat camera calibration. To make this practical for intraoperative use, the system will be extended to support zoom position interpolation over a discrete space of pre-calibrated camera intrinsic parameters. Much like the procedure itself, the restricted workspace and colinearity of instruments enforced by the transanal approach make probe manipulation a challenge, but the planned development and integration of a transanal robotic device will facilitate large-scale survey of the entire lumen. However, even with an accurate sub-surface measurement capability, this does not in itself guarantee completely negative radial and deep margins. Future integration of probe-based confocal laser endomicroscopy will allow immediate post-excision inspection.

Procedurally, transanal endoscopic microsurgery has not changed significantly since its original introduction in the 1980s. Through the addition of live ultrasound overlay, this work represents a significant innovation, required in part to meet the growing demands of prevalent cancer screening programmes. Through the introduction of novel calibration and tracking techniques, detailed calibration and validation results show sufficient levels of measurement accuracy, repeatability, computational efficiency and robustness in the context of realistic scenarios. In combination with medically-approved materials and transducers, and the fact that preoperative workup includes transanal endosonography examination in which rectal wall lesions are initially diagnosed and staged, these prepare the way for immediate human clinical translation. Naturally, the methods described in this work are also directly applicable to other minimally invasive procedures, including robotically-assisted interventions.

References

1. Cataldo, P., Buess, G.: Transanal Endoscopic Microsurgery: Principles and Techniques. Springer (2009)
2. Stetten, G., Chib, V., Hildebrand, D., Bursee, J.: Real time tomographic reflection: Phantoms for calibration and biopsy. In: IEEE/ACM International Symposium on Augmented Reality, pp. 11–19 (2001)
3. Leven, J., Burschka, D., Kumar, R., Zhang, G., Blumenkranz, S., Dai, X., Awad, M., Hager, G., Marohn, M., Choti, M., Hasser, C., Taylor, R.: DaVinci Canvas: A Telerobotic Surgical System with Integrated, Robot-Assisted, Laparoscopic Ultrasound Capability. In: Duncan, J.S., Gerig, G. (eds.) MICCAI 2005, Part I. LNCS, vol. 3749, pp. 811–818. Springer, Heidelberg (2005)
4. Ali, A., Logeswaran, R.: A visual probe localization and calibration system for cost-effective computer-aided 3D ultrasound. Computers in Biology and Medicine 37, 1141–1147 (2007)
5. Cheung, C.L., Wedlake, C., Moore, J., Pautler, S.E., Peters, T.M.: Fused Video and Ultrasound Images for Minimally Invasive Partial Nephrectomy: A Phantom Study. In: Jiang, T., Navab, N., Pluim, J.P.W., Viergever, M.A. (eds.) MICCAI 2010, Part III. LNCS, vol. 6363, pp. 408–415. Springer, Heidelberg (2010)
6. Dressel, P., Feuerstein, M., Reichl, T., Kitasaka, T., Navab, N., Mori, K.: Direct Co-calibration of Endobronchial Ultrasound and Video. In: Liao, H., Eddie Edwards, P.J., Pan, X., Fan, Y., Yang, G.-Z. (eds.) MIAR 2010. LNCS, vol. 6326, pp. 513–520. Springer, Heidelberg (2010)
7. Langø, T., Vijayan, S., Rethy, A., Vâpenstad, C., Solberg, O.V., Mârvik, R., Johnsen, G., Hernes, T.: Navigated laparoscopic ultrasound in abdominal soft tissue surgery: technological overview and perspectives. International Journal of Computer Assisted Robotics and Surgery (2011)
8. Schneider, C., Guerrero, J., Nguan, C., Rohling, R., Salcudean, S.: Intra-operative "Pick-Up" Ultrasound for Robot Assisted Surgery with Vessel Extraction and Registration: A Feasibility Study. In: Taylor, R.H., Yang, G.-Z. (eds.) IPCAI 2011. LNCS, vol. 6689, pp. 122–132. Springer, Heidelberg (2011)
9. Chen, T., Thurston, A., Ellis, R., Abolmaesumi, P.: A real-time freehand ultrasound calibration system with automatic accuracy feedback and control. Ultrasound in Medicine and Biology 35(1), 79–93 (2009)
10. Zhang, Z.: A flexible new technique for camera calibration. IEEE Transactions on Pattern Analysis and Machine Intelligence 22(11), 1330–1334 (2000)
11. Horn, B.: Closed-form solution of absolute orientation using unit quaternions. Journal of the Optical Society of America A 4(4), 629–642 (1987)
12. Bradski, G., Kaehler, A.: Learning OpenCV: Computer Vision with the OpenCV Library. O'Reilly Media, Inc. (2008)
13. Shu, C., Brunton, A., Fiala, M.: A topological approach to finding grids in calibration patterns. Machine Vision and Applications 21, 949–957 (2010)

Robotic Path Planning for Surgeon Skill Evaluation in Minimally-Invasive Sinus Surgery

Narges Ahmidi[1], Gregory D. Hager[1], Lisa Ishii[2], Gary L. Gallia[3], and Masaru Ishii[2]

[1] Department of Computer Science, Johns Hopkins University, Baltimore, MD 21218
nahmidi1@jhu.edu, hager@cs.jhu.edu
[2] Department of Otolaryngology-Head & Neck Surgery,
Johns Hopkins School of Medicine, Baltimore, MD 21287
{learnes2,mishii3}@jhmi.edu
[3] Department of Neurosurgery, Johns Hopkins University School of Medicine,
Baltimore, MD 21287
ggallia1@jhmi.edu

Abstract. We observe that expert surgeons performing MIS learn to minimize their tool path length and avoid collisions with vital structures. We thus conjecture that an expert surgeon's tool paths can be predicted by minimizing an appropriate energy function. We hypothesize that this reference path will be closer to an expert with greater skill, as measured by an objective measurement instrument such as Objective Structured Assessment of Technical Skill (OSATS).

To test this hypothesis, we have developed a Surgical Path Planner (SPP) for Functional Endoscopic Sinus Surgery (FESS). We measure the similarity between an automatically generated reference path and surgical motions of subjects. We also develop a complementary similarity metric by translating tool motion to a coordinate-independent coding of motion, which we call the Descriptive Curve Coding (DCC) method.

We evaluate our methods on surgical motions recorded from FESS training tasks. The results show that the SPP reference path predicts the OSATS scores with 88% accuracy. We also show that motions coded with DCC predict OSATS scores with 90% accuracy. Finally, the combination of SPP and DCC identifies surgical skill with 93% accuracy.

Keywords: Robotic path planning, Skill evaluation, Motions curvature representation, Support Vector Machine, OSATS, Minimally invasive surgery.

1 Introduction

Hand-eye coordination is a crucial skill in Minimally-Invasive Surgeries (MIS). This is particularly true for Functional Endoscopic Sinus Surgeries (FESS), where surgeon performance is limited by indirect observation and highly constrained tool movements inside the sinus cavity. For surgeons in training, their overall expertise level is expected to rise (from novice to expert), but their actual skill at a given point in time may vary widely between subjects, between tasks and also between task executions (trials). Thus, time and experience are not necessarily predictors of skill. An alternative is Objective

N. Ayache et al. (Eds.): MICCAI 2012, Part I, LNCS 7510, pp. 471–478, 2012.

Structured Assessment of Technical Skills (OSATS) [1] where a committee of faculty surgeons ranks residents' surgical trials.

Past work on the automation of surgical skill assessment has primarily relied on

Table 1. The relationship between self-declared scores (Expert or Novice) and the corresponding OSATS scores (Level-3 is expert and level-0 is novice).

		OSATS scores			
		Level-0	Level-1	Level-2	Level-3
Self-declared scores	Expert	5%	6%	10%	79%
	Novice	45%	20%	19%	16%

self-declared skill [2] mainly using techniques based on Hidden Markov Models (HMM) [2-5]. But, is self-declared skill consistent with OSATS? To answer this question, we ran an experiment by asking two independent groups of faculty surgeons to grade two MIS datasets (da Vinci robotic surgery and FESS) based on OSATS (level-0 to 3). We grouped levels 0 and 1 as Novices and levels 2 and 3 as Experts and then calculated the mismatch rate between the OSATS and self-declared scores (25% of the time with p-value<0.0001) (Table 1).

We hypothesize that, most of the differentiation in OSATS scores arises from the complexity in manipulating tools in MIS (e.g. avoiding critical tissues and finding the correct passage). Thus, a plausible approach to OSATS evaluation for MIS may be to first compute an optimal path, and then to compare measured paths to them. The idea of motion planning for MIS procedures is not new [6-8], but there is no prior study on using these paths as a basis for skill assessment.

In this paper, we address the problem of automated OSATS evaluation of skill by exploring the following two questions: (1) Can comparison with an optimal surgical path be used to establish a measure for skill evaluation? and (2) Does quality of motion, independent of path, provide additional information? To answer these questions we develop a Surgical Path Planner (SPP) and measure its similarity to recorded data from surgeons in training. To improve the similarity metric, we introduce the Descriptive Curve Coding (DCC) method which translates motion from Cartesian space into a coded string. This DCC string efficiently describes surgeon motion in a way that amplifies differences due to skill. We evaluate both SPP and DCC on the FESS trials, and report the similarity of the measured scores with respect to the OSATS scores.

2   Experimental Setup

A group of 20 subjects participated in the data collection (self-declared: 7 experts and 13 novices). A nasal surgery simulator was developed for this study, which consisted of a partially dissected cadaver head, a high-resolution video tower, tracked sinus endoscopes and a straight tracked pointer. A calibration process is then performed to find the tool tip location from the initial location of the sensors attached to the outer end of the tools. Subjects were naïve to the nasal anatomy and performed the tasks in a random and untimed fashion. Each surgeon performed 3 different non-destructive tasks repeatedly over a two-day period. Test subjects were allowed to familiarize themselves with the data collection setup prior to the data collection process and care was taken to simulate the surgical environment typically encountered in an operating room as best as possible.

The targets were: right Maxillary Sinus (MS.r), right Eustachian Tube (ET.r), and left Lamina Papyracea (LP.l). The tool motions were recorded using an electromagnetic tracker (Fig. 1) from a total of 109 trials: 36 MS.r (19 Expert/17 Novice), 34 ET.r (20/14), 39 LP.l (24/15). Three supervising faculty surgeons independently scored each trial using two-level grades ("expert/1" and "novice/0") and the total of their scores is used as the 4-level OSATS score (0 to 3).

For the purposes of analysis, the recorded surgical motions are transformed to the CT coordinate system using a landmark-based rigid registration.

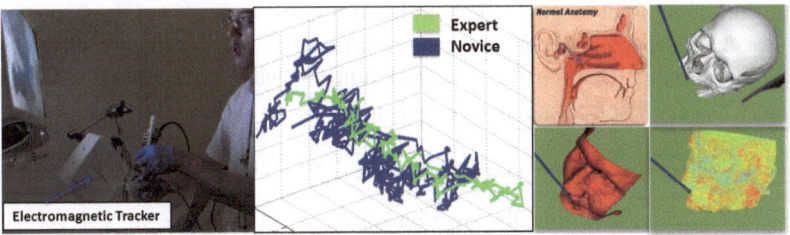

Fig. 1. (Left) Experiment setup. (Middle) Sample of tool motion in the Cartesian-space (Right) Sinus anatomy the bones/skin/soft tissue extracted from CT (blue line is the endoscopic)

3   Methodology

In this section, we introduce two methods: the Surgical Path Planner and the Descriptive Curve Coder. We then define how they are used to replicate OSATS scores (Fig. 2). Additionally, an OSATS-based HMM model is implemented using the algorithm reported in [4] on our dataset.

Surgical Path Planner (SPP): The nose is compact and contains many structures. Some of these structures like the middle and superior turbinate are involved in olfaction and are thus optimized to maximize surface area. This leaves few regions within the nose that are freely accessible with ballistic, collision-free paths; therefore a surgeon has to displace tissues to access many parts of the nose with a straight instrument. Our algorithm generates a surgical path optimized primarily to find the shortest path between the nostril and the target. It secondarily minimizes the number and extent of tissue-instrument collisions. Nasal anatomy was extracted from a CT of the paranasal sinuses. The stiffness of the obstacles is defined by the intensity of the CT voxels separated into 3 types: skin, bones and soft tissue. The endoscopic tool is modeled as a cylindrical robot of length $200mm$, radius $2mm$ with a 5DoF (degrees of freedom) with pose H in the CT coordinate system. The reference path (a sequence of H^t from start to goal over time t) is calculated by the following two steps:

(1) Probabilistic Road Map (PRM): Given the start and the goal point, we solve for the 3D translation motion of the tool tip using a PRM algorithm [9] with a uniform distribution. Dijkstra's algorithm then finds the shortest path toward the goal in the 3D Cartesian free-space. This initial path is used for the second step where we solve for the remaining 2DoF rotational motions of the robot.

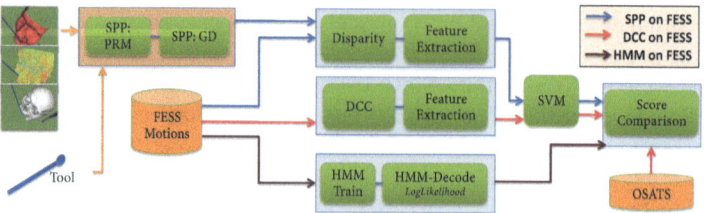

Fig. 2. The system components and the data flow for the SPP and DCC methods

(2) Gradient Descent: The robot starts to follow the initial path toward the goal (with an initial straight-to-goal orientation). If a collision happens, a numerical gradient descent approach [9] updates the robot orientation (the rotational components of H^t) by minimizing the collision cost function $\mathcal{F}$ (with higher/lower γ_j values for collision with bones/soft tissue, respectively):

$$\mathcal{F}(H^t) = \sum_{j=\{skin, softtissue, bones\}} \gamma_j * Collision_j(H^t)$$

where *Collision* is measuring the overlap of the robot with the jth CT layers. The minimization approach calculates the gradient of the repulsive forces α on the robot. Using the normalized α, the robot then moves away from the obstacles toward the position with the least collision with the tissue and updates its location:

$$H^{t+1} = H_\alpha^t = H^t * H_{\alpha_\varphi}^t * H_{\alpha_\theta}^t * H_{\alpha_x}^t * H_{\alpha_y}^t * H_{\alpha_z}^t$$

This procedure continues until the robot reaches the goal. To measure the disparity between the generated SPP path and each surgical trial, we measure the distance between each point on the surgical motion to its closest neighbor on the SPP path in Cartesian space. For each trial, we generate a feature vector containing the pairwise correlation between SPP path and the surgical path axes as well as the mean and the standard deviation of their disparities. Using these 11 dimension (9: correlation, 1: mean, 1: std) feature vectors, a Support Vector Machine (SVM) is trained (leave-one trial-out for test) to classify surgical trials to 4-classes (OSATS level for FESS). The expertise level of each trial is defined by its corresponding class label.

Descriptive Curve Coding (DCC): A drawback for skill evaluation methods based on Cartesian motions is that they do not describe the "texture" of the motion – i.e. coarseness, loops, sudden change of direction etc. – which appears to be highly correlated with skill. Hence, we introduce a new method for describing the geometrical curvature of a given 3D motion and investigate its success in skill evaluation. The idea of representing 3D curves based on their curvature has been heavily studied. For example, Frenet-Serret orthonormal frames [10] represent torsion and curvature of a non-degenerate curve, whereas authors in [11] measure the dissimilarity between two discrete curves by defining an orthogonal directional chain code. However, these methods were never used to represent surgical motions; we believe they can serve as an efficient vocabulary for motion coding.

The basic idea of our method (DCC) is to record the local curvature of the motion from the point of view of an observer traveling on the curve. The observer takes unit-size steps. Therefore, the next step on the curve is a change in direction toward left, right, up, down or continuing straight. We define a vocabulary for each of these changes (a code between 0 and 4) (Fig. 3).

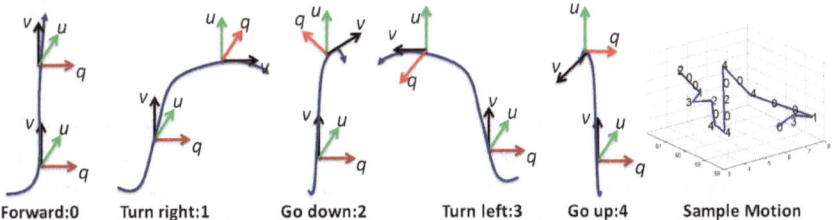

Forward:0   Turn right:1   Go down:2   Turn left:3   Go up:4   Sample Motion

Fig. 3. DCC vocabulary and changes in direction of the attached coordinate system

The DCC then traces changes of the orthonormal 3D coordinate system attached to the observer. The local coordinate system attached to the curve (r) at the step (s) is defined by its three orthonormal basis vectors: the unit tangent vector (v^s), the normal unit vector (u^s), and binormal unit vector (q^s). At each step s, the coordinate system is updated using the following equations:

$$v^s = (\|dr/ds\|^{-1})\frac{dr}{ds}$$
$$u^s = u^{s-1} \text{ if } c^{s-1} = 0, \qquad \text{otherwise } u^s = v^{s-1}$$
$$q^s = (\|u^s \times v^s\|^{-1})(u^s \times v^s)$$

where c^s is the code representing the tendency of the motion toward one of the 5 possible directions and is updated by projecting current v^s onto the previous orthonormal basis (x).

$$c^s = \operatorname*{argmax}_i \{v^s \cdot [x_i]\}, \qquad x = [v^{s-1}, q^{s-1}, u^{s-1}, -q^{s-1}, -u^{s-1}]$$

One advantage of the DCC is its flexibility in adding more vocabulary to the coding system, by simply adding new unit vectors in the projection function, e.g. instead of coding to four orthogonal directions we can refine the coding by adding 10 more vectors (a pairwise summation of each two projection units) to account for 45-degree changes of rotation.

Due to local interpretation of the curve, the strings generated from DCC are rotation and translation-invariant. Therefore, DCC-based skill evaluation methods are independent of the surgical site setup or the tracker reference point, whereas Cartesian-based models are sensitive to the location of the tracker and thus require registration with the tracker coordinate systems.

In this paper, from each trial's DCC string, we extract a 5-element feature vector, which is simply the normalized coding vocabulary histogram of that string. Using this feature vector, we use the same SVM configuration as described for SPP for the training and scoring of the surgical trials. We also augment the SPP feature vector with that of the DCC and explore its performance in skill evaluation.

4   Evaluation and Results

We evaluate the performance of each of the models by measuring the similarity be-tween their estimated scores ($\hat{S}$) for each surgical trial and their corresponding OSATS score (S_{OSATS}). In the 4-level OSATS score (scores=[0:3]), skill evaluation error is defined as

$$Error\ rate = |S_{OSATS} - \hat{S}|/l$$

where l is the normalization term (in our case $l=3$). This method credits partially cor-rect decisions (That is for a $S_{OSATS}=3$ an estimation of $\hat{S}=2$ is a closer decision than $\hat{S}=0$). We report the mean and standard deviation of the error rate - named OSATS Comparison Error Rate (OCER). We also include *Sim* the average similarity between the scores $\hat{S}$ and S_{OSATS}:

$$Sim = 1 - \mu_{OCER}$$

A method with a high performance has close-to-zero *OCER* and close-to-one *Sim* and Area Under the Curve (*AUC*). Fig 4 visualizes the results for the winner methods and a view from final location of the tool after hitting the goal in the presence of deformed tissue (visualization with VTK toolkit).

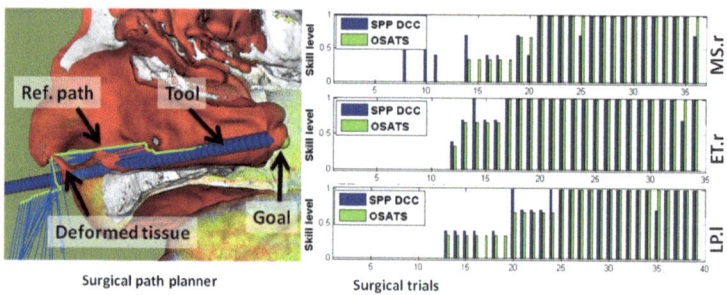

Fig. 4. (Left) Lateral clipped view of the sinus cavity where there is no straight collision-free path for tool to touch the goal. The tool follows the SPP reference path (green line) by opening its way toward the goal and putting minimum pressure on the soft tissue (blue lines). (Right) The resulting scores of SPP+DCC method (blue) and the corresponding OSATS score (green) for each trial (sorted by OSATS value, skill level of "zero" is novice and of "one" is expert).

As previously mentioned, there are no quantitative skills assessment studies that use OSATS for objective FESS evaluation. Authors in [4] represent a self-declared skill evaluation method with accuracy of 82.5% and 77.8% for expert and novice respectively. We implement their method and evaluate it against OSATS (HMM TCE in Table 2). The task ET.r was the most difficult one and resulted in a better discrimi-nation of the dexterity.

Comparing the average success rate (Table 2) of the different techniques via repli-cation scores (*sim*) shows the SPP (avg 88%) was better than the HMM (avg 75%) for all the tasks. The DCC method (invariant to translation and rotation of the surgical site) accurately graded the surgical trial skill (avg 87%) and performed similarly to the SPP method. The successful results of DCC show that there is a noticeable "texture" in the surgical trail, which differentiates experts from novices.

Finally, one could get the advantages of both techniques by concatenating their feature vectors (SPP+DCC) and then training the SVM classifier. In this case, we get even better classification (avg 93%). We note that the combined classification scheme has the most favorable area under the receiver operating curve and the smallest OCER of all techniques. The ROC graph for all methods and trials are shown in Fig. 5 to aid with the comparison process.

Table 2. Skill evaluation results (similarity, OSATS comparison error, Area under curve, and 95% confidence interval) for FESS tasks (MS.r, ET.r, and LP.l) from different methods (OSATS-based HMM [4], SPP, DCC, and their concatenation)

			Skill Evaluation Method			
			HMM TCE [4]	SPP	DCC	SPP + DCC
Endoscopic Task	MS.r	Sim	61.24%	83.60%	80.46%	**87.30%**
		OCER	0.38±0.31	0.16±0.30	0.19±0.31	**0.12±0.24**
		AUC	0.70	0.87	0.88	**0.98**
		95% CI	0.53 to 0.84	0.71 to 0.96	0.73 to 0.96	**0.87 to 1.00**
	ET.r	Sim	**79.35%**	**95.19%**	**92.15%**	**97.64%**
		OCER	0.20±0.28	0.04±0.13	0.07±0.20	**0.02±0.07**
		AUC	0.81	0.95	0.84	**0.96**
		95% CI	0.65 to 0.93	0.81 to 0.99	0.67 to 0.94	**0.833 to 0.99**
	LP .l	Sim	75.38%	**85.29%**	**88.37%**	**94.70%**
		OCER	0.24±0.26	0.14±0.26	0.11±0.18	**0.05±0.12**
		AUC	0.81	0.86	0.86	**0.95**
		95% CI	0.65 to 0.91	0.71 to 0.95	0.71 to 0.95	**0.83 to 0.99**

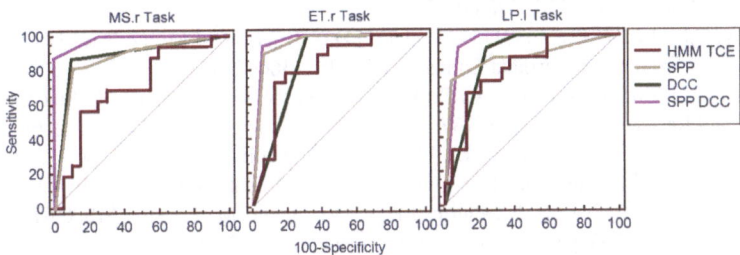

Fig. 5. ROC curves for different skill evaluation methods

5   Conclusion

In this paper, we introduced an automated skill assessment technique for Functional Endoscopic Sinus Surgeries (FESS). First, we showed that OSATS grading - the ground truth for evaluation of the resident surgical skills- is not consistent with the overall self-declared scores. Then, we introduced an OSATS-based automated skill evaluation technique. We believe that there is an optimal path for performing a FESS task which is close to what an expert surgeon would do in an ideal setup. The optimal path can be flexibly defined based on the faculty surgeon's approach in performing the surgery. Typically there is no collision-free path for FESS tasks, so here the reference path is optimized for the shortest distance to goal and least collision with the soft tissue. To explore the idea, we built a Surgical Path Planner (SPP) where the obstacles were extracted from CT. We then compared the SPP path to the one performed by the surgeons. Our results show the surgeons with higher OSATS are closer to the SPP path than the ones with lower scores. We then improved the skill assessment technique by translating the Cartesian-space motions to a coded domain using Descriptive Curve Coding (DCC). The new domain is rotation and translation-invariant and represents the "texture" of the motion. We showed that this representation amplifies the skill-related structures.

As the future work, we would like to investigate the success rate of the grammar-based DCC methods. For example, a substring with two sequential 4's might represents "retraction" which could be evaluated as a novice behavior. A sequence of zeros shows a clean and straight insertion. A substring of interleaved 2's and 3's reveals the jitter in the surgeon's hand.

Acknowledgments. This work was funded by NSF CDI-0941362. Any opinions, findings, conclusions or recommendations expressed in this material are those of the authors and do not necessarily reflect the views of the National Science Foundation.

References

1. Martin, J.A., Regehr, G., Reznick, R., MacRae, H., Murnaghan, J., Hutchison, C., Brown, M.: Objective Structured Assessment of Technical Skill for Surgical Residents. British Journal of Surgery 84, 273–278 (1997)
2. Reiley, C.E., Lin, H.C., Yuh, D.D., Hager, G.D.: A Review of Methods for Objective Surgical Skill Evaluation. Surgical Endoscopy 25, 356–366 (2011)
3. Padoy, N., Blum, T., Ahmadi, A., Feußner, H., Berger, M.O., Navab, N.: Statistical Modeling and Recognition of Surgical Workflow. J. Med. Image Analysis 16, 632–641 (2010)
4. Ahmidi, N., Hager, G.D., Ishii, L., Fichtinger, G., Gallia, G.L., Ishii, M.: Surgical Task and Skill Classification from Eye Tracking and Tool Motion in Minimally Invasive Surgery. In: Jiang, T., Navab, N., Pluim, J.P.W., Viergever, M.A. (eds.) MICCAI 2010, Part III. LNCS, vol. 6363, pp. 295–302. Springer, Heidelberg (2010)
5. Reiley, C.E., Hager, G.D.: Task versus Subtask Surgical Skill Evaluation of Robotic Minimally Invasive Surgery. In: Yang, G.-Z., Hawkes, D., Rueckert, D., Noble, A., Taylor, C. (eds.) MICCAI 2009, Part I. LNCS, vol. 5761, pp. 435–442. Springer, Heidelberg (2009)
6. Gayle, R., Segars, P., Lin, M.C., Manocha, D.: Path planning for deformable robots in complex environments. In: Robotics Systems and Science (2005)
7. Rilk, M., Wahl, F.M., Eichhorn, K.W.G., Wagner, I., Bootz, F.: Path Planning for Robot-Guided Endoscopes in Deformable Environments. J. Advances in Robotic, 263–274 (2009)
8. Nain, D., Haker, S., Kikinis, R., Eric, W., Grimson, L.: An Interactive Virtual Endoscopy Tool. In: IMIVA workshop, MICCAI (2001)
9. Choset, H., Lynch, K.M., Hutchinson, S., Kantor, G., Burgard, W., Kavraki, L.E., Thrun, S.: Principles of Robot Motion: Theory, Algorithms, and Implementations. MIT Press (2005)
10. Weisstein, E.W.: CRC encyclopedia of mathematics. CRC Press, Taylor & Francis (2009)
11. Bribiesca, E., Aguilar, W.: A Measure of Shape Dissimilarity for 3D Curves. Int. J. Contemp. Math. Sciences 1, 727–751 (2006)

Stereoscopic Scene Flow
for Robotic Assisted Minimally Invasive Surgery

Danail Stoyanov

Centre for Medical Image Computing
University College London, WC1E 8BT, UK
danail.stoyanov@ucl.ac.uk
http://cmic.cs.ucl.ac.uk

Abstract. Information about the 3D shape and motion of tissue surfaces at the surgical site during minimally invasive surgery is important for providing metric measurements that enable the deployment of image-guidance and enhanced robotic control. This article presents a scene flow algorithm that recovers the deformation and 3D structure of the surgical field-of-view from stereoscopic images by propagating information starting from a sparse set of candidate seed matches. By imposing spatial and temporal constraints the proposed algorithm is able to reconstruct dense 3D scene flow accurately and efficiently. Validation is performed using simulation data to evaluate the method against varying levels of image noise and results are also presented for benchmark phantom model data. The practical value of proposed method is shown by qualitative results for *in vivo* videos from robotic assisted procedures.

1 Introduction

Real-time information about the motion and 3D structure of the surgical site during Minimally Invasive Surgery (MIS) is important for enabling computer assisted interventions and robotic surgical systems with advanced capabilities for navigation and active control [1-4]. With robotic surgical systems, such as da Vinci® by Intuitive Surgical Inc., a stereoscopic laparoscope is used to provide the surgeon with depth perception of the operating field-of-view. The same stereo imaging device can also be used to compute real-time metric measurements from the surgical site using optics and without introducing additional hardware into the patient or the operating theatre [1,2,4]. However, vision-based shape reconstruction and motion tracking are challenging problems due to dynamics at the surgical site and large scale tissue deformation, occlusions from the surgical instruments and the complex scene illumination.

The feasibility of optical 3D reconstruction of the operating field using stereoscopic laparoscopes and computational stereo has previously been reported [5-7]. Preliminary validation studies on phantom models with ground truth data have shown promising results [6] but more comprehensive experimental analysis in complex scenes with realistic tissue reflectance need to be performed. Real-time performance reaching video frame rates for standard resolution images has also been reported [7]. Other optical systems that use active illumination such as structured light [8] and

N. Ayache et al. (Eds.): MICCAI 2012, Part I, LNCS 7510, pp. 479–486, 2012.

time-of-flight [9] have been demonstrated as promising especially when tissue surfaces are homogeneous [1]. These approaches compute a 3D reconstruction of the surgical site but do not retrieve any information about the temporal motion of tissues or instruments. Methods for combined temporal tracking and 3D reconstruction have been reported either using sparse salient features [10,11] or by using parametric surface models of the soft-tissue [12]. While such methods can operate in real-time and naturally enforce surface constraints on the tissue, it is not clear how they can accommodate large occlusions or surface discontinuities between instrument and tissue boundaries. A different approach to dense motion estimation has been investigated with monocular images by using optical flow estimation particularly for deriving the camera pose in diagnostic endoscopy [13-15]. With stereo laparoscopes the optical flow approach can be extended to 3D by computing the flow in both the left and right images and simultaneously estimating the stereo disparity [16, 17].

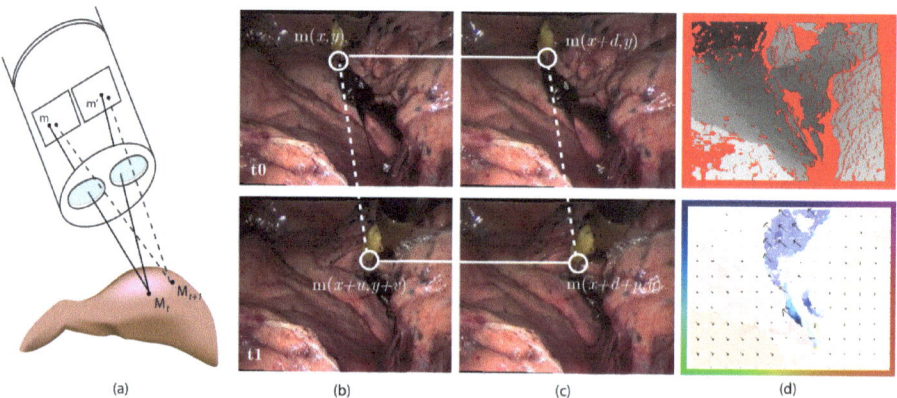

Fig. 1. (a) Schematic illustration of the stereo-laparoscope imaging a moving point on the tissue surface at two time instants; (b-c) rectified stereoscopic images obtained at two time points illustrating the constraints on scene flow motion in the images; (d) example depth map (lighter shade is closer to the camera and blue pixels are occluded) computed from the stereo pair in the top row and the optical flow image computed using scene flow between two time instants shown (color intensity represents magnitude of motion with white being no motion and deep color meaning more, the hue represents the direction as shown around the borders of the image.

In this study, we reports an algorithm for recovering the 3D scene flow at the surgical site by propagating information around a sparse set of corresponding points to both estimate the stereo disparity at each time frame and the temporal motion between consecutive frames. The advantage of this local technique is that it is easy to incorporate constraints on instrument motion and view invariant masking of highlights which can influence global optimization approaches. To the authors' knowledge this is the first work to report 3D scene flow in MIS where both the motion and the structure of the operating field are recovered in 3D. Validation using synthetic data and phantom models illustrates the performance of the method and qualitative results on *in vivo* videos from robotic assisted surgical procedures indicate that the method can potentially be used in clinical practice. An executable of the simulation environment used to generate synthetic validation data and the source code for algorithm reported in this study are available online[1].

2   Methods

This article reports a novel method for determining the 3D structure of the surgical site and its temporal motion. The technique involves determining the disparity at each time frame, estimating the 2D optical flow in the left and right views and subsequently determining a consistent 3D flow field and detecting occluded regions.

2.1   Disparity Estimation

The stereo laparoscope is assumed to be calibrated such that the intrinsic and extrinsic camera parameters are known and the toolbox used to perform the calibration is available online[1]. For each incoming stereoscopic image pair at time t the images are rectified to remove lens distortions and to align the epipolar geometry by using the known calibration parameters of the cameras [18]. From the rectified images the disparity $d(x,y,t)$ at an image pixel in the left image $\mathbf{m}_t^l = [x,y]^T$ provides the correspondence to the projection of the same world point in the right image as $\mathbf{m}_t^r = [x + d(x,y,t),y]^T$. The disparity map is estimated at each time frame by using the implementation of the algorithm in [6] which is also available online. This is based on a growing scheme [19] from an initial set of seed points that are matched across the stereoscopic view using a sparse matching algorithm [10]. The search space for growing is restricted to 1D by rectification and a symmetry constraint is added to ensure left-right disparity map consistency. We estimate the disparity map at every frame in order to decouple the flow and disparity computations and optimize each problem individually as has been reported to be effective for scene flow [17].

Any feature point detection and feature matching strategy can be used to generate seed points for the disparity growing scheme. We use simple corner features based on the image gradients as they can be computed efficiently and have previously been shown to work well for short-term tracking in MIS images with a stereoscopic tracking method [10]. More complex strategies and feature detectors or descriptors can be adapted to work within the proposed framework at the cost of additional computational load.

2.2   Scene Flow Estimation

The idea of scene flow is illustrated in Fig 1 where $\mathbf{m}_t^l$ and $\mathbf{m}_t^r$ are the pixel projection coordinates in the left and right stereo images of a point on the tissue surface $\mathbf{M}_t = [X,Y,Z]^T$ at time t. At time $t+1$ the point in the left image $\mathbf{m}_{t+1}^l$ corresponding to $\mathbf{m}_t^l$ can be written as $\mathbf{m}_{t+1}^l = [x + u(x,y,t),y + v(x,y,t)]^T$ and similarly for the right image the point corresponding to $\mathbf{m}_t^r$ can be written as $\mathbf{m}_{t+1}^r = [x + d(x,y,t) + p(x,y,t),y + v(x,y,t)]^T$. In 2D image space the optical

---

[1] http://www.cs.ucl.ac.uk/staff/dan.stoyanov/software.html

flow field for the left image is defined by $[u(x, y, t), v(x, y, t)]^T$ but because we have stereoscopic information we can derive the full scene flow for the 3D motion defined by $[u(x, y, t), v(x, y, t), p(x, y, t)]^T$ where the term $p(x, y, t)$ represents the change in disparity between t and $t + 1$. By computing the parameters $[u, v, p]^T$ (omitting image and time notation for clarity) we can calculate the full 3D scene flow.

For an incoming stereo image pair, given the disparity map generated at the previous time frame with the method in Section 2.1 we can make the several measurements to compute the flow information by measuring the similarity between image regions, we define:

$$\varepsilon_{ll} = \Theta\left(\mathbf{m}_t^l, \mathbf{m}_{t+1}^l\right) \quad \varepsilon_{rr} = \Theta\left(\mathbf{m}_t^r, \mathbf{m}_{t+1}^r\right) \quad \varepsilon_{lr} = \Theta\left(\mathbf{m}_{t+1}^l, \mathbf{m}_{t+1}^r\right) \tag{1}$$

Where the similarities of image regions denoted by ε are determined by the function Θ which is the zero mean normalized cross correlation measured between rectangular image windows centered at each point of interest. Using these measures it is possible to formulate the scene flow problem within a variation framework [13], however, this imposes smoothness priors that can be problematic in occluded areas or in regions with specular reflection. We therefore use a growing scheme similar to the one used for stereo matching in Section 2.1 and originally developed in [19] and recently adapted for scene flow in urban environments [16].

Starting from the set of candidate seed matches computed in Section 2.1 for both disparity and temporal motion we propagate information around each match using the best-first principle. The seeds are stored in a priority queue determined by their similarity scores from (1) and therefore obtaining the best seed to propagate at each step is performed by popping the queue. We perform the propagation independently in the left and right channels, which may seem redundant, but we exploit the redundancy to perform consistency and symmetry checking thus detecting occlusions in the flow as well as in the disparity. Furthermore, because the propagation is constrained by the epipolar geometry and by a disparity smoothness threshold, which we limit to one, there is an overlap of correlation computations which we can exploit for efficiency. Finally, we run the algorithm hierarchically starting with small correlation windows and then repeating with larger ones but using the earlier result as an initialization seed priority queue. The rejection scheme handles error propagation naturally in this case and the larger windows are able to fill in homogeneous regions more reliably.

3   Experiments and Results

The proposed method was implemented using C++ and, without specific optimization or parallelization, it is able to operate at approximately 1Hz for 360 x 288 images on a single core of an Intel i7 M620 2.76GHz mobile processor. For our simulation validation studies we used a custom simulation environment where textures are used with a surface model that can be augmented to simulate tissue deformations induced by the cardiac cycle and respiration. The environment is available online[2] and has a number of parameters that can be used to customize the virtual cameras, the amount of additive Gaussian noise and the type of deformation induced on the surface. We also

---

[2] http://www.cs.ucl.ac.uk/staff/dan.stoyanov/software.html

report results for the heart phantom datasets reported in [6] and made available by the Hamlyn Centre, Imperial College London[3]. Finally we show qualitative results on the *in vivo* data made available in [1,10].

3.1 Experiments with Synthetic Data

Ground truth information for 3D scene flow is not available in surgery and even for phantom experiments linking the temporal motion of dense surface points is not currently possible. Therefore we evaluate the stability and performance of the proposed method on synthetic data with varying levels of additive Gaussian noise with zero mean and increasing standard deviation. While simulation environments cannot render a fully photorealistic representation of the surgical site they allow testing the robustness of an approach against known ground truth information.

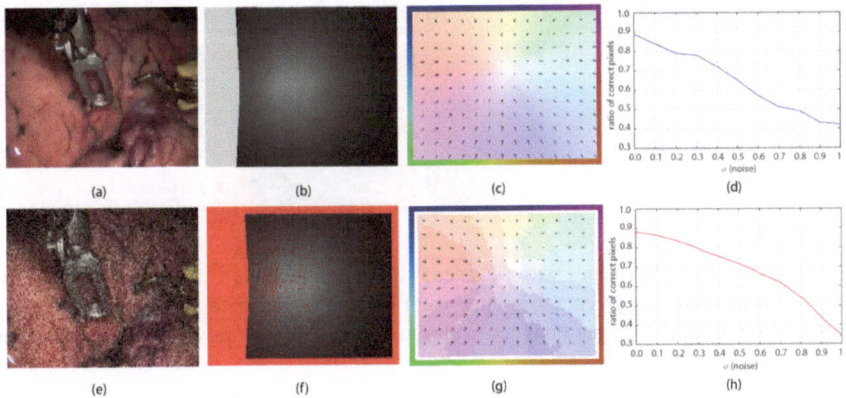

Fig. 2. (a,e) Images generated from the simulation environment with and without additive noise; (b, f) ground truth disparity map from the simulation and below the disparity generated with the proposed technique; (c, g) ground truth optical flow map in the left image (sub-pixel) and below the computed flow map using the proposed method; (d, h) plot of the error for disparity computation (blue) and optical flow (red) against varying levels of additive noise.

The results shown in Fig 2(g, h) indicate that the proposed method performs well on the synthetic data. We show ground truth disparity and flow images in Fig 2(b, c) and the corresponding example reconstructed disparity map in Fig 2(f, g) when additive image noise has been introduced to the image as shown in Fig 2(e). It is clear that there is good agreement between the ground truth and our results, however, our method operates only on integer values and therefore cannot match the sub-pixel quality of the ground truth. This results is banding of the results visible in the images but can be removed with a final subpixel refinement step. The plots in Fig 2(d) show the performance of our method against varying levels of noise where the deviation of additive noise is normalized in the 0-1 range.

---

[3] http://hamlyn.doc.ic.ac.uk/vision/

3.2   Experiments on Phantom Model Data

To evaluate the method proposed in this study against phantom model data we used the heart model data reported in [5]. The two datasets are of a beating heart phantom model with ground truth obtained using dynamic CT scanning to measure the geometry of the model. The data does not have temporal connectivity available and therefore evaluating the 3D scene flow we compute is not possible for this data. Hence we only compare the disparity results obtained with our technique to the ground truth disparity at each frame in the video sequences averaged over one cardiac cycle.

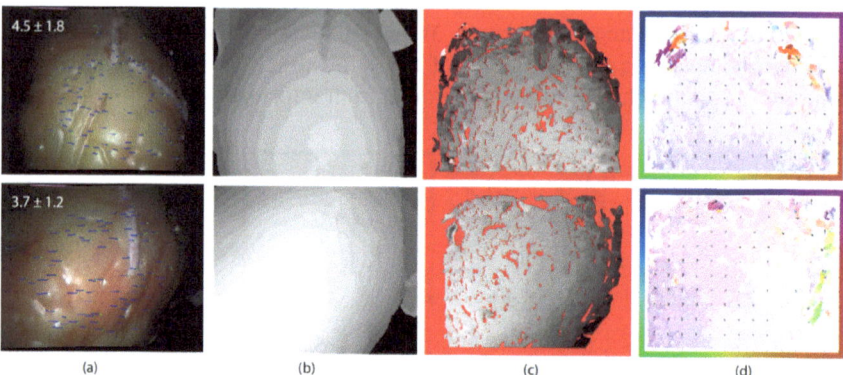

Fig. 3. (a) Two example images with seed feature tracks matched in stereo shown in blue and temporal tracks shown in green; (b) ground truth disparity images obtained from CT data; (c) corresponding disparity images obtained with our method; (d) the flow images corresponding to inter-frame motion

Fig 3 shows example images from the heart phantom with sparse feature tracks used to initialize our method overlaid on top of the video. The disparity maps resulting at a time frame generated by the proposed technique are shown in Fig 3(c) and visibly correspond well to the ground truth data. We ran our technique over both video sequences for a full cardiac cycle and the resulting disparity error and deviation are overlaid in Fig 3(a). The disparity error for each dataset was measured as 4.5±1.8 pixels and 3.7±1.2 pixels. The flow information shown has no ground truth but intuitively we observe larger motion close to the camera as the heart model simulates a cardiac cycle. While our errors are higher than reported in [6] it is important to note that we are computing disparity over the entire cycle of heart data and not on a single frame. This has a disadvantage because the video and dynamic CT data are not perfectly aligned in time and a conversion formula is used (please see the data's website).

3.3   Experiments with *in vivo* Data

We illustrate the practical value of the method proposed in this article by applying to several videos taken in vivo during robotic assisted surgery. The results shown in Fig 4 clearly capture the visual appearance of the 3D structures within the scene and perform well in terms of not mismatching occluded regions even with the presence of large instruments in the foreground.

It is more difficult to visualize the reconstructed 3D motion but qualitatively we can see that it corresponds to instrument motion where present and to different tissue surface planes in the scene. The motion data is best visualized using the video submitted as supplementary material for this submission. Naturally some errors are apparent and in the 3D reconstruction these are usually due to sharp discontinuities meanwhile in the motion fields they typically reflect sudden changes in motion direction

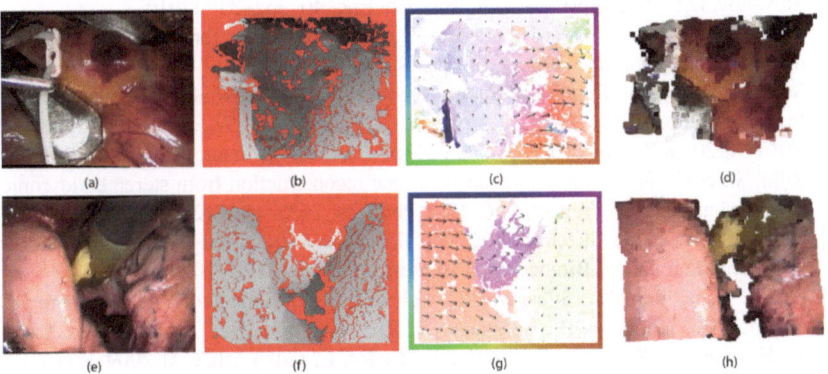

Fig. 4. (a, e) Example stereoscopic images from endoscopic beating heart surgery and a robotic procedure on the lung; (b, f) disparity images showing the 3D shape and (c, g) flow dynamics of the operating field; (d-h) renderings of the recovered 3D geometry of the surgical site without incorporated occluded regions

4   Discussion

In this article, we have presented stereoscopic framework for recovering the 3D structure and motion of the operating field during robotic assisted MIS. The method is robust as it uses a growing scheme that rejects outliers and ensures uniqueness and symmetry in the resulting disparity and flow estimates. We have shown that the method performs well against additive image noise on synthetic data and on benchmark phantom model data with known ground truth. Qualitative experiments on *in vivo* datasets from robotic assisted surgery also suggest that the method has practical value. We believe the method is capable of real-time performance with suitable code optimization and a hardware implementation utilizing parallelization. Furthermore the approach can be improved to provide subpixel results with a final refinement step. Our future work will focus on improving the computational performance of the technique and also on investigating more optimal propagation strategies with learned priors, occlusion boundaries and instrument detection.

Acknowledgements. We would like to acknowledge the data provided by Prof Guang-Zhong Yang and the Hamlyn Center, Imperial College London. This work was supported by a Royal Academy of Engineering/EPSRC Research Fellowship.

References

[1] Mountney, P., Yang, G.-Z.: Motion Compensated SLAM for Image Guided Surgery. In: Jiang, T., Navab, N., Pluim, J.P.W., Viergever, M.A. (eds.) MICCAI 2010, Part II. LNCS, vol. 6362, pp. 496–504. Springer, Heidelberg (2010)

[2] Mirota, D.J., et al.: Vision-Based Navigation in Image-Guided Interventions. Ann. Rev. Biomed. Eng. 13, 297–319 (2011)

[3] Hager, G., et al.: Surgical and interventional robotics: part III [Tutorial]. IEEE Robot. Autom. Mag. 15, 84–93 (2008)

[4] Stoyanov, D.: Surgical Vision. Ann. Biomed. Eng. 40, 332–334 (2012)

[5] Devernay, F., et al.: Towards endoscopic augmented reality for robotically assisted minimally invasive cardiac surgery. In: MIAR (2001)

[6] Stoyanov, D., et al.: Real-Time Stereo Reconstruction in Robotically Assisted Minimally Invasive Surgery. In: Jiang, T., Navab, N., Pluim, J.P.W., Viergever, M.A. (eds.) MICCAI 2010, Part II. LNCS, vol. 6362, pp. 275–282. Springer, Heidelberg (2010)

[7] Röhl, S., et al.: Dense GPU-enhanced surface reconstruction from stereo endoscopic images for intraoperative registration. Med. Phys. 39, 1632–1645 (2012)

[8] Clancy, N.T., et al.: Spectrally encoded fiber-based structured lighting probe for intraoperative 3D imaging. Biomed. Opt. Express. 11, 3119–3128 (2011)

[9] Penne, J., Höller, K., Stürmer, M., Schrauder, T., Schneider, A., Engelbrecht, R., Feußner, H., Schmauss, B., Hornegger, J.: Time-of-Flight 3-D Endoscopy. In: Yang, G.-Z., Hawkes, D., Rueckert, D., Noble, A., Taylor, C. (eds.) MICCAI 2009, Part I. LNCS, vol. 5761, pp. 467–474. Springer, Heidelberg (2009)

[10] Stoyanov, D., et al.: Soft-tissue Motion Tracking and Structure Estimation for Robotic Assisted MIS Procedures. In: Duncan, J.S., Gerig, G. (eds.) MICCAI 2005. LNCS, vol. 3749, pp. 139–146. Springer, Heidelberg (2005)

[11] Paul, P., et al.: A Surface Registration Method for Quantification of Intraoperative Brain Deformations in Image-Guided Neurosurgery. IEEE Trans. Inf. Tech. Biomed. 13, 976–983 (2009)

[12] Richa, R., et al.: Towards robust 3D visual tracking for motion compensation in beating heart surgery. Med. Image Anal. 15, 302–315 (2011)

[13] Deguchi, D., Mori, K., Suenaga, Y., Hasegawa, J.-I., Toriwaki, J.-I., Takabatake, H., Natori, H.: New Image Similarity Measure for Bronchoscope Tracking Based on Image Registration. In: Ellis, R.E., Peters, T.M. (eds.) MICCAI 2003. LNCS, vol. 2878, pp. 399–406. Springer, Heidelberg (2003)

[14] Jianfei, L., et al.: A stable optic-flow based method for tracking colonoscopy images. In: CVPRW, pp. 1–8 (2008)

[15] Mori, K., et al.: Tracking of a bronchoscope using epipolar geometry analysis and intensity-based image registration of real and virtual endoscopic images. Med. Imag. Anal. 6, 321–336 (2002)

[16] Cech, J., et al.: Scene flow estimation by growing correspondence seeds. In: CVPR, pp. 3129–3136 (2011)

[17] Wedel, A., et al.: Stereoscopic Scene Flow Computation for 3D Motion Understanding. Int. J. Comp. Vis. 95, 29–51 (2011)

[18] Hartley, R., Zisserman, A.: Multiple View Geometry in Computer Vision. Cambridge Press (2000)

[19] Lhuillier, M., et al.: Robust dense matching using local and global geometric constraints. In: ICPR, pp. 1968–1972 (2000)

Towards Computer-Assisted Deep Brain Stimulation Targeting with Multiple Active Contacts

Silvain Bériault, Yiming Xiao, Lara Bailey, D. Louis Collins,
Abbas F. Sadikot, and G. Bruce Pike

McConnell Brain Imaging Centre, Montreal Neurological Institute,
3801 University Street, Montreal, Quebec, H3A 2B4, Canada
silvain.beriault@mail.mcgill.ca

Abstract. We present a novel method for preoperative computer-assisted deep brain stimulation (DBS) electrode targeting that takes into account the multiplicity of available contacts and their polarity. Our framework automatically evaluates the efficacy of many possible electrode orientations to optimize the interplay between the extracellular electric field, created from distinct arrangements of active contacts, and anatomical structures responsible for therapeutic and potential side effects. Experimental results on subthalamic DBS cases suggest bipolar configurations provide more flexibility and control on the spread of electric field and, consequently, are most robust to targeting imprecision. Visualization of predicted efficacy maps provides surgeons with complementary feedback that can bridge the gap between insertion safety and optimal therapeutic efficacy. Overall, this work adds a new dimension to preoperative DBS planning and suggests new insights regarding multi-target stimulation.

Keywords: Deep brain stimulation, electric field modeling, Parkinson's disease, histological atlas, image-guided neurosurgery.

1   Introduction

Deep brain stimulation (DBS) is an increasingly important neurosurgical treatment for severe pharmacologically-resistant Parkinson's disease (PD), and other movement and affective disorders. The procedure involves the implantation of multi-contact stimulating electrodes in deep brain structures via minimally invasive image-guided neurosurgery (IGNS). Effective neuromodulation is highly dependent upon precise electrode targeting and programming to simultaneously maximize symptom relief and minimize side effects caused by stimulation of neighbouring anatomical structures. For example, bilateral high frequency DBS of the subthalamic nuclei (STN) is effective to reduce motor fluctuations, dyskinesias, rigidity, tremor and slowness of movement symptoms that characterize advanced PD. However, targeting inaccuracies can yield side effects due to the spread of extracellular electric field to the internal capsule (muscle contraction), the occulomotor nerve root (diplopia), the superior cerebellar peduncle (ataxia), the medial lemniscus and spinothalamic pathways (paresthesias) [1].

N. Ayache et al. (Eds.): MICCAI 2012, Part I, LNCS 7510, pp. 487–494, 2012.
© Springer-Verlag Berlin Heidelberg 2012

The most common clinical protocol for DBS targeting is carried in two phases. *Before the operation*, the neurosurgeon approximates the target position on the patient's preoperative MRI. However, typical DBS target sites, such as the STN, do not possess clear boundaries on clinical MRIs and the surgeon must often rely on the relative position of other anatomical landmarks (e.g. the AC-PC line) or on a stereotactic atlas of the basal ganglia that is deformed to the patient's datasets [2]. *During the operation*, micro-electrode recording (MER) of neuronal activity is used to refine the physiological extent of the targeted nucleus and neighbouring nuclei. Furthermore, monopolar (single contact) micro- and macro-stimulation is performed to determine salutary and untoward effects of stimulation.

Recently, several computer-assisted tools were developed to help neurosurgical teams with different aspects of the overall procedure. Some software platforms (e.g. [3-4]) were proposed to allow fusion of multi-modal MRI, automatic segmentation of key anatomical structures, registration to anatomical and functional atlases, and effective visualization of DBS lead trajectory. Advanced MRI techniques have also developed for direct visualization of the STN and other basal ganglia structures [5-6]. Probabilistic functional atlases, relating target sites to clinical outcome, have been used for semi-automatic or automatic target prediction [7-8]. Algorithms were also developed for automatic trajectory optimization to minimize hemorrhagic risks and loss of function (e.g. [9-10]).

However, current planning methods for preventing electric field propagation into neighbouring structures without compromising treatment efficacy are still performed intraoperatively, once the burr-hole has been made. An isotropic Gaussian model is often used to visualize the extent of cathodal (monopolar) stimulation and to build multi-subject probabilistic efficacy atlases [7-8]. A spherical shell kernel [11] was also proposed with the assumption that therapeutic effects arise from stimulating specific tissue located on an annulus, around the electrode, rather than the total volume of tissue activated. Finally, iterative finite element models (FEM) [12] have been proposed to account for the contact geometry and material, and anisotropic white matter conductivity, based diffusion tensor imaging (DTI). This latter approach is particularly useful for *a posteriori* optimization of the programming parameters given a final electrode position. However, the model is limited by the low spatial resolution of DTI datasets (typically 2x2x2-mm) and is computationally expensive for *a priori* planning.

This work presents a novel computer-assisted planning framework for *a priori* electrode targeting. A map of anatomical regions responsible for therapeutic and potential side effects is derived from a high-resolution basal ganglia histology atlas non-linearly registered to patient's T1w and susceptibility-based T2*w datasets acquired within a clinically acceptable time via a multi-echo MRI sequence. A fast practical model of the extracellular electric field is proposed to predict the spread into the target and neighbouring structures at increasing stimulation intensities, and to compute an overall efficacy measure for different arrangements of active contacts and polarities. Overall, we developed a new software simulation that mimics micro- and macro-stimulation preoperatively allowing many electrode orientations, depths and multi-contact configurations to be evaluated before entering the operating room.

2   Method

Our optimization framework relies on the interplay between the electric field generated from the stimulation of one or multiple active contacts and specific brain areas responsible for therapeutic and side effects. Section 2.1 describes the MRI acquisition protocol and registration to a high-resolution histology-derived atlas. Section 2.2 describes the analytical model used to describe the electric field and section 2.3 presents the novel planning and optimization algorithm.

2.1   MRI Acquisition and Image Processing

Multi-contrast MRI acquisition of the entire head is obtained from a 3D gradient echo MRI sequence with 0.95 mm isotropic resolution and 10 echoes (TR=30 ms, TEs={1.6; 4.1; 6.6; 9.1; 13.0; 16.0; 18.5; 21.0; 23.5; 26.0} ms, α=23°, BW=450Hz). The magnitude images from the first four echoes are averaged to provide suitable T1w contrast for neuronavigation. The magnitude images from the last five echoes are averaged to provide T2*w contrast and direct imaging of the STN. The total acquisition time is 7:05 min on a 3T Siemens TIM Trio scanner and a 32-channel coil. The T1w and T2*w datasets are intrinsically co-registered as they originate from the same acquisition.

A map of side effect areas is obtained from non-linear registration of the patient's T1w MRI with an existing high resolution (0.034x0.034x0.70-mm) histological atlas of the basal ganglia and thalamus (see Fig. 1a), using the Colin27 T1w average template as an intermediate volume [13]. For this prototype, the potential side effect regions were defined as the internal capsule, the superior cerebellar peduncle and the medial lemniscus pathways. To improve the registration accuracy of the small-size STN (not visible on T1w contrast), we used a similar non-linear registration method that integrates multiple MRI contrasts (T1w and T2*w) and an intensity inverted T2w Colin template as an intermediate volume (see [14] for implementation details and validation). The raw T1w and T2*w datasets are shown in Fig. 1b-c. Fig. 1d shows STN labeling over the T2*w dataset. Fig. 1e shows the final therapeutic and potential side effect regions overlaid on the T1w dataset.

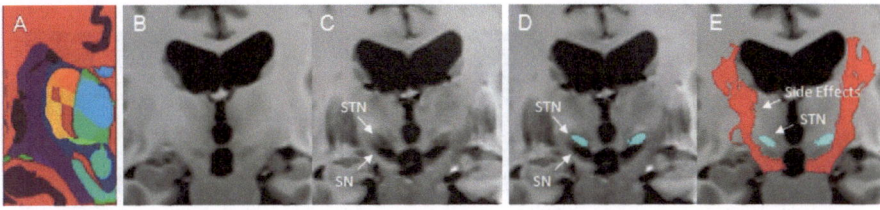

Fig. 1. (a) High resolution basal ganglia atlas (left side). (b) The T1w navigation dataset. (c) The T2*w dataset exhibiting STN and substantia nigra (SN) contrast. (d) Atlas-based warping of the STN label overlaid on the T2*w dataset. (e) Final therapeutic and side effects regions overlaid on the T1w navigation dataset.

2.2   Modeling the DBS Electric Field

Recently, Zhang and Grill [15] demonstrated that a point source model and a homogeneous brain tissue conductivity assumption yield comparable electric field and volume of tissue activated in comparison to a full FEM for small-sized contacts. This key observation enables the design of fast and representative analytical approximations of the extracellular electric field. Thus, for a point source delivering current I_0 (A), the current density $\vec{J}(r)\,(A/m^2)$ on a spherical surface of radius r (m) is given as the current divided by the surface area: $\vec{J}(r) = I_0 / 4\pi r^2$. From the generalized Ohm law ($\vec{J} = \sigma\vec{E}$) where σ is the tissue conductance (S/m) and $\vec{E}$ the electric field (V/m), or the negative gradient of the extracellular potential ($\vec{E} = -\nabla V$), the electric potential (V) at a distance r of the source is obtained from the following surface integration:

$$\int_0^r -\nabla V dr = \int_0^r \frac{-I_0}{4\pi\sigma r^2} dr \text{ , and } V = \frac{I_0}{4\pi\sigma r} \tag{1}$$

Eq. (1) describes the special case of single contact (monopolar) stimulation. Bipolar and other multi-contact configurations, often required for STN DBS [1] due to the proximity to the internal capsule, can be obtained using superposition. For example, the potential for bipolar stimulation becomes:

$$V = \frac{I_0}{4\pi\sigma}\left(\frac{1}{r_1} - \frac{1}{r_2}\right) \tag{2}$$

In Eq. (2), r_1 is the distance from the cathodal contact and r_2 the distance from the anodal contact. A similar expression is obtained for tripolar stimulation (not shown). Hence, monopolar stimulation is a special case of multi-contact DBS with $r_2=\infty$. Fig. 2 shows the potential and electric field distributions for monopolar and bipolar cases (with $I_0 = 4$ mA and $\sigma = 0.2$ S/m). The main advantage of bipolar stimulation is that the electrical field strength decays more rapidly, thus reducing the risk of stimulating neighbouring structures.

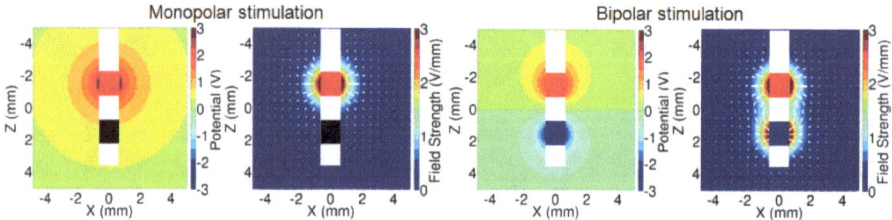

Fig. 2. Extracellular potential and electric field using point source contacts with I_0=4 mA, σ=0.2 S/m. For the monopolar case, lines of electric forces arising from the cathodal contact radiates isotropically. For the bipolar case, lines of electric forces are partially attracted to the anodal contact.

2.3   Preoperative Electrode Targeting Optimization

Using the therapeutic and side effects maps and the electric field model described in sections 2.1 and 2.2, we developed a software simulation that mimics micro- and macro-stimulation to evaluate many possible electrode orientations, depths and configurations preoperatively. To do so, we define an efficacy likelihood measure (EF) that modulates the interplay between a therapeutic effect profile (P_{TE}) and a side effect profile (P_{SE}). Fig. 3 shows the theoretical behavior of P_{TE} and P_{SE}. At low intensity (I), the likelihood of therapeutic and side effects is low. As the stimulation intensity increases, both P_{TE} and P_{SE} increase, because the stronger electric field will spread into more brain tissue. However, P_{TE} will typically increase faster then P_{SE}, because the electrode, unless off-target, is closer to the therapeutic areas than the side effects areas and will stabilize once the small-sized targeted nucleus is completely stimulated. Depending on the targeting accuracy, both P_{TE} and P_{SE} can be shifted to the left or right and our goal is to maximize the EF measure:

$$EF = \int_0^{I_{max}} P_{TE}(I)dI - \int_0^{I_{max}} P_{SE}(I)dI \tag{3}$$

For a given electrode orientation, depth, configuration of active contacts, and stimulation intensity, $P_{TE}(I)$ and $P_{SE}(I)$ relates to the sum of a voxel-wise activation likelihood (P_A) measured at specific voxels responsible for therapeutic and side effects:

$$P_A(x, y, z) = \begin{cases} 1 & E(x, y, z) > E_{max} \\ E(x, y, z)/E_{max} & E(x, y, z) < E_{max} \end{cases} \tag{4}$$

In Eq. (4), E_{max} is a user-defined parameter corresponding to electric field strength where activation is maximal ($P_A = 1.0$) with a 1:4 ratio for anodal contacts because anodic stimulation thresholds are consistently higher than cathodic thresholds [15]. Finally, P_{TE} and P_{SE} profiles are computed at increasing intensity (I) and the efficacy (EF) is computed via a discrete implementation of Eq. (3). The depth at which EF is maximal is kept for each evaluated electrode orientation and configuration.

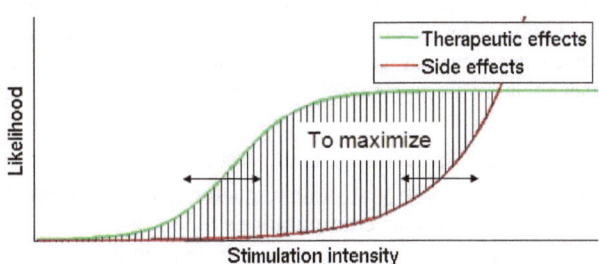

Fig. 3. Theoretical plot showing the interplay between the likelihood of therapeutic (P_{TE}) and possible side effects (P_{SE}) as the stimulation intensity increases. The goal is to maximize the efficacy (EF), which is modeled as the area between P_{TE} and P_{SE} curves and which can decrease and even become negative when the electrode is outside the targeted structure.

3   Results

A preliminary evaluation was performed on 3 PD patients (STN DBS). For each case, an initial search space of possible electrode orientations was defined from the identification of a tentative target point, within the dorsolateral STN (motor part) on the T2*w dataset, and a set of possible brain entry points, within the frontal lobe because it corresponds to typical insertion area for STN DBS. The search space was then automatically filtered [10] to exclude orientations yielding lead trajectories that approach sulci, ventricles and blood vessels at an unsafe distance. The remaining orientations were analyzed with our targeting optimization method and using the Medtronic 3389 electrode model (diameter: 1.27mm, contact height: 1.5 mm, contact spacing: 0.5 mm). Fig. 4 displays a color-coded map of the predicted efficacy, relatively to other orientations, for monopolar, wide bipolar and narrow bipolar. Fig. 5 plots the electric field at the predicted electrode depth for a specific orientation (subject 1). For all configurations, the cathodal contact responsible for most of tissue activation is well positioned within the dorsolateral STN.

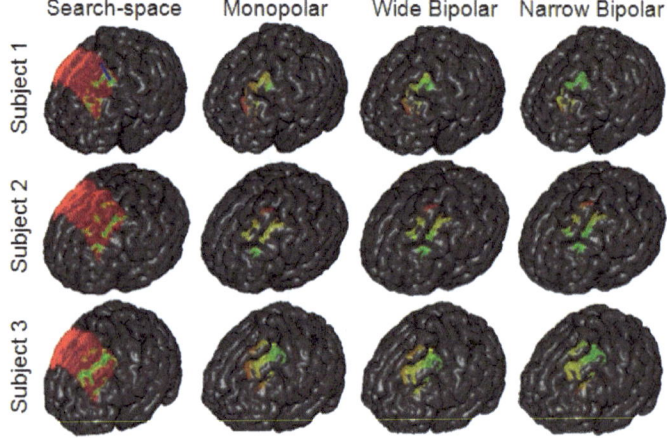

Fig. 4. Given an initial search space, our framework computes and allows immediate visualization of the computed efficacy for the different orientations and configurations of active contacts. Color scale for search-space column: green=safe, yellow=acceptable: red=rejected trajectories. Color scale for other columns: green=high, yellow=average, red=low predicted efficacy

Although more efficient in terms of battery consumption, monopolar STN DBS with optimal efficacy is concentrated onto a smaller patch of entry points (orientations) in comparison to the bipolar configurations (see Fig. 4). Furthermore, the narrow bipolar configuration provides the most control over to the spread of electric field into neighbouring structures, especially at high stimulation intensity, due to the small distance separating the cathodal and anodal contacts (see Fig. 5). Thus, this configuration is most robust to targeting imprecision. Interestingly, our software predicted anterior approaches for subject 2 and posterior approaches for subjects 1 and 3 yield superior efficacy. This can be attributed to the use of patient-specific search spaces, which take into account the high inter-subject variability of gyral patterns and ventricular size.

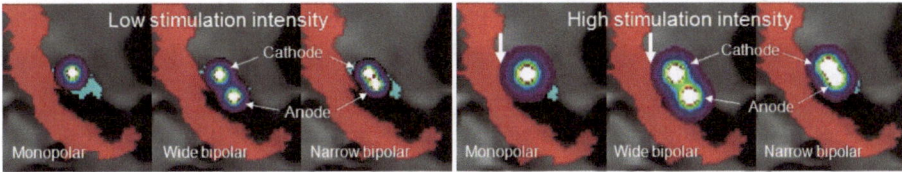

Fig. 5. Coronal view of the electric field for subject 1 on a specific electrode orientation (see blue marker on Fig. 4) at predicted depth for different configurations. At low stimulation intensity (4mA), any configuration can be used without propagation to the internal capsule. At high stimulation (10mA), the electric field overlaps with the internal capsule at the cathodal contact of both monopolar and wide bipolar configuration, hence increasing the risk of side effects.

4   Discussion and Conclusions

We presented a new electrode targeting optimization method that takes into account the multiplicity of available contacts on standard DBS lead. To our knowledge, this is the first published method that automatically computes an efficacy measure, for several possible electrode orientations, depths and configurations, based on the interplay between the created electric field and patient-specific maps of therapeutic and possible side effects. Within the context of automatic DBS targeting we also proposed the novel integration of a high-resolution basal ganglia histology atlas non-linearly registered to multi-contrast patient's datasets (T1w and T2*w) simultaneously acquired using a multi-echo MRI sequence. Our preliminary results reveal that our method provides the surgeon with high-level feedback, which is complementary to other planning considerations, and that can bridge the gap between lead insertion safety and optimal therapeutic efficacy.

Our modular framework also allows the use of alternate techniques for creating maps of therapeutic and possible side effects. Indeed, the small-sized STN could be segmented manually from the T2*w dataset, thus eliminating possible atlas registration inaccuracies. Otherwise, functional atlases constructed from a population of previous DBS surgeries could have also been used. However, recent advances in structural MRI pave the way to custom solutions based on the patient specific anatomy, and also enable simulated exploration of other anatomical targets and alternate DBS insertion strategies. Overall, the proposed software adds a new dimension to preoperative DBS planning and suggests new insights regarding multi-contact and multi-target stimulation, which may reveal essential as DBS becomes applicable to a wider variety of diseases and symptoms and with the increasing number of available contacts on new generations of lead models. For future work, we will calibrate the proposed therapeutic and side effect profiles using intraoperative micro- and macrostimulation recordings and we will incorporate a more accurate electrothermal model that takes into account white matter fiber orientation and presence of blood vessels via patient-specific DTI and SWI venography datasets.

References

1. Montgomery, E.B.: Deep Brain Stimulation Programming: Principles and Practice. Oxford University Press (2010)
2. Brunenberg, E.J., Platel, B., Hofman, P.A., Ter Haar Romeny, B.M., Visser-Vandewalle, V.: Magnetic resonance imaging techniques for visualization of the subthalamic nucleus. J. Neurosurg. 115, 971–984 (2011)
3. Nowinski, W.L., Yang, G.L., Yeo, T.T.: Computer-aided stereotactic functional neurosurgery enhanced by the use of the multiple brain atlas database. IEEE Trans. Med. Imaging 19, 62–69 (2000)
4. D'Haese, P.F., Pallavaram, S., Li, R., Remple, M.S., Kao, C., Neimat, J.S., Konrad, P.E., Dawant, B.M.: CranialVault and its CRAVE tools: A clinical computer assistance system for deep brain stimulation (DBS) therapy. Med. Image Anal. 16, 744–753 (2012)
5. Elolf, E., Bockermann, V., Gringel, T., Knauth, M., Dechent, P., Helms, G.: Improved visibility of the subthalamic nucleus on high-resolution stereotactic MR imaging by added susceptibility (T2*) contrast using multiple gradient echoes. Am. J. Neuroradiol. 28, 1093–1094 (2007)
6. Xiao, Y., Beriault, S., Pike, G.B., Collins, D.L.: Multi-contrast multi-echo FLASH MRI for targeting the subthalamic nucleus. Magn. Reson. Imaging 30, 627–640 (2012)
7. D'Haese, P.F., Cetinkaya, E., Konrad, P.E., Kao, C., Dawant, B.M.: Computer-aided placement of deep brain stimulators: from planning to intraoperative guidance. IEEE Trans. Med. Imaging 24, 1469–1478 (2005)
8. Guo, T., Parrent, A.G., Peters, T.M.: Surgical targeting accuracy analysis of six methods for subthalamic nucleus deep brain stimulation. Comput. Aided Surg. 12, 325–334 (2007)
9. Essert, C., Haegelen, C., Lalys, F., Abadie, A., Jannin, P.: Automatic computation of electrode trajectories for Deep Brain Stimulation: a hybrid symbolic and numerical approach. Int. J. Comput. Assist. Radiol. Surg. (2011)
10. Bériault, S., Al Subaie, F., Mok, K., Sadikot, A.F., Pike, G.B.: Automatic Trajectory Planning of DBS Neurosurgery from Multi-modal MRI Datasets. In: Fichtinger, G., Martel, A., Peters, T. (eds.) MICCAI 2011, Part I. LNCS, vol. 6891, pp. 259–266. Springer, Heidelberg (2011)
11. Pallavaram, S., D'Haese, P.-F., Kao, C., Yu, H., Remple, M., Neimat, J., Konrad, P., Dawant, B.: A New Method for Creating Electrophysiological Maps for DBS Surgery and Their Application to Surgical Guidance. In: Metaxas, D., Axel, L., Fichtinger, G., Székely, G. (eds.) MICCAI 2008, Part I. LNCS, vol. 5241, pp. 670–677. Springer, Heidelberg (2008)
12. McIntyre, C.C., Mori, S., Sherman, D.L., Thakor, N.V., Vitek, J.L.: Electric field and stimulating influence generated by deep brain stimulation of the subthalamic nucleus. Clin. Neurophysiol. 115, 589–595 (2004)
13. Chakravarty, M.M., Bertrand, G., Hodge, C.P., Sadikot, A.F., Collins, D.L.: The creation of a brain atlas for image guided neurosurgery using serial histological data. Neuroimage 30, 359–376 (2006)
14. Xiao, Y., Bailey, L., Mallar Chakravarty, M., Beriault, S., Sadikot, A.F., Pike, G.B., Collins, D.L.: Atlas-Based Segmentation of the Subthalamic Nucleus, Red Nucleus, and Substantia Nigra for Deep Brain Stimulation by Incorporating Multiple MRI Contrasts. In: Abolmaesumi, P., Joskowicz, L., Navab, N., Jannin, P. (eds.) IPCAI 2012. LNCS, vol. 7330, pp. 135–145. Springer, Heidelberg (2012)
15. Zhang, T.C., Grill, W.M.: Modeling deep brain stimulation: point source approximation versus realistic representation of the electrode. J. Neural. Eng. 7, 1–11 (2010)

Multi-object Spring Level Sets (MUSCLE)

Blake C. Lucas[1,2], Michael Kazhdan[2], and Russell H. Taylor[2]

[1] Johns Hopkins Applied Physics Laboratory, Laurel, MD, USA
[2] Johns Hopkins University, Baltimore, MD, USA
{blake,misha}@cs.jhu.edu, rht@jhu.edu

Abstract. A new data structure is presented for geometrically modeling multi-objects. The model can exhibit elastic and fluid-like behavior to enable interpretability between tasks that require both deformable registration and active contour segmentation. The data structure consists of a label mask, distance field, and springls (a constellation of disconnected triangles). The representation has sub-voxel precision, is parametric, re-meshes, tracks point correspondences, and guarantees no self-intersections, air-gaps, or overlaps between adjacent structures. In this work, we show how to apply existing registration algorithms and active contour segmentation to the data structure; and as a demonstration, the data structure is used to segment cortical and subcortical structures (74 total) in the human brain.

Keywords: registration, segmentation, tracking, active contour, level set, mesh.

1   Introduction

Deformable registration [1, 2] has become a popular technique for reliably and automatically segmenting multiple objects with little prior knowledge of anatomy or imaging technology. The output of the algorithm is a displacement field describing where voxel locations in the target image map to in the source image. This 3D-to-3D mapping allows any geometric structures identified in the source image to be warped into the target image to create a segmentation of the target [3]. To overcome the registration algorithm's lack of prior knowledge, there is a strong assumption that the target's anatomy is a smooth elastic deformation of the source's anatomy. This is rarely the case, leading to what is known as "atlas bias" where the warped source image still resembles the source image, possibly more than the target. One way to reduce bias is to repeat the registration with different source images and combine segmentations afterwards to create an "average" [4]. Methods that combine multiple segmentations produce "average" segmentations that are smoother than any individual segmentation [5]. Alternatively, one can reduce bias and increase the image segmentation's fidelity by following elastic registration with "fluid-like" segmentation [6, 7]. Segmentation reduces atlas bias from the registration phase because the deformation is driven by information in the target image alone. Traditional geometric data structures used to cascade registration and segmentation either lose information and / or do not preserve important geometric properties. We now review those data structures and the challenges each one poses.

N. Ayache et al. (Eds.): MICCAI 2012, Part I, LNCS 7510, pp. 495–503, 2012.
© Springer-Verlag Berlin Heidelberg 2012

2   Previous Work

Meshes. Triangle meshes have the ability to encode surface labels and track point correspondences. Displacement fields produced by registration can be directly applied to triangle meshes. Even though displacement fields represent smooth elastic deformations, the deformed triangle mesh can have sharp edges and cusps that were not present in the original mesh. To reduce artifacts, the mesh must be smoothed and re-sampled (re-meshed) to produce a higher quality mesh. Re-meshing is challenging and interferes with point correspondences in non-intuitive ways [8]. Re-meshing becomes more difficult when deformations are fluid-like, objects share boundaries or slide against each other, and practical geometric constraints are enforced. These constraints include: the mesh should not intersect adjacent structures or itself, and it should not create air-gaps between adjacent structures.

Level Sets. Objects can be represented with sub-voxel precision as level sets [9]. Level sets are functions of 3D space that are stored as images. A common choice for level set function is the signed distance field; in which, image intensities measure the minimum distance to the object's boundary. Level sets naturally enforce that structures do not self-intersect, and it is simple to enforce that they do not overlap or have air-gaps [10]. The drawback to level sets is that they do not maintain point correspondences or surface labels, and application of a displacement field requires re-sampling the level set image, which acts as a low-pass filter by smoothing underlying geometric structures.

Label Masks. It is common for objects to be manually segmented with a painting tool to produce binary masks. These masks are then merged together to create a label mask image. Displacement fields can be applied to labels by warping and re-sampling the label mask image. Re-sampling acts as a low-pass filter that smoothes underlying structures; and because label image values are region indicators, only nearest-neighbor interpolation can be used. Label masks have only voxel precision and have no ability to maintain point correspondences or surface labels.

Overview. Recently, a geometric data structure was presented that has properties of both meshes and level sets [11]. Spring Level Sets (SpringLS) couple a constellation of disconnected triangle surface elements (springls) with a level set. This work extends SpringLS to the multi-object case and shows how to use it for registration and segmentation. The new data structure is a combination of three existing data structures: a constellation of springls, a label mask, and a distance field. The new Multi-Object Level Set (MUSCLE) data structure is simultaneously all previously mentioned representations and addresses the drawbacks of each. To demonstrate, we cascade diffeomorphic Demons [12] registration and active contour segmentation [9] to segment and label 74 structures in MR images of the human brain.

3   Method

Representation. The Springl Constellation + Label Mask + Distance Field (MUSCLE) data structure is depicted in Fig. 1. A springl S_n is a triangular surface element consisting of a particle p_n and three springs connecting the particle to each of the triangle's vertices $q_{n,m}$ (Fig. 1a). Each springl maintains an object label $l_n \epsilon \mathcal{L} = \{1, \cdots, L\}$ and a correspondence point a_n that maps the particle p_n to a point on the original model. Each object has its own springl constellation that encloses the object's interior. Constellations for all objects (Fig. 1b) are merged into one constellation for storage and manipulation. The label mask $\chi: \Omega \longmapsto \mathcal{L}$ (Fig. 1c) maps each voxel in the image domain $\Omega \subset \mathcal{R}^3$ to an object label l. The distance field $\psi: \Omega \longmapsto \mathcal{R}$ (Fig. 1d) measures the distance of each voxel to the nearest object represented by level sets $\varphi_l: \Omega \longmapsto \mathcal{R}$ (i.e. $\psi(x) = \min_l |\varphi_l(x)|$). The signed distance φ_l for each object can be recovered at the boundary

$$\Lambda_l = \{x| \exists y \epsilon \mathcal{N}(x) \text{ s.t. } \sigma_l(x) \neq \sigma_l(y)\} \tag{1}$$

of each region l, where $\mathcal{N}(x)$ is the 6-connected neighborhood of voxel x and the sign $\sigma_l(x)$ is indicated by,

$$\sigma_l(x) = \begin{cases} -1 & \chi(x) = l \\ 1 & otherwise \end{cases}. \tag{2}$$

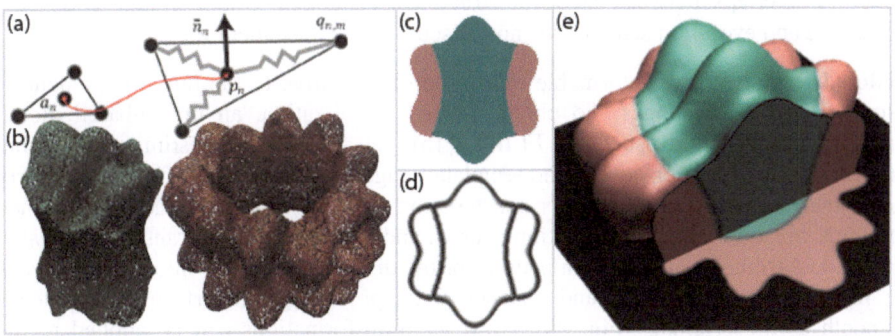

Fig. 1. (a) Diagram of springl. (b) Springl constellation for two objects. (c) label mask. (d) clamped distance field. (e) Raycast rendering of MUSCLE data structure.

We use the convention that distance measurements at locations inside the object have negative values and outside positive values. The partially reconstructed level set $\tilde{\varphi}_l : \Lambda_l \longmapsto \mathcal{R}$ is given by $\tilde{\varphi}_l(x) = \sigma_l(x) \psi(x)$. $\tilde{\varphi}_l$ measures the signed distance at the boundary (Λ_l) between objects and provides enough information to extract an iso-surface with marching cubes [13] or recover the entire signed distance field for each object with fast-marching [9]. More importantly, the "label mask + distance field" data structure avoids having to store and manipulate independent level set images for each object. For an $M \times M \times M$ image containing L objects, the amount of memory needed to store the MUSCLE data structure is $O(M^3 + LM^2)$. This is compared to $O(LM^2)$ for meshes, $O(LM^3)$ for independent level sets, and $O(M^3)$ for label masks.

Level Set Evolution. MUSCLE, like SpringLS, maintains a mesh and level set representation of the same geometry. To keep them consistent during deformation, level sets are evolved to minimize their distance to the constellation. This is accomplished by first constructing the clamped distance field for all springls:

$$\omega(x) = \min\{2d_{max}, d_1(x) \quad \ldots \quad d_N(x)\} \tag{3}$$

where $d_n(x)$ is the distance from location x to springl n, and $d_{max} = 0.5$ is the clamped distance. Level sets $\tilde{\varphi}_l$ are evolved to minimize the following:

$$E = \sum_l \int \left(\tfrac{1}{2}(\omega(x))^2 + \lambda|\nabla\tilde{\varphi}_l(x)|\right)\delta(\tilde{\varphi}_l(x))dx \tag{4}$$

where λ is a regularization weight that controls the model's smoothness. Solving the Euler-Lagrange equations, eq. 4 can be minimized with the following scheme:

$$\tilde{\varphi}_l^{z+1}(x) = \tilde{\varphi}_l^z(x) - \Delta t \delta_\varepsilon(\tilde{\varphi}_l^z(x))\left(\omega(x)\nabla\omega(x)\cdot\frac{\nabla\tilde{\varphi}_l^z(x)}{|\nabla\tilde{\varphi}_l^z(x)|} + \lambda\nabla\cdot\frac{\nabla\tilde{\varphi}_l^z(x)}{|\nabla\tilde{\varphi}_l^z(x)|}\right) \tag{5}$$

where $\delta_\varepsilon(d)$ is a compactly supported approximation to the dirac delta. The iterative scheme is implemented with Multi-Object Geodesic Active Contours (MOGAC) [14] because it uses the "label mask + distance field" data structure and does not create air-gaps or overlaps between adjacent structures. Equipped with the MUSCLE data structure and evolution scheme, we now discuss how to use them for registration.

Global Registration. Deformable registration is sensitive to the initial alignment of source and target images. To obtain a good initialization, an image-based global registration algorithm such as FLIRT [15] can be used to estimate an affine transformation between source and template images. The 4 × 4 transformation matrix A is then applied to the springls constellation (Fig. 2a), labels mask, and distance field. Nearest-neighbor interpolation is used, and must be used, to transform the label mask, and trilinear interpolation is used for the distance field. The interpolator acts as a filter on both the labels and distance field, producing iso-surfaces not quite as smooth as the originals (Fig. 2b). However, transformations can be applied to the constellation without interpolation. The label mask and distance field are then evolved to minimize the distance between their iso-surfaces and the constellation (eq. 5). Fig. 2c illustrates that this method is effective at boosting the fidelity of level sets that undergo global registration.

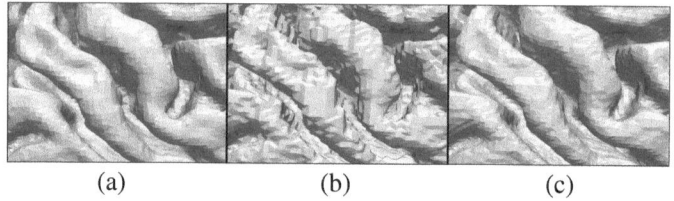

(a)　　　　　　　(b)　　　　　　　(c)

Fig. 2. Cortical surface after applying Affine transformation to (a) triangle mesh, (b) label mask and distance field (c) MUSCLE after 20 iterations of eq. 5 with $\lambda = 1$

Deformable Registration. Once source and target images have been roughly aligned with global registration, they are more precisely aligned with deformable registration.

Image based registration algorithms output a displacement field $\vec{v}_{ts}: \Omega \mapsto \mathcal{R}^3$ describing the offset of each location in the target image $I_t: \Omega \mapsto \mathcal{R}$ maps in the source image $I_s: \Omega \mapsto \mathcal{R}$. The source image, label mask, or distance field, can be transformed into the target via $I_t(\boldsymbol{x}) \doteq I_s(\boldsymbol{x} - \vec{v}_{ts}(\boldsymbol{x}))$. Displacements fields representing the forward mapping $\vec{v}_{st}: \Omega \mapsto \mathcal{R}^3$ can be applied to mesh vertices $q_{n,m}$ in the springls constellation to obtain new positions $\acute{q}_{n,m}$ via $\acute{q}_{n,m} = q_{n,m} + \vec{v}_{st}(q_{n,m})$. Unfortunately, most registration algorithms produce displacement fields that are not isomorphic (i.e. $\vec{v}_{st}(\boldsymbol{x} - \vec{v}_{ts}(\boldsymbol{x})) \neq \vec{v}_{ts}(\boldsymbol{x})$). A different procedure is needed for transforming label masks and distance fields so that their iso-surfaces are well aligned with springl constellations. To do so, springls are incrementally displaced along linear trajectories from source to target:

$$q_{n,m}(t) = q_{n,m}(0) + t\vec{v}_{st}\left(q_{n,m}(0)\right) \qquad (6)$$

where $t \in [0,1]$. After each displacement step k s.t. $t = k\Delta t$ for $k = 0, 1, \ldots, \lceil 1/\Delta t \rceil$, the label mask and distance field are evolved to track the moving mesh via eq. 5. The step size is chosen to be $\Delta t \leq d_{max}/\max_{n,m}\|\vec{v}_{st}(q_{n,m})\|$. The iterative scheme in eq. 5 is repeated 4 times per iteration of eq. 6. Fig. 3a illustrates that applying a displacement field to a mesh can create thin cusp structures that self-intersect. In the MUSCLE framework, the level set representation that is evolved with the mesh cannot develop self-intersections, but it can change topology (Fig. 3b). The simple-point test can be added to the level set method [16] to preserve the object's topology (Fig. 3c).

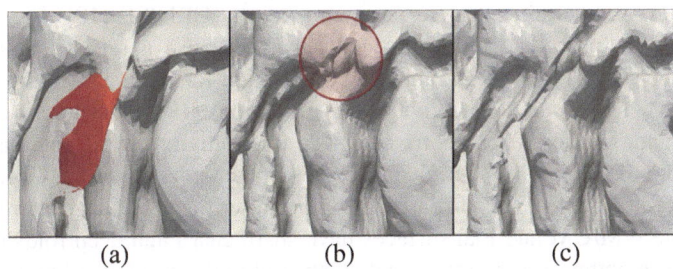

| (a) | (b) | (c) |

Fig. 3. Cortical surface after applying displacement field to (a) triangle mesh, (b) MUSCLE (c) MUSCLE with topology-preservation constraint. Back-face of the surface is shown in red, indicating self-intersection. Red circle indicates region with topology change.

Active Contour Segmentation. After registration, active contour methods are used to better align the model with anatomical boundaries visible in the target image. An active contour segmentation framework has been developed for SpringLS [11]. It consists of five phases: advection, relaxation, re-sampling, level set evolution, and hole filling. We extend the advection phase to multiple objects by considering advection equations of the following form,

$$\frac{dp_n}{dt} = \lambda_\rho\left(\rho_{l_n}(p_n) - \max_{\hat{l}\in\mathcal{N}(p_n) \text{ and } \hat{l}\neq l_n} \rho_{\hat{l}}(p_n)\right)\vec{n}_n + \lambda_\sigma\vec{\sigma}(p_n), \qquad (7)$$

where $\rho_l\colon \Omega \mapsto \mathcal{R}$ is the pressure for object l, $\vec{\sigma}\colon \Omega \mapsto \mathcal{R}^3$ is an external velocity field, and $\vec{n}_n$ is the outward pointing normal for springl n. The first term moves the boundary to classify location p_n as either inside or outside object l_n via the pressure difference between l_n and the maximum pressure from objects in the neighborhood $\mathcal{N}(p_n)$. The second term moves boundaries for all objects towards edges in the image, and $\lambda_\rho \setminus \lambda_\sigma$ control the relative contributions of each force to the movement of a springl. After all springls have been moved a small distance (less than d_{max}) via eq. 7, the relaxation phase uses inter-springl attraction forces to smooth and regularize the constellation (see Lucas et al. [11] for details). In MUSCLE, springls are only permitted to interact with springls that have the same label l during relaxation. The re-sampling phase removes springls with label l that are too far from $\tilde{\varphi}_l$'s zero iso-level or are too small. This includes removal of sharp edges and cusp structures (Fig. 3a) that lie far from any level set's zero iso-level. Level sets are then evolved to track the constellation. MUSCLE uses the multi-object level set method outlined in eqs. 3-5. In the final phase, large holes in the constellation are filled by adding springls, and point correspondences for new springls are interpolated based on point correspondences for neighboring springls. MUSCLE fills holes in the constellation with respect to each object individually as opposed to the union of all springls. The five phases are repeated in order until the iso-surfaces stop moving or the maximum number of iterations is reached.

4   Results and Discussion

A MUSCLE was constructed for the brain by extending gyral labels produced by FreeSurfer [17] with fast-marching [9] and combining them with sub-cortical labels and the level set for the central surface produced by CRUISE [18] (Fig. 4). It may seem unusual to parcellate the brain in this way because gyral structures are only present in the GM. However, an emerging application for brain parcellations is to use DTI fiber tracks to assess connectivity of gyral regions [19]. Fiber tracks can only be reliably found in the WM; so to establish connectivity, gyral regions must be extended into the WM. The central surface lies in the "middle" of the GM. We chose to use the central surface in our parcellation because it can be found more reliability [18], and the WM/GM and Pial surfaces have sharp cusps and deep folds that violate the uniform smoothness assumption that is inherent in the regularization of eq. 4.

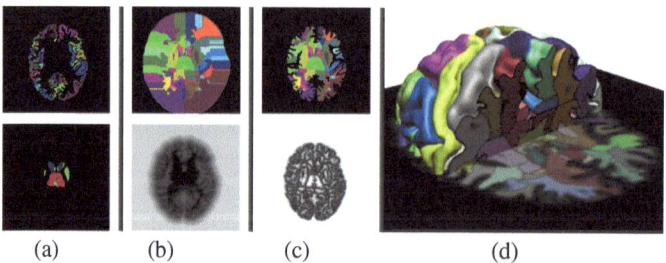

(a)   (b)   (c)   (d)

Fig. 4. (a) gyral labels (top), sub-cortical labels (bottom). (b) Sub-cortical + extended gyral labels (top), level set for central surface (bottom). (c) MUSCLE label mask for 74 structures (top), MUSCLE distance field (bottom). (d) Raycast rendering of MUSCLE parcellation.

MUSCLE brain parcellations were constructed for 10 subjects from the OASIS cross-sectional database [20]. Each parcellation was used to segment the other 9 subjects (90 experiments total) via the following pipeline: 1) each skull-stripped MRI was affine registered to the target; 2) The affine registered image was deformably registered to the target with diffeomorphic Demons [12]; 3) the displacement field and affine transformation were applied to the MUSCLE parcellation; 4) the MUSCLE parcellation was evolved with active contour methods to find the central surface produced by CRUISE. To find the central surface represented by level set $\psi_c : \Omega \mapsto \mathcal{R}$, we use $\rho_l(\boldsymbol{x}) = H_\varepsilon(\psi_c(\boldsymbol{x}))$ where $H_\varepsilon(x) = \mathrm{atan}(x/\varepsilon)$ with $\varepsilon = 0.25$, $\lambda_\rho = 1$, and $\lambda_\sigma = 0$. Fig. 5. shows one example of the registration + segmentation (reg+seg) pipeline. Table 1 compares the accuracy of several approaches. Labeling accuracy is measured with the extended Jaccard metric [7].

MUSCLE reg+seg and Hybrid Warp [6] have similar pipelines. MUSCLE augments Hybrid Warp by providing a data structure with which to represent full brain parcellations that can re-sample / re-mesh under geometric constraints (i.e. no self-intersections, air-gaps, or overlaps). CVS [7] uses a tetrahedral mesh (tet-mesh). Tet-meshes are difficult to use for registration because diffeomorphic deformations require safeguards to avoid tetrahedral inversion. MUSCLE places no restrictions on diffeomorphic deformations and has other useful geometric properties. For example, MUSCLE iso-surfaces are smooth, which is not always the case for meshes (Fig. 3) and rarely the case for iso-surfaces extracted from label masks. It is important to have smooth surfaces (along with point correspondences) because cortical surface analysis is often sensitive to surface curvature [17]. MUSCLE associates gyral labels with springls on the central surface instead of voxels in the GM, which partially explains why cortical labeling accuracy is higher for MUSCLE. In HAMMER and CVS, the sampling density of voxel-based gyral labels is affected by GM thickness. Regions where the GM is thin often report lower labeling accuracy because the Jaccard metric is sensitive to a labeled region's volume size. MUSCLE evenly samples the cortical surface with springls so that gyral labeling is unaffected by GM thickness. MUSCLE reg+seg produces less accurate subcortical segmentations than other works because it uses Demons instead of HAMMER. Subcortical segmentation with Demons and a label mask representation has an accuracy of 54.3±13.6%. MUSCLE's slightly lower accuracy (53.1±13.8%) is due to smoothing (eq. 4). Subcortical structures have sharper features than the central surface, so they should have a smaller smoothing weight (λ). To improve subcortical accuracy, one could use HAMMER for registration and disable / reduce smoothing in subcortical regions.

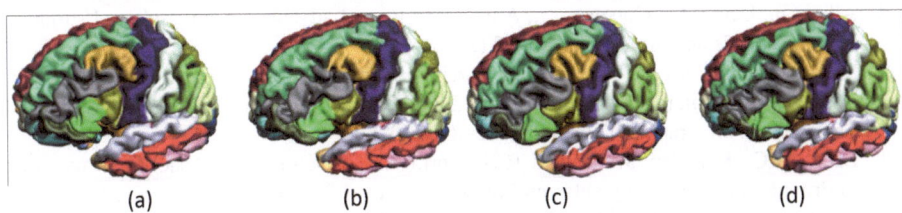

(a)   (b)   (c)   (d)

Fig. 5. MUSCLE parcellations for (a) source, (b) source after applying displacement field (18 sec) and affine transform (7 sec), (c) target, and (d) source after reg+seg (21 min total, 1.1M - 1.4M springls, 256^3 voxels, 100 active contour iterations). Computation times do not include FLIRT (10 min), Diffeomorphic Demons (1 hr), or CRUISE (2.5 hrs). Dual Intel E5630 (8 cores). Source code available at http://code.google.com/p/imagesci/.

Table 1. Performance summary. Distance measurements are for cortical surface only. Accuracies for referenced works do not reflect the same parcellations, datasets, or sample sizes.

Pipeline	Geometric Representation	Template to Subject	Subject to Template	Subcortical Label Acc.	Cortical Label Acc.
MUSCLE reg only	MUSCLE	1.29±0.45 mm	1.05±0.36 mm	53.1±13.8%	80.1±2.6%
MUSCLE reg + seg	MUSCLE	0.40±0.05 mm	0.25±0.01 mm	52.8±13.0%	81.2±2.7%
HAMMER [2, 7]	Label mask	--	--	66.8±6.7%	36.6±6.0%
Hybrid Warp [6]	Triangle mesh	0.45±0.05 mm	0.37±0.05 mm	--	--
CVS [7]	Tet-mesh	1.5 to 2.5 mm	--	70.5±4.6%	54.4±10%

Acknowledgments. This research was supported in part by a fellowship from the Johns Hopkins Applied Physics Laboratory.

References

1. Thirion, J.P.: Image matching as a diffusion process: an analogy with Maxwell's demons. Medical Image Analysis 2, 243–260 (1998)
2. Shen, D., Davatzikos, C.: HAMMER: hierarchical attribute matching mechanism for elastic registration. IEEE Trans. on Medical Imaging 21, 1421–1439 (2002)
3. Dawant, B.M., Hartmann, S., Thirion, J.P., Maes, F., Vandermeulen, D., Demaerel, P.: Automatic 3-D segmentation of internal structures of the head in MR images using a combination of similarity and free-form transformations. I. Methodology and validation on normal subjects. IEEE Transactions on Medical Imaging 18, 909–916 (1999)
4. Aljabar, P., Heckemann, R., Hammers, A., Hajnal, J., Rueckert, D.: Multi-atlas based segmentation of brain images: Atlas selection and its effect on accuracy. Neuroimage 46, 726–738 (2009)
5. Warfield, S.K., Zou, K.H., Wells, W.M.: Simultaneous truth and performance level estimation (STAPLE): an algorithm for the validation of image segmentation. IEEE Trans. on Medical Imaging 23, 903–921 (2004)
6. Liu, T., Shen, D., Davatzikos, C.: Deformable registration of cortical structures via hybrid volumetric and surface warping. Neuroimage 22, 1790–1801 (2004)
7. Postelnicu, G., Zollei, L., Fischl, B.: Combined volumetric and surface registration. IEEE Transactions on Medical Imaging 28, 508–522 (2009)
8. Alliez, P., Ucelli, G., Gotsman, C., Attene, M.: Recent advances in remeshing of surfaces. Shape Analysis and Structuring, 53–82 (2008)
9. Sethian, J.: Level set methods and fast marching methods. Cambridge Univ. Pr. (1999)
10. Losasso, F., Shinar, T., Selle, A., Fedkiw, R.: Multiple interacting liquids. ACM Transactions on Graphics (TOG) 25, 812–819 (2006)
11. Lucas, B.C., Kazhdan, M., Taylor, R.H.: SpringLS: A Deformable Model Representation to Provide Interoperability between Meshes and Level Sets. In: Fichtinger, G., Martel, A., Peters, T. (eds.) MICCAI 2011, Part II. LNCS, vol. 6892, pp. 442–450. Springer, Heidelberg (2011)
12. Vercauteren, T., Pennec, X., Perchant, A., Ayache, N.: Diffeomorphic demons: Efficient non-parametric image registration. Neuroimage 45, S61–S72 (2009)
13. Lorensen, W.E., Cline, H.E.: Marching cubes: A high resolution 3D surface construction algorithm. ACM Siggraph Computer Graphics 21, 163–169 (1987)

14. Lucas, B.C., Kazhdan, M., Taylor, R.H.: Multi-Object Geodesic Active Contours (MOGAC). In: MICCAI, Nice (2012)
15. Jenkinson, M., Smith, S.: A global optimisation method for robust affine registration of brain images. Medical Image Analysis 5, 143–156 (2001)
16. Han, X., Xu, C., Prince, J.: A Topology Preserving Level Set Method for Geometric Deformable Models. IEEE Trans. on Pattern Analysis and Machine Intelligence, 755–768 (2003)
17. Desikan, R.S., Ségonne, F., Fischl, B., Quinn, B.T., Dickerson, B.C., Blacker, D., Buckner, R.L., Dale, A.M., Maguire, R.P., Hyman, B.T.: An automated labeling system for subdividing the human cerebral cortex on MRI scans into gyral based regions of interest. Neuroimage 31, 968–980 (2006)
18. Han, X., Pham, D.L., Tosun, D., Rettmann, M.E., Xu, C., Prince, J.L.: CRUISE: cortical reconstruction using implicit surface evolution. Neuroimage 23, 997–1012 (2004)
19. Zalesky, A., Fornito, A., Harding, I.H., Cocchi, L., Yücel, M., Pantelis, C., Bullmore, E.T.: Whole-brain anatomical networks: Does the choice of nodes matter? Neuroimage 50, 970–983 (2010)
20. Marcus, D.S., Wang, T.H., Parker, J., Csernansky, J.G., Morris, J.C., Buckner, R.L.: Open Access Series of Imaging Studies (OASIS). J. of Cognitive Neuroscience 19, 1498–1507 (2007)

Combining CRF and Multi-hypothesis Detection for Accurate Lesion Segmentation in Breast Sonograms

Zhihui Hao, Qiang Wang, Yeong Kyeong Seong,
Jong-Ha Lee, Haibing Ren, and Ji-yeun Kim

Samsung Advanced Institute of Technology (SAIT), Samsung Electronics

Abstract. The implementation of lesion segmentation for breast ultrasound image relies on several diagnostic rules on intensity, texture, *etc.* In this paper, we propose a novel algorithm to achieve a comprehensive decision upon these rules by incorporating image over-segmentation and lesion detection in a pairwise CRF model, rather than a term-by-term translation. Multiple detection hypotheses are used to propagate object-level cues to segments and a unified classifier is trained based on the concatenated features. The experimental results show that our algorithm can avoid the drawbacks of separate detection or bottom-up segmentation, and can deal with very complicated cases.

1 Introduction

Breast cancer is the second leading cause of cancer death for women. Currently, early detection is the only solution to reduce the death rate. Ultrasonography is widely used in the diagnosis and observation of breast abnormality because of the convenience, safety and high accuracy rate [1]. However, it is also widely acknowledged that ultrasound image interpretation is highly reliant on medical expertise. Designing a computer-aided system to assist ultrasound practitioners in recognizing lesion and delineating the boundary is becoming necessary.

A typical breast ultrasound image is shown in the upper left of Fig. 1. Generally, object segmentation in ultrasound images is much more difficult than that in natural images due to the following aspects: poor quality of the image with low contrast and heavy speckle noise; large variation of lesion in shape and appearance, especially between the benign and the malignant; existence of similar tissues or acoustic shadows; irregular and poorly defined lesion boundaries.

In this paper, we put forward an automatic lesion segmentation algorithm. Unlike most previous works which solve the problem by translating the diagnostic rules into computer language term by term, we propose to achieve it in an integrated framework of all image cues. To this end, features from segments and multiple lesion detection hypotheses are combined together to train a single classifier. The lesion segmentation is then accomplished by optimizing a segment based CRF model. Fig. 1 gives an overview of our approach.

N. Ayache et al. (Eds.): MICCAI 2012, Part I, LNCS 7510, pp. 504–511, 2012.
© Springer-Verlag Berlin Heidelberg 2012

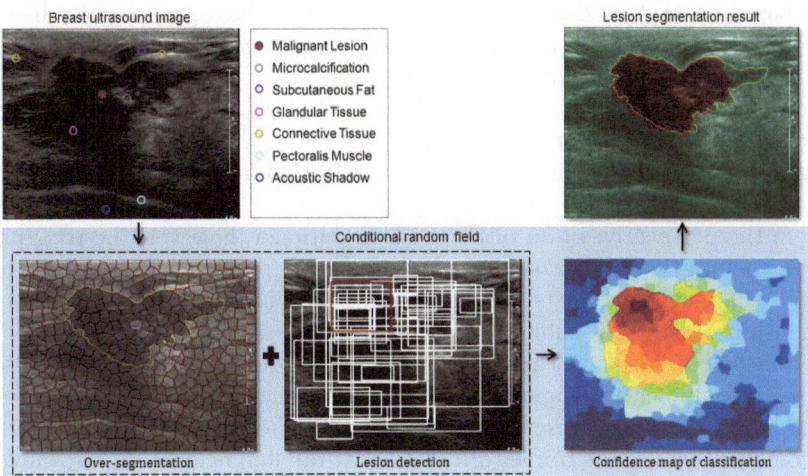

Fig. 1. An overview of the system. The process is depicted anticlockwise. The yellow contours show the groundtruth of lesion. Rectangles in the lower middle image show the detection windows, where the red one has the maximal confidence.

2   Motivations

A sound wave is sent by the sonographic transducer into the human breast, absorbed in or scattered from tissues and structures in it. The reflected wave is captured and processed into a sonogram by the ultrasonic instrument. Intensive research has been done in both fields of radiology and biomedicine [2] to distinguish lesions (both the benign and the cancerous) in ultrasound images from normalities and shadowing artifacts.

The diagnostic criteria can be generalized into the following terms [1]. First, the different echogenicity that nodule and the surrounding area show. A portion of fibrous lesions are hyperechoic with respect to isoechoic fat, while another portion of benign lesions and most of the malignant are markedly hypoechoic. And also, distinguishable internal echotexture can be observed in many cases. Second, the border and the shape of nodule. Benign nodules usually have a thin echogenic pseudocapsule with an ellipsoid shape or several gentle lobulations, and malignant nodules could show radially with spiculations and angular margins. Third, the position of the nodule. Most lesions appear in the middle mammary layer and shadows are produced under the nodules.

These criteria have been translated into computer vision language in many different ways for the design of computer-aided diagnosis system [2]. In [3], Madabhushi and Metaxas build probability distribution models for intensity and echotexture of lesion, based on which they estimate the seed point followed by a region growing procedure. To eliminate the spurious seeds, spatial arrangement together with other rules are then used. At last, the boundaries are located and shaped successively. In [4], Liu *etc.* divide the image into lattices and classify them based on texture descriptors. After that, they have to use rules like "lesions are more likely to be around the image center and occupy larger areas" to select the true regions of interest. Another common idea is towards deformable shape modeling, for example, the level set method [5]. The interior texture information can also be incorporated during the model deformation [6]. This type of algorithms usually requires a careful initialization and thus cannot avoid the selection of seed region.

From the perspective of an ultrasound practitioner, however, the recognition (and the delineation) of breast lesion in sonogram is perhaps not a product of an assembly line, which consists of several small and inaccurate rules with unclear relationships. Instead, it should be an integrated decision upon these rules. The importance of each rule is learned and adjusted through training and practicing with a large number of samples. A notable work comes from Siemens researchers recently [7]. They train discriminative models of both texture and boundary, and combine them in the framework of Markov random field. However, they still treat lesion detection and segmentation as two steps of one problem, and leave the situation that detection fails undiscussed.

We found that in practical applications, even the state-of-the-art lesion detector such as the deformable part based detection algorithm [8] still can not provide perfect detection result. So in this paper, we propose a novel algorithm to achieve a joint optimization of lesion detection and segmentation. Empirical rules are implicitly contained in different units. Specifically, rules about shape and structure are in the lesion detector, boundary and texture are in the image over-segmentation and the segment classifier, and position cues are in both of the sliding windows and segments.

The study on the combination of detection and segmentation is not new for computer vision community. In [9], Gao *et al.* augment the bounding box with internal cells to enrich the representation ability. Although outputting tighter masks, their motivation is still to improve the detection results by handling the problem of object occlusion. The most similar work to ours is [10], where bounding boxes are enforced as higher order potentials on the conditional random filed (CRF) model of image pixel. Detection hypothesis could be accepted or rejected depends on its agreement with confidences from pixels and segments. The difference of this paper is, we use over-redundant outputs of detection without considering their validity. We believe that many detection windows more than the true positive can provide higher level cues to the area they cover. These cues are collected and retrained with features from segments into a unified classification model, and thus the final segmentation is able to avoid the mistake which possibly occurs in lesion detection.

3   Algorithm

We define the problem of lesion segmentation on a pairwise CRF model. Let $\mathcal{X}$ denote the set of random variable which takes the label of either lesion or not, and $\mathcal{E}$ denote the set of edge which connects each pair of nodes. A typical pairwise

CRF is modeled as the sum of a unary potential ψ and a pairwise potential ϕ, and minimizes the energy function with the form of

$$E(\mathcal{C}|\mathcal{X}) = \sum_{x_i \in \mathcal{X}} \psi(c_i|x_i) + \mu \sum_{(x_i,x_j) \in \mathcal{E}} \phi(c_i, c_j|x_i, x_j), \qquad (1)$$

where c_i denotes the label (*i.e.* lesion or non-lesion) of the node x_i.

The node in the CRF model could correspond to a pixel or a segment in the image. We use the segment here. The over-segmentation tool we have used is a hierarchical method proposed by G. Mori [11]. The method starts with a normalized cut [12], and then builds the following layers iteratively by applying the k-means clustering on the premise of respecting the existing boundaries. The normalized cut tends to produce roughly equal size of patches and the k-means algorithm ensures a low internal variation of intensity. In this way, we obtain a set of segments with a multiple-layer structure. Features from different layers are collected together to enhance the representation ability. Other less time-consuming methods could be used for over-segmentation as well, for example, the quick shift [13], but the system performance would deteriorate with the loss of larger-scale information. We will show the related experiments in section 4.

The unary potential of the CRF model is defined based on the response of features of segment. Before solving the CRF problem, we will discuss first how the features are collected, especially from lesion detection.

3.1   Lesion Detection and Feature Propagation

When the image is broken into segments, some critical information of the lesion such as the shape or the context is possibly lost and can hardly be retrieved with this bottom-up fashion. Then the object detector becomes a complementary tool which is capable of providing higher-level supports. For this reason, we introduce the deformable part model (DPM) [8], one of the most successful detectors currently.

The deformable part-based detector produces over-complete sliding windows for potential lesion area. Many of them are retained after non-maximum suppression. Then, the MAP estimation is usually applied to select the window with maximum confidence and discard all of the others. For ultrasound image, the problem is becoming more difficult because of the existence of similar tissues and artifacts, which makes the detection confidence less reliable. So it is risky to select one of the windows as the bounding box of the lesion [7] before investigating the interior.

On the other hand, however, it is also difficult to re-rank the windows based on the ambiguous local cues. Here we propose a new mechanism to avoid the comparison. We propagate the information provided by these rectangular windows to amorphous segments. Specifically, the feature received by the segment x_i includes 4 pieces, *i.e.* $\mathbf{f}(x_i) = [\mathbf{f}_{rect}(x_i), \mathbf{f}_{dist}(x_i), \mathbf{f}_{prop}(x_i), \mathbf{f}_{acc}(x_i)]$.

$\mathbf{f}_{rect}(x_i) = [g(s_i), r(s_i), g(s_m), r(s_m)]$ records the original information of rectangles. s_i is the maximal confidence among the windows that cover x_i, and

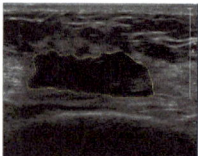 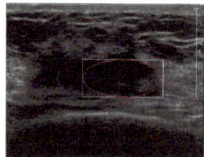 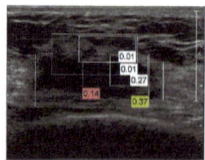 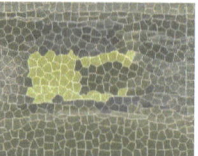

(a) Ultrasound image and groundtruth masks | (b) Foreground and background masks | (c) Detection windows with scores | (d) Score map of segments

Fig. 2. An illustration of how the intensity contrast score is computed and propagated to segments. 5 windows are shown in (c) where clearly, the window with the maximal score (in yellow) is not the one with the maximal detection confidence (in red).

$g(s_i) = 1/(1 + \exp(-2s_i))$. For ease of exposition, we call the detection window with s_i as the proxy of x_i. $r(s_i)$ contains the position and the size of the proxy, which are regularized by the format of the image. s_m is the maximal score in the full image.

$\mathbf{f}_{dist}(x_i) = [d(s_i), d(s_m)]$ records the distances from the segment to its proxy and the most supported window. Since tissues in windows usually appear as dense nodules, a segment around the center is more likely to inherit the property of the window. $d(s_i) = 2/(1 + \exp(2t))$ and $t = max(t_x, t_y)$, where t_x, t_y are the distances along x and y axes and regularized by the size of the window.

$\mathbf{f}_{prop}(x_i)$ contains the extended properties of detection window. Here we introduce the intensity contrast to measure the dissimilarity of a window to its surrounding area. The score equals to the Chi-square distance between their histograms of intensity. Different with [14], we modify the area masks from rectangle to ellipse and again pass on these scores from proxy windows to segments. See Fig. 2 as an example. Note that other objectness measures in [14] can be readily used as well.

$\mathbf{f}_{acc}(x_i)$ measures the total strength of detection confidence and intensity contrast score of all the windows covering x_i, and then regularized by the maximal value in the current image.

3.2   Problem Solving

We also extract the following features from segments: their positions in the image, histograms of intensity and texture descriptors derived from grey-level co-occurrence matrix [15]. These features and those propagated from detections are concatenated to train a segment classifier.

Finally, we solve the lesion segmentation problem by optimizing Eq. 1. The unary potential ψ in CRF model is defined based on the probability given by the output of the segment classifier: $\psi(c_i|x_i) = -\log(P(c_i|x_i))$. The pairwise potential ϕ is defined as

$$\phi(c_i, c_j|x_i, x_j) = \exp\left(-\frac{\|h_i - h_j\|^2}{2\sigma^2}L(x_i, x_j)\right)\delta(c_i \neq c_j), \qquad (2)$$

where $\|h_i - h_j\|$ is the distance between two histograms of intensity, and $L(x_i, x_j)$ is the strength of the shared boundary, which is set to infinity when x_i and x_j are not contiguous. $\delta(\pi)$ is a bool expression which takes 1 when π holds and 0 otherwise. The problem of minimizing Eq. 1 could be solved by using the popular min-cut/max-flow algorithm.

4 Experiments

We collect 480 breast ultrasound images to evaluate the proposed algorithm. All the ultrasound images are grayscale, produced by the ultrasound machine Philips IU22. 320 images are randomly selected for training, the other 160 for testing, but both of them covers all kinds of lesions presented in the full dataset. Lesion boundaries are delineated by experienced ultrasound practitioners.

We create about 400 segments for each image. The segment classifier is trained by support vector machines with RBF kernels. For the DPM detector, the number of parts is set to 8 and the minimal size of part template is 6×6. From several to dozens of detection windows are used for feature propagation depending on the complexity of the image.

To show the functionalities of different units, we have carefully designed two competitors. The first (**Fulkerson09**) is proposed in [16], where a segment based CRF model is used to solve the segmentation problem but without the intervention of any object detector. Segments are produced by the quick shift as in [16]. Another competitor (DPM-**Levelset**) is a cascade of lesion detection and level set segmentation. Similar to [7], the result of detection is used as the bounding box of the lesion to initialize the shape model of level set. The maximal number of dynamic iterations is set to 500.

For lesions with homogeneous appearance and distinct border, all these approaches perform well. We show some complicated cases with their results in Fig. 3. Lesions are benign in upper 4 rows and malignant in lower 4 rows. The proposed algorithm works best in these cases. The approach of **Fulkerson09** lacks of object-level information and thus has troubles in discriminating spurious segments and recovering the lesion boundary. Post-processing of these results is not straightforward. DPM-**Levelset** works quite well if the level set model is initialized properly, but it is totally confused when the lesion detection fails such as in the 4th and 8th cases. The proposed algorithm is able to find an optimal balance between the bottom-up and the top-down image cues, therefore avoids being trapped by any of these problems.

The segmentation performance is reported in Table 1. 10% outliers are removed for all methods as in [7]. Let S be the segmented lesion region and G be the lesion in groundtruth. The Jaccard coefficient is defined as $(S \cap G)/(S \cup G)$.

Table 1. Statistical results of lesion segmentation

	Fulkerson09	DPM-Levelset	The proposed
Average Jaccard	0.57 ± 0.24	0.69 ± 0.26	0.75 ± 0.17
Median Jaccard	0.65	0.76	0.81

Sonogram   Fulkerson09   DPM-Levelset   Proposed

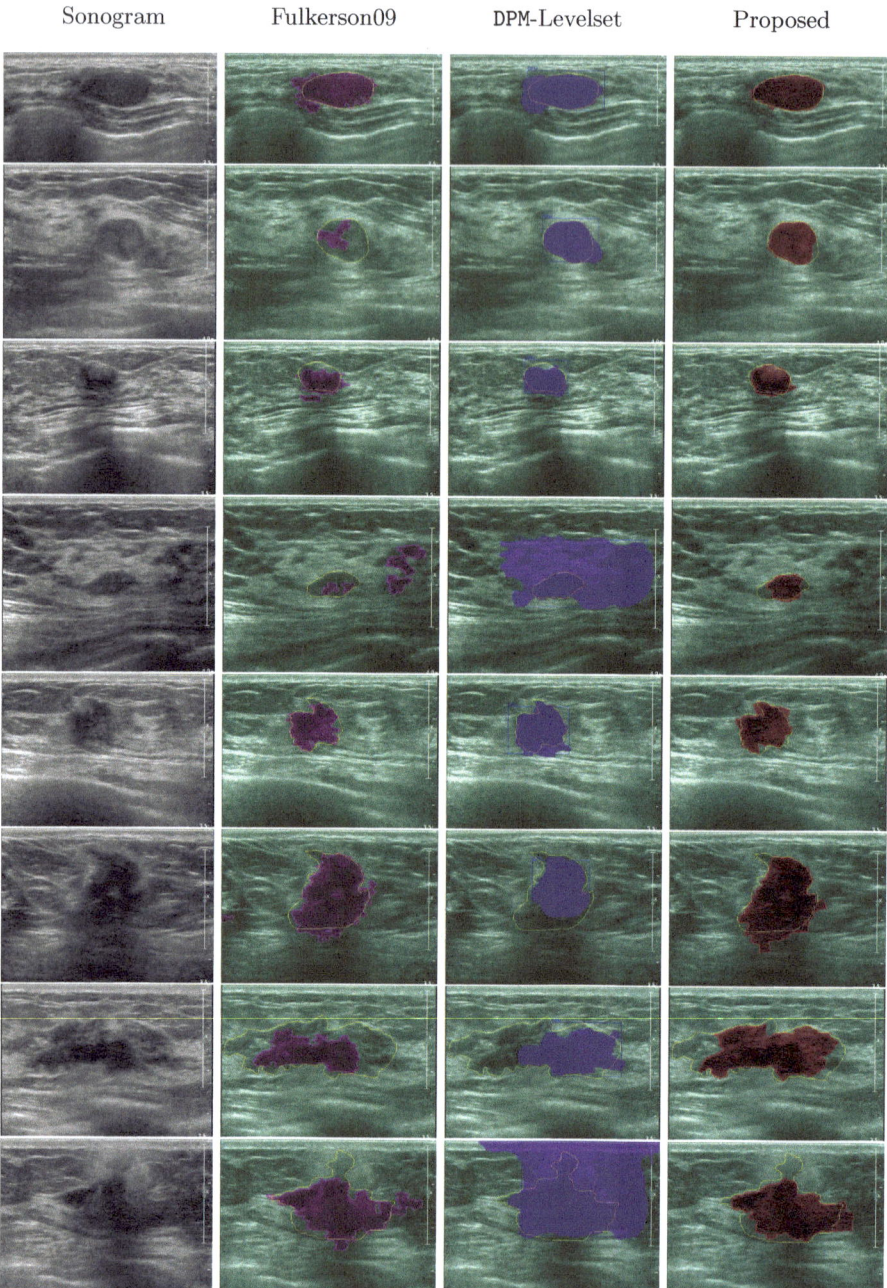

Fig. 3. Lesion segmentation results on breast ultrasound images. The upper 4 rows are benign cases and the lower 4 are malignant. Contours of groundtruth are shown in yellow. Detection windows of DPM with maximal confidences are shown as blue rectangles in the 3rd column. Note that the DPM detector works in both **DPM-Levelset** and the proposed algorithm. When it fails in the 4th and the last cases, the proposed algorithm ignores the detection mistakes and outperforms its counterparts.

5   Conclusion

We present a new algorithm for lesion segmentation in breast sonograms. The integration of image over-segmentation and lesion detection into a CRF model is proposed to achieve a comprehensive optimization on different diagnostic rules. The segmentation is driven by the segment-based CRF model and not aligned well with the local edge, which provides us a direction of the future work.

References

1. Stavros, A., Thickman, D., Rapp, C., Dennis, M., Parker, S., Sisney, G., et al.: Solid breast nodules: use of sonography to distinguish between benign and malignant lesions. Radiology 196(1), 123 (1995)
2. Noble, J., Boukerroui, D.: Ultrasound image segmentation: A survey. TMI 25(8), 987–1010 (2006)
3. Madabhushi, A., Metaxas, D.: Combining low-, high-level and empirical domain knowledge for automated segmentation of ultrasonic breast lesions. TMI 22(2), 155–169 (2003)
4. Liu, B., Cheng, H., Huang, J., Tian, J., Tang, X., Liu, J.: Fully automatic and segmentation-robust classification of breast tumors based on local texture analysis of ultrasound images. PR 43(1), 280–298 (2010)
5. Chan, T., Vese, L.: Active contours without edges. TIP 10(2), 266–277 (2001)
6. Huang, X., Metaxas, D.: Metamorphs: Deformable shape and appearance models. PAMI 30(8), 1444–1459 (2008)
7. Zhang, J., Zhou, S., Brunke, S., Lowery, C., Comaniciu, D.: Database-guided breast tumor detection and segmentation in 2d ultrasound images. In: SPIE Medical Imaging, vol. 7624, p. 3. Citeseer (2010)
8. Felzenszwalb, P., Girshick, R., McAllester, D., Ramanan, D.: Object detection with discriminatively trained part-based models. PAMI, 1627–1645 (2009)
9. Gao, T., Packer, B., Koller, D.: A segmentation-aware object detection model with occlusion handling. In: CVPR, pp. 1361–1368. IEEE (2011)
10. Ladický, Ľ., Sturgess, P., Alahari, K., Russell, C., Torr, P.H.S.: What, Where and How Many? Combining Object Detectors and CRFs. In: Daniilidis, K., Maragos, P., Paragios, N. (eds.) ECCV 2010, Part IV. LNCS, vol. 6314, pp. 424–437. Springer, Heidelberg (2010)
11. Mori, G.: Guiding model search using segmentation. In: ICCV, vol. 2, pp. 1417–1423. IEEE (2005)
12. Shi, J., Malik, J.: Normalized cuts and image segmentation. PAMI 22(8), 888–905 (2000)
13. Vedaldi, A., Soatto, S.: Quick Shift and Kernel Methods for Mode Seeking. In: Forsyth, D., Torr, P., Zisserman, A. (eds.) ECCV 2008, Part IV. LNCS, vol. 5305, pp. 705–718. Springer, Heidelberg (2008)
14. Alexe, B., Deselaers, T., Ferrari, V.: What is an object? In: CVPR, pp. 73–80. IEEE (2010)
15. Oliver, A., Freixenet, J., Martí, R., Zwiggelaar, R.: A Comparison of Breast Tissue Classification Techniques. In: Larsen, R., Nielsen, M., Sporring, J. (eds.) MICCAI 2006, Part II. LNCS, vol. 4191, pp. 872–879. Springer, Heidelberg (2006)
16. Fulkerson, B., Vedaldi, A., Soatto, S.: Class segmentation and object localization with superpixel neighborhoods. In: CVPR, pp. 670–677. IEEE (2009)

Hierarchical Manifold Learning

Kanwal K. Bhatia[1], Anil Rao[1], Anthony N. Price[2],
Robin Wolz[1], Jo Hajnal[2], and Daniel Rueckert[1]

[1] Biomedical Image Analysis Group,
Department of Computing, Imperial College London, London, UK
[2] Division of Imaging Sciences and Biomedical Engineering,
King's College London, London, UK[*]

Abstract. We present a novel method of Hierarchical Manifold Learning which aims to automatically discover regional variations within images. This involves constructing manifolds in a hierarchy of image patches of increasing granularity, while ensuring consistency between hierarchy levels. We demonstrate its utility in two very different settings: (1) to learn the regional correlations in motion within a sequence of time-resolved images of the thoracic cavity; (2) to find discriminative regions of 3D brain images in the classification of neurodegenerative disease.

1 Introduction

In recent years, the use of manifold learning has become increasingly widespread in medical imaging, being used to uncover underlying structure both within a subject [14][17], and across populations [2][9][11][15]. Manifold learning techniques aim to discover the intrinsic dimensionality of data: a low-dimensional embedding which retains local structure of the data. Typical methods operate on images as a whole, with an entire image represented by a single point in vector space. A single medical image, however, may consist of several anatomical structures, which may vary to different extents between subjects across a population or within a time sequence of, for example, images of the thoracic cavity. An automated manifold learning technique to investigate images on a regional basis, without any prior information, forms the goal of our work.

Prior work in this area has suggested dividing an image into regular patches and finding the embedding for all patches simultaneously [4]. This was shown to offer advantages over whole image, as well as independent patch embedding, in learning the cardiac and respiratory cycles in 2D time sequences of the heart. One issue with this method is that the patch size needs to be chosen in some way, reflecting the size of the structures of the data in order to be useful. In addition, the embedding requires the solution of a matrix of size *number of patches* ×

---

[*] We thank Marc Modat and M. Jorge Cardoso from the Centre for Medical Image Computing, University College London, for their advice and assistance. The work is partially funded under the 7th Framework Programme by the European Commission (http://cordis.europa.eu/ist/).

N. Ayache et al. (Eds.): MICCAI 2012, Part I, LNCS 7510, pp. 512–519, 2012.

number of images. This makes it unsuitable for large sets of 3D data or for analysis at finer scales. In our work, we continue the idea of patch embeddings; however, we take a multiscale approach to remove the need to choose patch size. This results in a hierarchy of low-dimensional embeddings created using large to successively smaller patch sizes. To ensure consistency of the embeddings across anatomy, we enforce similarity of the embeddings between hierarchy levels. We use this *hierarchical manifold learning* (HML) for the analysis of regional variations within the thoracic cavity. Additionally, we apply it to a population of 3D brain images. Using this, we are able to automatically detect regions in the brain relevant to the classification of neurodegenerative disease.

2 Background

Single Subject Analysis: Cardiac Image Analysis. Being able to learn the cardiac cycle from images is of great potential benefit. Previous work has used the manifold structure of the cardiac cycle as an aid to left ventricle segmentation [17]. Knowledge of the physical motion of the heart is also becoming of increasing interest in patient selection for cardiac resynchronisation therapy, with *mechanical* dyssynchrony derived from image data shown to be a better predictor of outcome in certain patients [7]. Being able to automatically determine the phase differences between different regions of the heart directly from image data could therefore prove clinically useful.

Cardiac image analysis is, however, complicated by the presence of respiratory motion. This can also be analysed using manifold learning and previous work has employed this for ultrasound gating [14] and for lung CT volume reconstruction [8]. Two techniques for measuring respiration are through respiratory bellows and free-breathing navigator-gated strategies. Bellows monitor the physical movement of the chest wall during breathing, while navigators measure the displacement of the diaphragm [12]. Both methods acquire surrogates for the respiratory motion at single physical locations which then need to be correlated with the motion of the heart. This motivates the investigation of how the physical movements at various locations within the abdominal/thoracic cavity are related, and how this can be learned directly from images.

We apply hierarchical manifold learning in order to learn the different motions occurring in a sequence of real-time cardiac MRI, obtaining spatially-varying respiratory and cardiac correlations.

Population Analysis: Feature Selection for Disease Classification. Manifold learning has been used to build efficient representations of large sets of brain images [9] [11]. Reducing the dimension in this way has shown, for example, to be of benefit in the classification of Alzheimer's disease [15]. Previous work, however, has solely focussed on whole images or specific segmented structures. We use HML to classify subjects from a population of subjects with Alzheimer's disease and normal controls. In addition to this, we show how our method can be used to automatically detect the most discriminative regions for classification.

3   Methods

3.1   Manifold Learning

Manifold learning algorithms are based on the premise that data are often of artificially high dimension. Indeed, they can be well-represented by a manifold of much lower dimensionality embedded in the high dimensional space. The aim of manifold learning algorithms (see [6] for a summary), is to discover the *embedding coordinates* approximating this manifold, thereby reducing the dimensionality of the data. In order to do this effectively, it is necessary to maintain the local structure of the data in the new embedding. This structure can be represented by constructing a graph $G(V, E)$, where the vertices V correspond to data samples and edges E represent neighbourhood (defined using k-nearest neighbour or ϵ-ball distance in the space of the original data) similarities between the data points. These similarities can be encapsulated in a similarity matrix $\mathbf{W}$ given by:

$$W_{ij} = \begin{cases} e^{-\frac{\|u_i - u_j\|^2}{2}} & \text{if } i,\, j \text{ neighbours;} \\ 0 & \text{otherwise.} \end{cases}$$

where $\|u_i - u_j\|^2$ represents the Euclidean (ℓ_2) distance between data points i and j. We can then define the graph Laplacian operator as $\mathbf{L} = \mathbf{D} - \mathbf{W}$ where $\mathbf{D}$ is a diagonal matrix with non-zero elements, $\mathbf{D}_{ii} = \sum_j W_{ij}$, representing the degree of the ith vertex.

Laplacian Eigenmaps. One commonly-used manifold learning technique is Laplacian Eigenmaps (LE) [5]. This preserves structure in the data by ensuring that data points which are "close" in the high-dimensional space remain "close" in the low-dimensional embedding. This is done by minimising the following cost function:

$$C(x) = \sum_{ij} (x_i - x_j)^2 W_{ij} \tag{1}$$

which minimises the weighted Euclidean distance between the embedding coordinates x_i and x_j of data points i and j, respectively, in the low-dimensional embedding. The measure of closeness between points i and j is defined by the weight, W_{ij}, which indicates their similarity. For medical imaging applications, these points can represent whole images or image patches. Some common similarity metrics include functions of the Euclidean norm distance (equivalent to sums-of-squared differences between the images) and the correlation coefficient [14] as well as those based on Gabor filter responses [13]. One advantage of LE over other manifold learning techniques is its capacity to additionally handle non-metric similarity measures such as Normalised Mutual Information [15]. The n-dimensional solution to (1) is given by the eigenvectors $\mathbf{x}$ of the generalised eigenvalue problem $\mathbf{Lx} = \lambda \mathbf{Dx}$, corresponding to the n smallest non-zero eigenvalues (λ).

3.2 Hierarchical Manifold Learning (HML)

Previous work on localised manifold learning [4] has shown that naively partitioning images into regular patches is insufficient: anatomical structures rarely
fall conveniently within a regular grid. To overcome this, the authors add a
weighting term between adjacent patches to keep their low-dimensional embeddings similar, thus utilising neighbourhood information in the construction of
the joint embeddings. One drawback of this approach is its inability to scale
to very large numbers of images or patches. Furthermore, it lacks a systematic
method of selecting patch size. Different regions may prove to be more or less
relevant at different scales and choosing a single scale may miss trends evident
at other levels. Hierarchical manifold learning aims to address these issues. In
our work we present our framework and show how it can be applied to cardiac
images at even very fine scales (2x2mm). In addition, we apply this to the classification of subjects with Alzheimer's disease and show how HML can be used
to automatically determine the best regions for classification.

The methodology is based on the idea of manifold alignment [10]. Given a
first level embedding $\bar{x}$ of the full image, we can then recursively subdivide the
image into equal smaller parts (for example, into four in a 2D image, or eight in
3D). As each subdivision is contained within the current level, we would expect
embeddings at successive levels to be similar in some way. We obtain the new
embedding x of one of these sub-parts by amending the LE cost function such
that the new embedding is also close to the embedding obtained at the previous
level, that is, we align the new embedding to its "parent" embedding $\bar{x}$.

$$C(x) = \sum_i \mu(x_i - \bar{x}_i)^2 + (1 - \mu) \sum_{ij} (x_i - x_j)^2 W_{ij} \qquad (2)$$

where μ is a weighting parameter to determine the influence of each term. Low
values for μ reduce the strength of the inter-manifold alignment and the embedding moves towards the embedding of individual patches. Higher values for μ,
in contrast, lead to closer aligned embeddings. Since the right-most term in Eq.
(2) is equivalent to $x^T L x$, it can be shown that the analytical solution to (2) is
given by the linear solution:

$$x = (\mu I + (1 - \mu)L)^{-1} \mu I \bar{x} \qquad (3)$$

Here, L is the graph laplacian for the particular patch under consideration, computed in the same way as in the standard LE formulation (and so has dimension
equal to the number of images). This avoids the need to solve eigenvalue problems of large, augmented laplacian matrices as in [4]. Additionally we can keep
recursively subdividing to very fine image scales to produce sensitive spatially-
varying embeddings. By keeping each embedding close to its previous level, we
avoid issues with smaller patches being dominated by noise.

This method requires calculating pairwise similarities between all images for
each patch at each level - but at each level this has the same number of operations
as a single level manifold embedding of the whole image. The linear equation [2]

is solved for every patch with the same complexity. The algorithm can therefore be applied at fine scales of large sets of 3D images.

4   Results

Application to Cardiac Image Analysis. Healthy volunteers were imaged using real time MR, using a balanced steady state free precession (SSFP) sequence with spatial resolution of 2x2x10mm and temporal resolution of 117ms per frame (FA/TE/TR = 20/1.2/2.4ms). Short axis, 2-chamber and 4-chamber cardiac views were acquired for 200 dynamics (the last 180 being used for analysis). Traces from respiratory bellows were recorded alongside sequence event markers in order to align images to physiological motion.

We apply HML to a time-varying sequence of 2D cardiac images. At each level, and at each patch, we construct a graph where each node represents part of a 2D frame at one point in time, in a similar way to the conventional method of manifold learning. Since we expect similar contrasts for all frames, we weight each pair of frames using the distance defined in Section 3.1, retaining the 24 nearest neighbours at each data point.

Reducing to two dimensions, we find that one dimension shows stronger correlation with the bellows trace and the other with the area of the left ventricle (a proxy for the cardiac cycle). Figure 1 shows the correlation coefficient, $\rho = \frac{Cov(X,Y)}{Var(X)Var(Y)}$, between the first dimension of the embedding coordinates for each patch and the respiratory bellows trace, for three different levels of the hierarchy. It can be seen that there is a strong correlation between the trace and, in particular, the motion of the liver. Figure 2 shows the correlation between the embedding coordinates for each patch and the area of the left ventricle in each frame. As expected, the best correlations can be found in the heart and also in areas with blood vessels. Additionally, as the embeddings are, by design, in alignment, we can correlate the embedding at any location with any other location, using their coordinates directly.

The weighting parameter μ dictates how strongly each embedding should be aligned to its parent embedding. A higher value keeps the embeddings closer, but may lead to a lower discernibility between patches. This can be seen in Figure 3, which shows the correlation coefficients between each patch and the bellows trace, where a high value of μ gives a more homogenous embedding.

Table 1 compares the computational time required for HML and the simultaneous embedding of [4], for varying patch sizes on a 2.4GHz processor. HML allows the embeddings of much smaller patch sizes to be efficiently computed.

Application to Feature Selection for Disease Classification. We have applied HML to the Alzheimer's Disease Neuroimaging Initiative (ADNI) [1] dataset of 429 subjects of size $160 \times 192 \times 160$ mm. This consists of 231 normal control subjects and 198 subjects with Alzheimer's disease. Skull-stripped images have been intensity-normalised and aligned to MNI space using affine registration. We apply HML to this dataset using $\mu = 0.1$ to allow for greater

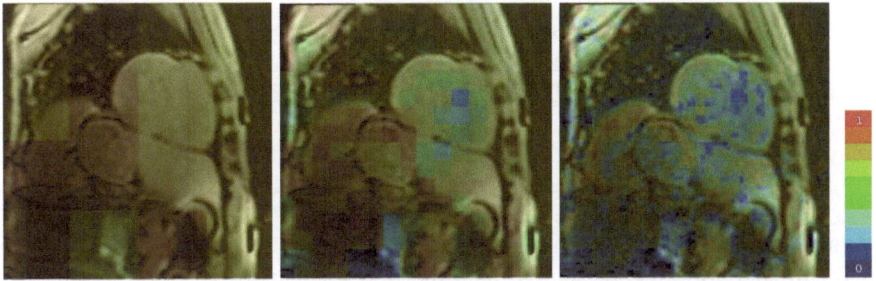

Fig. 1. Correlation with respiratory bellows trace at various resolution levels ($\mu = 0.5$)

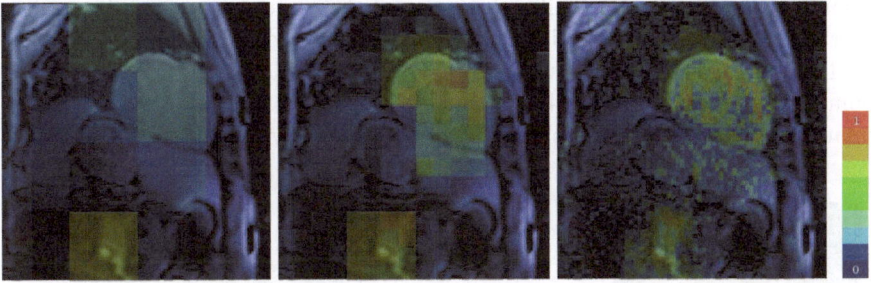

Fig. 2. Correlation with area of the left ventricle at various resolution levels ($\mu = 0.5$)

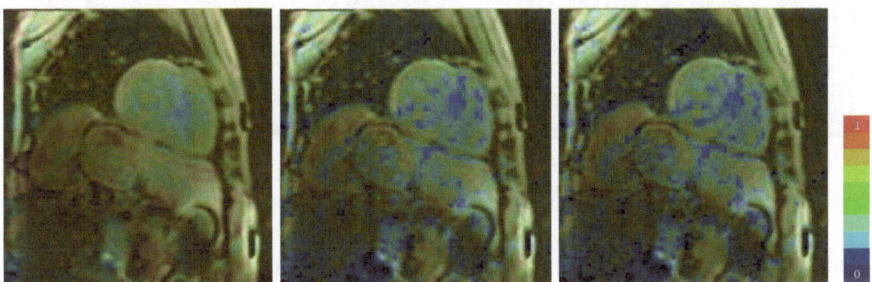

Fig. 3. Correlation with respiratory bellows trace using different weighting parameters μ. From left to right: $\mu = 0.9$, $\mu = 0.5$, $\mu = 0.1$.

discernability between patches and reduce the data to 20 dimensions. Similarity between patches is computed as specified in 3.1. The neighbourhood is selected to be as many neighbours as needed to keep the graph fully connected. At each level, we classify the patches using linear support vector machines on the embedding coordinates of each patch individually. Ten-fold cross validation is used, with the same folds used for each patch. This allows us to assess the discriminative power of each patch. Figure 4 shows the classification accuracy with the smallest patch size of 5x6x5mm. The most discriminative patches can be seen to

Table 1. Time in seconds to run each embedding for various patch sizes

Patch size (mm)	Hierarchical	Simultaneous [4]
64	1.23	0.22
32	1.80	16.1
16	3.46	4872

be concentrated around the hippocampus, in keeping with established results. HML can therefore also be viewed as a method for feature selection.

Table 2 shows the classification accuracy of the most discriminative patch with patch size (HML). The best value is comparable to classification rates obtained through manifold learning using segmented hippocampal volumes [16]. For comparison, we also show the classification rates of the same patches obtained when constructing a separate manifold for each patch independently (IND), using standard Laplacian Eigenmaps (that is, without any hierarchical alignment, while keeping all other parameters the same). It is likely that the neighbourhood information, implicit in HML embedding, helps to improve classification accuracy.

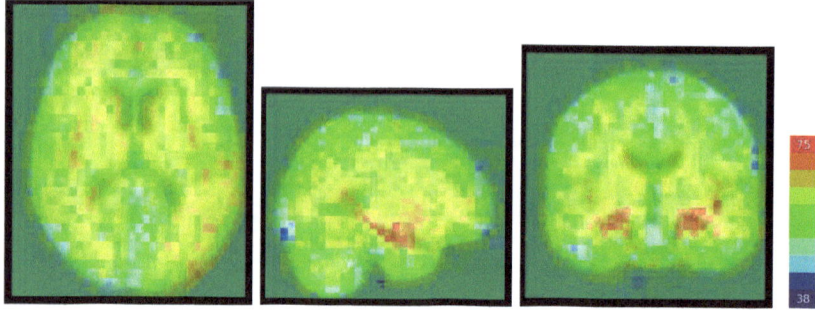

Fig. 4. Classification accuracy (%) of 5mm patches of Alzheimer's data

Table 2. Comparison of patch classification rates at various resolution levels using embeddings obtained from hierarchical manifold learning (HML) and independently, without linkage to coarser levels (IND)

Patch side length (mm)	160	80	40	20	10	5
Classification rate of most discriminative patch (HML) (%)	64	68	70	74	76	75
Classification rate of most discriminative patch (IND) (%)	64	66	68	66	68	69

5   Discussion

We have presented Hierarchical Manifold Learning to explore regional variations within image data. We have shown how it can be used to determine local correlations within the cardiac and respiratory cycles in image sequences of the thoracic cavity. The algorithm does not require pre-selecting regions of interest or patch size, and can be used to obtain embeddings even at very fine scales.

We have demonstrated the scalability of the algorithm by applying it to a population of 3D image datasets, in order to discover discriminative regions in the classification of Alzheimer's disease. In future work, we aim to investigate how to best combine these individual patch embeddings in more sophisticated ensemble classification schemes.

References

1. http://www.loni.ucla.edu/ADNI
2. Aljabar, P., et al.: A combined manifold learning analysis of shape and appearance to characterize neonatal brain development. IEEE TMI 30(12), 2072–2086 (2011)
3. Helm, R.H., Lardo, A.C.: Cardiac magnetic resonance assessment of mechanical dyssynchrony. Curr. Opin. Cardiol. 23, 440–446 (2008)
4. Bhatia, K.K., Price, A.N., Hajnal, J.V., Rueckert, D.: Localised manifold learning for cardiac image analysis. In: Haynor, D.R., Ourselin, S. (eds.) Proc. SPIE 2012 (2012)
5. Belkin, M., Niyogi, P.: Laplacian eigenmaps for dimensionality reduction and data representation. Neural Computation 15(6), 1373–1396 (2003)
6. Cayton, L.: Algorithms for Manifold Learning. Tech. report, UCSD (2005)
7. Delgado, V., Bax, J.J.: Assessment of systolic dyssynchrony for cardiac resynchronization therapy is clinically useful. Circulation 123, 640–655 (2011)
8. Georg, M., Souvenir, R., et al.: Manifold learning for 4D CT reconstruction of the lung. In: IEEE Computer Society Workshop MMBIA (2008)
9. Gerber, S., Tasdizen, T., Thomas Fletcher, P., Joshi, S., Whitaker, R., A.D.N.I.: Manifold modeling for brain population analysis. Med. Im. An. 14(5), 643–653 (2010)
10. Ham, J., Lee, D.D., Saul, L.K.: Semisupervised alignment of manifolds. AI and Statistics, 120–127 (2005)
11. Hamm, J., Davatzikos, C., Verma, R.: Efficient Large Deformation Registration via Geodesics on a Learned Manifold of Images. In: Yang, G.-Z., Hawkes, D., Rueckert, D., Noble, A., Taylor, C. (eds.) MICCAI 2009, Part I. LNCS, vol. 5761, pp. 680–687. Springer, Heidelberg (2009)
12. Savill, F., et al.: Assessment of input signal position for cardiac respiratory motion models during different breathing patterns. In: Proc. ISBI, pp. 1698–1701 (2011)
13. Souvenir, R., Pless, R.: Image distance functions for manifold learning. Image and Vision Computing 25(3), 365–373 (2007)
14. Wachinger, C., Yigitsoy, M., Navab, N.: Manifold Learning for Image-Based Breathing Gating with Application to 4D Ultrasound. In: Jiang, T., Navab, N., Pluim, J.P.W., Viergever, M.A. (eds.) MICCAI 2010, Part II. LNCS, vol. 6362, pp. 26–33. Springer, Heidelberg (2010)
15. Wolz, R., Aljabar, P., Hajnal, J.V., Rueckert, D.: Manifold Learning for Biomarker Discovery in MR Imaging. In: Wang, F., Yan, P., Suzuki, K., Shen, D. (eds.) MLMI 2010. LNCS, vol. 6357, pp. 116–123. Springer, Heidelberg (2010)
16. Wolz, R., et al.: Automatically determined hippocampal atrophy rates in ADNI. Alzheimer's and Dementia 6(4), S284 (2010)
17. Zhang, Q., Souvenir, R., Pless, R.: On manifold structure of cardiac MRI data: Application to segmentation. In: Proc. IEEE CVPR, vol. 1, pp. 1092–1098 (2006)

Vertebral Body Segmentation in MRI via Convex Relaxation and Distribution Matching

Ismail Ben Ayed[1], Kumaradevan Punithakumar[1], Rashid Minhas[1],
Rohit Joshi[2], and Gregory J. Garvin[2]

[1] GE Healthcare, London, ON, Canada
[2] The University of Western Ontario, London, ON, Canada

Abstract. We state vertebral body (VB) segmentation in MRI as a distribution-matching problem, and propose a convex-relaxation solution which is amenable to parallel computations. The proposed algorithm does not require a complex learning from a large manually-built training set, as is the case of the existing methods. From a very simple user input, which amounts to only three points for a whole volume, we compute a multi-dimensional model distribution of features that encode contextual information about the VBs. Then, we optimize a functional containing (1) a feature-based constraint which evaluates a similarity between distributions, and (2) a total-variation constraint which favors smooth surfaces. Our formulation leads to a challenging problem which is not directly amenable to convex-optimization techniques. To obtain a solution efficiently, we split the problem into a sequence of sub-problems, each can be solved exactly and globally via a convex relaxation and the augmented Lagrangian method. Our parallelized implementation on a graphics processing unit (GPU) demonstrates that the proposed solution can bring a substantial speed-up of more than 30 times for a typical 3D spine MRI volume. We report quantitative performance evaluations over 15 subjects, and demonstrate that the results correlate well with independent manual segmentations.

1 Introduction

Precise segmentation of the vertebral bodies (VBs) and intervertebral discs (IVDs) in MRI is an essential step towards thorough, reproducible and fast diagnosis of spine deformities [7,11]. Unlike CT, MRI scans depict soft-tissue structures, thereby allowing to characterize/quantify common spine disorders such as herniation [6] and disc degeneration [11]. However, most of related spine-segmentation works focused on CT, mainly because the latter affords high contrast for bony structures, e.g., [8,10,16], among others. In MRI, the problem is more challenging because of the intensity similarities and weak edges between the VBs and IVDs, the strong noise which results in intensity inhomogeneity within the VBs, and numerous acquisition protocols with different resolutions and noise types. Based on standard techniques such as adaptive-boosting learning combined with normalized cuts [7], active shape models [15], and fuzzy clustering

N. Ayache et al. (Eds.): MICCAI 2012, Part I, LNCS 7510, pp. 520–527, 2012.
© Springer-Verlag Berlin Heidelberg 2012

combined with atlas registration [11], existing MRI-based spine segmentation algorithms require an intensive learning from a large, manually-segmented training set and costly pose-estimation procedures. Furthermore, in some cases, they are difficult to extend beyond the 2D case, e.g., [7,11]. Although effective in some cases, training-based algorithms may have difficulty in capturing the substantial variations in a clinical context. The ensuing results are often bounded to the choice of a training set and a specific type of MRI data.

In this study, we state VB segmentation in MRI as a distribution-matching problem, and propose a convex-relaxation solution which is amenable to parallel computations. From a very simple user input, which amounts to only three points (clicks) for a whole 3D volume (cf. the example in Fig. 1), we compute a multi-dimensional model distribution of features that encode contextual information about the VBs and their neighboring structures. Then, we optimize a functional containing (1) a feature-based constraint which evaluates a similarity between distributions, and (2) a total-variation constraint which favors smooth surfaces. Our formulation leads to a challenging problem which is not directly amenable to convex-optimization techniques. We split the problem into a sequence of sub-problems, each can be solved globally via a convex relaxation and the augmented Lagrangian method. Unlike related graph-cut approaches [1,13], the proposed convex-relaxation solution can be parallelized to reduce substantially the computational time for 3D domains (or higher), extends directly to high dimensions, and does not have the grid-bias problem. The proposed algorithm does not require a complex learning from a large manually-segmented training set, as is the case of the existing spine-segmentation methods. Therefore, the ensuing results are independent of the choice of a training set and a specific type of MRI data. We report quantitative performance evaluations over 15 subjects, and demonstrate that the results correlate well with independent manual segmentations. Our parallelized implementation on a graphics processing unit (GPU) demonstrates that the proposed solution can bring a substantial speed-up of more than 30 times for a typical 3D spine MRI volume.

Distribution-matching formulations have recently attracted a significant interest in computer vision [1,12,13]. Several studies have shown that, in the context of 2D color segmentation [1,13], such global constraints can yield outstanding performances unattainable with standard segmentation algorithms. However, these works are based on either active contours [2,12] or iterative graph cuts [1,13]. The active contour solutions were obtained following standard gradient-descent procedures [12], which lead to computationally intensive algorithms [1,12], more so when the image dimension is high (3D or higher). The contour evolution ensuing from a distribution measure is incremental, and requires a large number of updates of computationally expensive integrals [1,12]. The recent graph cut solutions in [1,13] demonstrated significant improvements over active contours in regard to computational load/speed as well as optimality of the solution. Unfortunately, graph cuts are not amenable to parallel computations [18]. In practice, it is well known that graph cuts can yield an excellent performance in the case of 2D grids with 4-neighborhood systems [4]. However, the efficiency may decrease considerably when moving from 2D to 3D (or higher-dimensional) grids and when using larger-neighborhood grids [9]. Furthermore, the well-known grid bias is another limitation of graph-based approaches [14].

2   Formulation

Let $\mathbf{F} : \Omega \subset \mathbb{R}^n \to \mathcal{Z} \subset \mathbb{R}^k$ be a function which maps 3D (or higher-dimensional) domain Ω to a multi-dimensional (k-dimensional) space of contextual features $\mathcal{Z}$. For each point $\mathbf{x} \in \Omega$, $\mathbf{F}(\mathbf{x})$ is a vector containing image statistics within several box-shaped image patches of different orientations/scales (refer to the illustration in the left-hand side of Fig. 2). Such patch-based features can encode contextual knowledge about the region of interest and its neighboring structures (e.g., size, shape, orientation, relationships to neighboring structures, etc.). Let $\mathcal{M}$ denotes a k-dimensional model distribution of features learned from $\mathbf{F}$ within a rectangular approximation of one VB in a single 2D mid-sagittal slice of Ω (refer to the example in Fig. 1). Such approximation is obtained from a very simple user input which amounts to only three points (clicks). Given $\mathcal{M}$, we state VB segmentation as a distribution-matching problem. Our objective is to find an optimal region in Ω, so that (1) the distribution of the contextual features within the region most closely matches model $\mathcal{M}$ and (2) the surface of the region is smooth. We solve the following optimization problem:

$$\min_{u \in \{0,1\}} E(u) = \underbrace{- \sum_{\mathbf{z} \in \mathcal{Z}} \sqrt{\mathbf{P}_u(\mathbf{z}) \mathcal{M}(\mathbf{z})}}_{Contextual\ Distribution\ matching} + \underbrace{\lambda \int_{\Omega} |\nabla u(\mathbf{x})| \, d\mathbf{x}}_{Smoothness} \quad \text{where}$$

$$\mathbf{P}_u(\mathbf{z}) = \frac{\int_{\Omega} u(\mathbf{x}) K(\mathbf{F}(\mathbf{x}) - \mathbf{z}) d\mathbf{x}}{\int_{\Omega} u(\mathbf{x}) d\mathbf{x}} \quad \text{and} \quad K(\mathbf{y}) = \frac{1}{(2\pi\sigma^2)^{\frac{k}{2}}} exp^{-\frac{\|\mathbf{y}\|^2}{2\sigma^2}} \quad (1)$$

$u : \Omega \to \{0,1\}$ is binary function which defines a variable partition of Ω: $\{\mathbf{x} \in \Omega / u(\mathbf{x}) = 1\}$, corresponding to the target region, and $\{\mathbf{x} \in \Omega / u(\mathbf{x}) = 0\}$, corresponding to the complement of the target region in Ω. $\mathbf{P}_u$ is the kernel density estimate (KDE) of the k-dimensional distribution of features $\mathbf{F}$ within variable region $\{\mathbf{x} \in \Omega / u(x) = 1\}$. K is a Gaussian kernel (σ is the width of the kernel). The distribution-matching term in (1) measures the Bhattacharyya similarity between $\mathbf{P}_u$ and $\mathcal{M}$. This measure has a fixed (normalized) range which affords a conveniently practical appraisal of the similarity. This is not the case for the other common measures (e.g., the Kullback-Leibler divergence).

The smoothness term is a standard total-variation constraint which penalizes the occurrences of small, isolated regions in the solution. λ is a positive constant that balances the contribution of each term.

Direct computation of (1) is a challenging problem due to the high non-convexity of the distribution-matching term. To obtain a solution efficiently, we split the problem into a sequence of sub-problems, each of which can be solved globally via a convex relaxation and the augmented Lagrangian method.

Sub-problems: Rather than optimizing directly E, we optimize iteratively a sequence of instrumental functions, denoted $A(u, u^i)$, $i \geq 1$ (i is the iteration number), whose optimization is easier than E:

$$u^{i+1} = \min_{u \in \{0,1\}} A(u, u^i), \quad i \geq 1 \quad \text{s.t.} \tag{2a}$$

$$E(u) \leq A(u, u^i), \quad i \geq 1 \tag{2b}$$

$$E(u) = A(u, u) \quad \forall u : \Omega \to \{0, 1\} \tag{2c}$$

Using the constraints in (2b) and (2c), and by definition of minimum in (2a), one can show that the sequence of solutions in (2a) yields a decreasing sequence of E: $E(u^i) = A(u^i, u^i) \geq A(u^{i+1}, u^i) \geq E(u^{i+1})$. Furthermore, $E(u^i)$ is lower bounded and, therefore, converges to a minimum of E. Now, consider the following proposition [1]:

Proposition 1. *Given a fixed u^i, for any $u : \Omega \to \{0, 1\}$ verifying $\{\mathbf{x} \in \Omega / u(\mathbf{x}) = 1\} \subset \{\mathbf{x} \in \Omega / u^i(\mathbf{x}) = 1\}$ and $\forall \alpha \in [0, \frac{1}{2}]$, the following function verifies the constraints in (2b) and (2c) and, therefore, its iterative optimization yields a minimum of E (in the expression of A_α, $\mathbf{x}$ and $\mathbf{z}$ are omitted as arguments to simplify the notations):*

$$A_\alpha(u, u^i) = -(1 + \alpha) \sum_{\mathbf{z} \in \mathcal{Z}} \sqrt{\mathbf{P}_{u^i} \mathcal{M}} + \int_\Omega \{\alpha u g^i + (1 + \alpha)(1 - u)h^i + \lambda |\nabla u|\} d\mathbf{x}$$

$$\text{where } g^i = \frac{\sum_{\mathbf{z} \in \mathcal{Z}} \sqrt{\mathbf{P}_{u^i}(\mathbf{z}) \mathcal{M}(\mathbf{z})}}{\int_\Omega u^i d\mathbf{x}}; \quad h^i = \frac{u^i}{\int_\Omega u^i d\mathbf{x}} \sum_{\mathbf{z} \in \mathcal{Z}} K(\mathbf{z} - \mathbf{F}) \sqrt{\frac{\mathcal{M}(\mathbf{z})}{\mathbf{P}_{u^i}(\mathbf{z})}} \tag{3}$$

Convex Relaxation and Equivalent Constrained Problem: Now, we minimize A_α over $u \in \{0, 1\}$ via convex optimization. However, $\min_{u \in \{0,1\}} A_\alpha$ is still non-convex due to the binary-valued constraint $u \in \{0, 1\}$. We first relax such constraint to interval $[0, 1]$, thereby obtaining the following convex problem: $\min_{u \in [0,1]} A_\alpha$. Then, we propose the following result which allows us to obtain an exact and global minimum of A_α over $u \in \{0, 1\}$ via the multiplier-based augmented Lagrangian method (the proof follows the ideas of [17,18]):

Proposition 2. *The convex problem $\min_{u \in [0,1]} A_\alpha(u, u^i)$ is equivalent to the following constrained problem:*

$$\max_{p_h, p_g, p} \min_u \int_\Omega \{p_h + u(\operatorname{div} p - p_h + p_g)\} d\mathbf{x} \quad \text{s.t.}$$

$$p_h(\mathbf{x}) \leq (1 + \alpha)h^i(\mathbf{x}); \quad p_g(\mathbf{x}) \leq \alpha g^i(\mathbf{x}); \quad \text{and } |p(\mathbf{x})| \leq \lambda \text{ a.e. } \mathbf{x} \in \Omega \tag{4}$$

where u is viewed as the multiplier to constraint $\operatorname{div} p - p_h + p_g = 0$. $p : \Omega \to \mathbb{R}$, $p_h : \Omega \to \mathbb{R}$ and $p_g : \Omega \to \mathbb{R}$ are variables in the form of scalar functions. Furthermore, by simply thresholding the optimum $u^* \in [0, 1]$ of (4), we obtain an exact and global optimum of the non-convex problem $\min_{u \in \{0,1\}} A_\alpha(u, u^i)$.

---

[1] The proof is given in the supplemental material available at this link: http://externe.emt.inrs.ca/users/benayedi/BenAyed-Miccai12-Supp.pdf

The equivalence in proposition 2 is similar to the equivalence of the continuous max-flow/min-cut problem in [17,18]. This equivalence allows us to derive an efficient multiplier-based algorithm for optimizing E. The algorithm is based on the standard augmented Lagrangian method [3,17,18]. We define the following augmented Lagrangian function corresponding to the problem in (4) (multiplier u is replaced here by v to avoid confusion between inner and outer iterations in the algorithm presented next): $L_c(p_h, p_g, p, v) = \int_\Omega \{p_h + v(\operatorname{div} p - p_h + p_g) - \frac{c}{2}\|\operatorname{div} p - p_h + p_g\|^2\}d\mathbf{x}$. c is a positive constant. Here following a summary of the algorithm (i and j are the numbers of inner end outer iterations respectively).

Algorithm 1: Multiplier-based augmented-Lagrangian optimization

- Initialize u by $u^0(x) = 1$ ($i = 0$)
- **repeat**
  1. Update g^i and h^i according to (3)
  2. set $j = 0$, $p = p^0$, $p_h = p_h^0$, $p_g = p_g^0$ and $v = v^0$
  3. **repeat**
     - Optimize L_c with respect p:
       $$p^{j+1} = \max_{|p| \leq \lambda} -\frac{c}{2}\left\|\operatorname{div} p - p_h^j + p_g^j - \frac{v^j}{c}\right\|^2$$
       This can be solved by the Chambolle's algorithm [5].
     - Optimize L_c with respect to p_h (closed-form solution):
       $$p_h^{j+1} = \max_{p_h < (1+\alpha)h^i} \int_\Omega p_h - \frac{c}{2}\left\|\operatorname{div} p^{j+1} - p_h + p_g^j - \frac{v^j}{c}\right\|^2 d\mathbf{x}$$
     - Optimize L_c with respect to p_g (closed-form solution):
       $$p_g^{j+1} = \max_{p_g \leq \alpha g^i} -\frac{c}{2}\left\|\operatorname{div} p^{j+1} - p_h^{j+1} + p_g - \frac{v^j}{c}\right\|^2$$
     - Update multiplier v:
       $$v^{j+1} = v^j - c(\operatorname{div} p^{j+1} - p_h^{j+1} + p_g^{j+1})$$
     - Let $j = j + 1$
     until *Convergence*;
  4. Let $v*$ the solution obtained from the inner iterations above. Compute a binary solution by applying Otsu's thresholding to $v*$.
  5. Let $i = i + 1$
  6. Let u^i equal to the binary solution obtained at step 4.
  until *Convergence*;

---

3   Experiments

Description of the Features: The left-hand side of Fig. 2 depicts the contextual features we used in our experiments. For each point $\mathbf{x} \in \Omega$, we built a feature vector of dimension 3: $\mathbf{F}(\mathbf{x}) = (\mathbf{F}_1, \mathbf{F}_2, \mathbf{F}_3)$, with $\mathbf{F}_1$ the mean of intensity within a 21 x 7 x 1 rectangular-shaped, vertically-oriented patch, $\mathbf{F}_2$ the mean of intensity within a 7 x 21 x 1 rectangular-shaped, horizontally-oriented patch, and $\mathbf{F}_3$ the mean intensity within a 7 x 7 x 1 square-shaped patch, all centered at point $\mathbf{x}$. We used 32 bins to compute the feature distributions. Note that other features based on image gradients or texture can be used within the same framework.

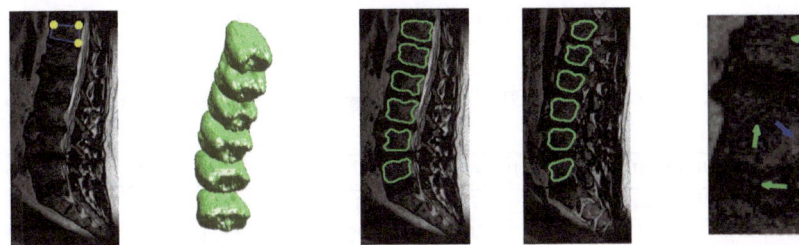

Fig. 1. A typical 3D example with a 320 x 150 x 80 volume. First column: three-point user input in a single 2D mid-sagittal slice (slice 35); second column: the obtained 3D surfaces of the lumbar (L1 to L5) and T12 VBs; third and fourth columns: the corresponding 2D-slice results (slices 35 and 25). Last column: an image patch from the user-input slice, which illustrates the difficulties inherent to spine MRI segmentation. The smoothness weight is set equal to one ($\lambda = 1$).

A Typical 3D Example: Fig. 1 depicts a typical example of the results using a 320 x 150 x 80 lumbar spine volume of the type T2-weighted. The first column shows the simple, three-point user input in a single 2D mid-sagittal slice (slice 35). The second column shows the obtained result, depicted by the 3D surfaces of the lumbar (L1 to L5) and T12 VBs. The third and fourth columns depict the corresponding 2D-slice results (slices 35 and 25). The last column is an image patch from the user-input slice, which illustrates the difficulties inherent to spine MRI segmentation. The red arrows point to weak edges between the VBs and IVDs, the green arrows to intensity similarities between the VBs and IVDs, and the blue arrow to strong image noise within the VBs.

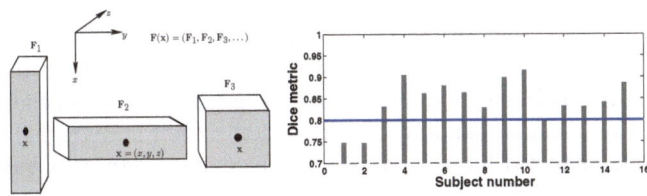

Fig. 2. Left: illustration of the contextual features; right: DM evaluations

Computational Evaluations: We further evaluated two implementations (with and without parallelization), one GPU based and the other CPU (central processing unit) based. The parallelized computations were run on an NVIDIA Quadro FX3700 with 112 Cuda cores, whereas the non-parallelized version was run on an E5440 quad core 2.83 GHz Xeon, with 3.25GB of RAM. Both versions were implemented in C. Table 1 reports the GPU/CPU times corresponding to the example in Fig. 1. For the 3D case, the parallelized version brought a substantial speed-up of more than 30 times. In the 2D case, the GPU version brought a less significant, but nonetheless important, speed-up of 13 times.

Table 1. Computational GPU/CPU times of the proposed solution

Implementation ($\lambda = 1$)	3D (320 x 150 x 80)	2D (320 x 150)
GPU (Parallelized)	143.08 s (< 3 min)	0.64 s
CPU	4.50×10^3 (≈ 75 min)	8.46 s

Table 2. Quantitative performance evaluations over 15 subjects

DM mean	DM std	Correlation coefficient (r)
0.85	0.051	0.98

Quantitative Evaluations: The evaluation was carried out over a data set of 15 mid-sagittal 2D MR spine scans acquired from 15 different subjects. We segmented automatically a total of 75 lumbar VBs starting from a simple three-point user input. We focused on lumbar VBs and MRI data of the type T2-weighted. However, the proposed method can be readily extended to IVDs and other MRI types, as it does not require any shape or image specific training. The results were compared to independent manual segmentations approved by an expert. We assessed the similarities between the ground truth and the obtained segmentations using two measures: the Dice metric (DM) and the correlation coefficient (r). DM is commonly used to measure the similarity (overlap) between the automatically detected and ground-truth regions: $DM = \frac{2S_{am}}{S_a + S_m}$, with S_a, S_m, and S_{am} corresponding respectively to the sizes of the segmented lumbar region (i.e., the region containing all the VBs from L1 to L5), the corresponding hand-labeled region, and the intersection between them. Table 2 reports for all the data analyzed the DM mean and standard deviation, as well as the correlation coefficient between manual and automatic region sizes. Fig. 2 (right) depicts the DM for the 15 analyzed lumbar regions (each region contains 5 VBs). We obtained a $DM > 0.80$ for 13 subjects (DM is about 0.75 for only two subjects). The proposed method also yielded a high correlation: $r = 0.98$.

4 Conclusion

We proposed a distribution-matching algorithm for VB segmentation in MRI and a convex-relaxation solution which is amenable to parallel computations. The algorithm removes the need for a complex learning from a large training set. We described quantitative performance evaluations over 15 subjects, and showed that a GPU-based implementation of our solution can bring a substantial speed-up of more than 30 times for a typical 3D spine MRI volume.

References

1. Ben Ayed, I., Chen, H.M., Punithakumar, K., Ross, I., Li, S.: Graph cut segmentation with a global constraint: Recovering region distribution via a bound of the bhattacharyya measure. In: CVPR, pp. 3288–3295 (2010)
2. Ben Ayed, I., Li, S., Ross, I.: A statistical overlap prior for variational image segmentation. International Journal of Computer Vision 85(1), 115–132 (2009)
3. Bertsekas, D.P.: Nonlinear Programming. Athena Scientific (1999)
4. Boykov, Y., Kolmogorov, V.: An experimental comparison of min-cut/max- flow algorithms for energy minimization in vision. IEEE Trans. on Pattern Analysis and Machine Intelligence 26(9), 1124–1137 (2004)
5. Chambolle, A.: An algorithm for total variation minimization and applications. Journal of Mathematical Imaging and Vision 20(1-2), 89–97 (2004)
6. Fardon, D.F., Milette, P.C.: Nomenclature and classification of lumbar disc pathology: Recommendations of the combined task forces of the north american spine society, american society of spine radiology, and american society of neuroradiology. spine 26(5), E93–E113 (2001)
7. Huang, S., Chu, Y., Lai, S., Novak, C.: Learning-based vertebra detection and iterative normalized-cut segmentation for spinal mri. IEEE Trans. on Medical Imaging 28(10), 1595–1605 (2009)
8. Klinder, T., Ostermann, J., Ehm, M., Franz, A., Kneser, R., Lorenz, C.: Automated model-based vertebra detection, identification, and segmentation in ct images. Medical Image Analysis 13(3), 471–482 (2009)
9. Klodt, M., Schoenemann, T., Kolev, K., Schikora, M., Cremers, D.: An Experimental Comparison of Discrete and Continuous Shape Optimization Methods. In: Forsyth, D., Torr, P., Zisserman, A. (eds.) ECCV 2008, Part I. LNCS, vol. 5302, pp. 332–345. Springer, Heidelberg (2008)
10. Mastmeyer, A., Engelke, K., Fuchs, C., Kalender, W.: A hierarchical 3d segmentation method and the definition of vertebral body coordinate systems for qct of the lumbar spine. Medical Image Analysis 10(4), 560–577 (2006)
11. Michopoulou, S., Costaridou, L., Panagiotopoulos, E., Speller, R., Panayiotakis, G., Todd-Pokropek, A.: Atlas-based segmentation of degenerated lumbar intervertebral discs from mr images of the spine. IEEE Trans. on Biomedical Engineering 56(9), 2225–2231 (2009)
12. Mitiche, A., Ben Ayed, I.: Variational and Level Set Methods in Image Segmentation, 1st edn. Springer (2010)
13. Pham, V.Q., Takahashi, K., Naemura, T.: Foreground-background segmentation using iterated distribution matching. In: CVPR (2011)
14. Pock, T., Chambolle, A., Cremers, D., Bischof, H.: A convex relaxation approach for computing minimal partitions. In: CVPR (2009)
15. Seifert, S., Wachter, I., Schmelzle, G., Dillmann, R.: A knowledge-based approach to soft tissue reconstruction of the cervical spine. IEEE Transactions on Medical Imaging 28(4), 494–507 (2009)
16. Shen, H., Litvin, A., Alvino, C.: Localized Priors for the Precise Segmentation of Individual Vertebras from CT Volume Data. In: Metaxas, D., Axel, L., Fichtinger, G., Székely, G. (eds.) MICCAI 2008, Part I. LNCS, vol. 5241, pp. 367–375. Springer, Heidelberg (2008)
17. Yuan, J., Bae, E., Tai, X.C., Boykov, Y.: A study on continuous max-flow and min-cut approaches. Part I: Binary labeling. Tech report CAM-10-61, UCLA (2010)
18. Yuan, J., Bae, E., Tai, X.C.: A study on continuous max-flow and min-cut approaches. In: CVPR (2010)

Evaluating Segmentation Error without Ground Truth

Timo Kohlberger[1], Vivek Singh[1], Chris Alvino[2],
Claus Bahlmann[1], and Leo Grady[3]

[1] Imaging and Computer Vision, Siemens Corp., Corporate Research and
Technology, Princeton, NJ, USA
[2] American Science and Engineering, Billerica, MA, USA
[3] HeartFlow, Inc., Redwood City, CA, USA

Abstract. The automatic delineation of the boundaries of organs and
other anatomical structures is a key component of many medical image
processing systems. In this paper we present a generic learning approach
based on a novel space of segmentation features, which can be trained to
predict the overlap error and Dice coefficient of an arbitrary organ segmentation without knowing the ground truth delineation. We show the
regressor to be much stronger a predictor of these error metrics than the
responses of Probabilistic Boosting Classifiers trained on the segmentation boundary. The presented approach not only allows us to build
reliable confidence measures and fidelity checks, but also to rank several
segmentation hypotheses against each other during online usage of the
segmentation algorithm in clinical practice.

1 Introduction

Measuring the quality of a segmentation produced by an algorithm is key to creating a deployable system and comparing the effectiveness of different algorithms
to address a particular application. In fact, segmentation quality measures form
the backbone for judging results of the segmentation challenges embraced by the
medical imaging community in recent years (e.g., [8]). Additionally, these quality
measures are key to publishing segmentation algorithms in order to demonstrate
improved effectiveness of a new algorithm. Recent studies have shown that standard quality measures used in the community (or combinations thereof) serve as
good proxies for human evaluation of segmentation quality in a clinical context
[5,7].

The basic procedure for applying the existing quality measures is to create
ground truth (manually segmented) structures and to compare those structures with algorithm-generated segmentations in terms of overlap or boundary
differences. Although this procedure is effective for developing and comparing
algorithms, there is no automated method for evaluating segmentation quality
after algorithm deployment since there is no ground truth available after deployment (if there were, then a segmentation algorithm would be unnecessary).
Consequently, in the field, our methods for evaluating segmentation quality are

N. Ayache et al. (Eds.): MICCAI 2012, Part I, LNCS 7510, pp. 528–536, 2012.
© Springer-Verlag Berlin Heidelberg 2012

not usable due to a lack of ground truth segmentations to compare with. Figure 1 illustrates this difference.

The evaluation of segmentation quality after deployment serves a very different purpose than the evaluation of segmentation quality during algorithm development. During development, the purpose of the evaluation is to compare different approaches or to optimize parameter settings. In contrast, on-line segmentation evaluation during deployment has several uses:

1. The evaluation can flag the user or system that a poor segmentation was obtained that requires particular manual review.
2. If a poor segmentation evaluation is obtained, the deployed system can try again to produce a better segmentation by re-running the segmentation with different algorithm parameters or a new algorithm entirely.
3. Every time a segmentation is required for a new dataset, several candidate segmentations may be generated on-line (e.g., in parallel) using different parameter settings and/or algorithms. The candidate segmentations are each evaluated and the segmentation with best evaluation score is then selected to return as output.

Several different types of popular segmentation algorithms are associated with measures that might be considered useful to evaluate segmentation in the absence of ground truth. For example, any of the family of optimization-based segmentation algorithms (e.g., level sets [17], graph cuts [2], random walker [9]) explicitly optimize an objective function to produce the desired segmentation. Therefore, a natural idea might be to use the energy of the output solution as an evaluation metric for segmentation quality. However, this energy of the minimal solution is unsuitable to evaluating segmentation quality since these algorithms are designed to compare *relative* energies of different segmentations and not to measure an *absolute* energy difference between a (possibly locally minimal) solution to the ground truth. Another class of popular segmentation algorithms utilizes learning to produce the segmentation. For these methods, a natural idea would be to use the outputs of the learning system as a confidence measure to perform on-line segmentation evaluation in the absence of ground truth. However, in Section 3 we demonstrate that the learning outputs of one popular learning algorithm, the Probabilistic Boosting Tree (PBT) [19], are poorly correlated with traditional measures of segmentation error when ground truth is known.

We adopt a hybrid approach to evaluating segmentation quality in the absence of ground truth. First, we calculate features to de-

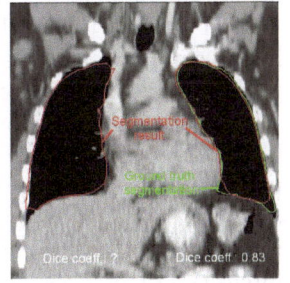

Fig. 1. With ground truth, quantifying the segmentation error is straightforward (left lung). This error relative to ground truth is essential during pre-development to select an algorithm and optimize parameters. In contrast, our method applies to the post-deployment situation where it is necessary to estimate error when no ground truth is available (right lung).

scribe the output segmentation which are derived from the optimization-based segmentation literature. Effectively, we choose features by adopting every generic term in an objective function that we could find from an optimization-based segmentation paper. Second, we train a regression algorithm to predict the conventional segmentation error with respect to a known ground truth. Once trained, the regression algorithm can be used to predict the segmentation error from the calculated features *in the absence of ground truth*.

2   Method

First we introduce a novel space of shape and appearance features to characterize a segmentation. We then use these features to learn a predictor of segmentation error by training on error with respect to ground truth.

2.1   Using Energy Terms as Segmentation Features

We propose the following 42 shape and appearance features, many of which can be found as building blocks of popular energy-based or graph-based segmentation approaches. Thereby we remain agnostic about which feature choices worked well for the final regressor. The features we used can be broken down into five major categories: (weighted or unweighted) geometric features, intensity features, gradient features, and ratio features.

Note that in the following descriptions, we will use three-dimensional (3-D) terminology such as voxels, volume, surface area, and mean curvature, but it is understood that when applied to 2-D problems, the appropriate 2-D counterparts are implied, without loss of generality. In addition, all weights in these descriptions refer to the Cauchy distribution function applied to the appropriate image intensities differences, i.e., $w(I_1, I_2) = \frac{1}{1+\beta(\frac{I_1-I_2}{M})^2}$, where I_1 and I_2 are two image intensities in question, β, which is set to 10^4 for all experiments, controls the sensitivity of the weight to intensity difference, and $M = \max_{(x,y) \in S} \|\nabla I(x,y)\|_1$ was the maximum L1 norm of all intensity gradients within the segmentation mask, S. The purpose of M is to normalize the weights. We will also define $w_+(I_1, I_2) = w(I_1, I_2)$ when $I_1 > I_2$ and $w_+(I_1, I_2) = 1$ otherwise. Likewise, we will define $w_-(I_1, I_2) = 1$ when $I_1 > I_2$ and $w_-(I_1, I_2) = w(I_1, I_2)$ otherwise.

Geometric features capture some measure of size of the segmentation mask $S \subset \mathbb{R}^3$, a concept dating back to some of the earliest works on image segmentation [1,16,4]. Of these, we chose: *volume*, defined as the number of voxels in the segmentation mask, $|S|$; *surface area*, the number of edges (assuming a graph structure with a 6-connected lattice) on the boundary of the segmentation, $\sum_{i,j:i \in S, j \in \bar{S}} 1$, where $\bar{S}$ is the set of voxels not in the segmentation mask; and *total curvature*, the sum of the mean curvature defined on the segmentation surface, $\sum_{i,j:i \in S, j \in \bar{S}} H(i,j)$, where $H(i,j)$ is the discretely computed mean curvature on the segmentation surface between voxels i and j and is locally computed as in [6].

Weighted geometric features are similar to the geometric features, but in addition the geometric measure is locally emphasized when intensity values are similar to each other and suppressed when local intensity values are dissimilar to each other. This concept has been pervasive in image segmentation since the work of Caselles *et al.* [3] and has been seen in many other recent works [9]. The geometric weights we use are based on local intensity in the image and are mapped via the Cauchy function $w(\cdot, \cdot)$ shown above. In the cases where we refer to voxel (or vertex $v \in V$) weight, we mean the average weight of all edges leaving that vertex, $w(v) = \frac{1}{D_v} \sum_{i:(v,i) \in E} w(I_v, I_i)$ where D_v is the degree of the vertex v. For weighted geometric features, we chose: *weighted volume*, the sum over the weights of all voxels, $\sum_{v \in S} w(v)$; *weighted cut*, the sum over the all edge weights along the boundary of the segmentation $\sum_{i,j:i \in S, j \in \bar{S}} w(I_i, I_j)$; *weighted curvature* $\sum_{i,j:i \in S, j \in \bar{S}} w(I_i, I_j) H(i, j)$, the sum of the mean curvature weighted by the local edge weight; *low-hi weighted cut*, $\sum_{i,j:i \in S, j \in \bar{S}} w_+(I_i, I_j)$; and *hi-low weighted cut* $\sum_{i,j:i \in S, j \in \bar{S}} w_-(I_i, I_j)$ along the segmentation boundary.

Intensity features use various measures of the direct image intensities. Of these, we chose: *mean intensity* defined as $\mu_I = \frac{1}{|S|} \sum_{v \in S} I_v$; *median intensity* defined as median$(\{I_v : v \in S\})$; *sum of intensities* $\sum_{v \in S} I_v$; *minimum intensity* $\min_{v \in S} I_v$; *maximum intensity* $\max_{v \in S} I_v$; *interquartile distance* (defined as half of the difference between the 75th percentile and the 25th percentile values) of intensities; and *standard deviation* of the intensities $\frac{1}{|S|-1} \sum_{v \in S} (I_v - \mu_I)^2$.

Gradient features use various measures of the intensity gradients (local intensity changes). All intensity derivatives comprising these gradients are computed via central differences. Of these, we chose: *sum of the L1 norms of the gradients,* $\sum_{v \in S} \|\nabla I(v)\|_1$; *sum of the L2 norms of the gradients,* $\sum_{v \in S} \|\nabla I(v)\|_2$; *mean of the L1 norms of the gradients* $\frac{1}{|S|} \sum_{v \in S} \|\nabla I(v)\|_1$; *mean of the L2 norm of gradients* $\mu_g = \frac{1}{|S|} \sum_{v \in S} \|\nabla I(v)\|_2$; *median of the L1 norms of gradients* median$(\{\|\nabla I(v)\|_1 : v \in S\})$; *minimum L1 norm of all gradients* $\min_{v \in S} \|\nabla I(v)\|_1$; *maximum L1 norm of all gradients* $\max_{v \in S} \|\nabla I(v)\|_1$; *interquartile distance of the L1 norms of the gradients*; *standard deviation of the L1 norms of gradients*; and *the standard deviation of the L2 norms of gradients* $\frac{1}{|S|-1} \sum_{v \in S} (\|\nabla I_v\|_2 - \mu_g)^2$.

We opt to explicitly include a selection of features that were ratios of our other features. The intent is not to be completely comprehensive, but rather to use domain knowledge of segmentation problems to explicitly choose combinations that the literature and our experience told us would be good indicators of segmentation performance. The ratio features are simply the ratio of two features above. We only include ratios that either we believe to be meaningful, or have appeared in the segmentation literature thus far. Several fall into the category of cut divided by volume, a concept that has appeared throughout the history of segmentation in various forms [13,10]. Of these, we chose: *all four weighted and unweighted combinations of cut divided by volume; all four combinations of low-hi weighted cut or hi-low weighted cut divided by unweighted or weighted volume; weighted cut divided by unweighted cut; all four combinations of low-hi weighted cut or hi-low weighted cut divided by unweighted or weighted cut; blur index* defined as *sum the L2 norms of the gradients* divided by *sum of the L1*

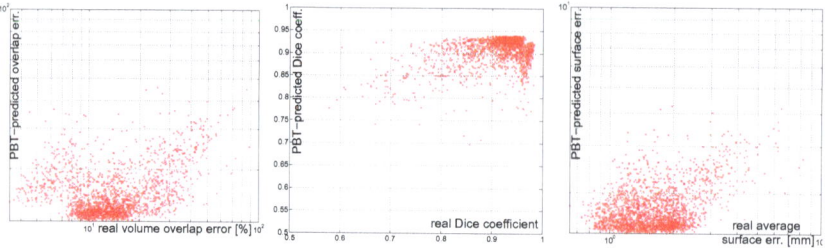

Fig. 2. Real segmentation errors (x-axis) versus linearly regressed PBT-probabilities (y-axis). Correlations coefficients (left to right): 0.45, 0.48, 0.49. Max. surf. err: 0.29. (Note that for readability we have adopted linear and log scaling where appropriate.)

norms of the gradients; *curvature over unweighted cut*; and *weighted curvature over unweighted cut*.

Some of the features, such as the geometric features and most of the intensity-based features, are not meant to be discriminative alone. Rather, they are intended to lend context about the expected values for some of the other more discriminative features for a given candidate segmentation. Our intention is to extract features that might be relevant *independent* of the classifier method, and then to let feature selection or the classifiers determine how the features would be used.

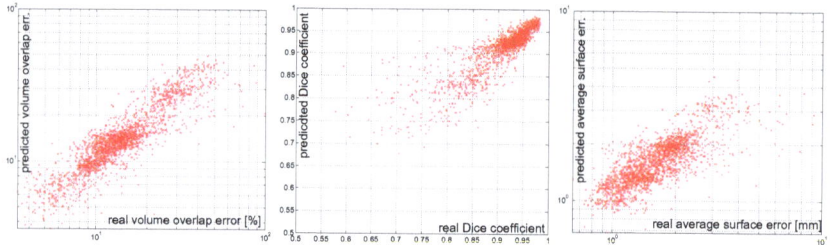

Fig. 3. Real segmentation errors (x-axis) versus SVM regressor-predicted ones (y-axis). Correlations coefficients (fr. l. to r.): 0.85, 0.79, 0.56. Max. surface error: 0.69.

2.2 Learning to Predict Segmentation Error

Based on this novel space of shape and appearance features, we propose to use nonlinear regressors in order to separately approximate different segmentation metrics. Specifically, we treat the 42 features as independent variables and each of the error metrics, which we will define below, as dependent variables.

In order to obtain a comprehensive quantification of the segmentation error relative to the ground truths, we employ four different error metrics. Let $G, S \subset \mathbb{R}^3$ denote the set of points of the ground truth segment and the computed segment, respectively. As first metric we use the popular *volumetric overlap error* [12]: $E_O(S, G) = 1 - (|S \cap G|)/(|S \cup G|)$, which is 0% for a perfect

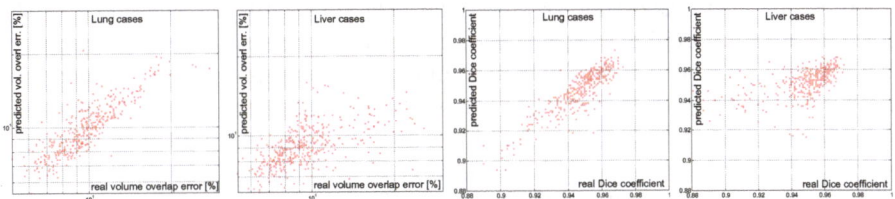

Fig. 4. Real segmentation errors (x-axis) versus predictions (y-axis) for 378 lung (left or right) and 411 liver segmentation from a level set approach [14] (ten-fold cross-validation).

segmentation (i.e. $S = G$) and 100% if the computed segment does not overlap with the ground truth at all. As a second volumetric measure we employ the *Dice coefficient*: $E_D = 2 |S \cap G| / (|S| + |G|)$, which is similar to the first one, and assigns 1 to a perfect segmentation and 0 to a completely failed one. In practice, S and G are typically represented as binary masks on a regular grid. In case segmentations are represented by surfaces, such masks can be obtained by voxelization. Besides these volumetric measures, we also compute the symmetric surface-to-surface metrics. In particular the well-known *Hausdorff distance*: $E_H = \max\{\sup_{x \in \partial S} \inf_{y \in \partial G} d(x, y),\ \sup_{x \in \partial G} \inf_{y \in \partial S} d(x, y)\}$, which measures the maximum of the Euclidean distance $(d(x, y) := |x - y|_{l^2})$ of each point on the computed segmentation surface ∂S to the ground truth surface ∂G and vice versa. Besides the maximum of the minimum per-vertex surface distances, we also gauge their mean by computing the *average surface error*: $E_S = \frac{1}{2}\left(\frac{1}{|\partial S|} \sum_{x \in \partial S} \min_{y \in \partial G} d(x, y) + \frac{1}{|\partial G|} \sum_{y \in \partial G} \min_{y \in \partial S} d(x, y)\right)$.

To perform the learning, we experimented with commonly known linear and non-linear regression approaches, all of which are available in the Weka tool [11]. Thereby we found an SVM regressor with a normalized polynomial kernel $\langle \mathbf{x}, \mathbf{y} \rangle / \sqrt{\langle \mathbf{x}, \mathbf{x} \rangle \langle \mathbf{y}, \mathbf{y} \rangle}$ with $\langle \mathbf{x}, \mathbf{y} \rangle = (1 + \mathbf{x} \cdot \mathbf{y})^2$ and an SMO-type optimizer [18] (with $C = 1$) to yield the highest correlations factors using a ten-fold-cross-validation.

3 Experiments

In this section we will address the following questions: Can the response of a commonly used boundary classifier be used to predict the above error metrics? How much better does the proposed regressor predict the segmentation errors than the boundary classifier probabilities? Can the new predictors estimate the error of a typical optimization based segmentation too? How do they perform on individual organs instead of of a whole collection? If we use the regressor to classify results into good and bad, how high is the error rate of this classification?

In order to address the first question, we used the machine learning-based organ segmentation approach described in [20] and [15] as reference. The last stage of this segmentation approach comprises a hierarchical boundary detection, where Probabilistic Boosting Tree boundary classifiers [19] are queried along the normals of an approximate segmentation mesh and the mesh vertices are then being placed at the location of maximum classifier response. We trained this method on eight different organs or organ parts (both referred to as "organs" in the following), for which we had the following number of ground truth segmentations: liver: 411, left lung: 187, right lung: 191, right kidney: 341, left kidney: 379, bladder: 311, prostate: 204, rectum: 149. All of those were generated by manual editing from a pool of 950 different CT scans that cover a variety of different patient anatomies, scanning protocols and parameters (slice resolution range: 1–5mm). For each ground truth segmentation, we applied the PBT and not only recorded the detected segmentation surface, but also the mean of the classifiers' probabilities over each segment surface. Subsequently, we used a linear regressor in order to fit the 2173 probability values to each of the four error metrics. See results in Figure 2. Surprisingly, the mean probabilities and any of the four metrics are only weakly correlated. This observation is in spite of the overall good segmentation accuracies of the system. Despite the individual boundary classifier responses provide a good prediction of the true boundary location on a local scale, in aggregation they seem to be a poor predictor for the overall accuracy of a segmentation shape.

By contrast, when training a regressor as described in Section 2.2, we observe significantly better correlations between the true and the predicted errors of the PBT-based segmentations, especially for the volume overlap error and the Dice coefficient. See results in Figure 3 using ten-fold cross-validation. In order to investigate a possible bias of the predictors towards PBT-type segmentation errors, we also ran them on segmentations generated by a level set approach [14], which relies on a volumetric shape representation. However, also for those segmentation results we observed very similar error prediction performances, with correlation coefficients being the same as for the PBT method up to the first decimal. In a next step, we trained and tested the regressors on different organ-specific subsets and discovered significant performance differences. For the lungs, for example, the real and predicted overlap and Dice errors are both correlated by a factor of 0.85 each, whereas for the liver only with 0.54, see Fig. 4. Finally, encouraged by the overall good correlation factors between the SVM regressor and the overlap error metric, we investigated the use of the former in classifying segmentations results into acceptable ($E_O \leq 10\%$) and non-acceptable segmentations ($E_O > 10\%$). Results in Table 1 show that the proposed method is capable of

Table 1. Confusion matrices when thresholding the regressor-predicted volume overlap error E_O. Left: for 2×2173 segmentations on all organs using results both from [15] and [14]. Right: for 377 left/right lung segmentations using [14] only.

# of true cases	# of predicted cases		# of true cases	# of predicted cases	
	$E_O \leq 10\%$	$E_O > 10\%$		$E_O \leq 10\%$	$E_O > 10\%$
$E_O \leq 10\%$	867	373	$E_O \leq 10\%$	178	39
$E_O > 10\%$	255	2851	$E_O > 10\%$	24	136

classifying into these two classes with low false positive rates (lower left entry) over all organ classes, as well as, e.g., for the lungs only.

4   Conclusion

We presented a method for predicting segmentation error *in the absence of ground truth* based on learning a classifier from errors measured against ground truth. Our method used a series of features derived from objective functions found in the literature for optimization-driven segmentation algorithms and trained our classifier to predict error measured against ground truth using standard error metrics used in the literature to compare segmentation quality. Despite training our classifier on segmentations for 8 very different organs, a strong correlation was observed between the predicted and actual errors when applied to an unseen test set. Furthermore, we demonstrated that a popular learning algorithm (PBT) does not provide the same power to predict segmentation quality.

A method for predicting segmentation error for on-line segmentations after deployment has many uses to improve final segmentation quality (by retrying poor segmentations or choosing the best segmentation from multiple algorithms run in parallel) or to request user review for a segmentation. We believe that the problem of predicting segmentation error without ground truth holds many future opportunities, such as the development of new feature sets, training across modalities and systems that can localize the source of segmentation error.

References

1. Blake, A., Zisserman, A.: Visual Reconstruction. MIT Press (1987)
2. Boykov, Y., Jolly, M.P.: Interactive Organ Segmentation Using Graph Cuts. In: Delp, S.L., DiGoia, A.M., Jaramaz, B. (eds.) MICCAI 2000. LNCS, vol. 1935, pp. 276–286. Springer, Heidelberg (2000)
3. Caselles, V., Kimmel, R., Sapiro, G.: Geodesic active contours. International Journal of Computer Vision 22, 61–79 (1997)
4. Caselles, V., Kimmel, R., Sapiro, G., Sbert, C.: Minimal surfaces based object segmentation. IEEE Trans. on Pat. Anal. and Mach. Int. 19(4), 394–398 (1997)
5. Deng, X., Zhu, L., Sun, Y., Xu, C., Song, L., Chen, J., Merges, R.D., Jolly, M.-P., Suehling, M., Xu, X.-D.: On Simulating Subjective Evaluation Using Combined Objective Metrics for Validation of 3D Tumor Segmentation. In: Ayache, N., Ourselin, S., Maeder, A. (eds.) MICCAI 2007, Part I. LNCS, vol. 4791, pp. 977–984. Springer, Heidelberg (2007)
6. El-Zehiry, N., Grady, L.: Fast global optimization of curvature. In: CVPR 2010, pp. 3257–3264. IEEE Computer Society (2010)
7. Frounchi, K., Briand, L.C., Grady, L., Labiche, Y., Subramanyan, R.: Automating image segmentation verification and validation by learning test oracles. Information and Software Technology 53(12), 1337–1348 (2011)
8. Ginneken, B.V., Heimann, T., Styner, M.: 3D segmentation in the clinic: A grand challenge. In: MICCAI Workshop 2007, pp. 7–15 (2007)
9. Grady, L.: Random walks for image segmentation. IEEE Trans. on Pat. Anal. and Mach. Int. 28(11), 1768–1783 (2006)

10. Grady, L., Schwartz, E.L.: Isoperimetric graph partitioning for image segmentation. IEEE Trans. on Pat. Anal. and Mach. Int. 28(3), 469–475 (2006)
11. Hall, M., Frank, E., Holmes, G., Pfahringer, B., Reutemann, P., Witten, I.: The WEKA Data Mining Software: An Update. SIGKDD Explorations 1(11)
12. Heimann, T., van Ginneken, B., Styner, M.: Comparison and evaluation of methods for liver segmentation from CT datasets. IEEE Trans. on Medical Imaging 28(8), 1251–1265 (2009)
13. Shi, J., Malik, J.: Normalized cuts and image segmentation. IEEE Trans. on Pat. Anal. and Mach. Int. 22(8), 888–905 (2000)
14. Kohlberger, T., Sofka, M., Zhang, J., Birkbeck, N., Wetzl, J., Kaftan, J., Declerck, J., Zhou, S.: Automatic Multi-organ Segmentation Using Learning-Based Segmentation and Level Set Optimization. In: Fichtinger, G., Martel, A., Peters, T. (eds.) MICCAI 2011, Part III. LNCS, vol. 6893, pp. 338–345. Springer, Heidelberg (2011)
15. Ling, H., Zhou, S., Zheng, Y., Georgescu, B., Suehling, M., Comaniciu, D.: Hierarchical, learning-based automatic liver segmentation. In: Proc. of CVPR 2008, pp. 1–8. IEEE Computer Society (2008)
16. Mumford, D., Shah, J.: Optimal approximations by piecewise smooth functions and associated variational problems. Comm. Pure and Appl. Math. 42, 577–685 (1989)
17. Sethian, J.A.: Level Set Methods and Fast Marching Methods. Cambridge University Press (1999)
18. Shevade, S., Keerthi, S., Bhattacharyya, C., Murthy, K.: Improvements to the SMO algorithm for SVM regression. IEEE Trans. on Neural Networks 11(5), 1188–1193 (2000)
19. Tu, Z.: Probabilistic boosting-tree: Learning discriminative models for classification, recognition, and clustering. In: Proc. of ICCV 2005, vol. 2, pp. 1589–1596. IEEE Computer Society (2005)
20. Zheng, Y., Barbu, A., Georgescu, B., Scheuering, M., Comaniciu, D.: Four-chamber heart modeling and automatic segmentation for 3-D cardiac CT volumes using marginal space learning and steerable features. IEEE Trans. on Medical Imaging 27(11), 1668–1681 (2008)

Rotational-Slice-Based Prostate Segmentation Using Level Set with Shape Constraint for 3D End-Firing TRUS Guided Biopsy

Wu Qiu, Jing Yuan, Eranga Ukwatta, David Tessier, and Aaron Fenster

Imaging Research Laboratories, Robarts Research Institute, 100 Perth, London, Ontario, Canada, N6A 5k8
{WQiu,JYuan,EUkwatta,DTessier,AFenster}@imaging.robarts.ca

Abstract. Prostate segmentation in 3D ultrasound images is an important step in the planning and treatment of 3D end-firing transrectal ultrasound (TRUS) guided prostate biopsy. A semi-automatic prostate segmentation method is presented in this paper, which integrates a modified distance regularization level set formulation with shape constraint to a rotational-slice-based 3D prostate segmentation method. Its performance, using different metrics, has been evaluated on a set of twenty 3D patient prostate images by comparison with expert delineations. The volume overlap ratio of $93.39 \pm 1.26\%$ and the mean absolute surface distance of $1.16 \pm 0.34mm$ were found in the quantitative validation result.

Keywords: prostate segmentation, 3D ultrasound, level set, shape constraint, rotational volume reslicing.

1 Introduction

Prostate cancer is the most frequent cancer in men in the United States and Europe with an incidence that reaches more than 25% of the new cases of cancers[14]. Transrectal ultrasound (TRUS) is currently the most commonly used imaging modality for image-guided biopsy and therapy of prostate cancer due to its real-time nature, low cost, and simplicity[4]. Moreover, accurate segmentation of the whole prostate from the TRUS image plays a key role in biopsy and therapy planning[3,18]. In addition, it allows for surface-based registration between the TRUS and other imaging modalities (e.g., MRI) during the image-guided intervention[6]. Although manual segmentation of the prostate boundary in 3D US images is possible, it is arduous and time consuming. However, automated and semi-automated prostate segmentation has challenges due to the presence of speckle noise, calcifications, nearby organs, missing edges or similarities between inner and outer texture of the prostate. In addition, prostate segmentation from 3D end-firing TRUS images is more challenging than from 3D side-firing TRUS images due to a few main reasons: (a) end-firing images are more inhomogeneous; (b) the prostate is located arbitrarily in the 3D volume, not just approximately in the center of the volume, thus, the localization uncertainty increases the difficulty of automatic and semi-automatic segmentation methods; and (c) the prostate is deformed differently in different images due to varying pressure of the end-firing transducer during the biopsy procedure.

N. Ayache et al. (Eds.): MICCAI 2012, Part I, LNCS 7510, pp. 537–544, 2012.

3D prostate segmentation methods can be categorized into two classes: direct 3D segmentation and propagation of the 2D slice-based segmentation. In terms of the first class, the user initializs a 3D deformable surface in multiple 2D slices of the prostate, then the initial 3D mesh is automatically refined by forces characterized by the image gradient and smoothness of the contour. Hu et al.[7] manually defined an ellipsoid that served as an initial guess. The estimated outline is then automatically deformed to better fit the prostate boundary. Abolmaesumi et al.[1] proposed to assimilate the prostate contour to the trajectory of a moving object that they tracked with an interacting multiple model probabilistic data association filter (IMM/PDAF). Following an initialization that consisted of selecting the base and apex axial slices, and seven landmarks. Mahadavi et al.[12] fitted a warped, tapered ellipsoid to the prostate using the edge points detected with the IMM/PDA filter. Carole et al.[5] presented a semi-automatic method based on discrete dynamic contour and optimal surface detection to segment the prostate in high intensity focused ultrasound(HIFU) therapy. This kind of method works well for high contrast 3D US images, but is time consuming and requires many user interactions that can lead to observer variability. Other methods are based on the slice-based propagation approach. Within slice-based segmentation, the result is iteratively propagated onto adjacent slices and then refined. Yan et al.[17] proposed a method combining local shape statistics and discrete deformable modal (DDM) to segment 2D video sequences of prostates. These approaches can give favorable results, however, they encounter difficulties in handling slices that are nearly tangent to the prostate surface (3D boundary), such as in the base and apex areas of the prostate. To overcome these issues, some researchers unfolded the 3D image in a rotational manner[11]. Wang et al.[16] resliced the 3D volume rotationally. All 2D slices pass through a common axis, approximately centered in the prostate, around which they are evenly radially spaced. DDM was then applied on each resliced image. Ding et al.[3] corrected them automatically by imposing a continuity constraint on the size of successive contours using an auto-regressive model. There does, however, remain the possibility that the contours may suffer from the accumulated error and "leak" at locations of weak edges[3].

To address the challenges involved with prostate segmentation, a level set based method is proposed in this paper, which has been used in the 3D side-firing TRUS guided prostate biopsy system. The key contribution of this study is that it incorporated the level set method with constraint shape information and high-level user interaction into a rotational-slice-based segmentation approach. It can potentially decrease the accumulated segmentation errors that occur in the propagation based method while preserving the accuracy .

2   Method

2.1   Overview of Approach

The proposed rotational-slice-based prostate 3D segmentation method is divided into three steps: first, selecting two points manually (red points in Fig.1(a)) on the long axis of the boundary on the coronal view of prostate. The initial slice and rotational axis is determined by these two points. The plane (blue slice in Fig. 1(a)) that includes these two points and is perpendicular to the coronal view is the approximate transverse view

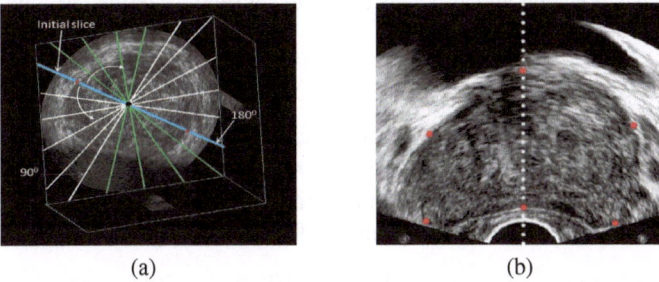

Fig. 1. Overview of approach. (a)reslicing the volume, (b)initializing boundary points.

of the prostate, which is assumed as the initial slice of the propagation method . The line on the transverse view perpendicularly bisecting the segment determined by those two selected points is identified as the rotational axis. Second, rotational reslicing of the 3D image of the prostate into N slices about the identified rotational axis is performed. All slices intersect along the axis approximately and have an equal angular spacing. The step angle was six degrees in our experiments resulting in a 3D volume that was resliced into 30 slices ($N = 30$). Third, four to eight initialization points (red points in Fig. 1(b))are manually chosen from the boundary of the prostate in the initial slice in which the initial contour is estimated using cardinal spline interpolation. A level set method is then used to deform this initial contour, which will be described in detail in section 2.2. Finally, the deformed contour in the initial slice is then propagated to its adjacent slice in a clockwise(green slices in Fig. 1(a)) and counter-clockwise (white slices in Fig. 1(a))direction, which is used as the initial contour before refining. This procedure is repeated until the contours in all 2D slices of the 3D image are segmented. A 3D prostate surface mesh is reconstructed from the contours in all 2D slices.

The detailed propagation will now be explained. The first segmented contour for the initial slice is used as the shape constraint for slice 1 to M and slice N to slice$N - M$ independently ($M = 3$ in our experiments). The resulting shapes $\{S_i | i = 1, .., M\}$ for the clockwise direction and $\{\hat{S}_i | i = N, .., N - M\}$ for the counter clockwise direction will be stored; the mean shape $\bar{S}_M$ and $\bar{\hat{S}}_M$ will be calculated, which is used as the shape constraint of the level set formulation for segmenting the next slice. From the slice $M + 1$, the obtained prostate contour will be added into set S_i, shape S_1 will be removed from set S_i, and the new mean shape $\bar{S}_M$ of S_i will be recalculated. The updated $\bar{S}_M$ will be given as the constraint shape for the next slice. This process is repeated until the segmentation is finished in the clockwise direction. The same procedure is conducted for the segmentation in the counter clockwise direction.

2.2 Segmentation Using Level Set

A distance regularization level set formulation (DRLSE)[10] method is modified to segment the prostate contour in each 2D slice. Let $\phi : \Omega \to \Re$ be a level set formulation (LSF) defined on a domain Ω. An energy functional $\varepsilon(\phi)$ is defined as:

$$\varepsilon(\phi) = \mu R_p(\phi) + \varepsilon_{ext}(\phi) \tag{1}$$

where $\mu > 0$ is a constant and $R_p(\phi)$ is the level set regularization term, defined by

$$R_p(\phi) \triangleq \int_\Omega p(|\nabla\phi|)dx \tag{2}$$

where p is a potential (or energy density) function $p : [0, \infty) \rightarrow \Re$. External energy term $\varepsilon_{ext}(\phi)$ is defined in the following. The minimization of the energy $\varepsilon(\phi)$ can be achieved by solving a level set evolution equation.

For an LSF $\phi : \Omega \rightarrow \Re$, an external energy function $\varepsilon_{ext}(\phi)$ is defined by

$$\varepsilon_{ext}(\phi) = \lambda L_g(\phi) + \alpha A_g(\phi) + \beta S(\phi) + \gamma T(\phi) + \nu A(\phi) \tag{3}$$

where $\lambda > 0$ and $\alpha \in \Re$ are the coefficients of the energy functionals $L_g(\phi)$ and $A_g(\phi)$, which are given by

$$L_g(\phi) \triangleq \int_\Omega g\delta(\phi)|\nabla\phi|dx \tag{4}$$

and

$$A_g(\phi) \triangleq \int_\Omega gH(-\phi)dx \tag{5}$$

where g is an edge indicator function defined by $g \triangleq \frac{1}{1+|\nabla G_\sigma * I|^2}$. The Dirac delta function δ and Heaviside function in H Eq.4 and Eq.5 are approximated by the following smooth function δ_ϵ and H_ϵ, respectively, as in many level set methods[2,13]. The energy $L_g(\phi)$ computes the line integral of the function g along the zero level contour of ϕ. The energy $A_g(\phi)$ calculates the weighted area of the region $\Omega_\phi^- \triangleq x : \phi(x) < 0$, which is introduced to speed up the motion of the zero level contour in the evolution process. $S(\phi)$, $A(\phi)$ and $T(\phi)$ are shape constraint energy, anchor point energy and local region-based energy, respectively.

Since the contour to be segmented is not far from the contour propagated from the previous slice, a shape constraint is imposed to discourage the evolved contour to leak in the region with a weak edge or without an edge. This shape constraint energy $S(\phi)$ [15]is defined by

$$S(\phi) = \int_\Omega \delta(\phi(x))B_S(x)dx \tag{6}$$

where

$$B_S(x) = \begin{cases} 0 & if \quad \min_{\hat{x}} D(x,\hat{x}) < d_S \\ D(x,\hat{x}) & otherwise \end{cases} \tag{7}$$

$D(x,\hat{x}) = \| x - \hat{x} \|$. $\hat{x} \in \Omega$ is an independent spatial variable, which is given by the constraint shape (described in section 2.1). d_S is the separation distance from the current evolving LSF to the constraint shape. This energy is nonzero when the evolving LSF moves farther from the constraint shape of any distance greater than d_S.

Let $\hat{y} \in \Omega$ be another independent spatial variable, the local region-based energy $T(\phi)$ [9]is

$$T(\phi(x)) = \int_\Omega \delta(\phi(x)) \int_\Omega B_L(x,\hat{y})[H(\phi(\hat{y}))(I(\hat{y})) - u_x)^2$$
$$+(1 - H(\phi(\hat{y})))(I(\hat{y})) - v_x)^2]d\hat{y}dx \tag{8}$$

where

$$B_L(x, \hat{y}) = \begin{cases} 1 & if \quad \| x - \hat{y} \| < r_L \\ 0 & otherwise \end{cases} \tag{9}$$

is used to define a circular-shaped local region with localizing radius r_L.
$u_x = \int_\Omega B_L(x, \hat{y}) H(\phi(\hat{y})) I(\hat{y}) d\hat{y} / \int_\Omega B_L(x, \hat{y}) H(\phi(\hat{y})) d\hat{y}$ and $v_x = \int_\Omega B_L(x, \hat{y})(1 - H(\phi(\hat{y}))) I(\hat{y}) d\hat{y} / \int_\Omega B_L(x, \hat{y})(1 - H(\phi(\hat{y}))) d\hat{y}$ are the mean image intensities of the interior and exterior of the active contour, respectively, within the region defined by $B_L(x, \hat{y})$. r_L determines the degree of blending local statistics around the boundary to global statistics of the image.

The energy $A(\phi)$ given by Eq. 10[15] encourages the evolving contour to pass through each anchor point x_A^i if the evolving contour is within a distance r_A to the anchor point. Anchor points in the first slice are the initial boundary points placed by users. During the propagation, two anchor points are selected, which act as the intersection points of the rotational axis and the segmented contour in the first slice. When the contour points are away from the anchor point by more than r_A, there is no influence by this energy.

$$A(\phi) = \sum_{i=1}^{N_p} \int_\Omega \delta(\phi(x)) B_A^i(x)(\phi(x) - \phi(x_A^i))^2 dx \tag{10}$$

where

$$B_A^i(x) = \begin{cases} 1 & if \quad \| x - x_A^i \| < r_A \\ 0 & otherwise \end{cases} \tag{11}$$

is used to define a circular-shaped region around the anchor point with radius r_A; N_p is the number of anchor points.

By taking the first variation of the Eq.1 with respect to ϕ, the following evolving equation will be obtained:

$$\frac{\partial \phi(x)}{\partial t} = \mu div(d_p(|\nabla \phi|)\nabla \phi) + \delta(\phi(x))\{\lambda div(g \frac{\nabla \phi}{|\nabla \phi|}) + \alpha g + \beta B_S(x)$$

$$+ \gamma \int_\Omega B_L(x, \hat{y}) \delta(\phi(\hat{y})[(I(\hat{y})) - u_x)^2 - (I(\hat{y})) - v_x)^2] d\hat{y} \tag{12}$$

$$+ \nu \sum_{i=1}^{N_p} B_A^i(x)(\phi(x) - \phi(x_A^i))\}$$

3   Experimental Results

All testing images were acquired with a rotational scanning 3D TRUS imaging system using a commercially available end-firing TRUS transducer (Philips, Bothell WA)[8], which is developed for 3D US guided prostate biopsy procedure. The size of each 3D image is $448 \times 448 \times 350$ voxels of size $0.19 \times 0.19 \times 0.19 mm^3$. Twenty five patient images were tested in this paper, which are divided into two sets. Five were used to optimize the parameter values of the algorithm, and the other twenty images were used

Table 1. Parameters and their optimized values

	λ	μ	α	β	γ	ν	d_S(pixels)	r_L(pixels)	r_A(pixels)
values	8	0.04	-5	10	5	5.5	8	20	5

to validate the proposed method. The parameter values were empirically chosen. Afterwards, the parameters were optimized sequentially by changing a single parameter at a time while holding other parameters fixed. Table.1 shows the optimized values of the parameters used in our experiments, which were kept constant during the validation experiments. The performance of the proposed method has been evaluated qualitatively by visual comparison with the expert-delineated contours. One reconstructed prostate surface (green surface after segmentation) is demonstrated in Fig. 2, which is superimposed on the manual surface (red one). Volume-based metrics: sensitivity(Se),

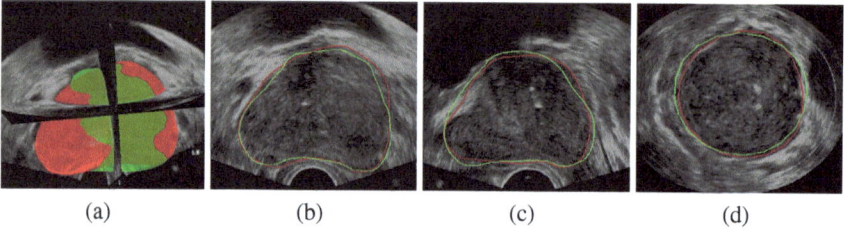

(a)   (b)   (c)   (d)

Fig. 2. Prostate segmentation result (green line) compared to manual segmentation(red line). (a)superimposed surface, (b)transverse view, (c)sagittal view, and (c) coronal view .

dice similarity coefficient (DSC) and volume difference (V_{diff}), and distance-based metrics: the mean absolute surface distance(MAD) and maximum absolute surface distance(MAXD) [5]were used to validate our segmentation method (M_{LS}) quantitatively compared to manual segmentation and other rotational-slice-based methods (Wang's method(M_{CW})[16] and Ding's method(M_{CCW})[3]). The coefficient of variation(CV) [19] of volume overlap rate was used to evaluate the intraobserver variability of our method.

The validation results in Table.2 show that our method can obtain a sensitivity of $94.28 \pm 2.18\%$ and a DSC of $93.39 \pm 1.26\%$ better than M_{CW} ($85.24 \pm 6.28\%$, $84.29 \pm 4.18\%$) and M_{CCW} ($88.33 \pm 4.58\%$, $87.18 \pm 3.37\%$). MAD of $1.16 \pm 0.34mm$ and $MAXD$ of $3.06 \pm 0.76mm$ of our method were obtained comparable to $1.95 \pm 0.74mm$ and $4.67 \pm 1.84mm$ of M_{CW}, $1.59 \pm 0.67mm$ and $4.2 \pm 1.56mm$ of M_{CCW}. The comparison with manual segmentation on volume difference (V_{diff}) demonstrates a volume error of $2.45 \pm 1.75cm^3$ on the entire prostate. The intraobserver variability experiments shows that our proposed method gave a CV of 2.5%. To validate the variability introduced by the manual initialization (initial slice and initial points), an inter-observer variability test was performed. Ten images were also segmented by three untrained observes who were blinded to patient identity. The proposed method yielded a DSC of $93.1 \pm 1.6\%$, $93.6 \pm 1.5\%$ and $92.4 \pm 1.7\%$, and a COV of 1.7%, 1.6% and 1.8%, respectively. The proposed method was developed in Matlab. The segmentation time of our method was found to be about 45s on a desktop computer with a core 2 CPU (2.66 GHz) in addition to 30s for initialization. A total segmentation time was found to be less than 1.5 minute.

Ten images randomly selected were used to test the sensitivity of our method to some parameters. The effect of d_s, r_L, and r_A on the segmentation accuracy (DSC) were only observed since they are dependent on the values of β, γ and ν that were kept constant (More details on how to choose these three parameters refer to [10]). As a result, DSC goes up slightly when d_s increases from 0 to 4 pixels, and it goes down when d_s is greater than 3 pixels. The range from 3 to 5 pixels for d_s is suggested. Our method presents the growth of DSC when the radius r_L of the local region increases from 0 to 10. It demonstrates less standard deviation of DSC at the expense of a decreasing DSC when r_L is greater than 20. In addition, DSC displays a downward trend with the growing radius of the anchor point. r_A varying from 0 to 5 pixels is capable of giving a good segmentation accuracy.

Table 2. Overall performance results

	Se(%)	DSC(%)	MAD(mm(vx))	MAXD(mm(vx))	$V_{diff}(cm^3)$
M_{LS}	94.28 ± 2.18	93.39 ± 1.26	1.16 ± 0.34 (6.13 ± 1.8)	3.06 ± 0.76 (16.1 ± 4.02)	2.45 ± 1.75
M_{CW}	85.24 ± 6.28	84.29 ± 4.18	1.95 ± 0.74 (10.25 ± 3.89)	4.67 ± 1.84 (24.56 ± 9.7)	5.8 ± 4.03
M_{CCW}	88.33 ± 4.58	87.18 ± 3.37	1.59 ± 0.67 (8.38 ± 3.54)	4.2 ± 1.56 (22.1 ± 8.2)	4.22 ± 3.95

4   Conclusion

A rotational-slice-based segmentation method, with a modified level set, has been proposed in this paper for a semi-automatic segmentation of the prostate in 3D end-firing TRUS images. It has been evaluated on a patient dataset obtained during a 3D end-firing TRUS guided prostate biopsy procedure. The resulting segmentations have been compared with manual expert delineations using different metrics (Se, DSC, MAD, MAXD, and volume difference). It is found that the proposed method is accurate, robust and computationally efficient.

References

1. Abolmaesumi, P., Sirouspour, M.R.: An interacting multiple model probabilistic data association filter for cavity boundary extraction from ultrasound images. IEEE Trans. Med. Imag. 23(6), 772–784 (2004)
2. Chan, T.F., Vese, L.A.: Active contours without edges. IEEE Trans Img. Process. 10(2), 266–277 (2001)
3. Ding, M., Chiu, B., Gyacskov, I., Yuan, X., Drangova, M., Downey, D.B., Fenster, A.: Fast prostate segmentation in 3d trus images based on continuity constraint using an autoregressive model. Med. Phys. 34(11), 4109–4125 (2007)

4. Fenster, A., Downey, D.B.: Three-dimensional ultrasound imaging and its use in quantifying organ and pathology volumes. Anal. Bioanal. Chem. 377(6), 982–989 (2003)
5. Garnier, C., Bellanger, J.J., Wu, K., Shu, H., Costet, N., Mathieu, R., de Crevoisier, R., Coatrieux, J.L.: Prostate segmentation in hifu therapy. IEEE Trans. Med. Imag. 30(3), 792–803 (2011)
6. Ghose, S., Oliver, A., Martí, R., Lladó, X., Freixenet, J., Vilanova, J.C., Meriaudeau, F.: Texture Guided Active Appearance Model Propagation for Prostate Segmentation. In: Madabhushi, A., Dowling, J., Yan, P., Fenster, A., Abolmaesumi, P., Hata, N. (eds.) MICCAI 2010. LNCS, vol. 6367, pp. 111–120. Springer, Heidelberg (2010)
7. Hu, N., Downey, D.B., Fenster, A., Ladak, H.M.: Prostate boundary segmentation from 3d ultrasound images. Med. Phys. 30(7), 1648–1659 (2003)
8. Bax, J., Cool, D., Gardi, L., Knight, K., Smith, D., Montreuil, J., Sherebrin, S., Romagnoli, C., Fenster, A.: Mechanically assisted 3d ultrasound guided prostate biopsy system. Med. Phys. 35(12), 5397, 5401 (2008)
9. Lankton, S., Tannenbaum, A.: Localizing region-based active contours. IEEE Trans. Imag. Process. 17(11), 2029–2039 (2008)
10. Li, C., Xu, C., Gui, C., Fox, M.D.: Distance regularized level set evolution and its application to image segmentation. IEEE Trans. Imag. Process. 19(12), 3243–3254 (2010)
11. Li, K., Wu, X., Chen, D.Z., Sonka, M.: Optimal surface segmentation in volumetric images-a graph-theoretic approach. IEEE Trans. Pattern Anal. Mach. Intell. 28(1), 119–134 (2006)
12. Mahdavi, S.S., Moradi, M., Wen, X., Morris, W.J., Salcudean, S.E.: Evaluation of visualization of the prostate gland in vibro-elastography images. Medical Image Analysis 15(4), 589–600 (2011)
13. Malladi, R., Sethian, J.A., Vemuri, B.C.: Shape modeling with front propagation: A level set approach. IEEE Trans. Pattern Anal. Mach. Intell. 17(2), 158–175 (1995)
14. Soc, A.C.: Cancer facts and figures (2010), http://www.cancer.org
15. Ukwatta, E., Awad, J., Ward, A.D., Buchanan, D., Samarabandu, J., Parraga, G., Fenster, A.: Three-dimensional ultrasound of carotid atherosclerosis: semiautomated segmentation using a level set-based method. Med. Phys. 38(5), 2479–2493 (2011)
16. Wang, Y., Cardinal, H.N., Downey, D.B., Fenster, A.: Semiautomatic three-dimensional segmentation of the prostate using two-dimensional ultrasound images. Med. Phys. 30(5), 887–897 (2003)
17. Yan, P., Xu, S., Turkbey, B., Kruecker, J.: Adaptively learning local shape statistics for prostate segmentation in ultrasound. IEEE Trans. Bio. Med. Eng. 58(3), 633–641 (2011)
18. Zhan, Y., Shen, D.: Deformable segmentation of 3-d ultrasound prostate images using statistical texture matching method. IEEE Trans. Med. Imag. 25(3), 256–272 (2006)
19. Zou, K.H., Mcdermott, M.P.: Higher-moment approaches to approximate interval estimation for a certain intraclass correlation coefficient. Statistics in Medicine 18(15), 2051–2061 (1999)

Segmentation of Biological Target Volumes on Multi-tracer PET Images Based on Information Fusion for Achieving Dose Painting in Radiotherapy

Benoît Lelandais[1], Isabelle Gardin[1,2], Laurent Mouchard[1],
Pierre Vera[1,2], and Su Ruan[1]

[1] University of Rouen, LITIS EA4108, QuantIF,
22 bd Gambetta, 76183 Rouen Cedex, France
{benoit.lelandais,laurent.mouchard,su.ruan}@univ-rouen.fr
http://www.litislab.eu/front-page/themes/quantif
[2] Centre Henri-Becquerel, Dept of Nuclear Medicine
1 rue d'Amiens, 76038 Rouen Cedex 1, France
{isabelle.gardin,pierre.vera}@chb.unicancer.fr

Abstract. Medical imaging plays an important role in radiotherapy. Dose painting consists in the application of a nonuniform dose prescription on a tumoral region, and is based on an efficient segmentation of Biological Target Volumes (BTV). It is derived from PET images, that highlight tumoral regions of enhanced glucose metabolism (FDG), cell proliferation (FLT) and hypoxia (FMiso). In this paper, a framework based on Belief Function Theory is proposed for BTV segmentation and for creating 3D parametric images for dose painting. We propose to take advantage of neighboring voxels for BTV segmentation, and also multi-tracer PET images using information fusion to create parametric images. The performances of BTV segmentation was evaluated on an anthropomorphic phantom and compared with two other methods. Quantitative results show the good performances of our method. It has been applied to data of five patients suffering from lung cancer. Parametric images show promising results by highlighting areas where a high frequency or dose escalation could be planned.

Keywords: Dose Painting, Positron Emission Tomography, Information Fusion, Segmentation, Belief Function Theory.

1 Introduction

Medical imaging plays an important role in radiotherapy for treatment planning with the delineation of Gross Tumor Volume on Computed Tomography (CT) images. Ling *et al.* [1] have proposed the concept of dose painting, consisting of the application of a nonuniform dose prescription based on the biological characteristics of the tumor. Positron Emission Tomography (PET) is used for sub-volumes definition, also called Biological Target Volumes (BTV)

N. Ayache et al. (Eds.): MICCAI 2012, Part I, LNCS 7510, pp. 545–552, 2012.
© Springer-Verlag Berlin Heidelberg 2012

corresponding, for instance, to tumoral regions. Different radiotracers are used for visualising specific properties: ^{18}F-FluoroDesoxyGlucose (FDG) for enhanced glucose metabolism, ^{18}F-FLuoroThymidine (FLT) for cell proliferation and ^{18}F-FluoroMisonidazol (FMiso) for hypoxic regions (lack of oxygen). An increase of the frequency of dose delivery on high proliferative cells could be planned, as well as a dose escalation on hypoxic regions regarding their radioresistance.

If the concept of dose painting is promising, it raises two methodological problems. First, it might be difficult to correctly segment BTVs because of the poor quality of PET images (significant noise), Partial Volume Effect (PVE) and possibly, a low contrast between normal and pathological tissues. Second, the large number of images that a radiation oncologist has at his disposal makes complex the decision-making when considering nonuniform dose prescription.

Although several algorithms have been proposed in the literature to delineate FDG-PET positive tissues, there is no consensus on this issue. One can quote thresholding methods [2], watershed algorithms [3], or methods based on probability measures [4] or membership degree estimation [5]. On the other side, few authors have proposed a method for the segmentation of FLT and FMiso-PET positive tissues. Even if, in first approximation, the level of noise, PVE and contrast between normal and pathological tissues can be considered in a same order of magnitude in FDG and FLT-PET images, performances of algorithms have to be evaluated on images of both tracers. Moreover, FMiso-PET images generally have a low contrast and an important noise. Here again, a specific validation is mandatory.

Our goal is to propose a framework based on Belief Function Theory (BFT) for the segmentation of BTV and creation of 3D parametric images to help the radiation oncologist for dose painting, in a context of noise, PVE, and muti-tracer images. In BFT, noise and PVE lead to partial knowledges and are considered as imperfect information. This theory was chosen for its ability to manage partial knowledge and to merge information coming from several sources [6–9]. To this end, we propose to benefit from neighborhood information in each image for BTV segmentation, and also to fuse multi-tracer PET images for 3D parametric images creation for dose painting.

2   Method

2.1   Belief Function Theory (BFT)

Frame of Discernment. Let $\Omega = \{\omega_1, \omega_2, \ldots, \omega_C\}$ be a finite set of classes, called *the frame of discernment*. Partial knowledge flowing out from information sources are taken into account using BFT by assigning masses, m, also called Basic Belief Assignments (BBAs), over different subsets of Ω. m is defined as a mapping of hypotheses from $2^\Omega = \{\emptyset, \{\omega_1\}, \{\omega_2\}, \ldots, \{\omega_C\}, \{\omega_1, \omega_2\}, \ldots, \Omega\}$ to $[0,1]$ verifying $\sum_{A \subseteq \Omega} m(A) = 1$. The mass $m(\Omega)$ represents the degree of ignorance ($m(\Omega) = 1$: total ignorance) and the mass $m(\emptyset)$ represents the conflict between sources.

In the hypotheses, one can distinguish singletons, such as $\{\omega_1\}$, from disjunctions, such as $\{\omega_1, \omega_2\}$ corresponding to a set of exclusive classes. Singletons allow to represent uncertainty as in probability theory. A BBA is considered as uncertain when masses are approximatively equals over singletons, corresponding to equiprobability in probability theory. Disjunctions allow to represent imprecision. A BBA is considered as imprecise when non-zero masses are assigned over disjunctions, meaning that we do not take part in favor of one class or an other.

Discounting. Having knowledge about the reliability of a source, the discounting process allows to reduce its reliability [7]. It consists in transferring a part of belief either on $X = \varnothing$ or $X = \Omega$ according to a coefficient α in $[0,1]$, such that:

$$m'(A) = \alpha.m(A), \quad \forall A \neq X \;,$$
$$m'(X) = 1 - \alpha\,(1 - m(X)) \;, \tag{1}$$

Information Fusion. When at least two sources contributing to the same BBA estimation are available, their fusion can be achieve using combination rules.

Let S_1 and S_2 be two information sources such that, at least, one is reliable. The disjunctive rule is given by:

$$m_{S_1 \textcircled{\tiny U} S_2}(A) = \sum_{B \cup C = A} m_1(B).m_2(C) \;. \tag{2}$$

It makes imprecision growing when sources are discordant, transferring masses over disjunctions.

Let S_1 and S_2 be two reliable sources of information. The conjunctive combination rule is given by:

$$m_{S_1 \textcircled{\tiny $\cap$} S_2}(A) = \sum_{B \cap C = A} m_1(B).m_2(C) \;. \tag{3}$$

It allows to reduce uncertainty and imprecision by transferring belief masses on intersections between hypotheses. When the information contained in sources are conflicting, non-zero masses are transfered on $\varnothing$. In order to satisfy $m(\varnothing) = 0$, the Dempster's rule is used [6] and consists in normalizing the conjunctive rule by $\kappa = m_{S_1 \textcircled{\tiny $\cap$} S_2}(\varnothing)$:

$$m_{S_1 \oplus S_2}(A) = \frac{1}{1 - \kappa} \sum_{B \cap C = A} m_1(B).m_2(C) \;. \tag{4}$$

2.2   Segmentation of Biological Target Volumes (BTV)

Frame of Discernment and Information Sources. We propose to represent mono-tracer PET images (FDG, FLT or FMiso) by two classes: one corresponds to low uptake (lu) region and the other, to high uptake (hu) region. Thus, the frame of discernment is represented by $\Omega = \{lu, hu\}$ and each voxel V_i is a source of information which is associated to a specific BBA represented by four masses: $m_{V_i}(\varnothing)$, $m_{V_i}(\{lu\})$, $m_{V_i}(\{hu\})$ and $m_{V_i}(\{lu, hu\})$.

BBA Estimation. This estimation can be separated in two steps leading each time to a set of BBAs.

At the first step, the BBAs of voxels according to $\{lu\}$, $\{hu\}$, and $\{lu, hu\}$ hypotheses are determined using a modified Fuzzy C-Means (FCM) algorithm [10]. The modification consists in integrating a disjunctive combination of neighboring voxels (Eq. 2) inside the iterative process. This combination tends firstly to transfer the masses over the disjunction $\{lu, hu\}$ for imperfect data due to the ambiguity of the information in the voxel environment, and secondly to represent BBAs corresponding only to non ambiguous knowledge over singletons. It results that the $\{lu\}$ and $\{hu\}$ centroids are updated iteratively in the FCM algorithm using only certain data. It allows to avoid bias induced by noise and PVE. Before the disjunctive combination, a discounting process (Eq. 1, $X = \varnothing$) is performed as follows. Let V_i be the considered voxel and V_k one of its neighbors. Because of the distance separating them, V_k provide less reliable information than V_i. We propose to discount each neighbor V_k according to a coefficient $\alpha_k = \exp\left(-(V_k - V_i)^2/\sigma^2\right)$ depending on the distance between V_i and V_k, with $\text{FWHM}^2 = 8\log 2.\sigma^2$ the Full Width at Half Maximum (= 6 mm) corresponding to the spatial resolution of the image.

The second step focuses on the reduction of imperfect data by combining neighboring voxels using Dempster's rule (Eq. 4). It tends to reduce the ambiguity brought by noise. Before doing this combination, the neighboring voxels are discounted in a same way as previously mentioned, with $X = \Omega$ (Eq. 1).

Segmentation. A labeling process is finally carried out by assigning, to each voxel, the $\{lu\}$ or $\{hu\}$ class having the highest belief mass.

2.3   Parametric Images for Dose Painting

Frame of Discernment and Information Sources. Now considering dose painting application from multi-tracer PET images, five classes are distinguished, namely Normal tissue $\{N\}$, those with an important glucose Metabolism $\{M\}$, an important cell Proliferation $\{P\}$, a significant Hypoxia $\{H\}$, and tissues with a Full uptake $\{F\}$: where tissues need an increasing of both the radiation therapy frequency and the dose. The frame of discernment for the three PET images is now: $\Omega = \{N, M, P, H, F\}$. For each voxel of the three modalities, BBAs are assigned to 32 hypotheses: $2^\Omega = \{\varnothing, \{N\}, \{M\}, \{P\}, \ldots, \{N, M\}, \ldots, \Omega\}$.

BBA Estimation. Considering separately each of the three PET images, BBA estimation as proposed in the previous section is first applied in order to assign to each voxel BBAs over $\{lu\}$, $\{hu\}$ and $\{lu, hu\}$. For dose painting, a new frame of discernment given in Table 1 is proposed according to medical interpretation of PET images. It assumes that a low uptake of FDG corresponds to a normal tissue, that a high uptake of FDG can possibly correspond to a high or low uptake of FLT or FMiso, and that a low uptake of FLT and FMiso leads not necessarily to the presence of normal tissue.

Table 1. Hypotheses considered after BBA estimation for multi-tracer PET images

Image	$\{lu\}$	$\{hu\}$	$\{lu,hu\}$
FDG	$\{N\}$	$\{M,P,H,F\}$	$\{N,M,P,H,F\}$
FLT	$\{N,M,H\}$	$\{P,F\}$	$\{N,M,P,H,F\}$
FMiso	$\{N,M,P\}$	$\{H,F\}$	$\{N,M,P,H,F\}$

Fusion of Multi-tracer PET Images for Parametric Image Construction.
First, a registration of the three CT scans is performed using mutual information [11]. Then, the obtained registration parameters are applied to PET images.
After BBA estimation, we propose to fuse each voxel of the three PET images
using conjunctive combination rule (Eq. 3). First, it allows to obtain the distinction between $\{M\}$, $\{P\}$, $\{H\}$ and $\{F\}$ hypotheses which are under consideration
regarding dose painting. The conflict corresponding to a high uptake of FLT or
FMiso and a low uptake of FDG is transfered on the empty set, allowing to
highlight areas of conflict between the different PET images.

Segmentation. A labeling process is carried out in the same way as presented in
the previous section, but considering $\{N\}$, $\{M\}$, $\{P\}$, $\{H\}$ and $\{F\}$ hypotheses.

3 Experiments and Results

The segmentation method was validated on PET images of an anthropomorphic
torso phantom (*Data Spectrum Corporation^{TM}, Hillsoborough, NC, USA*) filled
with organ inserts (liver, lungs and spine) and 15 spheres whose volumes vary
from 1 to 98 mL. The contrast varies from 4.7 to 10.1 (background), 1.9 to 4.1
(liver) and 30.2 to 65.2 (lung). Our method was compared with a classical FCM
[10] and with the Fuzzy Locally Adaptive Bayesian method (FLAB [4]). The
relative error rate is used as measure criterion, given by: $E = \left| 100 . \frac{V_s - V_a}{V_a} \right|$ (%),
where V_s and V_a are respectively the measured volume using one of the methods
and the actual volume of the sphere. Due to the large amount of spheres and
contrasts, mean and standard deviation are computed according to the contrasts
and several ranges of sphere volume. The results are given in Fig. 1. It can be seen
that our method gives, most of the time, better results than FCM, especially
for the smallest spheres. This is due to the centroid update using only non-
ambiguous data. Moreover, our method outperforms FLAB for spheres whose
volume is larger than 3 mL.

Our segmentation method and creation of parametric images for dose painting were carried out on 5 patients who underwent a curative radiotherapy for
paramediastinal non-small-cell lung cancer with no movement. The acquisition
of PET images (FDG, FLT, and FMiso) were performed on a *Biograph Sensation
16 Hi-Rez* PET/CT device (*SIEMENS Medical Solution, Knoxville, TN, USA*)
in a time interval less than 72 hours between each exam. Images were corrected

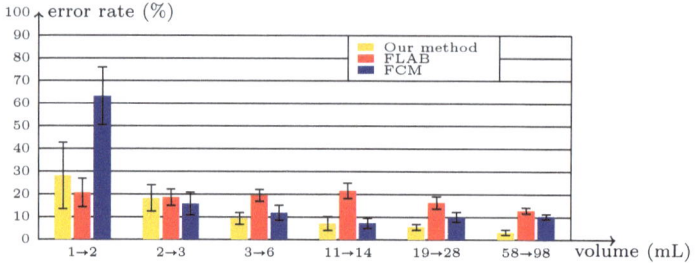

Fig. 1. Comparison of mean error rates according to different sphere volumes using our segmentation method, FLAB [4] and FCM [10]

for dead time, random, scatter and attenuation. The reconstruction was done using an attenuation weighted ordered subset expectation maximization algorithm (4 iterations, 8 subsets). A gaussian post filtering was applied (FWHM = 5 mm).

An example of results is given for one patient. Fig. 2 gives an illustration of the different steps of the segmentation process on FDG-PET image. Fig. 2(a) presents the primitive tumor localized in the Region Of Interest (ROI). The results obtained at the different steps of the algorithm are given in Fig. 2(b) to (h), as well as the final segmentation result. Using the first BBA estimation step, the belief masses are spread over the hypotheses $\{lu\}$, $\{hu\}$ and $\{lu, hu\}$ (Fig. 2(b), (c) and (d) respectively). The belief of each voxel for which the information is ambiguous in its neighborhood (noise, PVE) is mainly represented on the hypothesis $\{lu, hu\}$ (cf. Fig. 2(d)). The result of the segmentation after the second BBA estimation is given in Fig. 2(e), (f) and (g). This step provides high beliefs in favor of $\{lu\}$ and $\{hu\}$ because the uncertainty due to noise has been reduced by neighboring information fusion. The belief at the transitions between the two classes is mainly represented on the hypothesis $\{lu, hu\}$, where imprecision due to PVE is present. Finally, in order to segment $\{hu\}$, voxel labeling is done. The segmented tumor is given in Fig. 2(h).

Results on multi-tracer PET images of the same patient (FDG, FLT, and FMiso) are given Fig. 3(a), (b) and (c) respectively. First applying our BBA estimation method on each image, and then merging these multiple BBAs, we obtain the results as presented Fig. 3. It shows both the BBA corresponding

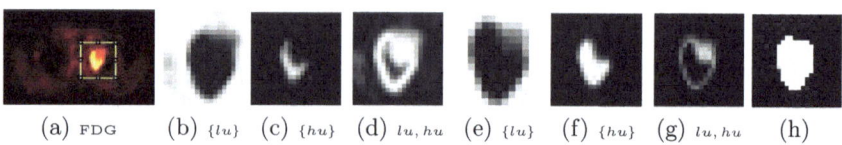

(a) FDG   (b) $\{lu\}$ (c) $\{hu\}$ (d) lu, hu (e) $\{lu\}$ (f) $\{hu\}$ (g) lu, hu (h)

Fig. 2. Illustration of the segmentation method on PET-FDG image. (a) is the initial image. (b), (c) and (d) show BBAs using the first step of the method in the ROI. (e), (f) and (g) show the BBAs using the second step. (h) presents segmentation result.

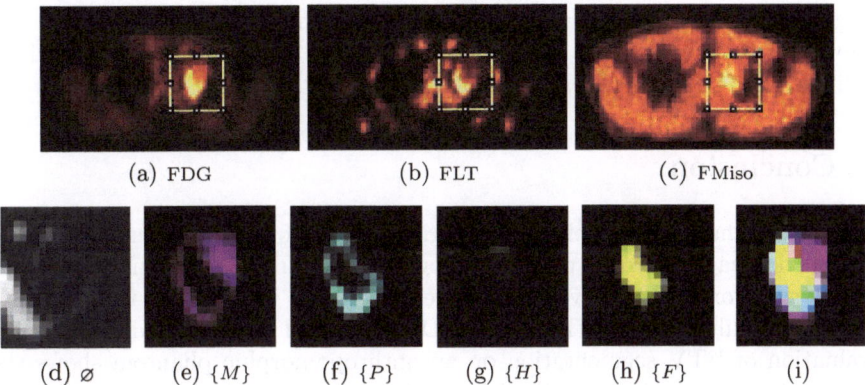

Fig. 3. Images showing results of the method of information fusion on multi-tracer PET images. (a), (b) and (c) are the initial images using FDG, FLT and FMiso tracers. (d), (e), (f), (g) and (h) are the parametric images applying first the BBA estimation of each ROI of each image and then fusing these BBAs. The final result presenting how to achieve dose painting is presented in (i) and corresponds to the segmented regions.

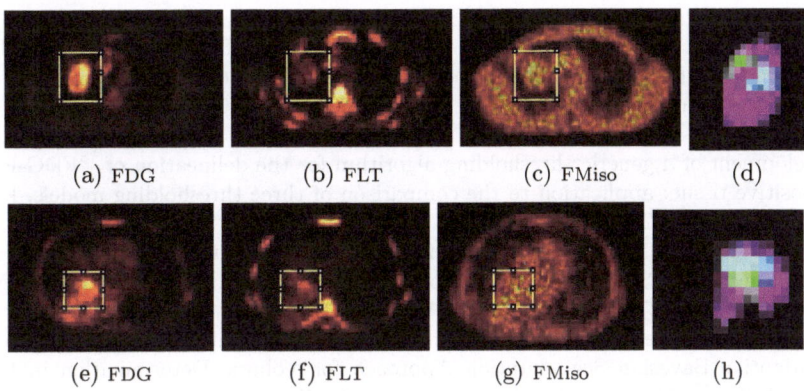

Fig. 4. Results of our information fusion method on multi-tracer PET images for two patients. (d) and (h) are the fusion results of (a), (b), (c) and (e), (f), (g) respectively.

to the conflict (Fig. 3(d)), and the BBAs corresponding to the hypotheses of interest: $\{M\}, \{P\}, \{H\}$ and $\{F\}$ (Fig. 3(e) to (h) respectively). Finally, Fig. 3(i) shows the parametric image which provides the distribution information about the three phenomena (glucose metabolism, cellular proliferation and hypoxia) over the pathological region.

The results using our fusion method for two other patients presenting high uptake of FDG, FLT and FMiso are given in Fig. 4. The parametric images given in Fig. 4(d) and (h), and also 3(i) can help radiation oncologist to decide if a classical treatment is needed or dose painting. As a clinical point of view, he can consider three radiotracers independently to delineate BTVs, or our parametric images in order to achieve a dose escalation on hypoxic region (green (H) and yellow (F) regions) as well as an increase of dose delivery frequency on high proliferative cells (blue (P) and yellow (F) regions).

4 Conclusion

A framework has been developed for segmentation of BTVs and creation of 3D parametric images for dose painting using BFT. An information fusion between neighboring voxels is achieved for segmentation. An information fusion is also done using multi-tracer PET images (FDG, FLT and FMiso) for dose painting. Evaluation of BTV segmentation on an anthropomorphic phantom shows the good performances of the method if compared to two other approaches based on fuzzy sets and probability theory. Even if these first results on 5 patient data are promising for dose painting, they have to be confirmed on a larger database. Nevertheless, the ability of belief function theory to merge information opens very interesting prospects in medical image processing.

References

1. Ling, C.C., Humm, J., Larson, S., Amols, H., Fuks, Z., Leibel, S., Koutcher, J.A.: Towards multidimensional radiotherapy (MD-CRT): biological imaging and biological conformality. Int. J. Radiat. Oncol. Biol. Phys. 47, 551–560 (2000)
2. Vauclin, S., Doyeux, K., Hapdey, S., Edet-Sanson, A., Vera, P., Gardin, I.: Development of a generic thresholding algorithm for the delineation of ^{18}FDG-PET-positive tissue: application to the comparison of three thresholding models. Phys. Med. Biol. 54(22), 6901–6916 (2009)
3. Geets, X., Lee, J.A., Bol, A., Lonneux, M.: A gradient-based method for segmenting FDG-PET images: methodologie and validation. Eur. J. Nucl. Med. Mol. Imaging 34, 1427–1438 (2007)
4. Hatt, M., Cheze-Le Rest, C., Turzo, A., Roux, C., Visvikis, D.: A Fuzzy Locally Adaptive Bayesian Segmentation Approach for Volume Determination in PET. IEEE Trans. Med. Imaging 28(6), 881–893 (2009)
5. Belhassen, S., Zaidi, H.: A novel fuzzy C-means algorithm for unsupervised heterogeneous tumor quantification in PET. Med. Phys. 37, 1309–1324 (2010)
6. Dempster, A.P.: Upper and lower probabilities induced by a multivalued mapping. Ann. Math. Stat. 38, 225–339 (1967)
7. Shafer, G.: A mathematical theory of evidence. Princeton University Press, Princeton (1976)
8. Smets, P., Kennes, R.: The Transferable Belief Model. Artif. Intell. 66, 191–234 (1994)
9. Bloch, I.: Defining belief functions using mathematical morphology - Application to image fusion under imprecision. Int. J. of Approx. Reason. 48(2), 437–465 (2008)
10. Bezdek, J.C.: Pattern Recognition with Fuzzy Objective Function Algorithms. Plenum Press, New York (1981)
11. Viola, P., Wells III, W.M.: Alignment by Maximization of Mutual Information. Int. J. Comput. Vision 24(2), 137–154 (1997)

Local Implicit Modeling of Blood Vessels
for Interactive Simulation

A. Yureidini[1,2,4], E. Kerrien[1,3], J. Dequidt[2,4],
Christian Duriez[2,4], and S. Cotin[2,4]

[1] Inria, Villers-lès-Nancy, F-54600, France
[2] Inria, Villeneuve d'Ascq, F-59650, France
[3] Université de Lorraine, Loria, UMR7503, Vandœuvre-lès-Nancy, F-54600, France
[4] Université Lille 1, Lifl, UMR8022, Villeneuve d'Ascq, F-59650, France

Abstract. In the context of computer-based simulation, contact management requires an accurate, smooth, but still efficient surface model for the blood vessels. A new implicit model is proposed, consisting of a tree of local implicit surfaces generated by skeletons (*blobby models*). The surface is reconstructed from data points by minimizing an energy, alternating with an original blob selection and subdivision scheme. The reconstructed models are very efficient for simulation and were shown to provide a sub-voxel approximation of the vessel surface on 5 patients.

1 Introduction

In the context of interventional radiology, interest is growing in the potential benefits of computer-based simulators. Overall, the expected benefit is a reduction of time: for training, operation and hospitalization; but also to promote new surgical devices and techniques. Such expectations are heightened in the intravascular treatment of brain aneurysms for which highly skilled practitioners are required. Recent works [2] attest the feasibility of real-time simulators for such procedures. However, a key requirement is the availability of the blood vessel surface. We propose in this paper an original blood vessel modeling algorithm, specifically suited to real-time simulation of the interventional gesture.

Vessel lumen segmentation can rely on a vast diversity of models [4]. Here, a catheter, or guide, is pushed through the vessels, interacting with their surface. The vessel surface model should enable a smooth motion of the tools and a precise and efficient collision detection. Implicit surface representations, where the surface is defined as the zero-level set of a known function f, are arguably well suited. First, C1-continuous models (with C0-continuous normal) allows for much smoother sliding contacts. Unwanted friction may occur with polyhedral surfaces or level-sets defined on a discrete grid. Second, implicit surfaces offer an improved collision management over parametric surfaces. Indeed, the implicit function value at a point tells whether this point is inside or outside the surface, detecting a collision in the latter case. Furthermore, the implicit function gradient gives a natural direction for the contact force used to handle this collision.

Implicit vessel modeling has been studied, in particular in the context of visualization [7]. A major problem is to handle unwanted blending between two

N. Ayache et al. (Eds.): MICCAI 2012, Part I, LNCS 7510, pp. 553–560, 2012.
© Springer-Verlag Berlin Heidelberg 2012

structures that are geometrically close, but topologically far from each other. Locally adapting the blending [1] has proven efficient, but is not a valid answer in the context of simulation because the simulated tool motion is discrete. The inclusion test might therefore remain successful even though a crossing over a small gap occurred during the time step. Since the seminal work of Masutani [5] the need for local models, based on the centerline of the vascular tree, has been recognized. Placing a graphics primitive at each point of the centerline [12], or using convolution [7] lacks precision where the vessel section is not circular (or elliptic), and does not correctly handle pathologies such as aneurysms. Schumann [8] addressed both problems and used Multi-level Partition of Unity (MPU) implicits, to get a locally defined model with large and general modeling capabilities. However, the blending issue is not addressed and the model is not related to the topology. Furthermore, MPU implicit gradient gives an appropriate contact direction close to the surface but could mislead contact forces elsewhere.

The proposed approach reconstructs the vessel surface as a tree of local implicit models: one local implicit model is placed at each point on the vessel centerline. Complex branching shapes such as the brain vasculature can thus be modeled in a way that is very efficient for interactive simulation. Implicit surfaces generated by skeletons were chosen for their locality and their genericity. Model fitting is defined as an energy minimization problem, alternating with a model refinement as in [11], but improving over this latter work. Our complete modeling algorithm is described in Section 2. Section 3 reports our results on a set of 5 3D rotational angiography (3DRA) patient data. Finally, we discuss our results and give a conclusion of our work in Section 4.

2   Modeling Algorithm

Our algorithm requires that the vessel centerline is extracted as a tree, not necessarily dense, and that a local vessel radius estimate is available at each point on this centerline. Many valuable methods can provide this initial structure [4]. Moreover, a set of points, located on the local vessel surface, should be associated with each point on the centerline. In practice, the results presented in Section 3 rely on [13]. However, should the vessel surface be available as a mesh, selecting the vertices in the vicinity of each point on the centerline should also provide such a point set. In this case, our method could be seen as a mesh implicitization. Our overall idea is to fit each local point set with an implicit surface generated by a point-set skeleton (Section 2.1). The local models are organized under the same tree structure as the point centerline (Section 2.2). Solving contact constraints at each point of the interventional tool, is performed using the appropriate local implicit model as the vessel surface (Section 2.3).

2.1   Local Implicit Modeling

Implicit Formulation. An implicit iso-surface generated by a point-set skeleton is expressed as the zero-level set of a function f, a sum of implicit spheres:

$$f(X;p) = T - \sum_{j=1}^{N_b} \alpha_j \phi \left(\frac{|X - C_j|}{\rho_j} \right).$$

T is the isosurface threshold, $\{\alpha_j\}$ are positive weights, and $\{C_j\}$ is the point set skeleton. Each implicit sphere $\#j$ is defined by a symmetric spherical function, centered on C_j, of width ρ_j. The local field function, or kernel, is a function $\phi : \mathbb{R} \to \mathbb{R}^+$, rapidly decreasing to 0 at infinity. For example, all results of Section 3 were produced using the 'Cauchy' kernel [9]: $\phi(x) = (1+x^2/5)^{-2}$ (dividing factor 5 normalizes the kernel such that $\phi''(1) = 0$).

Such objects were called differently depending on the kernel used [9]. Our method is not kernel-dependent, and was successfully used with the computationally less efficient Gaussian kernel. Muraki [6] was the first to use this type of model in the context of object reconstruction. Following this seminal work, we shall use the terms *blob* for an implicit sphere, and *blobby models* as a generic name for the implicit models.

In our particular simulation context, in order to help predict collisions, and have the function give a valid contact force direction, the algebraic value $f(X; p)$ at point X should relate monotonously to the geometric distance of X to the surface. We set $\alpha_j = \rho_j$, which obviously establishes the sought relation in the case of a single blob. Meanwhile, redundancy in the parameters of f is dismissed.

Energy Formulation. Fitting a surface to N points $\{P_i\}_{1 \leq i \leq N_p}$ can be written as an energy minimization problem [11,6]. We propose to combine 3 energy terms: $\mathcal{E} = \mathcal{E}_d + \alpha \mathcal{E}_c + \beta \mathcal{E}_a$ where $(\alpha, \beta) \in \mathbb{R}^{+2}$, and:

- $\mathcal{E}_d = 1/N_p \sum_i f(P_i; p)^2$
  translates the algebraic relation between data points and the zero-level set. It gives a raw expression of the approximation problem.
- $\mathcal{E}_c = 1/\left(N_b(N_b - 1)\right) \sum_{j \neq k} \left(\frac{s\sqrt{\rho_j \rho_k}}{|C_j - C_k|} \right)^{12} - 2 \left(\frac{s\sqrt{\rho_j \rho_k}}{|C_j - C_k|} \right)^6$
  is Lennard-Jones energy. Each term is minimal (with value -1) for $|C_j - C_k| = s\sqrt{\rho_j \rho_k}$, being repulsive for blobs closer than this distance, and attractive for blobs further away. It imposes some cohesion between neighboring blobs to avoid leakage where data points are missing, while preventing blobs from accumulating within the model.
- $\mathcal{E}_a = 1/N_p \sum_i \kappa(P_i)^2$
  $\kappa(P)$ is the mean curvature. It can be computed in a closed form at any point in space from the implicit formulation [3]

$$\kappa(P) = \frac{\nabla f^t H_f \nabla f - |\nabla f|^2 trace(H_f)}{2|\nabla f|^3}$$

where ∇f is the implicit function gradient and H_f its Hessian matrix, both computed at point P. This energy smoothes the surface according to the minimal area criterion. In particular, the wavy effect that could stem from modeling a tubular shape with implicit spheres, is reduced.

Behind the rather classical form given above for the energy terms, it is important to notice that the whole energy is known under a closed-form expression. As a consequence, closed-form expressions were derived for its gradients with respect to the blobby model paramaters $\{\rho_j\}$ and $\{C_j\}$.

Selection-Subdivision. The blob subdivision procedure proposed in the seminal work [6] was exhaustive and time consuming. A blob selection mechanism was added in [11], measuring the contribution of each blob to $\mathcal{E}_d$ in a user-defined window, and choosing the main contributor. User input is not an option in our context where thousands of blobby models are handled (see Section 3). Moreover, we experimentally noted that this technique was prone to favor small blobs, thus focusing on details, before dealing with areas roughly approximated by one large blob. This behavior is caused by this selection mechanism using the algebraic distance to the implicit surface. Our criterion relies upon the geometric distance approximation proposed by [10]. Point P_{i^*} farthest to the surface is such that:

$$i^* = \arg \max_{1 \leq i \leq N_p} \frac{|f(P_i; p)|}{|\nabla f(P_i; p)|} \tag{1}$$

The blob $\#j^*$ whose isosurface is the closest to P_{i^*} is selected (according to Taubin's distance). Note that this criterion is valid in large areas because we set $\alpha_j = \rho_j$ in the definition of f. The subdivision step then replaces this blob with two new ones. Their width ρ'_{j^*} is chosen such that two blobs, centered on C_{j^*}, of width ρ'_{j^*} would have the same isosurface as one blob centered on C_{j^*}, with width ρ_{j^*} (the formula depends on the kernel). The first new blob is centered on C_{j^*}, while the second is translated by $\rho_{j^*}/10$ towards P_{i^*}.

Optimization. Such a gradual subdivision procedure may lead to a dramatic increase in the number of blobs, and hence the size of the optimization problem. The locality of the kernel ϕ allows us to focus the optimization onto the newly created pair of blobs. More exactly, only the new blob that is slightly misplaced is optimized, the other blobs remaining constant. The energy is minimized using Polak-Ribiere conjugate gradient (PR) algorithm, taking advantage of the closed-form expressions of both the energy and its gradients. A single minimization loop consists in one PR minimization over the center (3 variables), followed by one on the width (1 variable). In practice, a maximum of 5 loops proved sufficient.

2.2   Global Implicit Modeling

The algorithm is initialized by placing two blobs at each node on the centerline that form an elongated shape along the vessel direction, with the same diameter as the vessel width. The local data point sets are concatenated so as to overlap with their neighbors, and generate smooth transition between adjacent blobby models. The following three steps are then applied on each blobby model:

1. A first energy minimization is performed over the full blobby model, with a single minimization loop (all centers then all widths of its blobs).
2. The subdivision process is applied, as described above. The process is stopped when a maximum number N_s of subdivisions is reached, or the distance between P_{i^*} and blob $\#j^*$ drops below a threshold t_g.
3. The model is fine tuned by a single energy minimization loop over the full blobby model, as in step 1.

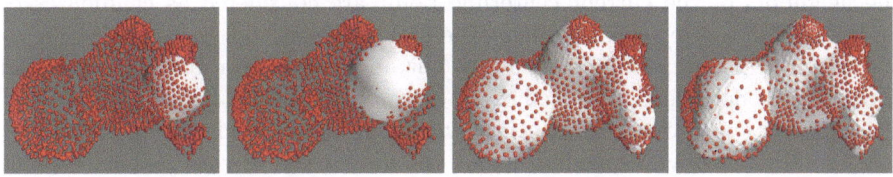

Fig. 1. Implicit modeling of an aneurysm. The points $\{P_i\}$ are in red. (From left to right) Initialization with a single blob ; after the first minimization ; after 25 subdivisions ; final result (100 subdivisions).

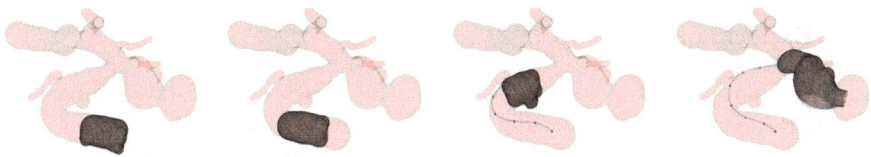

Fig. 2. Selection of a local blobby model during simulation. The current local blobby model surface used to solve the constraints at the tool tip is displayed in wireframe for 4 simulation steps. The overall vessel surface is shown in transparent red. Discrepancies with the blobby models might occur, due to this surface being simplified in order to minimize the CPU load devoted to visualization.

Redundant blobs are either ejected far away from the surface during the optimization over the centers, or their width is reduced to almost zero during the minimization over the widths. A simple clean-up procedure was applied after each minimization loop: blobs further than 20 mm from the node (twice the diameter of the largest artery), and blobs whose width was below 0.02 mm (10% of the voxel size) were removed from the blobby model. In combination with the subdivision process, this clean-up enables the algorithm to simulate large blob displacements, which is hardly possible with the local minimization, thereby adding robustness to poor initialization. Figure 1 illustrates the essential steps of this fitting algorithm and its capacity to model complex shapes, such as aneurysms, even from rough initialization.

Note that in this algorithm, each local blobby model is treated independently from the others, enabling a parallel computation.

2.3   Using the Local Models for Simulation

Most of the interventional tools are slender and their motion can be defined by that of longitudinal nodes. During a simulation step, contact with the vessel surface is detected and solved for each point on the tool. Each tool point is thus linked to its closest point on the centerline and the associated local blobby model is used as the surface constraint. In order to take into account the topology, only the neighbors of the current centerline point are considered as candidates to update the surface constraint during the motion of the tool (see Fig. 2).

Our model is adapted to simulation, but not to visualization. We translated the above model selection procedure to give a visual impression of the result in the next section: each local isosurface was first extracted with marching cubes, and was then cut by the median planes separating the current centerline point from each of its neighbors. No blending was performed between adjacent blobby models. The final surface presents as a stack of individual surfaces.

3   Results

3.1   Experimental Setup

A set of 5 patient data was used for validation. Each patient data set consisted of a 3DRA acquired on a vascular C-arm (Innova 4100, GE Healthcare) during the intra-arterial injection of the internal carotid artery. Each 3DRA volume is a 512^3 isotropic voxel cube, between 0.18-0.22 mm voxel size. For each patient, the vessels were tracked and points were extracted at their surface using [13].

The implicit modeling procedure was applied to all 5 datasets. The algorithm parameters were tuned on the carotid artery of one patient, and thereafter used for all patients. The 'Cauchy' kernel was chosen for its computational efficiency. The energy weights were tuned so the energy values are of the same order of magnitude, leading to $\alpha = 10^{-5}$ and $\beta = 10^{-3}$. For Lennard-Jones energy, s was set to 2 (natural distance between two blobs is twice the geometric mean of their width). The isolevel value T was set to 0.1. Indeed, since we set the weight of each blob equal to its width, blobs whose width is below T do not generate any isosurface (maximum function value is $\rho_j < T$). We therefore chose T to be approximately half the voxel size.

3.2   Geometric Precision Assessment

The geometric error of fit of a local blobby model with respect to a point set was estimated using Taubin's approximate distance. When measured at each data point, it provides a set of statistical samples for this error: the error of fit for a blobby model, d_{bm} was defined as the 90th percentile on this set, which is a more strict but also more robust measure than the mean. Table 1 reports the distribution, in percents, of d_{bm} measured on all 42840 blobby models. Four classes were considered: below 0.5, 1, 2 and over twice the voxel size (which varies between 0.18 and 0.22mm). Two parameters in particular have an impact on the geometric precision: the distance threshold t_g, expressing a targetted accuracy of fit, and the maximum number N_s of subdivision, expressing the maximum complexity allowed for the models. Measurements were performed for $t_g = 0.5, 0.3$ and 0.2 mm, $N_s = 100, 50, 30$ giving 9 algorithm configurations.

At most 1% of blobby models had an error of fit above 1 voxel. t_g appeared as the only parameter to impact the result and $t_g = 0.3$mm was the only case where

Table 1. Distribution in % of the blobby models according to the error of fit (d_{bm}, in voxels) in 4 classes (left column). 9 algorithm configurations were investigated depending on parameters t_g (targetted accuracy of fit) and N_s (maximum model complexity).

t_g	0.5mm			0.3mm			0.2mm		
N_s	30	50	100	30	50	100	30	50	100
$d_{bm} < 0.5$	47.44	47.18	47.29	60.28	65.07	70.52	89.86	90.07	90.14
$0.5 < d_{bm} < 1$	51.64	51.82	51.83	39.17	34.53	29.11	9.75	9.60	9.57
$1 < d_{bm} < 1.5$	0.85	0.96	0.83	0.48	0.34	0.32	0.32	0.26	0.23
$2 < d_{bm}$	0.06	0.04	0.04	0.06	0.06	0.05	0.08	0.07	0.06

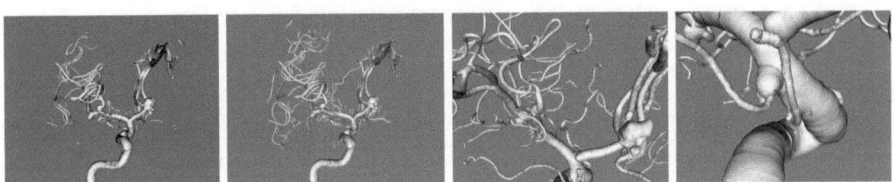

Fig. 3. Visible assessment (from left to right): isosurface from the raw data set ; isosurface from the blobby models (13956 models, 51272 blobs, $t_g = 0.3, N_s = 100$): much more vessels are visible; close-up showing smooth transitions between models ; close-up on a small artery branching onto the carotid: the connection is difficult to model

N_s had a noticeable influence. In our opinion, N_s only has an influence when t_g is adapted to the details to be modeled in the data: $t_g = 0.5$mm was too rough and $t_g = 0.2$mm led the blobby models to fit noisy data points. $t_g = 0.3$mm and $N_s = 100$ provided the best algorithm configuration.

3.3 Model Efficiency and Computation Time

The computation time to model one patient was between 15 and 30 minutes, depending on the number of nodes in the vascular tree (between 5461 and 13956 nodes). A sample result is shown on Figure 3, demonstrating a very good vessel resolution and smooth transitions between neighboring blobby models, except at some very isolated locations. Discontinuities between models do not depend on the kernel, but are mostly sensitive to inhomogeneities in the point set density. Despite discontinuities are below voxel size, we believe they prohibit using our model for blood flow simulation using Computational Fluid Dynamics (CFD). Therefore, direct reconstruction from image data is currently being investigated.

A rule of thumb to measure the efficiency of our model, is to count the number of primitives used. For each patient we compared the total number of blobs (with $t_g = 0.3$ and $N_s = 100$) to the number of triangles in a vessel isosurface mesh of a similar visual quality (see e.g. Fig. 3, left). The ratio #triangles/#blobs ranged from 7 to 13.8, with an average of 10.5. On a more local basis, the average number of blobs per local blobby model was 4.2 (min=3.7, max=4.6).

4   Conclusion

We have presented a patient-specific blood vessel surface reconstruction method that is particularly suited to the simulation of interventional radiology procedures. The final model presents as a tree of implicit surfaces generated by local skeletons. Each surface has a limited area of influence which overlaps with its topological neighbors to provide a smooth transition during the tool guidance. The model fitting is guided by the minimization of an energy, with a closed-form expression, alternating with an efficient blob selection and subdivision scheme. The reconstructed models provided a sub-voxel approximation of the vessel surface on 5 patient data. This model was integrated in our simulation software and preliminary tests proved the adequacy and efficiency of our model in that context. As a perspective, we aim at reconstructing directly from image data.

References

1. Bernhardt, A., Barthe, L., Cani, M.P., et al.: Implicit blending revisited. Comput. Graph. Forum 29(2), 367–375 (2010)
2. Dequidt, J., Duriez, C., Cotin, S., Kerrien, E.: Towards Interactive Planning of Coil Embolization in Brain Aneurysms. In: Yang, G.-Z., Hawkes, D., Rueckert, D., Noble, A., Taylor, C. (eds.) MICCAI 2009, Part I. LNCS, vol. 5761, pp. 377–385. Springer, Heidelberg (2009)
3. Goldman, R.: Curvature formulas for implicit curves and surfaces. Computer Aided Geometric Design 22, 632–658 (2005)
4. Lesage, D., Angelini, E., Bloch, I., et al.: A review of 3D vessel lumen segmentation techniques: Models, features and extraction schemes. Med. Image Anal. 13(6), 819–845 (2009)
5. Masutani, Y., Masamune, K., Dohi, T.: Region-growing Based Feature Extraction Algorithm for Tree-like Objects. In: Höhne, K.H., Kikinis, R. (eds.) VBC 1996. LNCS, vol. 1131, pp. 159–171. Springer, Heidelberg (1996)
6. Muraki, S.: Volumetric shape description of range data using blobby model. SIG-GRAPH Comput. Graph. 25, 227–235 (1991)
7. Preim, B., Oeltze, S.: 3D visualization of vasculature: An overview. In: Visualization in Medicine and Life Sciences. Math. and Vis., pp. 39–59. Springer (2008)
8. Schumann, C., Neugebauer, M., Bade, R., et al.: Implicit vessel surface reconstruction for visualization and CFD simulation. IJCARS 2(5), 275–286 (2008)
9. Sherstyuk, A.: Kernel functions in convolution surfaces: A comparative analysis. The Visual Computer 15(4), 171–182 (1999)
10. Taubin, G.: Estimation of planar curves, surfaces, and nonplanar space curves defined by implicit equations with applications to edge and range image segmentation. IEEE Trans. on PAMI 13, 1115–1138 (1991)
11. Tsingos, N., Bittar, E., Cani, M.P.: Implicit surfaces for semi-automatic medical organ reconstruction. In: Computer Graphics Internat (CGI 1995), pp. 3–15 (1995)
12. Tyrrell, J., di Tomaso, E., Fuja, D., et al.: Robust 3-D modeling of vasculature imagery using superellipsoids. IEEE Trans. Med. Imag. 26(2), 223–237 (2007)
13. Yureidini, A., Kerrien, E., Cotin, S.: Robust RANSAC-based blood vessel segmentation. In: SPIE Medical Imaging, vol. 8314, p. 83141M. SPIE (2012)

Real-Time 3D Image Segmentation by User-Constrained Template Deformation

Benoît Mory, Oudom Somphone, Raphael Prevost, and Roberto Ardon

Medisys, Philips Research, Suresnes, France

Abstract. We describe an algorithm for 3D interactive image segmentation by non-rigid implicit template deformation, with two main original features. First, our formulation incorporates user input as inside/outside labeled points to drive the deformation and improve both robustness and accuracy. This yields inequality constraints, solved using an Augmented Lagrangian approach. Secondly, a fast implementation of non-rigid template-to-image registration enables interactions with a real-time visual feedback. We validated this generic technique on 21 Contrast-Enhanced Ultrasound images of kidneys and obtained accurate segmentation results (Dice> 0.93) in less than 3 clicks in average.

1 Introduction

In medical applications, segmentation of anatomical structures in difficult conditions such as tissue inhomogeneities, noise, loss-of-contrast, can be significantly facilitated by the incorporation of prior knowledge. This approach has been extensively studied in terms of shape prior by constraining the solution to remain close to a predefined shape. For instance, statistical methods have been proposed to model shapes, such as the *active shape models* [1]. In the level-set framework, shape priors have also been used, penalizing the dissimilarity between the implicit object representation and the one embedding the prior shape, *via* an additive shape constraint [2–5]. These two approaches have been combined by embedding training shapes in distance functions and defining a statistical model for the shape term [6–9].

Template-to-image registration is a possible alternative, recently applied to medical applications such as liver segmentation in CT [10], in which segmentation is performed by geometrically deforming a binary template towards the image [10–12]. The prior is the template itself and the shape constraint consists in a regularization of the deformation.

Shape priors may be helpful but insufficient in pathological cases with extreme variability in image features and organ shapes; expert input is then essential to guide the segmentation. Few attempts to combine shape priors and interactivity have been made in 2D [13]. In 3D, the design of intuitive and fast interactive tools remains a key challenge. We propose a formulation of non-rigid template deformation that incorporates user constraints in the form of inside/outside labels and enables a live visual feedback of the surface evolution.

N. Ayache et al. (Eds.): MICCAI 2012, Part I, LNCS 7510, pp. 561–568, 2012.

2 Implicit Template Deformation

Region-based variational formulations of image segmentation consist in finding a partitioning of an image I that provides the best trade-off between classification error and boundary regularity. In the case of two regions, the optimal boundary is the surface $\mathcal{S}$ solution of:

$$\min_{\mathcal{S}} \left\{ \mathcal{R}(\mathcal{S}) + \int_{inside\ \mathcal{S}} r_1(\mathbf{x})\,d\mathbf{x} + \int_{outside\ \mathcal{S}} r_2(\mathbf{x})\,d\mathbf{x} \right\} \tag{1}$$

$\mathcal{R}(\mathcal{S})$ is a regularization term, commonly chosen as the surface area. r_1 and r_2 are classification error functions in the foreground and background regions, respectively. For instance, maximum-likelihood principles suggest the choice of log-likelihood terms $r_i(\mathbf{x}) = -\log p_i(I(\mathbf{x}))$ for known intensity distributions p_1 and p_2 [14].

An equivalent formulation can be derived for an implicit representation of $\mathcal{S}$, with a function $\Phi : \Omega \to \mathbb{R}$, positive inside $\mathcal{S}$ and satisfying $\Phi^{-1}(0) = \mathcal{S}$. Let H denote the Heaviside function ($H(a) = 1$ if $a > 0$, 0 otherwise); $H(\Phi)$ is the characteristic function of the region enclosed by $\mathcal{S}$ and (1) is equivalent to:

$$\min_{\Phi} \left\{ \mathcal{R}(\Phi) + \int_{\Omega} H(\Phi(\mathbf{x}))r(\mathbf{x})\,d\mathbf{x} \right\} \quad \text{with} \quad r(\mathbf{x}) = r_1(\mathbf{x}) - r_2(\mathbf{x}) \tag{2}$$

Regularization $\mathcal{R}(\Phi)$ can be complemented with an additional shape prior term that enforces the solution to remain close to a predefined implicit representation. For instance, if Φ is a distance function, the shape term can penalize the L_2-distance to a globally transformed template [2]. However, this technique does not guarantee that the zero level-set of the solution preserves the topology of the prior shape. Moreover, penalizing the surface area inevitably smooths out possible important details of the prior shape.

To cope with these problems, alternative approaches have been proposed [10–12] to define Φ as the deformation of a given implicit template Φ_0, defined in a referential Ω_0, with a geometric transformation ψ (see Fig. 1):

$$\Phi = \Phi_0 \circ \psi \tag{3}$$

The unknown becomes the transformation ψ and $\mathcal{R}(\Phi)$ in (2) is substituted with a shape term $\mathcal{R}(\psi)$, consisting in a regularization constraint acting on ψ.

Thus, a general formulation of image segmentation by implicit template deformation reads:

$$\min_{\psi} \left\{ E(\psi) = \mathcal{R}(\psi) + \int_{\Omega} H(\Phi_0 \circ \psi(\mathbf{x}))r(\mathbf{x})\,d\mathbf{x} \right\} \tag{4}$$

Compliance with the shape prior is determined by both the deformation model ψ and its associated constraint $\mathcal{R}(\psi)$. In the non-rigid case, Saddi *et al.* represented the deformation with a diffeomorphic fluid model [10], Somphone *et al.* proposed deformations based on finite elements [11], and Huang and Metaxas adopted Free Form Deformations in their *Metamorphs* [12].

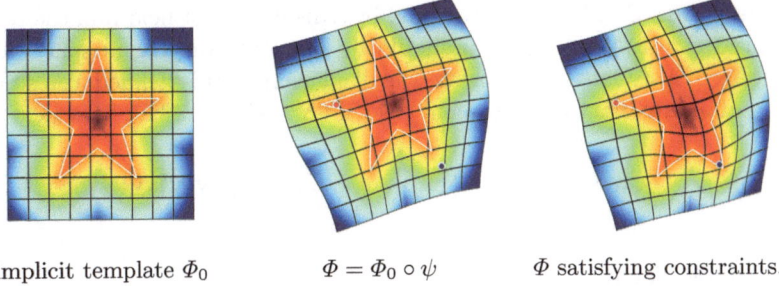

implicit template Φ_0 $\Phi = \Phi_0 \circ \psi$ Φ satisfying constraints.

Fig. 1. Deformation of a star-shaped template (white contour) implicitly represented with a signed distance function Φ_0, with inside (blue) and outside (red) constraints

3 Proposed Formulation

The aforementioned approaches of *template-to-image* registration do not consider possibilities for user interactions. Moreover, they are adapted from existing non-rigid *image-to-image* registration methods. Therefore, they inherit an algorithmic complexity that is incompatible with real-time feedback in 3D.

3.1 User Interactions as Inequality Constraints

Additional control can be obtained by letting the user locate specific points that lie inside/outside the object. Denoting $\{\mathbf{x}_k\}$ a set of N labeled points, this translates into N constraints on the sign of the transformed template at $\mathbf{x}_k$:

$$\forall k \in \{0, \dots, N-1\} \quad \gamma_k \Phi_0 \circ \psi(\mathbf{x}_k) \geq 0 \tag{5}$$

where $\gamma_k = 1$ (resp. -1) for inside (resp. outside) points, as illustrated in Fig. 1. Note that the surface $\{\Phi_0 \circ \psi = 0\}$ can also be enforced to go through a specific point by adding both inside and outside constraints at the same location.

3.2 Transformation Model

In the context of *template-to-image* registration, the choice of a transformation model ψ in (4) relates to the notion of *shape*. In particular, a *shape* should be invariant to geometric transforms such as rotation and scaling. We refer to such a global transformation as the *pose*. To separate pose from subsequent shape *deformation*, we define ψ as a *composition* of a global transformation $\mathcal{G}$ and a local transformation $\mathcal{L}$ [15]:

$$\psi = \mathcal{L} \circ \mathcal{G} \tag{6}$$

Pose. $\mathcal{G} : \Omega \to \Omega_0$ is chosen as a parametric transform that globally aligns the template with the target in the image. For anatomical structures, similarities (preserving aspect ratio) are particularly adapted. Thus, $\mathcal{G}$ is defined by a matrix in homogeneous coordinates, with 7 parameters $\mathbf{p} = \{p_i\}_{i=1\cdots 7}$.

Deformation. $\mathcal{L} : \Omega_0 \to \Omega_0$ is defined by a displacement field $\mathbf{u}$ in the template referential $\mathcal{L} = \mathbf{u} + \mathbf{Id}$, where $\mathbf{u}$ should be smoothly-varying in space. To take advantage of fast Gaussian filtering, the displacement $\mathbf{u}$ is defined as a smoothed version of an auxiliary displacement field $\mathbf{v}$ (K_σ is a Gaussian of scale σ):

$$\mathbf{u}(\mathbf{x}) = [K_\sigma * \mathbf{v}](\mathbf{x}) = \int_{\Omega_0} K_\sigma(\mathbf{x} - \mathbf{y})\mathbf{v}(\mathbf{y})d\mathbf{y} \tag{7}$$

3.3 Shape Term

Decomposing $\psi = \mathcal{L} \circ \mathcal{G}$ allows to define a shape term as a function of the shape deformation $\mathcal{L}$ only, regardless of the pose $\mathcal{G}$. Using the L_2 norm, we choose to constrain $\mathcal{L}$ towards the identity $\mathbf{Id}$:

$$\mathcal{R}(\mathcal{L}) = \frac{\lambda}{2}\|\mathcal{L} - \mathbf{Id}\|_2^2 = \frac{\lambda}{2}\int_{\Omega_0} \|\mathbf{u}(\mathbf{x})\|^2 d\mathbf{x} \tag{8}$$

where λ is a positive scalar parameter. $\mathcal{R}$ quantifies the deviation of the segmentation from the prior shape by a displacement magnitude in the template referential Ω_0. Finally, the constrained optimization problem to solve reads:

$$\min_{\mathbf{p},\mathbf{v}} \left\{ E(\psi_{\mathbf{p},\mathbf{v}}) = \frac{\lambda}{2}\int_{\Omega_0} \|K_\sigma * \mathbf{v}\|^2 + \int_{\Omega} H(\Phi_0 \circ \psi_{\mathbf{p},\mathbf{v}})r \right\} \tag{9}$$
$$\text{subject to} \qquad \gamma_k \Phi_0 \circ \psi_{\mathbf{p},\mathbf{v}}(\mathbf{x}_k) \geq 0, \quad \forall k \in 0..N-1$$

4 Augmented Lagrangian Scheme

To minimize the non-convex functional $E(\psi_{\mathbf{p},\mathbf{v}})$ under a set of N non-linear inequality constraints, we follow an Augmented Lagrangian methodology [16] and define an equivalent *unconstrained* problem. Problem (9) is equivalent to:

$$\min_{\psi_{\mathbf{p},\mathbf{v}}} \left\{ \tilde{E}(\psi_{\mathbf{p},\mathbf{v}}) = \max_{\boldsymbol{\alpha} \geq 0} \left\{ E(\psi_{\mathbf{p},\mathbf{v}}) - \sum_{k=0}^{N-1} \alpha_k c_k(\psi_{\mathbf{p},\mathbf{v}}) \right\} \right\} \tag{10}$$
$$\text{with} \quad c_k(\psi_{\mathbf{p},\mathbf{v}}) = \gamma_k \Phi_0 \circ \psi_{\mathbf{p},\mathbf{v}}(\mathbf{x}_k)$$

where α_k is the Lagrange multiplier associated to the kth constraint. (10) has the same set of solutions as the original Problem (9): if $\psi_{\mathbf{p},\mathbf{v}}$ satisfies all constraints c_k, then $\tilde{E}(\psi_{\mathbf{p},\mathbf{v}}) = E(\psi_{\mathbf{p},\mathbf{v}})$, otherwise $\tilde{E}(\psi_{\mathbf{p},\mathbf{v}}) = +\infty$. To avoid jumps of $\tilde{E}$ from finite to infinite values, a practical minimization requires to rely on a smooth approximation $\hat{E}$. In order to constrain the maximizers $\boldsymbol{\alpha} = \{\alpha_k\}$ to finite values during the iterative process, a quadratic penalty parameter μ and a set of multipliers $\boldsymbol{\alpha}^j$ (at the jth iteration) are explicitly introduced to define:

$$\hat{E}_\mu(\psi_{\mathbf{p},\mathbf{v}}, \boldsymbol{\alpha}^j) = \max_{\boldsymbol{\alpha} \geq 0} \left\{ E(\psi_{\mathbf{p},\mathbf{v}}) - \sum_{k=0}^{N-1} \alpha_k c_k(\psi_{\mathbf{p},\mathbf{v}}) - \frac{1}{2\mu}\sum_{k=0}^{N-1}\left(\alpha_k - \alpha_k^j\right)^2 \right\} \tag{11}$$

In (11), optimal Lagrange multipliers associated to each constraint $c_k(\psi_{\mathbf{p},\mathbf{v}})$ can be found as a function of previously estimated values:

$$
\alpha_k^{j+1} = \begin{cases} 0 & \text{if } \alpha_k^j - \mu c_k(\psi_{\mathbf{p},\mathbf{v}}) \leq 0 \\ \alpha_k^j - \mu c_k(\psi_{\mathbf{p},\mathbf{v}}) & \text{otherwise.} \end{cases} \tag{12}
$$

Substituting (12) in (11) yields the expression of the smooth approximation $\hat{E}_\mu$:

$$
\hat{E}_\mu(\psi_{\mathbf{p},\mathbf{v}}, \alpha^j) = E(\psi_{\mathbf{p},\mathbf{v}}) + \sum_{k=0}^{N-1} \Psi_\mu \left(c_k(\psi_{\mathbf{p},\mathbf{v}}), \alpha_k^j \right) \tag{13}
$$

$$
\text{with} \quad \Psi_\mu(a, b) = \begin{cases} -ab + \dfrac{\mu}{2} a^2 & \text{if } \mu a \leq b \\ -\dfrac{1}{2\mu} b^2 & \text{otherwise.} \end{cases} \tag{14}
$$

Finally, the alternate scheme below provides at convergence a local minimizer of (9) that satisfies all inequality constraints.

---

given starting penalty parameter μ^0, and $\alpha^0 = 0$,
repeat
    choose $\mu^t > \mu^{t-1}$,
    repeat
        (A) $\psi_{\mathbf{p},\mathbf{v}}$ fixed, update α^{j+1} as in (12)
        (B) α^j fixed, update $\psi_{\mathbf{p},\mathbf{v}}$ by minimizing (13)
    until *convergence*;
until *a local minimum of $E(\psi_{\mathbf{p},\mathbf{v}})$ satisfying $\forall k, c_k(\psi_{\mathbf{p},\mathbf{v}}) \geq 0$ is found*;

In our application, the effect of each interaction is visualized with a real-time display of the surface evolution. This relies on fast iterations of the minimization of (13) involved in step (B), jointly performed with respect to $\mathbf{p}$ and $\mathbf{v}$ by gradient descent of:

$$
\hat{E}(\mathbf{p}, \mathbf{v}) = E(\psi_{\mathbf{p},\mathbf{v}}) + \sum_{k=0}^{N-1} \Psi_\mu \left(c_k(\mathbf{p}, \mathbf{v}), \alpha_k^j \right) \tag{15}
$$

Evolution equations for each pose parameter p_i and the displacement field $\mathbf{v}$ are:

$$
\frac{\partial p_i}{\partial t} = -\frac{\partial \hat{E}}{\partial p_i} = \qquad -\int_{\Omega_0} \delta(\Phi_0 \circ \mathcal{L}) r \circ \mathcal{G}^{-1} \mathcal{A}_i - \sum_{k=0}^{N-1} b_k \mathcal{A}_i \circ \mathcal{G}(\mathbf{x}_k)
$$

$$
\frac{\partial \mathbf{v}}{\partial t} = -\frac{\partial \hat{E}}{\partial \mathbf{v}} = -K_\sigma * \left[\underbrace{\lambda \mathbf{u}}_{\text{shape}} + \underbrace{\left(\delta(\Phi_0 \circ \mathcal{L}) r \circ \mathcal{G}^{-1} \right.}_{\text{image force}} + \underbrace{\left. \sum_{k=0}^{N-1} b_k \delta_{\mathcal{G}(\mathbf{x}_k)} \right)}_{\text{constraints}} \nabla \Phi_0 \circ \mathcal{L} \right]
$$

$$
\tag{16}
$$

where $b_k = \gamma_k \dfrac{\partial \Psi_\mu}{\partial a}$, $\mathcal{A}_i(\mathbf{x}) = \left\langle \nabla \Phi_0 \circ \mathcal{L}(\mathbf{x}), \left(\mathbf{I} + \mathbf{J}_{\mathbf{u}(\mathbf{x})}\right) \dfrac{\partial \mathcal{G}}{\partial p_i} \circ \mathcal{G}^{-1}(\mathbf{x}) \right\rangle$ with $\mathbf{I}$ the Identity matrix and $\mathbf{J_u}$ the Jacobian matrix of $\mathbf{u}$, and $\delta_{\mathcal{G}(\mathbf{x}_k)}(\mathbf{x}) = \delta\left(\mathbf{x} - \mathcal{G}(\mathbf{x}_k)\right)$.

Let us now emphasize key properties of (16) that enable a fast implementation. First, interpolating $\Phi_0 \circ \mathcal{L}$ and $\nabla \Phi_0 \circ \mathcal{L}$ over the whole domain Ω_0 would be extremely time-consuming. Nevertheless, since it is multiplied either by $\delta(\Phi_0 \circ \mathcal{L})$ or $\delta_{\mathcal{G}(\mathbf{x}_k)}$, the warped gradient $\nabla \Phi_0 \circ \mathcal{L}$ is only needed on the set $\{\Phi_0 \circ \mathcal{L} = 0\}$ and at points $\{\mathbf{x}_k\}$ (Fig. 2.a) which highly reduces warped gradient computations.

Moreover, precise knowledge of the warped template $\Phi_0 \circ \mathcal{L}$ is only necessary near its zero level. Setting Φ_0 to a distance function to the prior shape allows a coarse-to-fine approach using octrees. At each level, decision is made to further refine each cell based on the distance value (Fig. 2.b) which also significantly reduces the warping complexity.

Finally, a benefit of the displacement model (7) is that image forces and constraints extrapolate to the whole space with a convolution with K_σ (Fig. 2.c).

Our 3D implementation supports about 100 time steps per second when discretizing Ω_0 on a lattice of 48^3 points, which allows a live response to constraints.

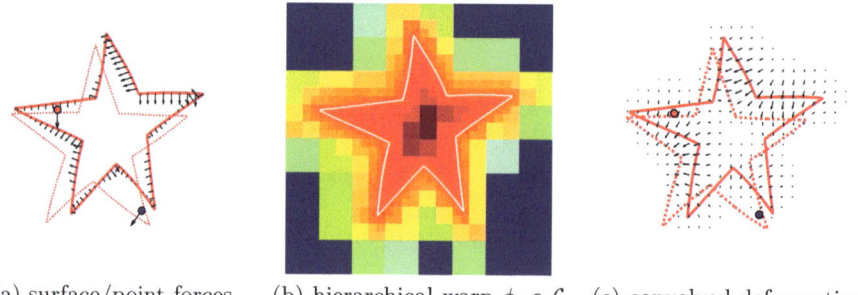

(a) surface/point forces   (b) hierarchical warp $\phi_0 \circ \mathcal{L}$ (c) convolved deformation

Fig. 2. Fast deformation of a distance function with hierarchical warp and convolution

5   Segmenting Kidneys in Contrast-Enhanced Ultrasound

We validated this method on 3D contrast-enhanced ultrasound (CEUS) images of kidneys. CEUS is a recent imaging modality that allows to visualize blood flow in real-time without any risk for the patient. However, segmenting kidneys in CEUS images is difficult : contrast agents generate noisy data, limited field of view of probes often prevents the acquisition of the whole kidney and lesions induce variations from the usual shape. Unlike in conventional ultrasound, very few methods have been reported for 3D CEUS segmentation.

Validation was performed on a representative dataset of 21 CEUS volumes acquired on a Philips iU22 ultrasound system with different probes (V6-2 and X6-1), resolutions and fields of view. Typical size of the images is $512 \times 320 \times 256$. For each case, ground truth segmentation was provided by a radiologist.

Template Φ_0 is set to an ellipsoid. Segmentation criterion is the image gradient flux across the boundary, which is equivalent to a region-based formulation such as (4) with $r(\mathbf{x}) = \Delta I(\mathbf{x})$ where Δ is the Laplacian operator. The scale σ of the deformation field in (7) is set to 25 mm.

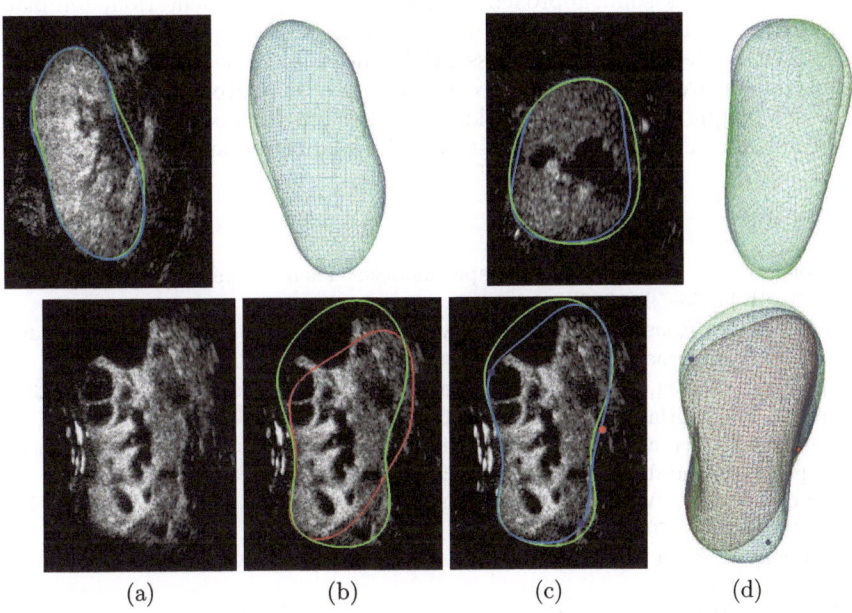

(a)   (b)   (c)   (d)

Fig. 3. Top: automatic segmentation (blue) and ground truth (green) for 2 patients. Bottom: segmentation with user interactions. (a) slice of the CEUS volume. (b) ground truth (green) and automatic segmentation (red). (c) corrected segmentation (blue) with 3 clicks. (d) ground truth (green), automatic (red) and after corrections (blue).

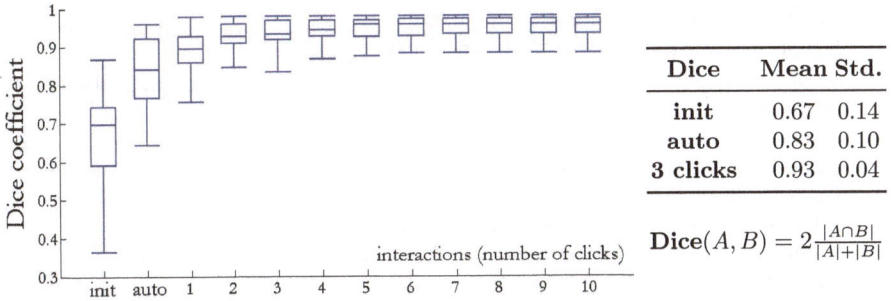

Dice	Mean	Std.
init	0.67	0.14
auto	0.83	0.10
3 clicks	0.93	0.04

$$\mathbf{Dice}(A, B) = 2\frac{|A \cap B|}{|A| + |B|}$$

Fig. 4. Comparison with ground truth, as a function of the number of interactions

While automatic segmentation is successful in some cases, difficult cases with cysts and partial visibility of the kidney (Fig. 3) inevitably require corrections. Fig. 4 summarizes the results obtained by a trained user and quantifies how segmentation performance improves with the number of interactions. In most cases, three clicks are sufficient to obtain a satisfactory result (Dice 0.93 ± 0.04).

6   Conclusion

Although proven a solid approach for medical image segmentation, template deformation is still unable to cope with the variety of shapes that pathologies generate. Reliable interactions are essential add-ons to these segmentation tools. In this context, we introduced user corrections in a template deformation framework with simple clicks inside/outside the object, with special care devoted to algorithmic efficiency to enable real-time 3D visualization and intuitive control.

References

1. Cootes, T.F., et al.: Active shape models: Their training and application. CVIU 61(1), 38–59 (1995)
2. Paragios, N., Rousson, M., Ramesh, V.: Matching Distance Functions: A Shape-to-Area Variational Approach for Global-to-Local Registration. In: Heyden, A., Sparr, G., Nielsen, M., Johansen, P. (eds.) ECCV 2002, Part II. LNCS, vol. 2351, pp. 775–789. Springer, Heidelberg (2002)
3. Cremers, D., et al.: Towards recognition-based variational segmentation using shape priors and dynamic labeling. In: Scale Space, pp. 388–400 (2003)
4. Chan, T.F., Zhu, W.: Level set based shape prior segmentation. In: IEEE CVPR, pp. II:1164–II:1170 (2005)
5. Foulonneau, A., et al.: Multi-reference shape priors for active contours. IJCV 81(1), 68–81 (2009)
6. Leventon, M.E., et al.: Statistical shape influence in geodesic active contours. In: IEEE CVPR, pp. 316–323 (2000)
7. Tsai, A., et al.: A shape-based approach to the segmentation of medical imagery using level sets. IEEE TMI 22(2), 137–154 (2003)
8. Bresson, X., et al.: A variational model for object segmentation using boundary information and shape prior driven by the Mumford-Shah functional. IJCV 68(2), 145–162 (2006)
9. Cremers, D., et al.: Shape statistics in kernel space for variational image segmentation. Pattern Recognition 36(9), 1929–1943 (2003)
10. Saddi, K.A., et al.: Global-to-local shape matching for liver segmentation in ct imaging. In: MICCAI (October 2007)
11. Somphone, O., Mory, B., Makram-Ebeid, S., Cohen, L.: Prior-Based Piecewise-Smooth Segmentation by Template Competitive Deformation Using Partitions of Unity. In: Forsyth, D., Torr, P., Zisserman, A. (eds.) ECCV 2008, Part III. LNCS, vol. 5304, pp. 628–641. Springer, Heidelberg (2008)
12. Huang, X., Metaxas, D.: Metamorphs: Deformable shape and appearance models. IEEE Trans. PAMI 30(8), 1444–1459 (2008)
13. Freedman, D., Zhang, T.: Interactive graph cut based segmentation with shape priors. In: CVPR, vol. 1, pp. 755–762 (June 2005)
14. Zhu, S.C., Yuille, A.: Region competition: Unifying snakes, region growing, and bayes/mdl for multiband image segmentation. PAMI 18(9), 884–900 (1996)
15. Yezzi, A., Soatto, S.: Deformotion: Deforming motion, shape average and the joint registration and approximation of structures in images. IJCV 53(2), 153–167 (2003)
16. Nocedal, J., Wright, S.J.: Numerical Optimization. Springer (August 1999)

Prior Knowledge, Random Walks and Human Skeletal Muscle Segmentation

P.-Y. Baudin[1−7], N. Azzabou[5−7], P.G. Carlier[5−7], and Nikos Paragios[2−4]

[1]SIEMENS Healthcare, Saint Denis, FR
[2]Center for Visual Computing, Ecole Centrale de Paris, FR
[3]Université Paris-Est, LIGM (UMR CNRS), Center for Visual Computing,
Ecole des Ponts ParisTech, FR
[4]Equipe Galen, INRIA Saclay, Ile-de-France, FR
[5]Institute of Myology, Paris, FR
[6]CEA, I[2]BM, MIRCen, IdM NMR Laboratory, Paris, FR
[7]UPMC University Paris 06, Paris, FR

Abstract. In this paper, we propose a novel approach for segmenting the skeletal muscles in MRI automatically. In order to deal with the absence of contrast between the different muscle classes, we proposed a principled mathematical formulation that integrates prior knowledge with a random walks graph-based formulation. Prior knowledge is represented using a statistical shape atlas that once coupled with the random walks segmentation leads to an efficient iterative linear optimization system. We reveal the potential of our approach on a challenging set of real clinical data.

1 Introduction

Segmentation of the skeletal muscles is of crucial interest when studding myopathies. Diseases understanding, patient monitoring, etc. rely on discriminating the muscles in anatomical images. However, delineating the muscle contours manually is an extremely long and tedious task, and thus often a bottleneck in clinical research. Simple automatic segmentation methods rely on finding discriminative visual properties between objects of interest, accurate contour detection or clinically interesting anatomical points. However, skeletal muscles show none of these features and as a result, automatic segmentation is a challenging problem. In spite of recent advances on segmentation methods, their application in clinical settings is difficult, and most of the times, manual segmentation/correction is still the only option.

Among the limited amount of work on this specific subject, in [1,2] a method based on deformable models was proposed to perform the segmentation of all the muscles in one limb. Deformable models are surface models which are fitted to the target image by minimizing a functional balancing a data term - pushing the model towards the target contours - and a regularization term - which imposes a smooth solution along the curve. Such models only reach a local optimum of the functional, which can be far from the desired solution, and depend heavily on

N. Ayache et al. (Eds.): MICCAI 2012, Part I, LNCS 7510, pp. 569–576, 2012.

their initial position. In [3], a more efficient shape representation was introduced where prior knowledge was encoded through diffusion wavelets to reduce the space of solutions and thus relax the smoothing constraints. The surface of one muscle was modeled through a hierarchical representation, and the set of allowed deformations at each scale was learned from an annotated training set. Modeling the surface of one muscle with landmark points is an efficient alternative, as proposed in [4] with a graph-based method. The shape variability was modeled through high-order pose-invariant priors and the data term relied on classification and detection of the landmark points. The graph-based framework allowed to perform an efficient non-local optimization, without initialization. However, such method requires to be able to learn consistent image features in order to detect the landmarks, which is difficult to insure in practice in the case of muscles. More generally, all surface models suffer from the absence of reliable contours in MRI images of skeletal muscles. Recently, in [5], a model-based method operating in the image domain with promising results was proposed. This approach consisted in modeling a segmentation though Principal Component Analysis in an Isometric Log-ratio space. Then, a gradient descent was performed with respect to the PCA coefficients to minimize an energy functional which allows label transition only along detected contours. In this method, contour detection is explicit, achieved in a pre-processing stage, and could be a weak link in the chain in cases of undetected or spurious contours.

Our approach builds upon the general Random Walker Segmentation algorithm proposed in [6]. The strength of this method relies on its robustness in the case of incomplete contours and its efficient optimization. While originally this method required manual interaction - an user had to annotate a few pixels of each desired object - the possibility of using prior knowledge based on intensity distribution was introduced in [7]. In this paper, we propose to build a prior model of the shape of the thigh muscles from a training data set, to be used in the RW framework. The prior term of our functional is derived from learning a Gaussian model of the RW unknown probability vector. We also propose to modulate the strength of the model constraints according to the strength of the contours found in the segmented image.

This paper is organized as follows: in section 2 we briefly recall the principle of the RW segmentation and detail the formulation of our model. Then, in section 3, we present segmentation results obtained on 3D MR volumes of the right thigh. Section 4 concludes the paper.

2   Random Walks Segmentation With Prior Knowledge

Notations Let us consider an image I with N pixels, and I_i the gray-level of pixel i. The segmentation is formulated as a labeling problem of an undirected weighted graph $\mathcal{G} = (\mathcal{V}, \mathcal{E})$, where $\mathcal{V}$ is the set of nodes and $\mathcal{E}$ is the set of edges. Given $\mathcal{S}$, a set of labels, we want to assign a label $s \in \mathcal{S}$ to each node $p \in \mathcal{V}$. In this framework, the node v_i is the i-th pixel, and to each label corresponds a muscle.

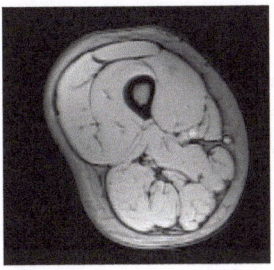 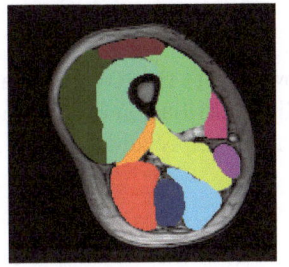 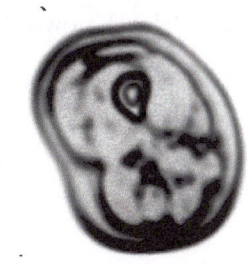

Fig. 1. (left) Cross-section of an MR volume of the thigh. (center) Manual segmentation of the muscles. (right) Confidence map.

2.1   Random Walks Formulation

Let us proceed with a review of the random walks algorithm for image segmentation. We refer the reader to [6] for an extensive description of this method.

The RW approach provides the probability x_i^s that the node $v_i \in \mathcal{V}$ is assigned to the label s. In its original formulation, one has to provide the algorithm with a few already labeled (marked) nodes, also called "seeds". Typically, the user will manually mark some pixels of each object to be segmented with a different label. Lets denote $\mathcal{V}_M$ the set of marked nodes and $\mathcal{V}_U$ the set of unmarked nodes, such that $\mathcal{V}_U \cap \mathcal{V}_M = \varnothing$ and $\mathcal{V}_U \cup \mathcal{V}_M = \mathcal{V}$. It was shown [6] that all *unknown* entries of $x^s = [x_1^s, x_2^s, \ldots, x_N^s]^T$ - i.e. the probabilities that each node $v_i \in \mathcal{V}_U$ is assigned to label s - can be obtained through the minimization of:

$$E_{\mathrm{RW}}^s (x^s) = x^{sT} L x^s \tag{1}$$

where the *known* entries of x^s (the seeds) are set as follow:

$$\forall v_i \in \mathcal{V}_M, \; x_i^s = \begin{cases} 1 & \text{if pixel } i \text{ is marked with label } s \\ 0 & \text{if pixel } i \text{ is marked with another label} \end{cases} \tag{2}$$

and where L is the combinatorial Laplacian matrix of the graph, defined as:

$$L_{i,j} = \begin{cases} \sum_k w_{kj} & \text{if } i = j \\ -w_{ij} & \text{if } i \neq j \\ 0 & \text{otherwise} \end{cases} \tag{3}$$

with

$$w_{ij} = \omega + \exp - \beta \left(I_i - I_j \right)^2 \tag{4}$$

where β is a scaling parameter to be set according to the contrast of the image, and ω is a regularization parameter which amounts to penalizing the gradient norm of x^s (no regularization if $\omega = 0$). After minimizing E_{RW}^s for each label s, the segmentation is obtained by retaining the label of maximum probability: $l_i = \arg\max_s x_i^s$.

2.2   Prior Knowledge

In [7], prior appearance knowledge to the RW formulation was introduced through an estimate of the probability distribution of the gray-level intensity for each label. A prior appearance term is simply added to the RW cost function, balanced by a parameter γ:

$$E_{\mathrm{RWP}}^s (x^s) = x^s\,^T L x^s + \gamma \left(x^{sT} D x^s - 2 x^{sT} d^s \right) \tag{5}$$

where $d^s (i)$ is the probability that the intensity at pixel i belongs to the intensity distribution for label s, and $D = \mathrm{diag}\left(\sum_s d^s\right)$ (we refer the reader to [7] for details). In the context of muscle segmentation, the intensity distributions of the labels (the muscles) are extremely similar resulting in an inefficient prior. Moreover, we could think of no other discernible and discriminative features (textures, remarkable points, etc.) to use within this framework. Thus, we decided to learn a pixel-based model of the shape based on previous segmentations of images in a training set $\mathcal{D}$.

Assume we know $\bar{x}_i^s$ and $\sigma_i^s\,^2$, respectively the mean and the variance of x_i^s. Our model simply penalizes the deviation of vector x_i^s from $\bar{x}_i^s$, weighted by the inverse of $\sigma_i^s\,^2$. In vector form, we obtain the following functional:

$$E_{\mathrm{model}}^s (x^s) = (x^s - \bar{x}^s)^T \Lambda_\sigma^s (x^s - \bar{x}^s) \tag{6}$$

where Λ_σ^s is a diagonal matrix such that $\Lambda_\sigma^s (i,i) = 1/\sigma_i^s\,^2$.

This is equivalent to modeling x_i^s as a random variable with Normal distribution $\mathcal{N}\left(\bar{x}_i^s, \sigma_i^s\,^2\right)$, and maximizing the log probability of x_i^s. Since x_i^s is a probability, such Gaussian modeling can only be a rough approximation. The mean and variance are estimated by computing, respectively, the empirical mean and the empirical variance over a training base of non-rigidly registered segmented images. When one owns only a small number of training examples, the empirical variance is known to be a particularly inefficient estimator. In [8], an improved locally-smooth estimator was proposed, for using as a similar shape prior in the level-set framework. The new estimate is computed, through a gradient descent, as the minimum of a functional which combines the log-likelihood of the training data and a spatial regularization term :

$$\tilde{\sigma}^s = \arg\min_\sigma \sum_{i=1}^N \left(\sum_{d \in \mathcal{D}} \log \sigma_i^2 + \frac{\left(x_{d,i}^s - \bar{x}_i^s\right)^2}{\sigma_i^2} \right) + \alpha \sum_{i,j=1}^N \delta_{i,j} \left(\sigma_i^2 - \sigma_j^2\right)^2 \tag{7}$$

where $x_{d,i}^s = 1$ if pixel i of training data d has label s ($x_{d,i}^s = 0$ otherwise), $\delta_{i,j} = 1$ if pixels i and j are neighbors ($\delta_{ij} = 0$ otherwise), and α is a weighting parameter setting the degree of smoothing.

We combine energy functionals (1) and (6) by introducing a balancing parameter λ^s:

$$E_{\mathrm{total1}}^s (x^s) = E_{\mathrm{RW}}^s (x) + \lambda^s E_{\mathrm{model}}^s (x) \tag{8}$$

It is possible to set a different value of λ^s for each label s, as some muscles may require a stronger influence from the prior model than others. The solution which minimizes (8) verifies:

$$(L + \lambda^s \Lambda^s_\sigma) x = \lambda^s \Lambda^s_\sigma \bar{x}^s \tag{9}$$

As noted in [7], when one adds such a prior term to the RW functional, it is no longer necessary to own pre-labeled nodes (seeds) in order to compute the segmentation. Indeed, the system of equations (9) is directly invertible, even when all entries of x are unknown. However, it is still possible - and useful - to use seeds to obtain more robust segmentations.

2.3   Confidence Map

As we saw previously , the functional $E^s_{\text{model}}(x^s)$ penalizes the deviation of x^s from the mean $\bar{x}^s$. Such prior is all the more useful as the local uncertainty of contour presence is large. One can impose such a condition by adjusting the influence of the model according to the strength of the contours in the test image: the *stronger* the contours, the *least* we should rely on the model. Assume we possess such a "confidence map" c, with values close to 0 on strong contours, and values close to 1 in homogeneous regions, we replace the term (6) by the following:

$$E^s_{\text{model}}(x^s) = (x^s - \bar{x}^s)^T \Lambda_c \Lambda^s_\sigma (x^s - \bar{x}^s)^T \tag{10}$$

where Λ_c is a diagonal matrix with c on the diagonal.

The local confidence of the image can be easily determined using a decreasing function inversely proportional to the image variance (see figure 1):

$$c_i = \exp -k_v \sigma_r^2(i) \tag{11}$$

where $\sigma_r^2(i)$ is the variance at pixel i computed on a patch with radius r, and k_v is a free parameter. The system to solve is now:

$$(L + \lambda^s \Lambda_c \Lambda^s_\sigma) x^s = \lambda^s \Lambda_c \Lambda^s_\sigma \bar{x}^s \tag{12}$$

3   Experimental Validation

Our data set comprises 14 3D volumes of the right thigh of healthy subjects, covering a wide range of morphologies, acquired with a 3T Siemens scanner and using 3pt Dixon sequence (TR=10ms, TE1=2.75 ms TE2=3.95 ms TE3=5.15 ms, rf flip angle =3°) of resolution: 1mm×1mm×5mm. We manually segmented each volume in order to evaluate the quality of the segmentation results. We focused our evaluation on clinically relevant muscles of the thigh (13 muscles). In order to compute the empirical mean $\bar{x}^s$ and the empirical variance $\sigma_i^{s\,2}$, we non-rigidly registered all the volumes and their segmentation map in the

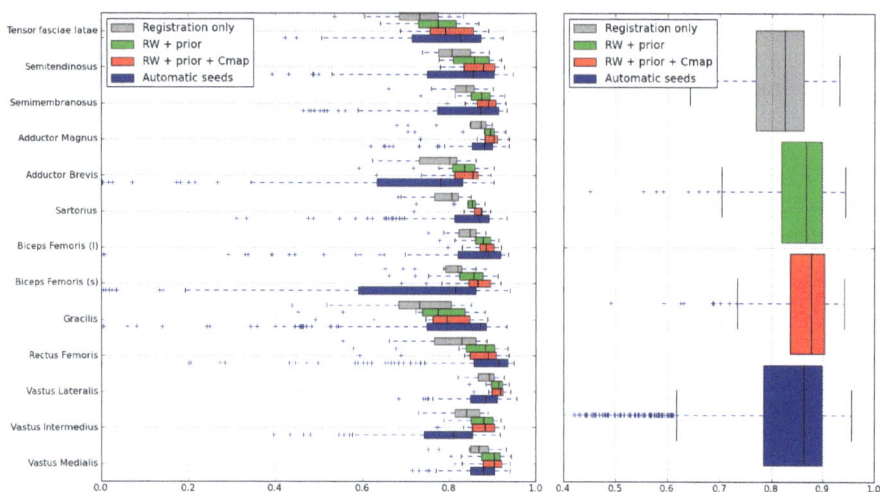

Fig. 2. Box-plot presentation of the Dice coefficients of our segmentation algorithm. (Right) Individual muscles; (Left) All muscles. Average dice values for: registration only: 0.81 ± 0.08; RW + shape prior: 0.84 ± 0.08; RW + shape prior + c. map: 0.86 ± 0.07; automatic seeds ([9]): 0.80 ± 0.19.

training set to the same target volume. The registration process is achieved using the method presented in [10] and the related registration software (Drop©, www.mrf-registration.net). We adopted a leave-one-out cross-validation protocol: each test volume is used as the target volume for the registration of the 13 other volumes. Then we computed the estimates of $\bar{x}^s$ and $\sigma_i^s{}^2$ on the 13 registered volumes, and perform the segmentation of the test volume. After the registration process, all volumes had the size: $191\times178\times63$. For solving the linear systems, we used iterative algorithms, such as Bi-conjugate Gradient. Computing the segmentation takes around 5 min on a 2.8 GHz Intel® processor with 4 GB of RAM. From a series of tests, we computed the best value for parameter $\lambda^s = 10^{-3}$, except for the Gracilis muscle which we had to constrain more: $\lambda^s = 10^{-1}$.

The quality of the segmentation is measured by computing Dice coefficients with the box-plot presentation [1] (See figure 2). The expression of the Dice coefficient is: $D = 2\,|T\cap R|\,/\,(|T| + |R|)$, where T and R are the pixel sets for the algorithm's output and the ground truth segmentation respectively. We also compared the different methods with p-values obtained using the non-parametric statistical test Wilcoxon rank-sum (cf. scipy.stats).

In figure 2, for comparision with a simple segmentation by atlas registration method, we computed the Dice coefficients of the segmentation which we obtain when retaining the label of maximum probability of the mean probability: $l_i =$

---

[1] Box-plot presentation: the boxes contain the middle 50% of the data and the median value, and the extremities of the lines indicate the min and max values, excluding the outliers (for more details, see the documentation of Matplotlib).

$\arg\max_s \bar{x}_i^s$. This method yielded inferior results as compared to our method without confidence map with a p-value of 2×10^{-10}. Adding the confidence map slightly improves the segmentation results as compared to not using it (p-value: 6.6×10^{-2}), yielding an average Dice coefficient value of 0.86 ± 0.07. We also compare our results with a previous method of ours [9]. This method consisted in automatically determining appropriate seed positions with respect to the different muscle classes. The output of this optimization process was then fed to the standard RW algorithm. We obtained inferior results to the method presented here (average Dice: 0.80 ± 0.19; p-value when compared to confidence map method: 7.0×10^{-4}).

In figure 3, we show cross-sections of segmentation results obtained with the RW method using the prior model and the confidence map. Segmentation errors tend to affect primarily small muscles (e.g. Gracilis) and muscles located on the extreme upper part of the volumes (e.g Tensor Fasciae Latae) which reveals the limitations of the mean model. These errors are due to the large registration errors on the same muscles. This shows that our model is too constraining, as it does not allow the segmentation to deviate enough from the mean. Due to the few number of training examples, we noted that the variance estimate had little influence on the results: replacing Λ_σ^s with the identity matrix gave us no significantly different results. This suggests that we should add more data to the training set in order to improve the statistical validity of our estimates.

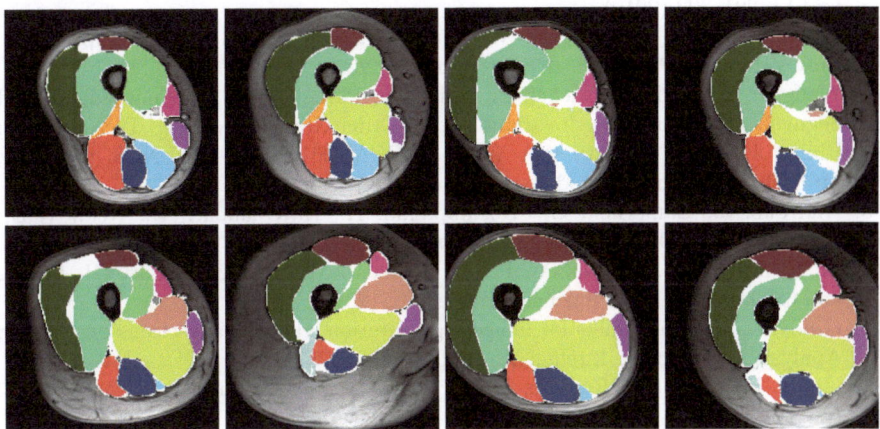

Fig. 3. Segmentation results obtained with the RW algorithm with shape prior and confidence map. Segmentation errors are shown in white.

4   Conclusion

The inherent difficulties of segmenting the skeletal muscles in MR images - namely: partial contours, no discernible texture differences, large variation inter-individuals and unremarkable shapes - render standard segmentation methods inoperative on this issue. One has to search for methods which perform robustly on inconsistent images cues (partial contours), and flexible models, allowing enough freedom to account for large inter-subject shape variations. We propose a prior model method, resting on the strengths of the Random Walks segmentation algorithm. Due to its robustness when faced with missing contours, the RW algorithm appears to be a good candidate for combination with a trained shape model. We believe to have achieved promising results which demonstrate the potential of our fully automatic approach.

Future work will consist in designing a model which allows more shape variability. We could obtain such model by building a low dimensional space through computing a PCA on the training base. Furthermore, the similarities between the RW algorithm and Markov Random Fields formulations let us envision applying the recent advances in MRF learning to the estimation of the Laplacian matrix.

References

1. Gilles, B., Pai, D.K.: Fast Musculoskeletal Registration Based on Shape Matching. In: Metaxas, D., Axel, L., Fichtinger, G., Székely, G. (eds.) MICCAI 2008, Part II. LNCS, vol. 5242, pp. 822–829. Springer, Heidelberg (2008)
2. Gilles, B., Magnenat-Thalmann, N.: Musculoskeletal MRI segmentation using multi-resolution simplex meshes with medial representations. Medical Image Analysis 14, 291–302 (2010)
3. Essafi, S., Langs, G., Paragios, N.: Hierarchical 3D diffusion wavelet shape priors. In: CVPR, pp. 1717–1724. IEEE (September 2009)
4. Wang, C., Teboul, O., Michel, F., Essafi, S., Paragios, N.: 3D Knowledge-Based Segmentation Using Pose-Invariant Higher-Order Graphs. In: Jiang, T., Navab, N., Pluim, J.P.W., Viergever, M.A. (eds.) MICCAI 2010, Part III. LNCS, vol. 6363, pp. 189–196. Springer, Heidelberg (2010)
5. Andrews, S., Hamarneh, G., Yazdanpanah, A., HajGhanbari, B., Reid, W.D.: Probabilistic Multi-shape Segmentation of Knee Extensor and Flexor Muscles. In: Fichtinger, G., Martel, A., Peters, T. (eds.) MICCAI 2011, Part III. LNCS, vol. 6893, pp. 651–658. Springer, Heidelberg (2011)
6. Grady, L.: Random walks for image segmentation. IEEE Transactions on Pattern Analysis and Machine Intelligence 28(11), 1768–1783 (2006)
7. Grady, L.: Multilabel Random Walker Image Segmentation Using Prior Models. In: CVPR, vol. 1, pp. 763–770 (2005)
8. Rousson, M., Paragios, N.: Prior knowledge, level set representations & visual grouping. International Journal of Computer Vision 76(3), 231–243 (2008)
9. Baudin, P.-Y., Azzabou, N., Carlier, P.G., Paragios, N.: Automatic Skeletal Muscle Segmentation Through Random Walks and Graph-Based Seed Placement. In: ISBI 2012 (in press, 2012)
10. Glocker, B., Komodakis, N., Tziritas, G., Navab, N., Paragios, N.: Dense image registration through MRFs and efficient linear programming. Medical Image Analysis 12, 731–741 (2008)

Similarity-Based Appearance-Prior
for Fitting a Subdivision Mesh
in Gene Expression Images

Yen H. Le[1], Uday Kurkure[1], Nikos Paragios[1,2],
Tao Ju[3], James P. Carson[4], and Ioannis A. Kakadiaris[1]

[1] Computational Biomedicine Lab, University of Houston, Houston, TX, USA
[2] Center for Visual Computing, Ecole Centrale de Paris, France
[3] Washington University in St. Louis, MO, USA
[4] Pacific Northwest National Laboratory, Richland, WA, USA

Abstract. Automated segmentation of multi-part anatomical objects in images is a challenging task. In this paper, we propose a similarity-based appearance-prior to fit a compartmental geometric atlas of the mouse brain in gene expression images. A subdivision mesh which is used to model the geometry is deformed using a Markov Random Field (MRF) framework. The proposed appearance-prior is computed as a function of the similarity between local patches at corresponding atlas locations from two images. In addition, we introduce a similarity-saliency score to select the mesh points that are relevant for the computation of the proposed prior. Our method significantly improves the accuracy of the atlas fitting, especially in the regions that are influenced by the selected similarity-salient points, and outperforms the previous subdivision mesh fitting methods for gene expression images.

Keywords: segmentation, gene expression image, subdivision mesh.

1 Introduction

Automated segmentation of the anatomical objects in images is a difficult task. It is even more challenging to segment multiple neighboring objects and/or multi-part objects. The use of appropriate and effective image appearance models plays a critical role in such segmentation tasks. Most of the existing approaches rely on the assumptions that the regions of interest are distinct (e.g., heart ventricles in MRI and contrast CT images) and have similar intensity patterns at particular locations (e.g., white and gray matter in the brain MRI images) across multiple images (images acquired from different subjects or the same subject at different time instances). However, these assumptions do not hold for gene expression images because of their complex appearance. The intensity at a pixel is related to the amount of precipitate in a cell, unlike in CT/MRI images, where it represents a particular tissue type. Therefore, the gene expression images provide incomplete anatomical information. Thus, the incorporation of appearance-prior in a segmentation method is non-trivial for gene expression images.

N. Ayache et al. (Eds.): MICCAI 2012, Part I, LNCS 7510, pp. 577–584, 2012.

Geometric model-to-image registration-based methods use soft shape constraints that are inherent to the model geometry which conforms with the object of interest. Various deformable model representations (e.g., simplex mesh [1], m-rep [2], subdivision mesh [3]) have been used to characterize the complex geometry of the structures. Of notable interest is the subdivision mesh-based representation that can compactly represent the complex, multi-part structures in a hierarchical manner using very few control points. A subdivision mesh-based geometric atlas has been used to segment the multi-part, mouse brain structures in the gene expression images [4–7]. Among those methods, an appearance-prior is employed weakly as a segmented brain boundary [4–7], anatomical landmarks [5, 6], or a texture of internal sub-region boundaries [5, 6]. Image-to-image registration-based approaches [8–11] use the deformation field to map the predefined segmentation labels from the reference image/atlas to the given image. However, these approaches require image warping at each iteration and can lead to nonphysical deformations to satisfy the energy constraints while recovering large deformations.

In this paper, we propose a novel approach for fitting the internal regions of a subdivision-based geometric atlas to anatomical structures. Our main contributions are: (i) we introduce a novel similarity-based appearance-prior for geometric atlas fitting in gene expression images, and (ii) we present a systematic method based on the modified similarity-saliency to identify the key vertices of the geometric atlas to be used to compute the appearance-prior during the deformation. Specifically, we modified the method proposed by Kurkure *et al.* [7] for model-to-image fitting of the subdivision atlas to include the proposed similarity-based appearance-prior. The main difference is that Kurkure *et al.* [7] did not include any appearance-prior as part of the framework, whereas our proposed prior enables fitting the geometric model to the internal regions of the brain (the main limitation of [7]). This is particularly important for this application where an accurate correspondence across gene expression images is needed to build a spatial database which can be queried for similarities in gene expression patterns to find potential interactive relationships between different genes in the same anatomical sub-region. Our proposed similarity-based appearance-prior is computed as a function of similarity of local patches at corresponding atlas locations between two images. Moreover, it can be used to fit other geometric models as a part of the energy/cost function (e.g., b-spline curve fitting on a vessel). Though we used mutual information as the similarity metric, it can be replaced with any suitable similarity measure depending on the properties of the images.

2   Background

Our segmentation method employs a Markov random field-based subdivision mesh fitting framework proposed by Kurkure *et al.* [7]. In that framework, the segmentation is performed by fitting a hybrid geometrical-anatomical atlas to the input image. The atlas is modeled by a subdivision mesh [4]. For any given input image, the fitting process deforms the subdivision mesh atlas based on the internal energy (of the mesh) and external energy (of the image), which includes energy build from our proposed similarity-based appearance-prior.

The subdivision mesh [4] is organized in a multi-resolution fashion, where the geometric mesh at the kth level is denoted by M^k. The mesh vertices at the coarsest level M^0 are referred to as control points whose locations completely determine the locations of the mesh points at higher resolution. The position of a mesh vertex i at the level k as $M^k(i)$ is computed as a linear combination of positions of the control points as, $M^k(i) = \sum_j \eta_j^k(i) M^0(j)$, where $\eta_j^k(i)$ denotes the influence of the control point $M^0(j)$ to the mesh vertex $M^k(i)$. The optimal fitting of the subdivision mesh is determined by estimating the optimal locations of the control points on the image.

The estimation of the optimal locations of the control points is formulated as a discrete label assignment problem, where the labels denote the discretized displacements of the control points. This label assignment problem is solved using MRF where an energy function is minimized. The energy function includes boundary-based (shape-based) energy, landmark-based energy, label regularization energy, and internal energy [7]. The label regularization and internal energy terms provide local geometric constraints, whereas the boundary-based (shape-based) and landmark-based energy terms provide global geometric constraints. Therefore, we categorize these energy terms as geometric priors, $E^G(f|I)$, where f denotes the labels of the displacements of the control points and I denotes the input image.

3   Similarity-Based Appearance-Prior

In this section, we provide details of our geometric atlas fitting approach. First, we introduce the proposed similarity-based appearance-prior. Then, we present the modified similarity-saliency measure and explain how it is used to select relevant appearance points. Finally, we describe the integration of the proposed appearance-prior in the MRF fitting framework [7].

3.1   Energy Function

Our appearance energy function is computed as the sum of similarities on selected pairs of *appearance points* from a reference image and the input image. Let R be the reference image, I be the input image, and S be the set of coordinates of appearance points, the appearance energy function E^A can be computed as: $E^A(I) = \sum_{s \in S} \psi(R(s), I(s))$, where $\psi(p, q)$ denotes the similarity metric between two image patches centered at point p and point q. In this paper, we use *normalized mutual information* (NMI) [12] as the similarity metric. The set of appearance points is determined by examining the pattern of the *similarity-saliency* on the set of training images.

Similarity-Saliency: Given two images I_1 and I_2, an image point u in I_1 is similarity-salient with respect to the image point v in I_2 if v exhibits higher similarity, than its neighbors, to u. The concept of this similarity-saliency is similar to the *mutual-saliency* used in [13] to perform *Gabor feature* selection and to weigh the similarity at each point to determine the corresponding points. However, we use the similarity-saliency to determine which mesh points are more reliable to use for the computation of the appearance-prior during mesh fitting. To compute the similarity-saliency, we define three types of regions in the neighborhood of the point v in the given image: (i) core neighborhood ($\mathcal{N}_C$), (ii) transitional neighborhood ($\mathcal{N}_T$, which is ignored in the computation because of smooth transition in degree of similarity), and (iii) peripheral neighborhood ($\mathcal{N}_P$) as illustrated in the left panel of Fig. 1. The similarity-saliency $\Upsilon(u,v)$ is then computed as: $\Upsilon(u,v) = \frac{\frac{1}{|\mathcal{N}_C(v)|}\sum_{m \in \mathcal{N}_C(v)} \psi(u,m)}{\frac{1}{|\mathcal{N}_P(v)|}\sum_{n \in \mathcal{N}_P(v)} \psi(u,n)}$.

Appearance Points Selection: In the gene expression images, all the genes typically do not express at the same level. Therefore, the gene expression images provide incomplete anatomical information. This issue leads to the weak similarity-saliency between some corresponding regions even when the two images have been properly aligned. In order to improve the robustness of the energy estimation, we select only a subset of all image points to compute the appearance energy function (the appearance points). The appearance points are determined from the pattern of similarity-saliency on a set of training images against the Nissl-stained image (NSI), which is also the template image used to fit test images. Since the NSI is generated using a universal gene probe to which all the cells in a tissue sample respond, it has maximum anatomical information and it exhibits the highest similarity to other gene expression images. Therefore, it is reasonable to introduce a MI-based similarity prior for mesh fitting in the gene expression images when using the NSI as the reference image. For each image in the training set, we manually align the subdivision mesh [4] to achieve point-to-

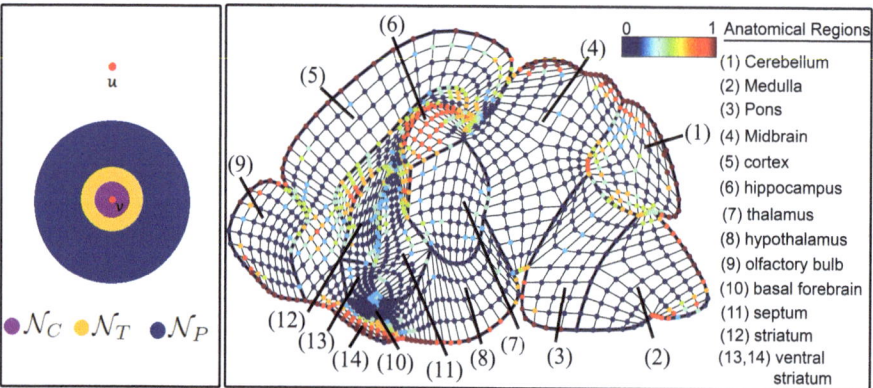

Fig. 1. Left: Illustration of mutual saliency definition for points v in image I_2 with respect to point u in image I_1. Right: A subdivision mesh, at subdivision 2, overlaid by average similarity-saliency scores of mesh vertices after scaling for visualization.

point correspondence across all training images. Then, we compute the average similarity-saliency score for each point u in the reference image (the NSI) by taking the average of the similarity-saliency between u and its corresponding points over all training images. For each point u, a high average similarity-saliency score expresses the high consistency of being a similarity salient point across most of the training images, and thus, it should be selected as an appearance point. The right panel of Fig. 1 depicts the color coded map of the average similarity-saliency score on the reference image. Note that most similarity-salient points are observed near the brain boundary, the hippocampus, the ventral striatum and the basal forebrain. Finally, we select similarity-salient points which have the average similarity-saliency score above a given threshold to be used as the appearance points.

3.2   Markov Random Field with an Appearance Energy Function

We integrate the proposed appearance energy function into the MRF-based subdivision mesh fitting framework proposed by [7]. In that framework, the fitting problem is modeled as a discrete labeling problem. From the subdivision mesh of the template image, a graph $\mathcal{G} = (\mathcal{V}, \mathcal{E})$ is created, where the set of N nodes $\mathcal{V}$ corresponds to the set of mesh control points M^0. A fitting solution of an input image to the template image is then represented as a configuration $f = \{f_1, f_2, ..., f_N\}$, where f_i is the discrete label of the displacements for node i. The configuration is then found by minimizing the total energy $E(f|I)$, which is the sum of the geometric energy $E^G(f|I)$ and the appearance energy $E^A(f|I)$ as follows: $E(f|I) = E^G(f|I) + E^A(f|I) = \sum_{c \in C} V_C^G(f|I) + \sum_{c \in C} V_C^A(f|I)$. The geometric energy $E^G(f|I)$ is the sum of clique potentials $V_C^G(f|I)$ over the set of all possible cliques C as described in [7]. The appearance energy $E^A(f|I)$ is derived from our appearance energy function presented in Section 3.1. Within the MRF framework, $E^A(f|I)$ is the sum of clique potentials $V_C^A(f|I)$, which is defined as the sum of pairwise potentials: $E^A(f|I) = \sum_{\{i,j\} \in \mathcal{E}} V_{ij}^A(f_i, f_j)$.

The set of graph edges $\mathcal{E}$ contains all the pairs of control points $\{i, j\}$ such that i and j influence the position of at least one common point in the image. For each pair $\{i, j\}$ with the corresponding label (f_i, f_j), its clique potential $V_{ij}^A(f_i, f_j)$ is computed as:

$$V_{ij}^A(f_i, f_j) = \sum_{M^k(m) \in \mathcal{S}} \hat{\eta}_{ij} \hat{\psi}\Big(R(M^k(m)), I(\hat{M}_{f_i,f_j}^k(m))\Big),$$

where $\hat{\psi}(p, q) = 2 - \psi(p, q)$ denotes the dissimilarity between two image patches centered at point p and point q. Here, we consider only image points that belong to both appearance points set and mesh vertices set at level k. By deforming the mesh template, the point $M^k(m)$ on the reference image is mapped to the point $\hat{M}_{f_i,f_j}^k(m)$ on the input image, which can be computed using the subdivision-basis coefficients as: $\hat{M}_{f_i,f_j}^k(m) = M^k(m) + \eta_i(m)d_{f_i} + \eta_j(m)d_{f_j}$, where d_{f_i} and d_{f_j} denote the discrete displacements with labels f_i and f_j respectively. The inverse weight coefficient, $\hat{\eta}_{ij}$ measures the influence of a mesh

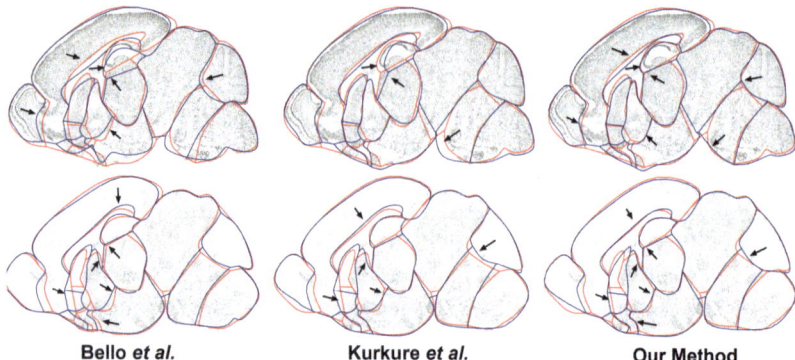

Bello *et al.*   **Kurkure *et al.***   **Our Method**

Fig. 2. The manually annotated boundaries (red) and the resulting boundaries (blue) of automatic segmentation on images of genes *Chrnb4* (top) and *Dscr3* (bottom). The arrows indicate the boundaries where our method achieved better alignment than the rest.

vertex m on the pairwise energy of control points i and j, and it is given by:
$\hat{\eta}_{ij}(m) = \dfrac{\eta_i(m) + \eta_j(m)}{\sum\limits_{a,b\in\mathcal{E}} (\eta_a(m) + \eta_b(m))}$. Note that, although the MRF graph is defined
by the mesh at the coarsest level (M^0), each configuration is evaluated based on the finer mesh at a higher subdivision level (M^k). This helps to reduce the size of the graph, enabling computation of the priors at a higher resolution. Also, the deformed meshes do not have non-smooth areas, thanks to the label regularization energy and the mesh internal energy.

4   Results

We evaluated our method on 100 gene expression images that depict sagittal sections of postnatal day 7 mouse brains at standard section 9 [6, 14]. Each image is 600×1000 pixels and is rigidly aligned to a reference Nissl-stained image. From the 100 test images, 40 images were included in the training set. The subdivision mesh has 93 control points. From 1,245 mesh points (at subidivision level $k = 2$), we manually selected 20 appearance points based on the similarity-saliency. Preference was given to the points on the internal boundaries. The radii for $\mathcal{N}_C$, $\mathcal{N}_T$ and $\mathcal{N}_P$ were set to 7, 3 and 5 pixels, respectively. The patch size to compute the mutual information was set to 41×41 pixels. Note that only a small number of points in the interior regions and in the regional boundaries have high scores (Fig. 1). This also demonstrates the lack of reliable anatomical information in the gene expression images. We did not include any points from the outer boundary as they are already taken into account in the boundary prior. We compare our method with the methods of Bello *et al.* [6] and Kurkure *et al.* [7], which also deform a subdivision mesh on the test images. The parameters of the competitive methods were selected as suggested by the original authors.

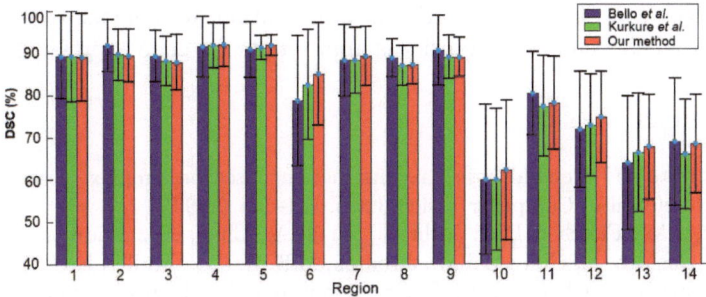

Fig. 3. A quantitative comparison of the mean and standard deviation of the DSC computed from the results of Bello *et al.* [6], Kurkure *et al.* [7], and our method

Figure 2 qualitatively indicates that our method results in better alignment of internal boundaries than [6] and [7]. The difference is mostly exhibited in regions 5-7, 10 and 14. For quantitative evaluation, we computed the region overlap ratio with respect to manual annotation using the Dice similarity coefficient (DSC). We plot the mean and standard deviation values of the DSC for all 14 regions in Fig. 3. At significance level of 0.05, our proposed appearance-prior improves the subdivision mesh fitting in seven regions: 5-7, 10 and 12-14 when compared to [7]. In regions that are highly influenced by the selected similarity-salient points (6, 10 and 14), the difference is remarkable since the mean DSC was improved by 3% using our method while the standard deviation was reduced. Our method improved the mesh alignment in the neighboring regions (5, 7, 11-13) as well because of the regularization. For the remaining regions, the results are comparable as they are not influenced by the selected similarity-salient points, hence the mesh in these regions is driven by the other priors. In comparison with Bello's [6] mesh fitting method, our method has higher mean DSC in regions 5-7 and 10-13. In the remaining regions, the mean DSCs from our method are comparable. However, our method has significantly lower standard deviation. This indicates that our method is more robust to the variations in the gene expression images.

5   Conclusions[1]

In this paper, we have proposed a similarity-based appearance-prior for fitting a geometric mesh model to a multi-part, structure of interest in the gene expression images. It has been incorporated into the Markov Random Field-based subdivision mesh fitting framework of [7]. We have also introduced a similarity-saliency score to select relevant mesh vertices appropriate to define the proposed

---

[1] This work was supported in part by NSF DBI0743691, NIH 1R21NS058553 and by the University of Houston (UH) Eckhard Pfeiffer Endowment Fund. All statements of fact, opinion, or conclusions contained herein are those of the authors and should not be construed as representing the official views or policies of NSF, NIH, or UH.

appearance-prior. Through experimental evaluation, we demonstrate that such a similarity-based appearance-prior is appropriate for gene expression images.

References

1. Delingette, H.: General object reconstruction based on simplex meshes. International Journal of Computer Vision 32(2), 111–146 (1999)
2. Pizer, S.M., Fletcher, P.T., Joshi, S., Thall, A., Chen, J.Z., Fridman, Y., Fritsch, D.S., Gash, A.G., Glotzer, J.M., Jiroutek, M.R., Lu, C., Muller, K.E., Tracton, G., Yushkevich, P., Chaney, E.L.: Deformable m-reps for 3D medical image segmentation. Int. J. Comput. Vision (IJCV) 55(2-3), 85–106 (2003)
3. Warren, J., Weimer, H.: Subdivision methods for geometric design: A constructive approach. Morgan Kaufmann (2001)
4. Ju, T., Warren, J., Eichele, G., Thaller, C., Chiu, W., Carson, J.: A geometric database for gene expression data. In: Proc. Eurographics Symposium on Geometry Processing, pp. 166–176 (July 2003)
5. Kakadiaris, I.A., Bello, M., Arunachalam, S., Kang, W., Ju, T., Warren, J., Carson, J., Chiu, W., Thaller, C., Eichele, G.: Landmark-Driven, Atlas-Based Segmentation of Mouse Brain Tissue Images Containing Gene Expression Data. In: Barillot, C., Haynor, D.R., Hellier, P. (eds.) MICCAI 2004, Part I. LNCS, vol. 3216, pp. 192–199. Springer, Heidelberg (2004)
6. Bello, M., Ju, T., Carson, J.P., Warren, J., Chiu, W., Kakadiaris, I.A.: Learning-based segmentation framework for tissue images containing gene expression data. IEEE Transactions on Medical Imaging 26, 728–744 (2007)
7. Kurkure, U., Le, Y., Paragios, N., Carson, J., Ju, T., Kakadiaris, I.: Markov random field-based fitting of a subdivision-based geometric atlas. In: Proc. IEEE (ICCV), Barcelona, Spain, November 6-13, pp. 2540–2547 (2011)
8. Ng, L., Pathak, S.D., Kuan, C., Lau, C., Dong, H., Sodt, A., Dang, C., Avants, B., Yushkevich, P., Gee, J.C., Haynor, D., Lein, E., Jones, A., Hawrylycz, M.: Neuroinformatics for genome-wide 3D gene expression mapping in the mouse Brain. IEEE/ACM Transactions on Computational Biology and Bioinformatics 4(3), 382–393 (2007)
9. Yi, Z., Soatto, S.: Correspondence transfer for the registration of multimodal images. In: Proc. IEEE ICCV, Rio de Janeiro, Brazil, October 14-21, pp. 1–8 (2007)
10. Sotiras, A., Ou, Y., Glocker, B., Davatzikos, C., Paragios, N.: Simultaneous Geometric - Iconic Registration. In: Jiang, T., Navab, N., Pluim, J.P.W., Viergever, M.A. (eds.) MICCAI 2010, Part II. LNCS, vol. 6362, pp. 676–683. Springer, Heidelberg (2010)
11. Kurkure, U., Le, Y.H., Paragios, N., Carson, J.P., Ju, T., Kakadiaris, I.A.: Landmark/image-based deformable registration of gene expression data. In: Proc. IEEE (CVPR), Colorado Springs, CO, June 21-23, pp. 1089–1096 (2011)
12. Maes, F., Collignon, A., Vandermeulen, D., Marchal, G., Suetens, P.: Multimodality image registration by maximization of mutual information. IEEE Transactions on Medical Imaging 16(2), 187–198 (1997)
13. Ou, Y., Davatzikos, C.: DRAMMS: Deformable Registration via Attribute Matching and Mutual-Saliency Weighting. In: Prince, J.L., Pham, D.L., Myers, K.J. (eds.) IPMI 2009. LNCS, vol. 5636, pp. 50–62. Springer, Heidelberg (2009)
14. Carson, J.P., Ju, T., Bello, M., Thaller, C., Warren, J., Kakadiaris, I.A., Chiu, W., Eichele, G.: Automated pipeline for atlas-based annotation of gene expression patterns: Application to postnatal day 7 mouse brain. Methods 50, 85–95 (2010)

Learning Context Cues
for Synapse Segmentation in EM Volumes

Carlos Becker*, Karim Ali, Graham Knott, and Pascal Fua

Computer Vision Lab, École Polytechnique Fédérale de Lausanne, Switzerland

Abstract. We present a new approach for the automated segmentation of excitatory synapses in image stacks acquired by electron microscopy. We rely on a large set of image features specifically designed to take spatial context into account and train a classifier that can effectively utilize cues such as the presence of a nearby post-synaptic region. As a result, our algorithm successfully distinguishes synapses from the numerous other organelles that appear within an EM volume, including those whose local textural properties are relatively similar. This enables us to achieve very high detection rates with very few false positives.

1 Introduction

New imaging technologies have been a key driver of recent advances in neuroscience. In particular, block face scanning electron microscopy (EM) can now deliver a $4nm$ nearly isotropic sampling and produce image stacks that reveal very fine structures. Stacks such as those of Fig. 1(a) can be used to analyze the size, shape and distribution of synapses, which in turn will lead to an understanding of the connection strength between neurons and, in time, brain circuits.

Currently, analysis is carried out by manually segmenting synapses using tools such as Fiji [1]. This is not only a tedious and time consuming process but also an error-prone one. Furthermore, the need for expert knowledge and the growing size of these datasets render manual segmentation intractable and not amenable to crowd-sourcing methods. There has been great interest in automating the process. However, current synapse segmentation methods either require first finding cell membranes [2] or operate on individual 2D slices [3], thus failing to leverage the 3D structure of the data. By contrast, the recent method of [4] operates entirely in 3D. However, it does not exploit the contextual clues that allow human experts to distinguish synapses from other structures, such as endoplasmic reticula, which exhibit similar textural properties, as depicted by Fig. 1(b).

In this work, we propose an approach designed to take contextual cues into account and emulate the human ability to distinguish synapses from regions that merely share a similar texture. Thus, we significantly outperform the method of [4]. Our algorithm relies on features which compute sums of various image properties over cubes placed in an extended 3D neighborhood surrounding the voxel to be classified, as shown in Fig. 1(c). It then uses AdaBoost [5] to select the most informative ones.

---

* This work was funded in part by the ERC MicroNano Grant.

N. Ayache et al. (Eds.): MICCAI 2012, Part I, LNCS 7510, pp. 585–592, 2012.

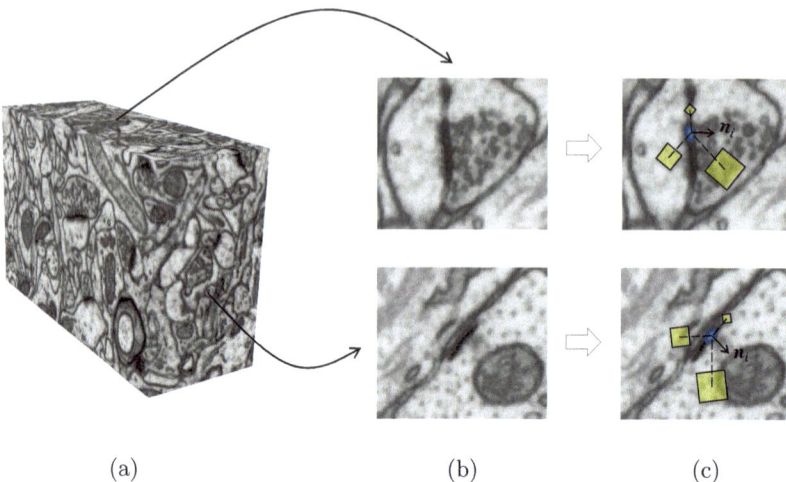

(a)   (b)   (c)

Fig. 1. Importance of context in synapse segmentation. The dark structures in the middle of both images look similar locally. However, only the ones in the top image constitute a synapse: the lack of vesicles in the bottom one is a indicative sign. The features we use are designed to capture this fact. To classify a voxel (blue), we consider sums over image cubes (shown as yellow squares) whose respective positions are defined relative to an estimated normal vector $\mathbf{n}_i$.

2   Related Work

Several fully automated approaches to reliable segmentation of organelles, such as mitochondria [6,7] or neuronal membranes [8,9], from 3D EM stacks have recently been proposed. However none of these methods exploit context in a meaningful way. Though features are extracted in a neighborhood around the voxel of interest, they are either pooled into global histograms [6,7] or computed at predetermined spatial locations [8,9]. The resulting classifier is therefore unable to hone in on arbitrary localized context cues. Along similar lines, a method for automated 3D segmentation of synapse in EM volumes using a Random Forest classifier has recently been proposed [4]. While this technique produces interesting results, it does not account for context as the features it uses simply measure various filter responses at the voxel of interest. The method is therefore unable to distinguish synaptic voxels from voxels exhibiting synapse-like textural properties. This is the limitation that our approach, specifically designed to utilize context cues, addresses. We run various filters over the EM stack but compute our features over arbitrarily sized cubes placed at arbitrary locations inside an extended neighborhood of the voxel to be classified. Next, we rely on a Boosting to select the relevant filter channels as well as the relevant cube locations and sizes. The resulting classifier is thus able to hone in on the presence of pre- and post-synaptic regions around the synapse. As a result, our method is shown to reduce the false alarm rate by a factor of 2 as compared to [4].

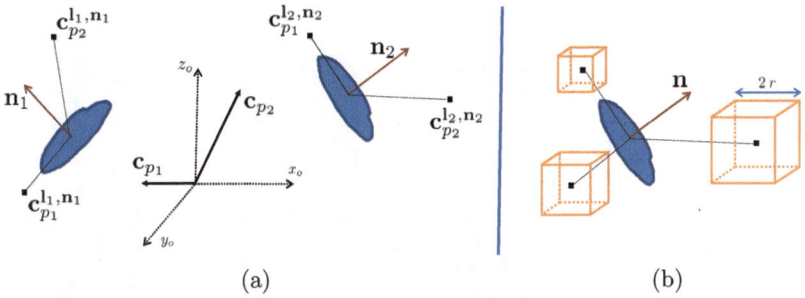

(a)   (b)

Fig. 2. (a) $\mathbf{c}_p^{l_i,\mathbf{n}_i}$ define consistent locations relative to differently located and oriented voxels. (b) Cubes over which sums are computed at consistent locations.

3   Method

As shown in Fig. 1(b), it can be difficult to distinguish synapses from other structures based solely on local texture evidence. Human experts confirm the presence of a synapse by looking nearby for post-synaptic densities and vesicles. This protocol cannot be emulated by measuring filter responses at the target voxel [4], pooling features into a global histogram [6,7] or relying on hand-determined locations for feature extraction [8,9]. To emulate the human ability to identify synapses, we design features, termed context cues, that can be extracted in any cube contained within a large volume centered on the voxel to be classified, as depicted by Fig. 2(b). They are computed in several channels using a number of Gaussian kernels, as shown in Fig. 3. As this yields a total of $40,000$ potential features, we rely on Boosting to select the most discriminative ones.

3.1   Contextual Features

Given that synapses have arbitrary 3D orientations, we ensure that our context cues are computed at consistent locations across differently oriented synapses. We rely on the pose-indexing framework of [10] to enforce this consistency.

Context Cue Location. Formally, let us consider voxel s_i, located at $\mathbf{l}_i$ and an associated unit vector $\mathbf{n}_i$. In practice, we take $\mathbf{n}_i$ to be the orientation of the eigenvector with largest eigenvalue of the Hessian operator, which can be expected to be normal to the synaptic cleft if there is one. Let

$$\mathbf{c}_p, \quad p = 1, \ldots, P \tag{1}$$

denote a set of P locations expressed in the common x_0, y_0, z_0 reference frame shown at the center of Fig. 2(a). These locations are translated and rotated to occur at consistent locations relative to a target voxel by defining,

$$\mathbf{c}_p^{l_i,\mathbf{n}_i} = \mathbf{l}_i + \mathbf{R}(\mathbf{n}_i)\mathbf{c}_p \tag{2}$$

where $\mathbf{R}(\mathbf{n}_i)$ is a rotation matrix such that $\mathbf{R}(\mathbf{n}_i)(0,0,1)^{\mathrm{T}} = \mathbf{n}_i$.

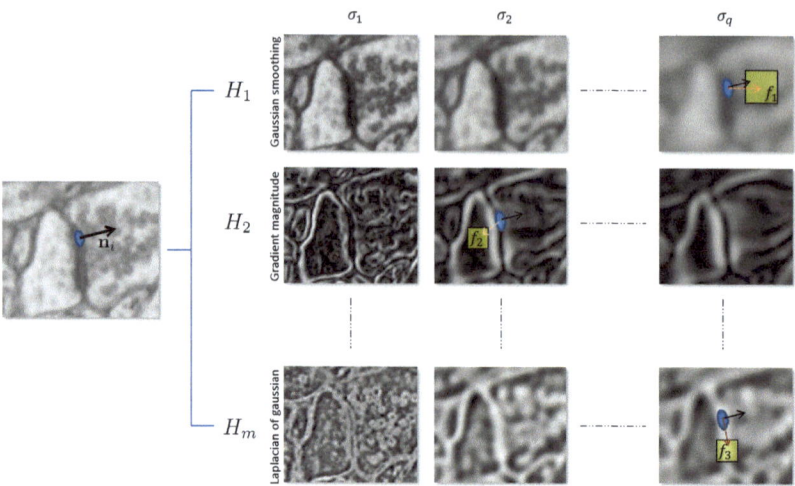

Fig. 3. Context cues. They are computed within the yellow rectangles whose coordinates are expressed with respect to the location of the voxel to be classified and the local orientation vector **n**. Each H_i line depicts a specific channel designed to capture different statistical characteristics.

Context Cue Features. Given the $\mathbf{c}_p^{l_i, \mathbf{n}_i}$ locations of Eq. 2, our goal now is to compute image statistics inside cubic neighborhoods $\mathcal{N}_r(\mathbf{c}_p^{l_i, \mathbf{n}_i})$ of edge length $2r$ centered around these locations, such as those depicted in Fig. 2(b).

To this end, we precompute gradient magnitudes, Laplacians of Gaussian and eigenvalues of structure tensors and Hessians everywhere in the EM volume. Each of the resulting cubes of data, in addition to the original one, is treated as a data channel m, $1 \leq m \leq 5$, and is smoothed using isotropic Gaussian kernels of increasing variance σ_n as in [4]. We denote the gray levels in the resulting data volumes as

$$H_{m, \sigma_n}(x, \mathbf{z}) \,, \tag{3}$$

where x is the original EM volume and $\mathbf{z}$ represents the 3D location. We take context cue features to be

$$f_{\mathbf{c}_p, m, \sigma_n, r}(x, l_i, \mathbf{n}_i) = \sum_{\mathbf{z} \in \mathcal{N}_r(\mathbf{c}_p^{l_i, \mathbf{n}_i})} H_{m, \sigma_n}(x, \mathbf{z}) \,. \tag{4}$$

In other words, we sum the smoothed channel output over the cubic boxes centered at all $\mathbf{c}_p$ for all possible values of m, σ_n, and r. This yields a set of $K = 40000$ features, which we will denote for simplicity

$$f_k(x, l_i, \mathbf{n}_i), \ k = 1, \ldots, K \,, \tag{5}$$

and which we use for classification purposes as discussed below.

3.2   Segmentation and Implementation Details

We create decision stumps by thresholding on the value of the f_k features of Eq. 5. These stumps are combined by a standard AdaBoost procedure [5] into a strong learner of the form

$$\varphi\left(x, \mathbf{l}_i, \mathbf{n}_i\right) = \sum_{t=1}^{T} \omega_t \mathbf{1}_{\{f_t(x, \mathbf{l}_i, \mathbf{n}_i) > \rho_t\}} . \tag{6}$$

Learning this classifier requires annotated training data. Since our contextual features are computed both for a given location and orientation, our training data must include both. As discussed above, we use the Hessian to compute the orientation for every voxel.

A potential difficulty arises from the fact that polarity also matters since pre- and post- synaptic regions look very different. We follow the pose-indexing methodology to exploit this structure. At training time, when dealing with synaptic voxels, we direct the orientation vector towards the pre-synaptic region in our positive examples and add the corresponding location with the flipped orientation vector to our list of negative examples. At run-time, we use the Hessian to compute $\mathbf{n}_i$, evaluate $\varphi(.)$ for both possible polarities, and retain the maximum response.

In practice, to speed-up the computation, we do not work on individual voxels of the EM volume. Instead, we group them into supervoxels that are regularly spaced small regions with relatively uniform gray level [11][1]. We then run our classification scheme on their centers.

4   Experiments

We now demonstrate our approach and compare its performance to that of [4] on two different volumes from the adult rat brain, one from the somatosensory cortex, and the other from striatum. Their respective sizes are $1500 \times 1125 \times 750$ and $1423 \times 872 \times 318$. The training set consists of 7 fully-labeled synapses in each volume plus negative samples labeled from non-synaptic voxels. For evaluation purposes, we labeled as synaptic or not each voxel in a somatosensory cortex subvolume of size $655 \times 429 \times 250$, which contains 24 synapses. It took approximately 40 minutes for each one, which highlights the need for automation. This voxel-wise ground truth allows for a robust quantitative evaluation and differs significantly from the protocol of [4], where synapses were annotated by an expert using a small sphere, making voxel-wise evaluation impossible.

Fig. 4 depicts the results of our quantitative evaluation on the ground-truth volume of the somatosensory cortex. We plot ROC curves, which show the True Positive Rate (TPR) as a function of the False Positive Rate (FPR). There are two parameters that we vary to obtain different sets of features f_k. The first is $r_{\max}$, the maximum possible size of the cubes over which sums are computed.

---

[1] Supervoxels source code available at `http://ivrg.epfl.ch/research/superpixels`

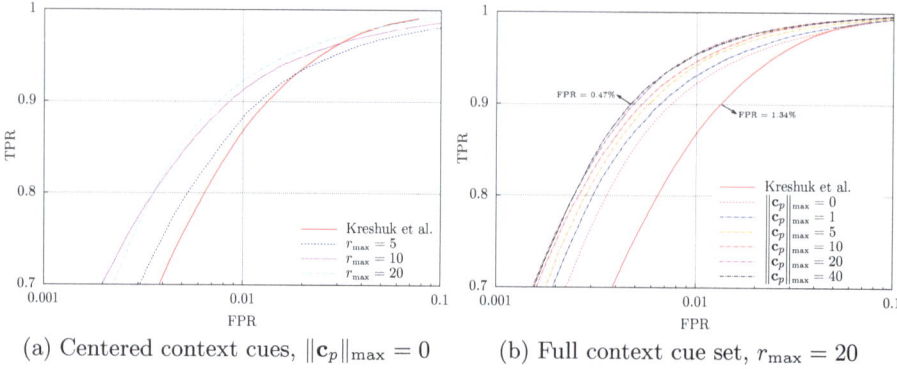

(a) Centered context cues, $\|\mathbf{c}_p\|_{\max} = 0$ (b) Full context cue set, $r_{\max} = 20$

Fig. 4. Voxel-wise classification ROC curves for different radii of the sphere within which the contextual features are computed

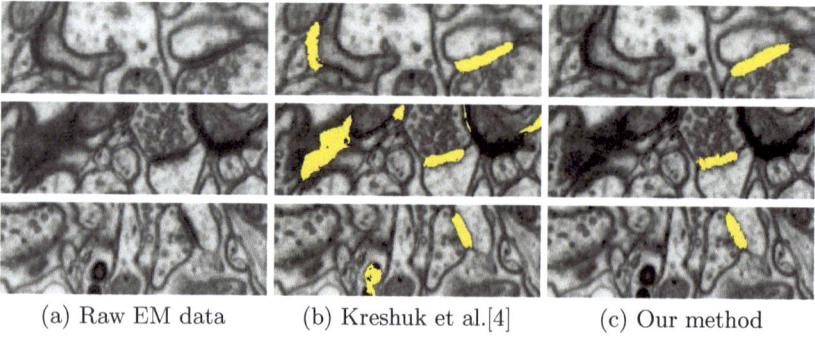

  (a) Raw EM data   (b) Kreshuk et al.[4]   (c) Our method

Fig. 5. Somatosensory cortex dataset results. Voxels labeled as synaptic by the method of [4] and ours overlaid in yellow. Threshold set to 90% TPR. Note the non-synaptic voxels found by [4] and correctly ignored by our method.

The second, $\|\mathbf{c}_p\|_{\max}$, is the radius of the sphere surrounding each voxel in which we extract our context features. Note that with $\|\mathbf{c}_p\|_{\max} = 0$ and $r_{\max} = 0$, our feature set essentially reduces to that of [4] where responses are measured at the target voxel, without exploiting context.

In Fig. 4(a), we set $\|\mathbf{c}_p\|_{\max} = 0$ and vary $r_{\max}$, meaning that the feature set only consists of cubes centered on the target voxel. As $r_{\max}$ grows, more context is taken into account and performance improves. At 90% TPR our method outperforms [4] in all cases. In Fig. 4(b), we set $r_{\max} = 20$ and vary $\|\mathbf{c}_p\|_{\max}$. In other words, we use our full feature set consisting of both centered and un-centered cubes. For $\|\mathbf{c}_p\|_{\max} = 40$, our approach yields a FPR almost three times smaller than the one of [4] at 90% TPR. Qualitatively, this difference in performance can be seen in Fig. 5 where the algorithm of [4] erroneously fires on non-synaptic tissue due to textural similarities.

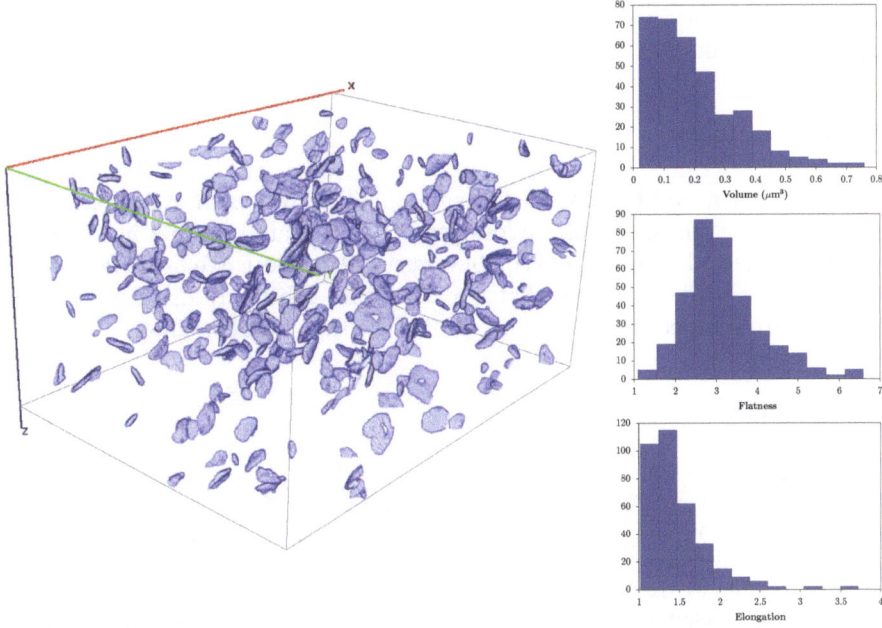

Fig. 6. 3D reconstruction of the detected synaptic voxels in the somatosensory cortex dataset. From our automated segmentation, various shape statistics can be computed for the purpose of analysis, such as the histograms on the right.

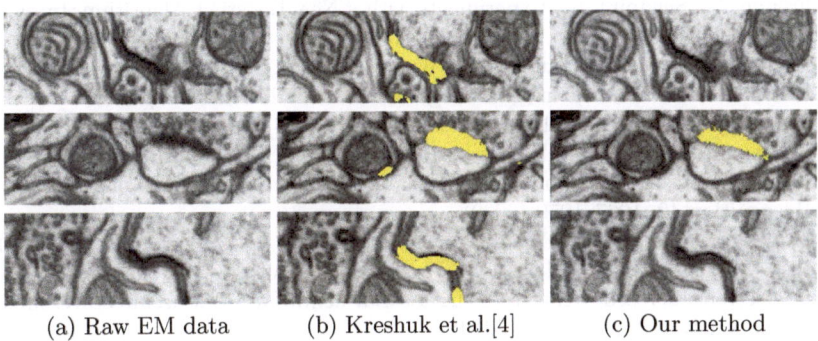

(a) Raw EM data   (b) Kreshuk et al.[4]   (c) Our method

Fig. 7. Striatum dataset results. Voxels labeled as synaptic by the method of [4] and ours overlaid in yellow. Threshold set to 90% TPR.

Performing this computation on the whole somatosensory volume and thresholding at 90% TPR yields the result depicted by Fig. 6, where connected regions of less than 2000 voxels were removed and a gaussian filter of $\sigma = 1$ was applied for visualization, as in [4]. The number of detected synapses is 358, which implies a density of 0.9 synapses per μm^3 and is in agreement with the expected density for the somatosensory cortex region (layer II) [12]. Finally, Fig. 7 depicts similar qualitative results for the striatum dataset.

5   Conclusion

We presented a novel approach to synapse segmentation. It relies on a large set of image features, specifically designed to take spatial context into account, which are selected, weighed and combined using AdaBoost. We used two different EM datasets to demonstrate that our algorithm effectively distinguishes true synapses from other organelles that exhibit the same local texture.

References

1. Schmid, B., Schindelin, J., Cardona, A., Longair, M., Heisenberg, M.: A high-level 3D visualization API for Java and ImageJ. BMC Bioinformatics 11, 274 (2010)
2. Mishchenko, Y., Hu, T., Spacek, J., Mendenhall, J., Harris, K.M., Chklovskii, D.B.: Ultrastructural analysis of hippocampal neuropil from the connectomics perspective. Neuron 67, 1009–1020 (2010)
3. Herold, J., Schubert, W., Nattkemper, T.W.: Automated detection and quantification of fluorescently labeled synapses in murine brain tissue sections for high throughput applications. Journal of Biotechnology 149, 299–309 (2010)
4. Kreshuk, A., Straehle, C., Sommer, C., Koethe, U., Knott, G., Hamprecht, F.: Automated segmentation of synapses in 3D EM data. In: 2011 IEEE International Symposium on Biomedical Imaging: From Nano to Macro, pp. 220–223 (2011)
5. Freund, Y., Schapire, R.: Experiments with a New Boosting Algorithm. In: ICML, pp. 148–156 (1996)
6. Lucchi, A., Smith, K., Achanta, R., Knott, G., Fua, P.: Supervoxel-based segmentation of mitochondria in EM image stacks with learned shape features. IEEE Transactions on Medical Imaging 31, 474–486 (2012)
7. Narasimha, R., Ouyang, H., Gray, A., McLaughlin, S.W., Subramaniam, S.: Automatic joint classification and segmentation of whole cell 3D images. Pattern Recognition 42, 1067–1079 (2009)
8. Jurrus, E., Paiva, A.R., Watanabe, S., Anderson, J.R., Jones, B.W., Whitaker, R.T., Jorgensen, E.M., Marc, R.E., Tasdizen, T.: Detection of neuron membranes in electron microscopy images using a serial neural network architecture. Medical Image Analysis 14, 770–783 (2010)
9. Venkataraju, K., Paiva, A., Jurrus, E., Tasdizen, T.: Automatic markup of neural cell membranes using boosted decision stumps. In: IEEE International Symposium on Biomedical Imaging: From Nano to Macro, pp. 1039–1042 (2009)
10. Fleuret, F., Geman, D.: Stationary Features and Cat Detection. JMLR 9, 2549–2578 (2008)
11. Achanta, R., Shaji, A., Smith, K., Lucchi, A., Fua, P., Suesstrunk, S.: SLIC Superpixels. Technical Report 149300, EPFL (2010)
12. DeFelipe, J., Marco, P., Busturia, I., Merchán-Pérez, A.: Estimation of the number of synapses in the cerebral cortex: Methodological considerations. Cerebral Cortex 9, 722–732 (1999)

Estimation of the Prior Distribution of Ground Truth in the STAPLE Algorithm: An Empirical Bayesian Approach

Alireza Akhondi-Asl and Simon K. Warfield

Computational Radiology Laboratory, Department of Radiology, Children's Hospital,
300 Longwood Avenue, Boston, MA, 02115, USA

Abstract. We present a new fusion algorithm for the segmentation and parcellation of magnetic resonance (MR) images of the brain. Our algorithm is a parametric empirical Bayesian extension of the STAPLE algorithm which uses the observations to accurately estimate the prior distribution of the hidden ground truth using an expectation maximization (EM) algorithm. We use IBSR dataset for the evaluation of our fusion algorithm. We segment 128 principle gray and white matter structures of the brain using our novel method and eight other state-of-the-art algorithms in the literature. Our prior distribution estimation strategy improves the accuracy of the fusion algorithm. It was shown that our new fusion algorithm has superior performance compared to the other state-of-the-art fusion methods in the literature.

1 Introduction

Fusion algorithms have been widely used in variety of medical image segmentation problems, in particular, in brain segmentation techniques. The key purpose of such algorithms is to match multiple templates to the target image and fuse their corresponding segmentations to have an estimate of the hidden ground truth. The simplest way to fuse the templates, known as majority voting, is to count the number of votes for each label and assign the label with the highest number of votes to the voxel. The key assumption in this method is that the votes are equally weighted, however, it is known that the templates or in the general case, raters, have different accuracies. Therefore, considering their performance variations may lead to a more accurate estimation of the hidden ground truth.

To this end, two categories of fusion methods have been introduced in the literature, that is, intensity based weighted voting methods and STAPLE algorithm with its extensions and variations. In the former approach, intensity similarity of the target image and templates are used to estimate the performance of the raters, where intensity similarities are considered as the weights of the decision of each template at each voxel. Moreover, mean square error and normalized cross correlation based methods are mainly used as the similarity metric in this type of approach. However, these algorithms can be very sensitive to the intensity

N. Ayache et al. (Eds.): MICCAI 2012, Part I, LNCS 7510, pp. 593–600, 2012.

normalization and cannot compensate some of the intrinsic weaknesses of the majority voting approach. [1–6].

In the latter method, the performance of the raters and the hidden ground truth are estimated iteratively using an Expectation-Maximization (EM) algorithm [7]. The method was first introduced for the estimation of the performance of the raters. Since then, it is being used in many applications as the fusion algorithm for the estimation of the hidden ground truth. There are many extensions of the algorithm, including SIMPLE, COLLATE, and STAPLER [8–10]. COLLATE algorithm is based on the STAPLE which considers the consensus level at each voxel for the estimation of the hidden ground truth. A similar concept was discussed by Rohlfing et al. and a simple solution was introduced, which is known as the STAPLE with assigned consensus region [11]. The idea discussed in [11] is to restrict the STAPLE algorithm to perform on the voxels where there is a disagreement between raters, otherwise, assign the corresponding label for the other voxels [11]. In this way, large consensus regions do not have any effect on the estimation of the performance parameters. STAPLER, another extension of the STAPLE, is designed to deal with the missing and also repeated segmentations. The algorithm uses training data to improve the estimation of the ground truth and performance parameters.

In the standard Bayesian analysis the prior distribution is assumed to be known and the observations do not re-scales the prior distribution. Therefore, in all of the STAPLE based algorithms, the prior on the ground truth needs to be set in the same manner. However, in practice this is usually discarded and the observations are used to estimate the prior distribution. While it is mentioned in the original STAPLE paper that the prior can be set using a probabilistic atlas, usually the decisions by the raters (observations) are used to estimate a global prior for each label.

In this paper we introduce a novel framework to estimate the prior using a parametric empirical Bayesian procedure. In our approach we estimate both performance parameters and hidden ground truth by updating the prior distribution of the ground truth using an EM algorithm. We show that this approach improves the accuracy of the fusion algorithm in the estimation of the hidden ground truth as well as the performance parameters.

2   Methods

Similar to any other fusion problem, we are interested in the estimation of $\mathbf{T}$, the hidden ground truth of the target image $\mathbf{I}$. It is assumed that T_i, the true label at voxel $i \in \{1, \ldots, i, \ldots, N\}$, is one of the labels $s \in \{1, \ldots, S\}$. In addition, we assume that J independent segmentation of the target image I are available where their performances are unknown. STAPLE is known to be one of the fusion methods that estimates the performance of the segmentations (raters) and utilize them in the estimation of the ground truth [7]. In the STAPLE algorithm, we are interested in the maximization of $f(\mathbf{D}, \mathbf{T} | \boldsymbol{\theta}, \boldsymbol{\rho})$, the probability density function of the complete data. In this formulation, $\boldsymbol{\theta} = \{\boldsymbol{\theta}_1, \ldots, \boldsymbol{\theta}_j, \ldots, \boldsymbol{\theta}_J\}$ indicates performance parameters where $\boldsymbol{\theta}_j$ is a matrix of size $S \times S$ and $\theta_{js's} = f(D_{ij} = s'|T_i = s)$. In addition, $\mathbf{D}$ is the decision matrix of size $N \times J$ where D_{ij} is the decision of rater j at voxel i. Also, $\boldsymbol{\rho}$ is the prior matrix of size $S \times N$ where $\rho_{si} = f(T_i = s)$ is the prior probability of the label s at voxel i.

In this formulation, both $\mathbf{T}$ and $\boldsymbol{\theta}$ are unknown. Thus, to estimate the unknown parameters the EM algorithm is used. In [7] authors assume that the prior $\rho = \hat{\rho}$ is known. They have suggested different approaches to estimate the prior and they have used the global or spatially fixed prior. However, in our new approach and using the empirical Bayesian approach, we assume that $\boldsymbol{\rho}$ is another set of unknown parameters which controls the shape of the prior distribution of the hidden ground truth. To solve the problem, we use the EM algorithm to iteratively estimate the ground truth, the performance parameters, and the prior distribution of the hidden ground truth. Using voxel-wise independence assumption and given $\boldsymbol{\theta}^t$ and $\boldsymbol{\rho}^t$, the estimation of the performance parameters and the distribution of the prior at the step t, the function Q is maximized iteratively:

$$Q(\boldsymbol{\theta}, \boldsymbol{\rho}|\boldsymbol{\theta}^t, \boldsymbol{\rho}^t) = E\left[\log f(\mathbf{D}, \mathbf{T}|\boldsymbol{\theta}^t, \boldsymbol{\rho}^t)\right]$$
$$= \sum_i \sum_{T_i} \log f(\mathbf{D}_i, T_i|\boldsymbol{\theta}, \boldsymbol{\rho}_i) f(T_i|\mathbf{D}_i, \boldsymbol{\theta}^t, \boldsymbol{\rho}_i^t) \tag{1}$$

The weight variable, W_{si}^t is computed using the following equation:

$$W_{si}^t = f(T_i = s|\mathbf{D}_i, \boldsymbol{\theta}^t, \boldsymbol{\rho}_i^t)$$

$$= \frac{\left[\prod_j f(D_{ij}|T_i = s, \boldsymbol{\theta}_j^t)\right] f(T_i = s|\boldsymbol{\rho}_i^t)}{\sum_{s'} \left\{\left[\prod_j f(D_{ij}|T_i = s', \boldsymbol{\theta}_j^t)\right] f(T_i = s'|\boldsymbol{\rho}_i^t)\right\}}$$

$$= \frac{\left[\prod_j \theta_{jD_{ij}s}^t\right] \rho_{si}^t}{\sum_{s'} \left\{\left[\prod_j \theta_{jD_{ij}s'}^t\right] \rho_{s'i}^t\right\}} \tag{2}$$

There are two sets of parameters that should be optimized. To this end, Eq. 1 is expanded as:

$$Q(\boldsymbol{\theta}, \boldsymbol{\rho}|\boldsymbol{\theta}^t, \boldsymbol{\rho}^t) = \sum_i \sum_{T_i} W_{si}^t \log f(\mathbf{D}_i, T_i|\boldsymbol{\theta}, \boldsymbol{\rho}_i) =$$

$$\sum_i \sum_s W_{si}^t \log \left[f(\mathbf{D}_i|T_i = s, \boldsymbol{\theta}) f(T_i = s|\boldsymbol{\rho}_i)\right] =$$

$$\sum_i \sum_s W_{si}^t \log(\prod_j \theta_{jD_{ij}s}) + \sum_i \sum_s W_{si}^t \log(\rho_{si}) \tag{3}$$

The first part of Eq. 3 is related to the performance parameters and is optimized using the constraint $\sum_{s'} \theta_{js's} = 1$. Thus, maximization of 3 with respect to the performance parameters lead to:

$$\theta_{js's}^{t+1} = \frac{\sum_{D_{ij}=s'} W_{si}}{\sum_i W_{si}} \tag{4}$$

For the prior distribution parameters, we have the constraint that $\sum_s \rho_{si} = 1$. Thus, using the Lagrange multiplier the following function is optimized with respect to the ρ_{si}:

$$Q'(\boldsymbol{\rho}_i, \lambda) = \sum_s W_{si}^t log(\rho_{si}) + \lambda \sum_s \rho_{si} \tag{5}$$

It can be seen that:

$$\frac{\partial Q'(\boldsymbol{\rho}_i, \lambda)}{\partial \rho_{si}} = \frac{W_{si}^t}{\rho_{si}} + \lambda = 0 \tag{6}$$

Using the constraint, it can be seen that $\lambda = -\sum_s W_{si} = -1$ which leads to the following estimation of the prior for the step $t+1$:

$$\rho_{si}^{t+1} = W_{si}^t \tag{7}$$

This means that the best estimation of the prior at each step is the estimated ground truth, given the performance and prior parameters at the previous step.

2.1 Relation to the Classic STAPLE

To see the relation to the classic STAPLE algorithm, we build a Maximum A Posteriori (MAP) formulation for the problem of estimation of the prior distribution. To this end, we consider a Beta distribution for each ρ_{si} with parameters α_{si} and β_{si} and reformulate Q' as follows:

$$Q'_{MAP}(\boldsymbol{\rho}_i, \lambda) = Q'(\boldsymbol{\rho}_i, \lambda) + \gamma \log \left(\prod_s \rho_{si}^{(\alpha_{si}-1)} (1 - \rho_{si})^{(\beta_{si}-1)} \right) \tag{8}$$

It is known that the Beta function takes its maximum at $\frac{\alpha_{si}-1}{\alpha_{si}+\beta_{si}-2}$. If $\hat{\rho}_{si}$ is the prior probability of T_i at voxel i for the label s in the classic STAPLE algorithm, we set the parameters of the Beta function to take its maximum at this point. In the other words,

$$\frac{\alpha_{si} - 1}{\beta_{si} - 1} = \frac{\hat{\rho}_{si}}{1 - \hat{\rho}_{si}} \tag{9}$$

Taking the derivative with respect to the ρ_{si} leads to:

$$\frac{\partial Q'_{MAP}(\boldsymbol{\rho}_i, \lambda)}{\partial \rho_{si}} = \frac{W_{si}^t}{\rho_{si}} + \lambda + \frac{\gamma(\alpha_{si} - 1)}{\rho_{si}} - \frac{\gamma(\beta_{si} - 1)}{1 - \rho_{si}} = 0 \tag{10}$$

Solving the equation for λ, leads to the following equation:

$$\rho_{si} = \frac{W_{si}^t + \gamma(\alpha_{si} + \beta_{si} - 2) + \gamma \frac{\beta_{si}-1}{\rho_{si}-1}}{1 + \sum_{n'} \gamma(\alpha_{n'i} + \beta_{n'i} - 2) + \sum_{n'} \gamma \frac{\beta_{n'i}-1}{\rho_{n'i}-1}} \tag{11}$$

Using the relation between α_{si} and β_{si} it is easy to see that:

$$\rho_{si} = \frac{W_{si}^t + \gamma \frac{(\beta_{si}-1)(\rho_{si}-\hat{\rho}_{si})}{(1-\hat{\rho}_{si})(\rho_{si}-1)}}{1 + \sum_{n'} \gamma \frac{(\beta_{n'i}-1)(\rho_{n'i}-\hat{\rho}_{n'i})}{(1-\hat{\rho}_{n'i})(\rho_{n'i}-1)}} \tag{12}$$

In the extreme situation, if $\gamma \to \infty$ and $\beta_{si} = K$, where K is a constant, it can be seen that $\rho_{si} = \hat{\rho}_{si}$ is the solution of the Eq. 12 which is similar to the classic STAPLE algorithm. In the other words, classic STAPLE is the MAP solution of our new algorithm when the prior weight is very large.

3   Results

We have evaluated our method and some of the state-of-the-art fusion algorithms for the automatic segmentation of Internet Brain Segmentation Repository (IBSR) MRI datasets. The database includes 18 T1-weighted volumetric images with slightly different voxel sizes and their corresponding manual segmentation and parcellation. The MR brain data sets and their manual segmentations were provided by the Center for Morphometric Analysis at Massachusetts General Hospital and are available at http://www.cma.mgh.harvard.edu/ibsr/. The volumetric images have been positionally normalized into the Talairach orientation (rotation only). In addition, bias field has been corrected for these data. There are two sets of manual segmentations for each one of the subjects: manual segmentation of 34 principle gray and white matter structures of the brain and parcellation results of 96 structures in Cerebral Cortex. Thus, for each subject combining these two manual segmentation sets leads to $34 - 2 + 96 = 128$ manually segmented structures.

We have used the leave-one-out strategy for the evaluation. In the other words, for each dataset, we have used the other 17 datasets (templates) for the segmentation of the 128 structures. To this end and in the first step, we registered all of the templates to the each one of the images (target images). Based on our experiments and within non-rigid-registration algorithms in the literature, SyN was chosen for the alignment of the templates to the target images [12]. For the next step, the output transformations of the non-rigid-registrations were applied to the corresponding label maps. The output of this step is fed in to the fusion algorithms. Finally, our novel method and some of the state-of-the-art fusion algorithms have been used for the segmentation of each one of the 128 structures. Methods that have been used for the comparison are: STAPLE with and without assigned consensus region, SIMPLE, STAPLER, COLLATE, methods of Sabuncu et al. and Artaechevarria et al [5–10].

For the STAPLE with and without assigned consensus region, we have used the implementations in http://crl.med.harvard.edu/software/STAPLE/. For the methods of SIMPLE, COLLATE, and STAPLER we have used implementations in http://www.nitrc.org/projects/masi-fusion/ with default settings. We have implemented methods of Sabuncu et al. and Artaechevarria et al. These two methods are sensitive to the intensity differences between the target image and

Table 1. Comparison of Dice coefficients for the proposed methods. Average segmentations of 128 brain structures for the IBSR datasets. M_1: our parametric empirical Bayesian approach, M_2: STAPLE with assigned consensus region [7], M_3: COLLATE [9], M_4: method proposed by Artaechevarria et al. [6], M_5: method proposed by Sabuncu et al. [5], M_6: Majority voting, M_7: SIMPLE [8], M_8: STAPLER [10], M_9: STAPLE without assigned consensus region [7].

	M1	M2	M3	M4	M5	M6	M7	M8	M9
1	**0.752**	0.743	0.731	0.711	0.704	0.697	0.690	0.685	0.638
2	0.697	0.697	0.678	0.687	0.685	0.678	0.674	0.622	0.580
3	**0.715**	0.707	0.697	0.685	0.688	0.679	0.666	0.662	0.622
4	**0.687**	0.679	0.675	0.652	0.656	0.644	0.651	0.642	0.605
5	**0.738**	0.732	0.719	0.709	0.707	0.702	0.695	0.669	0.623
6	**0.647**	0.645	0.638	0.606	0.600	0.598	0.590	0.609	0.576
7	0.726	**0.727**	0.708	0.695	0.694	0.686	0.669	0.670	0.632
8	0.691	0.691	0.680	0.673	0.663	0.654	0.651	0.641	0.603
9	**0.716**	0.713	0.701	0.698	0.699	0.688	0.683	0.644	0.600
10	**0.700**	0.693	0.688	0.686	0.676	0.668	0.655	0.640	0.600
11	0.696	**0.698**	0.678	0.661	0.661	0.652	0.642	0.654	0.616
12	**0.670**	0.669	0.657	0.644	0.638	0.627	0.621	0.640	0.606
13	**0.700**	0.699	0.698	0.674	0.676	0.663	0.664	0.640	0.601
14	**0.745**	0.739	0.727	0.716	0.717	0.707	0.702	0.664	0.615
15	**0.735**	0.732	0.734	0.703	0.709	0.693	0.687	0.665	0.618
16	**0.729**	0.721	0.713	0.701	0.698	0.687	0.689	0.661	0.618
17	**0.716**	0.714	0.716	0.682	0.684	0.668	0.675	0.657	0.614
18	0.724	0.724	0.712	0.683	0.678	0.675	0.672	0.666	0.625
Mean	**0.710**	0.707	0.697	0.681	0.680	0.670	0.665	0.652	0.611
STD	0.027	0.026	0.026	0.027	0.029	0.028	0.028	0.019	0.016
MAX	**0.752**	0.743	0.734	0.716	0.717	0.707	0.702	0.685	0.638
MIN	**0.647**	0.645	0.638	0.606	0.600	0.598	0.590	0.609	0.576
p-value		0.002	1e-06	1e-10	1e-9	1e-12	1e-12	1e-11	1e-13

atlases. To have a fair comparison we normalized intensities of each atlas using the histogram matching approach. In addition, we could not use some of the algorithms for the multi-category whole brain segmentation. Some of the algorithms perform well for the binary cases and implementations of some others were not applicable for the multi-category whole brain segmentation with 128 structures. To this end, we have used the fusion algorithm for each structure independently and compared the fusion results. Table 1 shows the comparison of nine methods using the average Dice coefficient of 128 strictures. It can be seen that our method outperforms the other fusion algorithms ($p < 0.002$). We also carried out a power analysis using a two-tailed paired t-test, for detecting an effect of the size we identified $(0.71 - 0.707)/0.0036 = 0.833)$ for a sample with $N = 18$, at the significance level of $\alpha = 5\%$. We found the power $(\beta) = 91\%$. Figure 1 shows the comparison of segmentation of a sample structure (pars triangularis (F3t)) using our method and the STAPLE with assigned consensus region in a coronal image of a representative IBSR dataset. It can be seen that using parametric empirical Bayesian framework to estimate the distribution of prior on the ground truth has substantial impact on the outcome of the fusion algorithm.

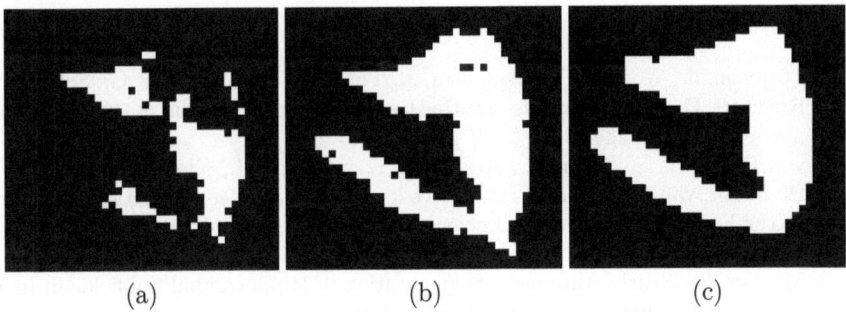

(a)   (b)   (c)

Fig. 1. Illustration of IBSR Multi-Atlas Segmentation Results. Comparison of segmentation of pars triangularis (F3t) generated by (a) STAPLE with assigned consensus region as the closest algorithm to our method [7]. (b) our method: parametric empirical Bayesian approach. (c) expert manual segmentation in a coronal image of a representative IBSR dataset. It can be seen that our method is superior to the classic STAPLE algorithm.

4 Conclusions

The prior has an important role in determining the local optimum to which the Expectation-Maximization algorithm converges. It has become conventional in usage of STAPLE to estimate the distribution of prior on the ground truth from the input data assuming all inputs are equally reliable. Obviously, when they are not all equally reliable, this can lead to poor performance. We have presented a new Expectation-Maximization algorithm to simultaneously estimate the ground truth and atlas performance from a set of segmentations by updating the prior distribution of the hidden ground truth using an empirical Bayesian approach. The introduced approach is effective when there is little information available from which to set the prior probability of the true labels. In our introduced method, the prior is updated iteratively which makes it less sensitive to the initialization of the prior distribution as compared to the classic STAPLE, where the prior distribution is fixed. 128 brain structures from IBSR dataset has been used for the evaluation of our algorithm and eight other state-of-the-art fusion methods in the literature. Our new algorithm is robust and has superior performance as compared to the other methods. Also, it was shown that the classic STAPLE algorithm is the MAP solution of our method when the weight of the prior is very large. It is possible to use the same idea in the STAPLE based algorithms such as COLLATE and local MAP STAPLE [13].

Acknowledgments. This investigation was supported in part by NIH grants R01 EB008015, R01 LM010033, R01 EB013248, and P30 HD018655 and by a research grant from the Boston Children's Hospital Translational Research Program.

References

1. Lötjonen, J., Wolz, R., Koikkalainen, J., Thurfjell, L., Waldemar, G., Soininen, H., Rueckert, D.: Fast and robust multi-atlas segmentation of brain magnetic resonance images. NeuroImage 49(3), 2352–2365 (2010)
2. van Rikxoort, E., Isgum, I., Arzhaeva, Y., Staring, M., Klein, S., Viergever, M., Pluim, J., van Ginneken, B.: Adaptive local multi-atlas segmentation: Application to the heart and the caudate nucleus. Medical Image Analysis 14(1), 39–49 (2010)
3. Yushkevich, P., Wang, H., Pluta, J., Das, S., Craige, C., Avants, B., Weiner, M., Mueller, S.: Nearly Automatic Segmentation of Hippocampal Subfields in In Vivo Focal T2-Weighted MRI. NeuroImage (2010)
4. Wang, H., Suh, J., Das, S., Pluta, J., Altinay, M., Yushkevich, P.: Regression-based label fusion for multi-atlas segmentation
5. Sabuncu, M., Yeo, B., Van Leemput, K., Fischl, B., Golland, P.: A generative model for image segmentation based on label fusion. IEEE Transactions on Medical Imaging 29(10), 1714–1729 (2010)
6. Artaechevarria, X., Munoz-Barrutia, A.: Combination strategies in multi-atlas image segmentation: Application to brain MR data. IEEE Transactions on Medical Imaging 28(8), 1266–1277 (2009)
7. Warfield, S., Zou, K., Wells, W.: Simultaneous truth and performance level estimation (STAPLE): an algorithm for the validation of image segmentation. IEEE Transactions on Medical Imaging 23(7), 903–921 (2004)
8. Langerak, T., van der Heide, U., Kotte, A., Viergever, M., van Vulpen, M., Pluim, J.: Label fusion in atlas-based segmentation using a selective and iterative method for performance level estimation (simple). IEEE Transactions on Medical Imaging 29(12), 2000–2008 (2010)
9. Asman, A., Landman, B.: Robust statistical label fusion through consensus level, labeler accuracy and truth estimation (collate). IEEE Transactions on Medical Imaging (99), 1779–1794 (2011)
10. Landman, B., Asman, A., Scoggins, A., Bogovic, J., Xing, F., Prince, J.: Robust statistical fusion of image labels. IEEE Transactions on Medical Imaging 31(2), 512–522 (2012)
11. Rohlfing, T., Russakoff, D.B., Maurer, C.R.: Expectation Maximization Strategies for Multi-atlas Multi-label Segmentation. In: Taylor, C.J., Noble, J.A. (eds.) IPMI 2003. LNCS, vol. 2732, pp. 210–221. Springer, Heidelberg (2003)
12. Avants, B., Yushkevich, P., Pluta, J., Minkoff, D., Korczykowski, M., Detre, J., Gee, J.: The optimal template effect in hippocampus studies of diseased populations. NeuroImage 49(3), 2457–2466 (2010)
13. Commowick, O., Akhondi-Asl, A., Warfield, S.K.: Estimating a reference standard segmentation with spatially varying performance parameters: Local map staple. IEEE Transactions on Medical Imaging (2012)

Unified Geometry and Topology Correction for Cortical Surface Reconstruction with Intrinsic Reeb Analysis*

Yonggang Shi[1], Rongjie Lai[2], and Arthur W. Toga[1]

[1] Lab. of Neuro Imaging, Dept. of Neurology, UCLA School of Medicine,
Los Angeles, CA, USA
[2] Dept. of Mathematics, University of Southern California, Los Angeles, CA, USA

Abstract. A key challenge in the accurate reconstruction of cortical surfaces is the automated correction of geometric and topological outliers in tissue boundaries. Conventionally these two types of errors are handled separately. In this work, we propose a unified analysis framework for the joint correction of geometric and topological outliers in cortical reconstruction. Using the Reeb graph of intrinsically defined Laplace-Beltrami eigenfunctions, our method automatically locates spurious branches, handles and holes on tissue boundaries and corrects them with image information and geometric regularity derived from paired boundary evolutions. In our experiments, we demonstrate on 200 MR images from two datasets that our method is much faster and achieves better performance than FreeSurfer in population studies.

1 Introduction

Automated reconstruction of cortical models from MR images is fundamental for large scale brain mapping. While many approaches were proposed [1–5], critical challenges remain in improving the accuracy, robustness, and speed of reconstruction algorithms. In this paper, we propose a unified analysis framework based on intrinsic Reeb graphs that jointly tackles the correction of geometric and topological outliers in cortical reconstruction. We demonstrate that our method can efficiently reconstruct accurate cortical surfaces and achieve better performance in large scale population studies [6, 7].

Cortical reconstruction is a complicated system development problem that requires the successful integration of various preprocessing steps including non-uniformity correction, skull stripping, non-linear registration, the labeling of subcortical structures, and tissue classification that classifies image intensities into white matter(WM), gray matter(GM) and cerebrospinal fluid(CSF). At the core of this system, though, is the generation of smooth and topologically correct mesh models of tissue boundaries. In previous works, smoothness is typically achieved with the incorporation of a global regularization in surface evolution. Topology correction, on the other hand, was handled separately with graph-based

---

* This work was supported by NIH grants K01EB013633 and 5P41RR013642.

N. Ayache et al. (Eds.): MICCAI 2012, Part I, LNCS 7510, pp. 601–608, 2012.

methods [3,4] or spherical mapping [2]. Using Laplace-Beltrami (LB) eigenfunctions [8–10] and their Reeb graphs, accurate surface reconstruction methods
were proposed recently [10, 12], but topological outliers were not considered.
Based on the theory of Morse functions and Reeb graphs, we propose in this
work a unified analysis framework that corrects both geometric and topological
outliers in cortical reconstruction. Using the Reeb graph of LB eigenfunctions,
our method can localize geometric and topological outliers and make decisions
about correction strategies with information from tissue classification and geometric regularity. After the correction, accurate surface models are generated
with adaptive interpolation.

The rest of the paper is organized as follows. In section 2, we develop a novel
approach for the construction of Reeb graph of LB eigenfunctions on triangular
meshes. The unified approach for topology and geometry correction is developed
in section 3. Experimental results are presented in section 4, where we demonstrate that our method can achieve better performance than FreeSurfer [2]. Finally conclusions are made in section 5.

2   Intrinsic Reeb Graph

For intrinsic shape analysis, the Reeb graphs of LB eigenfunctions have been
successfully applied for shape modeling and geometric outlier detection on genus-
zero surfaces [12]. In this section, we develop a novel and general method for
Reeb graph construction on surfaces of arbitrary topology. Instead of scanning
through all level sets on surfaces [11], our method is efficient and uses only level
sets in the neighborhood of saddle points.

Let $\mathcal{M} = (\mathcal{V}, \mathcal{T})$ be a triangular mesh, where $\mathcal{V}$ and $\mathcal{T}$ are the set of vertices
and triangles. Given a function $f : \mathcal{M} \to \mathbb{R}$, the Reeb graph $R(f)$ can be viewed
as a graph of critical points on meshes [11]. In this work, we choose the function
f as the intrinsically defined eigenfunctions of the Laplace-Beltrami operator on
surfaces, which have the advantage of being invariant to scale and pose variations.
Let $\mathcal{C} = \{c_1, c_2, \cdots, c_N\}$ be the set of critical points of f sorted according to the
critical values. For a vertex $\mathcal{V}_i \in \mathcal{V}$, its one-ring neighborhood is $N(\mathcal{V}_i)$. Let
$N_-(\mathcal{V}_i) = \{\mathcal{V}_j \in N(\mathcal{V}_i)|f(\mathcal{V}_j) < f(\mathcal{V}_i)\}$ and $N_+(\mathcal{V}_i) = \{\mathcal{V}_j \in N(\mathcal{V}_i)|f(\mathcal{V}_j) > f(\mathcal{V}_i)\}$ denote its lower and upper neighbors.

To construct the Reeb graph, we scan through all critical points sequentially.
If c_i is a minimum, we add a new, but incomplete, edge to $R(f)$ and set c_i as
the start node. If c_i is a saddle point, we define the isovalue of branches entering
and leaving this point so the critical points do not interfere with each other:

$$f_{iso}^-(c_i) = (f(c_i) + \max(f(c_{i-1}), \max_{\mathcal{V}_j \in N_-(c_i)} f(\mathcal{V}_j)))/2$$

$$f_{iso}^+(c_i) = (f(c_i) + \min(f(c_{i+1}), \min_{\mathcal{V}_j \in N_+(c_i)} f(\mathcal{V}_j)))/2. \quad (1)$$

For each component in $N_+(c_i)$, we trace a level contour $P = (\mathbf{p}_1, \mathbf{p}_2, \cdots, \mathbf{p}_N)$
at the value $f_{iso}^+(c_i)$ and add all intersecting points in P to the mesh $\mathcal{M}$ by
adding edges and splitting existing triangles in $\mathcal{M}$. A new, but incomplete, edge

in the Reeb graph is created with c_i as the start node. For all vertices in P, we label them as the starting vertices of this new edge. For each component in $N_-(c_i)$, we trace a level contour at the value $f_{iso}^-(c_i)$ on the mesh $\mathcal{M}$. Similarly, we augment the mesh with this set of new vertices and grow backward till we reach the starting vertices of an incomplete edge, which completes an edge in Reeb graph with c_i as the end node. If c_i is a maximum, we grow backward with it as the end node to complete an edge.

As an example, we show in Fig. 1 the construction of the Reeb graph on a double torus. In Fig.1(a), we can see one level contour crosses the lower neighborhood, and two level contours cross the upper neighborhood of the saddle point. The edges of the Reeb graph are shown in Fig.1 (b), where the graph structure is evident from the neighboring relation of the edges and we can see the loops in the graph captures the topology of the surface as suggested in Morse theory.

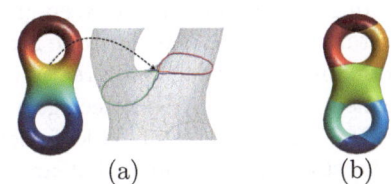

Fig. 1. Reeb graph of a LB eigenfunction on a double torus. (a) Level contours in the neighborhood of a saddle point. (b) Edges of the Reeb graph plotted in different colors.

3   Unified Geometry and Topology Correction

For the analysis of a 3D MR image, we denote the lattice of voxels as $A = \{(i,j,k) \in \mathbb{Z}^3 | 0 \leq i < I - 1, 0 \leq j < J - 1, 0 \leq k < K - 1\}$ and the 3D image as a function $A \to \mathbb{R}$. Following the preprocessing steps in [12], we can define an evolution speed F on the lattice A based on tissue classification of MR images, and use the fast evolution algorithm in [10,13] to find the boundary between two tissue types. Let A_o and A_b denote the object and background region, respectively, and their boundary be represented as a triangular mesh $\mathcal{M} = \{\mathcal{V}, \mathcal{T}\}$, where $\mathcal{V}$ and $\mathcal{T}$ are the set of vertices and triangles. For each face $\mathcal{T}_i \in \mathcal{T}$, we denote it as the intersection of two boundary voxels: the interior voxel $\mathbf{x}_o(\mathcal{T}_i) \in A_o$ and the exterior voxel $\mathbf{x}_b(\mathcal{T}_i) \in A_b$.

3.1   Paired Boundary Estimate

For topological analysis, we compute a pair of boundary estimates with the evolution speed F. The first boundary satisfies the genus-zero condition and is denoted as $\mathcal{M}^G = (\mathcal{T}^G, \mathcal{V}^G)$. The second boundary can have arbitrary topology and is denoted as $\mathcal{M}^F = (\mathcal{T}^F, \mathcal{V}^F)$, which is obtained by turning off the topology-preserving condition in the evolution algorithm. Let f be the first non-constant LB eigenfunction on $\mathcal{M}^F$, and $R(f) = (C, E)$ the Reeb graph of f on $\mathcal{M}^F$ that we build with the algorithm in section 2. Here C denotes the set of critical points, and E the set of edges. Each edge is represented as $E_i = (SC_i, EC_i, EV_i, LC_i^s, LC_i^e)$, where $SC_i, EC_i \in C$ are the start and end node, $EV_i \subset \mathcal{V}$ is the set of vertices belonging to this edge in $R(f)$, LC_i^s and LC_i^e are the level contours on the boundary of the edge. Using intrinsic Reeb analysis, we can locate outliers and correct them by modifying the evolution speed F to generate an accurate boundary estimation.

3.2   Geometric Outlier Correction

The degree of a node in the Reeb graph is the number of edges that it is either the start or the end node. A node is called a leaf node if its degree is one, and an internal node if its degree is greater than one. The edge connected to a leaf node is called a leaf edge. We detect geometric outliers from the set of leaf edges in the Reeb graph. Let E_i be a leaf edge, LC_i^s and LC_i^e denote the level contours at the start and end node that are used to generate the edge. Let $\mathcal{T}(EV_i)$ be the set of triangles connected to the vertices in EV_i, we consider this leaf edge as an outlier if it satisfies two conditions: (1) $length(LC_i^s) + length(LC_i^e) < \alpha$; (2) $Area(\mathcal{T}(EV_i))/(length(LC_i^s) + length(LC_i^e)) > \beta$, where the parameters α and β are thresholds selected to identify sharp and small outliers. To further localize geometric outliers, we project the mesh onto a subset of four LB eigenfunctions and calculate the area distortion of triangles to measure geometric regularity [10]. For each triangle in $\mathcal{T}^F$, its area distortion ratio is defined as $ADF(T_i^F) = Area(T_i^F)/Area(\hat{T}_i^F)$, where $\hat{T}_i^F$ is the corresponding triangle of T_i^F on the projected mesh $\hat{\mathcal{M}}^F$. For an outlier leaf edge, we define the set of outlier triangles as $Outlier(EV_i) = \{T_i^F \in \mathcal{T}(EV_i)|ADF(T_i^F) > \gamma\}$, where γ is a threshold for geometric regularity.

To remove the outlier, we modify the evolution speed F as follows. For each outlier edge E_i, we use the level contour LC_i^s and LC_i^e to compute:

$$H(E_i) = \int_{LC_i^s} < \mathbf{p}(s) - \bar{\mathbf{q}}_i^s, \mathbf{n}(\mathbf{p}(s)) > ds + \int_{LC_i^e} < \mathbf{p}(s) - \bar{\mathbf{q}}_i^e, \mathbf{n}(\mathbf{p}(s)) > ds \quad (2)$$

where $\mathbf{n}$ is the outward normal on the surface $\mathcal{M}^F$, $\mathbf{q}_i^s$ and $\mathbf{q}_i^e$ are the mean coordinates of points on LC_i^s and LC_i^e. If $H(E_i) > 0$, E_i is an outward leaf, we set $F(\mathbf{x}_o(T_i^F)) = -1$ for all $T_i^F \in Outlier(EV_i)$. If $H(E_i) < 0$, E_i is an inward leaf and we set $F(\mathbf{x}_b(T_i^F)) = 1$ for all $T_i^F \in Outlier(EV_i)$.

3.3   Topological Outlier Correction

For topological analysis, we first remove duplicated edges in $R(f)$. For any two edges with the same start and end node, we remove the one with smaller size from $R(f)$ and add it to the set of topological outlier which we denote as TO. After that, we represent the Reeb graph $R(f)$ as a matrix W. For any edge $E_i = (C_{i1}, C_{i2}, EV_i, LC_i^s, LC_i^e)$, we set $W(i1, i2) = \#(EV_i)$, which is the number of vertices on this edge.

For a node C_i in the directed graph W, we use breadth-first-search (BFS) to test if a handle or hole exists. Let $j_1, \cdots , j_K$ denote the set of neighboring nodes of C_i in $R(f)$. For each outgoing edge, we set $W(i, j_k) = 0$ and perform BFS with C_i as the starting node. This generates a spanning tree PAR_k of nodes reachable from C_i after the removal of the edge from C_i to C_{j_k}. By repeating this process for all outgoing edges at C_i, we generate a set of BFS trees $PAR_1, ..., PAR_K$. The intersection node $C_{J_{min}}$ of these trees is defined as the node with the smallest index j but in all spanning trees. Starting from $C_{J_{min}}$, we trace backward to the current node C_i on each tree PAR_k and pick the one with the smallest size as a topological outlier and add all edges on this path to TO.

For an edge $E_i \in TO$, we compute the feature $H(E_i)$ using (2). The edge E_i is classified as a handle if $H(E_i) > 0$ and a hole otherwise. For each handle or hole, we find a cutting path with minimal length. If E_i is a handle, we uniformly sample a set of level contours of the eigenfunction f between the start contour LC_i^s and end contour LC_i^e of E_i, and pick the one with the least length as the cutting path. For a hole, we combine two geodesic paths to form a cutting path. The first geodesic goes from the start to the end node inside the edge E_i. The second geodesic goes from the start to the end node without passing the edge.

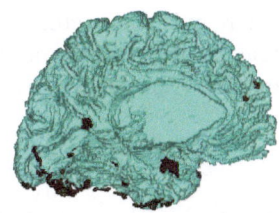

Fig. 2. Yellow: geometric outliers; Red: Topological outliers

To make cut or fill decisions about topological outliers, we find paired patches on $\mathcal{M}^G$ that jointly fill a hole or handle in $\mathcal{M}^F$. For all faces on $\mathcal{M}^G$ with their interior voxels in the background region of $\mathcal{M}^F$, we perform a connected component labeling and denote the set of patches as $CC^G = \{CC_1^G, CC_2^G, \cdots\}$. Triangles in different patches are paired if they share a common interior voxel. These triangle pairs are then grouped into paired components $PC^G = \{PC_1^G, PC_2^G, \cdots\}$ according to their paired patch labels in CC^G. For each paired patches, its interior voxels are $\mathbf{x}_o(PC_i^G)$ and they are filled inside $\mathcal{M}^G$ to satisfy the genus-zero constraint. A cut decision should be made if either conditions is met:

- Number of voxels $\mathbf{p} \in \mathbf{x}_o^T(PC_i^G)$ classified as CSF is greater than THD_{CSF}.
- Number of triangles $\mathcal{T}_j \in PC_i^G$ with $ADF(\mathcal{T}_j) > \gamma$ is greater than THD_{GEO}.

The first condition checks if filling a handle/hole needs voxels classified as CSF. The second condition measures the geometric regularity of the filling patches. To cut open a paired component in $\mathcal{M}^G$, we search for a handle or hole with the shortest cutting path that is connected to this paired component. Let CP_i denote the cutting path of this hole or handle and the set of triangles it passes on $\mathcal{M}^F$ as $\mathcal{T}^F(CP_i)$. To cut open this component, we modify the evolution speed as follows: $F(\mathbf{p}) = -1$ for $\mathbf{p} \in \mathbf{x}_o(\mathcal{T}^F(CP_i))$.

As an illustration, we plotted the detected outliers on a WM boundary with Reeb analysis in Fig. 2. By iteratively applying the steps in section 3.1, 3.2, 3.3, we can remove both geometric and topological outliers in a unified framework.

3.4   Sub-voxel Accuracy

Let M^G represent the genus-zero, triangular mesh representation of the boundary between high intensity tissue TM_h and low intensity tissue TM_l after the removal of outliers. The pair (TM_h, TM_l) could be (WM,GM) or (GM,CSF). To achieve sub-voxel accuracy, we estimate locally the isosurface location between the two tissue types at each vertex of $\mathcal{M}^G$. Let $s_\mathcal{V}$ denote the shift of all vertices to their locally estimated iso-surface location, we compute the final vertex coordinates by minimizing the energy

$$E = \| \mathbf{x} + S_\mathcal{V} - \hat{\mathbf{x}} \|^2 + \eta \| \Delta \hat{\mathbf{x}} \|^2 \tag{3}$$

where $\mathbf{x}$ is the vector of coordinates of all vertices, Δ is the discrete Laplacian matrix of the mesh, and η is a regularization parameter. The solution of this quadratic problem gives the coordinates of vertices on the final cortical surface:

$$\hat{\mathbf{x}} = (I + \eta \Delta' \Delta)^{-1}(\mathbf{x} + S_\mathcal{V}). \tag{4}$$

4   Experimental Results

In this section, we demonstrate our method and compare with FreeSurfer [2], which is widely used in brain imaging research, on two large datasets. The first dataset includes skull-stripped MR images of 50 normal controls(NC) and 50 Alzheimer's disease (AD) patients from ADNI [6]. The second dataset includes 100 skull-stripped MR images from ICBM [7] and it has a wide age range from 19 to 80. For all images, the same set of parameters are used in our method: $\alpha = 100mm, \beta = 5, \gamma = 100, THD_{CSF} = 5, THD_{GEO} = 5, \eta = 10$.

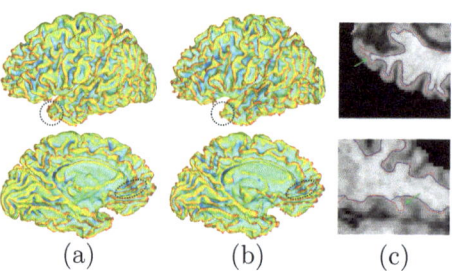

(a)   (b)   (c)

Fig. 3. A comparison of WM surfaces. (a) Our result. (b) FreeSurfer result. (c) Intersection of image slices with highlighted regions on surfaces. Red: our method. Blue: FreeSurer.

In the first experiment, we present detailed comparisons using one MR scan of an AD patient in ADNI. We applied our method and FreeSurfer to reconstruct the WM and GM surfaces on both hemispheres. Computationally our method took around 3 hours and is much more efficient than FreeSurfer, which took more than 10 hours. In Fig. 3, the left hemispherical WM surfaces reconstructed by both methods are plotted. In regions highlighted by the dashed curves, we can

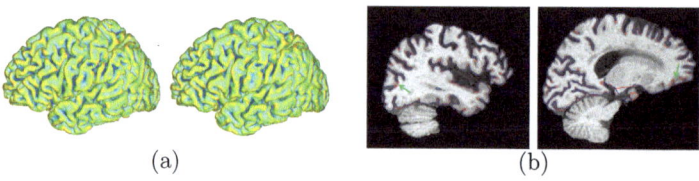

(a)   (b)

Fig. 4. A comparison of GM surfaces. (a) Left: Our result. Right: FreeSurfer result. (b) Intersection of sagittal slices with surfaces. Red: our method. Blue: FreeSurfer.

see that our method produces more complete reconstruction of the boundary, which is better illustrated with the intersections of surfaces and two axial slices shown in Fig. 3(c). The left hemispherical GM surfaces reconstructed with our method and FreeSurfer are plotted in Fig. 4(a). The intersections of the surfaces with two sagittal slices shown in Fig. 4(b) illustrate that our surface can better capture deep sulcal regions.

In the second experiment, we applied both our method and FreeSurfer to the MR images of 50 NC and 50 AD from ADNI. Using a general surface mapping algorithm [14], we projected the gyral labels of the LPBA40 atlas [15] to all left hemispherical surfaces. For each gyrus, we computed the average gray matter thickness and tested group differences between NC and AD using two tailed t-tests. The p-values from our method and FreeSurfer are plotted in Fig.5. Our method can achieve more significant p-values on 18 of the 24 gyral regions.

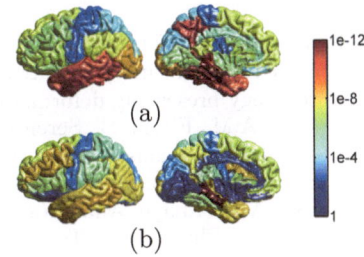

Fig. 5. P-value maps of gyrus-based thickness differences between NC and AD. (a) Our results. (b) FreeSurfer results.

In the third experiment, we applied our method and FreeSurfer to the 100 MR images from the ICBM database and used the results to model the decrease of gray matter thickness in normal aging. The reconstructed surfaces were first automatically labeled into gyral regions with the same approach in the second experiment. Regression analysis was then applied to the mean thickness of each gyrus against subject age. The results are shown in Fig. 6, where the rates of decrease are plotted in Fig. 6(a) and (b), and the p-values of the regression analysis are plotted in Fig. 6(c) and (d). We can see that our method can achieve statistically much more significant results on all gyral regions.

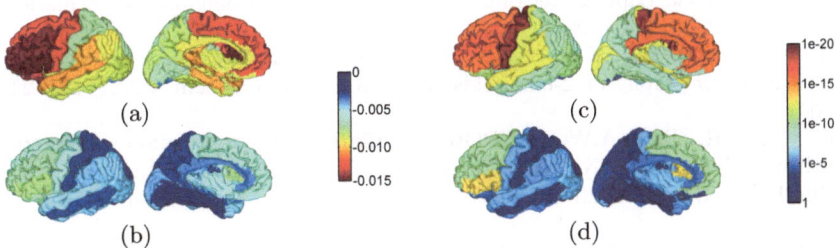

Fig. 6. Regression analysis of gray matter thickness and normal aging. (a) Rate of decrease from our results. (b) Rate of decrease from FreeSurfer results. (c) P-value maps of our results. (d) P-value maps of FreeSurfer results.

5   Conclusions

In this paper we developed a novel approach for the unified correction of geometric and topological outliers in cortical surface reconstruction. Comparisons with a state-of-the-art tool showed that our method is computationally more efficient and can achieve better performance in population studies. The Reeb analysis framework developed here is general and can be valuable for general surface reconstruction and analysis problems.

References

1. Mangin, J.F., Frouin, V., Bloch, I., Regis, J., Lopez-Krahe, J.: From 3D magnetic resonance images to structural representations of the cortex topography using topology preserving deformations. J. Math. Imaging. Vis. 5(4), 297–318 (1995)
2. Dale, A.M., Fischl, B., Sereno, M.I.: Cortical surface-based analysis i: segmentation and surface reconstruction. NeuroImage 9, 179–194 (1999)
3. Shattuck, D., Leahy, R.: BrainSuite: An automated cortical surface identification tool. Med. Image. Anal. 8(2), 129–142 (2002)
4. Han, X., Pham, D.L., Tosun, D., Rettmann, M.E., Xu, C., Prince, J.L.: CRUISE: Cortical reconstruction using implicit surface evolution. NeuroImage 23, 997–1012 (2004)
5. Li, G., Nie, J., Wu, G., Wang, Y., Shen, D.: Consistent reconstruction of cortical surfaces from longitudinal brain mr images. NeuroImage 59(4), 3805–3820 (2012)
6. Mueller, S., Weiner, M., Thal, L., Petersen, R.C., Jack, C., Jagust, W., Trojanowski, J., Toga, A., Beckett, L.: The Alzheimer's disease neuroimaging initiative. Clin. North Am. 15, 869–877 (2005) xi–xii
7. Mazziotta, J.C., Toga, A.W., Evans, A.C., et al.: A probabilistic atlas and reference system for the human brain: international consortium for brain mapping. Philos. Trans. R. Soc. Lond. B. Biol. Sci. 356, 1293–1322 (2001)
8. Reuter, M., Wolter, F.E., Shenton, M., Niethammer, M.: Laplace-beltrami eigenvalues and topological features of eigenfunctions for statistical shape analysis. Computer-Aided Design 41(10), 739–755 (2009)
9. Qiu, A., Bitouk, D., Miller, M.I.: Smooth functional and structural maps on the neocortex via orthonormal bases of the Laplace-Beltrami operator. IEEE Trans. Med. Imag. 25(10), 1296–1306 (2006)
10. Shi, Y., Lai, R., Morra, J., Dinov, I., Thompson, P., Toga, A.: Robust surface reconstruction via Laplace-Beltrami eigen-projection and boundary deformation. IEEE Trans. Med. Imag. 29(12), 2009–2022 (2010)
11. Cole-McLaughlin, K., Edelsbrunner, H., Harer, J., Natarajan, V., Pascucci, V.: Loops in Reeb graphs of 2 manifolds. Discrete Comput. Geom. 32(2), 231–244 (2004)
12. Shi, Y., Lai, R., Toga, A.W.: CoRPORATE: Cortical Reconstruction by Pruning Outliers with Reeb Analysis and Topology-Preserving Evolution. In: Székely, G., Hahn, H.K. (eds.) IPMI 2011. LNCS, vol. 6801, pp. 233–244. Springer, Heidelberg (2011)
13. Shi, Y., Karl, W.C.: A real-time algorithm for the approximation of level-set-based curve evolution. IEEE Trans. Image Processing 17(5), 645–657 (2008)
14. Shi, Y., Lai, R., Gill, R., Pelletier, D., Mohr, D., Sicotte, N., Toga, A.W.: Conformal Metric Optimization on Surface (CMOS) for Deformation and Mapping in Laplace-Beltrami Embedding Space. In: Fichtinger, G., Martel, A., Peters, T. (eds.) MICCAI 2011, Part II. LNCS, vol. 6892, pp. 327–334. Springer, Heidelberg (2011)
15. Shattuck, D., Mirza, M., Adisetiyo, V., Hojatkashani, C., Salamon, G., Narr, K., Poldrack, R., Bilder, R., Toga, A.: Construction of a 3D probabilistic atlas of human brain structures. NeuroImage 39(3), 1064–1080 (2008)

Automatic Detection and Classification of Teeth in CT Data

Nguyen The Duy, Hans Lamecker, Dagmar Kainmueller, and Stefan Zachow

Zuse-Institute Berlin, Germany
kainmueller@zib.de

Abstract. We propose a fully automatic method for tooth detection and classification in CT or cone-beam CT image data. First we compute an accurate segmentation of the maxilla bone. Based on this segmentation, our method computes a complete and optimal separation of the row of teeth into 16 subregions and classifies the resulting regions as existing or missing teeth. This serves as a prerequisite for further individual tooth segmentation. We show the robustness of our approach by providing extensive validation on 43 clinical head CT scans.

1 Introduction

Cone beam computed tomography (CBCT) is becoming a preferred imaging technique for three-dimensional diagnosis and therapy planning in dentistry as well as maxillofacial surgery. In dental implantology, for instance, surgical drill guides are individually manufactured based on CBCT data and rapid prototyping techniques. The accuracy of such drill guides highly depends on the quality of the 3D reconstructions of jaw structures. Such reconstructions often end up in tedious image segmentation tasks, in case dental fillings and brackets heavily degrade image quality due to the resulting shadowing artifacts within respective image slices. In most cases, only manual segmentation leads to useful results.

Research on jaw segmentation in CT data has mostly concentrated on the lower jaw [1–4], since the maxilla is generally more difficult to segment automatically. The maxilla exhibits thin bony structures (palate, sinus maxillaris, orbital walls), which are difficult to detect with intensity thresholds alone [5, 6]. To the best of our knowledge, only Kainmueller et al. [7] segment the maxillary bone as part of the midface. Tooth regions, however, are omitted in all previous studies due to the aforementioned artefacts. The problem of detecting teeth in medical images has been well studied for 2D radiographs, but sparsely researched for 3D images, since effects of metal artefacts are less severe in 2D than in 3D. Mahoor et al. [8], Nassar et al. [9] and Lin et al. [10] use a three-step approach consisting of tooth isolation in the row of teeth, independent classification of each isolated tooth and correction of the classification results. All three methods use *integral projection* to separate teeth. Then, each isolated tooth region is classified based on area features [9] or shape features [8, 10]. The latter need a segmentation of each tooth in the isolated region. After independent classification of each region,

N. Ayache et al. (Eds.): MICCAI 2012, Part I, LNCS 7510, pp. 609–616, 2012.

the result is corrected by considering tooth order. In this step, string alignment techniques are used. For 3D CT images, Gao et al. [11] and Hosntalab et al. [12] propose algorithms for segmentation, however, they do not perform a classification of teeth. The main limitation of these methods is that they require a segmentation of the tooth region as input. To the best of our knowledge, there exist no approaches which automatically detect teeth in 3D CT data.

This paper contributes an algorithm to reliably segment the maxillary bone and detect the individual dentition state in an automatic way. Therefore, we first perform an accurate and robust segmentation of the bony structure based on statistical shape model (SSM) adaptation, following the approach of [7]. Then, we use this segmentation to detect the 16 tooth regions by fitting 15 separation planes. Subsequently, we classify each separated region as "tooth" or "gap" via histogram analysis, yielding the individual dentition state. Fig. 1 depicts this algorithmic pipeline for an exemplary CT dataset.

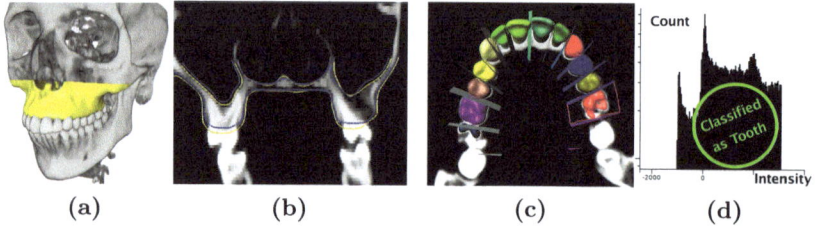

(a)   (b)   (c)   (d)

Fig. 1. Algorithmic pipeline in exemplary CT. (a) Maxilla segmentation, shown as yellow surface in volume rendering and (b) as yellow contour in coronal slice (vs. gold standard in blue). (c) Tooth region detection via separation planes. Gold standard teeth shown as colored surfaces. The red contour shows an individual tooth region that yields the intensity histogram (d) used for classification.

2   Maxilla Segmentation

For maxilla segmentation we follow the three-step approach proposed in [7], consisting of (1) initialisation of shape and pose of a statistical shape model (SSM) via the Generalized Hough Transform, (2) adaptation of the SSM governed by a heuristic bone intensity model, (3) refinement of SSM-based segmentation via locally regularized shape deformation. To cope with the specific properties of the maxilla, as well as the need to accurately reconstruct the tooth region for subsequent tooth separation and classification, we extend this framework as described in the following.

Automatic Bone Threshold Selection. The approach in [7] adapts an SSM to given image data by minimizing a cost-function that measures how well the model fits the data. A central parameter in this method is an image-specific threshold t_{Bone} characterizing typical bone intensities. For the segmentation of the lower jaw (mandible), a fixed threshold can be applied since the bony structure is rather compact and the cortical region is adequately sampled within the image data. However, for the upper jaw (maxilla), a fixed threshold is insufficient, because thin structures, such as the palate and the walls of the maxillary sinuses are typically undersampled in consecutive image slices. Here, partial volume effects lead to reduced intensities of thin bone structures. Thus, we propose to automatically determine t_{Bone} by analyzing the intensity histogram $h(x)$ in the vicinity of the initialised SSM. It exhibits a characteristic peak corresponding to air voxels at about $-1000\,HU$ and another one corresponding to soft tissue around $0\,HU$. We model the shape of each peak by a Gaussian function $g_i(x) = a_i \exp\left(\frac{(x-\mu_i)^2}{\sigma_i^2}\right), i \in \{1,2\}$ with mean μ_i, standard deviation σ_i, and scale a_i, and the remaining intensity occurrences with a constant C. The final function fitted to the histogram is $f(x) = g_1(x) + g_2(x) + C$. The problem of fitting $f(x)$ to $h(x)$ by determining the optimal parameter set $\Theta^* = (a_1, a_2, \mu_1, \mu_2, \sigma_1, \sigma_2, C) = \arg\min_\Theta (h(x) - f(x))^2$ can be solved via Levenberg-Marquardt optimization. Using Θ^*, we set the bone threshold as $t_{Bone} = \mu_2 + 2\sigma_2$, i.e., roughly above 85% of the intensities captured by the soft tissue peak.

Segmentation Strategy for the Tooth Region. The key idea of the algorithm in [7] is to analyze intensity profiles P sampled in direction of the surface normal on each vertex of the SSM to drive the segmentation process. To segment the bone region, we propose to decide for each intensity profile on the tooth region whether it contains a bone-soft tissue interface or not. After binary classification, we apply an individual segmentation strategy for each class. Using histogram analysis as described above, we heuristically determine lower intensity thresholds of soft tissue $t_{Tissue} = \frac{\mu_1 + \mu_2}{2}$ (inbetween air- and soft-tissue mean) and teeth $t_{Teeth} = \arg\min_x \frac{d}{dx} h(x) \wedge x > 1000HU$, i.e. the steepest descent above 1000HU. The latter can be interpreted as an upper threshold to bone, and thus serves as a lower threshold to teeth. We use these thresholds to classify each sample point on an intensity profile P. Afterwards, a rule-based decision is made whether to analyze the profile with the bone intensity model (BIM) as employed in [7]: If there is (1) no region classified as tooth, or (2) one or two regions classified as tooth as well as a transition from bone-classified to air-classified sample points, the BIM is employed. In all other cases, a conservative strategy is employed that slightly prefers the mid-sample point on the profile (i.e. the current position of the respective vertex on the deformable surface) over all others.

3   Tooth Detection

After successful segmentation of the maxillary bone, we determine the volumetric image region containing the teeth as all voxels within a reasonable distance to the *tooth patch*, which is a predefined region on our maxilla SSM's surface. We propose the following scheme to detect/classify teeth within that region: In a first step, the region is divided into 16 plausible subregions, each containing either single teeth or representing missing teeth. In a second step, the individual dentition state is classified.

Separation. For decomposing the entire tooth region into subregions, we employ 15 separation planes. We propose to formulate the task of finding a suitable position and orientation for each of these planes as a graph optimisation problem. This leads to a optimal solution with respect to an objective function as described in the following. First, we limit the number of possible positions and orientations for each plane to a finite set. Moreover, we limit the distances and angles between adjacent planes to plausible intervals which have been learnt a priori from the sizes of the respective teeth in training data. Hence, a feasible sequence of tooth separation planes (ID i next to ID $i+1$) defines a sequence of consecutive tooth cells corresponding to a sequential tooth numbering scheme.

For each potential separation plane P_i, we define a cost that encodes how likely it separates two teeth given the image data. This cost is derived from the average image intensity m_i and standard deviation s_i within the plane as well as the average directional derivative of the image perpendicular to the plane, g_i. Additionally, a penalty cost a_i is assigned to highly tilted planes as a regularizing term in case many consecutive teeth are missing. The cost c of P_i is then defined as a weighted sum

$$c(P_i) = \alpha \cdot m_i + \beta \cdot s_i + \gamma \cdot \frac{1}{g_i^2 + \epsilon} + \delta \cdot a_i \qquad (1)$$

where a small ϵ serves for avoiding divisions by zero. Note that the weights $(\alpha, \beta, \gamma, \delta)$ are fixed for all planes.

The costs are encoded within a graph: Each potential separation plane (i.e. combination of position and orientation) is represented by a graph node; Feasible neighboring separation planes are encoded via a graph edge between the respective nodes; Each graph node is weighted by the cost of the respective separation plane. The optimal path through this graph, computed with Dijkstra's algorithm, yields our optimal set of separation planes:

$$\left\{ \widehat{P}_i, i = 1 \ldots 15 \right\} = \underset{\{P_i, i=1\ldots15\}}{\arg\min} \sum_{i=1}^{15} c(P_i) \text{ subj. to } (P_i, P_{i+1}) \in E \; \forall i < 15 \quad (2)$$

where E denotes the set of graph edges.

Classification. Having partitioned the entire tooth region into distinct cells, we can independently decide whether a cell contains a tooth or not. If we detect a tooth, we can classifiy it directly from the ID of the cell containing it. Since teeth are imaged with a high intensity value in CT images, we use the intensity histogram of the region as a feature for the decision whether a tooth is present or not. To this end, a support vector machine (SVM) is learnt from training data and employed as a binary classifier.

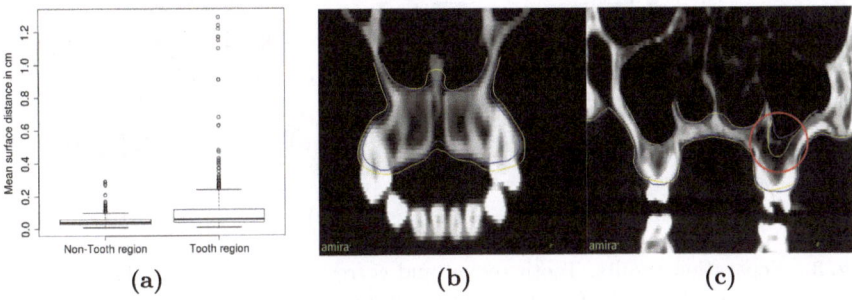

Fig. 2. Maxilla segmentation results. (a) Mean surface distances assessed in 43 datasets. (b,c) Exemplary automatic segmentation (yellow) vs. ground truth (blue). (c) Low intensity at sinus causes inaccuracy.

4   Results and Discussion

The data basis for our experiments consists of 43 clinical CT datasets, fully depicting the maxilla and the upper teeth. The individual maxillas differ in number of teeth and bone density. Moreover, the data basis contains "pathological" cases that occur in clinical practise, e.g. with dental prosthesis or metal artefacts due to fillings of implants.

Maxilla Segmentation. We assess the accuracy of maxilla segmentation in a leave-one-out evaluation. For each dataset, we use the ground truth shapes of the other 42 datasets to generate the SSM applied for segmentation. As quality measure for segmentation, we use mean surface distance to the ground truth. In order to evaluate the performance of the tooth region segmentation strategy, we separately measured mean surface distances for tooth and non-tooth region. Fig. 2 plots the resulting error measures and shows exemplary segmentation results. The median mean surface distance is below $1\,mm$ for both tooth- and non-tooth regions. Slightly higher errors for the tooth region can be attributed to a lack of image features within teeth, as well as a stronger influence of metal artefacts which occur mainly in the tooth region.

Tooth Separation. In order to test our tooth separation approach, we perform a ten-fold cross validation. We learn the tooth sizes in the training set, and apply our separation algorithm to the test set using these size parameters.

As for the weights $(\alpha, \beta, \gamma, \delta)$ of the per-plane costs that build the separation cost function (cf. Eq. 1), we set $\alpha = 1$ and determine the best set of remaining weights ("best" w.r.t. volume overlap averaged over all teeth and datasets) via exhaustive search. We had to exclude this search from the cross validation framework for performance reasons, and hence performed it just once, w.r.t. the whole data set, instead of for each training set, in violation of a strict separation between training- and test data.

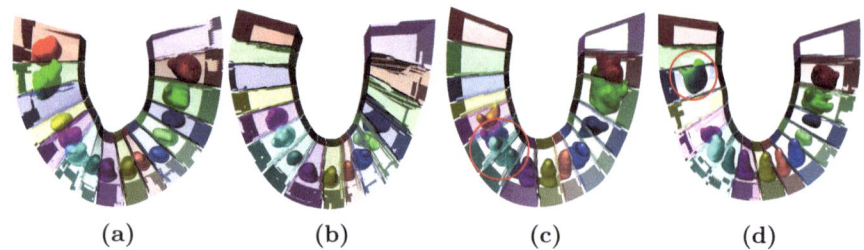

(a)   (b)   (c)   (d)

Fig. 3. Separation results. Tooth region and corresponding gold standard tooth are shown in same color. (a,b) Good results despite gaps. (c) Two regions contain three teeth - correspondence error is propagated. (d) One tooth in wrong region.

We measure the separation quality of each tooth region by volume overlap of the respective gold standard tooth: Let $T_i \subset \mathbf{R}^3$ be the i-th gold standard tooth and $R_i \subset \mathbf{R}^3$ the respective tooth region as determined by our separation algorithm. The volume overlap for this region is then computed as $(T_i \cap R_i)/T_i$. Table 1(a) lists the results for all datasets containing teeth, which are 27 out of the total 43. In 22 of these 27 datasets, *all* tooth regions determined by fully automatic separation contain at least 70% of the corresponding gold standard tooth (Table 1(a), 2nd row).

The tooth separation algorithm achieves high volume overlap when the row of teeth is complete or only solitary gaps exist inbetween. The method can even deal with larger gaps when they do not split off solitary teeth (Fig. 3(a,b)). If, however, one solitary tooth is split from the remaining row of teeth by a gap significantly larger than a single tooth, the separation algorithm runs the risk of placing it in a non-corresponding region (Fig. 3(d)). This might be partly due to a solitary tooth's naturally enlarged freedom to move. Furthermore, in case subsequent teeth are relatively slim and densely packed, they might be split into too few regions (Fig. 3(c)).

Tooth Classification. To evaluate classification performance, we first run a ten-fold cross-validation on "ideal" regions which perfectly separate teeth. These

Table 1. (a) Tooth separation results on 27 datasets. (b) Tooth classification results based on ideal (top) and automatic (bottom) separation. 61% of ground truth regions contain teeth; 39% contain gaps.

(a)

Overlap threshold	Number of datasets with					
	0	1	2	3	4	5
	teeth below threshold					
< 50%	25	1	0	1	0	0
< 70%	22	4	0	1	0	0
< 90%	8	9	4	5	0	1

(b)

		Ground truth	
		Tooth	No tooth
Auto, ideal sep.	Tooth	61%	1%
	No tooth	0%	38%
Auto, auto sep.	Tooth	58%	2%
	No tooth	3%	37%

"ground truth" regions are created from ground truth tooth segmentations. In a second experiment, we run another cross validation on the "real-world" regions computed by our tooth separation method. Table 1(b) lists the results. For ideal separation, 99% of auto-classifications are correct, while we have 0% false negatives and 1% false positives. For automatic separation, 95% of auto-classifications are correct, while we have 3% false negatives and 2% false positives.

In case classification fails, in the "real-world" scenario, it can be attributed mostly to previous errors in the automatic tooth separation step, where either correspondence between tooth and region does not apply (cf. Fig. 3(c,d)), or a tooth is split into two parts, one located in the region which is not supposed to contain a tooth. There are also individual cases where the patient has metal implants in the jaw which have intensity values similar to teeth and are therefore classified as tooth (cf. Fig. 4).

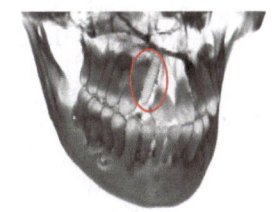

Fig. 4. Metal implant has same intensity as teeth

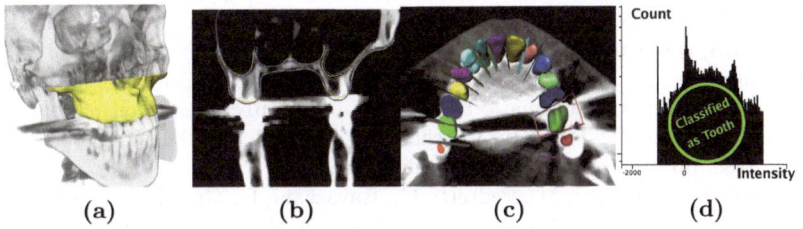

| (a) | (b) | (c) | (d) |

Fig. 5. Exemplary CT with dental fillings: Whole pipeline of segmentation (a,b), separation (c) and classification (d) successful despite strong metal artefacts

5   Conclusion

We propose a method which is able to segment the maxillary bone and detect and classify upper jaw teeth in CT images. Contrary to previous work, our segmentation approach specifically deals with the tooth regions and thus allows for subsequent tooth detection and classification. Our experiments provide evidence of the robustness of our approach on 43 clinical data sets. Even datasets with strong metal artefacts are processed successfully (cf. Fig. 5).

However, in challenging regions like the thin walls and sinus floor where polyps often occur, maxilla segmentation may still be improved, e.g. via locally adaptive threshold estimation. Furthermore, we observe that our classification scheme for bone/tooth profiles in some cases leaves us with too few profiles to drive the segmentation correctly. This may be overcome by a denser sampling of the tooth region on the SSM.

As for tooth classification, we expect that the use of volumetric information instead of intensity histograms as feature vectors would reduce false positive classifications. To this end, future work may integrate shape features, e.g. SSMs of individual teeth, into both tooth separation and classification. Most importantly, our tooth detection pipeline, together with tooth-specific SSMs, may serve as input for accurate automatic segmentation of individual teeth.

References

1. Lilja, M., Vuorio, V., Antila, K., Setal, H., Jarnstedt, J., Pollari, M.: Automatic Segmentation of the Mandible From Limited-Angle Dental X-Ray Tomography Reconstructions. In: ISBI: From Nano to Macro, pp. 964–967 (2007)
2. Rueda, S., Gil, J.A., Pichery, R., Alcañiz, M.: Automatic Segmentation of Jaw Tissues in CT Using Active Appearance Models and Semi-automatic Landmarking. In: Larsen, R., Nielsen, M., Sporring, J. (eds.) MICCAI 2006, Part I. LNCS, vol. 4190, pp. 167–174. Springer, Heidelberg (2006)
3. Lamecker, H., Zachow, S., Wittmers, A., Weber, B., Hege, H., Elsholtz, B., Stiller, M.: Automatic segmentation of mandibles in low-dose CT-data. Int. J. of Comp. Ass. Rad. Surg. 1, 393 (2006)
4. Kainmueller, D., Lamecker, H., Seim, H., Zinser, M., Zachow, S.: Automatic Extraction of Mandibular Nerve and Bone from Cone-Beam CT Data. In: Yang, G.-Z., Hawkes, D., Rueckert, D., Noble, A., Taylor, C. (eds.) MICCAI 2009, Part II. LNCS, vol. 5762, pp. 76–83. Springer, Heidelberg (2009)
5. Barandiaran, I., Macía, I., Berckmann, E., Wald, D., Dupillier, M.P., Paloc, C., Graña, M.: An Automatic Segmentation and Reconstruction of Mandibular Structures from CT-Data. In: Corchado, E., Yin, H. (eds.) IDEAL 2009. LNCS, vol. 5788, pp. 649–655. Springer, Heidelberg (2009)
6. Tognola, G., Parazzini, M., Pedretti, G., Ravazzani, P., Grandori, F., Pesatori, A., Norgia, M., Svelto, C.: Novel 3D Reconstruction Method for Mandibular Distraction Planning. In: IST 2006 - International Workshop on Imaging Systems and Techniques Minori, Italy, April 29, pp. 3–6 (2006)
7. Kainmueller, D., Lamecker, H., Seim, H., Zachow, S.: Multi-object Segmentation of Head Bones. MIDAS Journal, Contribution to MICCAI Workshop Head and Neck Auto-Segmentation Challenge, 1–11 (2009)
8. Mahoor, M., Abdelmottaleb, M.: Classification and numbering of teeth in dental bitewing images. Pattern Recognition 38(4), 577–586 (2005)
9. Nassar, D., Abaza, A., Ammar, H.: Automatic Construction of Dental Charts for Postmortem Identification. IEEE Transactions on Information Forensics and Security 3(2), 234–246 (2008)
10. Lin, P., Lai, Y., Huang, P.: An effective classification and numbering system for dental bitewing radiographs using teeth region and contour information. Pattern Recognition 43(4), 1380–1392 (2010)
11. Gao, H., Chae, O.: Automatic Tooth Region Separation for Dental CT Images. In: 2008 Int. Conf. on Conv. and Hybrid Inf. Tech., pp. 897–901 (2008)
12. Hosntalab, M., Aghaeizadeh Zoroofi, R., Abbaspour Tehrani-Fard, A., Shirani, G.: Segmentation of teeth in CT volumetric dataset by panoramic projection and variational level set. Int. J. of Comp. Ass. Rad. Surg. 3(3-4), 257–265 (2008)

Strain-Based Regional Nonlinear Cardiac Material Properties Estimation from Medical Images

Ken C. L. Wong[1,2], Jatin Relan[2], Linwei Wang[1], Maxime Sermesant[2],
Hervé Delingette[2], Nicholas Ayache[2], and Pengcheng Shi[1]

[1] Computational Biomedicine Laboratory, Rochester Institute of Technology, Rochester, USA
{chun.lok.wong,linwei.wang,pengcheng.shi}@rit.edu
[2] ASCLEPIOS Research Project, INRIA Sophia Antipolis, France
{jatin.relan,maxime.sermesant,herve.delingette,
nicholas.ayache}@inria.fr

Abstract. Model personalization is essential for model-based surgical planning
and treatment assessment. As alteration in material elasticity is a fundamental
cause to various cardiac pathologies, estimation of material properties is important to model personalization. Although the myocardium is heterogeneous, hyperelastic, and orthotropic, existing image-based estimation frameworks treat the
tissue as either heterogeneous but linear, or hyperelastic but homogeneous. In
view of these, we present a physiology-based framework for estimating regional,
hyperelastic, and orthotropic material properties. A cardiac physiological model
is adopted to describe the macroscopic cardiac physiology. By using a strain-
based objective function which properly reflects the change of material constants,
the regional material properties of a hyperelastic and orthotropic constitutive law
are estimated using derivative-free optimization. Experiments were performed on
synthetic and real data to show the characteristics of the framework.

1 Introduction

Estimation of subject-specific cardiac deformation has been an active research area for
decades as it provides useful information for verifying location and extent of cardiac
diseases [1]. Nevertheless, for model-based surgical planning, treatment assessment,
and cardiology study, retrieval of subject-specific cardiac physiological parameters is
necessary [2]. As alterations in myocardial fiber structure and material elasticity are
the more fundamental causes to various cardiac pathologies [3], estimation of material
properties is important for model personalization.

Although many works have studied myocardial material characteristics through
biomechanics [3], estimation of *in vivo* and subject-specific material properties is better realized through medical images. In [4], homogeneous, piecewise linear, and transversely isotropic material constants were estimated together with active stresses using
tagged magnetic resonance images (MRI). In [5], a simultaneous motion and material properties estimation framework was developed to estimate heterogeneous, linear,
and isotropic material constants from phase contrast and tagged MRI. Although these
works show physiologically and clinically interesting results, the use of linear material models may be physiologically implausible as the myocardial tissue is hyperelastic

N. Ayache et al. (Eds.): MICCAI 2012, Part I, LNCS 7510, pp. 617–624, 2012.
© Springer-Verlag Berlin Heidelberg 2012

and orthotropic [3], [6]. The estimation of hyperelastic material constants from images was unavailable until recently. In [7], [8], homogeneous, hyperelastic, and transversely isotropic material properties were estimated. A finite deformation elasticity problem was solved for early diastolic filling to simulate the passive mechanics of the left ventricle, and the estimation was performed by matching the predicted motion of material points derived from tagged MRI. Nevertheless, homogeneous properties are insufficient for model personalization. Furthermore, the interaction with active contraction was not accounted for in [5], [7], [8], and all frameworks used displacements as measurements.

In view of these issues, we present a physiology-based framework of estimating regional, hyperelastic, and orthotropic material properties from medical images. A cardiac physiological model comprising electric wave propagation and biomechanics is adopted [9]. Using a strain-based objective function which properly reflects the change of material constants, the regional exponential material constants of a hyperelastic and orthotropic constitutive law [6] are estimated through the BOBYQA algorithm for bound constrained optimization [10]. Although a cardiac cycle involves the interactions between active contraction, passive mechanics, and boundary conditions, to simplify the problem, we assume that the fibrous-sheet structure, active contraction, and boundary conditions are given and to be investigated in other papers. Experiments were performed on synthetic and real data to show the characteristics of the framework.

2   Cardiac Material Properties Estimation

2.1   Cardiac Physiological Model

The cardiac physiological model comprises electric wave propagation and biomechanics, which relates active contraction with cardiac deformation through given material properties and boundary conditions. The total-Lagrangian dynamics is utilized [9]:

$$\mathbf{M\ddot{U}} + \mathbf{C\dot{U}} + \mathbf{K}\Delta\mathbf{U} = \mathbf{F} \tag{1}$$

where $\mathbf{M}$, $\mathbf{C}$, and $\mathbf{K}$ are the mass, damping, and stiffness matrices respectively. $\mathbf{F}$ comprises active forces from electric wave propagation [11], internal stresses caused by finite deformation, and also the displacement boundary conditions. $\mathbf{\ddot{U}}$, $\mathbf{\dot{U}}$ and $\Delta\mathbf{U}$ are the respective acceleration, velocity and incremental displacement vectors respectively. With (1), the cardiac deformation can be related to the material properties in $\mathbf{K}$.

2.2   Strain Energy Function

The material properties in $\mathbf{K}$ are characterized by the strain energy function in [6]:

$$\Psi(\epsilon) = \kappa(J \ln J - J + 1) + \frac{1}{2}a(e^Q - 1) \tag{2}$$

where
$$\begin{aligned} Q = & b_{ff}\bar{\epsilon}_{ff}^2 + b_{ss}\bar{\epsilon}_{ss}^2 + b_{nn}\bar{\epsilon}_{nn}^2 \\ & + b_{fs}\left(\bar{\epsilon}_{fs}^2 + \bar{\epsilon}_{sf}^2\right) + b_{fn}\left(\bar{\epsilon}_{fn}^2 + \bar{\epsilon}_{nf}^2\right) + b_{sn}\left(\bar{\epsilon}_{sn}^2 + \bar{\epsilon}_{ns}^2\right) \end{aligned} \tag{3}$$

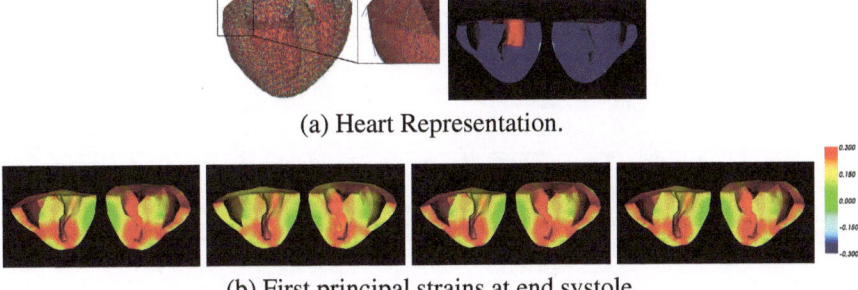

(a) Heart Representation.

(b) First principal strains at end systole.

Fig. 1. Synthetic data. (a) Left: heart geometry and tissue structure (f,s,n: fiber, sheet, sheet normal: blue, yellow, cyan). Right: infarcted region shown in red. (b) Left to right: simulated ground truth, simulations with initial parameters, with parameters from MI-based metric, and with parameters from MSE-based metric.

with J the determinant of deformation gradient, and κ the penalty factor for tissue incompressibility. $\bar{\epsilon}_{ij}$ are the isovolumetric components of the Green-Lagrange strain tensor ϵ. a (kPa) and b_{ij} (unitless) are the material constants. The f-s-n coordinate system represents the fibrous-sheet structure. With (2), the stress tensor and elasticity tensor can be derived and embedded into the cardiac electromechanical dynamics. Because of the difficulty in separating a from b_{ij} [6,8], only b_{ij} are estimated in this paper.

2.3   Strain-Based Derivative-Free Optimization

As realistic cardiac material properties are nonlinear [3], estimating material constants from deformation is a nonlinear optimization problem. In [11], the adjoint method was used to estimate the local active contractility from cardiac deformation. In [5], a simultaneous motion and material properties estimation framework based upon the maximum a posteriori estimation principles was realized through the extended Kalman smoother. These frameworks linearize the objective functions through approximations and assumptions, which may reduce the physiological plausibility and stability of the system dynamics. Furthermore, as each change of the material constants affects the whole cardiac cycle, frame-to-frame updates of material constants in [5] may reduce the physiological plausibility of the estimation.

In consequence, the BOBYQA algorithm for derivative-free bound constrained optimization is utilized [10]. With θ the parameters to be estimated, this algorithm approximates the objective function $\mathcal{F}(\theta)$ as a quadratic function, which is updated iteratively to search for the minimum within the given boundaries. As no linearization is performed, the intact nonlinearity of the model can be preserved. Furthermore, without the tedious derivation of the objective function gradient, more complicated but appropriate functions can be investigated. Our objective function is given as:

$$\mathcal{F}(\theta) = \sum_f \sum_r \sum_i \sum_j g_r \left(\bar{\epsilon}_{ij}, \epsilon_{ij}(\theta) \right) \qquad (4)$$

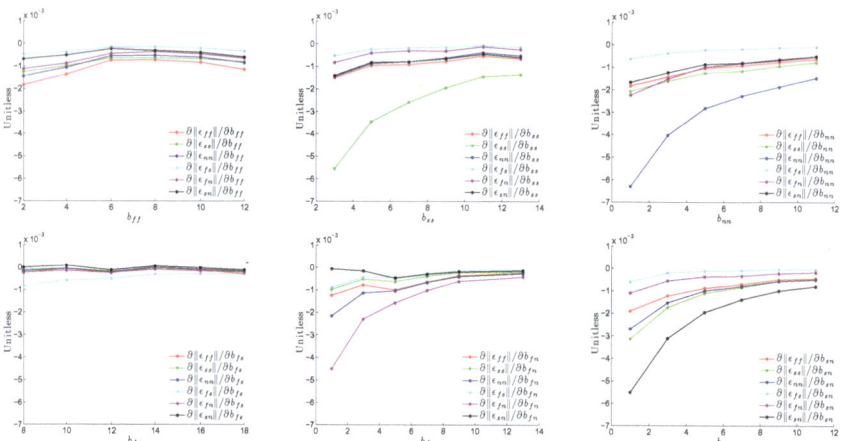

Fig. 2. Sensitivity analysis on synthetic data. Sensitivities of f-s-n Green-Lagrange strains with respect to b_{ij}. $\|\epsilon_{ij}\|$ are the mean strain magnitudes in a cardiac cycle.

Table 1. Synthetic data. Ground-truth parameters and estimated parameters. $a = 0.8$ kPa at the LV and RV and $a = 1.2$ kPa at the infarcted region.

	Ground truth						MI-based						MSE-based					
	b_{ff}	b_{ss}	b_{nn}	b_{fs}	b_{fn}	b_{sn}	b_{ff}	b_{ss}	b_{nn}	b_{fs}	b_{fn}	b_{sn}	b_{ff}	b_{ss}	b_{nn}	b_{fs}	b_{fn}	b_{sn}
LV	6.0	7.0	3.0	10.0	4.0	5.0	6.3	7.0	3.1	7.6	3.8	4.9	5.5	8.0	3.9	7.6	3.9	6.2
RV	5.0	6.0	2.0	9.0	3.0	4.0	5.0	6.2	1.6	8.3	3.5	3.8	3.4	6.8	2.2	8.7	3.0	4.1
Infarcted	8.0	9.0	5.0	12.0	6.0	7.0	8.4	8.2	5.7	10.8	5.5	6.8	7.6	7.4	6.8	8.1	6.3	7.4

with f and r the frames and regions used respectively. $\bar{\epsilon}_{ij}$ are the strain measurements from image-based cardiac motion recovery under the local f-s-n basis at region r [9], and $\epsilon_{ij}(\boldsymbol{\theta})$ are the corresponding strains simulated using (1). This strain-based objective function better reflects the change of b_{ij} as shown in the sensitivity analysis in Section 3.1. $g_r(\bullet)$ computes the similarity between the measured and simulated strains in region r, for which the mean-squared-error-based (MSE-based) and the mutual-information-based (MI-based) metrics were investigated (Section 3.2 and 3.3). The MSE-based metric minimizes the absolute difference, while the MI-based metric minimizes the difference between patterns regardless of the local contrasts. With (4), assuming the active contraction and boundary conditions are given, b_{ij} are estimated simultaneously.

3   Experiments

3.1   Sensitivity Analysis

Strains ϵ_{ij} are direct components of strain energy functions (e.g. (3)) comprising spatial derivatives of displacements, thus are more appropriate for material properties estimation. To show the relations between ϵ_{ij} and b_{ij} under the local f-s-n basis, a sensitivity analysis was performed. The heart architecture from the University of Auckland was

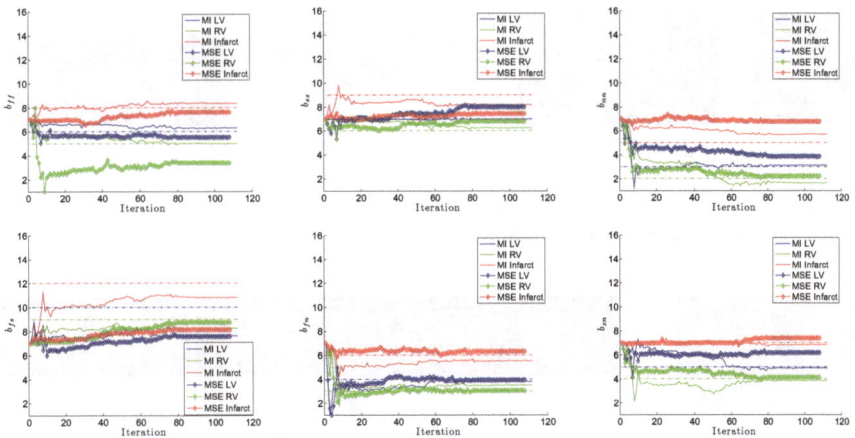

Fig. 3. Synthetic data. Parameter estimation using MI-based and MSE-based metrics. Blue, green, and red dash-dot lines represent the ground truths of LV, RV, and infarct.

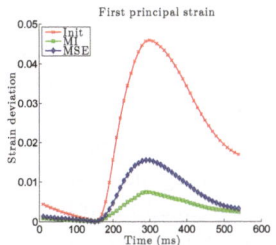

Fig. 4. Synthetic data. Mean deviations of first principal strains from the ground truth.

used to provide the anatomical cardiac geometry and tissue structure for the experiments [12] (Fig. 1(a)). With the parameters obtained from [6] ($a = 0.88$ kPa, $b_{ff} = 6$, $b_{ss} = 7$, $b_{nn} = 3$, $b_{fs} = 12$, $b_{fn} = 3$, $b_{sn} = 3$), cardiac cycles with different parameters were simulated with normal electrical propagation through (1) for the one-at-a-time sensitivity analysis (Fig. 2) [13]. The results show that ϵ_{ij} are most sensitive when the corresponding b_{ij} changes, thus strain-based objective function is a proper choice for material properties estimation.

3.2 Synthetic Data

Experimental Setup. The heart architecture from the University of Auckland was used (Fig. 1(a)). The heart was partitioned into regions of LV, RV, and infarct (Fig. 1(a)), with parameters shown in Table 1. A cardiac cycle of 550 ms was simulated using the cardiac physiological model as the ground truth, and the resulted strains were used as the measurements. The MI-based and MSE-based metrics of g_r in (4) were tested. In the experiments, a is known, and b_{ij} were initialized as 7 and were estimated simultaneously using the measurements from the whole cardiac cycle.

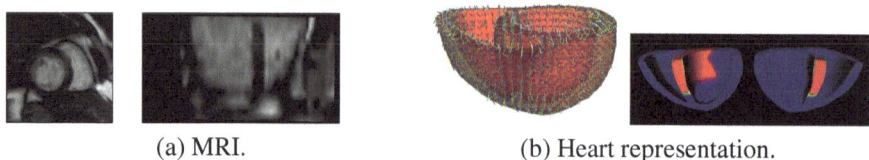

(a) MRI.   (b) Heart representation.

Fig. 5. Real data. (a) MRI. (b) Left: tissue structures (f,s,n: fiber, sheet, sheet normal: blue, yellow, cyan). Right: infarcted region shown in red.

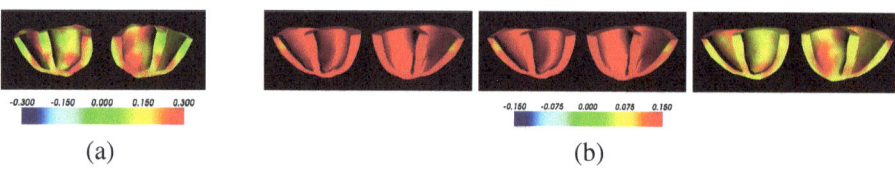

(a)   (b)

Fig. 6. Real data. First principal strains at end systole. (a) Recovered cardiac deformation from MRI. (b) Left to right: simulations with initial parameters, with parameters from MI-based metric, and with parameters from MSE-based metric.

Results. Fig. 3 shows the material constants at each iteration during optimization, and Table 1 shows the estimated material constants. Comparing between the MI-based and MSE-based metrics, they have similar numbers of iterations before convergence, but the MI-based metric gives better parameter identification. For both metrics, except b_{fs}, the estimated b_{ij} maintain the correct regional orders. Such orders appeared at the early iterations, and the latter iterations refined the results. The performance of estimating b_{fs} can be inferred from the sensitivity analysis (Fig. 2), in which the strains are less sensitive to b_{fs}. Fig. 1(b) shows the cardiac deformation at end systole. Although the MSE-based metric has less accurate estimation, the simulation using the corresponding parameters is very close to the ground truth, and is similar to the simulation using the parameters estimated by the MI-based metric (Fig. 4).

3.3   Real Data

Experimental Setup. To investigate the behaviors of the proposed framework in reality when the tissue structure, active contraction, and boundary conditions are not ideal, experiments were performed on human data sets from patients with acute myocardial infarction [14]. Because of the page limits, only the results of Case 2 are presented. Case 2 contains a human short-axis MRI sequence of 16 frames (50 ms/frame), 13 slices/frame, 8 mm inter-slice spacing, and in-plane resolution 1.32 mm/pixel (Fig. 5(a)). Segmentation was performed to obtain the initial heart geometry, with the fibrous-sheet structure mapped from the Auckland heart architecture using nonrigid registration (Fig. 5(b)). The expert-identified infarcted region is shown in Fig. 5(b), and the heart geometry was partitioned into LV, RV, and infarct accordingly. The cardiac deformation was estimated from the MRI sequence using the framework in [9] to provide the strain inputs for the material properties estimation. Active contraction parameters were adopted from the literature [3,11] but manually calibrated using the recovered cardiac cycle with the initial

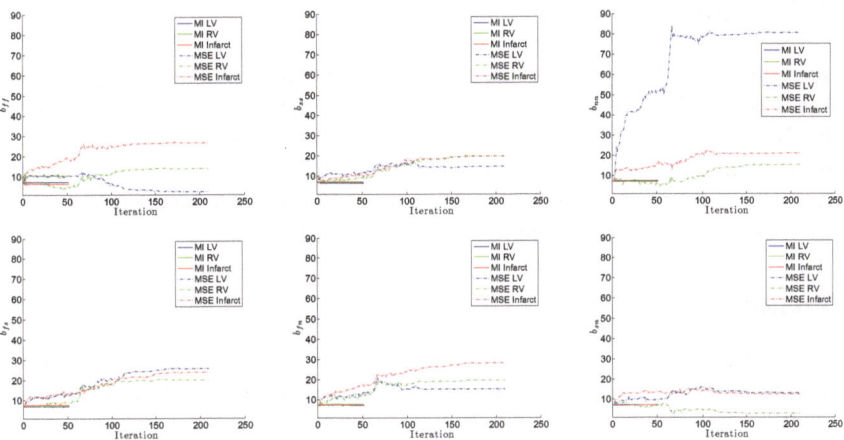

Fig. 7. Real data. Parameter estimation using MI-based and MSE-based metrics.

Table 2. Real data. Estimated parameters. $a = 0.88$ kPa at all regions.

	MI-based						MSE-based					
	b_{ff}	b_{ss}	b_{nn}	b_{fs}	b_{fn}	b_{sn}	b_{ff}	b_{ss}	b_{nn}	b_{fs}	b_{fn}	b_{sn}
LV	7.2	6.4	7.3	6.9	7.2	7.1	2.6	14.7	80.5	25.7	15.3	13.1
RV	10.3	7.1	6.9	7.1	7.7	7.1	13.9	19.7	15.2	20.1	19.6	2.8
Infarcted	6.3	6.8	7.5	7.6	7.3	7.1	26.6	19.7	20.9	23.9	28.2	12.6

material constants. $a = 0.88$ kPa at all regions, and b_{ij} were initialized as 7 and were estimated simultaneously.

Results. Fig. 7 shows the material constants at each iteration during optimization, and Table 2 shows the estimated material constants. For the real data, the performances between the MI-based and MSE-based metrics are very different. The MI-based metric did not have proper estimation of parameters, which only slightly fluctuate around the initial value of 7 until convergence. On the other hand, the MSE-based metric performed much better. Except the outlier of b_{nn} at the LV which is probably caused by the unrealistic active contraction and boundary conditions, other parameters evolved in the range similar to those in other researches [7], [8], and the estimated parameters can partially reflect the properties of the infarcted region. Fig. 6 shows the visual comparisons at end systole. The simulated strain pattern using the parameters from the MI-based metric is very similar to that of the initialization which deviates a lot from the measured strain from the MRI. On the other hand, although the strain simulated using the parameters from the MSE-based metric is only halved of that of the measurements, the strain pattern properly accounts for the infarcted region.

4   Discussions

The experiments on the synthetic data show that in the ideal situation, the performance of MSE-based and MI-based metrics are similar, and the MI-based metric gives better results. Nevertheless, the results on the real data show that when the discrepancies between simulations and measurements are large because of the improper tissue structure, active contraction, and boundary conditions, the use of MI-based metric is less robust, though more experiments are required to confirm this justification.

References

1. Frangi, A.J., Niessen, W.J., Viergever, M.A.: Three-dimensional modeling for functional analysis of cardiac images: a review. IEEE Transactions on Medical Imaging 20(1), 2–25 (2001)
2. Hunter, P.J.: Modeling human physiology: the IUPS/EMBS physiome project. Proceedings of the IEEE 94(4), 678–691 (2006)
3. Glass, L., Hunter, P., McCulloch, A. (eds.): Theory of Heart: Biomechanics, Biophysics, and Nonlinear Dynamics of Cardiac Function. Springer (1991)
4. Hu, Z., Metaxas, D., Axel, L.: *In vivo* strain and stress estimation of the heart left and right ventricles from MRI images. Medical Image Analysis 7(4), 435–444 (2003)
5. Liu, H., Shi, P.: Maximum a posteriori strategy for the simultaneous motion and material property estimation of the heart. IEEE Transactions on Biomedical Engineering 56(2), 378–389 (2009)
6. Usyk, T.P., Mazhari, R., McCulloch, A.D.: Effect of laminar orthotropic myofiber architecture on regional stress and strain in the canine left ventricle. Journal of Elasticity 61, 143–164 (2000)
7. Wang, V.Y., Lam, H.I., Ennis, D.B., Cowan, B.R., Young, A.A., Nash, M.P.: Modelling passive diastolic mechanics with quantitative MRI of cardiac structure and function. Medical Image Analysis 13(5), 773–784 (2009)
8. Xi, J., Lamata, P., Shi, W., Niederer, S., Land, S., Rueckert, D., Duckett, S.G., Shetty, A.K., Rinaldi, C.A., Razavi, R., Smith, N.: An Automatic Data Assimilation Framework for Patient-Specific Myocardial Mechanical Parameter Estimation. In: Metaxas, D.N., Axel, L. (eds.) FIMH 2011. LNCS, vol. 6666, pp. 392–400. Springer, Heidelberg (2011)
9. Wong, K.C.L., Wang, L., Zhang, H., Liu, H., Shi, P.: Physiological fusion of functional and structural images for cardiac deformation recovery. IEEE Transactions on Medical Imaging 30(4), 990–1000 (2011)
10. Powell, M.J.D.: The BOBYQA algorithm for bound constrained optimization without derivatives. Technical report, DAMTP, University of Cambridge (2009)
11. Sermesant, M., Moireau, P., Camara, O., Sainte-Marie, J., Andriantsimiavona, R., Cimrman, R., Hill, D.L.G., Chapelle, D., Razavi, R.: Cardiac function estimation from MRI using a heart model and data assimilation: advances and difficulties. Medical Image Analysis 10, 642–656 (2006)
12. LeGrice, I.J., Smaill, B.H., Chai, L.Z., Edgar, S.G., Gavin, J.B., Hunter, P.J.: Laminar structure of the heart: ventricular myocyte arrangement and connective tissue architecture in the dog. Am. J. Physiol. Heart Circ. Physiol. 269, H571–H582 (1995)
13. Saltelli, A., Ratto, M., Andres, T., Campolongo, F., Cariboni, J., Gatelli, D., Saisana, M., Tarantola, S.: Global Sensitivity Analysis: The Primer. John Wiley & Sons Ltd. (2008)
14. PhysioNet/Computers in Cardiology challenge 2007: electrocardiographic imaging of myocardial infarction (2007), http://www.physionet.org/challenge/2007/

Frangi Goes US : Multiscale Tubular Structure Detection Adapted to 3D Ultrasound

Paulo Waelkens, Seyed-Ahmad Ahmadi, and Nassir Navab

Computer Aided Medical Procedures, Technische Universität München, Germany

Abstract. We propose a Hessian matrix based multiscale tubular structure detection (TSD) algorithm adapted to 3D B-mode vascular US images. The algorithm is designed to highlight blood vessel centerline points and yield an estimate of the cross-section radius at each centerline point. It can be combined with a simple centerline extraction scheme, yielding precise, fast and fully automatic lumen segmentation initializations.

TSD algorithms designed with CTA and MRA datasets in mind, e.g. the Frangi Filter [3], are not capable of reliably distinguishing centerline points from other points in vascular US datasets, since some assumptions underlying these algorithms are not reasonable for US datasets. The algorithm we propose, does not have these shortcomings and performs significantly better on vascular US datasets.

We propose a statistic to evaluate how well a TSD algorithm is able to distinguish centerline points from other points. Based on this statistic, we compare the Frangi Filter to various versions of our new algorithm, on 11 3D US carotid datasets.

1 Introduction and Medical Motivation

In recent years, tracked freehand ultrasound (3D US) emerged as a viable and low-cost (compared to CT and MRI) 3D imaging modality. 3D US shows a lot of potential, especially for vascular imaging (e.g. of the carotid arteries).

Today, when considering serious procedures, e.g. a carotid endarterectomy, vascular surgeons request CT or MRI angiographies (CTA and MRA)[1] to get a clear 3D visualization of the diseased vascular tree. However, angiographies have serious drawbacks: they are expensive, time consuming and present health hazards, in particular for elderly patients.

If it becomes possible to automatically and reliably extract more clinically relevant information from vascular 3D US, one would expect the need for angiographies to decline. We hope the TSD algorithm proposed in this paper is a first step in this direction.

Characteristics of Vascular US. In figure 1, left column, an US image of the cross-section of a common carotid artery is shown. The vessel lumen cross-section

---

[1] Intravascular ultrasound (IVUS) is not used for carotid imaging, as the US probe might rupture atheromas. We thus do not consider it an alternative to CTA/MRA.

N. Ayache et al. (Eds.): MICCAI 2012, Part I, LNCS 7510, pp. 625–633, 2012.

can be identified by its size, shape (roughly circular), signal response (uniformly low) and surroundings (a narrow ring of higher signal response points). One can also notice the influence the US beam direction has on the US signal response strength: edges orthogonal to the beam direction reflect the sound waves better (leading to a higher response) than edges with other orientations. The closer the edge comes to being parallel to the beam direction, the lower the reflection and the US response will be. During a freehand US scan, the practitioner has limited possibilities of where to locate and how to orient the probe. Thus, usually only a few beam directions can be used to generate the US response of a given voxel, and a strong direction dependency will be present in the reconstructed 3D dataset, in contrast to CT and MRI (and IVUS) datasets.

This is why, whilst assuming the symmetry of vessel features around centerlines is reasonable in CTA and MRA, the same does not apply for 3D US datasets.

Related Works. Guerrero *et al* [4] and Carvalho *et al* [2] propose centerline detection and tracking algorithms for sequences of tracked 2D vascular freehand US images. On each image they attempt to fit an ellipse to the vessel cross-section, and connect this 2D information with the spatial information provided by the tracking system. In [2], the direction dependency of US images is considered. Their approaches are inherently 2D, while we focus on less restrictive 3D approaches.

Among 3D algorithms, we point especially to the Frangi Filter, a multiscale TSD algorithm proposed by Frangi in [3]. Works published by Krissian *et al*, e.g. [5], and Pock *et al*, e.g. [7], among others, present similar and related ideas. All these authors use the information provided by the Hessian matrix of the smoothed data: Frangi proposes a vesselness measure as a function of the eigenvalues of the Hessian matrix; Krissian *et al* propose to combine the Hessian matrix with the structure tensor, and base their measure on the eigenvalues and eigenvectors of this combined descriptor; Pock *et al* propose a medialness function, which is evaluated on the plane spanned by the two largest principal curvatures of the Hessian matrix. To normalize their results over multiple scales, the authors of [3], [5] and [7] point to the scale-space theory proposed by Lindeberg [6], i.e. smoothing with Gaussian kernels and using γ-normalized partial derivatives.

To the best of our knowledge, the TSD algorithms proposed by all cited authors assume symmetry of features around centerlines.

We focus only on multiscale Hessian based approaches, as they allow the automatic detection of an arbitrary number of vessels, of arbitrary lengths and orientations over multiple scales; in contrast to more restrictive approaches like statistical shape models, or semi-automatic methods (e.g. Aylward *et al* [1]).

Contributions. We propose a Hessian matrix based multiscale tubular structure detection (TSD) algorithm adapted to 3D B-mode vascular US images. Without loss of generality (WLOG), we sort the Hessian's eigenvalues $|\lambda_1| \leq |\lambda_2| \leq |\lambda_3|$. WLOG the associated eigenvectors v_1, v_2 and v_3 are normalized: $\|v_i\| = 1$.

We propose 4 changes, which will be described in more detail in the next section, on Frangi's vesselness algorithm:

- *Ideal lumen model and associated kernel:* We propose the use of a non-Gaussian smoothing kernel, whose second partial derivatives better fit the expected lumen shape
- *Beam direction dependency:* At a centerline point, we assume the direction of highest curvature ($= v_3$) will be parallel to the US beam direction
- *Intensity prior:* We integrate the information that the vessel interior, i.e. the neighborhood of a vessel centerline point, has low US signal response
- *Vessel feature assymetry:* At a centerline point, we expect $\frac{|\lambda_2|}{|\lambda_3|} < 1$, i.e. we expect assymetry of the depicted vessel features and compensate for this fact

2   Materials and Methods

Basic Algorithm for CTA and MRA. We describe the basic workings of the Frangi Filter. WLOG assume a dark lumen surrounded by brighter tissue. Consider the Hessian matrix of the smoothed data at a point p,

$$smoothData_r(p) := (kernel(\zeta_r) * data)(p)$$

where ζ_r is the kernel parameter, a function of the scale parameter r. Recall that λ_i corresponds to the second directional derivative of the smoothed data in the direction v_i ($i = \{1, 2, 3\}$), and $\{v_1, v_2, v_3\}$ is an orthonormal basis of $\mathbb{R}^3$. If p is a lumen centerline point with cross-section radius r, Frangi assumes

$$\lambda_1 \approx 0 \qquad\qquad sign(\lambda_2) = sign(\lambda_3) = 1$$
$$|\lambda_2| >> 0 \qquad\qquad \lambda_2 = \lambda_3$$

i.e. at a centerline point, the curvature of the smoothed data in the directions v_2 and v_3 is large, and the curvature in the direction v_1 is small. v_2 and v_3 span the cross-section plane and v_1 is the centerline tangent direction.

He proposes a vesselness measure that is higher at points where his assumptions are satisfied. The assumption $\lambda_2 = \lambda_3$ is not reasonable for US datasets, due to direction dependency. Also, only the Gaussian kernel is considered for multiscale smoothing, following the scale-space theory proposed by Lindeberg [6].

Ideal Lumen Model. We assume an idealized model for the vessel lumen in our framework. The lumen is represented by a dark cylinder (in 3D) or a dark disc (in 2D cross-sections) of a given radius r. The lumen is surrounded by a white ring of a given thickness $th(r)$, which represents the vessel wall's echo-response and echogenicities in close proximity to the vessel. Based on the observation of 16 3D US carotid datasets, we chose $th(r) = 0.6r$. The tissue outside the white ring can have arbitrary response patterns and is thus represented by noise. The idealized model is illustrated in figure 1. It serves two purposes:

1) it provides a model of the shape that the algorithm is expected to find, i.e. it allows us to build an adequate smoothing convolution kernel and

2) the model is used to provide a reference vesselness value for centerline points of tubular structures at the scale r; for the scale r, this value is defined as the vesselness value at a centerline point of the ideal model for this scale.

Multiscale Normalization Scheme. For each scale r_i the algorithm iterates over, we obtain the reference vesselness value. Vesselness results for the scale r_i are normalized (i.e. divided) by the associated reference value.

Design of the Smoothing Kernel. At the appropriate scale r, λ_2 and λ_3 should be high at a vessel's centerline point c. Thus, based on the ideal lumen model for the scale r, $iLum(r)$, the kernel should be selected so that

$$[\frac{\partial^2}{\partial k^2}(kernel(\zeta_r) * iLum(r))](c) = [(\frac{\partial^2}{\partial k^2} kernel(\zeta_r)) * iLum(r)](c) \qquad (1)$$

is as large as possible, where k is the second or third coordinate in the coordinate system $\{v_1, v_2, v_3\}$ (i.e. expression (1) $= \lambda_2$ or λ_3). In particular, the expression should be larger at centerline points than at all other points.

Additionally, an acceptable smoothing kernel must be spherically symmetric, unimodal, non-negative and add up to 1. It follows that the first and second partial derivatives of the kernel add to 0.

By symmetry it suffices to define the kernel on a half-line starting from 0. Let $\mathbb{1}_S$ denote the indicator function of a set S. Notice from equation (1) that convolutions and differentiations commute. Intuitively, an ideal kernel would be defined by the function $g : \mathbb{R}_+ \to \mathbb{R}_+$, where

$$\frac{d^2}{dt^2} g(t; r, th) = \frac{1}{K}[-\mathbb{1}_{\{0 \leq t < r\}} + \frac{r}{th} \mathbb{1}_{\{r \leq t < (r+th)\}}] \qquad (2)$$

and $K > 0$. The one dimensional kernel generated, $ker_g : \mathbb{R} \to \mathbb{R}_+$, would be:

$$ker_g(t; r, th) = \mathbb{1}_{\{t<0\}} g(-t; r, th) + \mathbb{1}_{\{t \geq 0\}} g(t; r, th) \qquad (3)$$

K is chosen so ker_g adds up to 1. At a centerline point, $\frac{d^2}{dt^2} ker_g$ gives negative weights to the lumen, positive weights to the white ring and ignores the noise: an ideal match to the ideal lumen model in one dimension. However, g is not a smooth function. For performance reasons, convolutions in $\mathbb{R}^3$ are done in the frequency domain. To avoid aliasing, all functions involved should be smooth. So, instead of g, we use a smooth function of similar shape, $g^* : \mathbb{R}_+ \to \mathbb{R}_+$:

$$g^*(t; \zeta_r) = \frac{1}{K} e^{P_{12}^*(t;\zeta_r)} \qquad (4)$$

Where the polynomial P_{12}^* is given by

$$P_{12}^*(t; \zeta_r) = -0.5(c_{12}(\frac{t \cdot 0.408}{\zeta_r})^{12} + c_{10}(\frac{t \cdot 0.408}{\zeta_r})^{10} + c_8(\frac{t \cdot 0.408}{\zeta_r})^8$$
$$+ c_6(\frac{t \cdot 0.408}{\zeta_r})^6 + c_4(\frac{t \cdot 0.408}{\zeta_r})^4 + c_2(\frac{t \cdot 0.408}{\zeta_r})^2)$$

with $c_{12} = 1$, $c_{10} = 409.6$, $c_8 = 128$, $c_6 = 42.66$, $c_4 = 16$ and $c_2 = 8$.
The generated $\mathbb{R}^3$ kernel is given by:

$$kernel^*(t; \zeta_r) = \frac{1}{\left| e^{P_{12}^*(t; \zeta_r)} \right|_1} e^{P_{12}^*(t; \zeta_r)} \tag{5}$$

where t is the distance from the origin (recall: spherical symmetry) and $| \cdot |_1$ denotes the $\mathscr{L}^1$ norm. To obtain the link between ζ_r and r: fix a positive value of r^* (e.g. $r^* = 1$) and find ζ^* that maximizes

$$\max_{\zeta^* > 0} \frac{1}{\left| \frac{\partial^2}{\partial k^2} kernel(\zeta^*) \right|_1} \left(\frac{\partial^2}{\partial k^2} kernel(\zeta^*) * iLum(r^*) \right)(c) \tag{6}$$

where k is the second or third coordinate in the coordinate system $\{v_1, v_2, v_3\}$. The link will be given by

$$\zeta_r = \frac{\zeta^*}{r^*} r$$

Expression (6) is maximized for the kernel parameter ζ^* that minimizes the proportion of wrong associations of $\frac{\partial^2}{\partial k^2} kernel(\zeta^*)$ values to vessel features, i.e. when the proportion of low and negative weights for white ring voxels is kept at a minimum. For the 3D version of $kernel^*$ we numerically obtained $\zeta_r = 0.95r$. For the 3D Gaussian kernel, we numerically obtained $(\sigma_r =) \zeta_r = 0.575r$.

Notice g has 2 parameters to define its size, r and th, whilst g^* only has ζ_r. g^* was designed so that $\frac{d^2}{dt^2} g^*$ fit $\frac{d^2}{dt^2} g$ with $th = 0.6r$. For thicker walls choose polynomials of lower degree (e.g. Gaussian kernel); for narrower walls, higher.

The Gaussian kernel only has 1 parameter, σ_r, to define its size, which implies it fits g for a specific ratio $\frac{th}{r}$: $th(r) \approx 3r$. This does not match the selected ideal lumen model as well as $kernel^*$. The Gaussian kernel $\frac{d^2}{dt^2}$ either gives significant importance to the noise component and possibly negative weights to white ring points, or, alternatively, associates low weights to white ring points, yielding low values of λ_2 and λ_3 at c. In short, the Gaussian is not always the ideal choice as smoothing kernel for Hessian-based algorithms. Figure 1 illustrates this fact:

Beam Direction Dependency. Due to the physics behind US imaging, the ultrasound echo reponse will be higher at vessel wall sections which are oriented perpendicularly to the US beam than at vessel wall sections with different orientations, since sections perpendicular to the US beam reflect more of it directly back to the emitter (this effect is visible on the US image depicted in figure 1). For a lumen centerline point, this fact translates to the highest curvature being in the US beam direction. Thus, at a centerline point, we expect the direction of highest curvature (by definition, the eigenvector v_3) to be parallel to the US beam. To evaluate if this assumption is met, we propose the measure:

$$BDD = | < v_3, beamDirection > | \in [0; 1] \tag{7}$$

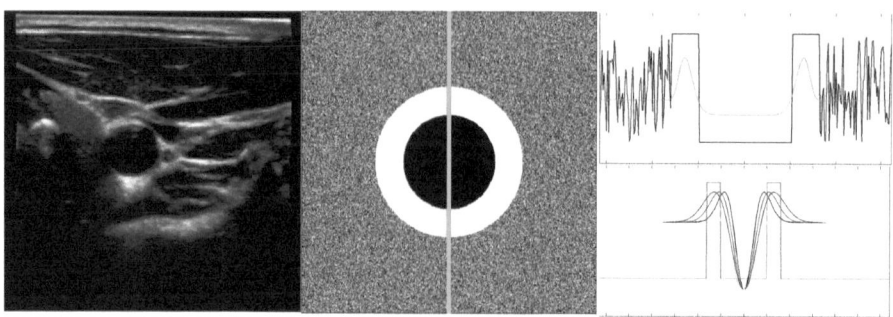

Fig. 1. Left: Common carotid artery cross-section; Middle: Ideal lumen cross-section with line segment overlaid; Right: Line segment of ideal lumen cross-section with $\frac{\partial^2}{\partial k^2}$ *kernel* overlaid: proposed kernel (top, in green), multiple attempts to fit the gaussian kernel (bottom; noise removed for better visualization)

Intensity Prior. We assume that the vessel lumen has a uniformly low US signal response (=dark), and is surrounded by higher signal response regions(=bright). For a given lumen radius r, the data smoothed with a Gaussian kernel with, e.g., $\sigma = 5r$, $smoothData_{IP}$ (IP = intensity prior) will still be dark at a centerline point, but brighter at lumen points closer to the lumen boundaries. So, to better distinguish centerline points from other lumen points, we propose the measure:

$$iPrior = \frac{1}{1 + ip \cdot smoothData_{IP}} \tag{8}$$

where $ip \geq 0$ guides this measure's importance. An added advantage is that bright regions, even with high values of λ_2 and λ_3, are also penalized.

Vessel Feature Assymetry. For the reasons described in section "Beam direction dependency", at a centerline point we also expect $\lambda_2 < \lambda_3$. But, we still expect $\frac{\lambda_2}{\lambda_3} >> 0$. Thus, we set a threshold $thresh_{quo}$ for acceptable values of $\frac{\lambda_2}{\lambda_3}$ and propose the compensated eigenvalue quotient measure:

$$cQuo = \begin{cases} 1 & \text{if } \frac{|\lambda_2|}{|\lambda_3|} \geq thresh_{quo} \\ \frac{\lambda_2}{\lambda_3} & \text{otherwise.} \end{cases} \tag{9}$$

We estimate a value for $thresh_{quo}$ experimentally (see "Parameter selection").

Remaining Statistics. Similar to Frangi in [3], we use a blobness measure:

$$R_B = \frac{|\lambda_1|}{\sqrt{|\lambda_2 \lambda_3|}} \tag{10}$$

and a measure of the relative significance of the information in the eigenvalues

$$S = \sqrt{|\lambda_2|^2 + |\lambda_3|^2} \tag{11}$$

New Overall Vesselness Measure. Our modified vesselness measure is:

$$vess = \begin{cases} 0 & \text{,if } (\lambda_2 \leq 0) \vee (\lambda_3 \leq 0) \\ iPrior \cdot BDD^\alpha \cdot cQuo^\beta \cdot e^{-\gamma R_B} \cdot (e^{\delta S} - 1) & \text{,otherwise} \end{cases} \quad (12)$$

3   Experiments and Results

Parameter selection $\alpha = 1$, $\beta = 1$ and $\gamma = 1$. For numerical stability reasons, we take $\delta = 0.1$. We choose ip so that the results are halved at very bright voxels: the data range is $[0, 255]$, so we take $ip = \frac{1}{255}$.

$thresh_{quo}$, should be as high as possible, but low enough to yield good results at lumen centerline points. We perform supervised learning on 15 manually segmented cross-section planes from 5 3D US carotid datasets. For each plane, we choose the highest value of $tresh_{quo}$ that maximizes the vesselness at the marked centerline point. We test 26 equally spaced possible values of $tresh_{quo}$ in $[0.01, 1]$. The average threshold obtained was 0.3921, the lowest threshold was 0.089. We select the first quartile as the threshold value, i.e. $thresh_{quo} = 0.2674$.

Comparison to Frangi Filter. We measure if the proposed modifications improve the algorithm's capability to distinguish centerline points (=high vesselness) from all other points. We manually segment 4 centerline points for each dataset and consider the statistic:

$$quality = \frac{\sum_{i=1}^{4} |vess(c_i) - \bar{X}_{vess}|}{\sigma_{vess}} \quad (13)$$

where c_i is a centerline point, $\bar{X}_{vess}$ is the average vesselness value and σ_{vess} the standard deviation of the vesselness. Higher values of $quality$ indicate a better capability to distinguish centerline points from the background.

The statistic is evaluated on 11 3D US carotid datasets. We mark 2 centerline points below and 2 above the bifurcation. We run 5 variations of the algorithm, adding a new feature for each variant: no modifications (as a proxy to the Frangi Filter); (+) the new kernel; (+) beam direction dependency; (+) intensity prior; (+) vessel feature assymetry. Results can be seen in figure 2.

4   Discussion and Conclusion

We proposed a novel TSD algorithm adapted to US imaging properties, based on Frangi's Hessian matrix based multiscale vesselness algorithm. We identified which assumptions of Frangi's original formulation are unsuitable for vascular US, adapted them and added new assumptions based on prior knowledge of the expected lumen shape and of the physics underlying US imaging.

We also used a non-Gaussian smoothing kernel in the context of a multiscale algorithm. Our good results suggest that there are viable alternatives to the

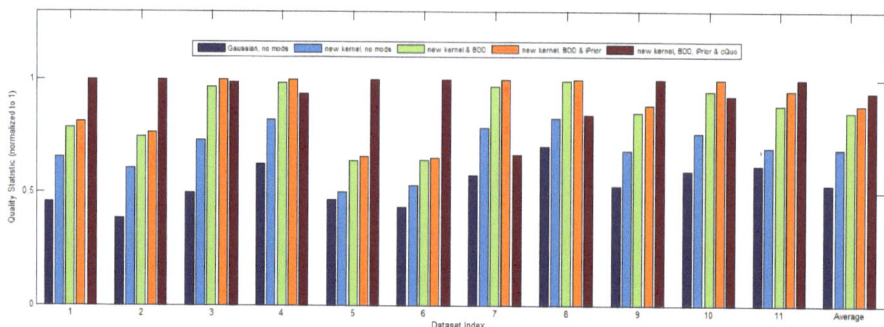

Fig. 2. *quality* statistic evaluated on 11 3D US carotid datasets; we tested 5 variations of the algorithm. Dark blue represents the results for the Frangi filter.

multiscale approach proposed in Lindeberg's work [6], especially if the expected shape of the feature of interest is already known.

All 4 modifications we proposed improved the algorithm's results, as measured by our *quality* statistic (see figure 2). The new kernel, the beam direction dependency and the intensity prior made the vesselness more stringent in general, while keeping the vesselness at centerline points unaltered. The vessel feature assymetry increased the vesselness at centerline points, but made the vesselness less stringent in general. While, on average, the results for this variant were better, significant decreases in the *quality* are possible (see datasets 7 and 8).

The algorithm can be parallelized extremely well. Using CUDA on a GTX 560ti, the computation time for 256^3 voxels was < 30 secs, per scale.

As our promising results show, the suggested changes are important contributions to the knowledge on vessel detection in 3D US, bringing us closer to a robust, fast (with GPUs) and fully automatic vessel tree detection and segmentation initialization algorithm, for clinical applications in the future.

References

1. Aylward, S., Bullitt, E.: Initialization, noise, singularities, and scale in height ridge traversal for tubular object centerline extraction. IEEE Transactions on Medical Imaging 21(2), 61–75 (2002)
2. Carvalho, D.D., Klein, S., Akkus, Z., ten Kate, G.L., Schinkel, A.F., Bosch, J.G., van der Lugt, A., Niessen, W.J.: Estimating 3D lumen centerlines of carotid arteries in free-hand acquisition ultrasound. Int. J. Comput. Assist. Radiol. Surg. 7(2), 207–215 (2012)
3. Frangi, A.F.: Three-Dimensional Model-Based Analysis of Vascular and Cardiac Images. Ph.D. thesis, Universiteit Utrecht (2001)
4. Guerrero, J., Salcudean, S.E., McEwen, J.A., Masri, B.A., Nicolaou, S.: Real-time vessel segmentation and tracking for ultrasound imaging applications. IEEE Trans. Med. Imaging 26(8), 1079–1090 (2007)

5. Krissian, K., Ellsmere, J., Vosburgh, K., Kikinis, R., Westin, C.F.: Multiscale Segmentation of the Aorta in 3D Ultrasound Images. In: 25th Annual Int. Conf. of the IEEE EMBS, pp. 638–641 (2003)
6. Lindeberg, T.: Scale-space theory: a basic tool for analyzing structures at different scales. Journal of Applied Statistics 21(1-2), 225–270 (1994)
7. Pock, T., Beichel, R., Bischof, H.: A Novel Robust Tube Detection Filter for 3D Centerline Extraction. In: Kalviainen, H., Parkkinen, J., Kaarna, A. (eds.) SCIA 2005. LNCS, vol. 3540, pp. 481–490. Springer, Heidelberg (2005)

Limited Angle C-Arm Tomography and Segmentation for Guidance of Atrial Fibrillation Ablation Procedures

Dirk Schäfer[1], Carsten Meyer[1], Roland Bullens[2],
Axel Saalbach[1], and Peter Eshuis[2]

[1] Philips Research, Röntgenstraße 24-26, 22335 Hamburg, Germany
[2] Philips Healthcare, Veenpluis 6, 5684 PC Best, The Netherlands
dirk.schaefer@philips.com

Abstract. Angiographic projections of the left atrium (LA) and the pulmonary veins (PV) acquired with a rotational C-arm system are used for 3D image reconstruction and subsequent automatic segmentation of the LA and PV to be used as roadmap in fluoroscopy guided LA ablation procedures. Acquisition of projections at high oblique angulations may be problematic due to increased collision danger of the detector with the right shoulder of the patient. We investigate the accuracy of image reconstruction and model based roadmap segmentation using limited angle C-arm tomography. The reduction of the angular range from 200° to 150° leads only to a moderate increase of the segmentation error from 1.5 mm to 2.0 mm if matched conditions are used in the segmentation, i.e. the model based segmentation is trained on images reconstructed with the same angular range as the test images. The minor decrease in accuracy may be outweighed by clinical workflow improvement, gained when large C-arm angulations can be avoided.

Keywords: Atrial fibrillation, ablation guidance, 3D roadmap.

1 Introduction

Electric isolation of the pulmonary veins (PV) by ablation is a standard procedure for treatment of atrial fibrillation (AF). Patient specific 3D surface models of the left atrium (LA) are used as roadmap overlay to support the fluoroscopy guided intervention. The roadmap can either be integrated from a segmentation of a pre-interventional CT or MR scan, or it can be generated directly on the C-arm system with a 3D Atriography scan (3D-ATG) [1]. A 3D-ATG acquisition consists of a rotational acquisition covering an angular range of 200 degree from 100° RAO (right anterior oblique) to 100° LAO (left anterior oblique). The left atrium and the pulmonary veins (LAPV) are filled with contrast agent and are positioned in the iso-center of the C-arm system. The acquired angiograms are used for 3D image reconstruction which is followed by automatic model based segmentation.

N. Ayache et al. (Eds.): MICCAI 2012, Part I, LNCS 7510, pp. 634–641, 2012.
© Springer-Verlag Berlin Heidelberg 2012

The patient is shifted asymmetrically to the right with respect to the C-arm system in order to position the LA in the iso-center. In this setup, the acquisition of the projections between $\approx 60°$RAO and $100°$RAO may be problematic due to increased collision danger of the detector with the patient shoulder.

Hence, reconstructions from a limited tomographic angle are desired. However, filtered back-projection (FBP) reconstructions from limited angles suffer from decreased sharpness and image blur along the direction perpendicular to the missing projection directions. This problem has been adressed using iterative reconstruction techniques with edge preserving regularization [2] or minimization of the total variation norm [3]. In the case of C-arm imaging additional problems arise due to the limited detector size and the lateral truncation of the projections. The incomplete projection data can be handeled in iterative algorithms by reconstructing very large image sizes [4], which is depreciated for interventional use due to time constraints. Furthermore iterative methods are known to be more sensitive to inconsistencies due to motion or varying contrast agent filling.

Therefore, we keep the FBP method and optimize the segmentation method with respect to the given clinical task. By focussing on the clinical needs Bachar et al. [5] showed e.g. for interventional head and neck C-arm imaging sufficient image quality in terms of the localization accuracy. They obtained a localization error of several features representing different contrast levels below 2.5 mm for tomographic angles $\geq 90°$ using standard FBP. In this work, we concentrate on the clinical need of delineation of the LA and PV combined with improved workflow of limited angle tomography. The issue of limited angle tomography is adressed by matched learning of the segmentation algorithm using standard FBP reconstruction. We investigate the accuracy of 3D-ATG image reconstruction and subsequent model based segmentation of the LAPV using rotational acquisitions with reduced angular ranges to minimize the collision danger and hence improve the clinical workflow. In particular, we present a detailed quantitative evaluation of the segmentation performance in matched and mismatched training and test conditions, acquired with different angular ranges.

2   Methods

2.1   3D Rotational Angiography

All intra-procedural imaging was performed using a flat-detector C-arm system (Allura Xper FD10, Philips Medical Systems, Inc., Best, The Netherlands). The contrast agent (CA) is either administered by a right-sided or a left sided injection. A right sided injection is performed by administration of CA into the right atrium (RA) or pulmonary artery (PA) with a delay of the X-ray scan of $3 - 5$ seconds by manual-triggering accounting for the time needed for the CA to arrive in the left atrium. A left sided injection is performed directly into the left atrium together with hyper-pacing or administration of adenosine to disable the pumping of the heart and maintain the CA inside the LA. During injection, patients were instructed to hold their breath at end-expiration until completion of the rotational run. The rotational X-ray data sets are acquired with 116 projections on $\approx 200°$ from $100°$ RAO to $100°$ LAO over 4 seconds at a sampling rate of 30 frames/s. For our investigation, we reduce the angular range of the acquisition by skipping some projections at the endings of the source trajectory.

2.2   Image Reconstruction

The flat detector is fixed at maximum distance from the X-ray source with a fan angle of $9°$ and rotated in propeller mode around the patient along a calibrated circular arc, which is parameterized by the path length $\lambda \in \Lambda$. The angular range Δ of the source path Λ covers $200°$ from $100°$ RAO to $100°$ LAO in the full acquisition and is symmetrically reduced to four different settings $\Delta = 170°, 150°, 130°, 110°$. The distance between source $\mathbf{S}$ and the detector center $\mathbf{D}$ is given by D. The normalized vector $\hat{\mathbf{d}}(\lambda)$ points from $\mathbf{D}(\lambda)$ to the source. The detector v-axis is parallel to the rotational axis and the u-axis is parallel to the trajectory tangent vector. The cone beam projection data of the object f_0 is denoted by $\mathcal{X}(u, v, \lambda)$:

$$\mathcal{X}(u, v, \lambda) = \int_0^\infty f_0(\mathbf{S}(\lambda) + l\hat{\mathbf{e}}(u, v, \lambda))\mathrm{d}l,$$

where $\hat{\mathbf{e}}(u, v, \lambda)$ is the unit vector from the source position $\mathbf{S}(\lambda)$ to the detector element $\mathbf{E}(u, v, \lambda)$. The corresponding length is denoted by $\overline{SE}$. The projection data is extended prior to filtering using the Lewitt-method to mitigate truncation artifacts. The 3D image f is reconstructed using cone-beam filtered back-projection [6]:

$$f(\mathbf{x}) = \int_\Lambda \frac{D}{|(\mathbf{x} - \mathbf{S}) \cdot \hat{\mathbf{d}}|^2} \int_{-\infty}^\infty w(\lambda, u') \frac{D}{\overline{SE}(\mathbf{x})} \mathcal{X}(u', v, \lambda)\, h_R(u - u')\, \mathrm{d}u'\mathrm{d}\lambda,$$

where h_R is the ramp filter and u, v are the detector coordinates of the forward projected point $\mathbf{x}$. The weighting function $w(\lambda, u)$ is given by the short scan Parker weights in case of $\Delta = 200°$. If Δ is reduced, w is given by $w = \frac{\pi}{\int_{\Lambda(\Delta)} \mathrm{d}\lambda}$ to correct for the decreasing brightness in the reconstructed image when using less projections.

2.3   Model Based Segmentation

We use a model-based segmentation framework developed for segmenting the left atrium and pulmonary veins [1]. Mesh adaptation is performed after initial automatic localization by iterating two steps until the mesh reaches a steady state [7]. First, boundaries are detected. Then, the mesh is deformed by minimizing the weighted sum of an external energy E_{ext} and an internal energy E_{int}. The external energy pulls the mesh to the detected boundaries. The internal energy penalizes deformations which deviate from a reference shape (e.g., mean shape) undergoing a geometric transformation (e.g., rigid or affine) accounting for pose and shape variability.

Image Intensity Calibration: To compensate for image intensity variations across images in 3D-ATG data, we compute the image histogram and determine the low and high 2% percentiles. The intensity values within the remaining histogram are then linearly re-scaled to a suitable reference interval, e.g., $[0, 1]$.

The LAPV + trachea model: We use a deforming mesh consisting of an LAPV part and a trachea part shown in Fig. 2. The trachea has been added to facilitate carina-based registration of the 3D model overlay to the live fluoroscopic projections during intervention [8]. The LAPV part represents the endocardial surface of the LA and the surface of the four main PV trunks. This mesh part is made of 1330 vertices which form 2717 triangles. The trachea part consists of 1076 nodes forming 2148 triangles. With this mesh topology, a reference (ground truth) mesh was obtained semi-automatically using a bootstrapping approach, i.e. a sequence of intermediate models was created based on a subset of the available volumes. Using these models, segmentations were obtained for each of the 57 3D-ATG data sets and then refined by a clinical expert by manual adaptation to match the observable image boundaries as closely as possible.

Multi-stage segmentation: A multi-stage adaptation framework is applied to increase robustness. The first step is the initialization of the barycenter of the model based on a generalized Hough transform (GHT) [9]. In a second step, the mesh is deformed parametrically, by applying individual similarity transformations for the LAPV and the trachea mesh parts to minimize the external energy E_{ext}. This compensates for pose misalignment as well as for variations in the relative orientation of the LAPV and the trachea between patients. Finally, a deformable adaptation step is performed as described above (including E_{int}) to account for more local variations of the patients anatomy.

Optimized Boundary Detection: Since vertex correspondence is preserved during mesh adaptation, we can assign a locally optimal boundary detection function to each mesh triangle using the Simulated Search approach [10]. Specifically, the magnitude of the image gradient (projected onto the triangle normal vector) together with several additional constraints on the gray values and image characteristics across the boundary are used for boundary detection. Suitable candidates for the constraints (e.g. gray values left or right of the boundary) and reasonable acceptance intervals for the constraints are estimated from the training images. The simulated search selects the optimal boundary detection function for each triangle from all candidates.

Assessment of Segmentation Accuracy and Mesh Comparison: The segmentation accuracy is assessed by measuring the Euclidean surface-to-patch distance $\epsilon_{i,n}$ between the automatic segmentation of the 3D-ATG data and the corresponding reference mesh. $\epsilon_{i,n}$ is defined as the distance between triangle center i of the adapted 3D-ATG mesh for patient n to an anatomically corresponding patch of maximum geodesic radius $r = 10\,\mathrm{mm}$ of the reference mesh and vice versa [7]. Averaging over triangles i gives the error ϵ_n per patient, and further averaging over the 57 patients gives the mean error ϵ_{mean}. The triangle positions near the artificial cut-planes which define the distal bounds of the truncated pulmonary veins and those of the trachea are excluded from the error measurement [11].

3   Results

In this study, 57 rotational ATG data sets have been used, which were acquired at three different clinical sites in Europe and the USA according to the protocol described in Section 2.1.Each data set has been reconstructed by restricting the projections to the 5 different angular ranges $\Delta =200°,170°,150°,130°,110°$. For each angular range Δ, a separate model for automatic segmentation has been generated, i.e. optimal boundary detection features and a GHT (see Sec. 2.3) have been trained on the corresponding reconstructed images. For training and evaluation of the model, 10-fold cross-validation has been used. In addition, each trained model has been evaluated on the reconstructions of the corresponding test patients with the other angular ranges, to assess the effect of a mismatch between the angular range used in training and testing. A summary of the mean segmentation error ϵ_{mean} with respect to the reference meshes (see Sec. 2.3) for the various scenarios is given in Table 1 and visualized in Fig. 1.

Table 1. Average segmentation error ϵ_{mean} of the whole mesh in [mm] for various training and test angular ranges

			Test on		
Training on	200°	170°	150°	130°	110°
200°	*1.51*	1.61	2.53	4.35	5.82
170°	**1.48**	**1.59**	2.41	3.86	5.30
150°	1.59	1.66	**1.98**	3.33	4.86
130°	2.11	1.86	2.05	*3.00*	3.58
110°	1.98	1.92	2.24	**2.94**	**3.22**

For each angular range used for reconstructing the test image, the optimal training model (leading to the minimal test error) is highlighted by bold numbers in Table 1. For three angular ranges ($\Delta = 170°,150°,110°$), this minimal error is obtained for matched conditions, i.e., a model trained on the same angular range as used in the test. For the remaining two ranges the difference to the minimal error is very small (bold and italic numbers). In the case of train and test with 200°, the segmentation error of 1.5 mm is similar to other published results [1][12].

The following conclusions can be drawn: First, a reduction of the angular range from 200° to 170° has — if at all — only a minimal influence on the segmentation performance (from 1.5 mm to 1.6 mm). Second, if smaller angular ranges ($<$ 170°) are used in the test images, segmentation performance decreases significantly (Figure 1). Better segmentation performance can be obtained by using a segmentation model trained in matched conditions, i.e., on images reconstructed with the same angular range as the test image. Thereby, for 150° reconstructions, a segmentation error of about 2 mm is obtained. Third, these findings hold for the whole LAPV plus trachea mesh, but also for the individual anatomical structures of the mesh, as shown in Table 2. Fourth, if the reconstruction angle is further reduced to 130° or 110°, a segmentation error of about 3 mm is obtained in matched conditions. Models trained on low reconstruction angles are generally more robust in mismatched test conditions, while not being optimal for large reconstruction angles.

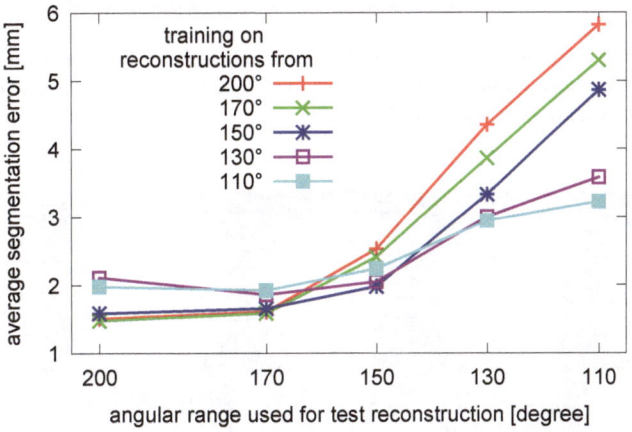

Fig. 1. Average segmentation error ϵ_{mean} of the whole mesh for various training and test angular ranges

Table 2. Average segmentation error of the individual mesh parts in [mm] for various training and test angular ranges

	Test on 200°			Test on 170°			Test on 150°		
	Train: 200°	Train: 170°	Train: 150°	Train: 200°	Train: 170°	Train: 150°	Train: 200°	Train: 170°	Train: 150°
Whole mesh	1.51	**1.48**	1.59	1.61	**1.59**	1.66	2.53	2.41	**1.98**
Left atrium	1.58	**1.49**	1.61	1.74	**1.63**	1.76	2.17	2.30	**2.04**
Inf. Left PV	**1.87**	1.88	2.00	1.99	**1.83**	1.88	2.65	2.81	**2.20**
Inf. Right PV	1.87	**1.81**	1.94	1.85	1.85	**1.77**	2.33	2.60	**2.31**
Sup. Left PV	1.41	**1.38**	1.65	1.65	**1.41**	1.70	2.11	2.13	**2.08**
Sup. Right PV	1.67	**1.65**	1.68	1.73	**1.61**	1.63	1.99	1.93	**1.84**
Trachea	**1.35**	1.36	1.46	**1.38**	1.51	1.52	3.00	2.55	**1.86**

These findings are also confirmed by visual inspection of the mesh outline as overlay on angiograms (Fig. 2) and slices of the reconstructed images (Fig. 3). The decreasing depth resolution in anterior-posterior direction can be observed in the transaxial slices for $\Delta = 130°, 110°$ resulting in mesh deformations and larger segmentation errors.

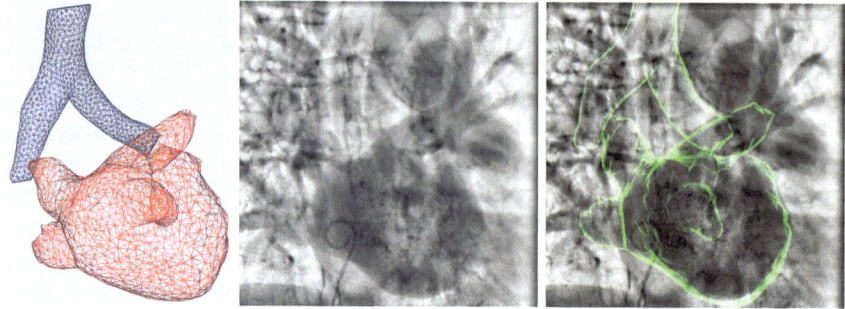

Fig. 2. Oblique view on the joint LAPV and trachea model as wire rendering (left), angiogram of the case shown in Fig. 3 post-processed by local contrast enhancement (middle), and overlay of corresponding adapted model trained on 200° (right)

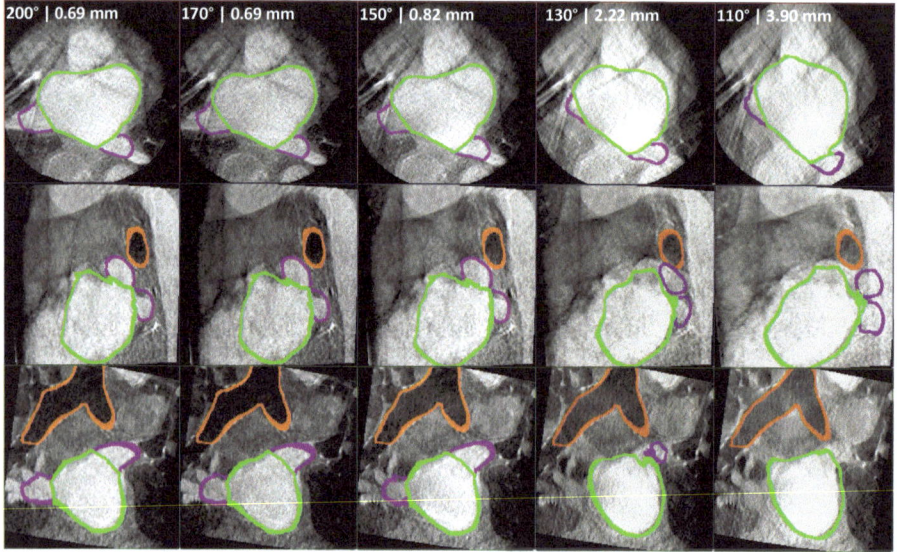

Fig. 3. Example overlay of segmentation results on the corresponding test data reconstructions using the trained model from 150° with 10-fold cross-correlation. Transaxial slices (top), sagittal (middle), coronal (bottom). In the top row the angular range Δ and the error ϵ_{mean} is given for the corresponding column.

4   Summary and Conclusions

A reduction of the angular range from 200° to 170° has only a minimal influence on the segmentation performance (from 1.5mm to 1.6mm). If smaller angular ranges are used in the test images, the decrease in segmentation performance can be partly compensated by using a segmentation model trained in matched conditions. Thereby, for 150° reconstructions, a segmentation error of about 2 mm is obtained. Hence, accepting this minor decrease in segmentation performance, the clinical workflow can be substantially simplified by avoiding large C-arm angulations between 60° RAO and 100° RAO.

References

1. Manzke, R., Meyer, C., Ecabert, O., Peters, J., Noordhoek, N.J., Thiagalingam, A., Reddy, V.Y., Chan, R.C., Weese, J.: Automatic Segmentation of Rotational X-Ray Images for Anatomic Intra-Procedural Surface Generation in Atrial Fibrillation Ablation Procedures. IEEE Trans. Med. Imag. 29(2), 260–272 (2010)
2. Delaney, A.H., Bresler, Y.: Globally Convergent Edge-Preserving Regularized Reconstruction: An Application to Limited-Angle Tomography. IEEE Trans. Imag. Proc. 7(2), 204–221 (1998)
3. Persson, M., Bone, D., Elmqvist, H.: Total variation norm for three-dimensional iterative reconstruction in limited view angle tomography. Phys. Med. Biol. 46, 853–866 (2001)
4. Snyder, D.L., O'Sullivan, J.A., Murphy, R.J., Politte, D.G., Whiting, B.R., Williamson, J.F.: Image reconstruction for transmission tomography when projection data are incomplete. Phys. Med. Biol. 51, 5603–5619 (2006)
5. Bachar, G., Siewerdsen, J.H., Daly, M.J., Jaffray, D.A., Irish, J.C.: Image quality and localization accuracy in C-arm tomosynthesis-guided head and neck surgery. Med. Phys. 34, 4664–4677 (2007)
6. Feldkamp, L., Davis, L., Kress, J.: Practical cone-beam algorithm. J. Opt. Soc. Am. A 1, 612–619 (1984)
7. Ecabert, O., Peters, J., Schramm, H., Lorenz, C., von Berg, J., Walker, M., Vembar, M., Olszewski, M., Subramanyan, K., Lavi, G., Weese, J.: Automatic model-based segmentation of the heart in CT images. IEEE Trans. Med. Imag. 27(9), 1189–1201 (2008)
8. Li, J.H., Haim, M., Movassaghi, B., Mendel, J.B., Chaudhry, G.M., Haffajee, C.I., Orlov, M.V.: Segmentation and registration of three-dimensional rotational angiogram on live fluoroscopy to guide atrial fibrillation ablation: A new online imaging tool. Heart Rhythm 6(2), 231–237 (2009)
9. Saalbach, A., Wächter-Stehle, I., Kneser, R., Mollus, S., Peters, J., Weese, J.: Optimizing GHT-Based Heart Localization in an Automatic Segmentation Chain. In: Fichtinger, G., Martel, A., Peters, T. (eds.) MICCAI 2011, Part III. LNCS, vol. 6893, pp. 463–470. Springer, Heidelberg (2011)
10. Peters, J., Ecabert, O., Meyer, C., Kneser, R., Weese, J.: Optimizing boundary detection via Simulated Search with applications to multi-modal heart segmentation. Medical Image Analysis 14(1), 70–84 (2010)
11. Meyer, C., Manzke, R., Peters, J., Ecabert, O., Kneser, R., Reddy, V.Y., Chan, R.C., Weese, J.: Automatic Intra-operative Generation of Geometric Left Atrium/Pulmonary Vein Models from Rotational X-Ray Angiography. In: Metaxas, D., Axel, L., Fichtinger, G., Székely, G. (eds.) MICCAI 2008, Part II. LNCS, vol. 5242, pp. 61–69. Springer, Heidelberg (2008)
12. Zheng, Y., Wang, T., John, M., Zhou, S.K., Boese, J., Comaniciu, D.: Multi-part Left Atrium Modeling and Segmentation in C-Arm CT Volumes for Atrial Fibrillation Ablation. In: Fichtinger, G., Martel, A., Peters, T. (eds.) MICCAI 2011, Part III. LNCS, vol. 6893, pp. 487–495. Springer, Heidelberg (2011)

Automatic Non-rigid Temporal Alignment of IVUS Sequences

Marina Alberti[1,2], Simone Balocco[1,2], Xavier Carrillo[3],
Josepa Mauri[3], and Petia Radeva[1,2,*]

[1] Dept. of Applied Mathematics and Analysis, University of Barcelona, Spain
[2] Computer Vision Center, Campus UAB, Bellaterra, Barcelona, Spain
[3] University Hospital "Germans Trias i Pujol", Badalona, Spain
malberti@cvc.uab.es

Abstract. Clinical studies on atherosclerosis regression/progression performed by Intravascular Ultrasound analysis require the alignment of pullbacks of the same patient before and after clinical interventions. In this paper, a methodology for the automatic alignment of IVUS sequences based on the Dynamic Time Warping technique is proposed. The method is adapted to the specific IVUS alignment task by applying the non-rigid alignment technique to multidimensional morphological signals, and by introducing a sliding window approach together with a regularization term. To show the effectiveness of our method, an extensive validation is performed both on synthetic data and *in-vivo* IVUS sequences. The proposed method is robust to stent deployment and post dilation surgery and reaches an alignment error of approximately 0.7 *mm* for *in-vivo* data, which is comparable to the inter-observer variability.

1 Introduction

Intravascular Ultrasound (IVUS) is a catheter-based imaging technique used for diagnostic purposes and for planning and validation of Percutaneous Coronary Intervention (PCI). IVUS sequences are acquired by dragging an ultrasound emitter carried by a catheter, at constant speed, inside the arterial vessel, from the distal to the proximal position (pullbacks). The image alignment of the same vessel from different IVUS pullbacks is important from a clinical viewpoint. After performing PCI, frame alignment allows physicians to assess the intervention outcome (i.e., evaluate final lumen dimensions and blood flow restoration, detect stent malapposition and inspect side-branch occlusion by deployed stent). At follow-up, it is crucial to monitor restenosis and the evolution of plaque composition. Currently, in plaque regression studies, the longitudinal correspondence of coronary artery segments is manually determined by identifying common landmarks, such as bifurcations [1, 2]. To our knowledge, no method for the automatic alignment of IVUS sequences has been published in literature.

---

* This work is supported by TIN2009-14404-C02 and CONSOLIDER INGENIO CSD 2007-00018.

N. Ayache et al. (Eds.): MICCAI 2012, Part I, LNCS 7510, pp. 642–650, 2012.

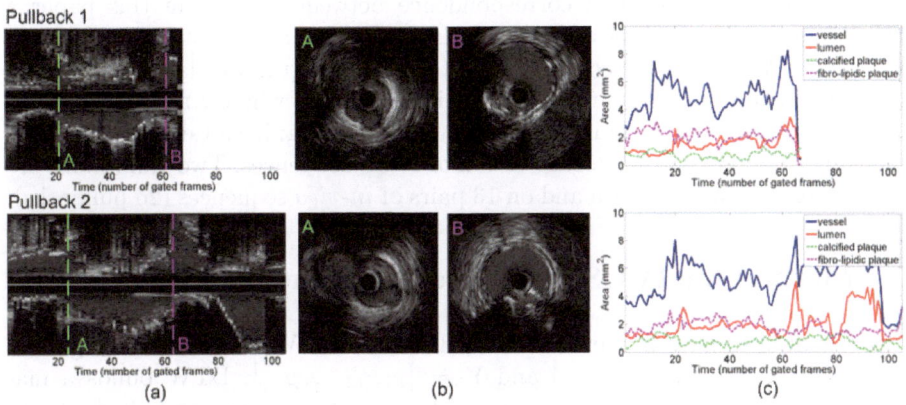

Fig. 1. Pair of IVUS sequences of the same vessel: (a) longitudinal views, (b) corresponding frames, (c) temporal signals describing the pullbacks

Despite the constant catheter speed, an automatic alignment is hampered by several obstacles: (1) the heart beating causes a non-rigid deformation of the vessel, (2) the catheter and the heart motion generate acquisition artifacts, such as the catheter longitudinal swinging and the roto-translation of successive frames (see Figure 1(b)), (3) the catheter can follow different trajectories inside the vessel, therefore the acquired image sections might not be orthogonal to the vessel walls, (4) the probe can remain stuck in the vessel for some time and then accelerate, (5) different initial and end spatial positions of the pullbacks cause partial overlapping (see Figure 1(a)) and (6) the vessel morphology can significantly change after the intervention or evolve at follow-up. Consequently, there is no one-to-one correspondence between frames of the two pullbacks, thus making image-based alignment approaches inaccurate. Hence, instead of using an image-based description, in this study the morphological content of the artery is exploited. IVUS sequences can be described by temporal morphological signals, i.e., side-branch location, vessel, lumen and plaque areas (see Figure 1(c)). Thus, the IVUS alignment task is addressed as a temporal alignment problem.

In different applications, such as speech recognition, activity recognition, shape matching, several methods have been developed for non-rigid signal alignment, like Dynamic Time Warping (DTW), Canonical Time Warping (CTW) and Correlation Optimized Warping (COW) [3–5]. DTW [3] minimizes the Euclidean distance of corresponding points of the signals. Canonical Time Warping (CTW) [4] improves DTW by combining it with Canonical Correlation Analysis (CCA), thus adding a feature weighting mechanism. The optimization process requires the application of CCA at successive iterations. Correlation Optimized Warping (COW) [5] is a piecewise data alignment method which allows limited changes in segment lengths and performs a segment-wise correlation optimization by means of dynamic programming.

To address the non-rigid correspondence between frames, in this paper a DTW-based framework is adapted to the specific clinical task and compared vs. the CTW and COW techniques. To tackle the partial overlapping problem, the alignment algorithms are integrated into a sliding window approach. Moreover, a regularization term is introduced to penalize significant differences in the global temporal expansion/compression of IVUS sequences. Two validations are presented, on synthetic data and on 13 pairs of *in-vivo* sequences (26 pullbacks).

2   Method for IVUS Sequences Alignment

The signal alignment framework is based on the DTW technique. To align two sequences $X = [x_1, x_2, \ldots x_{n_x}]$ and $Y = [y_1, y_2, \ldots y_{n_y}]$, DTW builds a matrix $d_{(n_x \times n_y)}$, where $d(i, j)$ ($1 \leq i \leq n_x; 1 \leq j \leq n_y$) represents a dissimilarity measure between $X(i)$ and $Y(j)$ [3]. In the classical DTW formulation, $d(i, j)$ is computed as the Euclidean distance $d_E(i, j)$. Successively, the algorithm finds the *warping path* (i.e., a mapping of the time axes of X and Y on a common time axis, $\mathbf{f} = \langle [i(k), j(k)] \, | k = 1, \ldots, K \rangle$) with the minimum cumulative distance (MCD). The MCD of the path leading to the entry (i, j) is computed by dynamic programming as: $D(i, j) = d(i, j) + min(D(i - 1, j), D(i - 1, j - 1), D(i, j - 1))$. Finally, the *matching cost* is calculated as $\Phi(X, Y) = \underset{\mathbf{f}}{argmin} \sum_{k=1}^{K} d(i(k), j(k))$.

2.1   Multidimensional Profiles Extraction

Profile Framework: A pair of corresponding IVUS sequences is described by temporal morphological profiles (i.e., signals describing the evolution of morphological measurements along the vessel) and defined as a pair of time series $X \in \mathbb{R}^{m \times n_x}$ and $Y \in \mathbb{R}^{m \times n_y}$, of length n_x, n_y and dimensionality m. The profiles are invariant to frame rotation, thus making the method independent from the catheter torsion. The use of multiple features is aimed to increase the robustness with respect to 1-D alignment. The following morphological measurements are proposed in this study: (1) vessel area, defined as the area inside the media-adventitia border [6], (2) lumen area [7], (3) area of calcified plaque [8], (4) area of fibro-lipidic plaque [8], (5) angular extension of bifurcations [9]. It is worth noticing that the framework could potentially provide similar results using a different set of profiles and it is independent from the technique employed for the measurements.

Gating Preprocessing: To limit the morphological variations due to vessel pulsation and catheter swinging effect, an image-based gating algorithm [10] is applied to the pullbacks in order to select the frames belonging to the end-diastolic phase. The selected images provide coherent morphological measures, since the arterial tissues are subject to the same blood pressure. Moreover, the preprocessing assures that the frames are consecutive in the direction of the catheter movement.

2.2   IVUS Alignment Framework

Sliding Window (SW) Approach: The DTW approach suffers from a limitation: it attempts to compute a global matching between all the frames of the two sequences, even in presence of partial overlapping (see Figure 1(a)). Hence, the alignment algorithm is integrated into a sliding window approach. The two sequences are iteratively slided one along the other and for each step the alignment between the overlapping subsegments is identified. The optimal iteration is selected by minimizing a *matching cost* $\Phi_{NORM}(X_{iter}, Y_{iter}) = \Phi(X_{iter}, Y_{iter})/l_{iter}$, where X_{iter} and Y_{iter} are the overlapping subsegments and l_{iter} is the length of the overlapping window at iteration *iter*. In order to decrease the computational cost, the allowed overlap ranges from $n_s - w_{elast}$ to n_s, where n_s is the length of the shortest sequence.

Regularization Cost (RC): In the classical version of DTW [3], an arbitrary *band constraint* is employed to guide the *warping path* by limiting its acceptable domain to a band around the diagonal of the dissimilarity matrix d. In this paper, a regularization term, described by a continuous formulation, is introduced to favor *warping paths* closer to the diagonal. Such improvement automatically penalizes an excessive and non-physiological compression/expansion of the two sequences. In the $DTW+SW$ framework, the dissimilarity measure $d(i,j)$ is computed as: $d(i,j) = d_E(i,j) + w_R \cdot d_R(i,j)$, where $d_R(i,j) = |i - j|$ is the *regularization cost* (see Figure 2(d)) and w_R represents the penalization weight. The regularization is aimed to reduce the alignment error when the profiles are affected by noise corruption, as shown in Figure 2(a)-(c).

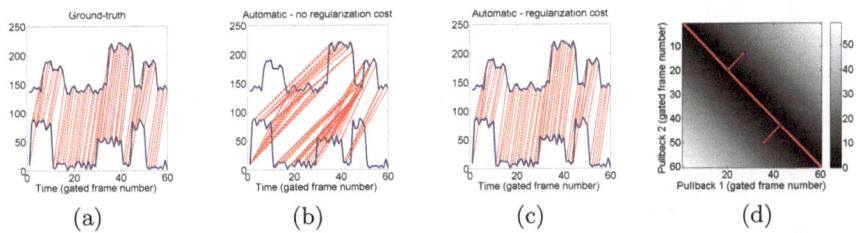

(a)   (b)   (c)   (d)

Fig. 2. Example of alignment of noise-corrupted signals. In (b) incorrect alignment by classical DTW, in (c) correct alignment by applying RC, in (d) *regularization cost* matrix d_R, where the red arrows indicate the penalization increase. In (a), (b), (c), blue lines represent the signals and red lines represent correspondences between frames.

3   Experimental Results

Our dataset consists of 26 *in-vivo* IVUS sequences from human coronary arteries. The acquisitions have been performed both preoperatively and after intervention (stent deployment, post dilation), by using an iLab IVUS Imaging System (Boston Scientific). The performance of DTW is fairly compared with two other *state-of-the-art* techniques, CTW and COW, (1) adapting the classical formulation to multidimensional signals, using the same weight for the different features, (2) integrating into the SW approach and (3) additionally applying the regularization term $(SW+RC)$. It is worth noticing that both DTW and CTW are fully automatic, while COW requires the setting of two parameters, the initial segment length *Seg* and the maximum segment length variation *Slack*. Additionally, two new parameters related to the developed IVUS framework are introduced for each alignment method, w_{elast} and w_R, for SW and RC, respectively. The *alignment error* E is defined as the average distance between the reference and the output *warping path*, expressed in number of gated frames.

3.1   Experiments on Synthetic Data

Synthetic Morphological Signals: Pairs of sequences (X, Y) are synthetically generated by modifying the morphological profiles extracted from the 26 *in-vivo* pullbacks. The scheme in Figure 3 summarizes the applied types of distortion:

1. Amplitude distortion: additive zero-mean random noise is applied to the morphological profiles. The noise amplitude w_1 is computed as a percentage of the mean value of the signal (Figure 3(a)).
2. Partial overlapping: a portion of the original sequence is selected, whose length is a percentage w_2 of the initial profile (Figure 3(b)).
3. Temporal distortion: a temporal expansion/compression generates vertical or horizontal transitions in the *warping path*, i.e., multiple correspondences between the frames of X and Y. We distinguish three cases, in which we randomly introduce: (a) the same number (w_3) of multiple correspondences from X to Y and vice-versa (Figure 3(c)); (b) additional multiple correspondences from X to Y (Figure 3(d)); (c) additional multiple correspondences from Y to X (Figure 3(e)).

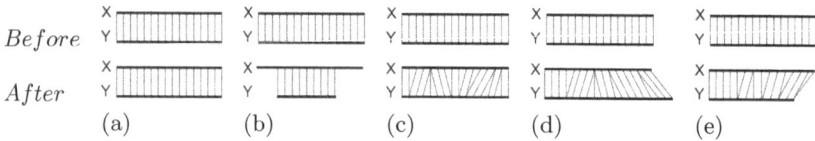

$$\begin{array}{ccccc} & (a) & (b) & (c) & (d) & (e) \end{array}$$

Fig. 3. Idealized pairs of sequences (X, Y) (continuous lines), and frame-to-frame correspondences (dotted lines), before and after the distortion simulation

The parameters w_1, w_2, w_3, w_4, w_5 model the signal distortion simulation. Their default values and ranges, which represent average *in-vivo* conditions and realistic variations, respectively, are suggested by a medical expert and empirically measured on the whole ground-truth: $w_1 = (100 \pm 100)\%$, $w_2 = (75 \pm 25)\%$, $w_3 = 60\ (0-120)$ frames, $w_4 = 5\ (0-15)$ frames, $w_5 = 0\ (0-15)$ frames. The tuning of the parameters of the alignment methods, $w_{elast}, w_R, Seg, Slack$, is performed by minimizing the mean of E over $N_{iter} = 40$ experiments, setting

Table 1. Quantitative results ($MEAN \pm STD$) for E on synthetic data, as a function of m, and on *in-vivo* data. For the *in-vivo* experiments, bifurcation profiles are not used.

	Synthetic					In − vivo
	$m = 1$	$m = 2$	$m = 3$	$m = 4$	$m = 5$	$m = 4$
DTW	9.21 ± 9.28	4.37 ± 3.89	2.78 ± 2.85	1.88 ± 0.93	1.5 ± 0.58	3 ± 2.68
DTW + SW	7.05 ± 9.31	3.38 ± 4.84	2.04 ± 3.49	1.21 ± 0.68	0.96 ± 0.5	3.29 ± 5.16
DTW + SW + RC	3.98 ± 5.09	1.98 ± 1.65	1.37 ± 0.71	1.1 ± 0.51	$\mathbf{0.93 \pm 0.44}$	1.43 ± 0.68
CTW	9.57 ± 9.39	4.33 ± 3.72	2.79 ± 2.3	2.14 ± 0.93	1.8 ± 0.74	3.94 ± 3.91
CTW + SW	6.59 ± 8.95	2.62 ± 2.48	1.76 ± 0.91	1.38 ± 0.66	1.06 ± 0.47	2.54 ± 1.96
CTW + SW + RC	5.72 ± 7.75	2.29 ± 2.2	1.64 ± 0.99	1.29 ± 0.57	$\mathbf{1.07 \pm 0.46}$	1.62 ± 0.82
COW	8.77 ± 3.91	9.69 ± 3.86	9.71 ± 4.02	9.85 ± 4.29	9.7 ± 4.34	7.54 ± 5.61
COW + SW	4.4 ± 5.31	2.6 ± 1.38	2.35 ± 1.07	2.36 ± 1.01	2.41 ± 0.93	2.68 ± 1.71
COW + SW + RC	4.4 ± 5.17	2.53 ± 1.48	2.24 ± 0.89	2.21 ± 0.92	2.3 ± 1.22	$\mathbf{2.46 \pm 1.5}$
inter − observer						$\mathbf{1.2 \pm 1.41}$

the distortion parameters to default values. The parameters are estimated by exhaustive search: $w_{elast} \in [0, 35]$, $w_R \in [0, 0.003]$ for DTW/CTW, $w_R \in [0, 0.1]$ for COW, $Seg \in [16, 30]$ and $Slack \in [6, Seg - 9]$.

Relevance of the Multidimensional Alignment: In order to evaluate the robustness of the framework as a function of the number of morphological profiles, E is computed over $N_{iter} = 40$ experiments, for $m = 1, \ldots, 5$. Pairs of synthetic signals are generated by setting w_1, w_2, w_3, w_4, w_5 to default values. As expected, Table 1 shows that E decreases as m increases. The error reduction is particularly high when more than one signal are considered, confirming the interest of a multidimensional extension of the method.

Feature Relevance Estimation: From the previous experiment, the relevance of the different morphological profiles is assessed. To this aim, the feature occurrence in the *optimal* feature combinations, minimizing E, is determined. The following rank for relevance is obtained: (1) calcified plaque area, (2) bifurcation extension, (3) fibro-lipidic plaque area, (4) lumen area, (5) vessel area.

Robustness to Signal Noise and Distortion: In the second set of experiments, the robustness to noise and distortion is evaluated (see Figure 4). When one of the distortion parameters is varied in the chosen range, the others are set to default values. This experiment demonstrates that the SW approach is useful since DTW, CTW and COW are robust to partial overlapping only when integrated in the SW framework (see Figure 4 (first row, middle)). SW and RC are generally advantageous (see Figure 4 (first row)) except when w_4 and w_5 are very high (see Figure 4 (second row)). COW always shows the highest error, indicating that a segment-wise alignment is not suited for the IVUS problem.

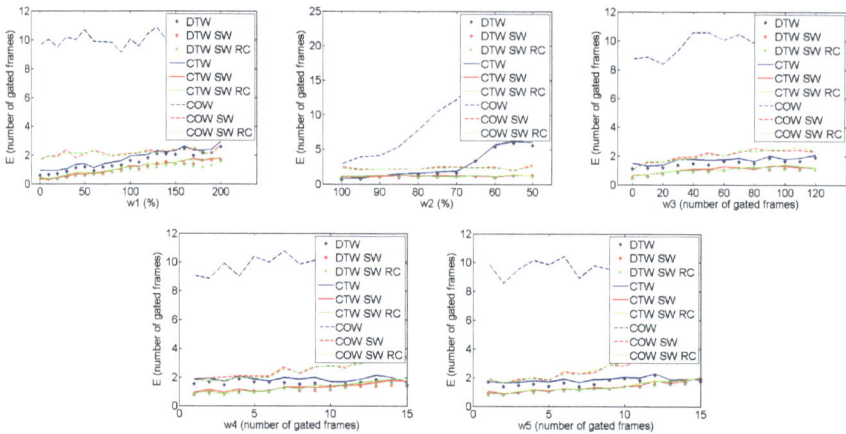

Fig. 4. E as a function of amplitude distortion (w_1), partial overlapping (w_2), temporal distortions (w_3, w_4, w_5)

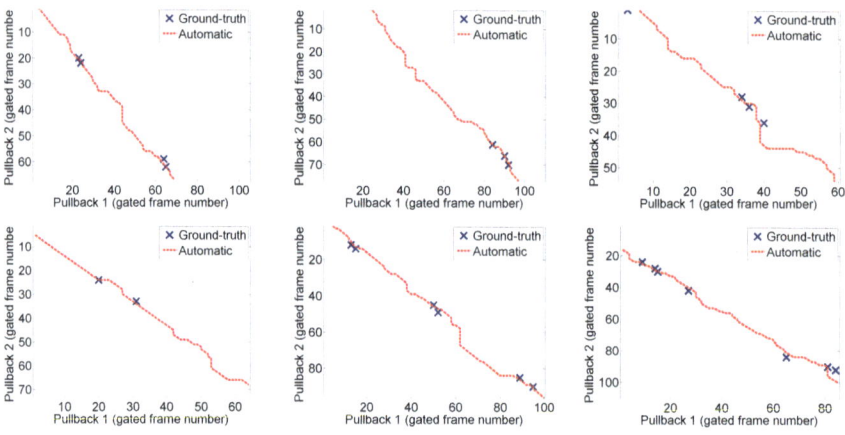

Fig. 5. Ground-truth and automatic *warping path* , computed by $DTW+SW+RC$

3.2 Experiments on In-vivo Data

The performance of the proposed approach is evaluated over 13 pairs of corresponding pullbacks, all characterized by morphological changes due to intervention. Following the same strategy employed in [1], corresponding bifurcation locations (initial and end positions) are used as ground-truth. Manual annotations are performed by two physicians. Indeed side branches are the only immutable landmarks, since lumen and media size, stent and plaque might vary due to surgical artery dilatation or stent deployment. Hence, in this experiment, the signal of bifurcation extension is excluded from the alignment framework. The parameter tuning is performed by means of *Leave-One-Patient-Out* (LOPO) technique: given the number of correspondences, one of them is iteratively used as test set, and the parameters are optimized by minimizing E over all the other correspondances. As observed in Table 1 (seventh column), the $SW+RC$ framework always reaches the lowest error. The Wilcoxon test proves that with a significance level $\alpha = 0.1$, the performance of $DTW+SW+RC$ is significantly better than $COW+SW+RC$ and comparable to $CTW+SW+RC$ and to the inter-observer variability. The mean value for E by $DTW+SW+RC$ - 1.43 gated frames - can be estimated around 0.7 mm. In Figure 5, ground-truth and output *warping paths* for pairs of corresponding pullbacks are illustrated. The only significant errors are close to the extremes of the sliding window (Figure 5 (third column)).

4   Discussion and Conclusion

This paper presents, for the first time, a fully automatic framework for the temporal alignment of IVUS pullbacks. The proposed method is robust to morphological changes induced by stent deployment and post dilation, and is invariant to the catheter or imaging system employed. Extensive experiments show that the use of multiple morphological profiles along with the sliding window approach and regularization term enhance the result. Future work will address the application of this framework on intra-modality alignments, for instance, IVUS and Optical Coherence Tomography sequences. Furthermore, the proposed method will be evaluated on follow up cases. Finally, the application of feature weights based on the feature relevance will be investigated.

References

1. Diletti, R., Garcia-Garcia, H.M., Gomez-Lara, J., Brugaletta, S., Wykrzykowska, J.J., van Ditzhuijzen, N., van Geuns, R.J., Regar, E., Ambrosio, G., Serruys, P.W.: Assessment of coronary atherosclerosis progression and regression at bifurcations using combined ivus and oct. JACC Cardiovasc. Imaging 4, 774–780 (2011)
2. Kovarnik, T., Wahle, A., Downe, R.W., Sonka, M.: IVUS Role in Studies Assessing Atherosclerosis Development. In: Intrvascular Ultrasound, pp. 53–68. InTech (2012)
3. Sakoe, H., Chiba, S.: Dynamic programming algorithm optimization for spoken word recognition. IEEE TASSP 26, 43–49 (1978)
4. Zhou, F., de la Torre, F.: Canonical time warping for alignment of human behavior. In: NIPS, pp. 2286–2294 (2009)
5. Nielsen, N.P.V., Carstensen, J.M., Smedsgaard, J.: Aligning of single and multiple wavelength chromatographic profiles for chemometric data analysis using correlation optimised warping. Journal of Chromatography 805, 17–35 (1998)
6. Ciompi, F., Pujol, O., Gatta, C., Carrillo, X., Mauri, J., Radeva, P.: A *Holistic* Approach for the Detection of Media-Adventitia Border in IVUS. In: Fichtinger, G., Martel, A., Peters, T. (eds.) MICCAI 2011, Part III. LNCS, vol. 6893, pp. 411–419. Springer, Heidelberg (2011)
7. Balocco, S., Gatta, C., Ciompi, F., Pujol, O., Carrillo, X., Mauri, J., Radeva, P.: Combining Growcut and Temporal Correlation for IVUS Lumen Segmentation. In: Vitrià, J., Sanches, J.M., Hernández, M. (eds.) IbPRIA 2011. LNCS, vol. 6669, pp. 556–563. Springer, Heidelberg (2011)

8. Ciompi, F., Pujol, O., Gatta, C., Leor, O.R., Ferre, J.M., Radeva, P.: Fusing in-vitro and in.vivo intravascular ultrasound data for plaque characterization. International Journal of Cardiovascular Imaging 26, 763–779 (2010)

9. Alberti, M., Gatta, C., Balocco, S., Ciompi, F., Pujol, O., Silva, J., Carrillo, X., Radeva, P.: Automatic Branching Detection in IVUS Sequences. In: Vitrià, J., Sanches, J.M., Hernández, M. (eds.) IbPRIA 2011. LNCS, vol. 6669, pp. 126–133. Springer, Heidelberg (2011)

10. Gatta, C., Balocco, S., Ciompi, F., Hemetsberger, R., Leor, O.R., Radeva, P.: Real-Time Gating of IVUS Sequences Based on Motion Blur Analysis: Method and Quantitative Validation. In: Jiang, T., Navab, N., Pluim, J.P.W., Viergever, M.A. (eds.) MICCAI 2010, Part II. LNCS, vol. 6362, pp. 59–67. Springer, Heidelberg (2010)

Stochastic 3D Motion Compensation of Coronary Arteries from Monoplane Angiograms

Jonathan Hadida*, Christian Desrosiers, and Luc Duong

École de Technologie Supérieure, 1100 Notre-Dame Ouest, Montréal, Canada
jonathan.hadida.1@ens.etsmtl.ca,
{christian.desrosiers,luc.duong}@etsmtl.ca

Abstract. Image-based navigation during percutaneous coronary interventions is highly challenging since it involves estimating the 3D motion of a complex topology using 2D angiographic views. A static coronary tree segmented in a pre-operative CT-scan can be overlaid on top of the angiographic frames to outline the coronary vessels, but this overlay does not account for coronary motion, which has to be mentally compensated by the cardiologist. In this paper, we propose a new approach to the motion estimation problem, where the temporal evolution of the coronary deformation over the cardiac cycle is modeled as a stochastic process. The sequence of angiographic frames is interpreted as a probabilistic evidence of the succession of unknown deformation states, which can be optimized using particle filtering. Iterative and non-rigid registration is performed in a projective manner, and relies on a feature-based similarity measure. Experiments show promising results in terms of registration accuracy, learning capability and computation time.

1 Introduction

Percutaneous coronary intervention (PCI) is a routine procedure in cardiology aimed at providing revascularization of coronary vessels. Such interventions remain highly challenging since cardiologists must rely on occasional contrast injection to assess coronary motion and topology on 2D X-ray angiographic frames. CT-based navigation was proposed [1] to outline coronary vessels even when contrast agent is not present, but these techniques provide only static guidance. The task of intra-vascular navigation through the coronary arteries is impeded by the complexity of their topology, their constant motion composed of sudden movements, and the fact that they can often be observed only one angle at a time. An accurate estimation of this motion would be a step further towards efficient motion compensation techniques, or augmented reality solutions, where angiographic frames would be overlaid with interactive catheter roadmaps. This problem is difficult for several reasons: first, the coronary motion is a complex combination of rigid and non-rigid deformations caused by both cardiac and respiratory activities. Second, the topology of the coronary arteries is remarkably

---

* This research was supported by NSERC Discovery Grant.

N. Ayache et al. (Eds.): MICCAI 2012, Part I, LNCS 7510, pp. 651–658, 2012.
© Springer-Verlag Berlin Heidelberg 2012

complex and varies significantly from one patient to another. Third, because we aim for an intra-operative application, computational costs have to remain low. Last, the estimation of 3D motion from 2D temporal projections is notably known as an *ill-posed* problem, therefore difficult by essence.

1.1   Related Works

The goal of 3D/2D registration methods is to find a geometric transformation that brings a 3D pre-operative patient dataset into the best spatial correspondence with 2D intra-operative datasets [2]. Such methods can be roughly grouped in three separate categories. The first category proposes simple rigid deformation models and focuses on the *registration criterion*, implicitly seeking a smooth criterion to be optimized [3]. The second category derives from the work on active shape models, and focuses on the *deformation model* using statistical atlases [4, 5]. These methods rely on the assumption that an average topology can be drawn from multiple segmentations, and that patient-specific structures can later be consistently described as deviations from this mean topology. In our case, this assumption does not apply since the topology of the coronary arteries varies too much from one patient to another. Recently, [6] proposed a graph-based non-rigid deformation model showing good results despite the important number of parameters and the heavy computational costs. Other attempts at motion compensation in the field of 3D reconstruction require multiple views and generally propose heavily parameterized deformation models [7–9]. Finally, the methods in the third category put their attention on the *optimization strategy* [10, 11], arguing that the ill-posedness of 3D/2D registration calls for the use of robust optimization techniques allowing multiple hypothesis to coexist during the search, such as techniques based on Monte-Carlo sampling. Nevertheless, very few of the works in the literature explicitly consider temporal consistency in the problem of coronary motion estimation. Furthermore, when included, such temporal constraints are usually applied between consecutive frames only, instead of considering a stable and coherent deformation over the entire cardiac cycle – a point that is stressed out in the discussion of [8].

1.2   Contributions

We propose a novel probabilistic approach to describe and predict the 3D deformations of the coronary arteries from 2D monoplane angiogram. The originality and advantages of this approach, with respect to existing methods for the problem of 3D/2D registration of coronary arteries, are the following:

- As opposed to current methods, our approach enforces temporal consistency over the entire sequence by using a Hidden Markov Model, which enables a more robust and accurate registration;
- Unlike deterministic registration methods, our probabilistic approach considers multiple hypotheses simultaneously during the optimization process, thereby avoiding the problem of local optima;

– Since its deformation model has few parameters and the optimization process, based on particle filtering, is highly parallelizable, it is computationally efficient and could eventually be used in a real-time registration setting.

The rest of this paper is divided as follows. The next section presents our method and the probabilistic model on which it is based. In the experimental section, we evaluate the accuracy of this method on simulated and real patients angiograms. Finally, we conclude this paper by summarizing our contributions and experimental results, and provide possible extensions of this work.

2 Proposed Method

The 3D/2D coronary registration problem can be formulated as follows. Let $I_{1..K}$ be a sequence of K segmented binary angiographic images, where image I_k is taken at time t_k, and denote by X_0 the set of points forming the centerline of the reference 3D coronary tree. As mentioned above, this reference data is acquired prior to the registration process, for instance, by segmenting vessel centerlines from a CT-scan. The goal is to find the sequence of deformed 3D centerline points $X_{1..K}$ that best corresponds to the sequence of observed images, once projected in the image plane. In practice, optimizing every deformed centerline coordinate directly, at each instant, is not feasible due to the largeness of the resulting search space. Instead, we suppose that these coordinates are fully determined by the parameters θ of a deformation model $f_d(X_0; \theta)$, and search for the most likely sequence of parameters $\theta_{1..K}$. In the next section, we describe a probabilistic model that offers a simple yet realistic description of the coronary motion.

2.1 Probabilistic Generative Model

The general tracking approach proposed by [12] was adapted to the problem of coronary motion compensation by including a model of cardiac motion based on Hidden Markov Models (HMM). This model, illustrated in Figure 1, receives at each instant t_k an estimate $\hat{\phi}_k$ of the 2π-period phase of the cardiac cycle, and describes the evolution of the unknown cardiac deformations as follows[1]:

$$p(\theta_k \mid \theta_{k-1}, v_{k-1}) \sim \delta(\theta_k, \theta_{k-1} + (t_k - t_{k-1}) v_{k-1}) \tag{1}$$

$$p(v_k \mid v_{k-1}, \phi_k) \sim \mathcal{N}((1-\alpha) v_{k-1} + \alpha v_e(\phi_k), \Sigma_v) \tag{2}$$

$$p(\phi_k) \sim \mathcal{N}(\hat{\phi}_k, \sigma_\phi^2) \tag{3}$$

Instead of estimating directly the deformation parameters θ_k, we evaluate their instantaneous variations v_k, using a time-linear approximation (Equation 1). By constraining the variations instead of the actual parameters, we obtain smoother and more realistic movements. Moreover, the transition model of these parameter variations, as defined in Equation 2, is constrained in two important ways. First, we consider a temporal constraint that acts as an *inertial factor* on the movement. Again, this allows to focus on regular, jitter-free movements.

---

[1] δ is the Kronecker delta such that $\delta(x, y) = 1$ if $x = y$, and 0 otherwise.

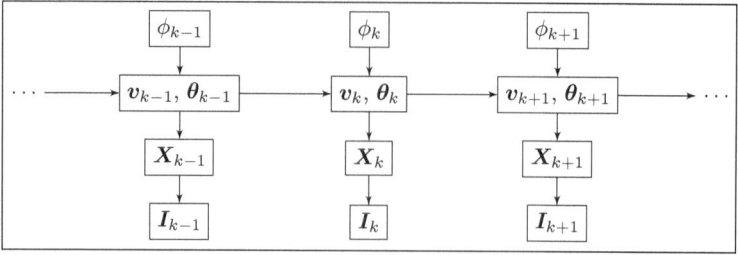

Fig. 1. Graphical model (HMM) of the image generation process

However, because the cardiac motion contains sudden movements caused by ventricular contractions, we also inject *prior knowledge*, which enables the model to anticipate and follow such movements. Thus, v_k also depends on an empirical model (or *template*) of the cardiac motion, given by the continuous function v_e. Since the cardiac motion is cyclic, v_e is defined as a 2π-periodic function of the cardiac phase ϕ_k. To control the trade-off between having a purely inertial model or a model based only on empirical knowledge, we use the parameter $\alpha \in [0,1]$. Moreover, covariance matrix Σ_v is used to model the inherent uncertainty of the estimation and the possible temporal correlation between the deformation parameters. In Section 2.5, we describe how v_e and Σ_v can be learned.

Finally, as expressed in Equation 3, we suppose the measured phase values to be noisy estimates of the real values, and use parameter σ_ϕ^2 to model this noise. In practice, the cardiac cycle phase can be estimated from the ECG signal by synchronizing $(\phi_k \bmod 2\pi) = 0$ with end-diastolic phases. Interestingly, this latter assumption allows for the exploration of a wider range of deformations at contraction time. Indeed, for a given phase uncertainty, a larger range of values can be found in the template function v_e in regions where this function has greater variations. Additionally, slower component of the cardiac motion (e.g., the respiratory component) can be implicitly captured by this model, due to the first-order inertial constraints allowing small, potentially directed velocity increments throughout the sequence.

2.2 Cardiac Deformation Model

The unknown 3D deformed centerline points at time t_k are assumed to be fully determined once the parameters θ_k of the deformation model f_d are estimated:

$$p(\boldsymbol{X}_k | \boldsymbol{\theta}_k) \;=\; \delta(\boldsymbol{X}_k, \, f_d(\boldsymbol{X}_0, \, \boldsymbol{\theta}_k)) \tag{4}$$

The choice of f_d is critical to the efficiency and accuracy of registrations. Such model should have the following two properties: *i*) be expressive enough to allow realistic deformations, and *ii*) have a limited number of parameters to reduce the search space at registration time. For this work, we chose the *planispheric* deformation model defined in [13], which is presented as a compromise between spherical and cylindrical models, and provides a convenient affine formulation to non-rigid deformations in a transformed coordinates system. This system relies on a geometrical model of the left ventricle, and can be conceived as a spherical frame shifting along a portion of the long axis. Our deformation model comprised 6 rigid parameters (rotations and translations), and 5 non-rigid parameters.

2.3   Image Generation and Likelihood

The last component of our probabilistic model describes how 2D images I_k are generated from the deformed 3D centerline points X_k, and how their likelihood $p(I_k|X_k)$ is evaluated. We considered a feature-based similarity measure involving a Frangi *et al.* vesselness filter [14] followed by a graylevel thresholding of angiographic frames $I_{1..K}$ to obtain binary images of the coronary vessels. In order to diffuse the information of proximity to the target vessels, we use a distance transform mapping each pixel i of the original image to a value $1/(1 + d_i^\gamma)$, where d_i is the distance from i to its nearest centerline pixel in the image, and $\gamma \geq 0$ is a diffusion factor. From preliminary tests, we found $\gamma = 0.5$ to give optimal results and used this value for our experiments. Given a predicted deformation θ_k, a 2D predicted image $\hat{I}_k$ is then generated by projecting the 3D deformed centerlines points X_k, and compared to the target image using a cosine similarity:

$$p(I_k|X_k) \;=\; \cos(I_k, \hat{I}_k) \;=\; \frac{\sum_{i,j} I_k(i,j) \cdot \hat{I}_k(i,j)}{\left(\sum_{i,j} I_k^2(i,j)\right)^{1/2} \cdot \left(\sum_{i,j} \hat{I}_k^2(i,j)\right)^{1/2}} \qquad (5)$$

2.4   Deformation Parameters Optimization

To find the most likely sequence of parameters $\theta_{1..K}$, given the observed images and measured phase values, we use particle filtering [15]. Essentially, a set of candidate deformations (the *particles*) are extended using the transition model and resampled according to their observation likelihood (Equation 5). At each frame, the deformation used for registration is the one having the highest likelihood. While well-known approaches, such as Kalman filtering, exist to compute the *a posterori* distribution directly, we have selected particle filtering for three important reasons. First, unlike Kalman filters, particle filters can learn multi-modal distributions, which allows one to consider several hypotheses simultaneously. Secondly, it is highly parallelizable and, therefore, a good candidate for real-time registration. Finally, it allows one to use probability models that can not be expressed in closed form, such as our image generation process.

2.5   Learning v_e and $\sum_v$

The empirical knowledge v_e and the covariance matrix Σ_v play important roles in our model, respectively guiding the search, and controling its range during optimization. However, when these values are unknown, our model can still be used with purely inertial transitions ($\alpha = 0$), compensating for the loss of *prior* by increasing manually the search space controled by Σ_v, and increasing the number of particles accordingly, at the expense of longer computation times. In turn, this allows one to estimate both parameters from multiple registrations performed without empirical knowledge.

3   Results and Discussion

Our dataset contained the 3D coronary centerlines – extracted from pre-operative CT-scans – and associated intra-operative biplane angiographic sequences of 7 patients (5 left coronary arteries, 2 right, sequences from 10 to 18 frames). The projection matrices were computed from the geometric parameters of the imaging systems. Although not necessary, covariance matrix Σ_v was assumed to be diagonal to simplify the configuration and learning steps of our experiments. The registration was performed in a coarse-to-fine manner, dividing the search of the deformation parameters in two steps. The first step looked for rigid deformations using N_1 particles, while the second step looked for both rigid and non-rigid deformations with N_2 particles. Target-to-registration errors were used to evaluate the accuracy of the compensation, in 3D (TRE 3D) during the simulations, and in 2D (TRE 2D) for both simulations and real patient datasets. For the latter, the TRE 2D was computed, with knowledge of the pixel-spacing, as the average pixel-wise product between an Euclidian distance transform computed on the target binary image, and the registered binary projection of the centerline.

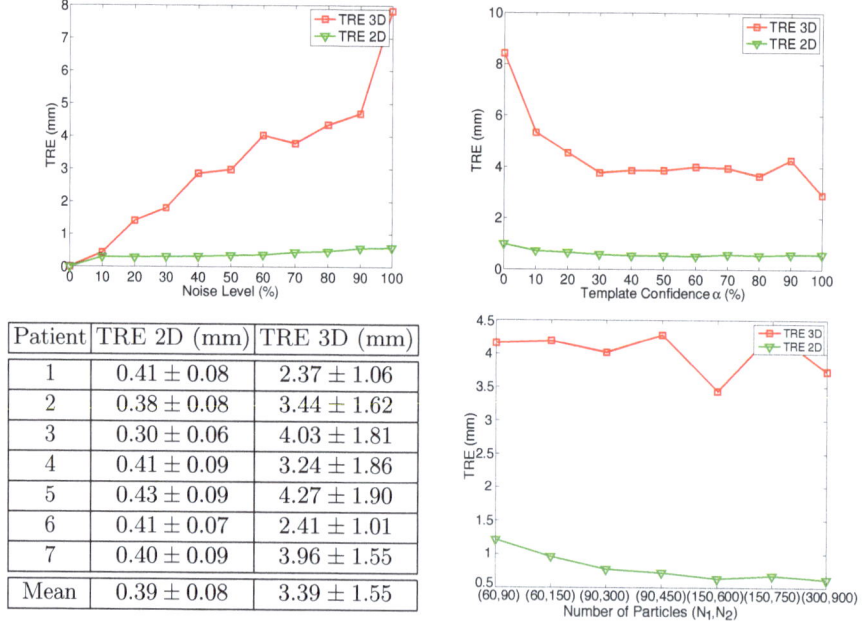

Patient	TRE 2D (mm)	TRE 3D (mm)
1	0.41 ± 0.08	2.37 ± 1.06
2	0.38 ± 0.08	3.44 ± 1.62
3	0.30 ± 0.06	4.03 ± 1.81
4	0.41 ± 0.09	3.24 ± 1.86
5	0.43 ± 0.09	4.27 ± 1.90
6	0.41 ± 0.07	2.41 ± 1.01
7	0.40 ± 0.09	3.96 ± 1.55
Mean	0.39 ± 0.08	3.39 ± 1.55

Fig. 2. TRE 3D (red squares) and 2D (green triangles) for simulations under the influence of noise level (top left, with $N_1 = 150$, $N_2 = 600$, $\alpha = 80\%$); template confidence (top right, with $N_1 = 90$, $N_2 = 300$, 60% noise); coronary topology (bottom left, mean $\pm$ std, with $N_1 = 150$, $N_2 = 600$, $\alpha = 80\%$, 30% noise); and number of particles (bottom-right, with $\alpha = 50\%$, 70% noise)

3.1   Evaluation on Synthetic Sequences

For these experiments, matrix $\boldsymbol{\Sigma}_v$ and function $\boldsymbol{v}_e$ were configured manually to randomly sample visually realistic deformation sequences with motion noise. The deformed centerlines were projected on binary images, and thickened prior to the distance transform, to better simulate thresholded, vesselness-filtered angiographic images. Four experiments were carried out, respectively, to evaluate the influence of: template confidence, noise, coronary topology, and number of particles on the registration accuracy (see Figure 2). The TRE 2D was less than 1.2 mm for all experiments, and as expected, degraded with increasing noise, and decreased with increasing prior knowledge or number of particles. On the other hand, the TRE 3D was somewhat higher (average of 4 mm), due to the fact that only one projection plane was used to assess the 3D motion.

3.2   Evaluation on Real Sequences

These experiments were designed to estimate both the applicability of our method to clinical datasets, and the ability of our method to learn parameters $\boldsymbol{\Sigma}_v$ and $\boldsymbol{v}_e$ as presented in Section 2.5. For this purpose, we used a leave-one-out approach, registering six out of the seven sequences using both planes, with $\alpha = 0$, $N_1 = 600$ and $N_2 = 1200$ particles. These registrations were used to estimate $\boldsymbol{\Sigma}_v$ and $\boldsymbol{v}_e$, which were then injected in our model (with $N_1 = 60$ and $N_2 = 150$) for the single-plane registration of the remaining sequence, with learned template ($\alpha = 0.8$) and without ($\alpha = 0$). The mean TRE 2D were respectively 2.75 ± 1.15 mm and 3.61 ± 2.10 mm (24% improvement in accuracy, 46% in deviation), for a mean computation time of 5.2 seconds per image using Matlab.

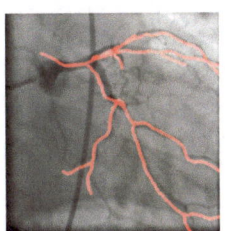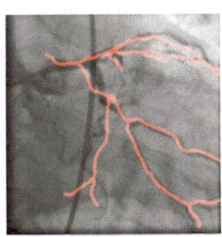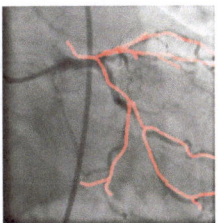

Fig. 3. Motion-compensated CT-centerline overlaid on top of angiographic images at different cardiac phases; end-diastole, early systole and systolic peak (from left to right)

4   Conclusion

This study presented a novel motion compensation technique based on a stochastic temporal model of 3D coronary centerline deformations. While generic, this approach allows one to learn patient-specific knowledge on coronary motion, which is used to improve the accuracy, robustness and efficiency of the registration. Motion can be learned and generalized from a large database of patients undergoing coronary intervention. This could be further investigated in future works to provide a more personalized model of coronary motion.

References

1. Duong, L., Liao, R., Sundar, H., Tailhades, B., Meyer, A., Xu, C.: Curve-based 2D-3D registration of coronary vessels for image guided procedure. In: SPIE Medical Imaging, vol. 7261 (2009)
2. Markelj, P., Tomazevic, D., Likar, B., Pernus, F.: A review of 3D/2D registration methods for image-guided interventions. Medical Image Analysis (2010)
3. McLaughlin, R., Hipwell, J., Hawkes, D., Noble, J., Byrne, J., Cox, T.: A Comparison of 2D-3D Intensity-Based Registration and Feature-Based Registration for Neurointerventions. In: Dohi, T., Kikinis, R. (eds.) MICCAI 2002, Part II. LNCS, vol. 2489, pp. 517–524. Springer, Heidelberg (2002)
4. Tang, T.S.Y., Ellis, R.E.: 2D/3D Deformable Registration Using a Hybrid Atlas. In: Duncan, J.S., Gerig, G. (eds.) MICCAI 2005, Part II. LNCS, vol. 3750, pp. 223–230. Springer, Heidelberg (2005)
5. Chen, X., Graham, J., Hutchinson, C., Muir, L.: Inferring 3D Kinematics of Carpal Bones from Single View Fluoroscopic Sequences. In: Fichtinger, G., Martel, A., Peters, T. (eds.) MICCAI 2011, Part II. LNCS, vol. 6892, pp. 680–687. Springer, Heidelberg (2011)
6. Groher, M., Zikic, D., Navab, N.: Deformable 2D-3D registration of vascular structures in a one view scenario. IEEE Trans. on Medical Imaging 28(6) (2009)
7. Blondel, C., Malandain, G., Vaillant, R., Devernay, F., Coste-Manière, È., Ayache, N.: 4D Tomographic Representation of Coronary Arteries from One Rotational X-Ray Sequence. In: Ellis, R.E., Peters, T.M. (eds.) MICCAI 2003. LNCS, vol. 2878, pp. 416–423. Springer, Heidelberg (2003)
8. Shechter, G., Devernay, F., Coste-Maniere, E., Quyyumi, A., McVeigh, E.: Three-dimensional motion tracking of coronary arteries in biplane cineangiograms. IEEE Trans. on Medical Imaging 22(4), 493–503 (2003)
9. Rohkohl, C., Lauritsch, G., Prümmer, M., Hornegger, J.: Interventional 4D Motion Estimation and Reconstruction of Cardiac Vasculature without Motion Periodicity Assumption. In: Yang, G.-Z., Hawkes, D., Rueckert, D., Noble, A., Taylor, C. (eds.) MICCAI 2009, Part I. LNCS, vol. 5761, pp. 132–139. Springer, Heidelberg (2009)
10. Florin, C., Williams, J., Khamene, A., Paragios, N.: Registration of 3D Angiographic and X-Ray Images Using Sequential Monte Carlo Sampling. In: Liu, Y., Jiang, T.-Z., Zhang, C. (eds.) CVBIA 2005. LNCS, vol. 3765, pp. 427–436. Springer, Heidelberg (2005)
11. Ruijters, D., ter Haar Romeny, B., Suetens, P.: Vesselness-based 2D-3D registration of the coronary arteries. Int. J. CARS 4(4), 391–397 (2009)
12. Sidenbladh, H., Black, M.J., Fleet, D.J.: Stochastic Tracking of 3D Human Figures Using 2D Image Motion. In: Vernon, D. (ed.) ECCV 2000, Part II. LNCS, vol. 1843, pp. 702–718. Springer, Heidelberg (2000)
13. Declerck, J., Feldmar, J., Ayache, N.: Definition of a four-dimensional continuous planispheric transformation for the tracking and the analysis of left-ventricle motion. Medical Image Analysis 2(2), 197–213 (1998)
14. Frangi, A., Niessen, W., Vincken, K., Viergever, M.: Multiscale Vessel Enhancement Filtering. In: Wells, W.M., Colchester, A.C.F., Delp, S.L. (eds.) MICCAI 1998. LNCS, vol. 1496, pp. 130–137. Springer, Heidelberg (1998)
15. Djuric, P., Kotecha, J., Zhang, J., Huang, Y., Ghirmai, T., Bugallo, M., Miguez, J.: Particle filtering. IEEE Signal Processing Magazine 20(5), 19–38 (2003)

A Fast Convex Optimization Approach to Segmenting 3D Scar Tissue from Delayed-Enhancement Cardiac MR Images

Martin Rajchl[1,2,*], Jing Yuan[1], James A. White[1,3], Cyrus M.S. Nambakhsh[1,2], Eranga Ukwatta[1,2], Feng Li[1,2], John Stirrat[1], and Terry M. Peters[1,2]

[1] Imaging Laboratories, Robarts Research Institute, London, ON
[2] Department of Biomedical Engineering, Western University, London, ON
[3] Division of Cardiology, Department of Medicine, Western, University, London, ON
mrajchl@robarts.ca

Abstract. We propose a novel multi-region segmentation approach through a *partially-ordered Potts (POP) model* to segment myocardial scar tissue solely from 3D cardiac delayed-enhancement MR images (DE-MRI). The algorithm makes use of prior knowledge of anatomical spatial consistency and employs customized label ordering to constrain the segmentation without prior knowledge of geometric representation. The proposed method eliminates the need for regional constraint segmentations, thus reduces processing time and potential sources of error. We solve the proposed optimization problem by means of convex relaxation and introduce its duality: the *hierarchical continuous max-flow (HMF) model*, which amounts to an efficient numerical solver to the resulting convex optimization problem. Experiments are performed over ten DE-MRI data sets. The results are compared to a FWHM (full-width at half-maximum) method and the inter- and intra-operator variabilities assessed.

Keywords: Image segmentation, DE-MRI, Convex relaxation.

1 Introduction

Clinical interest in myocardial scar imaging using delayed enhancement magnetic resonance imaging (DE-MRI) has expanded over the past decade. A potential for DE-MRI to guide cardiovascular procedures, such as ablative therapies for elimination of atrial or ventricular arrhythmias and the optimal placement of pacemaker leads to treat heart failure (Cardiac Resynchronization Therapy), is now being appreciated [1,2]. However, ability to translate this information into the procedural environment is a significant challenge. The recent validation of high-resolution isotropic 3D DE-MRI techniques provides superior spatial characterization of scar compared to its 2D predecessor[1]. Further, this dataset provides an unprecedented capacity to accurately represent scar within volumetric models to guide cardiac intervention. However, the efficient and accurate

---

* Corresponding author.

N. Ayache et al. (Eds.): MICCAI 2012, Part I, LNCS 7510, pp. 659–666, 2012.

segmentation of scar signal from these datasets presents a significant challenge. Recently, several approaches [2,3] were proposed to segment the 3D scar tissue, which employ additional information from other images to constrain the search for scar tissue within the myocardium geometrically. Additional myocardial segmentations [4], or registrations [5] to other images is time consuming and a potential source of error.

Contributions. In this study, we propose a novel multi-region segmentation method to extract myocardial 3D scar tissue from high-resolution DE-MRI volume data sets. For this purpose, we introduce a *POP model* which uses prior knowledge of the anatomical spatial consistency of cardiac structures as additional constraints, rather than geometry. In particular, we solve the formulated non-convex optimization problem in terms of convex relaxation, by proposing a new *HMF formulation* and demonstrate its duality to the *convex relaxed POP model*. We show that such a *convex HMF model* allows for a fast algorithm in modern convex optimization theory, which can be implemented on parallel computation platforms to reduce processing time using commercially available graphics hardware. The technique was tested using 3D DE-MRI datasets (N=10) obtained at 3 Tesla in patients with prior myocardial infarction.

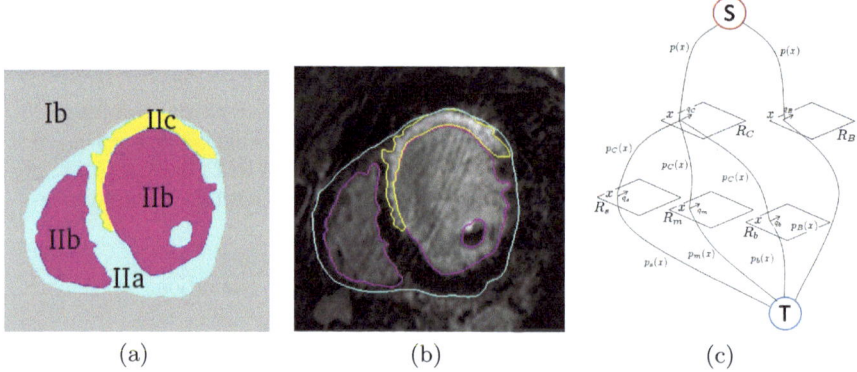

                    (a)   (b)   (c)

Fig. 1. Proposed label ordering based on anatomic spatial consistency (a) and contours overlaid on a DE-MRI slice (b). The region constraining the heart Ia) is split up in three subregions: IIa) myocardium, IIb) blood and IIc) scar tissue. Ib) represents the thoracic background. The graph in 1(c) shows the respective regions and flow configuration.

2   Methods

In the DE-MRI volume, we can clearly identify several compartments (see Fig. 1(a)): the cardiac region and Ib) thoracic background, where the cardiac compartment further contains three spatially coherent sub-regions: IIa) myocardium, IIb) blood volume and IIc) scar tissue; each of the three cardiac sub-regions has its distinct appearance model, which constitutes the complex appearance model of cardiac anatomy in DE-MRI. In this paper, we employ such a complex appearance model to assist segmenting the cardiac region accurately, which, in turn, automatically helps to identify the inherent sub-region of scar tissue. In fact, [6] shows the application of such complex appearance model significantly improves the segmentation accuracy for imaging which can not be simply modeled by independent and identically distributed random variables. We introduce the *POP model* to multi-region cardiac segmentation, which properly encodes prior information of label order.

2.1   Partially-Ordered Potts Model and Convex Relaxation

We segment the given DE-MRI volume Ω into multiple regions such that

$$\Omega = \Omega_C \cup \Omega_B \tag{1}$$

and

$$\Omega_C = \Omega_s \cup \Omega_m \cup \Omega_b \tag{2}$$

where Ω_C and Ω_B represent the two disjoint regions: Ia) the cardiac region and Ib) the thorical background; $\Omega_{s,m,b}$ represent the sub-regions of scar tissue, myocardium and blood respectively, which are disjoint from each other. To simplify our notations, we define the label sets: $L = \{C, B\}$ and $C = \{s, m, b\}$. Clearly, (2) states a partial order of regions, which can be incorporated into Potts model such that:

$$\min_{\Omega_{C,B}, \Omega_{s,m,b}} \sum_{l \in L \cup C} \int_{\Omega_l} \rho(l, x) \, dx + \sum_{l \in L \cup C} |\partial \Omega_l| \tag{3}$$

subject to the region constraints (1) and (2), where $\rho(l, x)$ gives the cost to label the pixel x by $l \in L \cup C$ and $|\partial \Omega_l|$ represents the weighted length of the region Ω_l. In practice, the cost for labeling the cardiac region can be fixed to 0, i.e. $\rho(C, x) = 0$; such that the cost for the cardiac region equals to the total cost of its contained three sub-regions: scar tissue, myocardium and blood. In this paper, we call (3) the *POP model*. Let $u_l(x) \in \{0, 1\}, l \in L \cup C$, be the indicator function of the corresponding region Ω_l and $\omega_l(x)$ its regularization weight. Then the POP model (3) can be rewritten as

$$\min_{u_l \in L \cup C} \sum_{l \in L \cup C} \int_\Omega u_l(x) \rho(l, x) \, dx + \sum_{l \in L \cup C} \int_\Omega \omega_l(x) |\nabla u_l| \, dx \tag{4}$$

subject to the constraints of the labeling functions $u_l(x)$ such that

$$u_C(x) + u_B(x) = 1, \quad \sum_{l \in C} u_l(x) = u_C(x); \quad u_{l \in L \cup C}(x) \in \{0, 1\} \tag{5}$$

for each $\forall x \in \Omega$. Clearly, (5) just corresponds to (1) and (2). In this work, we solve the POP model (4) by its convex relaxation:

$$\min_{u_l \in L \cup C} \sum_{l \in L \cup C} \int_\Omega u_l(x) \rho(l, x) \, dx + \sum_{l \in L \cup C} \int_\Omega \omega_l(x) |\nabla u_l| \, dx \tag{6}$$

subject to the convex constraints

$$u_C(x) + u_B(x) = 1, \quad \sum_{l \in C} u_l(x) = u_C(x); \quad u_{l \in L \cup C}(x) \in [0, 1]. \quad (7)$$

The binary constraints for $u_l(x)$, $l \in L \cup C$, in (5) are relaxed into their convex version in (7). The formulation (6), thereafter, boils down to a convex optimization problem, namely the *convex relaxed POP model*.

2.2   Hierarchical Continuous Max-Flow Model

We introduce a new *continuous HMF model* which is dual to the convex relaxed POP model. For this, we introduce the two-level flow-maximization configurations in a spatially continuous settings (see Fig. 1(c)): in addition to the source and sink terminals s and t, we put 2 copies R_C and R_B of the image domain Ω in parallel at the upper level; and put 3 copies R_l, $l \in C$ i.e. $\{s, m, b\}$, of Ω in parallel at the bottom level. We link s to the same pixel x at each upper-level domain R_C and R_B and define the unique flow $p_s(x)$ along the link from s to x; link x at R_C to the same pixel x at each domain of R_l, $l \in C$, and define the unique flow $p_C(x)$ along the links; link each pixel of R_B and R_l, $l \in C$, to the sink terminal t, and define the flows $p_B(x)$ and $p_l(x)$, $l \in C$. Additionally, the spatial flow fields $q_l(x)$, $l \in L \cup C$, are defined within each domain Ω_l.

Hierarchical Continuous Max-Flow Model. Based on the above settings, we set up the flow capacity and conservation conditions: for domains at the upper level, we define the flow capacity constraints:

$$|q_l(x)| \le \omega_l(x), \quad l = \{C, B\}; \quad p_B(x) \le \rho(B, x), \quad (8)$$

and the flow conservation constraints, i.e. the flow residues $G_l(x)$ vanish:

$$G_l(x) := (\operatorname{div} q_l - p_s + p_l)(x) = 0, \quad l = \{C, B\}; \quad (9)$$

for the domains at the bottom level, we define the flow capacity constraints

$$|q_l(x)| \le \omega_l(x), \quad p_l(x) \le \rho(l, x), \quad l = \{s, m, b\}, \quad (10)$$

and the flow conservation constraints, i.e. the flow residues $G_l(x)$ vanish:

$$G_l(x) := (\operatorname{div} q_l - p_C + p_l)(x) = 0, \quad l = \{s, m, b\}. \quad (11)$$

We propose the *continuous HMF model* which maximizes the total flow streaming from the source s to the sink t, i.e.

$$\max_{p,q} \int_\Omega p_s(x) \, dx \quad (12)$$

subject to the flow constraints (8), (9), (10) and (11). There is no constraint for the flow functions $p_s(x)$ and $p_C(x)$.

Following the same analytical steps as [7], we can prove the duality between the continuous HMF model (12) and the convex relaxed POP model (6), where the labeling functions $u_l(x)$, $l \in L \cup C$, work as the optimum multipliers to the respective flow conservation constraints of (9) and (11).

2.3 Hierarchical Continuous Max-Flow Algorithm

The continuous HMF model proposes a convex optimization problem with a linear energy function subject to the linear equality constraints (9) and (11), besides the constraints (8) and (10) on flow values, i.e. flow capacities. Thereafter, an efficient augmented Lagrangian based algorithm, namely the continuous HMF algorithm, can be derived, which iteratively optimizes the following augmented Lagrangian function:

$$\max_{p,q} \min_u L_c(u;p,q) := \int_\Omega p_s \, dx + \sum_{l \in L \cup C} \langle u_l, G_l \rangle - \frac{c}{2} \sum_{l \in L \cup C} \|G_l\|^2$$

subject to the flow capacity constraints (8) and (10).

Similar as the continuous max-flow algorithm proposed in [8,7], the continuous HMF algorithm explores two sequential steps at each k-th iteration:

- Maximize the augmented Lagrangian function $L_c(u;p,q)$ over the flow functions $p_s(x)$, $p_l(x)$ and $q_l(x)$ where $l \in L \cup C$ subject to the flow capacity constraints (8) and (10).
- Update the labeling functions $u_l(x)$, where $l \in L \cup C$, by

$$u_l^{k+1} = u_l^k - c\,G_l(x), \quad l \in L \cup C.$$

To achieve computation efficiency, a one-step projected gradient strategy is applied to the maximization over each flow function, which shows a fast and steady convergence in practice.

3 Experiments

We developed a graphical user interface for the proposed method and implemented the optimization algorithm on a parallel computing architecture (CUDA, nVidia Corp., Santa Clara, CA.) for a significant increase in computation speed. The user can place seeds for regions on three orthogonal slice views corresponding to one of the labels shown in Fig 1(a). From all the seeded regions, we obtain a cost from each sample histogram with a maximum log-likelihood calculation [9] and add these costs as data fidelity terms $D(x) = -\log P(I(x)|l_i)$. Additionally, we use seeds as hard constraint costs. This approach provides the ability to correct for intensity inconsistencies, such as artifacts or uncertain regions. The label IIc) representing the scar tissue will be component-thresholded to all connected components containing seeds. This ensures that only marked tissue is classified as scar while other regions of fibrous tissue (for example from the mitral valvular apparatus) are excluded (see Fig. 2(b)). For both label groups I) and II), the total variation penalties α and β (Eq. (6)) were designed in the form $\alpha, \beta = \lambda_1 + \lambda_2 \exp(-\lambda_3 |\nabla I(x)|^2)$. λ_1 and λ_2 may be varied by the user, and λ_3 was fixed to the value of 10 during these experiments. Using this interface, users were asked to segment 10 DE-MRI data sets of different levels of

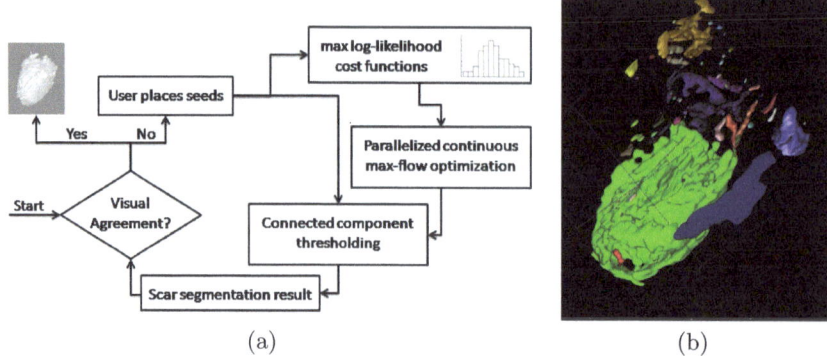

(a)   (b)

Fig. 2. (a) Proposed interactive segmentation pipeline. (b) Rendered example of intermediate segmentation result before connected component thresholding. While the image shows 38 separate components, only one of these components (*green*) represents scar tissue.

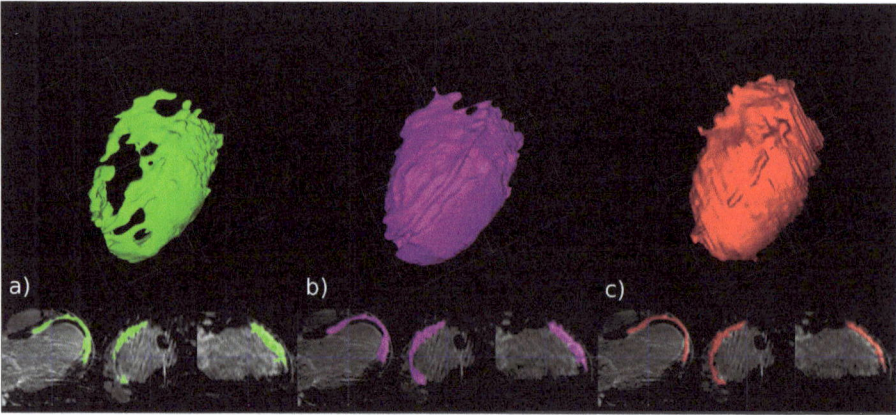

Fig. 3. Rendered example segmentation (*top row*) after *a)* the first and *b)* three recomputations. Rendered gold standard manual segmentation *c)* of the same scar tissue volume and respective slice views of segmentation on DE-MRI (*bottom*).

image quality containing scar volumes. The user places seeds for each label and computes the max-flow to obtain a segmentation result, and we record the time and the result, compared to a manually segmented ground truth of the scar. To assess robustness towards initialization and variability between operators, three users were asked to segment the same data set three times until they were satisfied with the result. Additionally we compared the segmentation results to those of the FWHM method. Constraining myocardial segmentations needed for the FWHM method were performed manually by a single expert and introduced a regional measure of overlap in form of a Dice coefficient (DSC) and a root mean squared surface error (RMSE) to measure the agreement of segmentation results to a single expert user manual segmentations.

4   Results

Intermediate visual results of the segmentation pipeline after one and three interactions are shown in Fig. 3.

Numerical results are shown in Table 1. We observe an increase in mean overlap and at the same time a decrease in mean surface error as well as a decrease in their standard deviations. The proposed method outperforms a manually initialized FWHM method in every metric. Furthermore, the results of repeated segmentations (N=3) from three users are stated in Table 1. In this study, the users segmented the same randomly chosen images until they were satisfied with the results.

Table 1. Numerical results for proposed HMF method on data base (N=10) (*left*) and intra-/interoperator variabilities on the randomly-selected data set(*right*). A comparsion between FHWM and HMF-based segmentation is shown on the bottom.

Interactions	DSC [0,1]	RMSE [mm]	userID	DSC [0,1]	RMSE [mm]
1	0.55 ± 0.17	3.80 ± 4.90	1	0.77 ± 0.02	0.91 ± 0.04
2	0.66 ± 0.14	3.03 ± 4.90	2	0.75 ± 0.02	1.05 ± 0.18
3	0.69 ± 0.14	2.77 ± 4.79	3	0.74 ± 0.01	1.12 ± 0.06
4	0.71 ± 0.06	1.44 ± 0.62			
5	0.74 ± 0.04	1.40 ± 0.62	All	0.75 ± 0.02	1.02 ± 0.14

Method	DSC [0,1]	RMSE [mm]	Scar volume [ml]	volume error [%]
HMF	0.78 ± 0.03	1.06 ± 0.16	46.37 ± 12.87	0.19 ± 0.12
FWHM	0.47 ± 0.10	2.12 ± 0.86	14.42 ± 4.73	-0.62 ± 0.15

5   Discussion and Conclusion

We developed a segmentation framework based on a novel POP model approach to GPU-based convex relaxation, to segment 3D myocardial scar tissue from high-resolution DE-MRI volume data. Testing on 10 data sets of different quality showed that after a few interactions all error metrics decrease. The final segmentation results in the RMSE plus one standard deviation lie within the maximum image resolution of 1.3 mm and the user was able to get outliers from two data sets under control by correcting in critical regions. The performance of FWHM suggests that it is underestimating volumes from 3D DE-MRI. This might be due the increased variability of an intensity maximum occuring with increased sample size due to the additional spatial dimension. This might further lead to a threshold shift greatly underestimating scar extent. The GPU-based optimizer running on a Geforce 580 GTX provides high speed computations in less than 5 seconds. On average, it required 9±2 minutes to extract the 3D scar volume from images. Inter- and intra-operator variability are both within ±2% suggesting robustness towards initialization from different users. The observed performance and robustness suggests that the proposed segmentation method is suitable for clinical purposes, especially for the planning and guidance of interventional procedures reliant upon accurate spatial representation of myocardial scar tissue.

Acknowlegdements. We want to thank Dr. Aaron Ward and Eli Gibson for fruitful discussions and input on this topic. This project is supported by Canada Foundation for Innovation (CFI) grant #20994, Canadian Institutes of Health Research (CIHR) grant MOP 179298 and ORF - RE-02-038. Martin Rajchl is enrolled in the CIHR Strategic Training Program in Vascular Research at Western University, London, ON.

References

1. White, J.A., Fine, N., Gula, L.J., Yee, R., Al-Admawi, M., Zhang, Q., Krahn, A., Skanes, A., MacDonald, A., Peters, T., Drangova, M.: Fused whole-heart coronary and myocardial scar imaging using 3-t cmr. implications for planning of cardiac resynchronization therapy and coronary revascularization. JACC. Cardiovascular Imaging 3(9), 921–930 (2010)
2. Andreu, D., Berruezo, A., Ortiz-Pérez, J., Silva, E., Mont, L., Borràs, R., de Caralt, T., Perea, R., Fernández-Armenta, J., Zeljko, H., Brugada, J.: Integration of 3d electroanatomic maps and magnetic resonance scar characterization into the navigation system to guide ventricular tachycardia ablation. Circulation. Arrhythmia and electrophysiology 4(5), 674–683 (2011)
3. Neizel, M., Boering, Y., Bönner, F., Balzer, J., Kelm, M., Sievers, B.: A fully automatic cardiac model with integrated scar tissue information for improved assessment of viability. Journal of Cardiovascular Magnetic Resonance 14(suppl. 1), M12 (2012)
4. Folkesson, F., Samset, E., Kwong, R., Westin, C.F.: Unifying statistical classification and geodesic active regions for segmentation of cardiac mri. IEEE Transactions on Information Technology in Biomedicine 12(3), 328–334 (2008)
5. Lehmann, H., Kneser, R., Neizel, M., Peters, J., Ecabert, O., Kühl, H., Kelm, M., Weese, J.: Integrating Viability Information into a Cardiac Model for Interventional Guidance. In: Ayache, N., Delingette, H., Sermesant, M. (eds.) FIMH 2009. LNCS, vol. 5528, pp. 312–320. Springer, Heidelberg (2009)
6. Delong, A., Gorelick, L., Schmidt, F.R., Veksler, O., Boykov, Y.: Interactive Segmentation with Super-Labels. In: Boykov, Y., Kahl, F., Lempitsky, V., Schmidt, F.R. (eds.) EMMCVPR 2011. LNCS, vol. 6819, pp. 147–162. Springer, Heidelberg (2011)
7. Yuan, J., Bae, E., Tai, X.-C., Boykov, Y.: A Continuous Max-Flow Approach to Potts Model. In: Daniilidis, K., Maragos, P., Paragios, N. (eds.) ECCV 2010, Part VI. LNCS, vol. 6316, pp. 379–392. Springer, Heidelberg (2010)
8. Yuan, J., Bae, E., Tai, X.: A study on continuous max-flow and min-cut approaches. In: CVPR 2010 (2010)
9. Boykov, Y., Jolly, M.: Interactive Graph Cuts for Optimal Boundary & Region Segmentation of Objects in N-D Images. In: ICCV, pp. 105–111 (2001)

Robust Motion Correction
in the Frequency Domain
of Cardiac MR Stress Perfusion Sequences

Vikas Gupta[1,2,*], Martijn van de Giessen[1,2,*], Hortense Kirişli[3],
Sharon W. Kirschbaum[4], Wiro J. Niessen[3,5], and Boudewijn P.F. Lelieveldt[1,2]

[1] Division of Image Processing, Leiden University Medical Center, The Netherlands
[2] Department of Intelligent Systems, Delft University of Technology, The Netherlands
[3] Biomedical Imaging Group Rotterdam, Erasmus MC Rotterdam, The Netherlands
[4] Dept. of Radiology and Cardiology, Erasmus MC Rotterdam, The Netherlands
[5] Quantitative Imaging Group, Delft University of Technology, The Netherlands
m.vandegiessen@lumc.nl

Abstract. First-pass cardiac MR perfusion (CMRP) imaging allows
identification of hypo-perfused areas in the myocardium and therefore
helps in early detection of coronary artery disease (CAD). However,
its efficacy is often limited by respiratory motion artifacts, especially in
stress-induced sequences. These distortions lead to unreliable estimates
of perfusion linked parameters, such as the myocardial perfusion reserve
index (MPRI). We propose a novel, robust motion correction method
that suppresses motion artifacts in the frequency domain. The method
is validated using rest and stress perfusion datasets of 10 patients and
is compared to a state-of-the-art independent component analysis based
method. Contrary to the latter, the proposed method reduces the remaining motion to less than the pixel size and allows the reliable computation
of the MPRI. The strong agreement between perfusion parameters based
on expert contours and after applying the proposed method enables the
near-automated quantitative analyses of stress MR perfusion sequences
in a clinical setting.

1 Introduction

Coronary artery disease (CAD) often entails a cascade of events [1] that lead to
the deterioration of myocardial tissue. To detect perfusion abnormalities at an
early stage of CAD, myocardial perfusion is assessed by analyzing cardiac MR
perfusion (CMRP) images. Clinical interest is moving towards a combination
of both rest and stress-induced perfusion [2,3] to quantify parameters such as
the myocardial perfusion reserve index (MPRI), a measure for the ability of the
heart to adapt to physical exercise.

However, in many cases, especially in stress MR acquisitions, the inability of a
patient to breath-hold adequately during the image acquisition leads to misalignments between subsequent frames of an image acquisition [4] and MPRI, which

---

* These authors contributed equally to this work.

N. Ayache et al. (Eds.): MICCAI 2012, Part I, LNCS 7510, pp. 667–674, 2012.
© Springer-Verlag Berlin Heidelberg 2012

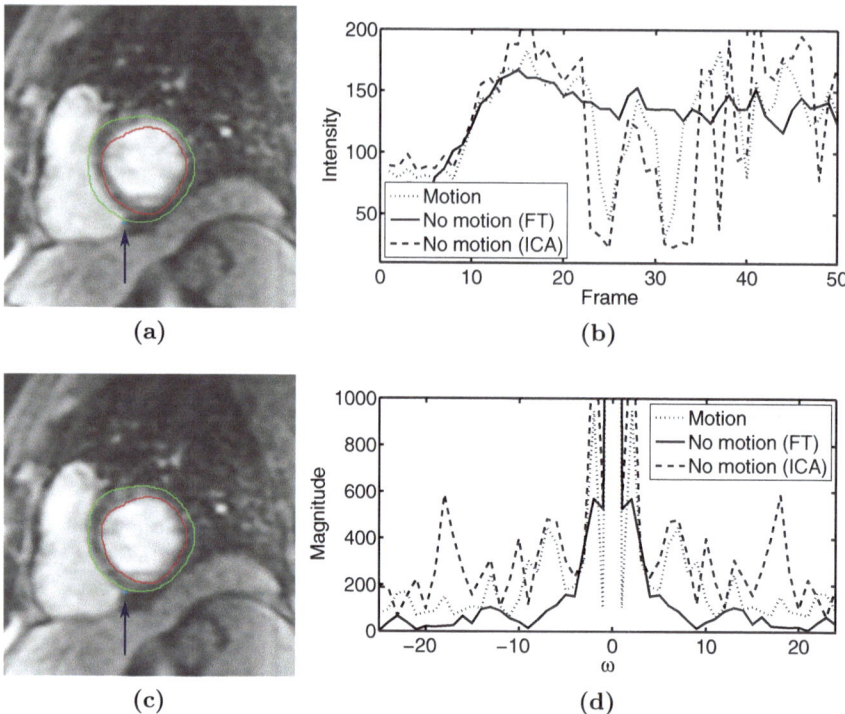

Fig. 1. Typical frames of cardiac sequences before (a) and after (c) motion correction (with FT). The frames are annotated with epi- and endocardial contours. + (near arrows) indicates the RV insertion point. (b) Example time-intensity curves in the time domain and (d) in the frequency domain. The motion artifacts visible in the time domain show up as additional high-frequency content in the frequency domain.

is based on dynamic contrast uptake (upslope), cannot be measured reliably. In this paper, we propose a novel motion correction method which is especially aimed at robustness.

Many methods have been proposed to eliminate CMRP motion artifacts, but predominantly in rest sequences. An in-depth overview of these algorithms is given in [5]. A group of algorithms that was shown to outperform most other approaches was based on independent component analysis ICA [6,7]. The efficacy of this method, however, is constrained by its dependence on the correct identification of component images and their corresponding weights to generate a reference image. A similar approach, which adds robustness to motion in a free breathing acquisition, was used by [8] but its applicability is limited by an inherent assumption of quasi-periodicity in these sequences.

Although the existing strategies succeed in achieving desired results for rest image sequences, their efficacy on stress images from patients suspected of CAD has not been proven yet. As the motion in stress images differs considerably from motion in rest images both in its extent and variability, we found that methods based on estimates of global components, such as [6,7] are likely to fail because initial component estimates are too unreliable. Instead of explicitly estimating the time-intensity curves for different regions, our approach aims to minimize the sudden changes in intensity that are characteristic for motion artifacts. To this end we iteratively minimize the high frequency content in the time-intensity curves by concurrently realigning the frames in the cardiac sequence. The proposed frequency domain approach is aimed to be robust against large and irregular patient motion and therefore makes very few assumptions on the expected scan data. Furthermore the algorithm is computationally inexpensive and inherently robust to time-shifts in the acquisition.

The proposed algorithm is validated on rest and stress sequences of 10 patients and compared to an ICA based method [6] that was shown to be more robust in comparison to the other methods in literature, including the standard registration methods.

2   Method

Motion artifacts manifest themselves as sudden intensity changes that typically only last a single frame. Such sudden changes show up as undesired high frequency content (See Figure 1). Using a high pass filter, this content can be separated from the frequencies present in a sequence without motion artifacts. We propose to write the high frequency content as a cost function of the translations of all the frames in the sequence. Minimizing this cost function concurrently over all frames then should remove the motion artifacts.

Let us denote the intensity profile of a pixel at coordinates x and y in input image sequence I with N frames as $I_{x,y}(t)$. The frequency content of this time-intensity curve is then given by the discrete Fourier transform (DFT):

$$\hat{I}_{x,y}(\omega) = \mathscr{F}[I_{x,y}(t)] = \sum_{t=0}^{N-1} I_{x,y}(t)e^{-j2\pi\omega t/N} \tag{1}$$

where t and ω refer to time (in this work frame number) and frequency, respectively.

We define a high pass filter $H(\omega)$ that passes the high frequency components due to motion artifacts. The filtered signal in the frequency domain is complex, however, and therefore the energy spectral density of the signal is used to form the cost for the intensity profile at $I_{x,y}$:

$$C_{x,y} = \frac{1}{2\pi} \sum_{\omega} \left(H(\omega)\hat{I}_{x,y}(\omega)\right)\left(H(\omega)\hat{I}_{x,y}(\omega)\right)^{*} \tag{2}$$

where * denotes the complex conjugate. The total cost within a region of interest Ω is then given by

$$C_{total} = \sum_{(x,y)\in\Omega} C_{x,y} \tag{3}$$

Using Vandermonde matrices F to compute the DFT and vector $\mathbf{h}_\omega$ and $\mathbf{i}_{x,y}$ for the filter $H(\omega)$ and time-intensity profile $I_{x,y}(t)$, respectively the cost $C_{x,y}$ can be evaluated inexpensively as

$$C_{x,y} = \mathbf{i}_{x,y}^T F^* \mathbf{h}_\omega^* \mathbf{h}_\omega F \mathbf{i}_{x,y} \equiv \mathbf{i}_{x,y}^T W \mathbf{i}_{x,y} \tag{4}$$

where W is the same for each intensity profile, as it only depends on the number of frames. Each intensity value in $\mathbf{i}_{x,y}$ can be considered as a function of the transformation of the respective slice. For translations $s_{x,t}$ and $s_{y,t}$ for frame t in the x and y directions, respectively, the gradient of the cost to these translations is given by

$$\frac{\partial C_{x,y}}{\partial s_{x,t}} = \frac{\partial C_{x,y}}{\partial \mathbf{i}_{x,y}} \frac{\partial \mathbf{i}_{x,y}}{\partial s_{x,t}} = 2\mathbf{i}_{x,y}^T W \frac{\partial \mathbf{i}_{x,y}}{\partial s_{x,t}} \tag{5}$$

where $\frac{\partial \mathbf{i}_{x,y}}{\partial s_{x,t}}$ is the negative image intensity derivative in the x direction. A similar equation holds for the y direction.

Using a constant high-pass filter $H(\omega)$ that blocks the frequencies present in motion-less time intensity curves, the complete motion correction procedure consists of two steps:

1. Select a region of interest (ROI) Ω containing the left and right ventricles.
2. Minimize (3) using a gradient-descent algorithm.

To avoid the trivial solution of moving all high frequency content out of the ROI Ω, the sums of all translations in the x direction and all translations in the y direction are kept 0.

3   Data

A dataset comprising rest and stress images from 10 patients with suspected CAD and normal left ventricular ejection fraction was used to validate the proposed method. All the images were acquired using a 1.5 Tesla MRI scanner (Signa CV/i, GE Medical Systems, Milwaukee, Wisconsin, USA), with a cardiac eight-element phased-array receiver coil placed over the thorax. The acquisition was performed using a steady-state free precession technique (FIESTA) and with Gd-DTPA (Magnevist, Schering, Germany) as the contrast agent. The temporal resolution per slice of 120 ms allowed imaging of 3-6 slices per R-R interval. Stress images were acquired 15 minutes after the acquisition of rest images using adenosine as the vasodilator. Both rest and stress images were acquired using the same pulse sequence and orientations.

4   Experiments

The following experiments validate the proposed method in terms of registration accuracy as well as two clinically relevant perfusion parameters: relative upslope and myocardial perfusion reserve index (MPRI). These parameters are widely

Table 1. Comparison of motion in unregistered sequences, in sequences registered using ICA, and in sequences registered using the proposed method (FT). Results for both rest and stress sequences of the same patient are presented.

	Rest			Stress		
Pat.	Unregistered	ICA	FT	Unregistered	ICA	FT
1	3.14 ± 9.98	0.39 ± 1.20	0.06 ± 0.43	2.77 ± 5.18	6.51 ± 13.81	0.22 ± 1.00
2	0.39 ± 1.04	0.06 ± 0.43	0.02 ± 0.11	2.48 ± 16.00	3.05 ± 6.16	0.11 ± 0.40
3	1.15 ± 2.91	1.04 ± 2.70	0.20 ± 0.51	1.58 ± 3.42	5.61 ± 13.65	0.06 ± 0.36
4	4.34 ± 12.81	10.53 ± 26.12	0.14 ± 0.60	7.29 ± 18.24	9.16 ± 12.51	0.11 ± 0.43
5	0.75 ± 2.06	0.47 ± 1.47	0.01 ± 0.08	3.37 ± 6.09	2.39 ± 3.43	0.61 ± 2.57
6	0.17 ± 0.67	0.23 ± 0.66	0.03 ± 0.14	5.54 ± 8.69	2.19 ± 2.37	0.06 ± 0.23
7	4.09 ± 9.91	0.48 ± 1.10	0.17 ± 0.67	7.33 ± 12.64	8.71 ± 15.37	0.36 ± 2.22
8	0.04 ± 0.29	0.00 ± 0.00	0.00 ± 0.00	7.62 ± 13.40	6.31 ± 21.84	0.07 ± 0.35
9	4.01 ± 16.87	1.28 ± 4.67	0.68 ± 4.78	3.40 ± 9.48	1.67 ± 2.46	0.14 ± 0.67
10	6.60 ± 13.84	2.53 ± 8.08	0.19 ± 0.88	7.07 ± 13.95	5.22 ± 13.06	0.57 ± 2.46

accepted as reliable indices [2,3] These outcomes are compared to the existing ICA based algorithm for motion correction in [6,7].

From ten patients, the basal slices of both a rest and a stress sequence of approximately 50 frames were used for validation. All frames were annotated by an expert with epi- and endocardial contours as well as a landmark at the inferior RV insertion point (See Figure 1). This landmark is normally used to determine the orientation of the myocardium. The annotated landmarks serve as ground truth for the motion correction, while the ground truth (expert) perfusion parameters are computed based on the annotated contours.

All rest and stress sequences were registered using the ICA based algorithm and the proposed Fourier transform (FT) based algorithm. For the evaluation of ICA and FT based algorithms, only one pair of contours was drawn on the first frame, which were propagated to the subsequent frames after motion correction. For all three sets (expert, ICA and FT), the relative upslopes were computed using the MASS software package [9].

5   Results

5.1   Motion Correction

The means and standard deviations of the annotated RV insertion points in the unregistered and registered sequences (with ICA and FT) from all patients are shown in Table 1, expressed in pixels (Average pixel size 1.52 ± 0.05 mm isotropic). These values describe the Euclidean distances between the landmarks in consecutive frames. The mean motion in the unregistered images was 2.46 ± 7.04 pixels in rest and 4.85 ± 10.71 pixels in stress sequences. After the ICA based registration, these values reduced to 1.76 ± 4.64 and 5.08 ± 10.46 pixels, respectively. However, the motion in images registered using the proposed FT method was 0.15 ± 0.82 pixels (rest) and 0.23 ± 1.06 pixels (stress).

Table 2. MPRI values for expert annotation and after FT motion correction

Patient	1	2	3	4	5	6	7	8	9	10
Expert	1.11	4.04	3.84	1.72	1.53	1.52	1.39	2.73	1.24	0.62
FT	1.07	3.65	3.31	1.73	1.58	1.58	1.68	2.55	1.15	0.60

The relatively bad performance of the ICA based motion correction, especially in the stress sequences, can be attributed to the incorrect identification of the components on which its correction algorithm relies. These components now mainly captured motion artifacts instead of time-intensity perfusion information. For four patients the FT algorithm had standard deviations higher than a pixel. In these cases single frames, with very low contrast in the myocardial region were misregistered. The large error for ICA in the rest sequence of patient 4 was due to flickering intensity variations between consecutive frames. The FT algorithm is apparently robust against these artifacts. The robustness of the proposed algorithm clearly follows from the sub-pixel mean values in Table 1.

5.2 Perfusion Parameters

Based on the registered sequences, the relative upslope is defined as the ratio of the absolute upslopes of the myocardium and the LV blood pool, where the absolute up-slope is given by the maximum value of the first order derivative of time-intensity curve within the ROI. Only the initial ascent of the contrast agent's first pass is considered for this computation. MPRI is computed as the ratio of the relative upslope values obtained under stress and at rest.

Figure 2 shows the relative upslopes (for both rest and stress) as estimated after motion correction using ICA and FT and compared to the upslopes based on the contours annotated by the expert. For both ICA and FT, the rest upslopes did not differ statistically significant ($P < 0.05$) from the expert annotations. However, the stress upslope estimates after ICA motion correction were significantly different ($P = 0.0255$). Furthermore it can be observed in Figure 2 that, using ICA, the relative upslope tends to be overestimated. This is to be expected, due to high first order derivatives caused by motion artifacts.

As both the rest and stress upslopes for FT did not differ significantly from the expert values, MPRI values based on these can be considered meaningful and they are compared to the expert values in Table 2.

5.3 Computation Time

Our experiments show that sequences of 50 frames can be automatically registered in 20 seconds compared to approximately 1 minute required by ICA and 10 minutes required for manual annotation. This shows the substantial reduction in processing time achievable for registering large CMRP image datasets when using the proposed registration method.

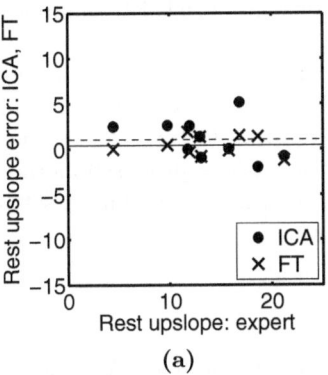 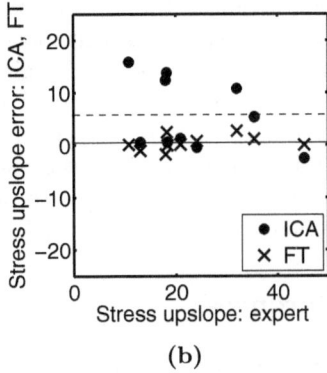

(a)   (b)

Fig. 2. Bland-Altman plots with ICA and FT estimates of relative upslopes in (a) rest and (b) stress sequences, compared to expert annotations. The means are denoted with a dashed line for ICA and a solid line for FT. For clarity, confidence boundaries have been left out.

6   Discussion and Conclusion

We have presented a robust method that eliminates motion artifacts in rest and stress CMRP images by correcting for translations due to respiratory motion, which is particularly apparent in stress sequences. The method was validated on datasets from 10 patients prone to CAD and it compared favorably to a state-of-the-art ICA based method [6,7], especially in stress sequences. Particularly encouraging were the mean registration errors of less than a pixel in both rest and stress sequences and the agreement between the perfusion parameters based on expert contours and the proposed method. The differences between them were found to be statistically insignificant, which shows that translations alone were sufficient to remove motion artifacts.

By minimizing motion artifacts in the frequency domain using a high-pass filter, the motion correction problem became a simple quadratic function of time-intensity profiles that can be solved efficiently. Furthermore, the algorithm is inherently robust to time-shifts in the acquisition. Although not explicitly shown in the results, the method does not suffer from drift, as relative displacements between all frames influence the cost to be minimized.

No failure cases were observed in our datasets but large in/through plane motion could, in principle, induce inter-frame shape variations that introduce higher frequency content similar to motion artifacts. Another drawback from the current implementation is that it is semi-automatic as user input is required for the selection of an ROI that encompasses both the RV and the LV. Future work will therefore focus on: a) including a transformation model with more degrees of freedom, and b) detecting the ROI automatically.

However, selecting an ROI in a single frame requires minimal user-interaction, while previously the amount of manual adjustments needed to compensate for large and frequent patient motion were prohibitive. Since the correction of deformations using non-rigid registration only slightly improves the motion compensation when compared to rigid registration [10], the absence of through plane motion correction is also not a significantly limiting factor. To our knowledge, the minimal effort, combined with the robustness of the proposed method make it feasible for the first time to process stress sequences in a clinical setting and using parameters such as MPRI in patient care.

References

1. Kaandorp, T., Lamb, H., Bax, J., van der Wall, E., de Roos, A.: Magnetic resonance imaging of coronary arteries, the ischemic cascade, and myocardial infarction. American Heart Journal 149(2), 200–208 (2005)
2. Al-Saadi, N., Gross, M., Bornstedt, A., Schnackenburg, B., Klein, C., Fleck, E., Nagel, E.: Comparison of various parameters for determining an index of myocardial perfusion reserve in detecting coronary stenosis with cardiovascular magnetic resonance tomography. Zeitschrift für Kardiologie 90(11), 824 (2001)
3. Jerosch-Herold, M., Seethamraju, R., Swingen, C., Wilke, N., Stillman, A.: Analysis of myocardial perfusion MRI. Journal of Magnetic Resonance Imaging 19(6), 758–770 (2004)
4. McLeish, K., Hill, D., Atkinson, D., Blackall, J., Razavi, R.: A study of the motion and deformation of the heart due to respiration. IEEE Transactions on Medical Imaging 21(9), 1142–1150 (2002)
5. Gupta, V., Kirişli, H.A., Hendriks, E.A., van der Geest, R.J., van de Giessen, M., Niessen, W., Reiber, J.H.C., Lelieveldt, B.P.F.: Cardiac MR perfusion image processing techniques: A survey. Medical Image Analysis 16(4), 767–785
6. Milles, J., van der Geest, R.J., Jerosch-Herold, M., Reiber, J.H.C., Lelieveldt, B.P.F.: Fully automated motion correction in first-pass myocardial perfusion MR image sequences. IEEE Transactions on Medical Imaging 27(11), 1611–1621 (2008)
7. Gupta, V., Hendriks, E.A., Milles, J., van der Geest, R.J., Jerosch-Herold, M., Reiber, J.H.C., Lelieveldt, B.P.F.: Fully Automatic Registration and Segmentation of First-Pass Myocardial Perfusion MR Image Sequences. Academic Radiology 17(11), 1375–1385 (2010)
8. Wollny, G., Ledesma-Carbayo, M.J., Kellman, P., Santos, A.: Exploiting quasiperiodicity in motion correction of free-breathing myocardial perfusion MRI. IEEE Transactions on Medical Imaging 29(8), 1516–1527 (2010)
9. Van der Geest, R.J., Lelieveldt, B.P.F., Angelie, E., Danilouchkine, M., Sonka, M., Reiber, J.H.C.: Evaluation of a new method for automated detection of left ventricular contours in time series of Magnetic Resonance Images using an Active Appearance Motion Mode. Journal of Cardiovascular Magnetic Resonance 6(3), 609–617 (2004)
10. Xue, H., Guehring, J., Srinivasan, L., Zuehlsdorff, S., Saddi, K., Chefdhotel, C., Hajnal, J.V., Rueckert, D.: Evaluation of Rigid and Non-rigid Motion Compensation of Cardiac Perfusion MRI. In: Metaxas, D., Axel, L., Fichtinger, G., Székely, G. (eds.) MICCAI 2008, Part II. LNCS, vol. 5242, pp. 35–43. Springer, Heidelberg (2008)

Localization of Sparse Transmural Excitation Stimuli from Surface Mapping

Jingjia Xu, Azar Rahimi Dehaghani, Fei Gao, and Linwei Wang

Computational Biomedicine Laboratory, Golisano College of Computing and
Information Sciences, Rochester Institute of Technology, Rochester, NY, 14623, USA

Abstract. As *in-silico* 3D electrophysiological (EP) models start to play
an essential role in revealing transmural EP characteristics and diseased
substrates in individual hearts, there arises a critical challenge to properly initialize these models, i.e., determine the location of excitation
stimuli without a trial-and-error process. In this paper, we present a
novel method to localize transmural stimuli based on their spatial sparsity using surface mapping data. In order to overcome the mathematical
ill-posedness caused by the limited measurement data, a neighborhood-
smoothness constraint is used to first obtain a low-resolution estimation
of sparse solution. This is then used to initialize an iterative, re-weighted
minimum-norm regularization to enforce a sparse solution and thereby
overcome the physical ill-posedness of the electromagnetic inverse problem. Phantom experiments are performed on a human heart-torso model
to evaluate this method in localizing excitation stimuli at different regions and depths within the ventricles, as well as to test its feasibility in
differentiating multiple remotely or close distributed stimuli. Real-data
experiments are performed on a healthy and an infarcted porcine heart,
where activation isochronous simulated with the reconstructed stimuli
are significantly closer to the catheterized mapping data than other stimuli configurations. This method has the potential to benefit the current
research in subject-specific EP modeling as well as to facilitate clinical
decisions involving device pacing and ectopic foci.

Keywords: transmural electrophysiology, *in silico* electrophysiological
models, sparse excitation stimuli, surface mapping.

1   Introduction

Disruption to the path of electrical propagation in the heart can lead to life-
threatening situations and sudden cardiac death [1]. However, current clinical
routines measure cardiac electrophysiological (EP) activity by surface mapping
data, *i.e.*, body-surface electrocardiograms (ECG) or heart-surface catheterized
mapping, which provides a poor surface surrogate for transmural EP activities
across the depth of the myocardium [2]. Recent research has seen promising
progress towards this challenge, where these surface mapping data are combined
with 3D *in silico* EP models via different mathematical methods to get an estimation of the individualized transmural EP characteristics, such as the *maximum*

N. Ayache et al. (Eds.): MICCAI 2012, Part I, LNCS 7510, pp. 675–682, 2012.
© Springer-Verlag Berlin Heidelberg 2012

a posteriori (MAP) of 3D action potential [3,4] and the estimation of conduction velocity[5,4]. These different methods of subject-special EP modeling have the potential to improve the early diagnosis and prevention of malignant arrhythmia, and to predict patient response to different therapeutic interventions.

However, these studies face the common challenge of properly initializing the EP models, *i.e.*, setting the locations of excitation stimuli, which will directly impact the calibration of EP models. In diseased ventricles, such as hearts with focal arrhythmia, the excitation may not start at regular Purkinje end-terminals. Even in healthy ventricles, there is a lack of practical means to measure the locations of subject-specific Purkinje end-terminals that may vary from subject to subject. How to obtain accurate locations for the ventricular stimuli becomes a critical issue for subject-specific EP modeling, and some initial efforts include personalizing Purkinje end-terminals from surface optical mapping data [6].

Excitation stimuli, the starting points of electrical propagation, are typically sparse in space no matter whether the ventricles are under sinus-rhythm or pacing (external stimulus, foci, etc) conditions. In this paper, we exploit this spatial sparsity of EP stimuli to solve the problem of transmural stimuli localization using surface mapping data. We present a two-step algorithm where a neighborhood-smoothness constrained minimum-norm solution is first obtained to overcome the *mathematical ill-posedness* of the problem caused by the limited number of surface data. This solution provides a low-resolution estimation of the spatial distribution of excitation stimuli, which is then used to initialize an iterative re-weighted regularization method that, based on the stimuli sparsity in space, prunes the initial estimation of the stimuli into a sparse solution that pinpoints the locations of stimuli. Phantom experiments are perform on a human heart-torso model to evaluate this method in localizing single stimulus ($n = 175$) at different longitudinal, circumferential, and transmural regions within the ventricles and to further test its feasibility in differentiating multiple, closely or remotely distributed stimuli. Real-data experiments are performed on a healthy and an infarcted porcine heart, where the activation isochrones simulated with the reconstructed stimuli are significantly more consistent with the measured catheter maps than other stimuli configurations. Pinpointing transmural excitation stimuli from noninvasive or minimally-invasive surface data, this method is potentially beneficial to subject-specific EP modeling research as well as clinical decisions involving external device pacing and ectopic foci.

2   Method

The relationship between the excitation stimuli and surface mapping data can be described by a quasi-static simplification of Maxwell's equation on an image-derived discrete, anatomically-detailed model for any individual subject [7]:

$$\mathbf{\Phi} = \mathbf{Hu} + \mathbf{n} \tag{1}$$

where $\mathbf{\Phi}_{m \times 1}$ represents the surface mapping potential and $\mathbf{u}_{n \times 1}$ the value of active electrical sources distributed within the 3D myocardium. At the begin of electrical propagation, only very few locations are excited while the majority of the myocardium are at the resting stage, $i.e.$, $\mathbf{u}$ is a sparse vector where the majority of the elements has the value 0. Transfer matrix $\mathbf{H}_{m \times n}$ ($m \ll n$) encodes the geometrical and conductivity information of the individual. $\mathbf{n}$ is added to represent uncertainty caused by measurement and modeling error.

The inverse problem of inferring $\mathbf{u}$ from $\mathbf{\Phi}$ is plagued by two types of non-uniqueness [7], and we present a two-step algorithm to overcome the two challenges step by step:

1. First, to overcome the *mathematical* ill-posedness caused by the limited number of surface data compared to the number of unknowns in the heart, a neighborhood-smoothness constraint is imposed to achieve the effect of reducing the number of unknowns and to obtain a low-resolution solution of $\hat{\mathbf{u}}$. At this moment, the solution $\hat{\mathbf{u}}$ is not sparse.
2. Second, this inverse problem is further afflicted with the *physical* ill-posedness associated with the electromagnetic field, where adjacent stimuli can produce the same potential distribution on the surface. To overcome this problem, we present a sparsity-based, iterative re-weight minimum-norm regularization which, initialized by the solution from the first step, will pinpoint the exact location of excitation stimuli by achieving a sparse solution of $\hat{\mathbf{u}}$.

Neighborhood-Smoothness Estimation: The inverse solution derived at the first step overcomes the *mathematical* ill-posedness by imposing a neighborhood-smoothness constraint [8] on a minimum norm cost function. It thus considers the neighborhood as one region to reduce the number of unknown variables:

$$\min_{\mathbf{u}} \| \mathcal{S}\mathbf{u} \|^2, \qquad s.t : \|\mathbf{\Phi} - \mathbf{H}\mathbf{u}\| \leq \sigma^2 \qquad (2)$$

where $\mathcal{S}$ is the neighborhood-smoothness term and σ^2 the variance of the noise.

The design of $\mathcal{S} = \mathbf{\Omega} \bigotimes \mathbf{I}\mathbf{\Psi}$ takes into account two factors: The first factor (diagonal weight matrix $\mathbf{\Omega}$) considers the contribution of each region to the surface recordings: $\Omega_{ii} = \sqrt{\mathbf{h}_{i,:}\mathbf{h}_{i,:}^T}$, $\mathbf{h}_{i,:}$ being the i-th row of the forward mapping matrix $\mathbf{H}$; The second factor $\mathbf{\Psi} = (\psi_1^T, \psi_2^T, ..., \psi_n^T)^T$ decides the size of neighborhood for the smoothness constraint and is defined as:

$$\psi_i = \frac{1}{N^2}\left(\frac{\sum_b \varphi_b}{\sum_b \varphi_b + 1} - \varphi_i\right), \qquad s.t : \| \mathbf{r}_i - \mathbf{r}_b \| \leq N \qquad (3)$$

where φ is value of $\mathbf{u}$ weighted by $\mathbf{\Omega}$, and $\mathbf{r}_i$ and $\mathbf{r}_b$ are the coordinates for the nodes. In other words, we define the spatial neighborhood by radius N, combined with boundary conditions so that boundary points only have a partial sphere.

Sparse Source Reconstruction: Within the "smoothest" solution from first step as *a priori*, the sparse stimuli is reconstructed in the second step with a re-weight minimum norm algorithm [9] that performs an iterative procedure of energy localization to overcome the *physical* ill-posedness problem:

$$\min_{\mathbf{q}_k} \| \mathbf{q}_k \|, \qquad s.t : \|\mathbf{H}\mathbf{W}_k\mathbf{q}_k - \mathbf{\Phi}\| \leq \sigma^2 \qquad (4)$$

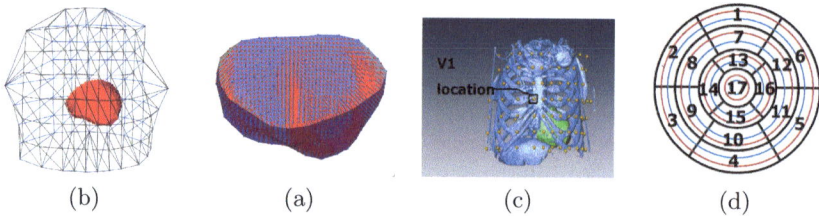

| (b) | (a) | (c) | (d) |

Fig. 1. (a) and (b): Boundary-element represented torso model with coupled meshfree nodes represented ventricular model; (c) Body-surface 120 leads with electrodes covering both the front and back of the body surface; (d) 17×3 segment of the LV where 17 is the standard AHA segments plus 3 transmural layers

where a weighted minimum-norm $||\mathbf{q}_k = \mathbf{W}_k^{-1}\mathbf{u}_k||$ is performed in each iteration, and the diagonal weight matrix $\mathbf{W}_k$ at iteration k has elements from the previous solution $\mathbf{u}_{k-1}$. The relatively large entries in W reduce the contribution of the corresponding elements of $\mathbf{u}$ in the cost function, and vice versa. By an iterative procedure, a sparse solution is achieved by adjust the weight matrix and, as a result, the most-likely candidate of stimuli will have its signal value strengthened when the rest candidates will have their values weakened to 0.

This optimization problem (4) is solved through an adaptive regularization:

$$\mathbf{u}_k = diag(\mathbf{u}_{k-1}) \cdot \arg\min_{\mathbf{q}_k}\{\| \ \mathbf{\Phi} - \mathbf{H}diag(\mathbf{u}_{k-1})\mathbf{q}_k \ \|_2 + \lambda \ \| \ \mathbf{q}_k \ \|\} \qquad (5)$$

where λ is a regularization parameter, determined by L-curve in this study.

Combining the two-step process, the initial $\mathbf{u}_0$ is provided by neighborhood-smoothness solution to start the iterative, re-weighted minimum norm regularization. The iteration terminates when the difference between two successive solutions is smaller than the pre-defined tolerance, and a sparse and unique distribution of excitation stimuli will be achieved.

3   Results

3.1   Phantom Experiment

Phantom experiments are conducted on a human anatomical heart-torso model, derived from $3mm$ whole-body CT scans. Fig. 1 shows the heart-torso model(a) with coupled ventricular model(b); (c) shows the set up of body-surface 120 leads which cover both the front and back of the body surface. We evaluate our method on 1) localizing single stimulus at different locations and depths of the ventricles, and 2) localizing and differentiating multiple stimuli distributed close or remotely with each other. In each case, *true* stimuli locations are set to simulate 120-lead body-surface ECG, which are then corrupted with 20-dB white Gaussian noise as inputs for localizing the stimuli. Localization errors are quantified by the Euclidean distance between the reconstructed and *true* stimuli.

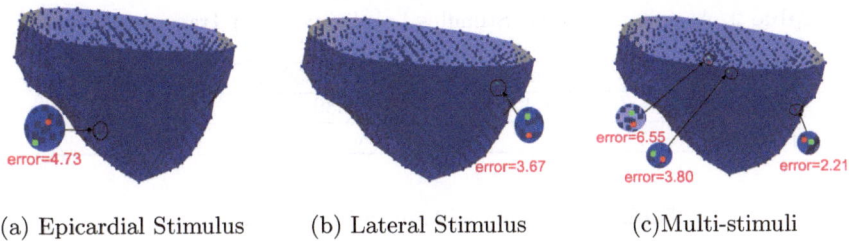

(a) Epicardial Stimulus   (b) Lateral Stimulus   (c)Multi-stimuli

Fig. 2. (a) Single stimulus in epicardial-septal LV. (b) Single stimulus in endocardial-lateral LV. (c) 3 remotely distributed stimuli at septal-endocardial and lateral-intramural LV: average error=3.58mm.

Table 1. Accuracy of Single Stimulus Localization at Different Regions

Segment	Anterior (n=28)	Inferior (n=28)	Apex (n=6)	Lateral (n=49)	Septal (n=49)	RV (n=15)
Error (mm)	0.11 ± 0.60	0.23 ± 0.85	0.53 ± 1.30	0.56 ± 1.72	1.05 ± 2.46	2.44 ± 4.34
Missed %	3.57%	0%	0%	2.04%	0%	6.67%

A. Single Stimulus of Different Locations: To evaluate the accuracy in localizing stimulus at different locations of the ventricles, we consider the location by 17×3 segment of the LV where 17 is the standard AHA segments along longitudinal and circumferential directions plus 3 transmural layers (epicardial, endocardial, and intramural) (Fig.1(d)). By selecting a single excitation stimulus in these 51 segments, with 3-4 cases in each segment, altogether we have 160 cases of single stimulus covering different areas of LV and 15 randomly selected cases within the RV. For all the 175 cases, the neighborhood radius N is set to be $7mm$ and the iterative regularization takes in average 6.2 iterations to converge. Fig. 2 shows two examples of a single stimulus at the epicardial-septal LV (a) and at the endocardial-lateral LV (b), with superimposed *true* stimuli (red) and reconstructed stimuli (green). Table 1 compares the accuracy of stimuli location at different ventricular regions, and Table 2 compares the accuracy of stimuli location at different transmural layers. Note *missed* case means that the reconstructedû has no physiological meanings. From Table 1 & 2, we found that accuracy of stimuli location has some correlation with the physical locations of stimuli in the myocardium: anterior, inferior and apical stimuli can be localized with the highest accuracy because of the coverage of recording leads on the front and back of the body surface, followed by stimuli in lateral and septal region. Compared to LV stimuli, localization of RV stimuli is more difficult with an average error of $2.44 \pm 4.34mm$, most likely because they are more *hidden* from body-surface recordings. Similar reasons apply to the accurate localization of epicardial stimuli, followed in accuracy by intramural and endocardial stimuli.

Table 2. Accuracy of Single Stimulus Localization at 3 Transmural Layers

Segment	Epicardial(n=55)	Intramural (n=59)	Endocardial (n=61)
Error (mm)	0.18 ± 1.12	0.88 ± 2.39	1.12 ± 2.51
Missed %	0%	0%	3.57%

Table 3. Accuracy of Multi-Stimuli Localization

Types	Two close (n=10)	Two remotely (n=10)	Three close (n=10)	Three remotely (n=10)
Average Distance (mm)	4.2 ± 0.82	68.82 ± 12.56	5.45 ± 1.89	50.67 ± 10.34
Error (mm)	1.09 ± 1.82	2.79 ± 3.26	4.02 ± 3.87	3.35 ± 3.08
Iteration number	6.4	7.6	11.6	9.2

B. Randomly Selected Multiple Stimuli: We further test the feasibility of our algorithm in localizing and differentiating multiple stimuli by setting 4 types of stimuli configurations within both the LV and RV (Table 3): 1) two close distributed with each other; 2) two remotely; 3) three close; and 4) three remotely. In total, we perform 40 experiments and parameter N is set to be 5mm. Table 3 summarizes the results that show high localization accuracy of our method at the presence of multiple excitation stimuli, and not seem to be influenced by the distance between the stimuli. As an example, Fig.2 (c) shows the *true* and reconstructed locations of 3 stimuli distributed at septal-endocardial and lateral-intramural layers, with an averaged localization errors = $3.58mm$.

3.2   Real Data

Real data experiments are performed on two porcine datasets. Case 1 is a health porcine heart, and case 2 is a porcine heart with chronic infarction. For each porcine heart, a comprehensive dataset of *in vivo* CARTO mapping (Biosense Webster, Inc., Diamond Bar, CA) and *ex vivo* DW-MR (1.5T GE Signa-Excite scanner) are provided. Here, we use the first two time frames of the epicardial CARTO unipolar electrogram and the image-derived ventricular model as input data to localize the excitation stimuli. Because the exact locations of excitation stimuli are not directly available, validations are performed by simulating transmural EP dynamics with the *Aliev-Panfilov* model [10] using the reconstructed stimuli locations, and comparing the resulting activation isochrone with the CARTO mapping. Fig 3 (a) and Fig 4 (a) show the epicardial isochrone maps of the healthy and infarcted heart, respectively, measured by CARTO and projected to the MR-derived ventricular model.

For the healthy heart, parameter N is set to be 5mm and iteration times is 7. Two stimuli are identified, one localized in anterior-basal RV and the other in apical LV. Fig. 3 (c) shows the activation isochrone simulated with sinus-rhythm excitation at normal Purkinje end-terminals for human hearts experimentally determined in [11], which almost shows an opposite conduction pattern compared

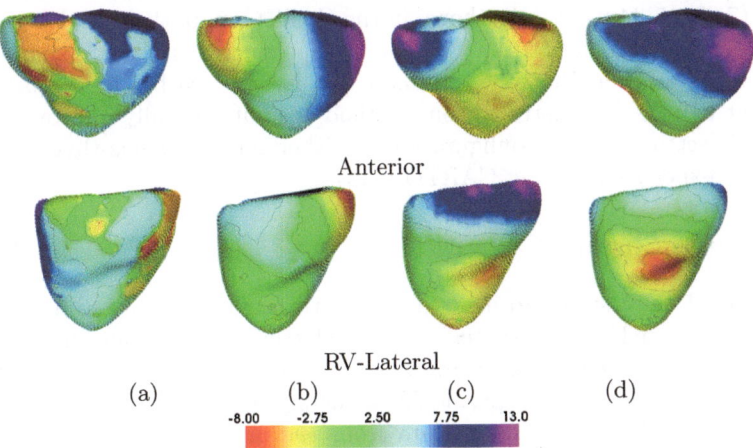

Fig. 3. Epicardial isochrone maps in healthy porcine heart. (a) CARTO-mapping, (b) Simulation with reconstructed stimuli, (c) Simulation with sinus-rhythm excitation from common Purkinje end-terminals, (d) Simulation with expert suggested stimuli.

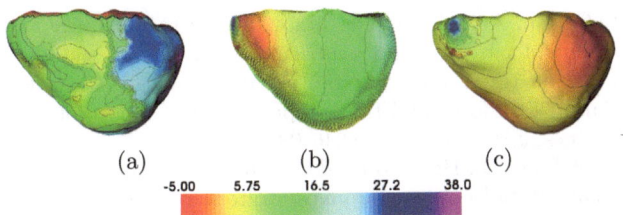

Fig. 4. Epicardial isochrone maps in the infarct porcine heart, (a) CARTO-mapping, (b) Simulation with reconstructed stimuli, (c) Simulation with sinus-rhythm excitation from common Purkinje end-terminals

to the CARTO maps (a). This may be because the porcine Purkinje structure is known to be different from human. Fig 3 (d) shows the isochrone simulated with an expert-suggested stimuli configuration based on examining CARTO maps (one stimuli at LV apex and the other at RV apex). While it captures the RV-to-LV activation pattern, it fails to reproduce the local activation features especially that around RV. The averaged absolute error in activation time compared to CARTO data is $4.92 \pm 5.12ms$. Fig. 3 (b) shows the isochrone simulated with our result, which closely captures the early activation at anterior RV as well as the RV-to-LV activation with an absolute error $3.63 \pm 2.47ms$.

For the infarcted heart, parameter N is set as 5mm and iteration time is 10. The DW-MR enhanced scar is centered at middle-anterolateral LV and is incorporated into the simulation. Fig. 4 compares the epicardial CARTO isochrone map (a) with that simulated with stimuli configured at common Purkinje end-terminals (error = $11.52 \pm 8.76ms$) (c) and that simulated with the reconstructed stimuli $(7.89 \pm 5.34ms)$(b). As shown in the CARTO map, there is also a RV-to-LV activation in this heart that can not be reproduced with the assumption of common excitation at Purkinje terminals, but is captured by the reconstructed stimuli at RV. As demonstrated, our method can substantially improve current practice in setting stimuli configuration by either common sinus-rhythm excitation or by experts examining CARTO maps.

4   Discussion and Conclusion

We presented a two-step algorithm to localize transmural excitation stimuli from surface data based on the spatial sparsity of stimuli. Phantom and real data experiments demonstrate the accuracy as well as the usefulness of this method in relevant research in subject-specific EP modeling. In the current study, stimuli localization considers only input data from one or two time instants. Future investigation will focus on the possibility to combine temporal information to the proposed sparse source reconstruction. In future studies, we will also investigate the impact of neighborhood size N on the final solutions.

References

1. Zipes, D.P., Camm, A.J., Borggrefe, M., et al.: ACC/AHA/ESC 2006 guidelines for management of patients with ventricular arrhythmias and the prevention of sudden cardiac death: A report of the american college of cardiology/american heart association task force and the european society of cardiology committee for practice guidlines. JACC 48, e247–e346 (2006)
2. Wijnmaalen, A.P., et al.: Head-to-head comparison of contrast-enhanced magnetic resonance imaging and electroanatomical voltage mapping to assess post-infarct scar characteristics in patients with ventricular tachycardias: Real-time image integration and reversed registration. European Heart Journal 32, 104–114 (2011)
3. Wang, L., et al.: Noninvasive computational imaging of cardiac electrophysiology for 3-d infarct. Trans. Biomed. Eng. 58(4), 1033–1043 (2011)
4. Camara, O., Sermasant, M., et al.: Inter-model consistency and complementarity: Learning from ex-vivo imaging and electrophysiological data towards an integrated understanding of cardiac physiology. Prog. Bio. Mol. Biol., 122–133 (2011)
5. Relan, J., Sermesant, M., et al.: Parameter estimation of a 3d cardiac electrophysiology model including the restitution curve using optical and mr data. In: WC on Medical Physics and Biomedical Engineering, pp. 1716–1719. Springer (2010)
6. Camara, O., Pashaei, et al.: Personalization of fast conduction purkinje system in eikonal-based electrophysiological models with optical mapping data. In: STACOM, pp. 281–290 (2010)
7. Plonsey, R.: Bioelectric phenonmena. McGraw Hill, New York (1969)
8. Pascual-Marqui, R., Michel, C., Lehmann, D.: Low resolution electromagnetic tomography. Int. J. Psychophysiol. 18(1), 49–65 (1994)
9. Gorodnitsky, I.F., Rao, B.D.: Sparse signal reconstruction from limited data using focuss: A re-weighted minimum norm algorithm. IEEE Trans. Signal Processing 45(3), 600–616 (1997)
10. Aliev, R.R., et al.: A simple two-variable model of cardiac excitation. Chaos, Solitions & Fractals 7(3), 293–301 (1996)

Automated Intraventricular Septum Segmentation Using Non-local Spatio-temporal Priors

Mithun Das Gupta[1], Sheshadri Thiruvenkadam[1],
Navneeth Subramanian[1], and Satish Govind[2]

[1] John F. Welch Technology Center, GE Global Research, Bangalore, India
[2] Narayana Hrudayalaya, Bangalore, India
{mithun.dasgupta,sheshadri.thiruvenkadam,navneeth.s}@ge.com,
drsatishgovind@yahoo.com

Abstract. Automated robust segmentation of intra-ventricular septum (IVS) from B-mode echocardiographic images is an enabler for early quantification of cardiac disease. Segmentation of septum from ultrasound images is very challenging due to variations in intensity/contrast in and around the septum, speckle noise and non-rigid shape variations of the septum boundary. In this work, we effectively address these challenges using an approach that merges novel computer vision ideas with physiological markers present in cardiac scans. Specifically, we contribute towards the following: 1) A novel 1-D active contour segmentation approach that utilizes non-local (NL) temporal cues, 2) Robust initialization of the active contour framework, based on NL-means de-noising, and MRF based clustering that incorporates physiological cues. We validate our claims using cardiac measurement results on ~30 cardiac scan videos (~2000 ultrasound frames in total). Our method is fully automatic and near real time (0.1sec/frame) implementation.

1 Introduction

In echo-cardiography, wall and chamber dimensions are used as screening parameters for early indication of cardiac diseases. In this work, we address the inter-ventricular septum thickness (IVSd), which is accepted as a screening parameter for septal hypertrophy and has also shown a correlation to 24 hour ambulatory blood pressure. Unfortunately, the manual measurement of these parameters on echo-cardiograms suffers from large inter and intra observer variability based on the experience and expertise of the cardiologist. An end-to-end IVSd measurement in accordance with the American Society of Echocardiography (ASE) guidelines [1] involves segmentation of the septum, identification of mitral valve tip, and measurement of the thickness orthogonal to septum centerline.

Automation of septum segmentation from ultrasound images faces several challenges. First, the intensity in and around the septum region has a multimodal distribution, precluding simple schemes based on intensity alone. Second,

N. Ayache et al. (Eds.): MICCAI 2012, Part I, LNCS 7510, pp. 683–690, 2012.

the speckle noise inherent in ultrasound images makes edge-based methods unreliable. These methods are sensitive to initialization and are plagued by the
near-field haze which leads to low contrast at the upper part of the septum. For
any approach to segment the septum across several frames reliably, robustness
to noise and initialization is needed.

Region based active contour approaches [2,3] typically offer robustness to initialization and noise. Due to very low contrast at the upper part of the septum,
purely region based methods are likely to get trapped in local minima leading
to the introduction of shape priors [4]. Given the large inter-patient shape variability and non rigid deformations across frames, it is infeasible to build a shape
atlas of the septum. In Subramanian et al. [5], a region based active contour approach with a width prior for the septum is proposed. Constraining the width of
the septum, makes the resulting segmentation robust to noise/inhomogeneities
induced by near field haze. However, the width constraint is suited for advancing
the profiles closer to the septum boundary and fails in cases where the septum
boundary has low contrast. Further, [5] relies on a reasonable guess for the contour in the first frame, and in the absence of temporal cues, the segmentation is
most likely to drift away in cases of large non-rigid motion between frames.

Cardiac ultrasound data has rich temporal information in terms of continuity
of motion of structures which could provide reliable information on the location of the boundary under boundary gaps and low-contrast regions. Hence, it
seems natural to model either velocity/acceleration using previous frames [6].
Consequently, we introduce temporal constraints to the segmentation cost functional. We constrain acceleration of boundary points to be similar in a non-local
neighborhood around each boundary location. The non-local temporal penalty
differentiates our work from the state-of-the-art [5], and is key in robust prediction of the septum location in the absence of strong contrast for the segmentation
functional. The second part of our work deals the important aspect of initializing the 1D contours for the segmentation technique. We propose to mitigate
the non-trivial problem of initializing the septum boundary using physiological
cues. We propose a robust routine based on non-local (NL)-means de-noising,
and Markov Random field (MRF) based clustering.

This paper is organized as follows. In Sec. 2, we describe the details of algorithms pertaining to each of the individual pieces. In Sec. 3, we present our
results on 32 patients, and our conclusions are listed in Sec. 4.

2   Methods

In a typical echocardiography scan, usually 3 cardiac loops are captured, where
one loop is defined as end-diastolic frame to the next end-diastolic frame. Based
on the frame rate of the scanner usually about 100 frames are captured in this
loop. In this work we look at the parasternal long axis (PLAX) view. The mitral
valve tip detection is handled identical to the method proposed by Subramanian
et al. [5].

2.1 1D Active Contour Formulation Using Non-local Temporal Priors

Similar to [5], we propose an energy based formulation with a search space of pairs of smooth 1D profiles (representing the top and bottom boundaries of the septum). This representation enables easy access to regional statistics in and around the septum, and model interactions between the top and bottom septum boundaries. Further, the simplified representation makes the approach faster than 2D active contour approaches, making it feasible for real time tracking. The main contribution of this work is to incorporate temporal cues into the above framework to improve robustness to noise, gaps, and large motion.

For image $I : \Omega \to R$, $\Omega = [a, b] \times [c, d]$, we look for two smooth 1D functions $g, f : [a, b] \to [c, d]$, whose profiles represent the top and bottom parts of the septum. We denote the septum region between the 1D profiles of f and g, as R^s. We denote the neighborhood region above the septum as R^{up}, i.e. between profiles of g and $g + \Delta$, where Δ is some pre-defined interval. Similarly, the neighborhood below the septum is R^{dn}, between profiles of $f - \Delta$ and f. We make a piece wise constant assumption of intensity in and around a neighborhood of the septum. Consequently, we divide $(a, b) = \bigcup_{i=1}^{K}(a_i, b_i)$ into K disjoint intervals and seek for f, g that give homogeneous distributions in regions $R_i^{up} = R^{up} \cap ([a_i, b_i] \times [c, d])$, $R_i^{dn} = R^{dn} \cap ([a_i, b_i] \times [c, d])$ and $R_i^s = R^s \cap ([a_i, b_i] \times [c, d])$.

The following energy is minimized over the space of smooth 1D functions $f, g : [a, b] \to [c, d]$ and mean statistics $\mu^{up}, \mu^s, \mu^{dn}$:

$$E_{frm}(f, g, \mu^{up}, \mu^s, \mu^{dn}) =$$

$$\sum_{i=1}^{K} \left[\int_{R_i^s} (I - \mu_i^s)^2 dydx + \int_{R_i^{up}} (I - \mu_i^{up})^2 dydx + \int_{R_i^{dn}} (I - \mu_i^{dn})^2 dydx \right]$$

$$+ \lambda_{width} \int_a^b (f + w - g)^2 dx + \lambda_{smooth} \int_a^b \left(\sqrt{1 + (f')^2} + \sqrt{1 + (g')^2} \right) dx \quad (1)$$

The data term drives f, g to take piece wise constant values in each of R_i^s, R_i^{up}, R_i^{dn}. The smoothness terms for f and g are governed by parameter $\lambda_{smooth}(0.08)$. The width term constrains the width of R^s to be close to the expected septum width (w) and is balanced by $\lambda_{width}(\sim 1.0\text{cm})$. In most cases, because of strong contrast between the septum and blood pool, the bottom boundary f of the septum is reliably segmented and the width term drives the top boundary g out of local minima closer to the actual boundary. From here, contrast close to the septum boundary takes over and drives the segmentation. In low contrast cases, one would expect the evolution to be dominated by the smoothness and width terms and be drawn to arbitrary minima.

We now augment the above energy with temporal priors computed from previous frames. The septum being an elastic structure exhibits motion that is correlated across different locations, which can be captured through temporal priors resulting in robust prediction of the septum in the absence of strong contrast. Given the large shape variations and complex non-rigid motion of the septum, it seems natural to model either velocity/acceleration using previous frames similar to [6]. If f^{n-2}, f^{n-1}, f^n are the profiles at frames $n-2, n-1, n$, one could penalize velocity $V^n = f^n - f^{n-1}$ using $\int_a^b (\frac{dV^n}{dx})^2 dx$, or penalize acceleration $A^n = f^{n-2} - 2f^{n-1} + f^n$ using $\int_a^b (\frac{dA^n}{dx})^2 dx$. Here, we look at a non-local penalty for acceleration defined by $\int_a^b \int_a^b w(x,y)(A^n(x) - A^n(y))^2 dx dy$, where w is a weight function for the pair (x,y). The choice of non-local priors is physically intuitive in that velocity interactions between pixels extend beyond local neighborhoods and modeling these non-local interactions might give better robustness to noise/boundary gaps. The Euler Lagrange equations of the above acceleration penalty is $A^n - w * A^n = 0$ or in terms of velocity $V^n - w * V^n = V^{n-1} - w * V^{n-1}$. Thus velocity at each point on the profile f is updated using relative velocities learnt in the previous frame and velocities of non-local neighboring points. As for the choice of w, for simplicity we use $w(x,y) = G_\sigma(|x-y|)$, thus the above equations involve only convolutions and would be fast to compute. Alternatively, one could consider intensity/contrast dependent terms for w to down-select points to learn relative velocities. Note that in the work proposed by Snare et al. [7], the motion prior is local wherein, motion models at neighboring control points do not interact with each other. Thus if a control point falls in a poor contrast/signal dropout location, for a couple of frames, the segmentation will drift away. We modify Eq. 1 to include the temporal term. For each frame n, denote $A^n = f^{n-2} - 2f^{n-1} + f^n$ and $B^n = g^{n-2} - 2g^{n-1} + g^n$. We minimize:

$$E_{temp}^n = E_{frm} + \lambda_T \int_a^b \int_a^b w(x,y)((A^n(x) - A^n(y))^2 + (B^n(x) - B^n(y))^2) dx dy$$

$$(2)$$

Given profiles from previous time points f^j, g^j, $j = n-2, n-1$, E_{frm} is minimized, using descent on the Euler Lagrange equations for Eq. 2, using an explicit finite difference scheme. The following synthetic results show the robustness of the temporal prior. In Fig. 1, the goal is to segment the current frame (III) from two clean previous frames shown in (I), (II). In these experiments, segmentation results are shown in Red, and the ground truth is in Green.

In the noisy (white noise) experiment shown in Fig. 1 (top row), (a) is the noisy frame, (b) is the result without temporal information, (c) is the result using non-local temporal priors (proposed approach). In (d), even for really high levels of noise, a reasonable segmentation is computed. In the second experiment Fig. 1 (bottom row), on segmenting in the presence of gaps, (e), (f) show results without temporal priors. The kink in the lower and upper boundaries is lost, and the missing pieces are completed with straight lines because of the smoothness term. In (g)-(i) using our approach, for increasing size of the gap, the kink is seen to be preserved. The reasoning is that at a location with poor contrast, gap or high noise, a non-local neighbor where the contrast is possibly good, directly contributes to the update at the location using relative velocities learnt from previous frames.

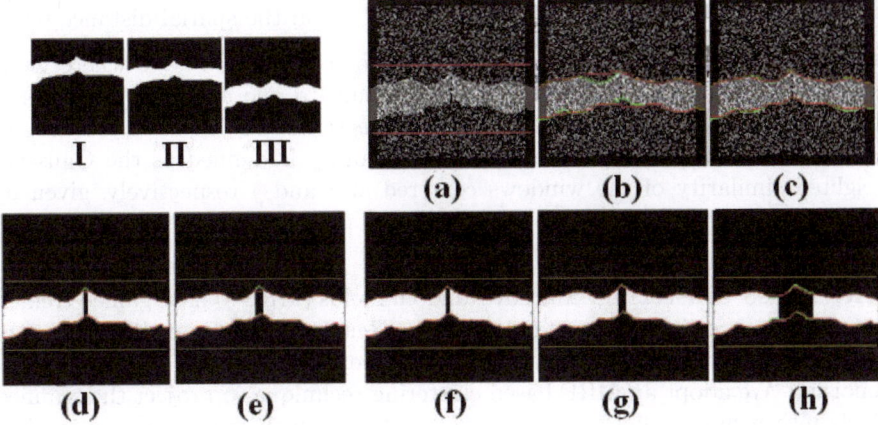

Fig. 1. Synthetic Experiments: (I) Frame n-2 (II) Frame n-1 (III) Current Frame n. Top Row: Noise Robustness: (a) Noisy image with initialization (b) Result w/o temporal prior (c) Result using temporal approach. Bottom Row: Robustness to Gaps: (d)-(e) Results w/o temporal prior (f)-(h) Results using temporal approach. Groundtruth is in green and the algorithm output is shown in red.

2.2   Active Contour Initialization Using Blood Pool Detection

One of the primary drawbacks of active contour based methods [5] for segmentation is the inherent need for correct initialization. The initial contour needs positioned reasonably close to the final contour to guarantee convergence. For completely automated system required to work for large patient populations, initialization has to be driven by physiological cues such that patient variability can be properly captured [8]. The LV blood pool is an "anechoic" region (no oscillating sources in it) and hence it appears completely dark under ultrasound. Based on this key observation, we propose to detect the LV blood pool to infer an estimate for the lower boundary of the septum and initialize the curves. The first step in our approach is a denoising algorithm using Non-Local means, and the second is an MRF based clustering technique to find the maximum width of the blood pool. Once the blood pool is identified, the septum is its immediate neighbor towards the ultrasound probe position. This knowledge can now be used to initialize an active contour method for segmentation.

Neighborhood Based Non-local Smoothing. The key intuition for non-local (NL) means based filtering, as proposed by Buades et al. [9] is that the denoised value at location x is a mean of the values of all points within the image domain whose Gaussian neighborhood is similar to the neighborhood of x. Given a discrete noisy image $\mathbf{v} = \{v(i)|i \in I\}$, the estimated value $NL(\mathbf{v})(i)$ is computed as a weighted average of all the pixels in the image $\mathbf{I}$, given by $NL(\mathbf{v})(i) = \sum_{j \in \mathbf{I}} w(i,j)v(j)$, where the weights $w(i,j)$ quantify the similarity between the pixels i and j and satisfy the conditions $0 \leq w(i,j) \leq 1$ and

$\sum_j w(i,j) = 1$. To decouple the similarity term from the spatial distance term, [9] propose the weighting function to be $w(i,j) = \frac{1}{Z_i} e^{-\frac{sim(i,j)}{h^2}}$, where Z_i is a normalization term such that the weights sum to one and the parameter h controls the spatial decay of the exponential function. Defining a window around pixel i as $\mathcal{N}_i$, the similarity between pixel i and j is defined as the Gaussian weighted similarity of the windows centered at i and j respectively, given by $sim(i,j) = \sum_k e^{-\frac{(\mathcal{N}_i(k) - \mathcal{N}_j(k))^2}{\sigma^2}}$.

MRF Based Clustering. Markov Random Fields (MRF's) have gained tremendous importance since the seminal paper by Geman and Geman [10] that introduced the idea of denoising as a labeling problem and used an MRF model for denoising. We adopt an MRF based clustering technique to project the scanned pixels into a finite label space $\{L : |L| \ll 255\}$ which is the maximum pixel range for 8 bit image data. The observation field Y is fixed and is assumed to be non-interacting. The label field X is evolved with iterations minimizing the following cost function

$$E(L) = \sum_{p \in \mathcal{X}} D_p(L_p) + \sum_{q \in \mathcal{N}_p} V_{p,q}(L_p, L_q) \tag{3}$$

where $\mathcal{N}_p$ represents the neighborhood for a particular node p. The MRF model balances the two cost terms in Eq. 3 to generate the possible label for the target node. The first term constrains the label to be close to the observation. If the cluster center intensities are pre-specified, then this term can be simply evaluated as $I(p) - C_i$ over all labels $i = \{1, 2, \ldots, L\}$, where $I(p)$ is the pixel intensity at location p. For our experiments we typically set $|L| = 5$.

Lateral Cluster Projection. The NL-means filtering and clustering, leaves us with an image where the blood pool is certain to be one of darkest clusters (Fig. 2 (left panel)) in the label map. We compute the radial histogram of the pixels with bins centred at the probe location as our feature. This essentially leads to counting pixels radially for each label class and results in an 1D curve with as many points as the image depth for each bin. To identify the LV blood pool, the two darkest clusters (red and pink colors in Fig. 2 right panel) are considered. The initialization estimate is then, a radial curve at the maximal bin index corresponding to the blood pool cluster.

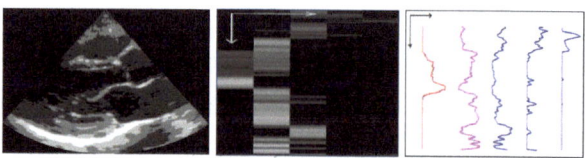

Fig. 2. Left to right: MRF based pixel clusters, label histogram, histogram for individual label classes

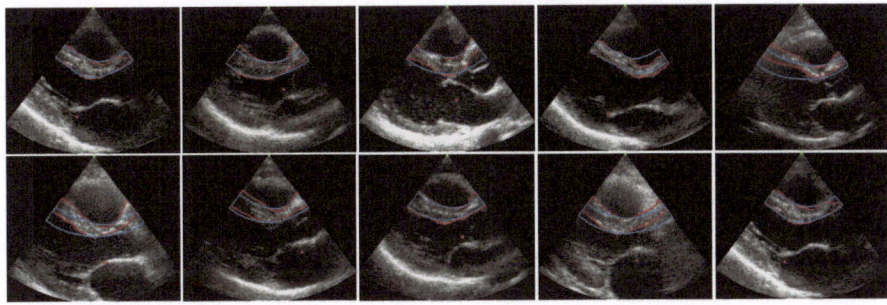

Fig. 3. Comparative Results. Red curve: proposed method. Blue curve: Subramanian et al. [5]. The red dot shows the mitral valve tip.

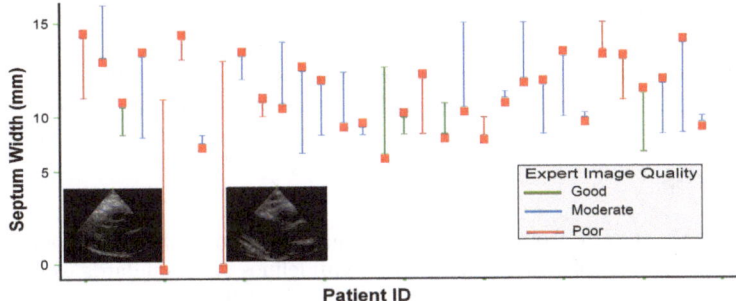

Fig. 4. Quantitative comparisons. Quantitative comparison of automated vs expert measurements on 32 cases. The height of the bar denotes the error in measurement (one end ground truth and the other end algorithm output). Red markers denote the algorithm output. Inset images correspond to the two failure cases with poor image quality.

3   Results

We evaluated our method on B-mode PLAX recordings, representing a total of 32 different patients with has ≈3 cycles/recording. The subjects with varied clinical background, normal chamber dimensions and systolic function underwent routine echocardiography (commercially available Vivid 7, GE) with ECG gating. The patient data used in our validation included normal and hypertrophic patients. We present comparative visual results against the method proposed in [5] for cardiac segmentation and tracking in Fig. 3. Our method runs in near real-time, with an average computation time of 0.1 sec/frame on a 2.6GHZ PC with 2GB RAM.

The performance of the method was quantitatively evaluated by comparing the thickness measurement, as generated by the segmentation, with the cardiologist's measurement. Fig. 4 shows the measurement error for each dataset. We observe that the method performs favorably, with the exception of two cases rated as having poor image quality. In these cases, both the segmentation and mitral valve estimation fail (Fig. 4). Discarding these two cases, which are extremely poor quality, we report a mean error = 1.8949mm, variance = 3.609mm, maximum error bound = [-1.173mm, 6.0042mm] for our proposed method.

4   Conclusions

We have developed an automatic approach for cardiac segmentation that is robust to the image noise, haze and cardiac motion typical in ultrasound. 1D curve evolutions based on regional statistics and constrained by temporal priors are shown to be well suited for segmentation of rapidly moving cardiac structures. Additionally, the non-trivial step of robust initialization to enhance convergence of active contours is addressed. Our framework was validated on 32 B-mode PLAX recordings and compared favourably with the true boundary on an average of 93% of the cases, making it attractive for clinical application. In the future, we would like to evaluate the performance of the framework to segment and track other cardiac structures, such as, the posterior wall and LV cavity.

References

1. Lang, R.M., et al.: Recommendations for chamber quantification: a report from the American Society of Echocardiography's Guidelines and Standards Committee. J. American Soc. Echocardiography 18, 1440–1463 (2005) [1]
2. Lankton, S., Tannenbaum, A.: Localizing region-based active contours. IEEE Trans. Image Processing 17, 2029–2039 (2008) [2]
3. Chan, T.F., Vese, L.A.: Active contours without edges. IEEE Trans. Image Processing 10, 266–277 (2001) [2]
4. Leventon, M., Grimson, W.L., Faugeras, O.: Statistical shape influence in geodesic active contours. In: CVPR, vol. 1, pp. 316–323 (2000) [2]
5. Subramanian, N., Padfield, D., Thiruvenkadam, S., Narasimhamurthy, A., Frigstad, S.: Automated Interventricular Septum Thickness Measurement from B-Mode Echocardiograms. In: Jiang, T., Navab, N., Pluim, J.P.W., Viergever, M.A. (eds.) MICCAI 2010, Part I. LNCS, vol. 6361, pp. 510–517. Springer, Heidelberg (2010) [2], [3], [4], [7]
6. Niethammer, M., Tannenbaum, A.: Dynamic geodesic snakes for visual tracking. In: IEEE CVPR (2004) [2], [3]
7. Snare, S.R., Mjølstad, O.C., Orderud, F., Dalen, H., Torp, H.: Automated septum thickness measurement–A kalman filter approach. Computer Methods and Programs in Biomedicine (2011) [4]
8. van Stralen, M., et al.: Time Continuous Detection of the Left Ventricular Long Axis and the Mitral Valve Plane in 3-D Echocardiography. Ultrasound in Medicine and Biology 34, 196–207 (2008) [5]
9. Buades, A., Coll, B., Morel, J.M.: A review of image denoising methods, with a new one. In: Multiscale Modeling and Simulation, vol. 4, pp. 490–530 (2006) [5]
10. Geman, S., Geman, D.: Stochastic relaxation, gibbs distributions, and the bayesian restoration of images. IEEE Trans. Pattern Anal. Machine Intelligence 6, 721–741 (1984) [6]

Active Shape Model with Inter-profile Modeling Paradigm for Cardiac Right Ventricle Segmentation

Mohammed S. ElBaz[1,2] and Ahmed S. Fahmy[1,3]

[1] Medical Imaging and Image processing Lab., Center for Informatics Science,
Nile University, Cairo, Egypt
[2] Division of Image Processing, Department of Radiology,
Leiden University Medical Center, Leiden, The Netherlands
[3] Systems and Biomedical Engineering Department, Cairo University, Cairo, Egypt
m.s.m.m.el_baz@lumc.nl

Abstract. In this work, a novel active shape model (ASM) paradigm is proposed to segment the right ventricle (RV) in cardiac magnetic resonance image sequences. The proposed paradigm includes modifications to two fundamental steps in the ASM algorithm. The first modification includes employing the 2D-Principal Component Analysis (PCA) to capture the inter-profile relations among shape's neighboring landmarks and then model the inter-profile variations between the training set. The second modification is based on using a multi-stage searching algorithm to find the best profile match based on the best maintained profile's relations and thus the best shape fitting in an iterative manner. The developed methods are validated using a database of short axis cine bright blood MRI images for 30 subjects with total of 90 images. Our results show that the segmentation error can be reduced by about 0.4 mm and contour overlap increased by about 4% compared to the classical ASM technique with paired Student's t-test indicates statistical significance to a high degree for our results. Furthermore, comparison with literature shows that the proposed method decreases the RV segmentation error significantly.

1 Introduction

Segmentation of the right ventricle (RV) has recently gained a lot of the clinical research focus. This is due to new findings that confirm the relationship between the RV function and a number of cardiac diseases such as heart failure, RV myocardial infarction, congenital heart disease and pulmonary hypertension [1,2]. Since manual segmentation of the RV borders throughout the cardiac cycle is tedious process and may suffer from personal bias, and inter-observer variations; accurate computer-aided segmentation methods are required. One of the increasingly popular and successful segmentation approaches is the Active Shape Model (ASM) introduced by Cootes et.al [3,4]. ASMs have been used for many segmentation tasks including medical images [3,4]. The classic ASM paradigm [4] represent the object of interest by a set of labeled points called landmarks, these landmarks define the shape of the object. The global statistics of the shape variation is then examined from number of examples in

N. Ayache et al. (Eds.): MICCAI 2012, Part I, LNCS 7510, pp. 691–698, 2012.

the training dataset by applying the Principal Component Analysis (PCA) on the landmarks of the training shapes to model the ways in which the points of the shape tends to move together through the training set [4]. Then, the gray-level appearance model that describes the typical image structure around each landmark is modeled by sampling a grey-level profile around each landmark then applies PCA on the training shapes profiles to model the profile appearance of each landmark in the shape independently. Throughout the image search, starting from the mean shape and initial model pose parameters (landmarks position, rotation and scaling), shapes are fitted in an iterative manner by fitting the appearance model of each landmark separately i.e. using local search. The shortcoming of the classical ASM paradigm is that while it models the global statistics of the shape variations, it merely builds a separate gray-level appearance model for each landmark in the shape. That is, the appearance model does not include any global information about the relationships among the appearance profiles of the different landmarks. Furthermore, searching for the best profile fit for each landmark independently might cause the contour to stick to local minimum.

In this work, we propose a novel appearance profile modeling paradigm to overcome these shortcomings. The proposed paradigm called inter-profile modeling in which for each shape in the training set, the appearance profiles are set in matrix form and the Two Dimensional Principal Component Analysis (2DPCA) [6] is applied to capture the inter-profile relations among the shape's landmarks and then to model the inter-profile variations between the different training shapes. Compared with PCA, 2DPCA algorithm is more efficient to deal with the proposed 2D profile matrices, as 2DPCA works directly on the 2D matrices without pre-transformation to 1D vector as required by PCA. This yields that 2DPCA constructs much smaller covariance matrix compared with PCA which gives 2DPCA a significant computational advantage [6,7]. Additionally, 2DPCA preserves the 2D integral structure and the spatial information of the input 2D matrices as opposed to the PCA which breakup this 2D integral through the 2D matrix to 1D vector transformation. Additionally, Multi-stage searching algorithm is also proposed to employ the modeled inter-profile variation to find the best profile match.

2   Methodology

Following from the active shape model algorithm [4], we apply the same shape modeling step. Then, for the profile modeling step we use a new profile-modeling paradigm as follows:

2.1   Inter-profile Appearance Modeling

We define the Inter-profile modeling as the process of capturing the profile modes of variation by the ways in which all shape appearance profiles tend to change together through the training set. In order to achieve this modeling, we start by constructing a grey level appearance profiles matrix (shortly we will refer to it as profiles matrix) for each shape (where similar to the ASM [4], each profile is perpendicular on the contour and sampled with length of n_s pixels on either side of the contour). The profiles matrix holds all shape profiles together. That is, given a training set of **K** shapes, **M** landmarks and intensity profile of length **N** at each landmark, then $\mathbf{G_i}$ (**i**=1,2,...,**K**) is given by,

$$
\mathbf{G_i} =
\begin{bmatrix}
L_{11}, L_{12} \ldots, L_{1N} \\
L_{21}, L_{22} \ldots, L_{2N} \\
\cdot \\
\cdot \\
\cdot \\
L_{M1}, L_{M2} \ldots, L_{MN}
\end{bmatrix}
\tag{1}
$$

Each row (i.e. grey-level profile) is normalized by the maximum value in the row to compensate for the illumination differences.

2.2   Capturing the Inter-profile Variations Using 2D-PCA

In order to capture the modes-of-variations of the inter-profile matrices of the training database, two-dimensional PCA (2DPCA) is employed [7] with its two versions (horizontal and vertical) [8] to capture both the horizontal and vertical inter-profile variations. For the horizontal 2DPCA version, the mean profile matrix $\overline{\mathbf{G}}_h$ and covariance matrix $\mathbf{C_t}$ are computed as

$$
\overline{G}_h = \frac{1}{K} \sum_{i=1}^{K} G_i \quad (2) \qquad \text{and} \qquad C_t = \frac{1}{K} \sum_{i=1}^{K} (G_i - \overline{G}_h)^T (G_i - \overline{G}_h) \tag{3}
$$

The grey-level variation around the mean profile $\overline{\mathbf{G}}_h$ is expressed by matrix ,$\mathbf{P_{gh}}$, of size N×D. That is $\mathbf{P_{gh}}$ contains the **D** eigenvectors of $\mathbf{C_t}$ corresponding to the **D** largest eigenvalues $\Lambda_1, \Lambda_2, \ldots, \Lambda_D$. The horizontal-based new profiles matrix approximation can be computed as

$$
G_i \approx \overline{G}_h + \left(P_{gh} b_{gh}\right)^T \tag{4}
$$

Contarary to the classical ASM vector model parameters, here, the model parameters are expressed by the matrix $\mathbf{b_{gh}}$ of size **D×M** computed as

$$
b_{gh} = P_{gh}^{\ T} (G_i - \overline{G}_h)^T \tag{5}
$$

Thus $\mathbf{b_{gh}}$ captures the horizontal inter-profile relations between the landmarks profiles. We apply constraints to the parameter $\mathbf{b_{gh}}$ to ensure plausible profiles (e.g. $|\mathbf{b_{gh}}| < 3\sqrt{\Lambda}$). To capture the grey-level modes of variation using the vertical 2DPCA, the same procedure discussed above is followed except that the input to the vertical 2DPCA is the transpose of the profiles matrix $\mathbf{G_i}$. This yields a model defined by the matrices: $\mathbf{P_{gv}}$ and $\mathbf{b_{gv}}$. During the search for the object that best fits the constructed shape model; some goodness-of-fit measure is needed. In the proposed modeling paradigm, the inter-profile model is given by the matrices $\overline{\mathbf{G}}_h$ and $\mathbf{P_{gh}}$ (assuming horizontal 2DPCA). The parameters required to best fit the horizontal model to $\mathbf{G_i}$ is given by the matrix $\mathbf{b_{gh}}$ computed by (5). To measure how well the model fits the profiles matrix $\mathbf{G_i}$, the Frobenius-norm of the parameter matrix $\mathbf{b_{gh}}$ is used as a distance measure. The Frobenius-norm, $\mathbf{F_h}$, is given by,

$$F_h = \|b_{gh}\|_{Frobenius} = \sqrt{\Sigma_{x,y}[b_{gh}(x,y)]^2} \qquad (6)$$

It is worth noting that $\mathbf{F_h}$ tends to zero as the quality of fit improves.

2.3   Iterative Multi-stage Bidirectional 2DPCA-Based Best Profile Search Algorithm

We define the best profile match as the profile which together with all other profiles in the profiles matrix yields maximum matrix fit. That is, the best profile match (fit) includes all shape's profiles information in the fitting procedure. Following the classical ASM procedure, starting from the mean shape, each landmark is moved along the direction perpendicular to the contour to, $\mathbf{n_s}$, different positions on either side, evaluating a total of $2\mathbf{n_s}+1$ positions. However, to employ the 2DPCA- based inter-profile modeled variations, we propose two stage searching algorithm to find the best profile fit. In the first stage, the target is to reach to a combination of candidate profiles which have good inter-profile relations with each other. So, we start by initializing the profile's matrix by the mean profile's matrix (i.e $\mathbf{G} = \overline{\mathbf{G}}$). Then, for each landmark, the $2\mathbf{n_s}+1$ candidate positions is evaluated, for each evaluation, all rows of $\mathbf{G}$ remain the same except the row corresponding to the current landmark which is replaced by the current profile under evaluation(i.e. this row is replaced $2\mathbf{n_s}+1$ times) and the profile with minimum $\mathbf{F}$ is the best profile fit for this landmark. This process is repeated for each landmark and at each time , the matrix $\mathbf{G}$ is re-initialized by $\overline{\mathbf{G}}$. Here, we should note that even we replace only the landmark's corresponding row in $\mathbf{G}$ at each time, the resultant profile after each landmark evaluation is the profile that increases the overall inter-profile relation among the matrix (shape) profiles because in the calculation of ,F, (Eqn.6) all profiles in the matrix are included in the evaluation. Profiles constraints are applied on $\mathbf{b_{gh}}$ (or $\mathbf{b_{gv}}$ in the vertical modeling case) (e.g. $|\mathbf{b_{gh}}| < 3\sqrt{\lambda}$) to ensure plausible profiles. The result of this stage is matrix $\mathbf{G_{min}}$ that holds the resultant best profiles (e.g. first row in $\mathbf{G_{min}}$ holds the profile that gave the minimum $\mathbf{F}$ during first landmark fitting). In the second stage, $\mathbf{G}$ is initialized by $\mathbf{G_{min}}$, then similar to the first stage, for each landmark ,we evaluate for the best fit out of $2\mathbf{n_s}+1$ candidate profiles using minimum $\mathbf{F}$ as the best fit criterion. Contrary to the first stage, after each landmark fit, we update the corresponding row in $\mathbf{G}$ by the profile that gives the minimum $\mathbf{F}$ (so, not to reinitialize $\mathbf{G} = \overline{\mathbf{G}}$ after each landmark evaluation). Then, the updated matrix $\mathbf{G}$ is used in the evaluation of the next landmark best fit. This ensures that each landmark update or fit is considering the best of other shape landmarks profiles leading to fitting the whole shape towards the shape that maintains the best inter-profile relations. The second stage is iterated predefined number of times until either convergence (e.g. stop when 90% or more of the best found pixel along the search profile is within the central 50 % of the profile length) or completing the number of predefined iterations. The same two stage procedure is applied in case of the vertical fitting. Furthermore, bidirectional fitting procedure is applied to maintain both the horizontal and vertical inter-profile variations.

That is, for each candidate position we compute both the horizontal (the two-stages) followed by vertical fitting and also, the vertical followed by the horizontal fitting. Then we admit the fitting with the smaller final $\mathbf{F}$ to be the best fit for the current landmark in the current iteration. Additionally, similar to the classical ASM algorithm we may build the aforementioned inter-profile models for multiple resolutions; this may improve the speed and the robustness of the algorithm.

3   Experimental Setup

The dataset used in this study is the York dataset of short axis cardiac MR images [8]; this dataset was constructed by studying 33 subjects to mainly evaluate the LV segmentation results. In our experiments we have excluded three subjects (5, 6 and 27) from the dataset due to their low signal to noise ratio, resulting in 30 subjects (image sets) for our experiments. In each image set, three end-diastolic, mid-ventricular slices were selected for the total of 90 images of 256 X 256 pixels; pixel sizes: 1.1719–1.6406 mm. For all of the 90 images, RV is manually outlined to be used as ground truth for automatic segmentation performance validation. Initial pilot experiments were performed to find the best ASMs parameters, fixed settings were selected that yielded good performance. The same parameters are used for both the classical and the proposed ASM. Training images are used to build the right ventricle specific statistical shape model. The shape model was built with 119 landmarks ($\mathbf{M}$=119) which were distributed equally over the model contour. The first 16 modes (eigenvectors) are retained describing 99% of shape variations of the train-ing dataset. For the construction of the gray-level appearance models, the grey level profile length chosen to be 2 pixels on either side of the landmarks ($\mathbf{N}$=5); 98% of the appearance variation is explained, that represented by the first 4 eigenvectors for the vertical 2DPCA, and by 53 to 74 eigenvectors for the horizontal 2DPCA which varies based on the resolution level and training shapes included in the current cross-validation iteration. Furthermore, two resolution levels are used for modeling. To compare segmentation performance between the classical ASM and our proposed method, overlap measure and point to curve error measure (P2C) are used which cal-culated as follows:

$$\text{Overlap} \quad \Omega = \frac{TP}{TP+FP+FN} \tag{7}$$

where TP stands for the true positive, FP for false positive and FN for false negative, Ω=1 for perfect overlap and Ω=0 if there is no overlap at all.

$$P2C(C_a, C_m) = \frac{1}{N_a} \sum_{i=1}^{N_a} \min_j \ d(p_a^i, p_m^j) \tag{8}$$

Where $\mathbf{C_a}$ denoting the automatically resulted contour, $\mathbf{C_m}$ denoting the manual deli-neated contour (ground truth), $\mathbf{p_a^i}$ is a point on $\mathbf{C_a}$, $\mathbf{p_m^j}$ is a point on $\mathbf{C_m}$ and $\mathbf{d}(...)$ represents the Euclidean distance between two points, if P2C=0 then there is perfect match between the automatic and manual contours while P2C=1 means total mis-match. To test the proposed algorithm performance, rough good shape parameters (position and orientation) initialization is manually determined which the same for both algorithms under comparison.

Table 1. Overlap and P2C measure results of the Classical ASM and the proposed method

	Overlap $\mu \pm \sigma$	Overlap median	P2C $\mu \pm \sigma$ (mm)	P2C Median (mm)
Classic ASM	0.74 ± 0.11	0.76	1.13 ± 0.79	0.88
Our method	0.78 ± 0.06	0.79	0.73 ± 0.37	0.62

Table 2. Mean segmentation errors reported in the literature and for our method

Authors	No. subj.	%P	Slice no.	Error (mm)
Mitchell 01 [9]	54	45	3 Mid	2.46 ± 1.39^a
Lorenzo 04[10]	10	100	3 Mid	2.26 ± 2.13
Grosgeorget 10[11]	59	100	6–10 Mid	2.27 ± 2.02
Lötjönen 04 [12]	25	100	4-5	2.37 ± 0.5^c
Abi-Nahed 06 [13]	13	-	-	1.1^b
Sun et al. 10[14]	40	75	8-12	1.19 ± 0.28
proposed method	30	93	3 Mid	0.73 ± 0.37

%P percentage of pathological subjects.
[a] RMS error. [b] No standard deviation provided. [c] Surface to surface error measure.

4   Results

In order to avoid bias, segmentation performance is evaluated using 5-fold cross-validation strategy, the original dataset (n=90 images) is partitioned into 5 subsets with 18 images for each subset. Of the 5 subsets, a single subset is retained as the validation set for testing the model, and the remaining 4 subsets are used as training data. The cross-validation process is then repeated 5 times. To show the performance of our method, all results are compared with the classical ASM-based RV Segmentation method. The mean contour overlap measure and P2C error measure results of the experiment are given in Table 1. Furthermore, Table 2 presents the Point to curve (P2C) errors of our method along with segmentation errors collected from the literature for the right ventricle segmentation. A paired Student's t-test was carried out to determine the level of statistical significance between the proposed method and the classical ASM which resulted in high significance for the P2C with $p < 7.68 \times 10^{-10}$ and also for the overlap with $p < 2.22 \times 10^{-15}$. Figure 2 shows an example of our proposed method segmentation performance in comparison with the classical ASM.

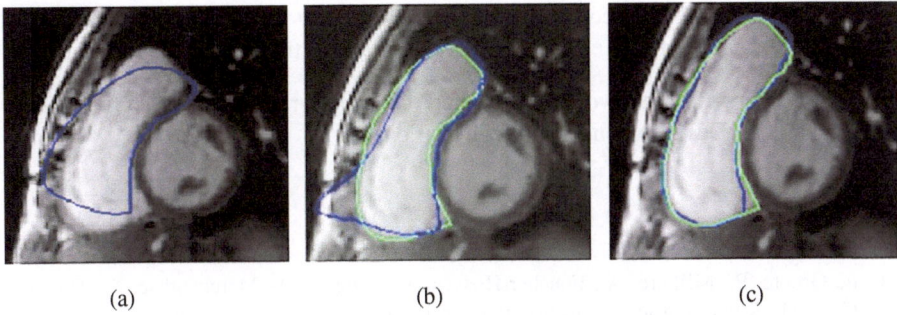

(a)   (b)   (c)

Fig. 1. (a) initial contour, (b) classic ASM result (green contour is ground truth and the blue contour is the segmentation result, (c) proposed ASM paradigm result

5   Discussion and Conclusion

Our results show that the proposed ASM with inter-profile modeling paradigm is rather accurate relative to the classical ASM with P2C errors around 0.7 mm. Table 1 shows that ASM with inter-profile modeling method improves the segmentation overlap measure between the automatic segmentation and the manual segmentation by about 4% than the classical ASM method with high statistical significance of $p< 2.22 \times 10^{-15}$ using paired t-test. Meanwhile, it shows that our method minimized the P2C error by about 0.4 mm in comparison with the classical ASM P2C error with high statistical significance of $p< 7.68 \times 10^{-10}$ using paired t-test. In building the shape model, shapes were aligned for rotation and translation while no scaling was included in the alignment step. In addition, For measuring how well the model fits the profile matrix (Eqn. 6), we have tested many norm evaluation methods including L1-norm,L2-norm , infinity- norm and frobenius-norm. However, the frobenius-norm has given the best results. It is worth noting that although the maximum number of allowed iteration for the second stage in the search algorithm was set to 6 in all our experiments, a value of only 3 or 4 was sufficient to achieve reasonable results. Table 2 shows that the performance of our ASM with inter-profile modeling method substantially outperforms the recently published literature results. Herein, we should note that many of the presented literature results were obtained using 3D segmentation algorithms [9,10, 12, 13, 14], whereas our approach is a 2D based method. Although, it is required to be cautious when trying to compare techniques that use different MRI sequences, different segmentation protocols and different error criteria; the high statistical significance of the proposed paradigm compared to the classical ASM and the difference between proposed method and other literature results should be encouraging. Matlab implementations for both the classical ASM and ASM with inter-profile modeling using 2.00 GHz Intel Core 2 Duo laptop are used to compare the speed of both algorithms. For the classical ASM, it required about 710 seconds for the segmentation of the whole 90 Images while for our method it required about 1015 seconds. The proposed method is relatively more computationally expensive than the classical ASM but this difference seems to be acceptable due to the significant improvement compared to the classical ASM. In conclusion, the new ASM with inter-profile modeling paradigm introduced in this paper substantially improves the original ASM method performance and an effective method to segment the cardiac Right Ventricle.

Acknowledgements. This work is supported in part by grant #1979 from the Science and Technology Development Fund (STDF), Egypt.

References

1. de Groote, P., Millaire, A., Foucher-Hossein, C., Nugue, O., Marchandise, X., Ducloux, G., et al.: Right ventricular ejection fraction is an independent predictor of survival in patients with moderate heart failure. J. Am. Coll. Cardiol. 32, 948–954 (1998)
2. Matthews, J.C., Dardas, T.F., Dorsch, M.P., Aaronson, K.D.: Right sided heart failure: diagnosis and treatment strategies. Curr. Treat. Options Cardiovasc. Med. 10, 329–341 (2008)
3. Cootes, T., Taylor, C.J., Cooper, D.H., Graham, J.: Active shape models – their training and application. CVIU 61(1), 38–59 (1995)
4. Cootes, T., Hill, A., Taylor, C., Haslam, J.: The use of active shape models for locating structures in medical images. Image Vis. Comput. 12, 355–366 (1994)
5. Sirovich, L., Kirby, M.: Low-dimensional procedure for characterization of human faces. J. Opt. Soc. Amer. 4, 519–524 (1987)
6. Yang, J., Zhang, D., Frangi, A.F., Yang, J.Y.: Two-dimensional PCA: A new approach to face representation and recognition. IEEE Trans. Pattern Anal. Mach. Intell. 26(1), 131–137 (2004)
7. Yang, J., Liu, C.: Horizontal and vertical 2DPCA-based discriminant analysis for face verification on a large-scale database. IEEE Trans. Information Forensics and Security 2(4), 781–792 (2007)
8. Andreopoulos, A., Tsotsos, J.K.: Efficient and generalizable statistical models of shape and appearance for analysis of cardiac mri. Med. Image Anal. 12(3), 335–357 (2008)
9. Mitchell, S., Lelieveldt, B., van der Geest, R., Bosch, J., Reiber, J., Sonka, M.: Multistage hybrid active appearance model matching: segmentation of left and right ventricles in cardiac MR images. IEEE Trans. Med. Imaging 20(5), 415–423 (2001)
10. Lorenzo-Valdes, M., Sanchez-Ortiz, G., Elkington, A., Mohiaddin, R., Rueckert, D.: Segmentation of 4D cardiac MR images using a probabilistic atlas and the EM algorithm. Med. Image Anal. 8(3), 255–256 (2004)
11. Grosgeorge, D., Petitjean, C., Caudron, J., Fares, J., Dacher, J.N.: Automatic cardiac ventricle segmentation in MR images: a validation study. International Journal of Computer Assisted Radiology and Surgery 6(5), 573–581 (2011)
12. Lötjönen, J., Kivistö, S., Koikkalainen, J., Smutek, D., Lauerma, K.: Statistical shape model of atria, ventricles and epicardium from short- and long-axis MR images. Med. Image Anal. 8(3), 371–386 (2004)
13. de Bruijne, M., Lund, M.T., Tankó, L.B., Pettersen, P.P., Nielsen, M.: Quantitative Vertebral Morphometry Using Neighbor-Conditional Shape Models. In: Larsen, R., Nielsen, M., Sporring, J. (eds.) MICCAI 2006, Part I. LNCS, vol. 4190, pp. 1–8. Springer, Heidelberg (2006)
14. Sun, H., Frangi, A.F., Wang, H., Sukno, F.M., Tobon-Gomez, C., Yushkevich, P.A.: Automatic Cardiac MRI Segmentation Using a Biventricular Deformable Medial Model. In: Jiang, T., Navab, N., Pluim, J.P.W., Viergever, M.A. (eds.) MICCAI 2010, Part I. LNCS, vol. 6361, pp. 468–475. Springer, Heidelberg (2010)

Tractometer: Online Evaluation System for Tractography

Marc-Alexandre Côté, Arnaud Boré, Gabriel Girard,
Jean-Christophe Houde, and Maxime Descoteaux

Sherbrooke Connectivity Imaging Laboratory (SCIL), Computer Science Department,
Université de Sherbrooke, Sherbrooke, Canada

Abstract. We have developed a Tractometer: an online evaluation system for tractography processing pipelines. One can now evaluate the end effects on fiber tracts of different acquisition parameters (b-value, number of directions, denoising or not, averaging or not), different local estimation techniques (tensor, q-ball, spherical deconvolution, spherical wavelets) and to different tractography parameters (masking, seeding, stopping criteria). At this stage, the system is solely based on a revised FiberCup analysis, but we hope that the community gets involved and provides us with new phantoms, new algorithms, third party libraries and new geometrical metrics, to name a few. We believe that the new connectivity analysis and tractography characteristics proposed can highlight limits of the algorithms and contribute in elucidating the open questions in fiber tracking: from raw data to connectivity analysis.

1 Introduction

Diffusion MRI and fiber tractography have gained importance in the medical imaging community for the last decade. The neuroscience community often uses fiber tractography as a black box, and its limits are ignored by most. The diffusion community has done a good job in the last years to highlight the limitations of diffusion tensor imaging (DTI) in crossings and high curvature areas. Thus, numerous new high angular resolution diffusion imaging (HARDI) tractography techniques have been proposed. Several groups have studied the effect of interpolation, step size, stopping criteria, but mostly on toy simulated data or qualitatively [1] on large tracts or inter-hemispheric connections. Validation of fiber tractography remains an open question and a challenge on real data.

A first attempt has been done with the FiberCup phantom dataset [2], which was made public and is now used by the community for quantitative evaluation of tracking algorithms. However, in our opinion, two important drawbacks of the FiberCup are the seed points given and the quantitative metric used to compare with ground truth. Only 16 seeds are given here and there in the dataset, close to boundaries and in the middle of structures. These 16 seeds result in 16 individual tracts that are compared with the ground truth in terms of spatial, tangent to the tract and a curvature distance. These measures are local and do not capture well the global connectivity profile of the tractography algorithm. Other

N. Ayache et al. (Eds.): MICCAI 2012, Part I, LNCS 7510, pp. 699–706, 2012.

problems are that each participant of [2] performed his own analysis and that the implementations used are not available to the community.

In this paper, we propose a revised FiberCup analysis that is in closer spirit to brain connectivity analysis. In brain connectivity, the importance is *connectivity*. Does region A connect to B as expected? Does region A connect to unexpected regions of the brain? Therefore, instead of using local seeds and local point-by-point distances for evaluation, we propose a global view of the dataset and the *tractogram* (the fiber tractography output). We developed a tractogram evaluation method to compare tracts and evaluate the number of found and not found fiber bundles, the proportion of tracts part of existent and non-existent bundles, and the proportion of incomplete tracts. Since these tractogram characteristics have a direct impact on connectivity analysis, having a tractogram evaluation tool is crucial in the era of the human connectome studies [3].

This paper is thus aimed at providing a framework to encourage the community to rigorously choose a tractography processing pipeline and report the known limitations of their technique. Therefore, in the rest of the paper, we describe our new online system (**url: *scil.dinf.usherbrooke.ca/tractometer***) to evaluate and rank pipelines. At this stage, a user has the choice of providing 3 things to the system: 1) A diffusion dataset corrected with the user's best algorithm, 2) a field of ODFs coming from the user's best algorithm, or 3) a tractogram. The user can then obtain a ranking against the current database of state-of-the-art techniques. Presently, in this database, we have $N = 1152$ different tractograms coming from our in-house tools, *MRtrix* [1] and *TrackVis* (`trackvis.org`) using one of the acquisitions or the averaged, local estimation techniques (tensor, q-ball, constant solid angle q-ball, spherical deconvolution and wavelets), masking from a complete phantom mask or regions of interest (ROIs), multiple seeding strategies and different stopping criteria.

2   A Revised FiberCup Analysis

Fig. 1 illustrates the FiberCup dataset mimicking a coronal slice of the human brain. The phantom was built following the procedure of [4] for the MICCAI FiberCup workshop held in 2009, which resulted in a group publication in [2]. In our opinion, the metrics proposed in [2] are too local and vulnerable to the seeds given and, as a result, do not capture the global *connectivity* behavior of the tractography technique. To better reflect brain connectivity studies, especially in terms of seeding and performance evaluation, we revisit the FiberCup analysis. The main difference is to consider two different starting configurations: 1) From a complete mask of the phantom mimicking a brain white matter (WM) mask, as seen in Fig. 1b), or 2) From ROIs mimicking gray/white matter interface, as seen in Fig. 1c). Hence, the tractogram from a resulting tractography algorithm (Fig. 1e)) can be filtered by the ROIs at the end of bundles to quantify the global success (Fig. 1f)) and errors present in the tractogram.

Definitions and Rationale. We performed a survey with neurosurgeons and neurologists at our institute concerning true and false connections of tractograms.

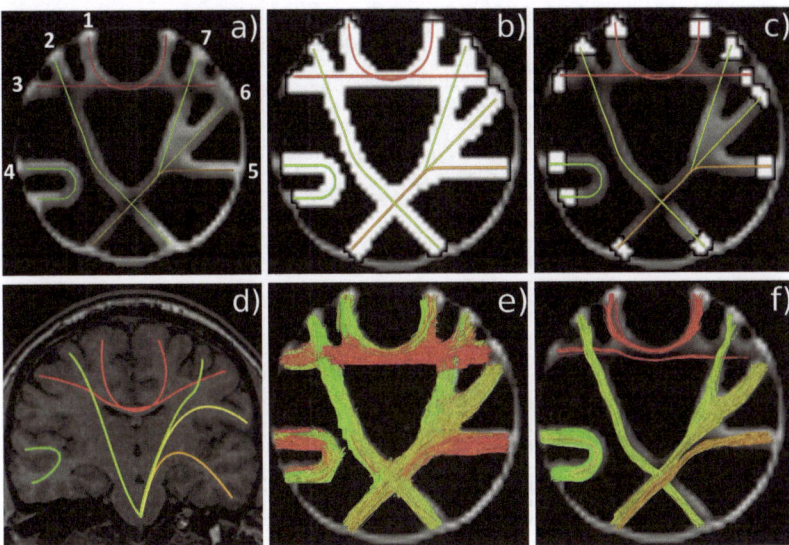

Fig. 1. a) FiberCup mimicking a brain in coronal slice d). b) Fibercup's white matter mask and c) regions of interest (ROIs) similar to white/gray matter interface on the cortex. e) Full tractogram (45,000 tracts) and f) tracts passing through ROIs of c).

We concluded that these terms were not the best choice for connectivity analysis purposes. Therefore, we define the following five new terms:

- *True Connections (TC)*: tracts connecting expected ROIs. This is illustrated by tracts in Fig. 1f). TC will be reported in percentage of true connections.
- *False but Plausible Connections (FPC)*: tracts connecting unexpected ROIs. These tracts are spatially coherent, have managed to connect ROIs, but do not agree with the ground truth (see Fig. 2a)). It is reported in %. According to our survey with clinicians, these are problematic tracts as they "look anatomically good" but are in fact non-existent from *a priori* knowledge.
- *Wrong Connections (WC)*: tracts that simply do not connect two ROIs. Depending on how the tractography algorithm handles stopping criteria, these tracts either stop prematurely due to stopping criteria or, most often, hit the boundaries of the tracking mask, as illustrated in Fig. 2b), c), e), f).
- *True Bundles (TB)*: bundle connecting expected ROIs. Figure 1a) shows the true bundles. TB is reported in bundle counts, from 0 to 7 for the FiberCup.
- *False but Plausible Bundles (FPB)*: bundle connecting unexpected ROIs. As TB, FPB is reported in bundle counts. Figure 2a) and d) show that bundles 1, 3 are mismatched, but look plausible, had we not known the ground truth.

Tractography. For this paper, we have focused only on the 3 mm isotropic, 64 directions, $b = 1500$ s/mm^2 dataset as 9/10 participants of [2] used this dataset). At the acquisition level, two measurements of the raw data are available. Hence, either one acquisition or an averaged were tested. For local estimation, diffusion

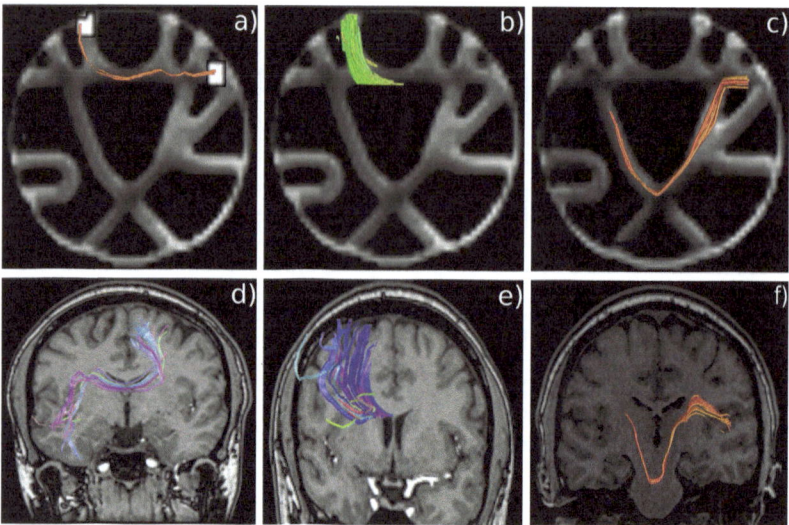

Fig. 2. a) A FPC between 2 ROIs of gray matter (FiberCup) and a real data analogy in d). In b), c), e) and f), we see WC due to many collisions with the tracking mask.

tensors were estimated using our in-house log-Euclidean implementation [5], the one from *TrackVis* or from *MRtrix* (public softwares). Otherwise, the diffusion orientation distribution function (ODF) from analytical q-ball of [6] (a-ODF) and normalized version with constant solid angle of [7] (csa-ODF) were implemented for several spherical harmonics (SH) order. Here, we report order 4 (r4) because it is the best for the FiberCup data. Next, a spherical wavelet (SW) decomposition based on [8] was performed at order 8. Moreover, spherical deconvolution (SD) techniques were tested at order 4 (r4), 6 (r6) and 8 (r8). We have an in-house implementation of [9] as well as the estimation of MRtrix to recover the fiber ODF (fODF). These local estimations are illustrated in Fig. 3.

As mentioned before, tracking is performed in a complete tracking mask shown in Fig. 1b), but seeding is either started from everywhere in that mask or from the ROIs (Fig. 1c)). Using these seeding options, we tested multiseeding with our implementation of [3] covering all possible maxima when seeding in crossing voxels, random multiseeding of *MRtrix* and the one from *TrackVis*. Finally, we used deterministic streamline option from *MRtrix*, *TrackVis* and our in-house tools (similar to [3]), as well as the probabilistic option of *MRtrix*. For DTI, tensorline, streamline, FACT and Runge-Kutta (rk) options of *TrackVis* were tested as well as our in-house tensorline and streamline algorithms.

Ranking system, database and website. To compute the TC, FPC, WC, TB and FPB from the tractograms, we use *MRtrix* (filter_tracks) to filter the resulting tracts of pipelines using different sets of ROIs. For each subset of tracts that corresponds to a specific connection between ROIs, the metrics are updated and sent to a database. Once all metrics are computed for all tractography pipelines,

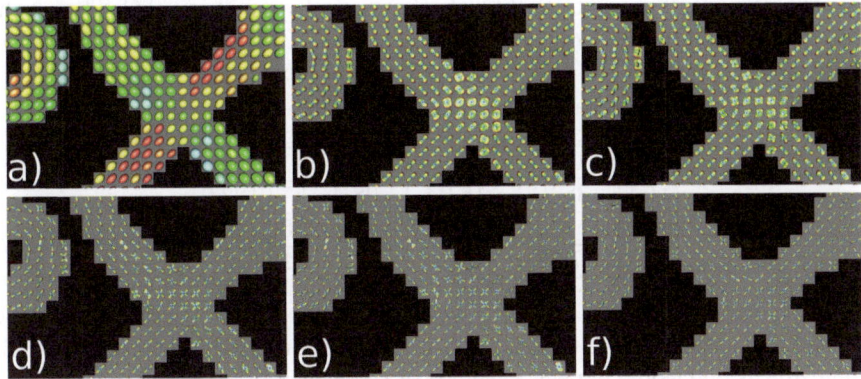

Fig. 3. Different local estimation methods provided in the Tractometer. a) DTI, b) a-ODF-r4, c) csa-ODF-r4, d) SD-r6, e) SD-r8 and f) SW-r8.

each once is ranked in 5 columns according to TC, FPC, WC, TB and FPB. The website allows one to submit his dataset(s) (modified diffusion dataset, fields of ODF, or tractogram) and a short description in order to compare it against what others have proposed. In the case of a diffusion dataset or fields of ODF submissions, our framework will automatically combine the submitted data with other pipelines already implemented in the database. Doing so, it will show the impacts of new contributions to tractography pipelines. As the website grows, more features will be added like new algorithms, the possibility to submit third party libraries, new geometrical metrics and other phantoms, to name a few.

3 Results and Discussion

Here is an overview of different results and messages that come out of the new analysis of the $N = 1152$ tractograms in the database. We advise the reader to have the new definitions of TC, FPC, WC, TB and FPB in mind before reading this section. Bold entries in tables represent "best" results. Firstly, not all methods are able to retrieve all the 7 out of 7 (7/7) TB.

TB (%)	0/7	1/7	2/7	3/7	4/7	5/7	6/7	7/7
DTI	0.0	0.7	6.2	11.8	54.9	19.4	6.9	0.0
a-ODF	0.0	0.0	0.0	0.0	4.2	12.5	37.5	45.8
csa-ODF	0.0	4.2	6.2	2.1	10.4	16.7	31.2	29.2
SD	0.0	2.1	0.0	0.0	2.1	8.3	16.7	**70.8**
SW	0.0	0.0	4.2	0.0	4.2	16.7	20.8	54.2
Total	0.0	1.4	3.3	2.8	15.1	14.7	22.6	40.0

Sharp angular distributions have more success at recovering 7/7 TB, from SD, SW and then csa-ODFs and a-ODFs. DTI never recovers 7/7 TB. Secondly, it may seem easy to obtain TB from the FiberCup dataset. However, we note that there is only a small percentage of tracts that actually result in a TC. The results show that less than 38.2% of recovered tracts are TC! Hence, the major part of fiber tracts are either FPC or WC, as seen in the next table:

	TC (%)	FPC (%)	WC (%)	TB	FPB
Min	0.2	0.0	57.6	1.0	0.0
Max	38.2	15.2	98.4	7.0	22.0
μ	14.6	3.8	81.6	5.5	9.2
σ	7.8	3.2	9.2	1.6	4.5

Overall, between 57%-98% of tracts are WC and the remaining tracts are FPC (0% to 15%). These FPC account for 0 to 22 FPB out of the possible 39 FPB.

Thirdly, as one would expect, each TB of the FiberCup has a different success rate depending on its complexity, as seen in the following table:

Local Estimation \ No. Bundle	1	2	3	4	5	6	7
DTI	81.9	8.3	34.7	83.3	82.6	92.4	23.6
a-ODF	87.5	70.8	45.8	**100.0**	91.7	91.7	52.1
csa-ODF	**100.0**	70.8	75.0	**100.0**	**100.0**	**100.0**	79.2
SD	93.8	85.4	**84.9**	99.0	97.4	97.9	**89.6**
SW	79.2	**91.7**	79.2	**100.0**	95.8	**100.0**	66.7

In fact, bundles 2 and 7 are harder to track than their homologue bundle in the brain because they go through several complex fiber crossing regions, whereas bundles 1, 4, 5, and 6 are most often tracked successfully by HARDI techniques.

Next, the following table shows that the more tracking seeds used, the more success the pipeline has in reaching the target ROI and thus increasing the % of pipelines scoring 7/7 TB. However, this also increases the chance to find FPB.

Nb. Seeds \ Mean (%)	TC	FPC	WC	TB	FPB	(7/7)
1	14.2	**3.7**	82.1	4.7	**5.4**	15.7
9	14.6	3.8	81.6	5.6	9.3	**42.6**
17	**14.8**	3.8	**81.4**	5.8	10.6	50.0
33	**14.8**	3.9	**81.4**	**5.9**	11.5	52.8

Hence, one can see that TC, FPC and WC remain constant as multiseeding increases. Meaning that one must be careful when using aggressive multiseeding.

The next table compares *MRtrix*'s deterministic and probabilistic tracking based on a field of fODFs. All techniques recover, on average, the same number of TB and make low FPC. However, we note that the percentage of TC and WC seem to advantage deterministic tracking (i.e. better TC while keeping the WC and FPB lower). This highlights a limitation of probabilistic tracking, in that it explores the whole shape of the fODF but may take wrong turns and follow peaks that are part of different fiber bundles. This is something one should consider and further explore, especially in large-scale connectivity analysis studies.

| MRtrix Pipelines | | TC (%) | FPC (%) | WC (%) | TB | FPB |
Local Estimation	Tracking					
SD-r6	Deterministic	**18.3**	3.2	**78.5**	**6.8**	10.1
SD-r6	Probabilistic	5.5	2.0	92.5	6.7	17.6
SD-r8	Deterministic	14.9	**1.6**	83.5	6.7	**8.0**
SD-r8	Probabilistic	7.0	**1.6**	91.4	**6.8**	16.4

Finally, in the following table, we explore the *decoupling* of fODF estimation from the tracking algorithm itself, between our in-house tools and *MRtrix*:

| Pipelines | | TC (%) | FPC (%) | WC (%) | TB | FPB |
Local Estimation	Tracking (Det.)					
csa-ODF(in-house)	in-house	16.3	1.9	81.8	6.2	8.2
SD-r6 (in-house)	in-house	14.1	1.4	84.6	6.2	8.7
SW-r8 (in-house)	in-house	15.1	1.5	83.4	6.1	10.2
SD-r6 (MRtrix)	MRtrix	18.3	3.2	78.5	**6.8**	10.1
ODF-rk2 (TrackVis)	TrackVis	3.0	**0.1**	96.9	5.3	**3.4**
SD-r6(MRtrix)	in-house	**24.5**	3.4	**72.1**	6.5	10.5

As seen in this table, *MRtrix* has, on average, the best success at recovering 7/7 TB. However, we also see that the best results *TrackVis*, based a Runge-Kutta interpolation of the qball ODF field, has a very low FPC and FPB. Moreover, we finally see that fODFs from *MRtrix* combined with our tracking has the best compromise between TC and WC. We believe that this is especially owed to the seeding strategy that differs between the two tracking techniques. Carefully covering all multiple orientations in a seed voxel when there are many (as done in our in-house tools and as opposed to random seeding done in *MRtrix*), achieves more TC and less WC. This needs to be further investigated and motivates the fact of *decoupling* tracking steps (seeding, masking, interpolation and stopping).

A conclusion based on available techniques in the database is that the current best tractography pipeline configuration for optimal trade-off between TC, FPC, WC, TB and FPB is using the averaged dataset, a sharp local estimation (e.g. spherical deconvolution), a multiseeding strategy, is starting from the ROIs and uses a tracking algorithm handling fiber crossings such as [3] and *MRtrix*.

Limitations. The current Tractometer system has limitations. Currently, only a single dataset has been included in the database. Of course, one has to be careful not to develop or tune his fiber tractography algorithm to best perform solely on the FiberCup dataset. As mentioned in [2], this phantom data is not perfect and can privilege a certain class of techniques such as streamline techniques based on an angular distribution content of the DW-MRI data. Raw signal modeling-based approaches are disadvantaged (such as implemented in FSL) and not well suited for the FiberCup [2]. Moreover, the FiberCup phantom does not provide a real 3D space example and is limited to the 2D plane. Other phantoms should take into account more complex bundles. Or, ideally, new techniques should be developed to compare tracts bundles within a brain. Finally, we have currently focused on the global TC, FPC, WC, TB and FPB metrics but other geometrical metrics could be incorporated to get a more complete ranking system.

4 Conclusion

We have developed a new Tractometer to evaluate tractography pipelines. Overall, we have shown that *MRtrix* and our in-house tools based on SD currently provide the best rankings. *Trackvis* is based on q-ball ODFs or DTI, and thus, does not perform as well, just as our in-house tracking based on q-ball and DTI. Of course, there are limitations to this system but we believe that, as the community contributes to the system with more, and better phantoms, this new system can have a positive impact on the dMRI community. Just as the machine learning and computer vision communities have used benchmarks to move forward in algorithm design and evaluation, the dMRI community needs to do the same to answer open questions. Only then can new tractography algorithms be compared to the state-of-the-art and their contributions quantified.

Send us your corrected raw diffusion data, your ODFs or your fiber tracts and you will be compared and ranked against other state-of-the-art techniques!

References

1. Tournier, J.D., Calamante, F., Connelly, A.: MRtrix: Diffusion tractography in crossing fiber regions. International Journal of Imaging Systems and Technology 22(1), 53–66 (2012)
2. Fillard, P., Descoteaux, M., Goh, A., Gouttard, S., Jeurissen, B., Malcolm, J., Ramirez-Manzanares, A., Reisert, M., Sakaie, K., Tensaouti, F., Yo, T., Mangin, J.F., Poupon, C.: Quantitative evaluation of 10 tractography algorithms on a realistic diffusion mr phantom. NeuroImage 56(1), 220–234 (2011)
3. Hagmann, P., Cammoun, L., Gigandet, X., Meuli, R., Honey, C.J., Wedeen, V.J., Sporns, O.: Mapping the structural core of human cerebral cortex. PLoS Biology 6(7), e159 (2008)
4. Poupon, C., Rieul, B., Kezele, I., Perrin, M., Poupon, F., Mangin, J.F.: New diffusion phantoms dedicated to the study and validation of hardi models. Magnetic Resonance in Medicine 60, 1276–1283 (2008)
5. Arsigny, V., Fillard, P., Pennec, X., Ayache, N.: Log-euclidean metrics for fast and simple calculus on diffusion tensors. Magnetic Resonance in Medicine 56(2), 411–421 (2006)
6. Descoteaux, M., Angelino, E., Fitzgibbons, S., Deriche, R.: Regularized, fast, and robust analytical q-ball imaging. Magnetic Resonance in Medicine 58(3), 497–510 (2007)
7. Tristán-Vega, A., Aja-Fernández, S.: Dwi filtering using joint information for dti and hardi. Medical Image Analysis 14(2), 205–218 (2010)
8. Kezele, I., Descoteaux, M., Poupon, C., Poupon, F., Mangin, J.F.: Spherical wavelet transform for odf sharpening. Medical Image Analysis 14(3), 332–342 (2010)
9. Tournier, J.D., Calamante, F., Connelly, A.: Robust determination of the fibre orientation distribution in diffusion mri: Non-negativity constrained super-resolved spherical deconvolution. NeuroImage 35(4), 1459–1472 (2007)

A Novel Sparse Graphical Approach
for Multimodal Brain Connectivity Inference

Bernard Ng, Gaël Varoquaux, Jean-Baptiste Poline, and Bertrand Thirion

Parietal Team, Neurospin, INRIA Saclay-Ile-de-France, France
bernardyng@gmail.com

Abstract. Despite the clear potential benefits of combining fMRI and diffusion MRI in learning the neural pathways that underlie brain functions, little methodological progress has been made in this direction. In this paper, we propose a novel multimodal integration approach based on sparse Gaussian graphical model for estimating brain connectivity. Casting functional connectivity estimation as a sparse inverse covariance learning problem, we adapt the level of sparse penalization on each connection based on its anatomical capacity for functional interactions. Functional connections with little anatomical support are thus more heavily penalized. For validation, we showed on real data collected from a cohort of 60 subjects that additionally modeling anatomical capacity significantly increases subject consistency in the detected connection patterns. Moreover, we demonstrated that incorporating a connectivity prior learned with our multimodal connectivity estimation approach improves activation detection.

Keywords: brain connectivity, diffusion MRI, fMRI, multimodal integration.

1   Introduction

Recent evidence suggests that the effects of many neurological diseases are manifested through abnormal changes in brain connectivity [1]. Techniques for inferring connectivity from functional magnetic resonance imaging (fMRI) data can be largely divided into two categories. One category comprises techniques, such as the seed-based approach and independent component analysis (ICA) [1], which group brain areas into networks. The other category includes techniques that estimate the connectivity between brain areas [2] and apply graph-theoretic measures to characterize the estimated connection structure. We focus on connectivity estimation in this work.

The strong noise inherent in fMRI data and its high dimensionality given the typically small sample sizes pose major challenges to reliable connectivity estimation [2]. Since neural dynamics is largely shaped by the structure of the underlying fiber pathways [3, 4], informing connectivity estimation with anatomical information extracted from e.g. diffusion MRI (dMRI) data should prove beneficial. Past studies that jointly examined dMRI and fMRI data have primarily focused on comparing connectivity measures estimated from each modality separately [3, 4]. The general finding is that brain areas with high anatomical connectivity typically exhibit high functional

N. Ayache et al. (Eds.): MICCAI 2012, Part I, LNCS 7510, pp. 707–714, 2012.

connectivity [3, 4], but the converse does not necessarily hold due to factors, such as noise-induced correlations in fMRI observations, indirect functional connections, and tractography errors [4]. Other widely-used approaches for multimodal analysis include employing fMRI to guide seed selection in tractography [3, 4]. The use of fiber bundle shapes to predict activated brain areas has also been explored [5]. A major limitation to the aforementioned approaches is that pooling information extracted independently from each modality does not capitalize on the complementary information that a joint analysis of the two modalities would facilitate. To exploit the joint information in dMRI and fMRI data, variants of ICA and canonical correlation analysis [6] have been proposed for identifying brain areas that display high correlations between anatomical and functional attributes, such as fractional anisotropy and activation effects. Recently, a probabilistic model has been put forth for combining dMRI and fMRI data in detecting group differences in brain connection structure [7].

In this paper, we propose a novel multimodal integration approach based on sparse Gaussian graphical model (SGGM) for estimating intra-subject brain connectivity. Specifically, we cast connectivity estimation as a sparse inverse covariance learning problem [8]. Since elements of the inverse covariance matrix are proportional to the partial correlations between the associated variable pairs, zero entry would indicate conditional independence [8]. Using SGGM thus enables simultaneous estimation of connection strength and structure. To integrate anatomical information into functional connectivity estimation, we adapt the degree of sparse penalization on each functional link based on its anatomical capacity. Functional connections with less anatomical support are thus more heavily penalized, which helps reduce false detection of noise-induced functional connections. Also, using partial correlations as a measure of functional connectivity reduces the effects of indirect interactions. Furthermore, although larger penalizations are exerted on functional connections with no anatomical support, if ample evidence from fMRI data suggest the presence of such links, these connections will not necessarily be assigned zero connectivity. Our approach hence provides some tolerances to the inconsistencies between dMRI and fMRI-derived connectivity measures that hinder integration of these modalities. On a large dataset of 60 subjects, we showed that applying our multimodal approach significantly increases subject consistency in the detected connection structure over analyzing fMRI data alone. Enhanced group activation detection was also obtained by incorporating a connectivity prior [9] learned with our proposed approach, thus demonstrating the gain of integrating anatomical and functional information in brain connectivity estimation.

2   Methods

In this work, we focus on integrating dMRI with resting state (RS) fMRI for estimating brain connectivity. For this, we propose a SGGM-based approach (Section 2.1). Critical to the estimation is the choice on sparsity level, which we optimize using cross validation with a refined grid search strategy (Section 2.2). We validate our approach based on subject consistency and group activation detection (Section 2.3).

2.1   Sparse Gaussian Graphical Model

Let $\mathbf{S}$ be a $d{\times}d$ sample covariance matrix computed from data that are assumed to follow a centered multivariate Gaussian distribution. In the present context of brain connectivity estimation, $\mathbf{S}$ corresponds to correlations between the RS-fMRI observations of d brain areas of a given subject. To learn a well-conditioned sparse inverse covariance matrix, $\hat{\mathbf{\Lambda}}$, we minimize the negative log data likelihood over the space of positive definite (p.d.) matrices, $\mathbf{\Lambda} > 0$, with an l_1 penalty imposed on $\mathbf{\Lambda}$ [8]:

$$\hat{\mathbf{\Lambda}} = \arg \min_{\mathbf{\Lambda}>0} tr(\mathbf{S}\mathbf{\Lambda}) - \log \det(\mathbf{\Lambda}) + \lambda \sum_{i=1}^{d} \sum_{j=1}^{d} \mathbf{W}_{ij} |\mathbf{\Lambda}_{ij}|, \tag{1}$$

where λ governs the overall level of sparsity and $\mathbf{W}_{ij}$ differentially weights the amount of sparse penalization on each connection based on its anatomical capacity:

$$\mathbf{W}_{ij} = \begin{cases} \exp(-\mathbf{K}_{ij}/\sigma) & i \neq j \\ 0 & i = j \end{cases}, \tag{2}$$

where $\mathbf{K}_{ij}$ corresponds to some measures of anatomical capacity. We set $\mathbf{K}_{ij}$ as the fiber count between brain areas i and j [3, 4] with the amount of penalization saturating to zero for $\mathbf{K}_{ij} \gg \sigma$, modeling how the additional fibers may reflect redundant wiring. Other decreasing functions of $\mathbf{K}_{ij}$ can also serve as $\mathbf{W}_{ij}$. We defer the selection of $\mathbf{W}_{ij}$ for future work. σ is learned from data (Section 2.2). In accordance to past findings [3, 4], $\mathbf{\Lambda}_{ij}$ associated with brain areas that have fewer connecting fibers are more strongly penalized. Note that we have explicitly set $\mathbf{W}_{ij}$ to 0 for $i = j$, which has been theoretically proven and empirically shown to provide more accurate solutions of (1) [10]. To solve (1), we employ a recent second-order algorithm [8] that facilitates efficient computation of Newton steps with iterates guaranteed to remain p.d. This algorithm provides substantially faster convergence rate than current gradient-based methods. We define convergence as having a duality gap, η, below 10^{-5} [10]:

$$\eta = tr(\mathbf{S}\mathbf{\Lambda}) + \lambda \sum_{i=1}^{d} \sum_{j=1}^{d} \mathbf{W}_{ij} |\mathbf{\Lambda}_{ij}| - d. \tag{3}$$

2.2   Parameter Selection

The estimated connection structure critically depends on λ. To learn the optimal λ and σ data-drivenly for each subject, we combine cross validation with a refined grid search strategy, as summarized in Algorithm 1. The algorithm requires the following inputs: $\mathbf{Z}$ = an $t{\times}d$ matrix containing RS-fMRI time courses of d brain areas, $\mathbf{K}$ = fiber count matrix, λ_{lb} and λ_{ub} = initial lower and upper bounds of the λ search range, σ_{lb} and σ_{ub} = lower and upper bounds of the σ search range, R = number of refinement levels, F = number of grid points for λ, G = number of grid points for σ, and C = number of cross validation folds. We set λ_{ub} to $\max|\mathbf{S}_{ij}|$, $i \neq j$, which corresponds to the maximum λ beyond which $\hat{\mathbf{\Lambda}}_{ij}$ is guaranteed to shrink to 0 [10]. As for λ_{lb}, we empirically found that setting λ_{lb} to $\lambda_{ub}/100$ assigns non-zero value to >90% of the elements in $\hat{\Lambda}$ in the case of uniform sparse penalization. We fix σ_{lb} and σ_{ub} to the 25th and 75th percentile of the fiber count distribution. R, F, G, and C are set to 3, 5, 5, and 3, respectively.

Algorithm 1. Refined Grid Search for λ_{opt} and σ_{opt}

1: Input: $\mathbf{Z}$, $\mathbf{K}$, λ_{lb}, λ_{ub}, σ_{lb}, σ_{ub}, R, F, G, C
2: Output: λ_{opt}, σ_{opt}
3: Temporally divide $\mathbf{Z}$ into C folds
4: Set σ_{grid} to a log grid with G grid points between σ_{lb} and σ_{ub}
5: **for** $r = 1$ to R
6:      Set λ_{grid} to a log grid with F grid points between λ_{lb} and λ_{ub} in decreasing order
7:      **for** $f = 1$ to F, $g = 1$ to G, and $c = 1$ to C
10:         Estimate sample covariance, $\mathbf{S}_{train}$, with all folds of $\mathbf{Z}$ except the cth fold
11:         Estimate sample covariance, $\mathbf{S}_{test}$, with the cth fold of $\mathbf{Z}$
12:         Solve (1) to find Λ_{train} with $\lambda = \lambda_{grid}(f)$, $\sigma = \sigma_{grid}(g)$
13:         Compute data likelihood, $dl(f,g,c)$, of $\mathbf{S}_{test}$ given Λ_{train}, based on (1)
14:             without the sparse penalization term
17:     **end**
18:     Find λ_{opt} and σ_{opt} based on maximum of the average $dl(f,g,c)$ over C folds
19:     **if** $\lambda_{opt} == \lambda_{grid}(1)$
20:         Set λ_{lb} to $\lambda_{grid}(2)$, set λ_{ub} to $\lambda_{grid}(1)$
22:     **else if** $\lambda_{opt} == \lambda_{grid}(F)$
23:         Set λ_{lb} to $\lambda_{grid}(F)/10$, set λ_{ub} to $\lambda_{grid}(F-1)$
25:     **else**
26:         Find f_{opt} corresponding to λ_{opt}
27:         Set λ_{lb} to $\lambda_{grid}(f_{opt}-1)$, set λ_{lb} to $\lambda_{grid}(f_{opt}+1)$
29:     **end**
30: **end**

2.3 Validation

We base our validation on: 1) increased subject consistency in the support of $\hat{\Lambda}$ and 2) increased group activation detection. The rationale behind the first criterion is that subjects within the same population should have similar brain connection structure [2]. As for the second criterion, we have shown in a previous work [9] that incorporating a RS-connectivity prior improves group activation detection. Thus, greater increase in group activation detection presumably implies that the corresponding connectivity estimates better reflect the underlying neural circuitry.

Subject Consistency. For each pair of subjects in our dataset (Section 3), we compare the support of their $\hat{\Lambda}$'s using the Dice Similarity Coefficient (DSC), defined as TPR / (2TPR + FPR + FNR), with each subject alternately taken as the reference. TPR, FPR, and FNR are the true positive rate, false positive rate, and false negative rate, respectively. Both connections commonly present in each pair of subjects as well as those in one subject but not the other are thus accounted for in our chosen metric.

Group Activation Detection. Our previously proposed connectivity-informed activation model [9] is summarized below:

$$\mathbf{Y} \sim N(\mathbf{AX}, \mathbf{V}_1) = \frac{1}{\left|2\pi\mathbf{V}_1\right|^{\frac{n}{2}}} \exp\left(-\frac{1}{2}tr\left((\mathbf{Y}-\mathbf{AX})^T \mathbf{V}_1^{-1}(\mathbf{Y}-\mathbf{AX})\right)\right), \tag{4}$$

$$\mathbf{A} \sim MN\left(0, \mathbf{V}_2, \alpha\mathbf{XX}^T\right) = \frac{\left|\alpha\mathbf{XX}^T\right|^{\frac{d}{2}}}{\left|2\pi\mathbf{V}_2\right|^{\frac{m}{2}}} \exp\left(-\frac{\alpha}{2}tr\left(\mathbf{X}^T\mathbf{A}^T\mathbf{V}_2^{-1}\mathbf{AX}\right)\right), \tag{5}$$

where $\mathbf{Y}$ is a $d{\times}n$ matrix containing task fMRI time courses of d brain areas of a given subject. $\mathbf{X}$ is a $m{\times}n$ regressor matrix [11]. $\mathbf{A}$ is a $d{\times}m$ activation effect matrix to be estimated. $\mathbf{V}_1$ and $\mathbf{V}_2$ are $d{\times}d$ covariance matrices of $\mathbf{Y}$ and $\mathbf{A}$, respectively. $\mathbf{XX}^T$ models the correlations between the m experimental conditions. $MN(0, \mathbf{V}_2, \alpha\mathbf{XX}^T)$ denotes the matrix normal distribution, which serves as a conjugate prior of (4) with α controlling the influence of this prior on $\mathbf{A}$. We assume $\mathbf{V}_1 = I_{d{\times}d}$ as conventionally done. $\mathbf{V}_2$ is set to the connectivity estimates learned with our proposed approach.

3   Materials

fMRI Data. Task fMRI data were collected from 60 healthy subjects at multiple imaging centers. Each subject performed 10 language, computation, and sensorimotor tasks similar to those in [12] over a period of ~5 min. RS-fMRI data of ~7 min were also collected. Data were acquired using 3T scanners from multiple manufacturers with TR = 2200 ms, TE = 30 ms, and flip angle = 75°. Standard preprocessing, including slice timing correction, motion correction, temporal detrending, and spatial normalization, was performed on the task fMRI data using the SPM8 software. Similar preprocessing was performed on the RS-fMRI data except a band-pass filter with cutoff frequencies at 0.01 to 0.1 Hz was applied. White matter and cerebrospinal fluid confounds were regressed out from the gray matter voxel time courses.

dMRI Data. dMRI data were collected from the same 60 subjects. Acquisition sequence similar to [13] was used with TR = 15000 ms, TE = 104 ms, flip angle = 90°, 32 gradient directions, and b-value = 1300 s/mm^2. MedINRIA was employed for tensor estimation and fiber tractography [14]. We warped our brain parcel template (described below) onto each subject's B$_0$ volume to facilitate fiber count computation.

Brain Parcellation. We divided the brain into P parcels (P set to 500) to enable finer brain partitioning than facilitated by standard brain atlases (typically $P < 150$). This choice of P provides a balance between functional localization and robustness to subject variability in tractography [7]. Parcellation was performed by concatenating RS-fMRI time courses across subjects and applying Ward clustering [15]. Parcel time courses were then generated by averaging the voxel time courses within each parcel, and normalized by subtracting the mean and dividing by the standard deviation.

4   Results and Discussion

To explore the gain in learning connectivity jointly from dMRI and RS-fMRI data, we compared based on DSC the subject consistency in the support of $\hat{\Lambda}_{ij}$ as estimated using our SGGM-based approach with anatomical capacity-weighted sparse penalization (SGGM-A) versus uniform sparse penalization without anatomical information (SGGM-U). To establish a baseline for comparison, we permuted 200 times the columns and rows of $\hat{\Lambda}_{ij}$ learned with SGGM-A to generate a null distribution of DSC. The average DSC of both SGGM-A and SGGM-U (Fig. 1(a)) were significantly greater than that of the null distribution based on a Wilcoxon signed rank test (p-value < 0.05). Hence, the observed subject consistency was significantly above chance. Moreover, DSC of SGGM-A was significantly higher than that of SGGM-U (p-values < 0.05), thus demonstrating the benefits of multimodal integration for connectivity estimation. In addition, we compared the sensitivity in group activation detection using: 1) ordinary least square (OLS) [11] without any connectivity prior, 2) ridge regression to control overfitting [9], connectivity-informed activation model [9] with connectivity prior learned by applying 3) oracle approximating shrinkage (OAS) on RS-fMRI data only [16], 4) SGGM-U on RS-fMRI data only, and 5) SGGM-A on dMRI and RS-fMRI data jointly. We examined 21 contrasts between the 10 experimental conditions. To enforce strict control over FPR so that we can safely base our validation on increased group activation detection, max-t permutation test [17] was used. Fig. 1(b) shows the percentage of parcels detected with significant activation averaged over contrasts. In agreement with [9], adding a connectivity prior substantially improved activation detection over OLS and ridge regression. More importantly, SGGM-A was found to outperform both SGGM-U and OAS. To assess whether the enhanced detection was statistically significant, we used a permutation test. Specifically, for each permutation, we first randomly selected half of the parcels and exchanged the labels (active or non-active) assigned by SGGM-A and each of the contrasted methods in turn for a given p-value threshold. We then computed the difference in the average number of detected parcels, and performed this procedure 10,000 times to generate a null distribution. For all p-value thresholds in Fig. 1(b), the original difference in the number of detected parcels was found to be greater than the 95th percentile of the corresponding null distribution. Hence, the detection improvement was statistically significant. Qualitatively, our approach additionally detected relevant areas adjacent to those found by considering functional information alone (Fig. 1(c)).

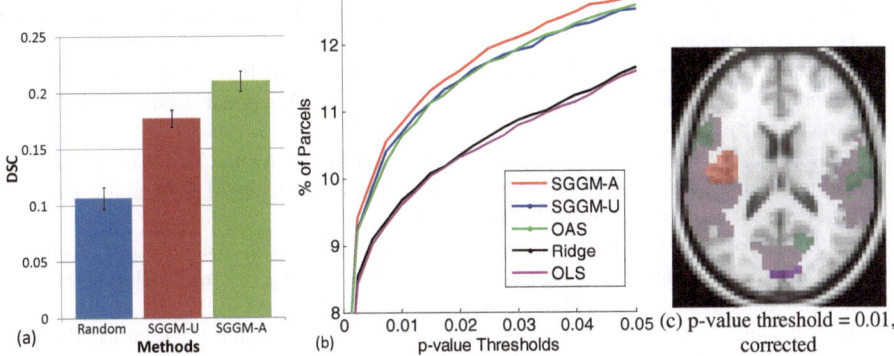

Fig. 1. Real data results. (a) Subject consistency based on DSC. (b) Percentage of parcels with significant activation averaged over contrasts vs. *p*-value thresholds. (c) Parcels detected for auditory tasks. Red = detected by SGGM-A only. Purple = detected by SGGM-A and SGGM-U. Green = detected by SGGM-A, SGGM-U, and OAS. Violet = detected by all methods.

5   Conclusions

We proposed a novel SGGM-based approach for multimodal brain connectivity inference. We showed that integrating dMRI and RS-fMRI data significantly increases subject consistency in the learned connection structure compared to analyzing RS-fMRI data alone. Enhanced group activation detection was also demonstrated. Our results thus suggest that connectivity estimated by combining anatomical and functional information may better resemble the underlying neural pathways than solely relying on functional information. A particularly important byproduct of this work is that our multimodal connectivity estimation approach in combination with our connectivity-informed activation model [9] provides a statistically-rigorous test bench for comparing different dMRI processing strategies. Quantitative evaluation, as opposed to qualitative assessment as often used in most dMRI studies, is thus facilitated.

Acknowledgments. This work was supported by the ANR grant, BrainPedia ANR-10-JCJC 1408-01, and the Berkeley INRIA Stanford grant. The data were acquired within the IMAGEN project. Jean Baptiste Poline was partly funded by the IMAGEN project, which receives funding from the E.U. Community's FP6, LSHM-CT-2007-037286. This manuscript reflects only the authors' views and the Community is not liable for any use that may be made of the information contained therein.

References

1. Fox, M.D., Greicius, M.D.: Clincial Applications of Resting State Functional Connectivity. Front. Syst. Neurosci. 4, 19 (2010)
2. Varoquaux, G., Gramfort, A., Poline, J.B., Thirion, B.: Brain Covariance Selection: Better Individual Functional Connectivity Models Using Population Prior. In: Advances in Neural Information Processing Systems, vol. 23, pp. 2334–2342 (2010)

3. Honey, C.J., Thivierge, J.P., Sporns, O.: Can Structure Predict Function in the Human Brain. NeuroImage 52, 766–776 (2010)
4. Damoiseaux, J.S., Greicius, M.D.: Greater than the Sum of its Parts: A Review of Studies Combining Structural Connectivity and Resting-state Functional Connectivity. Brain Struct. Funct. 213, 525–533 (2009)
5. Zhu, D., Li, K., Faraco, C.C., Deng, F., Zhang, D., Guo, L., Miller, L.S., Liu, T.: Optimization of Functional Brain ROIs via Maximization of Consistency of Structural Connectivity Profiles. NeuroImage 59, 1382–1393 (2012)
6. Si, J., Pearlson, G., Caprihan, A., Adali, T., Kiehl, K.A., Liu, J., Yamamoto, J., Calhoun, V.D.: Discriminating Schizophrenia and Bipolar Disorder by Fusing fMRI and DTI in a Multimodal CCA + joint ICA Model. NeuroImage 57, 839–855 (2011)
7. Venkataraman, A., Rathi, Y., Kubicki, M., Westin, C.F., Golland, P.: Joint Modeling of Anatomical and Functional Connectivity for Population Studies. IEEE Trans. Med. Imaging 31, 164–182 (2012)
8. Hsieh, C.J., Sustik, M.A., Dhillon, I.S., Ravikumar, P.: Sparse Invers Covariance Matrix Estimation Using Quadratic Approximation. In: Advances in Neural Information Processing Systems, vol. 24, pp. 2330–2338 (2011)
9. Ng, B., Abugharbieh, R., Varoquaux, G., Poline, J.B., Thirion, B.: Connectivity-Informed fMRI Activation Detection. In: Fichtinger, G., Martel, A., Peters, T. (eds.) MICCAI 2011, Part II. LNCS, vol. 6892, pp. 285–292. Springer, Heidelberg (2011)
10. Duchi, J., Gould, S., Koller, D.: Projected Subgradient Methods for Learning Sparse Gaussions. In: Int. Conf. Uncertainty in Artificial Intelligence (2008)
11. Friston, K.J., Holmes, A.P., Worsley, K.J., Poline, J.B., Frith, C.D., Frackowiak, R.S.J.: Statistical Parametric Maps in Functional Imaging: A General Linear Approach. Hum. Brain Mapp. 2, 189–210 (1995)
12. Pinel, P., Thirion, B., Meriaux, S., Jober, A., Serres, J., Le Bihan, D., Poline, J.B., Dehaene, S.: Fast Reproducible Identification and Large-scale Databasing of Individual Functional Cognitive Networks. BioMed. Central Neurosci. 8, 91 (2007)
13. Jones, D.K., Williams, S.C.R., Gasston, D., Horsfield, M.A., Simmons, A., Howard, R.: Isotropic Resolution Diffusion Tensor Imaging with Whole Brain Acquisition in a Clinically Acceptable Time. Human Brain Mapping 15, 216–230 (2002)
14. Toussaint, N., Souplet, J.C., Fillard, P.: MedINRIA: Medical Image Navigation and Research Tool by INRIA. In: MICCAI Workshop on Interaction in Medical Image Analysis and Visualization, pp. 1–8 (2007)
15. Michel, V., Gramfort, A., Varoquaux, G., Eger, E., Keribin, C., Thirion, B.: A Supervised Clustering Approach for fMRI-based Inference of Brain States. Patt. Recog. 45, 2041–2049 (2012)
16. Chen, Y., Wiesel, A., Eldar, Y.C., Hero, A.O.: Shrinkage Algorithms for MMSE Covariance Estimation. IEEE Trans. Sig. Proc. 58, 5016–5029 (2010)
17. Nichols, T., Hayasaka, S.: Controlling the Familywise Error Rate in Functional Neuroimaging: a Comparative Review. Stat. Methods Med. Research 12, 419–446 (2003)

From Brain Connectivity Models
to Identifying Foci of a Neurological Disorder

Archana Venkataraman[1], Marek Kubicki[2], and Polina Golland[1]

[1] MIT Computer Science and Artificial Intelligence Laboratory, Cambridge, MA
[2] Psychiatry Neuroimaging Laboratory, Harvard Medical School, Boston, MA

Abstract. We propose a novel approach to identify the foci of a neurological disorder based on anatomical and functional connectivity information. Specifically, we formulate a generative model that characterizes the network of abnormal functional connectivity emanating from the affected foci. We employ the variational EM algorithm to fit the model and to identify both the afflicted regions and the differences in connectivity induced by the disorder. We demonstrate our method on a population study of schizophrenia.

1 Introduction

Aberrations in functional connectivity inform us about neuropsychiatric disorders. Functional connectivity is measured via temporal correlations in resting-state functional Magnetic Resonance Imaging (fMRI) data [1]. Univariate tests and random effects analysis are commonly used in population studies of connectivity [2]. This approach relies on a statistical score, computed independently for each functional correlation, to determine significantly different connections within a clinical population. Multi-pattern analysis of functional connectivity has also been explored for clinical applications [3–5]. Although these studies identify functional connections affected by the disease, connectivity results are difficult to interpret and validate. Specifically, the bulk of our knowledge about the brain is organized around regions (i.e., functional localization, tissue properties, morphometry) and not the connections between them. Moreover, it is nearly impossible to design non-invasive experiments that target a particular connection between two brain regions.

In contrast to prior work, we propose a novel framework that pinpoints regions, which we call "foci", whose functional connectivity patterns are the most disrupted by the disorder. Using a probabilistic setting, we define a latent (hidden) graph that characterizes the network of abnormal functional connectivity emanating from the affected brain regions. This generates population differences in the observed fMRI correlations. We employ the variational EM algorithm to fit the model to the observed data. Our algorithm jointly infers the regions affected by the disease and the induced connectivity differences.

We use neural anatomy as a substrate for modeling functional connectivity. In particular, we rely on Diffusion Weighted Imaging (DWI) tractography to

N. Ayache et al. (Eds.): MICCAI 2012, Part I, LNCS 7510, pp. 715–722, 2012.
© Springer-Verlag Berlin Heidelberg 2012

estimate the underlying white matter fibers in the brain. The latent anatomical connectivity inferred from these fibers constrains the graph of aberrant functional connections. Previous work in joint modeling of resting-state fMRI and DWI data [4, 6–8] suggests that a direct anatomical connection between two regions predicts a higher functional correlation; however, multi-stage pathways may explain some of the functional effects. Since neural communication in the brain is constrained by white matter fibers, we hypothesize that the strongest effects of a disorder will occur along direct anatomical connections. Hence, we model whole-brain functional connectivity but only use functional abnormalities between anatomically connected regions to identify the disease foci. We emphasize that our model can be readily applied to the complete graph of pairwise functional connections and need not incorporate anatomy.

We demonstrate that our method learns a stable set of afflicted regions on a population study of schizophrenia. Schizophrenia is a poorly understood disorder marked by impairments in widely-distributed functional and anatomical networks [2, 9]. Accordingly, we apply our model to whole-brain connectivity information. Our results identify the posterior cingulate and superior temporal gyri as most affected regions in schizophrenia.

2   Generative Model and Inference

The basic assumption of our model is that impairments of the disorder localize to a small subset of brain regions, which we call foci, and affect the neural signaling along pathways associated with these regions. Fig. 1 presents a network diagram of the brain and the corresponding graphical model.

The nodes in Fig. 1(a) correspond to regions in the brain. The green nodes are healthy, and the red nodes are diseased. The edges denote neural connections, which are captured by latent anatomical connectivity A_{ij}. Specifically, the presence or absence of edge $\langle i, j \rangle$ in the network is governed by the value of A_{ij}. The anatomical network structure is shared between the control and clinical populations. The regions in this work correspond to (large) Brodmann areas. Prior results in the field suggest that the anatomical differences between schizophrenia patients and normal controls are very small in this case.

Based on the region assignments, aberrant functional connectivity along anatomical pathways is defined using a simple set of rules: (1) a connection between two diseased regions is always abnormal (solid red lines in Fig. 1(a)), (2) a connection between two healthy regions is never abnormal (solid green lines), and (3) a connection between a healthy and a diseased region is abnormal with probability η (dashed lines). We use latent functional connectivity variables F_{ij} and $\bar{F}_{ij}$ to model the neural synchrony between two regions in the control and clinical populations, respectively. Ideally, $\bar{F}_{ij} \neq F_{ij}$ for abnormal connections and $\bar{F}_{ij} = F_{ij}$ for healthy connections. However, due to noise, we assume that the latent templates can deviate from the above rules with probability ϵ.

The observed DWI measurements D_{ij}^l and fMRI correlations B_{ij}^l provide noisy information about the latent network structure.

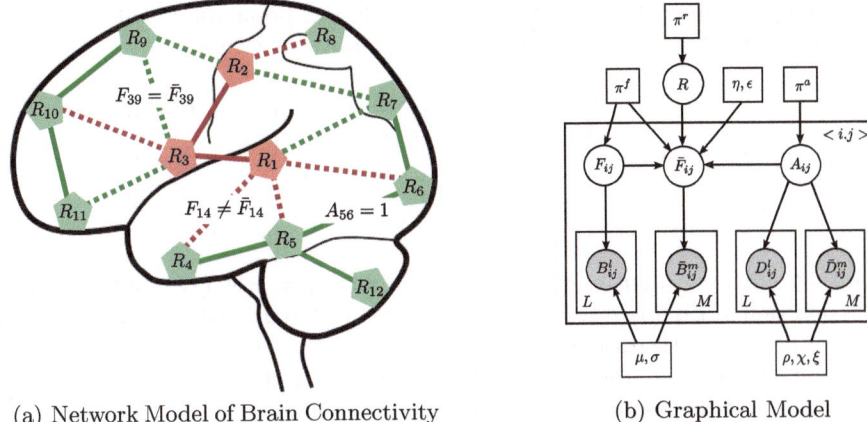

(a) Network Model of Brain Connectivity   (b) Graphical Model

Fig. 1. (a) A network model of connectivity. The nodes correspond to regions in the brain, and the lines denote anatomical connections between them. The green nodes and edges are normal. The red nodes are foci of the disease, and the red edges specify pathways of abnormal functional connectivity. The solid lines are deterministic given the region labels; the dashed lines are probabilistic. (b) Graphical model representation. Vector R specifies diseased regions. A_{ij} and F_{ij} represent the latent anatomical and functional connectivity, respectively, between regions i and j. D_{ij}^l and B_{ij}^l are the observed DWI and fMRI measurements in the lth subject. Variables associated with the diseased population are identified by an overbar. Boxes denote non-random parameters; circles indicate random variables; shaded variables are observed.

Disease Foci. The random variable $R = [R_1, \ldots, R_N]$ is a binary vector that indicates the state, healthy ($R_i = 0$) or diseased ($R_i = 1$), for each brain region i. We assume an *i.i.d.* Bernoulli prior for the elements of R:

$$P(R_i; \pi^r) = (\pi^r)^{R_i}(1 - \pi^r)^{1-R_i}, \tag{1}$$

where π^r is an unknown parameter shared by all nodes in the network.

Latent Connectivity. We model anatomical connectivity A_{ij} as a binary random variable with *a priori* probability π^a that a connection is present:

$$P(A_{ij}; \pi^a) = (\pi^a)^{A_{ij}}(1 - \pi^a)^{1-A_{ij}}. \tag{2}$$

Latent functional connectivity F_{ij} is modeled as a tri-state random variable drawn from a multinomial distribution with parameter π^f. These states represent little or no functional co-activation ($F_{ij} = 0$), positive functional synchrony ($F_{ij} = 1$), and negative functional synchrony ($F_{ij} = -1$). For convenience, we represent F_{ij} as a length-three indicator vector with exactly one of its elements $[F_{ij,-1} \quad F_{ij0} \quad F_{ij1}]$ equal to one:

$$P(F_{ij}; \pi^f) = \prod_{k=-1}^{1} \left(\pi_k^f\right)^{F_{ijk}}. \tag{3}$$

The latent functional connectivity $\bar{F}_{ij}$ of the clinical population is also tri-state and is based on F_{ij} and the healthy/diseased indicator vector R:

$$P(\bar{F}_{ij}|F_{ij}, R_i, R_j, A_{ij}) = \begin{cases} (1-\epsilon)^{F_{ij}^{\mathrm{T}}\bar{F}_{ij}} \left(\frac{\epsilon}{2}\right)^{1-F_{ij}^{\mathrm{T}}\bar{F}_{ij}}, & A_{ij}=1, R_i=R_j=0, \\ \epsilon^{F_{ij}^{\mathrm{T}}\bar{F}_{ij}} \left(\frac{1-\epsilon}{2}\right)^{1-F_{ij}^{\mathrm{T}}\bar{F}_{ij}}, & A_{ij}=1, R_i=R_j=1, \\ \epsilon_1^{F_{ij}^{\mathrm{T}}\bar{F}_{ij}} \left(\frac{1-\epsilon_1}{2}\right)^{1-F_{ij}^{\mathrm{T}}\bar{F}_{ij}}, & A_{ij}=1, R_i \neq R_j, \\ \mathcal{M}(\pi^f), & A_{ij}=0, \end{cases} \quad (4)$$

such that $\mathcal{M}(\cdot)$ is a multinomial distribution and $\epsilon_1 = \eta\epsilon + (1-\eta)(1-\epsilon)$. The first condition in Eq. (4) states that if there exists a latent anatomical connection ($A_{ij} = 1$) and if both regions are healthy ($R_i = R_j = 0$), then the edge $\langle i, j \rangle$ is healthy. Consequently, the functional connectivity of the clinical population is equal to that of the control population with probability $1 - \epsilon$, and it differs with probability ϵ. The second term is similarly obtained by replacing ϵ with $1 - \epsilon$. The probability ϵ_1 in the third condition reflects the coupling between η and ϵ when the region labels differ. The final term of Eq. (4) implies that $\bar{F}_{ij}$ is drawn from the prior π^f, irrespective of F_{ij} and R, if there is no anatomical connection between the regions i and j.

Data Likelihood. The DWI measurement D_{ij}^l for the lth subject in the control population is a noisy observation of the latent anatomical connectivity A_{ij}:

$$P(D_{ij}^l|A_{ij}; \{\rho,\chi,\xi^2\}) = \mathcal{P}_0(D_{ij}^l; \{\rho,\chi,\xi^2\})^{1-A_{ij}} \cdot \mathcal{P}_1(D_{ij}^l; \{\rho,\chi,\xi^2\})^{A_{ij}}, \quad (5)$$

where $\mathcal{P}_k(D_{ij}) = \rho_k\delta(D_{ij}) + (1-\rho_k)\mathcal{N}(D_{ij}; \chi_k, \xi_k^2)$ for $k = 0, 1$. ρ_k represents the probability of failing to find a tract between two regions, which corresponds to $D_{ij}^l = 0$. Otherwise, D_{ij}^l is drawn from a Gaussian distribution with mean χ_k and variance ξ_k^2 ($k = 0, 1$). The data $\bar{D}_{ij}^m$ for the clinical population follows the same likelihood.

The BOLD fMRI correlation B_{ij}^l is a noisy observation of the functional connectivity F_{ij}:

$$P(B_{ij}^l|F_{ij}; \{\mu,\sigma^2\}) = \prod_{k=-1}^{1} \mathcal{N}\left(B_{ij}^l; \mu_k, \sigma_k^2\right)^{F_{ijk}}. \quad (6)$$

We fix $\mu_0 = 0$ to center the parameter estimates. The likelihood for the clinical population $\bar{B}_{ij}^m$ has the same functional form and parameter values as Eq. (6) but uses the clinical template $\bar{F}_{ij}$ instead of the control template F_{ij}.

Using histograms of the data, we verified that the Gaussian distributions in Eqs. (5-6) provide reasonable approximations for the DWI and fMRI data. Pragmatically, they greatly simplify the learning/inference steps.

Variational EM. We employ a maximum likelihood (ML) framework to fit the model to the data. The region variable R induces a complex coupling between pairwise connections. Therefore, we use a variational approximation [10] for the latent posterior probability distribution when deriving the ML solution. Our variational posterior assumes the following form:

$$Q(R, A, F, \bar{F}) = Q^r(R) \cdot Q^c(A, F, \bar{F}) = Q^r(R) \prod_{<i,j>} Q_{ij}^c(A_{ij}, F_{ij}, \bar{F}_{ij}), \quad (7)$$

where $Q_{ij}^c(\cdot)$ is an 18-state multinomial distribution corresponding to all configurations of anatomical and functional connectivity. This factorization yields a tractable inference algorithm and also preserves the dependency between A_{ij}, F_{ij}, and $\bar{F}_{ij}$ given the region indicator vector R.

For a fixed setting of model parameters, we obtain the distribution $Q(\cdot)$ that minimizes the variational free energy by alternatively updating $Q^r(R)$ and $Q^c(A, F, \bar{F})$ until convergence. Due to space constraints, we omit the update rules. We emphasize that both the posterior distribution $Q(\cdot)$ and the model parameters are estimated directly from the observed data without tuning any auxiliary parameters.

Model Evaluation. The marginal posterior distribution $Q^r(R_i = 1)$ tells us how likely region i is to be diseased given the observed connectivity data. We estimate the marginal posterior by averaging across Gibbs samples $\mathcal{S}$:

$$q_i = Q^r(R_i = 1) = \frac{1}{S} \sum_{s=1}^{S} R_i^s. \quad (8)$$

We evaluate the significance of our model through non-parametric permutation tests. To construct the null distribution for $\{q_i\}$, we randomly permute the subject diagnosis labels (NC vs. SZ) 1,000 times. For each permutation, we fit the model and compute the statistic in Eq. (8). The significance of each region is equal to the proportion of permutations that yield a larger value of q_i than the true labeling. These uncorrected p-values confirm that a particular region is rarely selected. Since our inference algorithm estimates the joint posterior distribution over the entire vector R, and since none of the permutations return the same set of disease foci, it is unclear that element-wise correction provides any additional insight.

Based on the MAP estimate of each R_i and the ML estimates of the model parameters, we can also construct the graph of functional connectivity differences to gain insight into the behavior of individual connections.

Our framework enables us to estimate all unknown parameters. However, we further explore the solution space by specifying the expected number of diseased regions via the prior π^r. In particular, the evolution of disease foci across a range of prior values (in this work $\pi^r \in [0, 0.5]$) illustrates the stability of our model in explaining the data. Moreover, tuning π^r is an intuitive way to inject clinical knowledge into our framework and may be useful in certain applications.

Finally, we have run extensive simulations on synthetic data, which demonstrate that our model recovers the ground truth region labels. However, due to space constraints, we focus on real data in this paper.

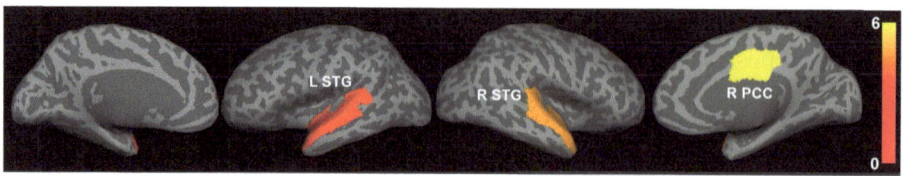

Fig. 2. Significant regions based on permutation tests ($q_i > 0.5$, uncorrected $p <$ 0.044). The colorbar corresponds to the negative log p-value. We present the lateral and medial viewpoints for each hemisphere. The highlighted regions are the posterior cingulate (R PCC) and the superior temporal gyrus (L STG & R STG).

3   Results

We demonstrate our model on a study of 19 male patients with chronic schizophrenia and 19 male healthy controls. For each subject, an anatomical scan (SPGR, $TE = 3ms$, $res = 1mm^3$), a diffusion-weighted scan (EPI, $TE = 78ms$, $res = 1.66 \times 1.66 \times 1.7mm$, 51 gradient directions with $b = 900s/mm^2$, 8 baseline) and a resting-state functional scan (EPI-BOLD, $TR = 3s$, $TE = 30ms$, $res = 1.875 \times 1.875 \times 3mm$) were acquired using a 3T GE Echospeed system.

We segment the anatomical images into 77 cortical and sub-cortical regions using FreeSurfer [11]. The DWI data is corrected for eddy-current distortions, and two-tensor tractography [12] is used to estimate the white matter fibers. The DWI measure D_{ij}^l is computed by averaging FA along all detected fibers between regions i and j. D_{ij}^l is set to zero if no tracts are found. We discard the first five fMRI time points and perform motion correction by rigid body alignment and slice timing correction using FSL [13]. The data is spatially smoothed using a $5mm$ kernel, temporally low-pass filtered with $0.08Hz$ cutoff, and motion corrected via linear regression. We also remove global contributions from the white matter, ventricles and the whole brain. The fMRI measure B_{ij}^l is the Pearson correlation coefficient between the mean time courses of regions i and j.

Significant Regions. Our method identifies three foci such that $q_i > 0.5$; the uncorrected p-value of each region is less than 0.044. Fig. 2 displays the significant regions, which we color according to $-\log(p)$. Our results implicate the right posterior cingulate ($q_i = 1, p < 0.004$), the right superior temporal gyrus ($q_i = 1, p < 0.014$), and the left superior temporal gyrus ($q_i = 1, p < 0.044$).

Prior studies have found abnormalities in the superior temporal gyri in schizophrenia [14]. These impairments correlate with clinical measures of auditory hallucination and attentional deficits. The default network has been implicated in resting-state fMRI studies [2]. Reduced connectivity in the posterior cingulate correlate with both positive and negative symptoms of schizophrenia.

In Fig. 3, we observe that functional abnormalities originating in the posterior cingulate project to the midbrain and frontal lobe, whereas abnormalities stemming from the right and left superior temporal gyri tend to span their

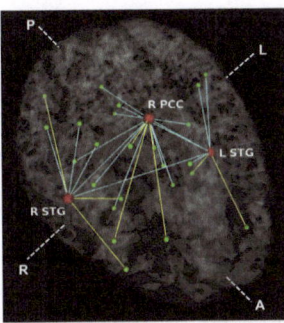

Fig. 3. Estimated graph of functional connectivity differences. The red nodes indicate the disease foci. Blue lines indicate reduced functional connectivity and yellow lines indicate increased functional connectivity in the schizophrenia population.

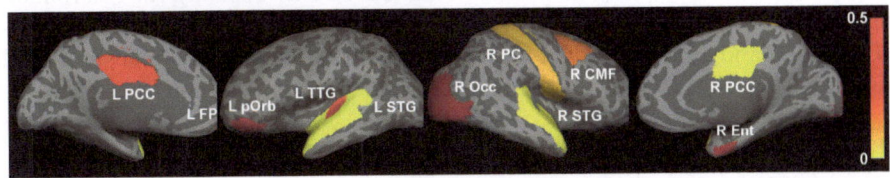

Fig. 4. Evolution of the disease foci when varying the region prior π^r. The color corresponds to the smallest value of π^r such that $q_i > 0.2$. The highlighted regions are the posterior cingulate (L PCC & R PCC), the superior temporal gyrus (L STG & R STG), the postcentral gyrus (R PC), the frontal pole (L FP), the caudal middle frontal gyrus (R CMF), the transverse temporal gyrus (L TTG), the pars orbitalis (L pOrb), the entorhinal cortex (R Ent) and the lateral occipital cortex (R LOcc).

respective hemispheres. Overall, schizophrenia patients exhibit reduced functional connectivity. Of notable exception are connections to the frontal lobe. This phenomenon has been reported in prior studies of schizophrenia [9] and is believed to interfere with perception by misdirecting attentional resources.

Effects of the Region Prior. Fig. 4 illustrates the results of varying the prior π^r for the region indicator vector R. Empirically, we observe that sets of regions affected by the disease form a nested structure as π^r increases. We color each of the selected regions according to the smallest value of π^r such that the marginal posterior $q_i > 0.2$. The yellow regions are always identified as foci, whereas the orange/red regions are selected for larger values of the prior π^r.

The nesting property is a highly desirable feature of our model. It suggests an initial set of disease foci, identical to the significant regions in Fig. 2. We can then tune a single scalar to progressively include regions that exhibit some functional abnormalities but are not as strongly implicated by the data.

4   Conclusion

We proposed a novel probabilistic framework for multimodal analysis of fMRI and DWI data that integrates population differences in connectivity to isolate

foci of a neurological disorder. This is achieved by defining a network of abnormal connectivity emanating from the affected regions. We demonstrate that
our method identifies a stable set of schizophrenia foci consisting of the right
posterior cingulate and the right and left superior temporal gyri. Prior clinical
studies have linked these regions to the effects of schizophrenia. Moreover, we
uncover additional regions by adjusting the prior on the number of disease foci.
These results establish the promise of our approach for aggregating connectivity
information to localize region effects.

Acknowledgments. This work was supported by the National Alliance for
Medical Image Computing (NIH NIBIB NAMIC U54-EB005149), the Neuroimaging Analysis Center (NIH NCRR NAC P41-RR13218 and NIH NIBIB NAC P41-
EB-015902) and NSF CAREER Grant 0642971. A. Venkataraman is supported
in part by the NIH Advanced Multimodal Neuroimaging Training Program.

References

1. Fox, M., Raichle, M.: Spontaneous fluctuations in brain activity observed with
   functional magnetic resonance imaging. Nature 8, 700–711 (2007)
2. Bluhm, R., et al.: Spontaneous low-frequency fluctuations in the bold signal in
   schizophrenic patients: Abnormalities in the default network. Schizophrenia Bul-
   letin, 1–9 (2007)
3. Jafri, M., et al.: A method for functional network connectivity among spatially
   independent resting-state components in schiz. NeuroImage 39, 1666–1681 (2008)
4. Venkataraman, A., et al.: Joint modeling of anatomical and functional connectivity
   for population studies. IEEE TMI 31, 164–182 (2012)
5. Venkataraman, A., et al.: Robust feature selection in resting-state fmri connectivity
   based on population studies. In: MMBIA, pp. 63–70 (2010)
6. Greicius, M., et al.: Resting-state functional connectivity reflects structural connectivity in the default mode network. Cerebral Cortex 19, 72–78 (2008)
7. Koch, M., et al.: An investigation of functional and anatomical connectivity using
   magnetic resonance imaging. NeuroImage 16, 241–250 (2002)
8. Deligianni, F., Varoquaux, G., Thirion, B., Robinson, E., Sharp, D.J., Edwards,
   A.D., Rueckert, D.: A Probabilistic Framework to Infer Brain Functional Connectivity from Anatomical Connections. In: Székely, G., Hahn, H.K. (eds.) IPMI 2011.
   LNCS, vol. 6801, pp. 296–307. Springer, Heidelberg (2011)
9. Gabrieli-Whitfield, S., et al.: Hyperactivity and hyperconnectivity of the default
   network in schizophrenia and in first-degree relatives of persons with schizophrenia.
   PNAS 106, 1279–1284 (2009)
10. Jordan, M., et al.: An introduction to variational methods for graphical models.
    Machine Learning 37, 183–233 (1999)
11. Fischl, B., et al.: Sequence-independent segmentation of magnetic resonance im-
    ages. NeuroImage 23, 69–84 (2004)
12. Malcolm, J., et al.: A filtered approach to neural tractography using the watson
    directional function. NeuroImage 14, 58–69 (2010)
13. Smith, S., et al.: Advances in functional and structural mr image analysis and
    implementation as fsl. NeuroImage 23(51), 208–219 (2004)
14. Lee, K., et al.: Increased diffusivity in superior temporal gyrus in patients with
    schizophrenia: A diffusion tensor imaging study. Schiz Research 104, 33–40 (2009)

Deriving Statistical Significance Maps for SVM Based Image Classification and Group Comparisons

Bilwaj Gaonkar and Christos Davatzikos

Section for Biomedical Image Analysis,
University of Pennsylvania, Philadelphia, PA 19104, USA

Abstract. Population based pattern analysis and classification for quantifying structural and functional differences between diverse groups has been shown to be a powerful tool for the study of a number of diseases, and is quite commonly used especially in neuroimaging. The alternative to these pattern analysis methods, namely mass univariate methods such as voxel based analysis and all related methods, cannot detect multivariate patterns associated with group differences, and are not particularly suitable for developing individual-based diagnostic and prognostic biomarkers. A commonly used pattern analysis tool is the support vector machine (SVM). Unlike univariate statistical frameworks for morphometry, analytical tools for statistical inference are unavailable for the SVM. In this paper, we show that null distributions ordinarily obtained by permutation tests using SVMs can be analytically approximated from the data. The analytical computation takes a small fraction of the time it takes to do an actual permutation test, thereby rendering it possible to quickly create statistical significance maps derived from SVMs. Such maps are critical for understanding imaging patterns of group differences and interpreting which anatomical regions are important in determining the classifier's decision.

1 Significance

Precise quantification of group differences using medical images central in scientific studies of the effects of disease on the human body. The dominant approach addressing this problem involves performing independent statistical testing either pixel/voxel-wise [1] or regions of interest (ROI-wise) in the image. It has been argued that such univariate analysis might miss group difference patterns that span multiple voxels or regions [2]. Hence, replacing univariate methods by multivariate methods such as SVMs [3] [4][5] has been discussed in literature. However, unlike univariate methods [1], SVMs do not naturally provide statistical tests (and corresponding p-values) associated with every voxel/region of an image. Permutation testing has been suggested for interpreting SVM output for such high dimensional data [6]. However, performing these tests is time consuming and computationally costly. Hence, we developed and validated an analytical approximation for SVM permutation tests that allows for tremendous

N. Ayache et al. (Eds.): MICCAI 2012, Part I, LNCS 7510, pp. 723–730, 2012.

computational speed up. Section 2 of this mauscript presents the theory that allows us to achieve this speed up. Section 3 presents experiments that validate the theory. Section 4 presents a brief discussion and possible avenues for further development.

2   Analysis

2.1   Support Vector Machines: Background

The support vector machine [7] is a powerful pattern classification engine that was first proposed in the nineties. In medical imaging it has been used to distinguish cognitively abnormal people from controls based on their brain MR images. For completeness we briefly explain the concept of the SVM next. To use SVMs we stack preprocessed image data into a large rectangular matrix $X \in R^{m \times p}$ whose rows $\mathbf{x}_i$ index individuals in the population, and columns index image voxels. Also, with every individual $\mathbf{x}_i$ we associate a binary label $y_i \in +1, -1$ which indicates the presence or absence of disease. Note that the $\mathbf{x}_i$ live in a Euclidean space of dimension p. The SVM finds the largest margin hyperplane parameterized by the direction $\mathbf{w}^* \in R^p$ that separates the patients from the controls (or two groups, in general). This concept is illustrated for 2-dimensional space in figure 1. The SVM is typically formulated as follows:

$$\mathbf{w}^*, b^* = min_{\mathbf{w},b} \frac{1}{2}||\mathbf{w}||^2 + C \sum_{i=1}^{m} \xi_i$$

$$subj.to. \ y_i(\mathbf{w}^T \mathbf{x}_i + b) \geq 1 - \xi_i$$

$$\xi_i \geq 0 \ \ i = 1, ..., m \tag{1}$$

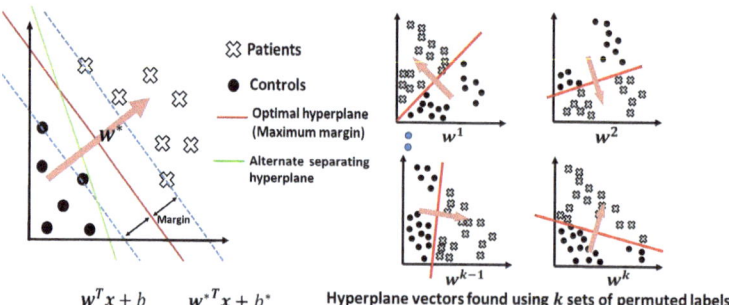

Fig. 1. Left: Concept of support vector machines in 2-D space Right: Permutation testing for support vector machines

For unseen data the SVM simply uses the position of the unseen data relative to the learnt hyperplane, $\mathbf{w}^*, b^*$ to decide upon disease status. Although SVM performance can be assessed by cross validation, it is equally important to be able to interpret which regions/features are important in deriving the classifier's decision. Such interpretations are particularly desirable by clinicians interested in understanding how disease affects anatomy and function and which features they should be attending to in interpreting medical images. Currently the only way to quantify importance of individual voxels to the SVM classification is through the use of permutation tests. The concept of permutation testing is illustrated in figure 1. Briefly, the data labels y_i are permuted randomly. For each random permutation an SVM is trained and a hyperplane $\mathbf{w}$ is found. After many permutations we can generate an approximation to the null distribution of each component of $\mathbf{w}$. Comparing the components of $\mathbf{w}^*$ with these null distributions allows for statistical inference. The inference procedure described above is based on [6]. Permutation testing is computationally expensive and becomes increasingly difficult as dataset size increases. In this paper we develop an analytical approximation of permutation testing using SVMs for medical imaging data.

2.2   The Analytical Approximation of Permutation Testing for SVMs

Key Assumption: The proposed analytic framework is based on one key observation about permutation testing with SVMs while using medical imaging data,as well as any high-dimensionality data observed via dramatically smaller number of samples. This observation is that for a great majority of the permutations, the number of support vectors(SVs) in the learnt models equal or almost equal the total number of training subjects themselves. This behavior and the corresponding assumption can be partly justified by appealing to a known generalization error bound for SVMs (See eqn 93 of [8])

$$E[P(Error)] \leq \frac{E[Number\ of\ support\ vectors]}{Number\ of\ training\ samples} \quad (2)$$

Here $E[P(Error)]$ is a measure of the generalization/test error of the SVM. Since most permutations are completely random, we do not expect the corresponding learnt models to generalize well to new training data. Thus, for most permutations the number of SVs tends to the total number of subjects themselves. This key assumption allows us to simplify the statistical analysis of SVMs while using medical imaging data. Using the theory developed under this assumption we are able to predict the nature of the null distribution for a variety of medical imaging datasets (see figure 2).

Theory: Note that VC-theory dictates that linear classifiers shatter high dimension low sample size data. Hence, for any permutation of $\mathbf{y}$ one can always find a separating hyperplane that perfectly separates the training data. Thus, we choose use the hard margin support vector machine formulation from [7] instead of (1) for further analysis in this paper. The hard margin support vector machine (see [7]) can then be written as:

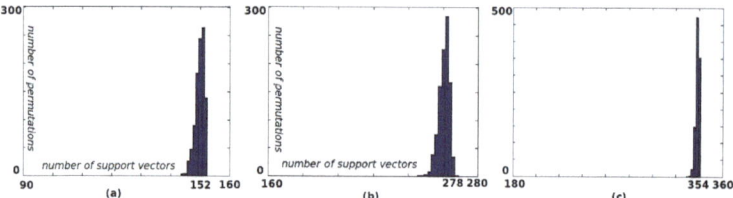

Fig. 2. For most permutations the number of support vectors in the learnt model is almost equal to the total number of samples (a) simulated dataset(b) real dataset with Alzheimer's patients and controls (c) real dataset with schizophrenia patients and controls

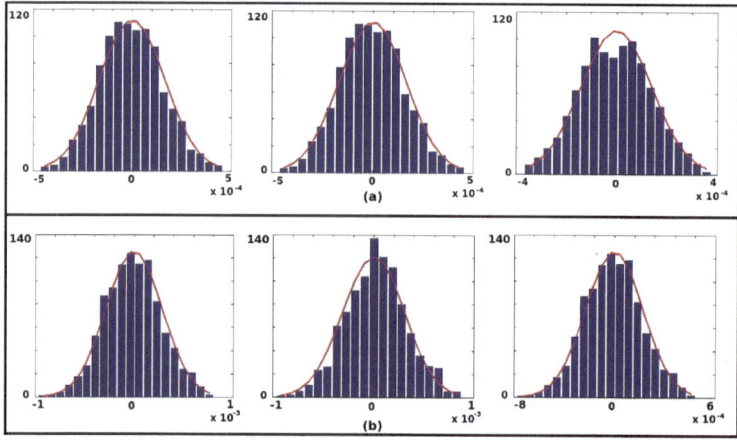

Fig. 3. Experimental(blue histogram) and theoretically predicted(red line) null distributions for two randomly chosen components of w in (a) real dataset with Alzheimer's patients and controls (b) simulated data

$$min_{\mathbf{w},b} \frac{1}{2}||\mathbf{w}||^2$$
$$subj.to.\ \ y_i(\mathbf{w}^T\mathbf{x}_i + b) \geq 1 \quad \forall i \in \{1,....,m\}$$

It is required (see [9]) that for the 'support vectors' (indexed by $j \in \{1, 2, .., n_{SV}\}$) we have $\mathbf{w}^T\mathbf{x}_j + b = y_j$ $\forall j$. Now, if all our data were support vectors this would allow us to write the constraints in optimization (3) as $\mathbf{Xw} + \mathbf{J}b = \mathbf{y}$ where $\mathbf{J}$ is a column matrix of ones and $\mathbf{X}$ is a super long matrix with each row representing one image. Since this is indeed the case for most of our permutation tests (figure 2), the optimization (3) becomes:

$$min_{\mathbf{w},b}||\mathbf{w}||^2$$
$$subj.to.\ \ \mathbf{Xw} + \mathbf{J}b = \mathbf{y} \tag{3}$$

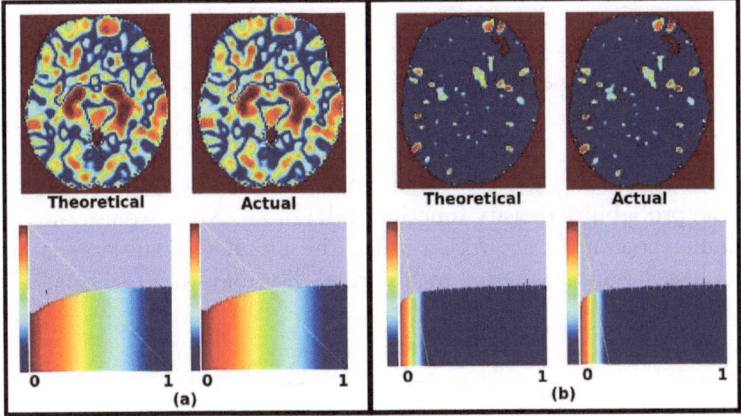

Fig. 4. Comparison of p-value maps(top row) with the corresponding image histograms(bottom row), generated using our theoretical framework and actual permutation tests (a) In real data pertaining to Alzheimer's disease (b) In simulated data

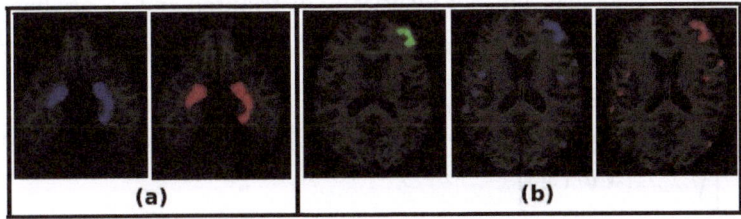

Fig. 5. Regions found by thresholding p-value maps at 0.05 a)in real data pertaining to Alzheimer's disease (left) theoretically predicted (right) actual permutation testing (b)in simulated data (left) ground truth region of introduced brain shrinkage (middle) found using theory (right) found using actual permutation testing

The above formulation is exactly the same as an LS-SVM [10]. This equivalence between the SVM and LS-SVM for high dimensional low sample size data was also previously noted in [11] where it was based on observations about the distribution of such data as elucidated in [12]. Since the LS-SVM, (4) can be solved in the closed form [10], we can now compute $\mathbf{w}$ as:

$$\mathbf{w} = \mathbf{X}^{\mathbf{T}}[(\mathbf{X}\mathbf{X}^{\mathbf{T}})^{-1} + (\mathbf{X}\mathbf{X}^{\mathbf{T}})^{-1}\mathbf{J}(-\mathbf{J}^{\mathbf{T}}(\mathbf{X}\mathbf{X}^{\mathbf{T}})^{-1}\mathbf{J})^{-1}\mathbf{J}^{\mathbf{T}}(\mathbf{X}\mathbf{X}^{\mathbf{T}})^{-1}]\mathbf{y} \qquad (4)$$

Note that this expresses each component w_j of $\mathbf{w}$ as a linear combination of y_j's. Thus, we can hypothesize about the probability distribution of the components of $\mathbf{w}$, given the distributions of y_j. If we let y_j attain any of the labels (either $+1$ or -1) with equal probability, we have a Bernoulli like distribution on y_j with $E(y_j) = 0$ and $Var(y_j) = 1$ (the theory can be readily extended in the case of unequal priors). Note that (5) expresses $\mathbf{w}$ as a linear combination of these y_j we have:

$$E(w_j) = 0 \qquad Var(w_j) = \sum_{i=1}^{m} C_{ij}^2 \qquad (5)$$

where C_{ij} are the components of the matrix $\mathbf{C}$, which is defined as:

$$\mathbf{C} \doteq \mathbf{X^T}[(\mathbf{XX^T})^{-1} + (\mathbf{XX^T})^{-1}\mathbf{J}(-\mathbf{J^T}(\mathbf{XX^T})^{-1}\mathbf{J})^{-1}\mathbf{J^T}(\mathbf{XX^T})^{-1}] \qquad (6)$$

At this point we know the expectation and the variance of w_j. We still need to uncover the probability density function (pdf) of w_j. Next, we use the Lyapunov central limit theorem to show that when the number of subjects is large, the p.d.f of w_j can be approximated by a normal distribution. To this end, from (5) and (7), we have:

$$w_j = \sum_{i=1}^{m} C_{ij} y_i = \sum_{i=1}^{m} z_i^j \qquad (7)$$

where we have defined a new random variable $z_i^j = C_{ij} y_i$ which is linearly dependent on y_i. We can infer the expectation and variance of z_i^j from y_j as:

$$\mathrm{E}(z_i^j) = 0 = \mu_i \quad Var(z_i^j) = C_{ij}^2 \qquad (8)$$

Thus, z_i^j are independent but not identically distributed and w_j are linear combinations of z_j^i. Then according to the Lyapunov central limit theorem(CLT) w_j is distributed normally if:

$$\lim_{m \to \infty} \frac{1}{\left[\sqrt{\sum_{i=1}^{m} Var(z_i^j)}\right]^{2+\delta}} \sum_{k=1}^{m} \mathrm{E}\left[|z_k^j - \mu_k|^{2+\delta}\right] = 0 \;\; for \; some \;\; \delta > 0 \qquad (9)$$

As is standard practice we check for $\delta = 1$.

$$E\left[|z_k^j - \mu_k|^{2+\delta}\right] = (1/2)|+C_{kj} - 0|^{2+\delta} + (1/2)|-C_{kj} - 0|^{2+\delta} = C_{kj}^3 \qquad (10)$$

Thus, we can write the limit in (10) as:

$$\lim_{m \to \infty} \frac{\sum_{k=1}^{m} C_{kj}^3}{\left[\sqrt{\sum_{i=1}^{m} C_{ij}^2}\right]^3} = \sum_{k=1}^{m} \left(\sqrt{\lim_{m \to \infty} \frac{C_{kj}^2}{\sum_{i=1}^{m} C_{ij}^2}}\right)^3 = 0 \qquad (11)$$

Hence, given an adequate number of subjects, the Lyanpunov CLT allows us to approximate the distribution of individual components of $\mathbf{w}$ using the normal distribution as:

$$w_j \xrightarrow{d} \mathcal{N}(0, \sum_{i=1}^{m} C_{ij}^2). \qquad (12)$$

These predicted distributions fit actual distributions obtained using permutation testing very well. Thus w_j's computed by an SVM model using true labels can now simply be compared to the distribution given by (13) and statistical inference can be made. Thus, (13) gives us a fast and efficient analytical alternative to actual permutation testing. In the next section we validate our analytical approximation using actual data.

3   Experiments and Results

In order to validate the theory proposed above we performed two experiments using brain imaging data. Both the experiments were done using tissue density maps (TDMs) generated after preprocessing of the raw images(these maps are commonly used in approaches like "modulated VBM" in which the Jacobian determinant multiplies the spatially normalized images). Tissue density maps were used because they inform us about the quantity of tissue present at each brain location in a common template space. These can be generated from registration fields warping a given subject to a template space. Since these maps are usually computed in template space a specific voxel location in a TDM corresponds to the same brain region across multiple subjects. Our two experiments were:

Experiment 1: Simulated data was generated as follows 1) grey matter tissue density maps were generated from brain images of 152 normal subjects 2)simulated brain shrinkage was introduced in the right frontal lobe of half of these images by a localized reduction in intensity of the corresponding TDMs. The vectorized TDM corresponding to each subject forms the superlong vector $\mathbf{x}_i$ of section 2.1.

Experiment 2: 278 TDMs were generated. This dataset contained 152 controls and 126 Alzheimer's patients. Grey matter (GM), white matter(WM) and ventricular(CSF) tissue density maps were computed. Maps corresponding to the ith subject are vectorized and the vectors of all 3 tissue types (each living in $R^{1 \times q}$) were concatenated into the super long vector $\mathbf{x}_i \in R^{1 \times 3q}$.

For both experiments we stacked the $\mathbf{x}_i$'s corresponding to controls and patients(either simulated or actual) into the matrix $\mathbf{X}$ as detailed in section 2.1. In both experiments, we performed permutation tests (1000 permutations) and also computed the predicted distribution using (13). Figure 3 shows how the predicted probability distribution function compares with the distribution obtained from the actual permutation tests. We also computed p-values at every voxel location according to the predicted and the actual distribution. These results are shown in figure 4. Notice that the predicted p-values are very close to the actual ones in both simulated and actual data. Furthermore a p-value threshold of 0.05 accurately demarcates the region of simulated brain shrinkage in the simulated data and the hippocampus in the real data (figure 5). The actual permutation tests took approximately 8 hours of computational time for Experiment 1 and 50 hours of computational time for Experiment 2 while the analytical approximation took less than a minute to compute for either experiment.

4   Discussion

An important issue that remains to be addressed is that of dataset size. This method assumes a large dataset size. So the natural question that occurs is "How big is big enough?" . This remains to be addressed as part of future work. Another perspective that needs to be explored is that of multiple comparisons.

"Do we need to correct for multiple comparisons?". If yes, how do we make such a correction? We intend to address both of these issues in future work.

Nevertheless, the current manuscript provides analytical machinery that potentially replaces computationally intensive permutation testing when using SVMs for multivariate image analysis and classification. This ability to easily associate voxel level statistical significance with the output of an SVM allows us to use it for easily discovering brain regions and networks associated with disease in addition to disease classification.

References

1. Ashburner, J., Friston, K.J.: Voxel-based morphometry–the methods. Neuroimage 11(6 pt. 1), 805–821 (2000)
2. Davatzikos, C.: Why voxel-based morphometric analysis should be used with great caution when characterizing group differences. Neuroimage 23(1), 17–20 (2004)
3. Mouro-Miranda, J., Bokde, A.L.W., Born, C., Hampel, H., Stetter, M.: Classifying brain states and determining the discriminating activation patterns: Support vector machine on functional mri data. Neuroimage 28(4), 980–995 (2005)
4. Wang, Z., Childress, A.R., Wang, J., Detre, J.A.: Support vector machine learning-based fmri data group analysis. Neuroimage 36(4), 1139–1151 (2007)
5. Klöppel, S., Stonnington, C.M., Chu, C., Draganski, B., Scahill, R.I., Rohrer, J.D., Fox, N.C., Jack Jr., C.R., Ashburner, J., Frackowiak, R.S.J.: Automatic classification of mr scans in alzheimer's disease. Brain 131(pt. 3), 681–689 (2008)
6. Hirschhorn, J.N., Daly, M.J.: Genome-wide association studies for common diseases and complex traits. Nat. Rev. Genet. 6(2), 95–108 (2005)
7. Vapnik, V.N.: The nature of statistical learning theory. Springer-Verlag New York, Inc., New York (1995)
8. Burges, C.J.C.: A tutorial on support vector machines for pattern recognition. Data Mining and Knowledge Discovery 2, 121–167 (1998)
9. Bishop, C.M.: Pattern Recognition and Machine Learning (Information Science and Statistics), 1st edn. (2006), corr. 2nd printing edn. Springer (October 2007)
10. Suykens, J.A.K., Vandewalle, J.: Least Squares Support Vector Machine Classifiers. Neural Processing Letters 9(3), 293–300 (1999)
11. Ye, J., Xiong, T.: Svm versus least squares svm. Journal of Machine Learning Research - Proceedings Track, 644–651 (2007)
12. Hall, P., Marron, J.S., Neeman, A.: Geometric representation of high dimension, low sample size data. Journal of the Royal Statistical Society: Series B (Statistical Methodology) 67(3), 427–444 (2005)

Analysis of Longitudinal Shape Variability via Subject Specific Growth Modeling

James Fishbaugh[1], Marcel Prastawa[1], Stanley Durrleman[2], Joseph Piven[3] for the IBIS Network[*], and Guido Gerig[1]

[1] Scientific Computing and Imaging Institute, University of Utah
[2] INRIA/ICM, Pitié Salpêtrière Hospital, Paris, France
[3] Carolina Institute for Developmental Disabilities, University of North Carolina

Abstract. Statistical analysis of longitudinal imaging data is crucial for understanding normal anatomical development as well as disease progression. This fundamental task is challenging due to the difficulty in modeling longitudinal changes, such as growth, and comparing changes across different populations. We propose a new approach for analyzing shape variability over time, and for quantifying spatiotemporal population differences. Our approach estimates 4D anatomical growth models for a reference population (an average model) and for individuals in different groups. We define a reference 4D space for our analysis as the average population model and measure shape variability through diffeomorphisms that map the reference to the individuals. Conducting our analysis on this 4D space enables straightforward statistical analysis of deformations as they are parameterized by momenta vectors that are located at homologous locations in space and time. We evaluate our method on a synthetic shape database and clinical data from a study that seeks to quantify brain growth differences in infants at risk for autism.

1 Introduction

Quantification of anatomical variability within a population and between populations are fundamental tasks in medical imaging studies. In many clinical applications, it is particularly crucial to quantify anatomical variability *over time* in order to determine disease progression and to isolate clinically important differences in both space and time. Such studies are designed around longitudinal imaging, where we acquire repeated measurements over time of the same

---

[*] The IBIS Network. Clinical Sites: University of North Carolina: J. Piven (IBIS Network PI), H.C. Hazlett, C. Chappell; University of Washington: S. Dager, A. Estes, D. Shaw; Washington University: K. Botteron, R. McKinstry, J. Constantino, J. Pruett; Childrens Hospital of Philadelphia: R. Schultz, S. Paterson; University of Alberta: L. Zwaigenbaum; Data Coordinating Center: Montreal Neurological Institute: A.C. Evans, D.L. Collins, G.B. Pike, P. Kostopoulos; Samir Das; Image Processing Core: University of Utah: G. Gerig; University of North Carolina: M. Styner; Statistical Analysis Core: University of North Carolina: H. Gu; Genetics Analysis Core: University of North Carolina: P. Sullivan, F. Wright.

N. Ayache et al. (Eds.): MICCAI 2012, Part I, LNCS 7510, pp. 731–738, 2012.

subject, which yields rich data for analysis. Statistical analysis of longitudinal anatomical data is a problem with significant challenges due to the difficulty in modeling anatomical changes, such as growth, and comparing changes across different populations.

Many methods have been proposed for the statistical analysis of cross-sectional time-series data, which do not contain repeated measurements of the same subject. Methods include the extension of kernel regression to Riemannian manifolds [1] or piecewise geodesic regression for image time-series [6]. Others have proposed higher order regression models, such as geodesic regression [9,4], regression based on stochastic perturbations of geodesic paths [11], or regression based on twice differential flows of deformation [3].

A method for the analysis of longitudinal anatomy was proposed recently in [2], where a longitudinal atlas is constructed by considering each individual subject as a spatiotemporal deformation of a mean scenario of growth. A single spatial deformation maps the geometry of the atlas onto the observed individual geometry, while a $1D$ time warp accounts for pacing differences between the atlas and subjects. In this framework, statistics are naturally performed on the initial momenta that parameterize the morphological deformation to each subject. However, this single deformation best explains how the *entire* evolution of the mean scenario maps to each individual. The analysis of shape variability at an arbitrary time point has not been explored.

Methods for constructing a longitudinal atlas for DTI [5] and images [7] have been introduced by combining subject specific growth modeling with cross-sectional atlas construction. As a first step, a continuous evolution is estimated for each subject using the standard piecewise geodesic regression model. The continuous evolution for all subjects is then used to compute a cross-sectional atlas. Lastly, subjects are registered to the atlas space by the same regression technique used to establish individual trajectories. Though subject specific growth trajectories are incorporated, the cross-sectional atlas building step is likely to smooth intra-subject variability, as only the images themselves are used for atlas construction; the trajectories are ignored.

In this paper, we propose a new approach for analyzing statistical variability of *shapes* over time, in the spirit of [5,7], which is based on combining cross-sectional atlas construction with subject specific growth modeling. The growth model used for shape regression naturally handles multiple shapes at each time point and does not require point correspondence between subjects, making the proposed framework both convenient and applicable to a wide range of clinical problems. We demonstrate the application of our modeling and analysis framework to a synthetic database of longitudinal shapes as well as a study that seeks to quantify growth differences in subjects at risk for autism.

2   Methods

The proposed framework consists of three steps, summarized in Fig. 1. First, a cross-sectional atlas is estimated by shape regression, which can be thought of

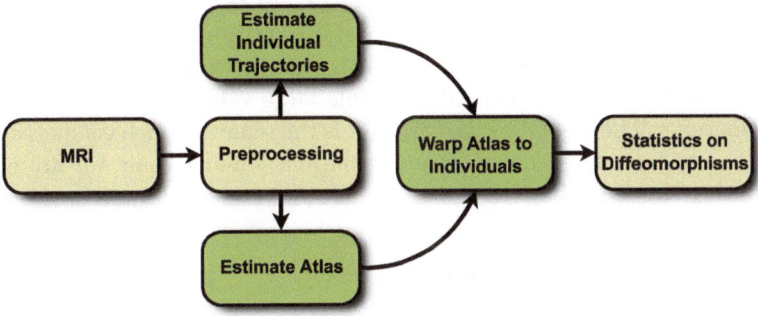

Fig. 1. Flowchart depicting the proposed method

as normative, reference evolution. Second, subject specific growth trajectories are estimated independently for each individual, accounting for intra-subject variability. Third, a homologous space for statistical analysis is obtained by warping the atlas to each individual at any time point of interest. The first two steps require the estimation of a growth model, the specifics of which are discussed in the next section.

2.1   Growth Model

The goal is to infer a continuous evolution of shape from a discrete set of shapes S_{t_i} observed at time t_i. Here we use the acceleration controlled growth model of [3], where shape evolution is modeled as a continuous flow of deformation. A baseline shape S_0, assumed to be observed at time t_0, is continuously deformed over time to match the target shapes. The estimation is posed as a variational problem balancing fidelity to data with regularity, described by the generic regression criterion

$$E = \sum_{t_i} d(\phi_{t_i}(S_0), S_{t_i})^2 + \gamma \mathrm{Reg}(\phi_t) \tag{1}$$

where ϕ_t is the time-varying deformation we wish to estimate, d is a measure of shape similarity, Reg is a regularity constraint on the flow of deformation, and γ is the trade-off parameter. The time-varying deformation ϕ_t is determined by integration of the 2nd-order ODE $\ddot{\phi}_t(x_i(t)) = a(x_i(t), t)$, where a is a time-varying acceleration field, and $x_i(t)$ are the location of shape points over time.

The parameterization by acceleration guarantees that the estimated evolution is temporally smooth. Furthermore, the acceleration controlled growth model is generic, with no constraint that the flow of deformation must follow a geodesic path, or close to a geodesic path.

For measuring shape similarity, we use the metric on currents [10]. This way, shapes are modeled as distributions, alleviating the need for explicit point correspondence between shapes. Regularity is enforced via a Hilbert space norm on acceleration, $||a||_V^2$ defined by the interpolating kernel.

The choice of metric and regularization leads to two intuitive parameters to control the estimation. First, λ_V controls the rigidity of the deformation. It is the scale that points in space move in a correlated manner. Small values of λ_V lead to highly non-linear deformations, while large values result in mostly rigid transformations. The second parameter, λ_W is the scale at which geometric shape differences are considered noise. Shape variations smaller than λ_W are ignored in computing shape similarity.

2.2 Matching Atlas to Individuals

We extract shape features, which are diffeomorphisms that map the reference atlas to each subject at a specific time point. This is accomplished by warping the atlas to each subject at the time point of interest using the registration framework of [10]. Due to regression, we can construct a shape from the atlas and from any individual at any time of interest. The warping from atlas space to each individual establishes homologous points between every subject. The flow of diffeomorphisms that match the atlas shape $A(t)$ to subject shape $S^s(t)$ at time t is found as the minimizer of

$$F(t) = d(\phi_t^s(A(t)), S^s(t))^2 + \gamma \mathrm{Reg}(\phi_t^s) \tag{2}$$

where d is the norm on currents, and regularity enforces smoothness on the time-varying velocity field, which is used to build the diffeomorphism.

2.3 Statistical Analysis

The flow of diffeomorphisms that warp the template shape to each individual subject shape are geodesic [8]. As a result, the initial momenta completely determine the entire deformation. Since the atlas is warped to each subject, every diffeomorphism ϕ_t^s starts from the same reference space. We can leverage this common vector space to compute intrinsic statistics. For example, a mean can be computed by simply taking the arithmetic mean of a collection of momenta fields. The mean momenta can then be applied to a shape via geodesic shooting.

3   Experiments

Synthetic Data: We first evaluate our framework with a database of synthetic longitudinal shape data. In this simple database, normative growth is modeled by a sphere which grows isotropically over time. We further consider two groups, A and B, with different patterns of growth. Group A starts as a small sphere, develops a protuberance in the negative x direction, and eventually evolves into a large sphere. Group B also starts from a small sphere, but develops a protuberance in the positive x direction, before evolving into a large sphere. Subjects from both groups contain 5 time points corresponding to 6, 10, 12, 18, and 24 months. We construct 12 subjects in each group by randomizing the amount

Group A

Normative Growth

Group B

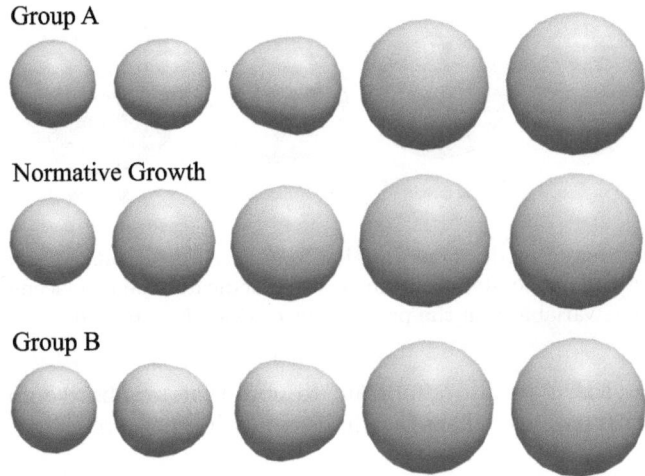

Fig. 2. The synthetic shape database with observations at 6, 10, 12, 18, and 24 months.
Top: Typical shape observations for a subject from group A. **Middle**: The normative
growth scenario. **Bottom**: Typical shape observations for a subject from group B.

of protuberance and also the amount of global scaling. A typical subject from
group A and group B as well as the normative reference growth are summarized
in Fig 2.

The normative reference atlas is estimated from a collection of spheres of
increasing radius using parameter values $\lambda_V = 0.5$ mm, $\lambda_W = 0.5$ mm, and $\gamma_R =$
0.0001. We further estimate individual growth models for all 24 subjects using
the same parameter values as for normative growth. The continuous evolution for
both the normative group and all individuals provides temporal correspondence,
as we can now generate shapes at any instant in time. The atlas shapes at time
points 7, 9, 12, 18, and 24 months are then warped to each individual via a
diffeomorphic mapping. First, we perform PCA on the momenta that warp the
normative atlas to each individual in group A. The first major mode of variation
is summarized in Fig 3 for several time points. This mode explains the variability
in group A with respect to the reference shapes. The bulge on the left side of
the shape is clearly identified along with variability in scale. A PCA on group B
produces similar results, however it captures the bulge on the right side of the
shape.

We also conduct hypothesis testing to determine if there are significant differences between group A and B. For each shape point, an independent t-test
is performed on the magnitude of initial momenta which parameterize the mapping from reference atlas to individuals. We are testing if the distribution of
momenta magnitude at each shape point is different between each group. Fig 4
shows the Bonferroni corrected p-values shown on the reference atlas at selected
time points. We observe significance on the left and right side of the shapes at
9, 12, and 16 months, corresponding to the bulge growing in opposite directions

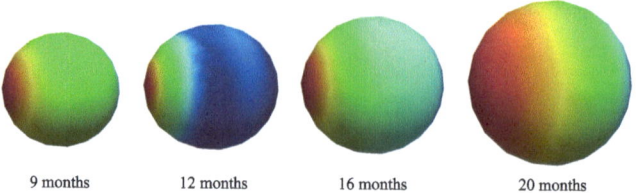

9 months   12 months   16 months   20 months

Fig. 3. The first major mode of deformation from PCA (mean plus one standard deviation) at selected time points for group A. Color indicates the displacement from the mean shape. The variability in the protuberance is clearly captured.

in group A and B. It is also important to note that we observe no significant differences at 20 months, where the shapes of each group are nearly identical.

Clinical Data: We also evaluate our method using a longitudinal database from an Autism Center of Excellence, part of the Infant Brain Imaging Study (IBIS). The study consists of high-risk infants as well as controls, scanned at approximately 6, 12, and 24 months. At 24 months, symptoms of autism spectrum disorder (ASD) were measured using the Autism Diagnostic Observation Schedule (ADOS). A positive ADOS score indicates the child has a high probability of later being diagnosed with autism. Finally, we have three groups: 15 high-risk subjects with positive ADOS (HR+), 40 high-risk subjects with negative ADOS (HR-), and 14 low-risk subjects with negative ADOS (LR-).

We perform a hierarchical, multi-scale rigid alignment to establish a common reference frame that preserves the relationship between anatomical structures in space and time. First, left/right hemisphere and cerebellum are segmented from rigidly aligned images. Next, for each individual, shape complexes are aligned across time. Finally, individual shapes are aligned across time for each subject.

First, we estimate a cross-sectional atlas of normative growth using all the data from the LR- group with parameters values $\lambda_V = 30$ mm, $\lambda_W = 10$ mm for each hemisphere and $\lambda_W = 8$ mm for the cerebellum, and $\gamma_R = 0.01$. Individual trajectories are estimated independently for each subject using the same parameter values. Finally, we investigate the shape variability at 7, 9, 12, 18, and 24

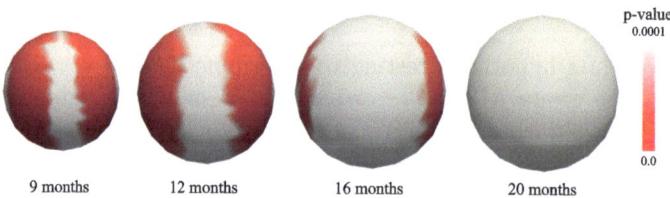

p-value
0.0001

9 months   12 months   16 months   20 months

0.0

Fig. 4. Significant differences in magnitude of momenta between group A and B at several time points, with p-values displayed on the surface of the reference atlas

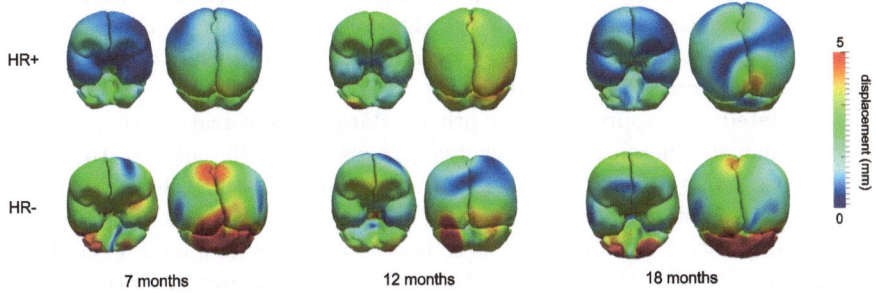

Fig. 5. The first mode from PCA (mean plus one standard deviation) at selected time points for the autism database. Color indicates displacement from the mean shape.

months by registering the atlas to every subject at the time points of interest, resulting in diffeomorphic mappings parameterized by initial momenta.

We investigate the shape variability in the HR+ and HR- groups by performing PCA on the initial momenta for each group. Recall that PCA is conducted using the momenta vectors that parameterize the mapping from atlas to subject at each selected time point. Therefore, the major modes of variability describe how each group varies from the normative growth scenario, shown in Fig. 5 for several time points of interest. There appears to be a difference in how each group deviates from the normative growth scenario, particularly in the cerebellum. This could be an interesting avenue to pursue for future research.

Hypothesis testing is conducted on the magnitude of initial momenta between groups. For each shape point, we perform a t-test on the distribution of momenta magnitude between each population. After correcting the p-value for multiple comparisons, using Bonferroni correction, we find no significant locations on the surfaces of the left/right hemisphere or cerebellum. This may be due to relatively small sample size. However, it may be the case that smaller scale anatomical surfaces, such as subcortical structures might lead to group discrimination due to hypothesized differences in brain growth.

It is important to stress that these results are intended to illustrate a potential application of our methodology. The results here are too preliminary to draw meaningful conclusions with respect to autism, due to the small sample size and the need to incorporate biostatistical modeling, that combines patient variables with our computational analysis.

4   Conclusions

We propose a new approach for analyzing shape variability over time, and for quantifying spatiotemporal population differences. Our approach estimates anatomical growth models over time for a reference population (an average model) and for individuals in different groups. We define a reference 4D space for our analysis as the average population model and measure shape variability through diffeomorphisms that map the average to the individuals. Conducting our analysis on this 4D space enables straightforward statistical analysis of deformations as they are parameterized by momenta vectors that are located at homologous locations in space and time.

We validated our approach on synthetic data, demonstrating that we can detect significant differences between two groups with different growth trajectories. Experiments on anatomical data from an autism study show that there is no significant difference in the brain development of high risk children with positive and negative ADOS scores, as compared to the development of controls. In the future, we plan to extend the framework by modeling the intra-subject variability in the reference population.

Acknowledgments. This work was supported by NIH grant RO1 HD055741 (ACE, project IBIS) and by NIH grant U54 EB005149 (NA-MIC).

References

1. Davis, B., Fletcher, P., Bullitt, E., Joshi, S.: Population shape regression from random design data. In: ICCV, pp. 1–7. IEEE (2007)
2. Durrleman, S., Pennec, X., Trouvé, A., Gerig, G., Ayache, N.: Spatiotemporal Atlas Estimation for Developmental Delay Detection in Longitudinal Datasets. In: Yang, G.-Z., Hawkes, D., Rueckert, D., Noble, A., Taylor, C. (eds.) MICCAI 2009, Part I. LNCS, vol. 5761, pp. 297–304. Springer, Heidelberg (2009)
3. Fishbaugh, J., Durrleman, S., Gerig, G.: Estimation of Smooth Growth Trajectories with Controlled Acceleration from Time Series Shape Data. In: Fichtinger, G., Martel, A., Peters, T. (eds.) MICCAI 2011, Part II. LNCS, vol. 6892, pp. 401–408. Springer, Heidelberg (2011)
4. Fletcher, P.: Geodesic Regression on Riemannian Manifolds. In: Pennec, X., Joshi, S., Nielsen, M. (eds.) MICCAI Workshop on Mathematical Foundations of Computational Anatomy, pp. 75–86 (2011)
5. Hart, G., Shi, Y., Zhu, H., Sanchez, M., Styner, M., Niethammer, M.: DTI longitudinal atlas construction as an average of growth models. In: Gerig, G., Fletcher, P., Pennec, X. (eds.) MICCAI Workshop on Spatiotemporal Image Analysis for Longitudinal and Time-Series Image Data (2010)
6. Khan, A., Beg, M.: Representation of time-varying shapes in the large deformation diffeomorphic framework. In: ISBI, pp. 1521–1524. IEEE (2008)
7. Liao, S., Jia, H., Wu, G., Shen, D.: A novel longitudinal atlas construction framework by groupwise registration of subject image sequences. NeuroImage 59(2), 1275–1289 (2012)
8. Miller, M.I., Trouvé, A., Younes, L.: On the metrics and Euler-Lagrange equations of Computational Anatomy. Annual Review of Biomedical Engineering 4, 375–405 (2002)
9. Niethammer, M., Huang, Y., Vialard, F.-X.: Geodesic Regression for Image Time-Series. In: Fichtinger, G., Martel, A., Peters, T. (eds.) MICCAI 2011, Part II. LNCS, vol. 6892, pp. 655–662. Springer, Heidelberg (2011)
10. Vaillant, M., Glaunès, J.: Surface atching via Currents. In: Christensen, G.E., Sonka, M. (eds.) IPMI 2005. LNCS, vol. 3565, pp. 381–392. Springer, Heidelberg (2005)
11. Vialard, F., Trouvé, A.: Shape splines and stochastic shape evolutions: A second-order point of view. Quarterly of Applied Mathematics 70, 219–251 (2012)

Regional Flux Analysis
of Longitudinal Atrophy in Alzheimer's Disease

Marco Lorenzi[1,2], Nicholas Ayache[1], and Xavier Pennec[1] for the Alzheimer's
Disease Neuroimaging Initiative*

[1] Project Team Asclepios, INRIA Sophia Antipolis, France
[2] LENITEM, IRCCS San Giovanni di Dio, Fatebenefratelli, Italy

Abstract. The longitudinal analysis of the brain morphology in Alzheimer's disease(AD) is fundamental for *understanding* and *quantifying*
the dynamics of the pathology. This study provides a new measure of
the brain longitudinal changes based on the Helmholtz decomposition
of deformation fields. We used the scalar pressure map associated to
the irrotational component in order to identify a consistent group-wise
set of areas of maximal volume change. The atrophy was then quantified in these areas for each subject by the probabilistic integration of
the flux of the longitudinal deformations across the boundaries. The
presented framework unifies voxel-based and regional approaches, and
robustly describes the longitudinal atrophy at group level as a spatial
process governed by consistently defined regions. Our experiments showed
that the resulting regional flux analysis is able to *detect* the differential
atrophy patterns across populations, and leads to precise and statistically powered *quantifications* of the longitudinal changes in AD, even in
mild/premorbid cases.

1   Introduction

The longitudinal analysis of the brain morphology in Alzheimer's disease(AD)
is fundamental for *understanding* and *quantifying* the dynamics of the pathology. The analysis of time series of MR images has been based on two different
paradigms: hypothesis free and regional analysis. In the former case, the longitudinal atrophy is modeled at fine scales on the whole brain such as in the
voxel/tensor based morphometry and cortical thickness analysis [1],[2]. These
methods are useful for exploratory purposes, but usually lack robustness for a
reliable quantification of the changes at the subject level, due to the high variability of the measurements and the multiple comparison problems. On the other
hand, the regional analysis is focused on the detection of significant changes on

* Data used in preparation of this article were obtained from the Alzheimer's Disease Neuroimaging Initiative (ADNI) database (`www.loni.ucla.edu/ADNI`). As such,
the investigators within the ADNI contributed to the design and implementation of ADNI and/or provided data but did not participate in analysis or writing of this report. A complete listing of ADNI investigators can be found at:
`www.loni.ucla.edu/ADNI/Collaboration/ADNI_Authorship_list.pdf`

N. Ayache et al. (Eds.): MICCAI 2012, Part I, LNCS 7510, pp. 739–746, 2012.
© Springer-Verlag Berlin Heidelberg 2012

regions which are usually identified thanks to segmentation. For instance, the boundary shift integral identifies the longitudinal atrophy as the shift of the segmented boundaries [3], and led to powered measure for the longitudinal hippocampal changes in Alzheimer [4]. However, this kind of approaches relies on strong a priori hypotheses on the localization of the dynamics of interest, and might fail to detect more complex patterns of changes which are likely to underly the evolution of the pathology. Providing a longitudinal measure which could at the same time identify, *consistently localize*, and *reliably quantify* the longitudinal changes is crucial for understanding the dynamics of the pathological evolution and to provide stable measures for the clinical setting.

Non rigid registration encodes the morphological changes between pairs of longitudinal MRIs as deformation fields. It has been employed for both whole brain exploratory analysis and regional quantification, for instance through the Jacobian determinant analysis. However, the regional quantification still relies on prior segmentation, and is still sensitive to the biases, for instance for the numerical derivative required for computing the Jacobian. The deformation fields implicitly encode the spatial location of relevant atrophy processes, and novel analysis techniques are required to consistently extract and analyze these features. It has been proposed in [5] to parametrize the deformations by irrotational and divergence-free components, according to the Helmholtz decomposition of vector fields. If we assume that the atrophy can be completely described by a change of volume, then it is completely encoded by the irrotational part, while the divergence-free one only accounts for the tissue reorganization. Thus, the maximal/minimal locations of the irrotational potential define the centers of expanding and contracting regions, and may represent a promising measure for morphometric studies. A different measure of volume change associated to the deformation field is the flux across surfaces [6], which is the mathematical formulation of the boundary shift. However flux-based analysis has been seldom used in morphometric studies, due to the complexity of reliably integrate vector normals on probabilistic segmentations of the surface boundaries.

In this study we propose the regional flux analysis, a new approach for the study of morphological changes based on the Helmholtz decomposition of vector fields. In Section 1 we introduce the Helmholtz theorem, and the relationship between pressure and flux of deformations. These measure are used in Section 2 to consistently define through a hierarchical model the subspace of regions involved in the atrophy processes . These regions are then used at the subject level for the probabilistic flux integration. Finally, the framework is applied in Section 3 on a large sample of longitudinal observation from the ADNI dataset [7], to *describe* and *quantify* the pathological changes at different clinical stages, from premorbid, to early and late Alzheimer stages.

2   Helmholtz Decomposition for Stationary Velocity Fields

The present work is based on the registration based on stationary velocity fields (SVF), which has been already applied for the longitudinal analysis of deformations [8], and for which an implementation of the log-Demons algorithm is easily available[1] [9].

Pressure Potential and Flux through a Region. The Helmholtz theorem states that, given a vector field v defined on $\mathbb{R}^3$ which vanishes when approaching to infinity, it can be uniquely factored as the sum of an irrotational and a divergence free component, $v = \nabla p + \nabla \times A$. The irrotational component ∇p is the gradient of a *scalar* pressure (potential) field p. Since $\nabla \times \nabla p = 0$, the component encodes the information concerning the volume change. On the other hand the divergence-free component is by definition such that $\nabla \cdot \nabla \times A = 0$ and therefore it describes the rotational part of the velocity. Finally, the flux of a stationary velocity field across a given surface ∂V is given by the Divergence (or Ostrogradsky's) theorem, and can be rewritten as $\oint_{\partial V} v \cdot n \, dS = \int_V \nabla \cdot v \, dV$. Recently the Helmholtz decomposition has been introduced in the Demons registration in order to estimate incompressible deformations [10]. Here we propose to use it on the contrary for the analysis of the compressible part, which encodes the observed matter loss as a smooth compression/expansion process. In such a model, the associated divergence quantifies the apparent anatomical changes as the flux of the estimated vector field across surfaces.

Topology of Pressure Fields. Theoretically, one could partition the whole space into *critical areas* of positive and negative divergence, each of them containing a critical point of local maximal/minimal pressure (Figure 1). From the divergence theorem, the flux across the boundaries of these areas is either flowing inward or outward. The saddle points for the pressure are on the boundaries of those regions, and identify a change in the flow.

The analysis of the critical points of a pressure map can be addressed by the *Morse-Smale* theory as a topological problem, leading to a complex of regions, boundaries, edges and vertices. Although intriguing, the application of such concepts to the medical imaging is still difficult, due to the missing statistical version of the Morse theory. In order to obtain a tractable approach to the problem, we propose to first focus on the definition of a consistent *subset* of critical regions across subjects, to robustly describe the atrophy processes at group level as a spatial process governed by key areas. This is a first step towards a topology definition and provides a sparse description of the deformation.

3   Flux-Based Analysis of Longitudinal Trajectories

The goal of this section is to estimate the group-wise set of critical regions, from the locations of maximal/minimal pressure. These regions are then used to evaluate the flux of the longitudinal deformations at the subject level.

---

[1] http://insight-journal.org/browse/publication/644

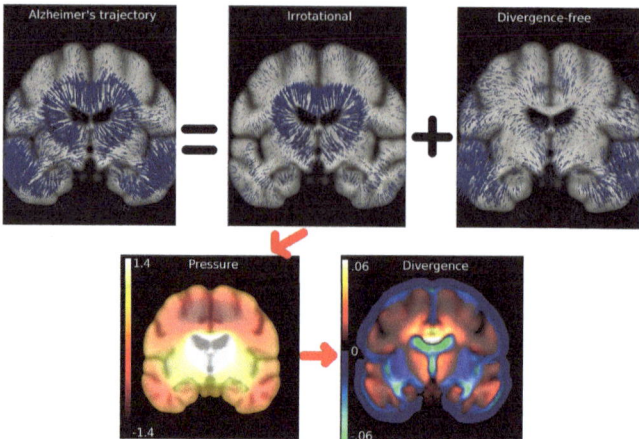

Fig. 1. Helmholtz decomposition of a longitudinal trajectory in Alzheimer's disease, and pressure potential and divergence maps associated to the irrotational component. The divergence describes the critical areas of local expansion and contraction.

Group-Wise Pressure Potential from Longitudinal SVFs. Consider the longitudinal observations from a group of subjects composed of baseline I_0^i and follow-up I_1^i brain scans. For each subject i, the log-Demons non rigid registration of the pair I_0^i, I_1^i estimates the longitudinal trajectory of changes as a diffeomorphism parametrized by stationary velocity field $\exp(v_i)$, such that $I_0^i \circ \exp(v_i) \simeq I_1^i$. The SVF v_i can then be decomposed according to the Helmholtz theorem in order to identify the corresponding pressure map p_i.

One interest in this decomposition is that the transport of each atrophy trajectory $\varphi_i = \exp(v_i) = \exp(\nabla p_i)$ through a subject-to-template deformation ψ_i can be obtained by simple scalar interpolation of the pressure field $\varphi_i^T = \exp(v_i^T) = \exp(\nabla(p_i \circ \psi_i))$, rather than parallel transporting vector quantities, $\varphi_i^T = \exp(\Pi^{\psi_i}(v_i))$, which generally leads to computationally intensive and potentially more unstable operations.

The pressure maps in the template space $p_i \circ \psi_i$ are integral quantities, and might differ by an arbitrary constant. However, an average pressure map can still be consistently defined either as $\bar{p} = \overline{p_i \circ \psi}$, or as the pressure map $\bar{p}$ associated to $\bar{v} = \overline{v_i^T} = \overline{\nabla(p_i \circ \psi_i)}$.[2]

Probabilistic Estimation of Group-Wise Critical Regions. Let $\{x_k\}$ be the set of critical points, maxima and minima, of $\bar{p}$. These points define the critical areas T_k of local expansion and contraction, i.e. of positive and negative divergence. Then, the probability of a point x to belong to a critical region depends on the proximity to the region T_k, and on the observed divergence. We can express this through the Bayes rule:

---

[2] In fact, if $p_i' = p_i \circ \psi_i + c_i$, with c_i constant, then $\bar{p} = \overline{p_i \circ \psi_i} + \bar{c}$ leads to $\bar{v} = \nabla \bar{p} = \overline{\nabla(p_i \circ \psi_i)}$.

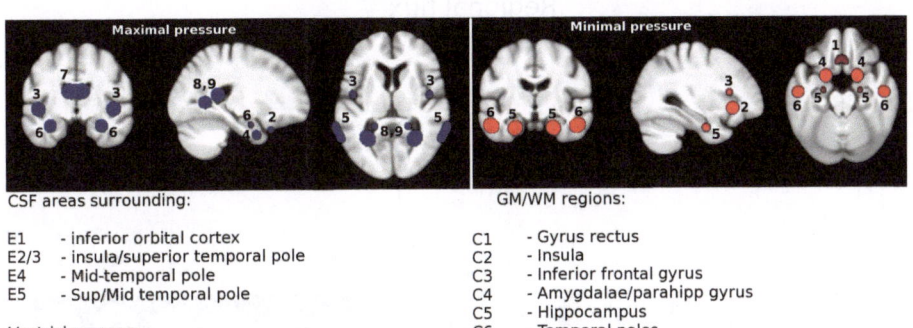

CSF areas surrounding:

E1	- inferior orbital cortex
E2/3	- insula/superior temporal pole
E4	- Mid-temporal pole
E5	- Sup/Mid temporal pole

Ventricles areas:

E6	- Temporal horn hippocampus
E7/8/9	- Ventricles

GM/WM regions:

C1	- Gyrus rectus
C2	- Insula
C3	- Inferior frontal gyrus
C4	- Amygdalae/parahipp gyrus
C5	- Hippocampus
C6	- Temporal poles

Fig. 2. Critical points associated to the Alzheimer's average pressure map

$$P(x \in T_k | \nabla \cdot v(x) = d) = \frac{P(\nabla \cdot v(x) = d | x \in T_k)P(x \in T_k)}{P(\nabla \cdot v(x) = d)} \qquad (1)$$

Since the denominator is a normalizing factor, in the following only the numerator is considered. The flux of the subject specific deformations $\exp(v_i)$ through the regions T_k can be easily estimated with (1) through a hierarchical model. At the first level, based on spatial priors for the location of the critical points, we can estimate a group-wise confidence map for the critical regions:

- Given a set of critical points $\{x_k\}$, define the spatial priors $P(x \in T_k) = \exp((x - x_k)^2/(2\sigma^2))$
- Define a group-wise prior $\overline{F_i^{\pm}}(x)$ for the critical areas as the group-wise average of the binary masks of positive/negative divergence $F_i^+ = \{x \in \Omega | \nabla \cdot v_i^T(x) > 0\}$, and $F_i^- = \{x \in \Omega | \nabla \cdot v_i^T(x) < 0\}$.
- From formula (1), define the confidence maps for the critical areas $P_k^{\pm}(x) = P(\nabla \cdot v_i^T(x) = d | x \in T_k)P(x \in T_k) = \overline{F^{\pm}}(x)\exp((x - x_k)^2/(2\sigma^2))$.

Finally, the group-wise confidence maps are reintroduced in (1) for the second level analysis :

- Transport the confidence maps $P_k^{\pm}$ in the subject space to obtain $P_{k,i}^{\pm} = P_k^{\pm} \circ \psi^{-1}$
- Apply (1) by considering $P(x \in T_k) = P_{k,i}^{\pm}$, and $F_i^{\pm} \circ \psi_i^{-1}$ as likelihood term.

Probabilistic Integration of the Regional Flux. The confidence maps in the subject space can then be used as weights for the integration of the divergence across the space Ω thanks to the Divergence theorem, to provide a measure of the subject specific flux across the critical regions T_k. The weighted integration of the divergence implicitly defines the critical regions in a maximum a posteriori approach through the posterior (1), therefore automatically accounting for the registration biases in the anatomical localization (e.g. due to the regularization).

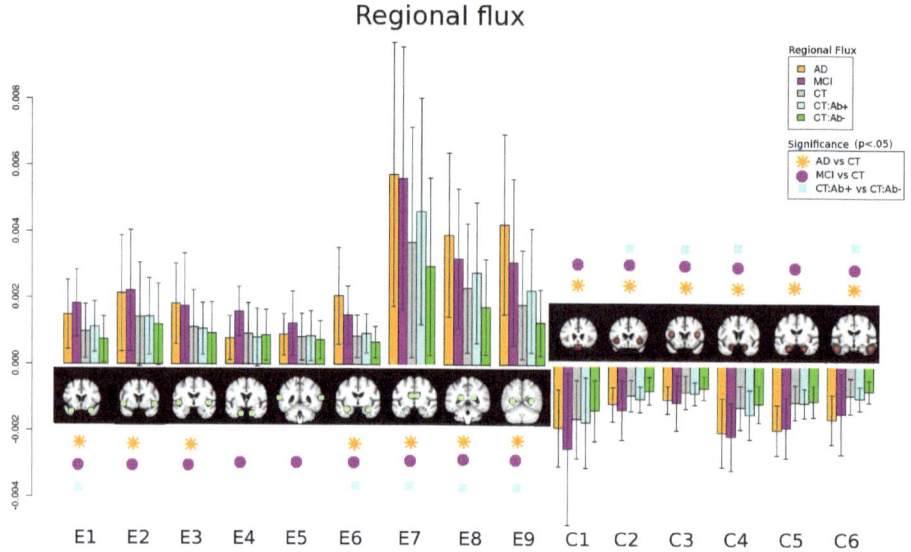

Fig. 3. Average regional flux for AD, MCI, healthy controls, and healthy $A\beta^+$ and $A\beta^-$ subgroups. E1 to E9: expanding regions. C1 to C6: contracting regions.

4 Apparent Gain and Loss of Matter in Alzheimer's Disease through Regional Flux Quantification

Baseline and one year follow-up brain scans of 200 healthy controls, 150 MCI, and 142 AD patients from the ADNI dataset were linearly aligned and non-rigidly registered with the log-Demons. The pressure maps p_i corresponding to the intra-subject longitudinal trajectories $\exp(v_i)$ were transported into a previously defined anatomical reference along the subject-to-template deformations ψ_i.

The set of local maxima and minima for the pressure in AD has been defined from the mean pressure map associated to the longitudinal deformations of 20 randomly selected AD patients. Of these sparse sets of points, 9 local minima and 6 local maxima have been manually labeled to define the set $\{x_k\}$ of critical points. The spatial priors T_k were defined through inflation (4 voxels neighborhood) and right/left symmetry (Figure 2).

The hierarchical model of Section 3 was used for the regional probabilistic integration of the flux for the remaining patients and the healthy controls. Moreover, the healthy population was stratified depending on the positivity to the CSF $A\beta_{42}$ marker (<192 pg/ml), and the flux analysis was performed to detect the effect of the positivity on the atrophy progression.

Figure 3 summarizes the group-wise regional flux. As we can see, the flux is higher for the ADs and MCIs with respect to the controls. Interestingly, the MCIs have larger flux than the ADs in some regions, which might indicate greater structural longitudinal changes at the early stages of the disease, or underline

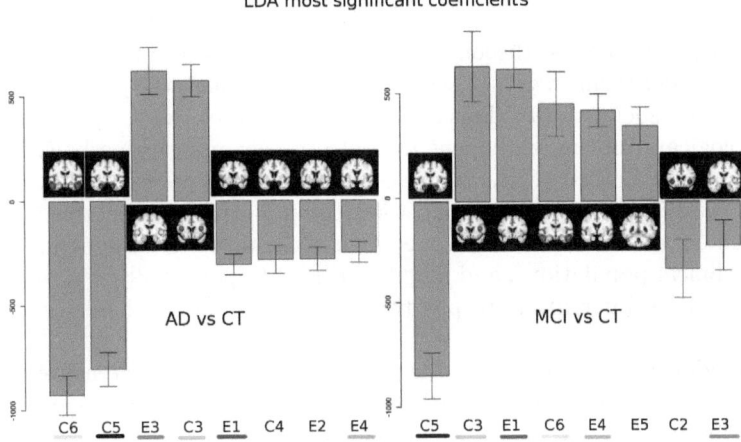

Fig. 4. LDA coefficients associated to the most discriminant critical regions for the longitudinal atrophy of the AD and MCI groups wrt normal aging. Among these regions, 6 of the 8 are common to both AD and MCI, and are indicated by the common colors.

different aspects of the heterogeneous MCI condition. The subgroup of healthy subject positive to the $A\beta42$ marker consistently show increased flux when compared to the negative, which is significant for several regions, and might suggest a possible effect of the $A\beta42$ marker on the future development of AD.

A power analysis based on the regional flux was performed to define the sample size required by an hypothetical 1-year clinical trial to detect a 25% difference of the progression of the measure with 80% power when considering the group alone, or by comparing with normal aging [4]. The regional measurements provided different sample size estimations[3]. To summarize, the lowest sample size for the AD group was provided by the flux across C5 (hippocampus): 38 (95% CI [33,44]) by considering the AD alone, and 203 [145,307] when controlling by normal aging. For the MCI group, the lowest sample size was given by the region E4 (mid-temporal pole): 54 [47,63] for the group alone and 307 [192,567] when controlled for normal aging.

Finally a linear discriminant analysis was performed to define the combination of such regions which maximises the flux differences for respectively AD and MCI vs healthy subjects. The analysis was carried out through a 2-folds cross-validation, with 1000 iterations (Figure 4). An additional power analysis was performed during the cross validation, to test the effectiveness of the LDA combination of the regional flux as a clinical measure. The average sample size (and average 95% CI) required for the LDA score when controlling for normal aging was 164 [106,290] for the AD group, and 277 [166,555] for the MCI.

---

[3] Supplementary material at http://www-sop.inria.fr/members/Marco.Lorenzi/Flux-MICCAI2012.pdf

5   Conclusions

We proposed to decompose the longitudinal trajectories according to the Helmholtz theorem, in order to analyze the atrophy processes through the pressure potential map and the associated flux. This new approach studies the temporal dynamics as a topological problem, and opens the path to new analysis methods based on graph and complex theory. The proposed work provided precise and statistically powered *quantifications* of the group-wise regional atrophy processes. Moreover the presented method *describes* and compares the patterns of dynamic changes between clinical populations, and might thus lead to potentially new anatomical findings, such as differential atrophy trajectories at different disease stages.

Acknowledgements. This work was partially funded by the French ANR "programme blanc" number ANR-09-BLAN-0332, and by the European Research Council through the ERC Advanced Grant MedYMA.

References

1. Fox, N., Crum, W., Scahill, R., Stevens, J., Janssen, J., Rossnor, M.: Imaging of onset and progression of Alzheimer's disease with voxel compression mapping of serial magnetic resonance images. Lancet 358, 201–205 (2001)
2. Thompson, P., Ayashi, K., Zubicaray, G., et al.: Dynamics of gray matter loss in Alzheimer's disease. The Journal of Neuroscience 23, 994–1005 (2003)
3. FreeBorough, P., Fox, N.: The boundary shift integral: An accurate and robust measure of cerebral volume changes from registered repeat MRI. TMI 16(5) (1997)
4. Leung, K.K., Barnes, J., Ridgway, G.R., et al.: Automated cross-sectional and longitudinal hippocampal volume measurement in mild cognitive impairment and Alzheimer's disease. NeuroImage 51(4), 1345–1359 (2010)
5. Hansen, M.S., Larsen, R., Christensen, N.V.: Curl-gradient image warping - introducing deformation potentials for medical image registration using Helmholtz decomposition. In: VISAPP 2009, vol. 1, pp. 179–185 (2009)
6. Chung, Worsley, Paus, et al.: A unified statistical approach to deformation-based morphometry. NeuroImage 14(3), 595–606 (2001)
7. Mueller, S., Weiner, M., Thal, L., et al.: The Alzheimer's disease neuroimaging initiative. Neuroimaging Clin 15, 869–877 (2005)
8. Lorenzi, M., Ayache, N., Frisoni, G.B., Pennec, X.: Mapping the Effects of $A\beta_1$-42 Levels on the Longitudinal Changes in Healthy Aging: Hierarchical Modeling Based on Stationary Velocity Fields. In: Fichtinger, G., Martel, A., Peters, T. (eds.) MICCAI 2011, Part II. LNCS, vol. 6892, pp. 663–670. Springer, Heidelberg (2011)
9. Vercauteren, T., Pennec, X., Perchant, A., Ayache, N.: Symmetric Log-Domain Diffeomorphic Registration: A Demons-Based Approach. In: Metaxas, D., Axel, L., Fichtinger, G., Székely, G. (eds.) MICCAI 2008, Part I. LNCS, vol. 5241, pp. 754–761. Springer, Heidelberg (2008)
10. Mansi, T., Pennec, X., Sermesant, M., Delingette, H., Ayache, N.: iLogDemons: A Demons-based registration algorithm for tracking incompressible elastic biological tissues. IJCV 9(30), 92–111 (2011)

Erratum: Localization of Sparse Transmural Excitation Stimuli from Surface Mapping

Jingjia Xu, Azar Rahimi Dehaghani, Fei Gao, and Linwei Wang

Computational Biomedicine Laboratory, Golisano College of Computing and
Information Sciences, Rochester Institute of Technology, Rochester, NY, 14623, USA

N. Ayache et al. (Eds.): MICCAI 2012, Part I, LNCS 7510, pp. 675–682, 2012.
© Springer-Verlag Berlin Heidelberg 2012

DOI 10.1007/978-3-642-33415-3_92

The authors of this paper would like to add an acknowledgement for the financial and data support of this study:

Acknowledgement: The authors would like to thank Rochester Institute of Technology's Junior Faculty Support and GCCIS FEAD Award for the financial support of this study. The authors would also like to thank Dr. Mihaela Pop and Dr. Graham Wright, both of Sunnybrook Research Institute (Toronto - Canada) for providing the EP-CARTO and DT-MRI data of the two animal models, and to Dr. Thomas Mansi (Siemens Corporate Research, Princeton, NJ, USA) and Dr. Maxime Sermesant (INRIA, Asclepios project - Sophia Antitpolis, France) for providing the anatomical mesh and fiber strcuture for the infarct heart and the healthy heart, respectively.

The original online version for this chapter can be found at
http://dx.doi.org/10.1007/978-3-642-33415-3_83

Author Index

Aach, Til   I-381
Abdillahi, Hannan   III-599
Abugharbieh, Rafeef   II-82
Acosta, Oscar   I-231
Adalsteinsson, Elfar   III-1
Adams, J.E.   III-361
Afifi, Ahmed   II-395
Afsari, Bijan   II-322
Afshin, Mariam   II-535
Ahmadi, Seyed-Ahmad   I-625,
   III-443
Ahmidi, Narges   I-471
Aichert, André   II-601
Aizenstein, Orna   II-179
Ajilore, Olusola   II-196, II-228
Akhondi-Asl, Alireza   I-593
Alber, Mark S.   I-373
Alberti, Marina   I-642
Alexander, Andrew L.   II-280
Ali, Karim   I-585, II-568
Allen, Peter K.   II-592
Alvino, Chris   I-528
Amunts, Katrin   I-206
An, Xing   I-340
André, Barbara   III-639
Annangi, Pavan   II-478
Arbel, Tal   II-379
Arbeláez, Pablo   III-345
Ardon, Roberto   I-561, III-66
Arienzo, Donatello   II-228
Arnold, Douglas L.   II-379
Arold, Oliver   I-414
Arridge, Simon   I-289
Arteta, Carlos   I-348
Arujuna, A.   II-25
Ashrafulla, S.   III-607
Asman, Andrew J.   III-426
Atkins, M. Stella   I-298, I-315
Aung, Tin   I-58
Avants, Brian   III-206
Awate, Suyash P.   III-189
Axel, Leon   I-281
Axer, Markus   I-206
Ayache, Nicholas   I-617, I-739, II-41

Aylward, Stephen   III-83
Azzabou, N.   I-569

Baccon, Jennifer   I-157
Bagci, Ulas   III-459
Baghani, Ali   I-42, II-617
Bahlmann, Claus   I-528
Bai, Junjie   I-239
Bai, Wenjia   II-659
Bailey, Lara   I-487
Balicki, Marcin   I-397
Balis, U.   I-365
Balocco, Simone   I-642
Bano, J.   I-91
Barillot, Christian   III-542
Bartlett, Adam   III-525
Bartoli, Adrien   II-634
Bartsch, I.   I-198
Batmanghelich, Kayhan   III-231
Baudin, P.-Y.   I-569
Bauer, Sebastian   I-414, II-576
Bayouth, J.   III-566
Becker, Carlos   I-585
Behrens, Timothy E.J.   II-188
Béjar Haro, Benjamín   I-34
Ben Ayed, Ismail   I-520, II-527, II-535
Ben-Bashat, Dafna   II-179
Benjelloun, Mohammed   II-446
Ben-Sira, Liat   II-179
Berger, Lorenz   III-329
Bériault, Silvain   I-487
Berkels, Benjamin   I-414
Bernardis, Elena   II-49, III-631
Betke, Margrit   I-389
Beymer, D.   III-501
Bhandarkar, Suchendra M.   II-502
Bhatia, Kanwal K.   I-512
Bicknell, Colin   II-560
Bilgic, Berkin   III-1
Birkbeck, Neil   II-462
Bismuth, Vincent   II-9
Bloy, Luke   II-254, III-231, III-468
Blumensath, Thomas   II-188
Boctor, Emad M.   II-552

Boese, Jan   II-544
Boettger, T.   III-566
Boettger, Thomas   II-462
Boetzel, Kai   III-443
Boisvert, Jonathan   II-446
Boré, Arnaud   I-699
Bouix, Sylvain   III-34
Bourgeat, Pierrick   II-220
Bourier, Felix   II-584
Bousleiman, Habib   I-66
Brady, Sir Michael   III-115
Brand, Alexander   II-609
Brost, Alexander   II-584
Brounstein, Anna   II-82
Buhmann, Joachim M.   I-323
Bullens, R.   II-25
Bullens, Roland   I-634
Burns, Joseph E.   III-509

Caballero, Jose   I-256
Cai, Weidong   I-74
Cai, Xiao   II-271
Callahan, M.J.   I-1
Cao, Yu   I-173
Cardoso, M. Jorge   I-289, II-262, III-26, III-256, III-289
Carlier, P.G.   I-569
Carrillo, Xavier   I-642
Carson, James P.   I-577
Caruyer, Emmanuel   III-10
Cash, David M.   III-289
Cattamanchi, Adithya   III-345
Ceklic, Lala   III-599
Cepek, Jeremy   I-455
Chaari, L.   III-180
Chang, Eric I-Chao   III-623
Chang, Jeannette   III-345
Chemouny, Stéphane   II-651
Chen, Chen   I-281
Chen, Danny Z.   I-373
Chen, Hanbo   II-271, III-297
Chen, Lei   III-272
Chen, Mei   I-307
Chen, Mingqing   I-239
Chen, Terrence   I-405, II-544
Chen, Tsuhan   I-272
Chen, Wufan   I-214
Cheng, Alexis   II-552
Cheng, Bo   I-82
Cheng, Jian   II-313

Cheung, Carol Y.   I-58
Chow, Ben   I-99
Choyke, Peter   III-582
Chronik, Blaine   I-455
Chu, Chengwen   I-10
Chung, Moo K.   II-280
Cifor, Amalia   II-667
Ciuciu, P.   III-180
Clarkson, Matthew J.   III-289
Cohen, Laurent D.   III-66
Cohen-Adad, Julien   III-1
Collins, D. Louis   I-487, II-379, III-91
Collins, Toby   II-634
Comaniciu, Dorin   I-405, I-438, II-17, II-33, II-486, II-544, III-566
Commowick, Olivier   II-163, III-313, III-476
Compas, Colin B.   III-58
Constantini, Shlomi   II-179
Cook, Philip A.   III-206
Cooklin, M.   II-25
Cootes, Timothy F.   III-156, III-353, III-361
Cormack, Robert A.   III-107
Côté, Marc-Alexandre   I-699
Cotin, Stéphane   I-50, I-91, I-553
Criminisi, Antonio   III-75, III-369, III-590
Cruz-Roa, Angel   I-157
Csapo, Istvan   III-280
Cuingnet, Rémi   III-66

Da Costa, Daniel   II-617
Damasio, H.   III-607
Darzi, Ara   I-463
Das, T.   III-369
Datteri, Ryan D.   III-139
Davatzikos, Christos   I-723, III-131
Davis, Brad   III-280
Davis, J. Lucian   III-345
Dawant, Benoît M.   III-139
Dawant, Benoît M.   II-421
Debats, Oscar   II-413
de Bruijne, Marleen   III-147
Declerck, J.   III-566
Dehaene-Lambertz, Ghislaine   III-172
Dehaghani, Azar Rahimi   I-675, E1
Delingette, Hervé   I-617, II-41
Demiralp, C.   III-369
Deng, Fan   III-214

Dennis, Emily L.   III-305
Depeursinge, Adrien   III-517
Dequidt, J.   I-553
Deriche, Rachid   II-313, II-339, III-10
Deroose, Christophe M.   I-107
Descoteaux, Maxime   I-699, II-288,
    II-339
Desjardins, Benoit   II-49
Desrosiers, Christian   I-651
de Zubicaray, Greig I.   III-305
Dhillon, Paramveer   III-206
Dickscheid, Timo   I-206
Di Marco, Aimee   I-463
Dinov, Ivo   II-138
Dione, Donald P.   III-58
Diotte, Benoit   I-18
Dirksen, Asger   III-147
Dohi, Takeyoshi   I-26
Doignon, C.   I-91
Donner, S.   I-198
Dore, Vincent   II-220
Dörfler, Arnd   II-511
Dössel, Olaf   II-1
Drew, Mark S.   I-315
Dries, Sebastian P.M.   II-1
Duché, Quentin   I-231
Duckett, Simon G.   II-41
Duffau, Hugues   II-651
Dufour, Pascal A.   III-599
Duin, Robert P.W.   III-550
Duncan, James S.   II-462, III-58
Duncan, John   III-26
Duong, D.   I-149
Duong, Luc   I-651
Duriez, Christian   I-50, I-553
Durlak, Peter   I-405
Durrleman, Stanley   I-731, III-223
Duy, Nguyen The   I-609
Dwivedi, Sarvesh   I-323

Edwards, Philip   II-659
Ehrhardt, Jan   II-74, II-347
El-Baz, Ayman   II-114
ElBaz, Mohammed S.   I-691
El-Ghar, Mohamed Abou   II-114
Ellison, David   I-157
Elnakib, Ahmed   II-114
Ennis, Daniel B.   II-494
Erat, Okan   II-609
Eshuis, Peter   I-634

Eskandari, Hani   II-617
Essler, Markus   I-430
Ettl, Svenja   I-414
Euler, Ekkehard   I-18, II-609
Everett, Allen   II-486

Fahmy, Ahmed S.   I-691
Fallavollita, Pascal   I-18, II-609
Fang, Ruogu   I-272
Fedorov, Andriy   III-107
Felblinger, Jacques   I-264
Feng, Dagan   I-74
Feng, Qianjin   I-214
Fenster, Aaron   I-455, I-537, II-643,
    III-377
Feragen, Aasa   III-147
Ferré, Jean-Christophe   III-542
Feulner, J.   III-590
Feusner, Jamie D.   II-196, II-228
Field, Aaron S.   II-280
Fillard, Pierre   II-57
Fishbaugh, James   I-731
Fleming, John O.   II-280
Fletcher, Daniel   III-345
Fletcher, P. Thomas   I-132, III-189
Fleury, Gilles   I-223
Foncubierta–Rodriguez, Antonio
    III-517
Forbes, F.   III-180
Fournier, Marc   III-172
Fox, Nick C.   II-262, III-289
Fragkiadaki, Katerina   III-631
Frangi, Alejandro F.   III-99
Freiman, M.   I-1
Fripp, Jurgen   II-220
Fua, Pascal   I-585, II-568, III-337
Fuerst, B.   III-566

GadElkarim, Johnson J.   II-196, II-228
Gahm, Jin Kyu   II-494
Galaro, Joseph   I-157
Gallia, Gary L.   I-471
Gambarota, Giulio   I-231
Gao, Fei   I-675, E1, III-558
Gao, Mingchen   II-387
Gao, Yaozong   III-385, III-451
Gaonkar, Bilwaj   I-723
Gardiazabal, José   III-42
Gardin, Isabelle   I-545

Garfinkel, Alan   II-494
Garvin, Gregory J.   I-520
Gateno, Jaime   I-99
Ge, Bao   III-485
Gee, James C.   III-206
George, Jose   I-107
Georgescu, B.   II-33
Gerig, Guido   I-731, III-223
Ghanbari, Yasser   III-231
Gibson, Eli   II-643
Gifford, René H.   II-421
Gijsbers, G.   II-25
Gill, J.   II-25
Gilmore, John H.   I-247
Gimel'farb, Georgy   II-114
Gioan, Emeric   III-533
Girard, Gabriel   I-699
Glaunés, Joan   II-57
Glocker, Ben   III-75, III-369, III-590
Goela, Aashish   II-527, II-535
Golby, Alexandra J.   III-123
Golland, Polina   I-715, III-410
González, Fabio   I-157
Gould, Stephen   I-357
Govind, Satish   I-683
Govind, Satish C.   II-478
Grady, Leo   I-528
Gramfort, Alexandre   II-288
GräI-ßel, David   I-206
Grebe, Reinhard   III-172
Greiser, Andreas   II-511
Grimbergen, Cornelis A.   II-155, III-164
Grimm, Robert   II-511
Grossman, Murray   III-206
Groth, Alexandra   II-1
Gubern-Mérida, Albert   II-371
Guevara, Pamela   II-57
Gunney, Roxanna   III-256
Guo, Lei   II-237, III-297, III-485
Gupta, Mithun Das   I-683, II-478
Gupta, Vikas   I-667
Gur, Ruben   II-254
Gurari, Danna   I-389
Guy, Pierre   II-82

Hacihaliloglu, Ilker   II-82
Hadida, Jonathan   I-651
Hagenah, Johann   III-272
Hager, Gregory D.   I-397, I-471, II-568
Hajnal, Jo   I-512

Hajnal, Joseph V.   I-256
Hamarneh, Ghassan   II-98
Hamm, Jihun   III-131
Hämmerle-Uhl, Jutta   III-574
Hammon, M.   I-438
Han, Junwei   II-237, III-485
Hanaoka, Shouhei   II-106
Hancock, J.   II-25
Handels, Heinz   II-74, II-347
Hansson, M.   I-422
Hao, Zhihui   I-504
Harder, Martin   I-141
Hartl, Alexander   I-430
Hartley, Richard   I-357
Harvey, Cameron W.   I-373
Hashizume, Makoto   I-26
Hayashi, Naoto   II-106
Haynor, D.R.   III-590
He, Qizhen   I-99
He, Ying   II-146
Heine, Martin   I-165
Heinrich, Mattias P.   III-115
Heisterkamp, A.   I-198
Herberich, Gerlind   I-381
Hipp, J.   I-365
Ho, Harvey   III-525
Hodgson, Antony   II-82
Hoffmann, Matthias   II-584
Hofmann, Hannes G.   II-511
Höller, Yvonne   III-574
Hong, Yi   III-197
Hontani, Hidekata   II-470
Hornegger, Joachim   I-414, II-511, II-576, II-584
Hosseinbor, A. Pasha   II-280
Hostettler, A.   I-91
Houde, Jean-Christophe   I-699
Housden, R.J.   II-25
Hu, Xintao   II-237, III-485
Huang, Heng   II-271
Huang, Junzhou   I-281, II-387
Huang, M.H.   I-91
Huang, Xiaojie   III-58
Huang, Xiaolei   II-387
Hughes, William E.   I-357
Huh, Seungil   I-331, III-615
Huisman, Henkjan   II-413
Hunter, Peter   III-525
Hutter, Jana   II-511
Hutton, Brian F.   I-289

Ieiri, Satoshi   I-26
Iglesias, Juan Eugenio   III-50
Iizuka, Tateyuki   I-66
Ingalhalikar, Madhura   II-254, III-468
Ionasec, Razvan   II-486, II-544
Ip, Horace H.S.   I-99
Ishii, Lisa   I-471
Ishii, Masaru   I-471
Ishikawa, Hiroshi   I-307
Islam, Ali   II-527, II-535
Itu, Lucian   II-486

Jagadeesh, Vignesh   III-321
Jahanshad, Neda   III-305
Jain, Anil K.   I-115
Jakob, Carolin   II-584
Janoos, Firdaus   III-107
Jena, R.   III-369
Jenkinson, Mark   III-115
Jerebko, Anna   I-438
Jiang, Tianzi   II-313
Jin, Changfeng   II-237, III-297
John, Matthias   II-17, II-544
Joshi, A.A.   III-607
Joshi, Rohit   I-520
Joshi, Sarang   I-132, III-197, III-223
Joshi, Shantanu H.   I-340
Joskowicz, Leo   II-179, II-363
Ju, Tao   I-577
Judkins, Alexander R.   I-157

Kainmueller, Dagmar   I-609
Kaizer, Markus   II-544
Kakadiaris, Ioannis A.   I-577, II-454
Kalkan, Habil   III-550
Kallenberg, Michiel   II-371
Kamen, A.   II-33, III-566
Kanade, Takeo   I-331, III-615
Kandasamy, Nagarajan   II-122
Kandel, Benjamin M.   III-206
Kang, Hakmook   II-246
Kang, Jin U.   II-552
Kapetanakis, S.   II-25
Karimaghaloo, Zahra   II-379
Karssemeijer, Nico   II-371, II-413
Kazemi, Kamran   III-172
Kazhdan, Michael   I-495, II-404
Keihaninejad, Shiva   III-26
Kelm, B.M.   I-438
Kendall, Giles S.   III-256

Ker, Dai Fei Elmer   I-331
Kerrien, E.   I-553
Khalifa, Fahmi   II-114
Khurd, P.   III-566
Kim, Ji-yeun   I-504
Kim, Minjeong   II-90
Kindlmann, Gordon   II-494
Kirişli, Hortense   I-667
Kirschbaum, Sharon W.   I-667
Kiselev, Valerij G.   II-297
Klein, T.   I-422
Kleiner, Melanie   I-206
Klinder, T.   I-198
Klug, William S.   II-494
Knott, Graham   I-585, III-337
Koch, Martin   II-584
Kohlberger, Timo   I-528, II-462
Kongolo, Guy   III-172
Kontos, Despina   II-437
Konukoglu, Ender   II-49, III-75, III-369, III-590
Korenberg, Julie R.   III-223
Kowal, Jens   III-599
Krawtschuk, Waldemar   II-486
Kronman, A.   II-363
Krueger, Martin W.   II-1
Krüger, A.   I-198
Kubicki, Marek   I-715
Kuklisova-Murgasova, Maria   II-667
Kumar, Anand   II-196, II-228
Kumar, R.   III-501
Kung, Geoffrey L.   II-494
Kurkure, Uday   I-577
Kurzidim, Klaus   II-584
Kutra, Dominik   II-1
Kuwana, Kenta   I-26
Kwitt, Roland   III-83
Kwon, Dongjin   III-131

Labadie, Robert F.   II-421
Labelle, Hubert   II-446
Ladikos, Alexander   II-601
Lahalle, Elisabeth   I-223
Lai, Maode   III-623
Lai, Rongjie   I-601
Lamecker, Hans   I-609
Landman, Bennett A.   II-246, III-426
Langet, Hélène   I-223
Laptev, Dmitry   I-323
Lasser, Tobias   I-430, III-42

Lathiff, Mohamed Nabil   II-617
Le, Yen H.   I-577
Leahy, R.M.   III-607
Le Bihan, Denis   II-57
Lecron, Fabian   II-446
Lee, Jong-Ha   I-504
Lee, Philip K.M.   I-99
Lee, Su-Lin   II-560
Lee, Tim K.   I-298, II-98
Lehmann, Helko   II-1
Lekadir, Karim   III-99
Lelandais, Benoît   I-545
Lelieveldt, Boudewijn P.F.   I-667
Lempitsky, Victor   I-348
Leow, Alex D.   II-196, II-228
Lepetit, Vincent   I-189
Lesage, David   III-66
Leube, Rudolf E.   I-381
Li, Fang   II-146
Li, Feng   I-659
Li, Junning   II-138
Li, Kaiming   II-237, III-297, III-485
Li, Lingjiang   II-237, III-297
Li, Ning   I-340
Li, Shuo   II-527, II-535
Li, Xiang   II-237
Lian, Jun   I-214
Liao, Shu   III-385, III-451
Lin, Ben A.   III-58
Lin, Shi   II-146
Lin, Stephen   I-58
Lin, Weili   I-247
Lindner, C.   III-353
Lindner, Uri   I-455
Linguraru, Marius George   III-418
Litjens, Geert   II-413
Liu, David   III-393
Liu, Huafeng   III-558
Liu, Jiang   I-58
Liu, Jun   III-264
Liu, Manhua   I-247, III-239
Liu, Peter   III-582
Liu, Tianming   II-237, II-271, II-502,
    III-214, III-297, III-485
Liu, Wei   III-189
Liu, Xiaomin   I-373
Liu, Yinxiao   I-124
Liu, Yu-Ying   I-307
Liu, Zhiwen   I-340
Lo, Pechin   III-147

Loeckx, Dirk   I-107
Loog, Marco   III-550
Lorenzi, Marco   I-739
Lourenço, Ana M.   II-122
Lu, Chao   II-462
Lucas, Blake C.   I-495, II-404
Lucas, D.   I-365
Lucchi, Aurelien   III-337
Lui, Harvey   I-298
Lui, Lok Ming   II-146
Lundstrom, Robert   III-501

Ma, Y.   II-25
Macq, Benoît   III-313
Madabhushi, Anant   I-157, I-365
Madooei, Ali   I-315
Mahmoudi, Saïd   II-446
Mahmoudzadeh, Mahdi   III-172
Malik, Jitendra   III-345
Mamaghani, Sina   II-544
Maneesh, Dewan   I-141
Mangin, Jean-François   II-57
Manjunath, B.S.   III-321
Mansi, T.   II-33, III-566
Marchesseau, Stéphanie   II-41
Marescaux, J.   I-91
Mariottini, Gian-Luca   II-625
Marlow, Neil   III-256
Martí, Robert   II-371
Martin, Nicholas G.   III-305
Masamune, Ken   I-26
Masutani, Yoshitaka   II-106
Matre, Knut   I-447
Matthies, Philipp   I-430
Maumet, Camille   III-542
Maurel, Pierre   III-542
Mauri, Josepa   I-642
McClure, Patrick   II-114
McKenzie, Charles A.   II-519
McLean, David   I-298
McMahon, Katie L.   III-305
McMillan, Corey T.   III-206
McNulty, Edward   III-501
Melbourne, Andrew   III-256, III-289
Mele, Katarina   I-357
Mendizabal-Ruiz, E. Gerardo   II-454
Menini, Anne   I-264
Merlet, Isabelle   I-231
Merlet, Sylvain   II-339, III-10
Mertins, Alfred   III-272

Metaxas, Dimitris N.   II-49, II-387, III-435
Meyer, Carsten   I-634
Mihalef, Viorel   II-486
Minhas, Rashid   I-520
Mirmehdi, Majid   III-329
Mirzaalian, Hengameh   II-98
Misawa, Kazunari   I-10
Modat, Marc   II-262, III-26, III-289
Mollura, Daniel J.   III-459
Monaco, James   I-365
Mori, Kensaku   I-10
Mory, Benoît   I-561, III-66
Mouchard, Laurent   I-545
Mountney, Peter   II-544
Mukhopadhyay, Anirban   II-502
Mulkern, R.V.   I-1
Müller, Henning   III-517
Müller, O.   I-198
Munoz, Hector   III-509

Nagao, Yoshihiro   I-26
Najman, Laurent   II-9
Nakaguchi, Toshiya   II-395
Nambakhsh, Cyrus M.S.   I-659
Nap, Marius   III-550
Napolitano, Raffaele   II-667
Navab, Nassir   I-18, I-422, I-430, I-625, II-486, II-601, II-609, III-42, III-443, III-566
Nemoto, Mitsutaka   II-106
Newton, Allen   II-246
Ng, Bernard   I-707
Nguyen, Kien   I-115
Nicolau, S.A.   I-91
Nie, Feiping   II-271
Niessen, Wiro J.   I-667
Niethammer, Marc   II-171, III-197, III-280
Nijhof, N.   II-25
Nitzken, Matthew   II-114
Noble, Jack H.   II-421
Noble, J. Alison   I-348, II-667, III-402
Nolte, Lutz-Peter   I-66
Nomura, Yukihiro   II-106
Nuyts, Johan   I-107

Odille, Freddy   I-264
O'Donnell, Lauren J.   III-123
Øye, Ola Kristoffer   I-447

Ohdaira, Takeshi   I-26
Ohtomo, Kuni   II-106
Okada, Kazunori   III-418
Okur, Aslı   I-430
O'Neill, M.   II-25
Ou, Yangming   II-49
Ourselin, Sebastien   I-289, II-262, III-26, III-256, III-289
Owen, Megan   III-147

Pallier, Christophe   III-248
Pan, Binbin   I-99
Papademetris, Xenophon   III-58
Papageorghiou, Aris   II-667
Papageorghiou, Aris T.   III-402
Paragios, Nikos   I-223, I-569, I-577, II-651
Parisot, Sarah   II-651
Parker, William A.   III-468
Pasternak, Ofer   II-305
Pauly, Olivier   III-443
Pavani, Sri-Kaushik   II-478
Pavlidis, I.   I-149
Payne, Christopher   I-463
Payne, Christopher J.   II-560
Pedemonte, Stefano   I-289
Pennec, Xavier   I-739, II-130
Perez-Rossello, J.M.   I-1
Peterlík, Igor   I-50
Peters, Jurriaan   III-313
Peters, Terry M.   I-659, II-519, II-535
Petersen, Jens   III-147
Philippe, Anne-Charlotte   II-339
Pietrzyk, Uwe   I-206
Pike, G. Bruce   I-487
Pinel, Philippe   III-248
Pinto, Peter   III-582
Piven, Joseph   I-731
Pizarro, Luis   II-659
Pjescic-Emedji, Natasa   III-337
Plate, Annika   III-443
Pohl, Kilian M.   II-49, III-131
Poline, Jean-Baptiste   I-707, III-248
Pop, M.   II-33
Poupon, Cyril   II-57, II-288
Prastawa, Marcel   I-731, III-223
Pratt, Philip   I-463
Prevost, Raphael   I-561, III-66
Price, Anthony N.   I-512
Price, S.J.   III-369

Prima, Sylvain   II-163
Puerto, Gustavo A.   II-625
Punithakumar, Kumaradevan   I-520,
    II-527
Pursley, Jennifer   III-107

Qian, Zhen   II-502
Qiu, Wu   I-537
Quaghebeur, Gerardine   II-667

Radeva, Petia   I-642
Rafii-Tari, Hedyeh   II-560
Rahmatullah, Bahbibi   III-402
Rajchl, Martin   I-659, III-377
Ralovich, Kristóf   II-486
Raniga, Parnesh   II-220
Rao, Anil   I-512
Rapaka, S.   II-33
Rathi, Yogesh   III-34
Razavi, Reza   II-25, II-41
Razzaque, Sharif   III-83
Reber, Clay   III-345
Reckfort, Julia   I-206
Reed, Sam   III-329
Rehg, James M.   I-307
Reichl, Tobias   II-601, III-42
Reisert, Marco   II-297
Reiter, Austin   II-592
Relan, Jatin   I-617
Ren, Haibing   I-504
Reyes, Mauricio   I-66, II-130
Rezatofighi, Seyed Hamid   I-357
Rhode, Kawal S.   II-25, II-41
Richa, Rogério   I-397, II-568
Riddell, Cyril   I-223
Riga, Celia   II-560
Rigamonti, Roberto   I-189
Rinaldi, C. Aldo   II-25, II-41
Rinehart, Sarah   II-502
Ringel, Richard   II-486
Risholm, Petter   III-107
Rivaz, Hassan   III-91
Roberts, M.G.   III-361
Roberts, Timothy P.L.   II-254, III-231,
    III-468
Robertson, Nicola J.   III-256
Roche, Alexis   II-355
Rohling, Robert   I-42, II-617
Romero, Eduardo   I-157

Rose, Kenneth   III-321
Rosenhahn, B.   I-198
Rowe, Christopher C.   II-220
Ruan, Su   I-545
Rueckert, Daniel   I-10, I-256, I-512,
    II-262, II-659
Rumpf, Martin   I-414

Saake, Marc   II-511
Saalbach, Axel   I-634, II-1
Sabuncu, Mert Rory   III-50
Sadeghi, Maryam   I-298, I-315
Sadikot, Abbas F.   I-487
Saha, Punam K.   I-124
Sahebjavaher, Ramin   II-617
Sahin, Mustafa   III-313
Saint-Jalmes, Hervé   I-231
Salcudean, Septimiu   I-42, II-617
Salvado, Olivier   I-231, II-220
Sanchez, Mar   III-197, III-280
Sanelli, Pina C.   I-272
Sankaranarayanan, Preethi   I-132
Sarkar, Anindya   I-115
Savadjiev, Peter   III-34
Savoire, Nicolas   III-639
Sawada, Yoshihide   II-470
Schäfer, Dirk   I-634
Scherrer, Benoît   III-313
Schmidt-Richberg, Alexander   II-74
Schmitt, Peter   II-511
Schnabel, Julia A.   II-667, III-115
Schneider, Caitlin   I-42
Schonfeld, Dan   II-196
Schultz, Thomas   III-493
Schuman, Joel S.   I-307
Schwab, Evan   II-322
Schwartz, Yannick   III-248
Seiler, Christof   I-66, II-130
Seong, Yeong Kyeong   I-504
Sermesant, Maxime   I-617, II-41
Setsompop, Kawin   III-1
Shackleford, James A.   II-122
Shakir, Dzhoshkun I.   I-430
Sharma, Puneet   II-486
Sharp, Gregory C.   II-122
Shastri, D.   I-149
Shattuck, D.W.   III-607
Shen, Dinggang   I-82, I-214, I-247, II-90,
    II-171, II-212, II-331, III-18,
    III-156, III-239, III-264, III-385, III-451

Shenton, Martha E.   II-305
Shi, Feng   I-247
Shi, Jianbo   III-631
Shi, Pengcheng   I-617, III-558
Shi, Wenzhe   II-659
Shi, Yonggang   I-340, I-601, II-138
Shi, Yundi   III-280
Shih, Min-Chi   III-321
Shofty, Ben   II-179
Shotton, J.   III-369
Shusharina, Nadya   II-122
Siless, Viviana   II-57
Simon, Tony J.   II-196
Singh, Nikhil   I-132
Singh, Vivek   I-528
Sinusas, Albert J.   III-58
Siochi, R. Alfredo C.   I-239
Skibbe, Henrik   II-297
Smith, Alex R.   II-254
Smith, S.   I-365
Smith, Stephen M.   II-188
Sokoll, Stefan   I-165
Sol, Kevin   III-533
Soler, L.   I-91
Soliman, Abraam S.   II-519
Soliman, Ahmed   II-114
Somphone, Oudom   I-561
Song, Yang   I-74
Sonke, Jan-Jakob   I-181
Sorrell, Keagan   III-525
Sosna, J.   II-363
Stamm, Aymeric   III-476
Steger, Sebastian   II-66
Stirrat, John   I-659
Stoyanov, Danail   I-479
Streekstra, Geert J.   II-155, III-164
Strobel, Norbert   II-584
Styner, Martin   III-197, III-280
Su, Hang   I-331, III-615
Subramanian, Navneeth   I-683, II-478
Subsol, Gérard   III-533
Suetens, Paul   I-107
Sühling, M.   I-438
Summers, Ronald M.   III-509, III-582
Sun, Zhenqiang   II-237
Suzuki, Miyuki   III-418
Switz, Neil   III-345
Syeda-Mahmood, Tanveer   III-501
Sznitman, Raphael   II-568, III-337

Talbot, Hugues   II-9
Tapley, Asa   III-345
Taquet, Maxime   III-313
Tavaré, Jeremy   III-329
Taylor, Russell H.   I-397, I-495, II-404,
    II-552, II-568
Tejpar, Sabine   I-107
Tempany, Clare   III-107
Tenenhaus, Arthur   I-223
Tessier, David   I-537
Thaller, Peter-Helmut   I-18, II-609
Thiagarajah, S.   III-353
Thirion, Bertrand   I-707, II-57, III-248
Thiruvenkadam, Sheshadri   I-683
Thomas, M.   II-25
Thomas, O.M.   III-369
Thompson, Paul M.   II-196, II-228,
    III-305
Thomsen, Laura H.   III-147
Tietjen, Christian   II-462
Toews, Matthew   II-204
Toga, Arthur W.   I-601, II-138, III-305
Tönnies, Klaus   I-165
Trachtenberg, John   I-455
Tran, Giang   II-138
Trousset, Yves   I-223
Trouvé, Alain   III-223
Tsiamyrtzis, P.   I-149
Tu, Zhuowen   III-623
Tung, Kai-Pin   II-659
Turkbey, Baris   III-582

Udupa, Jayaram K.   III-459
Uhl, Andreas   III-574
Ukwatta, Eranga   I-537, I-659, III-377
Ulvang, Dag Magne   I-447
Uzunbas, Mustafa   III-435

Vágvölgyi, Balázs   I-397
Vaillant, Régis   II-9
Van de Casteele, Elke   I-107
van de Giessen, Martijn   I-667, II-155,
    III-164
van de Ven, Wendy   II-413
Van de Ville, Dimitri   III-517
Van Leemput, Koen   III-50
van Vliet, Lucas J.   II-155, III-164
Varoquaux, Gaël   I-707, III-248
Vasconcelos, Nuno   III-83
Vécsei, Andreas   III-574

Venkataraman, Archana I-715
Vera, Pierre I-545
Vercauteren, Tom III-639
Verma, Ragini II-254, III-34, III-231, III-468
Vezhnevets, Alexander I-323
Vidal, René I-34, II-322
Villemagne, Victor L. II-220
Vincent, T. III-180
Viola, Ivan I-447
Vitanovski, Dime II-486
Vogel, Jakob III-42
Voros, Szilard II-502
Vos, Frans M. II-155, III-164
Voss, S.D. I-1
Vuissoz, Pierre-André I-264
Vunckx, Kathleen I-107

Wachinger, Christian III-410
Waelkens, Paulo I-625
Wald, Lawrence L. III-1
Wallis, G.A. III-353
Wallois, Fabrice III-172
Wang, Angela Y. I-132
Wang, Danny J.J. II-138
Wang, Defeng II-146
Wang, Fei III-501
Wang, Haitao I-373
Wang, Haiyan II-659
Wang, Hongzhi II-429
Wang, Lejing I-18, II-609
Wang, Li I-247
Wang, Lihong II-212
Wang, Linwei I-617, I-675, E1
Wang, Peng I-173, II-17
Wang, Qian II-90
Wang, Qiang I-504
Wang, Shijun III-582
Wang, Weiqi II-617
Wang, Yalin I-340
Wang, Yu I-405
Ward, Aaron D. II-643
Warfield, Simon K. I-1, I-593, III-313
Wasza, Jakob II-576
Wedeen, Van III-1
Wee, Chong-Yaw II-212
Weese, Jürgen II-1
Weidert, Simon I-18, II-609
Wein, Wolfgang I-447, II-601
Weinstein, Susan II-437

Weizman, Lior II-179
Wells III, William M. II-204, III-107, III-123
Wels, Michael I-438
Werner, René II-74
Wesarg, Stefan II-66
Westin, Carl-Fredrik II-305, III-34, III-123
White, James A. I-659, II-519
Wiest-Daesslé, Nicolas II-163
Wilkinson, J.M. III-353
Wille, Mathilde M.W. III-147
Wilms, Matthias II-347
Windoffer, Reinhard I-381
Winston, Gavin III-26
Wisniewski, Nicholas II-494
Wolf-Schnurrbusch, Ute III-599
Wollstein, Gadi I-307
Wolz, Robin I-10, I-512, II-262
Wong, Joyce Y. I-389
Wong, Ken C.L. I-617
Wong, Tien Yin I-58
Wright, G.A. II-33
Wright, Margaret J. III-305
Wu, Guorong I-214, I-247, II-90
Wu, H.S. I-91
Wu, Shandong II-437
Wu, Wen II-544
Wu, Yu-Chien II-280
Wu, Zheng I-389

Xia, James J. I-99
Xiao, Yiming I-487
Xu, Dong I-58
Xu, Jingjia I-675, E1
Xu, Yan III-623
Xu, Yanwu I-58
Xu, Ziyue I-124

Yang, Guang-Zhong I-463, II-560, III-99
Yang, Qi II-122
Yang, Xue II-246
Yao, Jianhua III-459, III-509
Yap, Pew-Thian I-214, II-171, II-212, II-331, III-18, III-156, III-239
Ye, Dong Hye III-131
Yin, Zhaozheng III-615
Yoshikawa, Takeharu II-106

Young, Brian   II-478
Yuan, Jing   I-537, I-659, II-519, III-377
Yuan, Peng   I-99
Yureidini, A.   I-553
Yushkevich, Paul A.   II-429

Zachow, Stefan   I-609
Zappella, Luca   I-34
Zhan, Liang   II-196, II-228
Zhan, Yiqiang   I-141, III-435
Zhang, Aifeng F.   II-196, II-228
Zhang, Daoqiang   I-82, II-212, III-239,
    III-264
Zhang, Hua   I-181
Zhang, Jianwen   III-566, III-623
Zhang, Jingdan   II-462
Zhang, Minqi   II-146
Zhang, Pei   II-171, III-156
Zhang, Shaoting   II-387, III-435
Zhang, Tuo   III-297, III-485
Zhang, Weiyu   III-631

Zhang, Xin   II-237
Zhang, Y.   III-501
Zhang, Yu   I-214, I-247
Zhao, Qun   II-237
Zhao, Tao   II-592
Zheng, Yefeng   I-239, II-17, II-462
Zhou, Luping   II-220
Zhou, S. Kevin   II-462, III-393
Zhou, Xiang Sean   I-141
Zhou, Xiaobo   I-99
Zhou, Yan   III-435
Zhou, Yun   I-74
Zhu, Dajiang   II-237, II-271, III-214,
    III-297, III-485
Zhuang, Xiahai   II-659
Ziegler, Sibylle I.   I-430
Zikic, Darko   III-75, III-369
Zisserman, Andrew   I-348
Zöllei, Lilla   II-204
Zuo, Siyang   I-26